MANAGEMENT OF THE
DIFFICULT
AND
FAILED AIRWAY

MANAGEMENT OF THE DIFFICULT AND FAILED AIRWAY

SECOND EDITION

ORLANDO HUNG, MD, FRCPC

Professor, Departments of Anesthesia, Surgery, and Pharmacology
Dalhousie University
Queen Elizabeth II Health Sciences Centre
Halifax, Nova Scotia, Canada

MICHAEL F. MURPHY, MD, FRCPC

Professor and Chair, Department of Anesthesiology and Pain Medicine
University of Alberta
Zone Chief of Anesthesiology
Edmonton, Alberta, Canada

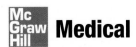

New York   Chicago   San Francisco   Lisbon   London   Madrid
Mexico City   Milan   New Delhi   San Juan   Seoul   Singapore   Sydney   Toronto

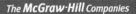

Management of the Difficult and Failed Airway, Second Edition

2 3 4 5 6 7 8 9 0   CTP/CTP   18 17 16 15

Set ISBN 978-0-07-162346-9; MHID 0-07-162346-9
Book ISBN 978-0-07-162344-5; MHID 0-07-162344-2
DVD ISBN 978-0-07-162345-2; MHID 0-07-162345-0

This book was set in Adobe Garamond by Cenveo Publisher Services.
The editors were Brian Belval and Peter J. Boyle.
The production supervisor was Sherri Souffrance.
Project management was provided by Vastavikta Sharma, Cenveo Publisher Services.
The illustration manager was Armen Ovsepyan.
The designer was Alan Barnett.
China Translation & Printing Services, Ltd., was printer and binder.

Cataloging-in-publication data for this title is on file at the Library of Congress.

McGraw-Hill books are available at special quantity discounts to use as premiums and sales promotions, or for use in corporate training programs. To contact a representative please e-mail us at bulksales@mcgraw-hill.com.

ASSOCIATE EDITORS

Thomas J. Coonan, MD, FRCPC
Professor, Departments of Anesthesia and Surgery
Dalhousie University
Queen Elizabeth II Health Sciences Centre
Halifax, Nova Scotia, Canada

J. Adam Law, BSc, MD, FRCPC
Professor, Departments of Anesthesia, and Surgery
Dalhousie University
Queen Elizabeth II Health Sciences Centre
Halifax, Nova Scotia, Canada

Ian R. Morris, BEng, MD, FRCPC, DABA, FACEP
Professor, Department of Anesthesia
Dalhousie University
Queen Elizabeth II Health Sciences Centre
Halifax, Nova Scotia, Canada

Ronald D. Stewart, MD
Professor Emeritus, Departments of Anesthesia, and
    Emergency Medicine
Queen Elizabeth II Health Sciences Centre
Halifax, Nova Scotia, Canada

We would like to dedicate this edition to our families,
Jeanette, Christopher, David, and Ana Hung,
as well as Debbie, Amanda, Ryan, and Teddy Murphy.
Without their continuing love and support,
it would not have been possible
to complete this book.

CONTENTS

Section 4. Practical Considerations in Difficult and Failed Airway Management

Contents of DVD of Airway Technique Videos

CONTRIBUTORS

David C. Abramson, MBChB, FFA(SA)
North Texas Children's Anesthesia
Dallas, Texas
Chapter 47

Aaron E. Bair, MD
Assistant Professor
Emergency Medicine
U.C. Davis Medical Centre
University of California
Sacramento, California
Chapter 25

Stephen Beed, MD, FRCPC, DipABA, Cert CCM
Associate Professor Anesthesia and Medicine
Dalhousie University
Attending Anesthesiologist and Critical Care Physician
Departments of Anesthesia and Critical Care Medicine
Queen Elizabeth II Health Sciences Centre
Halifax, Nova Scotia, Canada
Chapter 27

Phil Blum, MBBS, FANZCA
Senior Lecturer
Flinders University
Deputy Director
Department of Anaesthesia
Royal Darwin Hospital
Casuarina, Northern Territory, Australia
Chapter 56

Kerry B. Broderick, MD
Emergency Medicine
Denver Health Medical Centre
Denver, Colorado
Chapters 21, 22

David A. Caro, MD
Associate Residency Director
Assistant Professor
Department of Emergency Medicine
University of Florida Health Science Centre—Jacksonville
Jacksonville, Florida
Chapters 19, 25

Idena Carroll, CRNA, MS
Anesthesia Clinical and Educational Services, PA
Program Director
Nurse Anesthesia Program
Our Lady of the Lake College
Baton Rouge, Louisiana
Chapters 5, 18

Chris C. Christodoulou, MBChB, FRCPC
Assistant Professor in Anesthesia
Department of Anesthesia
University of Manitoba
I.H. Asper Clinical Research Institute
Winnipeg, Manitoba, Canada
Chapter 11

Thomas J. Coonan, MD, FRCPC
Professor, Departments of Anesthesia and Surgery
Dalhousie University
Queen Elizabeth II Health Sciences Centre
Halifax, Nova Scotia, Canada
Chapters 12, 56

Richard M. Cooper, BSc, MSc, MD, FRCPC
Professor
Department of Anesthesia
University of Toronto
Department of Anesthesia and Pain Management
Toronto General Hospital
Toronto, Ontario, Canada
Chapters 10, 28

Edward T. Crosby, MD, FRCPC
Department of Anesthesiology
Ottawa Hospital
Ottawa, Ontario, Canada
Chapters 2, 5, 15, 37

Jo Davies, MB BS, FRCA
Associate Professor
Department of Anesthesiology and Pain Medicine
University of Washington
Seattle, Washington
Chapter 61

D. John Doyle, MD, PhD, FRCPC
Professor of Anesthesiology and Staff Anesthesiologist
Department of General Anesthesiology
Cleveland Clinic Foundation
Cleveland, Ohio
Chapters 1, 57

Dennis Drapeau, BSc, MD, FRCPC
Dalhousie University
Department of Anesthesia
Queen Elizabeth II Health Sciences Centre
Halifax, Nova Scotia, Canada
Chapter 35

Laura V. Duggan, MD, FRCPC
Assistant Professor of Anesthesiology
Department of Anesthesiology, Pharmacology and Therapeutics
Faculty of Medicine
University of British Columbia
Vancouver, British Columbia, Canada
Chapter 42

Lorraine J. Foley, MD
Winchester Anesthesia Associates
Clinical Associate Professor of Anesthesia
Tufts School of Medicine
Department of Anesthesia
Winchester Hospital
Winchester, Massachusetts
Chapter 60

Ronald B. George, MD, FRCPC
Department of Anesthesia
Dalhousie University
Halifax, Nova Scotia, Canada
Chapters 4, 53

Steven A. Godwin, MD
Residency Director
Assistant Professor
Department of Emergency Medicine
University of Florida Health Science Centre—Jacksonville
Jacksonville, Florida
Chapter 19

Angelina Guzzo, MDCM, PhD, FRCPC
Department of Anesthesia
Montreal General Hospital
Montreal, Quebec, Canada
Chapter 31

Carin Hagberg, MD
Joseph C. Gabel Professor and Chair
Department of Anesthesiology
University of Texas Medical School at Houston
Houston, Texas
Chapter 39

Dietrich Henzler, MD, PhD, FRCPC
Professor of Anesthesiology and Physiology
Dalhousie University
Department of Anesthesia and Division of Critical Care
Queen Elizabeth II Health Sciences Centre
Halifax, Nova Scotia, Canada.
Chapter 29

Chris Hinkewich, MD
Resident, Department of Anesthesia
Dalhousie University
Queen Elizabeth II Health Sciences Centre
Halifax, Nova Scotia, Canada
Chapter 12

Wendy Howard, MD
Clinical Assistant Professor
Director of Anesthesia for ENT and Difficult Airways
Department of Anesthesiology
SUNY Upstate Medical University
Syracuse, New York
Chapter 41

Orlando R. Hung, MD, FRCPC
Departments of Anesthesia, Surgery, and Pharmacology
Dalhousie University
Queen Elizabeth II Health Sciences Centre
Department of Anesthesia
Halifax, Nova Scotia, Canada
Chapters 4, 6, 11, 12, 16, 17, 31, 35, 60

Narasimhan Jagannathan, MD
Department of Pediatric Anesthesia
Children's Memorial Hospital
Assistant Professor of Anesthesiology
Northwestern University Feinberg School of Medicine
Chicago, Illinois
Chapter 42

Andy Jagoda, MD, FACEP
Professor and Chair of Emergency Medicine
Mount Sinai School of Medicine
New York, New York
Chapter 15

Liane B. Johnson, MDCM, FRCSC
Department of Otolaryngology
Dalhousie University
Department of Pediatric Otolaryngology
IWK Health Centre
Halifax, Nova Scotia, Canada
Chapters 13, 31, 43, 44

Sara Kim, PhD
Associate Professor
Department of Medical Education and Bioinformatics
University of Washington
Seattle, Washington
Chapter 61

David Kirkpatrick, MD, FRCSC
Professor and Head
Department of Otolaryngology
Dalhousie University
Queen Elizabeth II Health Sciences Centre
Halifax, Nova Scotia, Canada
Chapter 26

George Kovacs, MD, FRCPC
Professor, Emergency Medicine
Dalhousie University
Attending Emergency Physician
Capital District Health Authority
Queen Elizabeth II Health Sciences Centre
Halifax, Nova Scotia, Canada
Chapters 7, 8

J. Adam Law, BSc, MD, FRCPC
Professor
Departments of Anesthesia, and Surgery
Dalhousie University
Queen Elizabeth II Health Sciences Centre
Halifax, Nova Scotia, Canada
Chapters 10, 15, 55, 56, 58

Gordon O. Launcelott, MD, FRCPC
Department of Anesthesia
Dalhousie University
Queen Elizabeth II Health Sciences Centre
Halifax, Nova Scotia, Canada
Chapters 13, 38

Richard M. Levitan, MD
Associate Professor, Emergency Medicine
Thomas Jefferson University
Philadelphia, Pennsylvania
Chapter 8

Robert C. Luten, MD
Professor, Pediatrics and Emergency Medicine
College of Medicine
University of Florida
Jacksonville, Florida
Chapter 48

Dolores M. McKeen, MD, MSc, FRCPC
Associate Professor, Department of Anesthesia
Dalhousie University
Halifax, Nova Scotia, Canada
Chapter 49

Genevieve MacKinnon, MD
Resident in Anesthesiology
Dalhousie University
Capital District Health Authority
Queen Elizabeth II Health Sciences Centre
Halifax, Nova Scotia, Canada
Chapter 24

Kirk J. MacQuarrie, MD, FRCPC
Associate Professor, Department of Anesthesia
Dalhousie University
Queen Elizabeth II Health Sciences Centre
Halifax, Nova Scotia, Canada
Chapter 26

Ian R. Morris, BEng, MD, FRCPC, DABA, FACEP
Professor, Department of Anesthesia
Dalhousie University
Queen Elizabeth II Health Sciences Centre
Halifax, Nova Scotia, Canada
Chapters 3, 9, 33, 34

Holly A. Muir, MD, FRCPC
Chief, Division of Women's Anesthesia
Vice Chair Clinical Operations
Director of Perioperative Leaders Group, DN OR
Assistant Professor of Anesthesia
Associate Professor of Obstetrics and Gynecology
Duke University Medical Centre
Durham, North Carolina
Chapters 51, 52

Michael F. Murphy, MD, FRCPC
Professor and Chair, Department of Anesthesiology and Pain
    Medicine
University of Alberta
Zone Chief of Anesthesiology
Edmonton Zone
Edmonton, Alberta, Canada
Chapters 1, 2, 6, 7, 14, 20, 24, 32, 54, 59, 60, 61

Joshua Nagler, MD
Assistant Professor of Pediatrics
Harvard Medical School
Fellowship Director
Pediatric Emergency Medicine
Children's Hospital Boston
Boston, Massachusetts
Chapter 48

Adeyemi J. Olufolabi, MBBS, DCH, FRCA
Division of Women's Anesthesia
Duke University Medical Centre
Durham, North Carolina
Chapters 51, 52

Steven Petrar, MD
Department of Anesthesia
Dalhousie University
Queen Elizabeth II Health Sciences Centre
Halifax, Nova Scotia, Canada
Chapter 6

David Petrie, MD, FRCPC
Associate Professor of Emergency Medicine
Dalhousie University
Attending Physician Emergency Medicine
Capital District Health Authority
Queen Elizabeth II Health Sciences Centre
Chapters 14, 24

Tom C. Phu, MD
Staff Anesthesiologist
Department of Anesthesia
University of British Columbia
Royal Columbian Hospital,
New Westminster, British Columbia, Canada
Chapter 16

Dmitry Portnoy, MD
Associate Professor, Department of Anesthesiology
University of Texas Medical School at Houston
Houston, Texas
Chapter 39

Saul Pytka, MD, FRCPC
Associate Professor of Anesthesiology (Clinical)
University of Calgary
Staff Anesthesiologist
Rockyview General Hospital
Referral Physician
STARS Air Ambulance
Calgary, Alberta, Canada
Chapters 5, 18, 59

Brian K. Ross, PhD, MD
Professor
Department of Anesthesiology
University of Washington
Seattle, Washington
Chapters 49, 50

Matthew G. Simms, MSc, MD, FRCPC
Staff Anesthesiologist
Department of Anesthesia
Dalhousie University
Queen Elizabeth II Health Sciences Centre
Halifax, Nova Scotia, Canada
Chapter 58

Christian M. Soder, MD, FRCPC
Chief, Department of Pediatric Critical Care
IWK Health Centre
Associate Professor of Anesthesia and Pediatrics
Department of Pediatric Critical Care
Dalhousie University
Halifax, Nova Scotia, Canada
Chapters 43, 46

Ronald D. Stewart, BA, BSc, MD, OC, ONS, DSc
Departments of Anesthesia and Emergency Medicine
Queen Elizabeth II Health Sciences Centre
Halifax, Nova Scotia, Canada
Chapter 16

John M. Tallon, MD, MSc, FRCPC
Associate Professor of Emergency Medicine, Surgery and
Community Health and Epidemiology
Dalhousie University
Attending Physician Emergency Medicine
Capital District Health Authority
Queen Elizabeth II Health Sciences
Halifax, Nova Scotia, Canada
Chapter 14

Narendra Vakharia, MD, FRCPC
Associate Professor, Dalhousie University
Victoria General Hospital Site
Halifax, Nova Scotia, Canada
Chapter 53

Robert J. Vissers, MD, FRCPC, FACEP
Director, Department of Emergency Medicine
Legacy Emanuel Hospital
Adjunct Associate Professor
Oregon Health Sciences University
Lake Oswego, Oregon
Chapter 23

Arnim Vlatten, MD
Assistant Professor of Anesthesia
Department of Anesthesia
Dalhousie University
Department of Pediatric Anesthesia
Department of Pediatric Critical Care
IWK Health Centre
Halifax, Nova Scotia, Canada
Chapter 45

Mark Vu, MD, FRCPC
Assistant Professor, Anesthesiology
University of British Columbia
Attending Anesthesiologist
Vancouver General Hospital
Vancouver, British Columbia
Chapters 14, 17

Sarah H. Wiser, MD
Department of Anesthesiology
Brigham and Women's Hospital
Harvard Medical School
Boston, Massachusetts
Chapter 41

Ron M. Walls, MD
Chairman Department of Emergency Medicine
Brigham and Women's Hospital
Professor of Medicine
Division of Emergency Medicine
Harvard Medical School
Boston, Massachusetts
Chapter 20

David T. Wong, MD
Associate Professor
University of Toronto
Department of Anesthesia
Toronto Western Hospital
Toronto, Ontario, Canada
Chapters 30, 40

Richard D. Zane, MD
Vice Chair, Department of Emergency Medicine
Brigham and Women's Hospital
Assistant Professor
Harvard Medical School
Boston, Massachusetts
Chapter 21

FOREWORD

Modern medicine can shepherd patients through profound injuries and physiological trespass, provided that they are never deprived of oxygen. Conversely, serious injuries often follow interruption of oxygen delivery, particularly in anesthetized patients. The most important aspect in the care of *any* patient is to assure the continued supply of oxygen, which requires a patent airway. Airway is the A of ABC.

Skilled airway management is the *sine qua non* of competence for an anesthesiologist. Anesthesiologists assist or control ventilation throughout the typical workday. Most are easily managed with airway maneuvers, positive pressure ventilation via a face mask, and occasional supplementation with an oral or nasal airway. If these are inadequate, anesthesiologists are facile with devices ranging from a simple laryngoscope and endotracheal tube to sophisticated videolaryngoscopes. This increasingly crowded spectrum of airway control devices includes the simple Eschmann introducer (bougie), lightwands, extraglottic devices, and surgical interventions, such as cricothyrotomy.

This spectrum of devices has grown so fast that no clinician has the time or resources to learn them all. How should the busy clinician decide which techniques to learn? How can he or she gain sufficient familiarity with a novel airway device to use it on patients without exposing them to risk, and subsequently use the device with confidence when the airway is compromised?

The second edition of *Management of the Difficult and Failed Airway* is the answer to these questions. This beautifully illustrated and extensively referenced textbook provides a comprehensive review of the available options for airway management. Written by experts, the book reviews the spectrum of airway management techniques. For the busy clinician, this book provides the most up-to-date review available of the many innovations that have been introduced in the past 10 years. This is accompanied by a thorough review of the pharmacology of airway management, helping clinicians understand how to give drugs to achieve the desired effects on ventilation and muscle strength.

The unique strength of the book is in the third section, "Case Studies in Difficult and Failed Airway Management." This section presents approximately 45 airway management vignettes, divided into prehospital care (arrest or trauma), patients in the emergency department, patients in the critical care unit, adult surgical patients, pediatric patients, and obstetrical patients. Each vignette is structured around a hypothetical patient:

- A six-year-old boy presents with Down syndrome and post-tonsillectomy bleeding.
- A young man drives into an unseen wire while he is snow-mobiling.
- A young woman presents to the emergency department two hours after the onset of lip swelling that has progressed to difficulty in breathing.
- A sixty-year-old man with chronic obstructive lung disease and limited exercise tolerance needs to be extubated five days after a difficult intubation for recent pneumonia.
- A morbidly obese patient receives muscle relaxants as part of the induction of anesthesia. The anesthesiologist then discovers he can neither intubate the trachea nor ventilate the patient's lungs.

To the experienced anesthesiologist these vignettes sound familiar, and haunting. They are the subject of lounge gossip and morbidity and mortality rounds. The expert management of these truly "textbook" airway cases illustrates contemporary approaches to difficult airways. These cases teach trainees the fundamental approaches to airway management, and include self-evaluation questions to reinforce the lessons. For experienced anesthesiologists, these cases present an opportunity to learn about recently introduced devices and techniques they may wish to incorporate into their clinical practice.

The utility of the book extends well beyond anesthesiologists. Two decades ago, an anesthesiologist was summoned whenever a patient abruptly encountered airway difficulty. That has changed in the past decade as healthcare has decentralized into the community, and patients have come to expect oblivion during invasive medical procedures. Every gastroenterologist, cardiologist, interventional radiologist, and office-based surgeon who administers sedation needs to understand the basics of airway management. Our colleagues in other specialties who commonly manage difficult airways, such as critical care and emergency room physicians, may choose to learn how to use extraglottic devices and videolaryngoscopes after reading the vignettes.

Hung, Murphy, and colleagues have produced their second outstanding textbook on airway management. Quoting from Dr. Archie Brain's introduction to the first edition: "the book you hold in your hands is an invaluable compendium of knowledge on the subject of airway management, and deserves a prominent place in your library."

Steven L. Shafer, MD
Columbia University
New York, NY
August 2011

PREFACE

Since the publication of the first edition, a plethora of airway devices have been introduced. Many of these devices have the potential of improving our ability to manage the patient's airway and improving the view of the larynx. They may even increase the success rate of tracheal intubation. While the clinical utility of these devices and techniques in managing patients with a difficult and failed airway remains to be determined, we firmly believe that the airway technique of choice depends not only on the patient's anatomy but on the situational context. This second edition emphasizes that airway management is "context-sensitive" and that selection of an airway technique must be determined by the clinical situation and environment. For instance, compared to an operating room setting, the airway management strategy would be quite different for a patient with a difficult airway in the prehospital setting, in the emergency department, or in the cardiac catheterization unit, where skill sets and limited resources play decisive roles. Furthermore, the airway approach might also be different if an urgent airway intervention is needed for a pregnant patient or for a small child who is uncooperative. Using the guiding principles of context-sensitivity, this second edition is designed to assist practitioners with the appropriate selection of airway devices and techniques for a wide range of clinical environments.

As in the first edition, this book is divided into four sections: the first section presents the foundational information in airway management; the second section reviews airway devices and techniques; the third section discusses airway management in different clinical situations, including prehospital care, in the emergency department, intensive care units, the operating room, the post-anesthetic care unit, as well as other parts of the hospital; and the last section highlights practical issues in airway management. To broaden the scope of discussion, a number of new chapters and clinical cases have been added to this new edition. For example, chapters discussing the basic principles of bag-mask-ventilation, single lung ventilation using double lumen tubes, airway management in austere environments, as well as airway education and simulation have been included.

It is our hope that the second edition, like the first edition, is embraced by clinicians as contributing a solid foundation of knowledge to the field of difficult and failed airway management.

ACKNOWLEDGMENTS

We would like to thank all the contributing authors for making this book possible. In particular, we would like to thank all the associate editors for their tireless efforts to ensure that the information in this book is clear and accurate. We wish to thank Sara Whynot for her editorial assistance and Christopher Hung and David Hung for the production of all the images and videos. We thank the continuing support of all the editorial staff at McGraw-Hill.

Orlando Hung, MD, FRCPC
Michael F. Murphy, MD, FRCPC

SECTION 1 Foundations of Difficult and Failed Airway Management

CHAPTER (1)

Evaluation of the Airway

Michael F. Murphy and D. John Doyle

1.1 INTRODUCTION

"Airway management" may be defined as the application of therapeutic interventions that are intended to affect gas exchange in patients. *Gas exchange* is the fundamental feature of this definition.[1] A number of devices and techniques are commonly employed in health-care settings to achieve this goal, for example, bag-mask-ventilation (BMV), extraglottic devices (EGDs), oral or nasal endotracheal intubation, and surgical airway management techniques.

The failure to adequately manage the airway has been identified as a major factor leading to poor outcomes in anesthesia, critical care, emergency medicine, and emergency medical services (EMS).[2,3] In fact, adverse respiratory events constituted the largest single cause of injury in the ASA Closed Claims Project.[4] Furthermore, it has been repeatedly shown that the single most important factor leading to a failed airway is the failure to predict the difficult airway.[3-5]

Screening tests designed to predict difficult laryngoscopic intubation in otherwise normal patients have proven to be so unreliable that airway practitioners need to be prepared to manage a failed airway every time they are faced with a patient in need of airway management.[6,7]

This chapter deals with the identification of the difficult and failed airway, particularly in an emergency, in which evaluation and management must be done concurrently in a compressed time frame and canceling the case or delaying management is not an option.

Successful airway management is generally governed by four intertwined factors:

- A clinical situation of varying urgency, venue, and resources
- Patient factors including airway anatomy and vital organ system reserve

- Available airway resources
- Skills of the airway practitioner

Because one must choose a method of airway management from an array of techniques, some degree of precision of language is essential. For example, a difficult oral laryngoscopy and intubation may not necessarily constitute a difficult airway if BMV is easily performed. Furthermore, a difficult laryngoscopic intubation does not mean a difficult intubation using a lightwand or using a video laryngoscope. In the same way, a failed intubation does not necessarily constitute a failed airway. A failed intubation, defined narrowly as the failure to intubate the trachea on three attempts,[6,8] may not constitute a failed airway if one is able to affect gas exchange with BMV or with an EGD. However, *intubation failure* ought to conjure a sense of urgency and mandates the airway practitioner to rapidly switch to a failed airway management sequence because such a situation may become life-threatening if gas exchange cannot be provided expeditiously and adequately by other means. Furthermore, the alternative airway technique employed must have the highest degree of success in the practitioner's skill set. It is inappropriate to make random disorganized attempts to manage the airway in the hope that one of the airway techniques might work. Rather, one should have a planned strategy (See the Algorithms in Chapter 2) including invasive techniques such as cricothyrotomy.[2-5]

Caveat:

Failure to Evaluate the Airway and Predict Difficulty is the Single Most Important Factor Leading to a Failed Airway.
(ASA Close Claims Database[4])

1.2   INCIDENCE OF DIFFICULT AND FAILED AIRWAY

1.2.1   How common are the difficult and failed airway?

Bag-mask-ventilation (BMV), the use of EGDs, endotracheal intubation, and surgical airway management constitute the four primary avenues by which gas exchange is provided in the event patients are unable to do so adequately for themselves. In each category, difficulty and failure may be encountered. Failure of all four, ordinarily, leads to the demise of the patient.

Until recently, the success or failure of airway management has been defined in terms of BMV and orotracheal intubation. The introduction of EGDs and the heightened profile of cricothyrotomy have broadened such concepts. Fortunately, tracheal intubation is usually straightforward, particularly in the elective setting of the operating room (OR). The same cannot be said for other venues.

Airways that are difficult to manage are fairly common in anesthesia and emergency medicine practice, with some estimates as high as 20% of all emergency intubations.[9-12] However, the incidence of intubation failure is quite uncommon (ranging 0.5%-2.5%), and the disastrous situation of being unable to intubate or ventilate rarely occurs (0.1%-0.05%).[2,9-17] This translates to a "can't intubate, can't ventilate" failure rate of about 1:1000 to 1:2000 patients in a general surgical population. The incidence is strikingly higher in the parturient undergoing cesarean section (1:280), an almost tenfold increase. In fact, half of the excess mortality (28 times) seen with general anesthesia for cesarean section over regional anesthesia is attributable to airway management failure.[18-20]

1.2.2   How do we avoid airway management failure?

Although circumstances can vary widely, the expectation is the same: timely, effective airway management executed without patient injury. In circumstances of multiple trauma, facial or airway swelling, abnormal upper airway anatomy, upper airway hemorrhage, or a myriad of other difficult airway scenarios, intubation may be difficult, or even impossible, and even BMV can fail. Nevertheless, the expectation remains that the patient's airway be promptly secured and oxygenation be maintained.

Responding to an identified need to reduce the incidence of airway management failure, the American Society of Anesthesiologists (ASA) issued guidelines and an algorithm for management of the difficult airway in 1993, with a revision in 2003.[6,21] The guidelines stressed the importance of performing an airway evaluation for difficulty prior to inducing anesthesia and paralyzing the patient. Planned awake intubation, awakening the patient in the presence of a failed airway, and acquiring skills in alternative airway-management techniques are hallmarks of the 1993 guidelines.[21] The 2003 guidelines reemphasize the importance of the airway evaluation and incorporate the laryngeal mask airway (LMA) as a discrete step in the algorithm, should failure occur. Unfortunately, the guidelines are less useful outside the operating room (OR), especially in circumstances in which tracheal intubation must be accomplished quickly and awakening the patient is not an option. Even in the OR setting, explicit guidelines for the rapid evaluation of an airway for occult difficulty and the prioritization of rescue maneuvers in the event of a mandated immediate intubation are not well handled by the ASA guidelines and algorithm (see Chapter 2). Furthermore, the ASA guidelines do not take into consideration patients who are uncooperative (eg, young children or mentally challenged patients) or different patient populations (eg, parturients).

Further complicating this issue are the many new, effective, and safe airway devices that have been introduced to assist with difficult and failed airway management. Flexible endoscopic and video-intubating bronchoscopes have become more portable and easier to use and have been joined by a collection of rigid fiberoptic scopes (Bullard Laryngoscope™, Upsher Laryngoscope™, etc), rigid fiberoptic stylets (eg, Shikani Optical Stylet™, Bonfils Stylet™, Levitan FPS Scope™, etc), and hybrid devices employing cameras or fiberoptics, such as video laryngoscopes (eg, GlideScope® and McGrath® video laryngoscope, see Chapter 10). The laryngeal mask airway (LMA) and intubating laryngeal mask airway (ILMA or LMA Fastrach™) have taken on a distinct role in the management of both the difficult and the failed airway. The Combitube™ has often been used as a lifesaving rescue device. Lighted stylet methods (eg, Trachlight™) may permit light-guided (transillumination) intubation in situations in which the vocal cords cannot be visualized. Certain airways are impossible to manage by any means other than surgical cricothyrotomy, a procedure of increasing importance for all airway practitioners.

The challenge for any airway practitioner is to be able to accurately predict when a difficult airway is present, to immediately recognize when an intubation failure has occurred, and to reliably and reproducibly secure continuous gas exchange in both of these unnerving circumstances.

1.3   STANDARD OF CARE

1.3.1   Is there a prevailing standard of care in managing the difficult and failed airway? How is it defined?

The growth in knowledge and evidence related to the practice of airway management is relentless. The challenge for the practitioner is to keep abreast of new information, new techniques, and the changing expectations by our colleagues and patients. Advances in airway management over the past decade have significantly improved patient outcome with a reduction in the incidence of death and disability.[22] Therefore, it is important for practitioners to keep abreast of these advances in airway management in their clinical practice.

Black's Law Dictionary[23] defines the "Standard of Care" as:

> The average degree of skill, care and diligence exercised by members of the same profession, practicing in the same or similar locality in light of the present state of medical and surgical science.

This definition incorporates several important features:

- Average degree of skill
- Same or similar locality
- Present state of knowledge

Taking these into consideration, the Standard of Care is the conduct and skill of an average and *prudent practitioner* that can be expected by a *reasonable patient*. A bad result due to a failure to meet the standard of care is generally considered to be malpractice. There are two main sources of information as to exactly what is the expected standard of care:

- The beliefs and opinions of experts in the field.
- The published scientific evidence, standards of care, practice guidelines, protocols.

Ultimately the standard of care is what a jury says it is!

Driven by the complex nature of this clinical dilemma and the need for successful solutions that are easily learned and maintained (and cost-effective), the standard of care in airway management is exceedingly dynamic. Continuing evolution of new devices and techniques, or ways of thinking, modify the existing standard of care on an ongoing basis. It is incumbent on practitioners to keep abreast of new devices and techniques and remain facile with existing rescue techniques. They can do so by continually perusing the literature and attending educational programs related to airway management.

1.3.2 What is the role of professional organizations in establishing the standard of care?

International, national, regional, and local professional organizations generally address issues relevant to airway management in a variety of ways. Most national societies, such as the American Society of Anesthesiologists (ASA), the Difficult Airway Society (UK), the American Association of Nurse Anesthetists (AANA), the American College of Emergency Physicians (ACEP), the Canadian Anesthesiologists' Society (CAS), and others, engage in crafting practice guidelines.[6,21,24,25]

In the event of an untoward outcome, the *reasonable patient* expects the published guidelines to be observed by the *prudent practitioner*. Organizations that craft and publish such practice guidelines are careful to stipulate that such guidelines do not constitute the Standard of Care.[6] Unfortunately, guidelines are often perceived as the standard of care, particularly in a medical–legal context.

Professional organizations often provide educational initiatives to ensure that their members practice at the prevailing standard. The

ASA, ACEP, and the Society for Airway Management (SAM) are good examples. SAM is an organization committed to advancing knowledge and improving the quality of airway care to our patients. This international society blends the expertise of anesthesia, otolaryngology, head and neck surgery, critical care, and emergency medicine to debate issues related to airway management. The SAM serves as a sounding board, not only for new devices and techniques but also for those wishing to challenge traditional dogma and advance new frontiers. Those with a specific interest in airway management are well advised to become involved in this organization.

1.3.3 How can we integrate the standard of care into our clinical practice?

Despite all these initiatives, the Standard of Care remains elusive, particularly when applied to the management of the difficult and failed airway. It means different things to different practitioners and is situation dependent. For example,

- To the plaintiff's attorney, it must be precisely defined in the most minute of detail
- To the practitioner, it is what they do every day
- To the defendant practitioner, it is consistent with their actions

It is perhaps easier to articulate what it is not:

- It is not so low as to consistently lead to bad outcomes.
- It is neither much better nor much worse care than that delivered on average by one's peers.
- It is not the same as the care provided by *experts* managing difficult and failed airways every day.
- It is not what ivory tower academic experts *think* it *ought to be*.
- It is not a single study published in a reputable journal last week, or a position advocated by *experts* in an editorial in a similarly reputable journal.

We do know that the Standard of Care is dynamic and our patients expect to receive it at a minimum.

Perhaps the best test with respect to difficult and failed airway management is to ask a specific question: "Should the average, reasonable, and prudent practitioner…"

- Be able to recognize and manage an anticipated difficult airway?
- Be able to manage an unanticipated difficult airway?
- Be able to use a flexible bronchoscope to intubate the trachea of a patient?
- Be able to recognize and manage the failed airway?
- Be facile with one or two rescue devices or techniques in the face of a failed airway?
- Be able to perform a surgical airway? Or at the least, transtracheal ventilation?

It is reasonable to expect that most practitioners charged with managing airways would answer yes to all of these questions and thereby define the standard of care.

1.4   DEVELOPMENT OF LARYNGOSCOPIC INTUBATION

1.4.1   How did the design of laryngoscopes and the basic technique of oral laryngoscopy evolve?

Herholdt and Rafn are generally credited with first describing blind oral intubation in 1796. Subsequently, Desault described blind nasal intubation in 1814. Although Sir William Macewen described direct vision oral intubation in 1880, it is generally accepted that the first description of laryngoscopic-aided oral intubation was by Kirsten in 1895. By 1907, Chevalier Jackson, an ENT surgeon of considerable renown, introduced distal lighting to the laryngoscope, and Janeway in 1913, innovated the insertion of electric batteries into the handle of a laryngoscope to facilitate the procedure. Magill and Rowbotham engineered the straight Magill blade in the 1920s by cutting a wedge out of the side of the blade of the ENT surgeon's anterior commissure laryngoscope to facilitate intubation (Figure 1-1). Across the Atlantic, this design (with minor modifications) became known as the Miller blade in the 1940s. The Macintosh blade was also introduced in the 1940s by Sir Robert Macintosh.[26]

Magill is credited with introducing the "retro-molar" or "para-glossal" approach, reasoning that placing the blade as far to the corner of the mouth as possible when attempting to bring the glottis into view (as opposed to being in the midline) ought to minimize the distance to the glottis and enhance the degree to which it is visible. This technique has recently been resurrected by Henderson.[27]

1.4.2   How did the design of endotracheal tubes evolve?

It was also Sir Ivan Magill (circa 1914) who recommended a left-sided bevel (Magill bevel) be created on the distal tip of an endotracheal tube (ETT) (Figure 1-2). At that time, blind nasal intubation using a non-beveled, gum-elastic tube was popular. Magill observed that, as the right nostril is usually largest and most anesthesia practitioners are right handed, nasotracheal intubation was usually first attempted through the right nostril. The natural tendency for a tube introduced through the right nostril was to deviate leftward as it transited the nasopharynx and oropharynx and to deflect off the left glottic structures into the left pyriform recess. Magill reasoned that the left-sided bevel would deflect the ETT into the glottis.[28] Left-side bevel ETTs continue to be the most commonly used tubes to this day.

Curare and succinylcholine were introduced into anesthetic practice during the 1940s. These drugs led to the need for positive pressure ventilation, a tracheal seal being achieved by packing gauze (at times oil soaked) around the glottic opening. A more effective seal could be obtained by incorporating a balloon (initially rubber, thick walled, high pressure, and removable) onto the ETT. However, the possibility that the beveled orifice of the distal tip could rest against the wall of the bronchus in the event of a right mainstem intubation permitting positive pressure inspiration but not passive expiration was noted. This led to the creation of the Murphy eye opposite the bevel orifice (ie, facing the right side).

The bulk of the ETT and balloon hindered its passage through the channel of laryngoscope blades, and this led the Eschmann Corporation to introduce the intubating stylet to facilitate a Seldinger-type intubation over the stylet in 1949.[29]

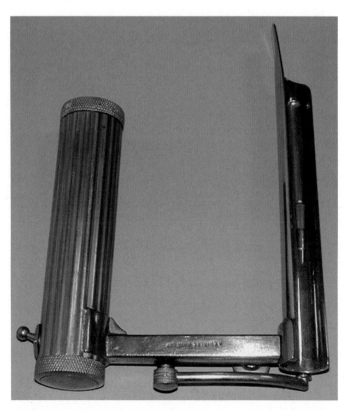

FIGURE 1-1. The Magill laryngoscope.

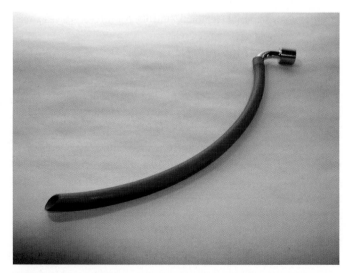

FIGURE 1-2. The left-sided Magill bevel on the endotracheal tube.

1.4.3 How has our understanding of how the difficult airway might be predicted developed over the years?

The use of neuromuscular blockade to facilitate orotracheal intubation followed the introduction of curare into anesthetic practice in the early 1940s and succinylcholine in the late 1940s. Up until that time, orotracheal intubation was largely performed with the patient ventilating spontaneously under inhalational anesthesia. The consequence of a failed intubation was mitigated by the fact that the patient continued to breathe spontaneously. The threat of failure to intubate in the face of neuromuscular blockade and apnea required anesthesia practitioners to evaluate the airway for difficulty, leading to a landmark publication by Cass in 1956.[30] This study identified those anatomical features that might predict difficult laryngoscopic intubation. Thus, the clinical use of neuromuscular blocking agents became inseparable from the ability to perform an airway evaluation and the ability to rescue the airway in the event of failure. Many practitioners still fail to recognize a difficult airway when one exists or they overlook the evaluation altogether.[4,6]

The literature regarding the difficult airway was relatively quiet until the mid-1980s when Patil offered the proposition that a thyromental distance of less than 6 cm was associated with orotracheal intubation difficulty.[31] During the 1990s, Savva did the same by using the sternomental distance.[32] The importance of Patil's dimension rests not in the distance described, or in its lack of sensitivity, specificity, or positive predictive value with respect to airway management difficulty, but in the fact that it alludes to the *geometry* of the airway. The thyromental line constitutes the hypotenuse of a right angle triangle (Figure 1-3). The axis is length of the floor of the mouth (a dimension of the mandibular space), and the abscissa locates the larynx in relation to the base of the tongue. The length of the oral axis affects the ease with which the glottis is exposed during conventional laryngoscopy: the glottis cannot be visualized beyond the horizon of visibility if it is too long; the larynx is shielded by the base of the tongue (anterior larynx) if it is too short. Likewise for the location of the larynx in relation to the base of the tongue: it is beyond the visible horizon if it is too far down the neck; it is tucked up under the base of the tongue if it is too high in the neck. Furthermore, the dimensions of the mandibular space (length, width, and depth; or volume) have important implications. The volume of the mandibular space must accommodate the tongue, a fluid-filled noncompressible structure, as it is displaced into this space during laryngoscopy to bring the glottis into view.

Mallampati in 1983 and 1985 created a scoring system,[33,34] modified by Samsoon in 1987,[35] that identified oral and pharyngeal access as an issue of importance in airway management (Figure 1-4). Although the score by itself had poor sensitivity, specificity, and positive predictive value, the notion that *access* is important became cemented.

It was during this time that Cormack and Lehane proposed their Laryngeal View Grade scoring system

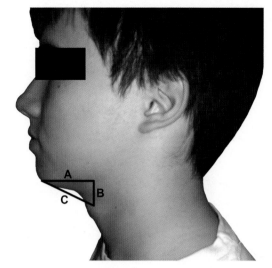

FIGURE 1-3. The Patil's triangle. (A) The second 3 of the evaluate 3-3-2; (B) The 2 of the evaluate 3-3-2; (C) The thyromental distance.

in an effort to provide some structure to the discussion of *difficult laryngoscopy* (Figure 1-5).[36] Although found to be subject to considerable interobserver variability, the scale has been embraced as a valid measure of difficulty; with Grade 3 and 4 views being equated with *difficult laryngoscopy*. By the late 1990s, other models with more reproducible scoring systems, such as Levitan's Percentage of Glottic Opening (POGO) visible, were proposed.[37-39] However, widespread adoption of these systems over the Cormack/Lehane (C/L) system has yet to occur (Figure 1-6).

By the late 1980s, it had become apparent that airway management failure was the most important contributor to poor patient outcome in anesthesia practice, lawsuits, and financial settlements.[4] The question facing airway practitioners became: Who should you not paralyze? A variety of investigators pursued univariate and multivariate systems of analysis that attempted to answer this question, but none with reliable success[40]:

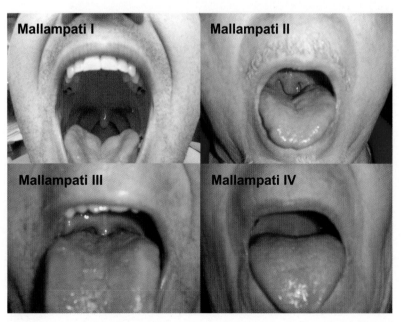

FIGURE 1-4. Mallampati scores.

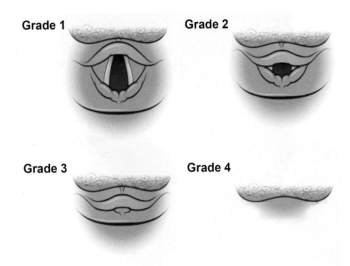

FIGURE 1-5. Cormack/Lehane Laryngeal View Grading Score.

- Wilson, 1988 (Wilson Risk Sum): Employed a weighted scoring system 0 to 2 incorporating body weight, head and neck movement, jaw movement, receding mandible, and prominent (buck) teeth.[41]
- Bellhouse, 1988: Used x-rays to evaluate for difficulty.[42-46]
- Rocke, 1992: Evaluated 1500 parturients using a combination of Mallampati, short neck, receding mandible, and buck teeth.[47]
- Savva, 1994: Identified a sternomental distance less than 12 cm as a risk for difficulty.[32]
- Tse, 1995: Combined Mallampati, head extension, and thyromental distance.[48]

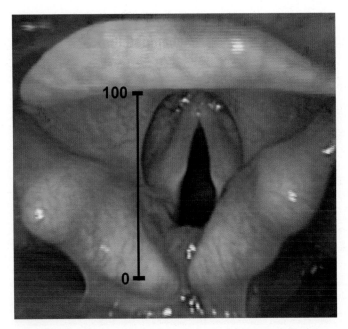

FIGURE 1-6. Levitan's Percent of Glottic Opening (POGO): 100—if the complete glottis can be seen; and 0—if no part of the glottis can be seen.

- El-Ganzouri, 1996: In a large study of 10,507 patients looked at mouth opening, Mallampati, neck movement, mandibular protrusion, body weight, and a positive history of airway management difficulty.[49]
- Karkouti, 2000: Evaluated 461 patients (38 difficult)—correlated mouth opening, chin protrusion, atlanto-occipital extension.[50]

Hot on the heels of the "Who should you not paralyze?" question is the dilemma: How is the airway best rescued in the event that intubation and/or ventilation is impossible, that is, a failed airway? In the past, BMV was viewed as the most commonly performed fallback technique. This technique, difficult to teach, learn, and perform, is being supplanted by more user friendly and easily performed EGDs. This has led to a reframing of the way we think about airway management: In the event laryngoscopy and intubation fails, is it likely that gas exchange can be maintained by BMV or one of these EGD devices? Furthermore, the recognition that while aspiration is undesirable, it is not usually a deadly occurrence, serves to emphasize the primacy of gas exchange over intubation and airway protection.

1.5   DEFINITIONS OF DIFFICULT AND FAILED AIRWAYS

The Difficult Airway is something you anticipate;
the Failed Airway is something you experience.

(Walls, 2002)

As noted earlier, this chapter explores the concepts of *the difficult* and *the failed* airway. The premise is that the pre-procedure recognition and management of the difficult airway should minimize the occurrence of a failed airway. Furthermore, recognizing the failed airway promptly ought to optimize the chances that failing techniques will be abandoned and replaced by techniques reasonably anticipated to succeed.

1.5.1   The difficult airway

When one is presented with a patient that requires tracheal intubation, the first decision is whether or not this airway needs to be managed immediately (typically, the *newly dead* or the *nearly dead crash airway*, see Chapter 2) and one simply proceeds to intervene in the airway. If it is not a crash airway, one must ask, "Is this a difficult airway?" Asking the question presumes that one has a framework to answer it!

As discussed above, and unlike the failed airway, the difficult airway is not so easily defined. Rather than a definition, in concept, the *difficult airway* has five dimensions[8]:

- Difficult BMV
- Difficult laryngoscopy
- Difficult intubation
- Difficult placement of a EGD
- Difficult cricothyrotomy

These five dimensions can be reduced to four technical operations:

- Difficult BMV
- Difficult laryngoscopy and intubation
- Difficult EGD
- Difficult cricothyrotomy

The evaluation of the airway for difficulty may be leisurely or urgent. In the latter circumstance, it must be done quickly with care taken not to omit anything important. Like well-constructed algorithms, mnemonics are efficient memory-aid strategies that lead to a complete, yet rapid, evaluation. One for each technical operation has been crafted to permit a rapid and complete evaluation, no matter the clinical circumstance.

1.5.2   The failed airway

The failed airway has been defined as[8]:

- Three failed attempts at orotracheal intubation by a skilled practitioner and/or
- Failure to maintain acceptable oxygen saturations, typically 90% or above, in otherwise normal individuals

The problem in everyday practice is not so much defining failure; it is recognizing failure once it has occurred, and then moving quickly to alternatives. Clinically, the failed airway presents itself in two ways:

1. You have time: "Can't intubate/can ventilate and oxygenate."
2. You have no time: "Can't intubate/can't ventilate or oxygenate" (CICV or CICO).

The intent is to minimize the chance of encountering a failed airway when one might have easily predicted a difficult intubation, difficult BMV, difficult EGD ventilation, or a difficult cricothyrotomy.

The adage in anesthesia practice with respect to neuromuscular blockade of a patient who has some effective spontaneous ventilation has always been "Don't take anything away from the patient that you can't replace." While such a rigid principle is not always consistent with the realities of airway management, it is a useful one to remember!

1.6   PREDICTION OF DIFFICULT AND FAILED AIRWAY

The most effective aids work well in all clinical situations, as everyday practice adjuncts. The following mnemonics fall into this category[8]:

1.6.1   Difficult bag-mask-ventilation: MOANS

The importance of BMV in airway management is not taken lightly by airway practitioners, particularly as a rescue maneuver when orotracheal intubation has failed. If the airway practitioner is

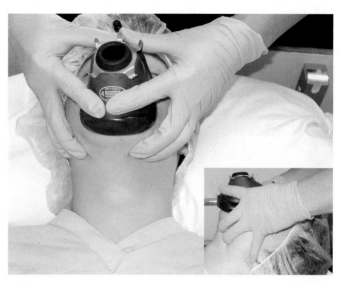

FIGURE 1-7. Optimum mask hold to achieve a mask seal using a two-hand technique.

uncertain that neuromuscular blockade facilitated tracheal intubation will be successful, they must be confident that BMV will be adequate, the use of an EGD will be successful, or at the very least, a successful cricothyrotomy can rapidly be performed.

The bag-mask devices most commonly used in resuscitation settings are capable of generating 50 to 100 cm of water pressure in the upper airway, provided that they do not have positive pressure relief valves, and an adequate mask seal can be obtained (Figure 1-7).

Pediatric and neonatal devices often incorporate positive pressure relief valves that can be easily defeated if needed. This degree of positive pressure is often sufficient to overcome the moderate degree of upper airway obstruction offered by redundant tissue (eg, the obese) or edematous tissue (eg, angioedema, croup, or epiglottitis). Research[51-59] has validated many of those anatomical features that over the years have been implicated in heralding difficult BMV (difficult mask ventilation or DMV). Those features can be grouped into five indicators that can be easily recalled by using the mnemonic **MOANS**[8]:

- *M*ask seal, high *M*allampati grades, *M*inimal jaw protrusion, or *M*ale gender: Bushy beards, crusted blood on the face, or a disruption of lower facial continuity are the commonest examples of conditions that may make an adequate mask seal difficult. Some recommend smearing a substance such as Vaseline or KY Jelly on a beard as a remedy to this problem. However, in the experience of the authors, it simply makes a bad situation worse in that the entire face becomes too slippery to hold the mask in place. Several studies have identified additional risk factors of difficult mask ventilation, including male sex, Mallampatti III or IV airways, and limited jaw protrusion[55,56,59].

- *O*bese or *O*bstructing lesions: Patients who are obese (defined by Langeron et al[57] as BMI >26 kg·m⁻² as opposed to the conventional definition of obese as 30-35 kg·m⁻²) are often difficult to ventilate adequately by bag and mask. BMV can also be difficult in parturients at term and in patients with upper-airway obstruction, angioedema, Ludwig angina, upper airway abscesses (eg, peritonsillar), and epiglottitis. There is a sense among experienced practitioners that edematous lesions (eg, angioedema, croup, epiglottitis, etc) are more amenable to bag-mask rescue should sudden obstruction occur or be induced, although the authors would not rely on this opinion. On the other hand, firm, immobile lesions such as hematomas, cancers, and foreign bodies usually cannot be circumvented by BMV. Total airway obstruction must be avoided in these patients, and care must be taken with airway manipulation (positioning, avoidance of bleeding, sedative hypnotic medications, etc).

- *Aged*: Age more than 55 is associated with a higher risk of difficult BMV, perhaps because of a loss of muscle and tissue tone in the upper airway.[52,57]

- *No teeth* or *Neck radiation*: An adequate mask seal may be difficult in the edentulous patient as the face tends to cave in. An option is to leave dentures in situ (if available) for BMV and remove them for intubation. Alternatively, gauze may be inserted in the cheeks to puff them out in an attempt to improve the seal (vigilance to prevent dislodgement into the airway is required). Radiation therapy in the past to the head and neck may hinder mask ventilation.[55]

- *Snores* or *Stiff*: For the former, this mnemonic affords one a reminder to check for sleep apnea, an increasingly important consideration in anesthetic practice today. BMV may be difficult or impossible in the face of substantial increases in airways resistance (eg, deadly asthma) or decreases in pulmonary compliance (eg, pulmonary edema).

As discussed in Chapter 8, several studies involving large patient populations have validated the above findings.[55,56,59] In a large study by Kheterpal et al involving over 53,000 adult patients receiving a general anesthetic at a tertiary care hospital, the reported incidence of *impossible* BMV (IMV) defined as "the inability to establish face-mask ventilation despite multiple airway adjuncts and two-hand mask ventilation" was 0.15%. Despite there being a diverse clinician group (trainees; nurse and physician anesthetists), having a junior anesthesia provider was not found to be an independent predictor for IMV. The presence of three or more predictors (neck radiation, male, OSA, Mallampati III or IV, beard) significantly increased the risk of IMV with an odds ratio of 8.9 compared to patients without these risk factors. Another important finding from this study is that of the IMV group, 25% were also difficult to intubate. It should be remembered, however, that these studies did not examine the incidence of DMV in patients requiring emergency airway management.

1.6.2 Difficult laryngoscopy and intubation: LEMON

Difficult laryngoscopy and intubation ordinarily implies that the operator had a poor view of the glottis. Cormack and Lehane[36] provided some clarity to the way we think of the *difficult airway* by parsing the act of intubation into its two subcomponents: laryngoscopy and intubation. They also introduced the most widely utilized system of categorizing the degree to which the glottis can be visualized during laryngoscopy (Figure 1-5). Cormack/Lehane view Grades 3 (epiglottis only visible) and 4 (no glottic structures at all visible) are often used as surrogates to define a difficult laryngoscopy and predict difficult intubation. View Grades 1

(visualization of the entire laryngeal aperture) and 2 (visualization of the posterior cords and arytenoids) are not typically associated with difficult intubation, though some Grade 2s may be difficult or impossible to intubate. Tough Grade 2s and 3s are *tailor-made* for intubating introducers such as the Eschmann Tracheal Introducer and Frova devices (see Sections 11.2.1 and 11.2.2).

As can be gleaned from the descriptions, the Cormack/Lehane grading system is insensitive to the degree to which the laryngeal aperture is visible during laryngoscopy: a little bit of it (Grade 2) or all of it (Grade 1). The question often asked is: How much of the cords must be viewed to assure intubation success? How much is enough? In attempting to provide a framework or an approach to answering this question, Levitan et al[37-39] devised a scoring system to quantify the POGO visible. While attractive in many ways, this scale has yet to gain wide acceptance (Figure 1-6).

The Cormack/Lehane grading system is predicated upon grading during the best attempt at conventional laryngoscopy, and best attempt in turn requires definition. Benumof[5] defines best attempt as being composed of six components:

1. Performance by a reasonably experienced practitioner
2. No significant muscle tone
3. The use of the optimal *sniffing* position
4. The use of external laryngeal manipulation (backward upward rightward pressure [BURP] or optimum external laryngeal manipulation [OELM])[60]
5. Length of the blade
6. Type of blade

Most times, an intubation demands that the first attempt be the best attempt, particularly in an emergency, although some compromises may be necessary (eg, residency training). Should an orotracheal intubation attempt fail and an additional attempt be contemplated, it seems reasonable to *change something* on the subsequent attempt to enhance the chances of success. That *something* may be one, some, or all of these factors. Reminding oneself of the components of the optimum or best attempt provides a framework to address "what to change?"

Optimization of all six components may not be in the patient's best interest in an emergency. For example, if difficulty is anticipated, it may not be advisable to paralyze the patient. Additionally, in the event the cervical spine is immobilized, it may not be possible to place them in the *sniffing* position. Most experts in airway management agree that positioning the head and neck is an important step in optimizing conventional laryngoscopy as a prelude to orotracheal intubation.[61]

If it is possible to consistently and precisely predict intubation failure, the initial selection of laryngoscopic oral intubation could be eliminated as a strategy and alternative techniques employed (eg, flexible bronchoscopic intubation, cricothyrotomy). However, they may be technically more challenging, risky, and time consuming. During the last several decades, this has not proven to be possible. Lists of anatomical features, radiologic findings, and complex scoring systems have all been explored without consistent success.

Therefore, we are left to assemble the known risks, match them to the skill, experience, and judgment of the practitioner, and make a decision: Does this airway meet the threshold of being sufficiently difficult to warrant using a Difficult Airway Algorithm, or am I safe to proceed directly to induction, paralysis, and intubation (eg, rapid sequence intubation or rapid sequence induction, commonly known as RSI)[8]

So, how do we quickly identify as many of the risks as possible? The mnemonic **LEMON** is a useful guide:

• *L*ook externally: If the airway looks difficult, it probably is (Figure 1-8). A litany of physical features have been associated with difficult laryngoscopy and intubation—a small mandible may indicate that the tongue is *retro-fitted* over the larynx; a large mandible elongates the pharyngeal axis serving to extend the distance to the larynx and perhaps move it beyond the horizon of view. Buck teeth block access to the oral cavity and elongate the length of the oral axis. A high, arched palate is often associated with a long, narrow oral cavity making access a problem. A short neck may mean the larynx is positioned higher in the neck relative to the base of the tongue making it more difficult to bring the glottis into view. Lower facial disruption is inconsistent with adequate mask seal and may make the glottis impossible to find. It is often said that when it comes to orotracheal intubation, the "tongue is your enemy" because it gets in your way and the "epiglottis is your friend" because once you find it, you ought to be able to find the glottic opening. In upper airway disruption, the tongue may actually be a friend as it leads to the epiglottis and the glottic opening.

• *E*valuate 3-3-2: Although there is no scientific basis to support the 3-3-2 rule, it serves to ensure that the relevant geometry of the upper airway is assessed adequately. The first *3* assesses the adequacy of oral access (Figure 1-9). One ought to be able to open one's mouth three of one's own finger breadths (approximately 5 cm).

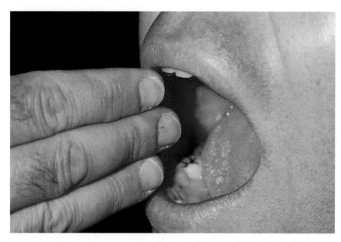

FIGURE 1-9. Airway evaluation: The first *3* of 3-3-2 evaluation indicates the extent of the mouth opening.

The second *3* and the *2* recognize the interplay of the geometric relationships among the various components of the upper airway as first articulated by Patil in 1983.[31] A thyromental distance of less than 6 cm was associated with difficult intubation (Figure 1-3). As described earlier, the thyromental distance is the hypotenuse of Patil's triangle (Figure 1-3), the base being the length of the mandible (Figure 1-10) and the third leg being the distance between the base of the tongue (neck–mandible junction at the level of the hyoid bone) and the top of the larynx (Figure 1-11). One ought to be able to accommodate three of one's own fingers (approximately 5 cm) between the tip of mentum and the mandible–neck junction (Figure 1-10) and fit two fingers between the mandible–neck junction and the thyroid notch (Figure 1-11). The second *3* steers one in assessing the capacity or volume of the mandibular space to accommodate the tongue on laryngoscopy. More than, or less than, three fingers (approximately 5 cm) are associated with greater degrees of difficulty in visualizing the larynx. The length of the oral axis is elongated if it is longer than three fingers, and the mandibular space may be too small to accommodate the tongue during laryngoscopy if it is shorter than three fingers, leaving

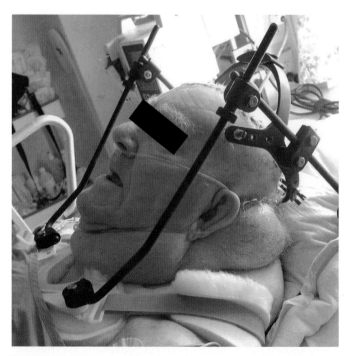

FIGURE 1-8. This patient provides an image recognizable instantly as a difficult airway.

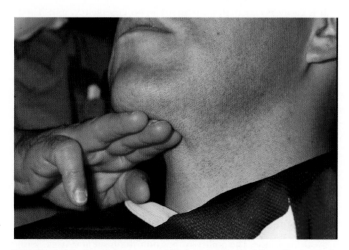

FIGURE 1-10. Airway evaluation: The second *3* of 3-3-2 evaluation indicates the length dimension of the mandibular space.

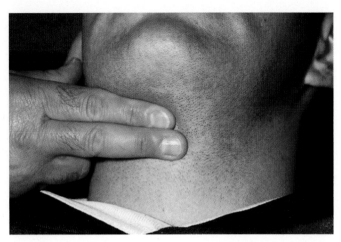

FIGURE 1-11. Airway evaluation: The *2* of 3-3-2 evaluation indicates the position of the larynx relative to the base of the tongue.

it to obscure the view of the glottis. This *volume* is determined by three dimensions: its length, its width, and its depth. The *2* identifies the location of the larynx in relation to the base of the tongue. If more than two fingers are accommodated, meaning the larynx is further below the base of the tongue, it may be difficult to visualize the glottis on laryngoscopy because it is too far down the neck and beyond the visual horizon. Fewer than two fingers may mean that the larynx is tucked up under the base of the tongue and may be difficult to expose. This condition is often called "anterior larynx."

- *Mallampati class:*[33,34] Mallampati studied the relationship between the visibility of the posterior oropharyngeal structures and success rate of laryngoscopic intubation. He had patients sit on the side of the bed, open their mouth as widely as possible, and protrude their tongue as far as possible, without phonating. Figure 1-4 depicts how the scale is constructed. Although Class I and II patients are associated with low intubation failure rates, circumspection with respect to the wisdom of utilizing neuromuscular blockade to facilitate intubation rests with those in Classes III and IV, particularly Class IV in which intubation failure rates may exceed 10%. This scale, by itself, is neither sensitive nor specific.[62] However, it is commonly used because it is easily performed, particularly in an emergency, and it may reveal important information about access to the oral cavity and potentially difficult glottic visualization.

- *Obstruction:* There are three cardinal signs of upper airway obstruction: muffled voice (*hot potato voice*); difficulty in swallowing secretions, either because of pain or obstruction; and stridor. The first two signs do not ordinarily herald imminent total upper airway obstruction. The presence of stridor generally indicates that the diameter of the airway has been reduced to 4.0 mm or less.[63] Upper airway obstruction should always be considered a difficult airway and managed with extreme care. The administration of small doses of opioids and benzodiazepines to manage anxiety may induce total obstruction as the stenting tone of the upper airway musculature relaxes.

- *Neck mobility:* The ability to position the head and neck is one of the six components of achieving an optimal view of the larynx on oral laryngoscopy. Although there is some dissention,[61] it has

long been taught that the "sniffing the morning air," or "sipping English tea" positioning (neck flexion, head extension) of the head and neck, when possible, is at least the best place to start. While cervical spine immobilization alone may not constitute a difficult laryngoscopy, airway practitioners should be cautious in managing patients with limited cervical spine movement.

1.6.3 Difficult use of an extraglottic device: RODS

The insertion of an EGD may be a planned backup maneuver (*Plan B*) when faced with a failed conventional orotracheal intubation. It may also serve as a bridging technique to reestablish gas exchange in a CICV setting while one prepares to perform a cricothyrotomy (see Chapter 2). To minimize the wasting of valuable time, airway practitioners should place the EGD concurrently while setting up to perform a surgical airway.

In the former case, when *Plan B* is an EGD, one ought to have performed an evaluation for difficult EGD placement before it is relied on as a primary or backup plan. While there are no prospective studies to evaluate predictors of difficult use of EGDs, there are many clinical reports of difficult use of EGDs, such as the LMA. **RODS** is a mnemonic that is intended to identify problem patients when an EGD is contemplated:

- *Restricted mouth opening:* Depending on the EGD to be employed, more or less oral access may be needed. For instance, at least 2 cm of mouth opening is required to accommodate an LMA Fastrach™.[64,65]

- *Obstruction:* Upper airway obstruction at the level of the larynx or below. An EGD will not bypass this obstruction. The use of an LMA can be potentially difficult in patients with lingual tonsillar hypertrophy.[66,67]

- *Disrupted or distorted airway:* At least in as much as the *seat and seal* of the EGD may be compromised.[68]

- *Stiff* lungs or *Stiff* cervical spine: Ventilation with an EGD may be difficult or impossible in the face of substantial increases in airway resistance (eg, deadly asthma) or decreases in pulmonary compliance (eg, pulmonary edema). Seal may be exceedingly difficult or impossible to achieve in the face of a fixed flexion deformity of the neck.[56] In addition, there are reports of difficult LMA insertion in patients with limited neck movement (eg, ankylosing spondylitis).[69,70]

1.6.4 Difficult cricothyrotomy: SHORT

There are no absolute contraindications to performing an emergency cricothyrotomy. However, some conditions may make it difficult or impossible to perform the procedure, making it imperative to identify those conditions upfront, particularly if one is relying on a rapidly performed cricothyrotomy as a rescue technique. Similarly, while there are no prospective trials to determine predictors of difficult cricothyrotomy, a number of clinical reports have identified situations associated with difficulties in performing a surgical airway. The mnemonic **SHORT** is used to quickly identify features that may indicate a difficult cricothyrotomy:

- *Surgery/disrupted airway:* The anatomy of the neck may be subtly or obviously distorted due to previous surgery, making the airway difficult to access. Patel reported a case of difficult surgical airway following a recent thyroidectomy.[71]

- *Hematoma or infection:* An infective process or hematoma in the pathway of the cricothyrotomy incision may make the procedure technically difficult but should never be considered a contraindication in a life-threatening situation.

- *Obese/access problem:* Obesity should be considered a surrogate for any problem that makes percutaneous access to the anterior neck problematic. A fixed flexion deformity of the cervical spine, halo traction, and other situations may also make access to the neck difficult. Patel reported a case of surgical airway failure in a patient with an obese and short neck.[71]

- *Radiation:* The tissue changes associated with past radiation therapy may alter tissues, making the procedure difficult.

- *Tumor:* Tumor either in or around the airway may present difficulty, both from an access perspective as well as bleeding.

1.7   SUMMARY

Failure to evaluate the airway and predict difficulty is the single most important factor leading to a failed airway. Despite decades of study, no system of evaluation is able to discern with certainty (100% reliability) those airways that can be managed with conventional laryngoscopic intubation and those where an alternative method is advisable. For this reason, each and every airway management episode must be approached with a view that some other device or technique may be necessary should the primary plan fail. Furthermore, the airway practitioner must evaluate the airway for difficulty relative to each of the alternatives contemplated. Once Plan A has failed, it is too late to suddenly realize that Plan B is also impossible because a factor which could have been detected had a prior evaluation for difficulty been conducted.

While not exhaustive in covering all of the features of a difficult airway, the mnemonics **MOANS**, **LEMON**, **RODS**, and **SHORT** provide guidance in evaluating all airways for difficulty, even though they are specifically designed to be employed rapidly in the face of an urgent or emergency clinical circumstance.

Finally, recognizing that one is in the midst of a failed airway is crucial in embarking on maneuvers that may rescue the airway. Persisting with a failing technique is a fundamental contributor to bad outcomes in airway management.

REFERENCES

1. Hung O, Murphy M. Unanticipated difficult intubation. *Curr Opin Anaesthesiol.* 2004;17:479-481.
2. Shiga T, Wajima Z, Inoue T, Sakamoto A. Predicting difficult intubation in apparently normal patients: a meta-analysis of bedside screening test performance. *Anesthesiology.* 2005;103:429-437.
3. Mort TC. Emergency tracheal intubation: complications associated with repeated laryngoscopic attempts. *Anesth Analg.* 2004;99: 607-613, table of contents.
4. Cheney FW, Posner KL, Caplan RA. Adverse respiratory events infrequently leading to malpractice suits. A closed claims analysis. *Anesthesiology.* 1991;75:932-939.
5. Benumof J. The ASA difficult airway algorithm: new thoughts and considerations. 51st Annual Refresher Course Lectures and Clinical Update Program, American Society of Anesthesiologists. 2000; 235.
6. Practice guidelines for management of the difficult airway: an updated report by the American Society of Anesthesiologists Task Force on Management of the Difficult Airway. *Anesthesiology.* 2003;98:1269-1277.
7. Wilson ME. Predicting difficult intubation. *Br J Anaesth.* 1993;71:333-334.
8. Walls RM, Murphy MF. Identification of the difficult and failed airway. In: Walls RM, Murphy MF, eds. *Manual of Emergency Airway Management.* 3rd ed. Philadelphia, PA: Lippincott, Williams and Wilkins; 2008.
9. Sakles JC, Laurin EG, Rantapaa AA, Panacek EA. Airway management in the emergency department: a one-year study of 610 tracheal intubations. *Ann Emerg Med.* 1998;31:325-332.
10. Bair AE, Filbin MR, Kulkarni RG, Walls RM. The failed intubation attempt in the emergency department: analysis of prevalence, rescue techniques, and personnel. *J Emerg Med.* 2002;23:131-140.
11. Sivilotti ML, Filbin MR, Murray HE, Slasor P, Walls RM. Does the sedative agent facilitate emergency rapid sequence intubation? *Acad Emerg Med.* 2003;10:612-620.
12. Sagarin MJ, Chiang V, Sakles JC, et al. Rapid sequence intubation for pediatric emergency airway management. *Pediatr Emerg Care.* 2002;18:417-423.
13. Benumof JL. The unanticipated difficult airway. *Can J Anaesth.* 1999;46:510-511.
14. Crosby E. The unanticipated difficult airway—evolving strategies for successful salvage. *Can J Anaesth.* 2005;52:562-567.
15. Hakala P, Randell T. Intubation difficulties in patients with rheumatoid arthritis. A retrospective analysis. *Acta Anaesthesiol Scand.* 1998;42:195-198.
16. Combes X, Le Roux B, Suen P, et al. Unanticipated difficult airway in anesthetized patients: prospective validation of a management algorithm. *Anesthesiology.* 2004;100:1146-1150.
17. Rose DK, Cohen MM. The airway: problems and predictions in 18,500 patients. *Can J Anaesth.* 1994;41:372-383.
18. Ross BK. ASA closed claims in obstetrics: lessons learned. *Anesthesiol Clin North Am.* 2003;21:183-197.
19. Ezri T, Szmuk P, Evron S, et al. Difficult airway in obstetric anesthesia: a review. *Obstet Gynecol Surv.* 2001;56:631-641.
20. Levack ID, Masson AH. Difficult tracheal intubation in obstetrics. *Anaesthesia.* 1985;40:384.
21. Practice guidelines for management of the difficult airway. A report by the American Society of Anesthesiologists Task Force on Management of the Difficult Airway. *Anesthesiology.* 1993;78:597-602.
22. Peterson GN, Domino KB, Caplan RA, Posner KL, Lee LA, Cheney FW. Management of the difficult airway: a closed claims analysis. *Anesthesiology.* 2005;103:33-39.
23. Black HC. *Black's Law Dictionary.* 7th ed. St Paul, MN: West Publishing Co; 1999.
24. Crosby ET, Cooper RM, Douglas MJ, et al. The unanticipated difficult airway with recommendations for management. *Can J Anaesth.* 1998;45:757-776.
25. Henderson JJ, Popat MT, Latto IP, Pearce AC. Difficult Airway Society guidelines for management of the unanticipated difficult intubation. *Anaesthesia.* 2004;59:675-694.
26. Stoller JK. The history of intubation, tracheostomy and airway appliances. *Respir Care.* 1999;44:595-603.
27. Henderson JJ. The use of paraglossal straight blade laryngoscopy in difficult tracheal intubation. *Anaesthesia.* 1997;52:552-560.
28. Virtual Museum of Equipment for Airway Equipment, Virtual Museum of Equipment for Airway Equipment.
29. Henderson JJ. Development of the 'gum-elastic bougie'. *Anaesthesia.* 2003;58:103-104.
30. Cass NM, James NR, Lines V. Difficult direct laryngoscopy complicating intubation for anaesthesia. *Br Med J.* 1956;1:488-489.
31. Patil VU, Stehling LC, Zauder HL. Predicting the difficulty of intubation utilizing an intubation guide. *Anesthesiology.* 1983;10:32.
32. Savva D. Sternomental distance—a useful predictor of difficult intubation in patients with cervical spine disease? *Anaesthesia.* 1996;51:284-285.
33. Mallampati SR. Clinical sign to predict difficult tracheal intubation (hypothesis). *Can Anaesth Soc J.* 1983;30:316-317.
34. Mallampati SR, Gatt SP, Gugino LD, et al. A clinical sign to predict difficult tracheal intubation: a prospective study. *Can Anaesth Soc J.* 1985;32:429-434.
35. Samsoon GL, Young JR. Difficult tracheal intubation: a retrospective study. *Anaesthesia.* 1987;42:487-490.
36. Cormack RS, Lehane J. Difficult tracheal intubation in obstetrics. *Anaesthesia.* 1984;39:1105-1111.

37. Levitan RM, Ochroch EA, Kush S, et al. Assessment of airway visualization: validation of the percentage of glottic opening (POGO) scale. *Acad Emerg Med*. 1998;5:919-923.

38. Ochroch EA, Hollander JE, Kush S, et al. Assessment of laryngeal view: percentage of glottic opening score vs Cormack and Lehane grading. *Can J Anaesth*. 1999;46:987-990.

39. Levitan RM, Hollander JE, Ochroch EA. A grading system for direct laryngoscopy. *Anaesthesia*. 1999;54:1009-1010.

40. Yentis SM. Predicting difficult intubation—worthwhile exercise or pointless ritual? *Anaesthesia*. 2002;57:105-109.

41. Wilson ME, Spiegelhalter D, Robertson JA, Lesser P. Predicting difficult intubation. *Br J Anaesth*. 1988;61:211-216.

42. Bellhouse CP. Prediction of difficult tracheal intubation. *Br J Anaesth*. 1995;74:490.

43. Bellhouse CP, Dore C. Criteria for estimating likelihood of difficulty of endotracheal intubation with the Macintosh laryngoscope. *Anaesth Intensive Care*. 1988;16:329-337.

44. Bellhouse CB. Predicting difficult intubation. *Br J Anaesth*. 1994;72:494.

45. Bellhouse CP. Predicting difficult intubation. *Anaesthesia*. 1992;47:440-441.

46. Bellhouse CP, Dore C. Predicting difficult intubation. *Br J Anaesth*. 1989;62:469.

47. Rocke DA, Murray WB, Rout CC, Gouws E. Relative risk analysis of factors associated with difficult intubation in obstetric anesthesia. *Anesthesiology*. 1992;77:67-73.

48. Tse JC, Rimm EB, Hussain A. Predicting difficult endotracheal intubation in surgical patients scheduled for general anesthesia: a prospective blind study. *Anesth Analg*. 1995;81:254-258.

49. El-Ganzouri AR, McCarthy RJ, Tuman KJ, Tanck EN, Ivankovich AD. Preoperative airway assessment: predictive value of a multivariate risk index. *Anesth Analg*. 1996;82:1197-1204.

50. Karkouti K, Rose DK, Wigglesworth D, Cohen MM. Predicting difficult intubation: a multivariable analysis. *Can J Anaesth*. 2000;47:730-739.

51. Adnet F. Difficult mask ventilation: an underestimated aspect of the problem of the difficult airway? *Anesthesiology*. 2000;92:1217-1218.

52. El-Orbany M, Woehlck HJ. Difficult mask ventilation. *Anesth Analg*. 2009;109:1870-1880.

53. Garewal DS, Johnson JO. Difficult mask ventilation. *Anesthesiology*. 2000;92:1199-1200.

54. Gautam P, Gaul TK, Luthra N. Prediction of difficult mask ventilation. *Eur J Anaesthesiol*. 2005;22:638-640.

55. Kheterpal S, Han R, Tremper KK, et al. Incidence and predictors of difficult and impossible mask ventilation. *Anesthesiology*. 2006;105:885-891.

56. Kheterpal S, Martin L, Shanks AM, Tremper KK. Prediction and outcomes of impossible mask ventilation: a review of 50,000 anesthetics. *Anesthesiology*. 2009;110:891-897.

57. Langeron O, Masso E, Huraux C, et al. Prediction of difficult mask ventilation. *Anesthesiology*. 2000;92:1229-1236.

58. Salem MR, Ovassapian A. Difficult mask ventilation: what needs improvement? *Anesth Analg*. 2009;109:1720-1722.

59. Yildiz TS, Solak M, Toker K. The incidence and risk factors of difficult mask ventilation. *J Anesth*. 2005;19:7-11.

60. Benumof JL, Cooper SD. Quantitative improvement in laryngoscopic view by optimal external laryngeal manipulation. *J Clin Anesth*. 1996;8:136-140.

61. Adnet F, Baillard C, Borron SW, et al. Randomized study comparing the "sniffing position" with simple head extension for laryngoscopic view in elective surgery patients. *Anesthesiology*. 2001;95:836-841.

62. Lee A, Fan LT, Gin T, et al. A systematic review (meta-analysis) of the accuracy of the Mallampati tests to predict the difficult airway. *Anesth Analg*. 2006;102:1867-1878.

63. Donlon JV. Anesthetic and airway management of laryngoscopy and bronchoscopy. In: Benumof J, ed. *Airway Management:Principles and Practice*. St Louis: Mosby; 1996: 666-685.

64. Preis C, Czerny C, Preis I, Zimpfer M. Variations in ILMA external diameters: another cause of device failure. *Can J Anaesth*. 2000;47:886-889.

65. Teoh WH, Lim Y. Comparison of the single use and reusable intubating laryngeal mask airway. *Anaesthesia*. 2007;62:381-384.

66. Fundingsland BW, Benumof JL. Difficulty using a laryngeal mask airway in a patient with lingual tonsil hyperplasia. *Anesthesiology*. 1996;84:1265-1266.

67. Parmet JL, Colonna-Romano P, Horrow JC, et al. The laryngeal mask airway reliably provides rescue ventilation in cases of unanticipated difficult tracheal intubation along with difficult mask ventilation. *Anesth Analg*. 1998;87: 661-665.

68. Buckham M, Brooker M, Brimacombe J, Keller C. A comparison of the reinforced and standard laryngeal mask airway: ease of insertion and the influence of head and neck position on oropharyngeal leak pressure and intracuff pressure. *Anaesth Intens Care*. 1999;27:628-631.

69. Ishimura H, Minami K, Sata T, et al. Impossible insertion of the laryngeal mask airway and oropharyngeal axes. *Anesthesiology*. 1995;83:867-869.

70. Olmez G, Nazaroglu H, Arslan SG, Ozyilmaz MA, Turghanoglu AD. Difficulties and failure of laryngeal mask insertion in a patient with ankylosing spondylitis. *Turk J Med*. 2004;34:349-352.

71. Patel RG. Percutaneous transtracheal jet ventilation: a safe, quick, and temporary way to provide oxygenation and ventilation when conventional methods are unsuccessful. *Chest*. 1999;116:1689-1694.

SELF-EVALUATION QUESTIONS

1.1. The most common factor leading to a failed airway is

A. morbid obesity

B. distorted airway anatomy

C. upper airway obstruction

D. failure to predict a difficult airway

E. not knowing enough rescue techniques well

1.2. The standard of care in airway management is related to all of the following **EXCEPT**:

A. the skill of an average practitioner

B. similar localities

C. procedures that give the best results

D. the expectations of the reasonable patient

E. opinions offered by experts

1.3. The standard of care expects that the average, reasonable airway practitioner ought to be able to do all of the following **EXCEPT**:

A. be able to manage an unanticipated difficult airway

B. be an expert and be able to use a flexible bronchoscope to intubate immediately in the face of a CICV airway

C. be facile with one or two rescue devices or techniques in the face of a failed airway

D. be able to perform a surgical airway

E. be able to recognize and manage a failed airway

CHAPTER (2)

The Algorithms

Michael F. Murphy and Edward T. Crosby

2.1   INTRODUCTION

2.1.1   What is the challenge of difficult and failed airway management?

Airway management is fundamental to the practice of anesthesia, emergency medicine, emergency medical services (EMS), critical care medicine, hospital medicine, and other areas of care. The focus of this chapter is the *management* of the difficult and failed airway in an emergency or urgent situation. Management of the predicted difficult intubation is dealt with in Chapter 3 and in Section II of this book.

The airway practitioner in this situation is faced with two particular challenges: to be able to accurately predict a difficult airway, and to be able to recognize when airway management has failed.[1] No matter the situation, reliably and reproducibly ensuring or establishing timely and effective oxygenation and ventilation is imperative.

Appropriate planning, selection of the correct device and technique, and calm execution based on learned methods and experience enhances success even in these most difficult cases. In an airway crisis, there is no question that having a logical and simple approach based on a planned strategy is most likely to be successful.

2.1.2   How reliably can we predict a difficult airway?

There are five ways by which effective gas exchange occurs:

- Spontaneous patient driven
- Bag-mask-ventilation (BMV)
- Extraglottic device (EGD)
- Laryngoscopy and endotracheal intubation
- Surgical airways

Four of these are *artificial* or nonnatural interventions, or methods of active airway management. In the event that a patient is unable to sustain adequate spontaneous gas exchange, or if in the course of therapy the patient's ability to maintain adequate gas exchange (eg, due to the use of medications) is compromised or eliminated, one of these four methods must be employed successfully to assure survival. They constitute the four dimensions of airway management. Hence, the assessment for difficulty is focussed on these four independent operations:

- Difficult bag-mask-ventilation
- Difficult EGD
- Difficult laryngoscopy and orotracheal intubation
- Difficult surgical airway

Health-care professionals are experts at evaluating whether or not a patient is adequately ventilating and oxygenating on their own and whether or not they will be able to sustain it in the near term (minutes to hours). It is therefore only reasonable to expect that if an airway practitioner is to intervene in such a manner that the spontaneous patient-driven method of gas exchange is to be hindered or eliminated, the practitioner must also be able to predict that an alternative artificial method of gas exchange will be successful.

In elective situations, difficulty with mask-ventilation is uncommon. Langeron prospectively reviewed the management of 1502 patients undergoing elective surgery under general anesthesia.[2] Difficult mask-ventilation was defined as (1) an inability to maintain SaO_2 greater than 92% while using 100% O_2 via the anesthesia circuit bag-mask unit; (2) significant gas leak around the face-mask; (3) a need to increase the fresh gas flow to rates greater than 15 L·min^{-1} and to use the flush valve more than twice; (4) no perceptible chest wall movement during ventilation; (5) the need to perform a two-handed mask technique; or (6) changing the operator. The anesthesia practitioner was asked to identify ventilation as difficult only if the difficulty was perceived to be clinically relevant, that is, potentially leading to a patient threat. In 5% of the patients ventilation was considered difficult, and in one patient ventilation was impossible. Following multivariate analysis, five criteria were recognized as independent factors for difficult mask-ventilation: age more than 55 years; BMI greater than 26 kg·m^{-2}; lack of teeth; presence of a beard; and a history of snoring (see Section 1.6.1).

Kheterpal et al[3,4] confirmed that obesity (BMI >30 kg·m^{-2}), snoring and sleep apnea, age (>56 years), and Mallampati of Grade III or IV were risk factors for difficult ventilation and, in addition, noted that a history of radiation therapy to the neck and severely limited jaw protrusion predicted difficult BMV (see Chapter 7 for a detailed discussion).

In the emergency situation, other factors may become relevant when considering whether difficulty with mask-ventilation is more likely to be encountered. Trauma to the face with resultant edema, bleeding or debris in the airway, and the need to maintain in-line C-spine immobilization where required may increase the degree of difficulty with mask-ventilation. In addition, the use of cricoid pressure, often perceived to be necessary in emergency intubations, is recognized to increase the likelihood of difficult mask-ventilation. Petito and Russell evaluated the impact of cricoid pressure on lung ventilation during bag-mask-ventilation (BMV).[5] Fifty patients were randomized to either with or without cricoid pressure applied during a 3-minute period of standardized mask-ventilation. Patients who had cricoid pressure applied were considered more difficult to ventilate (36% vs 12%), and these patients tended to have more air in the stomach than those patients considered easy to ventilate without applied cricoid pressure.

Most of the studies dealing with assessment of the airway in anticipation of tracheal intubation using a laryngoscope, including Cass' landmark paper in 1956,[6] and the Mallampati classification in the mid 1980s,[7,8] have little applicability to currently available alternative devices (eg, rigid fiberoptic devices, intubating EGDs, video laryngoscopes, etc). Modification of Mallampati's original schema,[9] as well as alternate strategies to assess the airway (see Section 1.6.2) have been proposed. These have ranged from using simple anatomical descriptors, ranking and summating anatomical

scoring systems, and using logistic regression to create predictive scales to derive performance indices. These strategies share some common characteristics: they have high sensitivity but low specificity and low positive predictive value with respect to predicting failure. For example, Shiga et al employing a meta analysis to assess combined Mallampati and temperomandibular joint displacement (TMD) scores found a positive association with difficult intubation of only 9.9%.[10] Additionally, many of the tests have only moderate interobserver reliability.[11,12] Such limitations may help to explain why these tests often fail to predict difficult tracheal intubation, and why perhaps some practitioners question the value of performing preanesthetic airway assessments.[13]

A number of new schemes and techniques used to predict potential airway difficulty have been described; their accuracy and widespread applicability are not yet determined. However, it is likely that they will have a low positive predictive value, similar to current strategies, because of the low incidence of airway difficulty.[13] Furthermore, we know that even with careful evaluation, difficulty will not be predicted in many instances.[14] Therefore, strategies to manage the unanticipated difficult airway should be preformulated and practiced to minimize adverse outcomes resulting from false-negative predictions.

2.2   AIRWAY EMERGENCIES

2.2.1   How is airway management in an emergency setting different?

Airway management in an emergency setting may be complicated by a multitude of factors. Trauma to the face and neck may distort anatomical features or obscure them with blood and debris. The requirement for in-line stabilization in patients with spinal injury or perceived to be at-risk for a spinal injury may make laryngoscopy more difficult.[15] Unprepared patients are often associated with a full stomach and are at a higher risk of regurgitation and aspiration of gastric contents. Although the literature is not consistent, the use of cricoid pressure to reduce the risk of regurgitation and aspiration likely makes laryngoscopy and tracheal intubation more difficult.[16-18] To make matters worse, there is no evidence that the risk of aspiration after RSI is decreased by the use of cricoid pressure.[19]

Smith evaluated the ease of rigid fiberoptic (WuScope System™) intubation in anesthetized adults receiving cricoid pressure.[20] Each patient had their trachea intubated under two conditions: with and without cricoid pressure. An easy intubation occurred in 91% of patients without cricoid pressure and in 66% of patients with cricoid pressure applied. Cricoid pressure compressed the vocal cords in 27% of patients and impeded tracheal tube placement in 15%. In three patients (9%), pressure had to be released in order to successfully intubate their tracheas. Hodgson assessed the effect of cricoid pressure on lightwand intubation success in 60 adult female patients presenting for abdominal hysterectomy.[21] All 30 patients allocated to intubation without cricoid pressure were intubated successfully on the first attempt with a median time of 28 seconds. Lightwand intubation with cricoid pressure was successful in 26 of 30 patients on the first attempt, but the median time to successful intubation was significantly longer at 48.5 seconds. Three patients required two attempts for successful intubation, and one could not be intubated with the lightwand while cricoid pressure was being applied. Shulman compared the Bullard laryngoscope (BL) with the flexible bronchoscope (FB) in a cervical spine injury model, using in-line stabilization with and without cricoid pressure.[22] The times for laryngoscopy and intubation were longer in the FB group than in the BL group. Further, there was a significantly lower rate of adequate laryngoscopic view in the FB group in the presence of cricoid pressure than in either of the BL groups, or in the FB no cricoid-pressure group. Shulman concluded that the BL is more reliable, quicker, and more resistant to the effect of cricoid pressure than is the FB when used in the setting of in-line stabilization with cricoid pressure applied.

In summary, cricoid pressure has a limited, and for the most part probably negative, impact on the success rate of airway interventions.

Emergency situations and hemodynamically unstable patients may contraindicate the use of drugs to facilitate laryngoscopy, resulting in intubation conditions which may be less than ideal. Finally, a chaotic emergency environment may distract the practitioner, making it more difficult to manage the airway.

2.3   DIFFICULT AND FAILED AIRWAY

2.3.1   What does experience tell us about rescuing the difficult airway?

Evidence has emerged that having automatic *default-to* strategies improves the success of rescue airway interventions and reduces the occurrence of adverse outcomes. Conversely, there are also data demonstrating that persisting with failing techniques rather than defaulting to rescue strategies results in higher rates of morbidity and mortality. Rose and Cohen reported that difficult laryngoscopy in anesthesia practice was most often managed with persistent attempts at direct laryngoscopy, and the use of alternative approaches to tracheal intubation was uncommon.[1] In these patients, there was a higher incidence of desaturation, esophageal intubation, dental damage, and unexpected ICU admissions.[1] Similarly, Mort, in reviewing the airway management of 2833 critically ill patients outside of the operating room, noted that the most common strategy implemented for managing difficult intubations was, again, repeated direct laryngoscopy.[23] There was a significant increase in the rate of airway-related complications as the number of laryngoscopic attempts increased (≤2 vs >2).[23,24] These complications included hypoxemia, regurgitation, aspiration, bradycardia, and cardiac arrest.[23-25]

Contrary to the experiences reported by Rose and Cohen and Mort, Hung noted that immediately choosing an alternate technique (lighted stylet) when direct laryngoscopy had failed was typically rewarded with rapid tracheal intubation.[26] Complications were both rare and minor and generally attributable to the preceding attempts at direct laryngoscopy. Heidegger reported on a protocol for management of both anticipated and unanticipated difficult intubations that emphasized defaulting to the flexible bronchoscope early when difficult laryngoscopy was anticipated or observed.[27] Applied in 13,248 intubations, the protocol failed in only six patients (0.045%); again this strategy was associated with minimal morbidity. Combes reported on the efficacy of an institutional protocol employing the intubating laryngeal mask and Eschmann Tracheal Introducer.[28] One hundred cases of unanticipated difficulties occurred among 11,257 tracheal intubations. There were three deviations from the protocol and two patients were wakened without further airway management. All patients managed by the protocol were successfully ventilated and intubated. Finally, Mort compared the outcomes of patients undergoing emergency tracheal intubation in his institution before and after the application of the American Society of Anesthesiologists (ASA) guidelines.[29] The rate of cardiac arrest during emergency intubation was reduced by 50%.

Connolly et al noted that alternatives to DL were far more likely to be successful than persistent use of DL in setting of multiple failed attempts.[30]

It is clear that early conversion to adjuncts and alternatives to direct-vision laryngoscopy when direct laryngoscopy proves difficult results in a higher salvage rate with low patient morbidity than does persistent use of the direct laryngoscope. The emerging evidence is that the choice of the alternative may be less important than the fact that it is a *practiced alternative* and chosen early in a planned approach when direct laryngoscopy has proven to be difficult or has actually failed.

2.3.2   Is there a pattern to the way airway practitioners behave in the face of a difficult or failed airway?

Tracheal intubation is still predominantly performed orally under direct laryngoscopy. Difficulties related to airway management largely involve failure to achieve tracheal intubation due to difficult direct laryngoscopy. A number of innovative new tools for tracheal intubation have been presented in recent years, which address many of the factors that give rise to difficult direct laryngoscopy.[31]

The direct laryngoscope is designed to facilitate tracheal intubation by establishing a line of sight from the mouth to the larynx. As has already been noted, there are multiple patient factors, which individually or in combination may conspire to obstruct a laryngeal view. The ability to predict all patients in whom it will be impossible to establish a line of sight during laryngoscopy is sufficiently imprecise that sole reliance on the laryngoscope to perform tracheal intubation is a precarious strategy.

It is likely that reliance on limited conventional airway techniques that are less than optimum is a risk-enhancing behavior, which predisposes patients to increased rates of morbidity and mortality. There is evidence that such behavior has been common among anesthesiologists. Rosenblatt surveyed a random sample of the active membership of the ASA.[32] The survey presented difficult airway scenarios involving cooperative adult patients who required tracheal intubation. Physicians were asked to identify their preferred management technique. In a scenario described as a patient with a history of previous difficult intubation, 60% of practitioners would induce general anesthesia and 59% would proceed with direct laryngoscopy. Experienced practitioners tended to use higher risk induction techniques and were more likely to use the laryngeal mask airway in situations commonly agreed to be unconventional or contraindicated. Use of alternative devices including the BL, lighted stylet, and other adjuncts was uncommon, occurring in less than 5% in all scenarios.

Jenkins surveyed 833 Canadian anesthesiologists to assess difficult airway management, training, and access to airway equipment.[33] Respondents were asked to indicate their management choices in 10 difficult airway scenarios. The direct laryngoscopy was the preferred technique overall, with FB being the second most commonly used device. More experienced, male, and older practitioners were more likely to choose asleep induction for high-risk scenarios, a finding similar to that of Rosenblatt. Respondents were not asked to indicate their degree of comfort in using the alternatives that were chosen to manage the clinical scenarios described in the survey. Wong et al surveyed Canadian anesthesiologists by mail regarding their management preferences in two situations: difficult intubation and cannot intubate, cannot ventilate. In the difficult intubation scenario, the preferred alternative airway devices were lighted stylet (45%), flexible bronchoscope (26%), and intubating laryngeal mask airway (20%). Only 57% of respondents had encountered a CICV situation in real life. In the CICV scenario, preferred invasive techniques were needle cricothyrotomy (51%), open cricothyrotomy (28%), and tracheotomy by surgeon (14%). In general, anesthesiologists had little experience with and were uncomfortable with open surgical airways, although those that had practiced on mannequins were more comfortable using them in patients.[34]

Kristensen similarly assessed airway management behavior, experience, and knowledge among Danish anesthesiologists by surveying all members of the Danish Society of Anesthesiologists.[35] Respondents were asked if they had experienced situations during anesthesia in which insufficient oxygenation had caused serious problems that could have been prevented by different airway management. About a quarter of those surveyed answered in the affirmative with 20% of registrars and 26% of specialists agreeing. When asked whether they would perform awake intubation if they expected a difficult intubation, 34% of registrars, 50% of senior registrars, but only 25% of specialists said that they would. Only 48% of registrars and 59% of specialists agreed that a previous difficult intubation was a reliable predictor of difficult intubation in the future. These high-risk attitudes and behaviors are especially concerning. Among the specialists, only 21% use a lighted stylet at least once a year, 11% a BL, and 7% a retrograde technique. Forty percent of specialists had intubated the trachea of an awake, spontaneously breathing patient 10 times or less in their career, and 23% of specialists had never done so using an FB. Finally, about half the registrars and a third of the specialists reported that they did not routinely have immediate access to an LMA when providing anesthesia.

Ezri's more recent survey of American anesthesiologists suggests that there may be an increasing willingness to use alternatives to the direct laryngoscope in airway scenarios perceived as high risk.[36] However, Ezri also observed that such a willingness persisted even when the anesthesiologists acknowledged that they were neither comfortable nor experienced with the alternate technology that they proposed using in these difficult situations.

2.3.3 What is the medical–legal experience with respect to airway management failure?

The largest series of published medical–legal cases involving airway management is that of the ASA Closed Claims Project. Data from the airway cases reviewed in the ASA Closed Claims Project were originally published in 1990, with additional publications in 1991, 2000, and 2005.[37,38] In the original (1990) report, respiratory claims accounted for 34% (522/1541) of all claims. Inadequate ventilation was the most common single event overall, accounting for 12.7% of all claims and more than a third of the respiratory claims. In the original report, esophageal intubation and difficult intubation claims occurred each at about half the rate of those for inadequate ventilation. Caplan et al[37] speculated that improved monitoring would reduce the incidence of inadequate ventilation and esophageal intubation and enhanced training would reduce the occurrence of difficult intubation and its sequelae.

In 2000, additional Closed Claims data was published in the ASA Newsletter.[39] Respiratory claims now accounted for 17.9% of total claims (798/4459), half the original proportion. Inadequate ventilation and esophageal intubation now accounted for considerably fewer claims than in the first report but claims for difficult intubation were now responsible for 6.4% of total claims, 14% higher than in the original report. In 48% of the difficult intubation claims, some difficulty was anticipated preoperatively by the anesthesiologist. Despite this expectation of difficulties, the most common (69% of instances) management strategy employed in these situations was induction of anesthesia followed by persistent attempts at oral laryngoscopic intubation. A similar strategy of multiple attempts orally was employed in scenarios in which difficulty was not anticipated but encountered. Of the cases in which difficulty was anticipated, 69% eventually deteriorated into a "can't intubate, can't ventilate" (CICV) situation. Airway management was deemed to be below the accepted *standard of care* in 49% of the cases reported in the update. This is significantly higher than that seen for other claims in the database.

An updated analysis of the closed claims relating to management of the difficult airway was published in 2005.[39] Two-thirds of the documented events took place during induction of anesthesia and the remaining third during surgery, extubation of the trachea, or recovery. Care was judged to be less than appropriate or substandard in nearly half of the difficult airway claims. In the claims with an anticipated difficult airway, the first strategy was still more likely to be intubation after induction of general anesthesia with ventilation ablated (61%) than awake intubation (32%). There was no difference in the outcome in claims when succinylcholine was used compared with those in which a nondepolarizing muscle relaxant was employed at induction. Awake intubation was attempted but unsuccessful in 12 claims, resulting in death or brain damage in 75% of these claims. In five of these 12 claims, airway difficulties arose when general anesthesia was induced after unsuccessful awake intubation. Finally, in claims in which an emergency airway situation developed, the outcome was worse with persistent attempts at intubation before attempting emergency nonsurgical ventilation or emergency surgical airway access.

Claims involving airway management are more likely to be associated with a permanent adverse outcome than others, and it is recognized that severe adverse outcomes can affect the judgment as to the *appropriateness of care*.[40] However, criticism of care may be well founded as a preoperative airway review was not conducted (or recorded as having been conducted) in 25% of cases, 28% of practitioner's had no explicit plan for dealing with anticipated difficulties, and 25% did not alter their conventional method of airway management despite recognizing the potential for difficulty. Furthermore, when difficulties were encountered, the most common management strategy was persistent nonsurgical attempts at tracheal intubation. In 69% of cases where difficulties were anticipated, a CICV situation arose. Finally, and significantly, no strategy for extubation was outlined in almost half of the cases in which the practitioner encountered difficulties intubating the trachea.[40]

Cook et al reported on the closed claims in the United Kingdom against the National Health Service between 1995 and 2007.[40] Of 841 relevant claims 366 (44%) were related to regional anesthesia, 245 (29%) obstetric anesthesia, 161 (19%) inadequate anesthesia, 95 (11%) dental damage, 71 (8%) airway (excluding dental damage), 62 (7%) drug related (excluding allergy), 31 (4%) drug allergy related, 31 (4%) positioning, 29 (3%) respiratory, 26 (3%) consent, 21 (2%) central venous cannulation, and 18 (2%) peripheral venous cannulation. Defining which cases are, from a medicolegal viewpoint, *high risk* is uncertain, but the clinical categories with the largest number of claims were regional anesthesia, obstetric anesthesia, inadequate anesthesia, dental damage, and airway, those with the highest overall cost were regional anesthesia, obstetric anesthesia, and airway, and those with the highest mean cost per closed claim were respiratory, central venous cannulation, and drug error excluding allergy. Although airway claims were relatively infrequent overall, they tended to be associated with some of the most severe outcomes and the highest costs to close. So we are not alone in North America!

2.4   AIRWAY ALGORITHMS

2.4.1   Why are algorithms useful in airway management?

Automatic responses are not typical when we are confronted by rare events such as the "cannot intubate, cannot ventilate" airway, or even many types of emergency airways. Therefore, fundamental to successfully managing the emergency or failed airway is the development of a systematic approach (*decision trees* or *algorithms*, mnemonics) to clinical situations rarely encountered in day-to-day practice. These algorithms must be evidence based and must be quickly and easily applied. It is fair to say that after years of formal medical education and practice, most of us harbor an aversion to *algorithms*. While it is recognized that rigidity stifles innovation and constrains personal preference, adherence to sensibly constructed decision trees minimizes variation, conserves valuable time, and has been shown to provide the greatest chance for success.

Decision aids such as algorithms and mnemonics are meant to *inform* rather than *dictate* to the practitioner. The practitioner is required to correctly identify the clinical problem (ie, a failed airway) before choosing the algorithm. The algorithm should be designed and validated to ensure a high degree of success, provided

that it is applied in the correct clinical situation. Many of these situations occur relatively infrequently in clinical practice, and it is unlikely that practitioners will have an opportunity to generate rules for managing the situations based on experience alone. By providing a limited number of likely-to-be successful options, the algorithm can increase the likelihood of a good outcome.

Reason has defined two basic mechanisms whereby practitioners deal with critical incidents. The first is a rule-based solution, whereby on recognizing the event for what it is, one identifies and applies a solution that experience has shown will likely be useful in solving the problem. Recognizing the event involves a process called "similarity-matching"; based on identifying that the characteristics of the events are similar to those of past events (in a sense, *pattern recognition*). The practitioner then decides upon a particular solution that is likely to be effective in solving the problem and resolving the threat. This presupposes that the practitioner has had sufficient experience with both the situation and the application of the rule to both immediately recognize the problem and to know which rule to apply. This ability constitutes what is called "expertise." Unfortunately, difficult and failed airways are encountered infrequently in practice, and the individual experiences of practitioners may have not been sufficient to earn them *expert* status.

The second mechanism for dealing with critical incidents is to apply a knowledge-based solution. This is a ground-up, first-principle strategy whereby the practitioner, without significant past experience with similar situations, attempts to find an appropriate solution. Not surprisingly, such strategies are time consuming, and when made under pressure of time, are more likely to fail.

Many airway practitioners will not have sufficient experience with difficult and failed airway scenarios to have, of themselves, created a rule-based, organized approach to these airway dilemmas for which knowledge-based solutions may be inadequate. For this reason, preformulated airway algorithms are helpful in these situations and deserve to be considered by all airway practitioners.

Coincident with the development of the decision trees (*strategies*) and vital to airway management success is skill in the application of an array of devices and techniques (*tactics*) that can optimize clinical outcomes. Techniques and devices advocated in this chapter, as in the case of the decision trees, are anchored by evidence and expert opinion, rather than personal preference.

Algorithms meant to guide practice in crisis situations must exhibit the following design elements:

- Entry and exit points are easily recognized.
- They are based on the best available evidence.
- Branch points are binary.
- There are a limited number of actions at each step.
- They are easy to remember and represent graphically.

2.4.2   What are the strengths and weaknesses of the ASA difficult airway algorithm?

The ASA, in an attempt to avert airway management disasters, has produced the *ASA Difficult Airway Algorithm* first in 1993 (Figure 2-1) and a revision in 2003 (Figure 2-2).[41,42] The ASA Difficult Airway Algorithm is derived from the *Practice Guidelines*

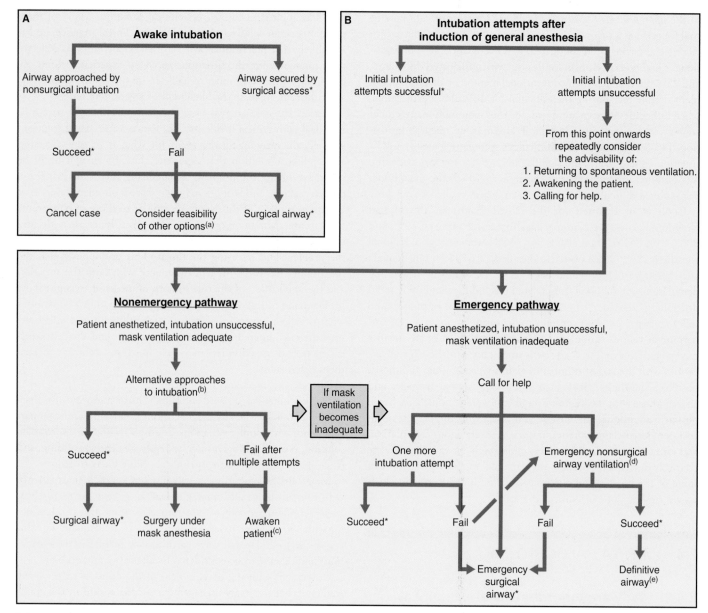

FIGURE 2-1. 1993 ASA Difficult Airway Management Algorithm.

for the Management of the Difficult Airway, developed by the ASA Task Force on Difficult Airway Management.

In both iterations, Panel A is directed at anticipating and managing the *difficult airway*, and Panel B deals with the *failed airway*. The algorithms guide management strategies when difficulty is predicted and recommend rescue tactics in the event of failure. They emphasize the importance of possessing expertise in more than one airway management technique and that each time an airway is managed the practitioner formulate a variety of backup plans should the primary plan fail (Plan B and Plan C).

As the ASA guidelines evolved from the first to the second iteration, a number of important changes were made. Guidance is now offered to those anatomic elements that may prove useful in the evaluation of the airway (Table 2-1), although no direction is given as to how to interpret the findings. The concept of a *reassuring* versus *nonreassuring* assessment is now included, with the recommendation that a *nonreassuring* assessment be a relevant factor in the construction of a plan for airway management. The need for the continuous application of oxygen to the patient during management of the difficult airway is emphasized in the second iteration. Finally, the laryngeal mask airway (LMA) for ventilation has been moved from the emergency pathway of Panel B to an entry point determining whether the emergency pathway is entered. This change is likely due to the worldwide recognition that the LMA is an effective rescue device.

A number of other groups have generated evidence-based consensus guidelines for the management of the difficult airway.[31,43] They differ from the ASA guidelines in being relevant only to the unanticipated difficult airway. They are similar to the ASA package in that they recognize the utility of alternatives to both BMV and direct laryngoscopy for intubation as well as emphasizing the role of salvage plans and physician training with the alternative devices.

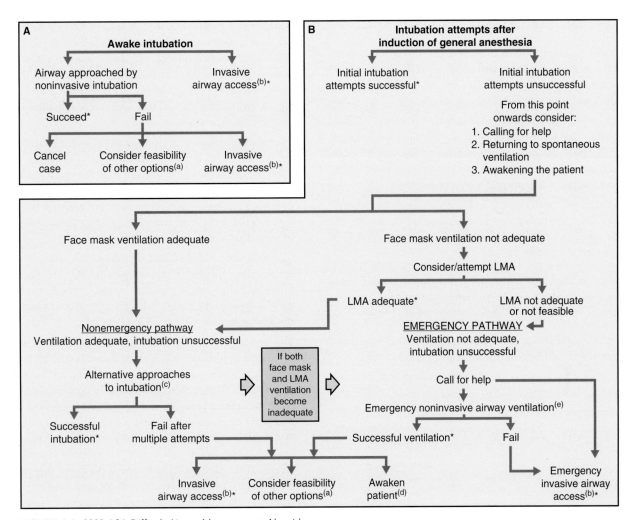

FIGURE 2-2. 2003 ASA Difficult Airway Management Algorithm.

TABLE 2-1*

Components of the Preoperative Airway Physical Examination

AIRWAY EXAM COMPONENT	NONREASSURING FINDING
Length or upper incisors	Relatively long
Relation of maxillary and mandibular incisors during normal jaw closure	Prominent overbite (maxillary incisors anterior)
Relation of incisors during protrusion of mandible	Overbite remains present
Interincisor distance	Less than 3.0 cm
Visibility of uvula (Mallampati class)	Not visible with tongue protruded, patient sitting (>II)
Shape of palate	High arched or narrow
Compliance of mandibular space	Stiff and indurated
Thyromental distance	Less than 3 fingerbreadths (5.0 cm)
Length of neck	Short
Thickness of neck	Thick
Range of motion of head on neck	Limited

*Adapted from: Caplan RA, Benumof JL, Berry FA, et al. Practice guidelines for management of the difficult airway. An updated report by the American Society of Anesthesiologists Task Force on Management of the Difficult Airway. Anesthesiology. 2003;98:1269-1277.

The essential messages of the ASA Difficult Airway Algorithms are:

- If difficulty is anticipated (a nonreassuring airway assessment) secure the airway awake. It is well appreciated that even following a careful assessment suggesting that an airway will not be difficult, some airways will be difficult to manage.

- If difficulty is encountered after induction of anesthesia awaken the patient. This is an option in an elective situation but may not be an option in an urgent or emergency situation or a case in which airway management is the clinical end point rather than a diagnostic or therapeutic intervention.

- Think ahead and have Plans B and C immediately available or in place. This implies that one has evaluated the airway for difficulty in performing Plans B and C *before* embarking on Plan A, as stressed in Chapter 1.

Additional essential messages from the ASA Closed Claims Project and the medical–legal experience accumulating in anesthesia include:

- If the airway evaluation is nonreassuring, the plan for airway management should be constructed reflecting this finding.

- When faced with a variety of effective intubation choices, do what you do best!!

- If the technique you do best has not worked, and is not working, after no more than three attempts, use some other technique. Do not persist with a technique already demonstrated to be inadequate.

The ASA Guidelines and Algorithm have served to highlight the importance of predicting and managing the difficult airway and have probably led to a reduction in adverse events related to airway management disasters in the operating room setting. However, several limitations are identified in a detailed study of the algorithm:

- The algorithm actually addresses both difficult and failed airway management, but does not explicitly identify the two pathways. Identifying when a *difficult airway* has progressed to a *failed* one is crucial in selecting management options that will avert a bad outcome.

- The nonbinary nature of the decision matrices and the multiplicity of pathways have limited the clinical usefulness of the algorithm in a crisis.

- Often, in real life, rescue maneuvers are contemplated and executed concurrently (eg, inserting an LMA at the same time preparations are underway to perform a surgical airway). The algorithm is silent in this regard.

- The algorithm does not provide for uncooperative patients (children, mentally challenged, and patients who refuse to cooperate with the planned airway management) and different patient populations (eg, obstetrical and pediatric patients).

- While surgical airway management is the cornerstone of failed airway management, anesthesia practitioners are often reluctant to undertake surgical airway management.[34] Most experts agree that all airway practitioners ought to be able to perform such an intervention. Failure of the practitioner to expeditiously perform a surgical airway is often leveled as a criticism by plaintiff experts in medicolegal actions. It follows then, that when faced with a failed airway, preparations for a surgical airway must begin immediately. Neither the 1993 nor the 2003 ASA algorithm reflect this thinking. Furthermore, the 2003 ASA algorithm inserts an additional LMA step, potentially delaying the performance of a surgical airway.

- The medicolegal context. The algorithm is intended to facilitate the management of the difficult airway and to reduce the likelihood of adverse outcomes and not to define the standard of care for such interventions. Although the determination of whether or not a practitioner met the standard of care will be judged in law, it is likely that reference to existing guidelines will be made in such determination.[29]

- The guidelines and algorithm are silent with respect to whether or not they ought to apply outside the operating room. However, when care is subject to audit by experts, the physician may be expected to comply with the algorithm no matter where the airway management is undertaken.[24,25]

- The option of *awakening the patient* is often not possible in a failed airway situation, particularly if the intubation is an emergency and the intubation is the actual and necessary clinical end point. This may seem elementary in concept, but the statement may pose a problem in medicolegal proceedings when the simplicity of *awakening the patient* is positioned by the plaintiff as *the* solution in the face of airway management failure, making the failure to do such a simple maneuver inexplicable and arcane. A simple statement by the Task Force that awakening the patient is not always feasible would go a long way in legally defending the appropriate actions of a practitioner in emergency airway situations.

- Despite any disclaimer, this document is likely to be referenced by medical experts in establishing the *standard of care* for difficult and failed airway management in anesthesia practice.

2.5   THE EMERGENCY AIRWAY ALGORITHMS[30]

2.5.1   Why do these algorithms work best in emergency situations?

The following Emergency Airway Management Algorithms adhere to the design elements of effective algorithms and are specifically intended to be applied in crisis situations in which actions must be intuitive and automatic to increase the changes of a good outcome. They are derived in a similar fashion to the ASA algorithm and are based on the same evidence. They describe a logical progression of *thinking* and *doing* when faced with the *crash* situation, the difficult airway, and the failed airway. An algorithm dealing with extubation of the difficult airway is also presented.

These algorithms are shown in Figures 2-3 to 2-6. The reader is encouraged to refer to the figures while reading the text descriptions

Start
Crash intubation?
Yes
Crash algorithm
Fails
No
Emergency intubation?
Yes
Difficult intubation?
Yes
Emergency difficult algorithm
Fails
Failed ("rescue") airway algorithm
No
Rapid sequence intubation
Fails
No
Difficult intubation?
Yes
Awake/sedated anesthetized method
Fails
No
Elective intubation
Fails

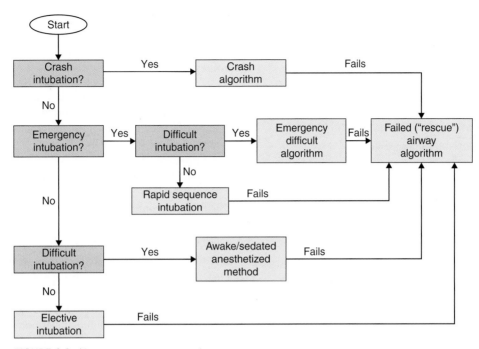

FIGURE 2-3. Airway management overview.

The crash airway algorithm
Crash airway
BMV or EGD
Attempt oral intubation
Successful?
Yes
Postintubation management
No
BMV or EGD successful?
No
Failed airway
Yes
Succinylcholine 2.0 mg/kg IVP
Repeat attempt at oral intubation
Successful?
Yes
Postintubation management
No
≤3 attempts by skilled intubator?
Yes
Failed airway
No

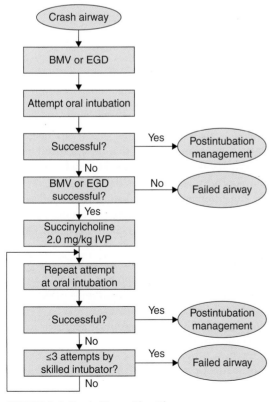

FIGURE 2-4. Crash Airway Algorithm.

The emergency difficult airway algorithm
Difficult airway predicted
Call for assistance
$S_pO_2 \geq 90\%$?
No
BMV or EGD maintains $S_pO_2 \geq 90\%$?
No
Failed airway
Yes
Yes
BMV or EGD predicted to be successful?
Yes
Intubation predicted to be successful?
Yes
RSI
No
No
Successful
"Awake" technique
PIM or RSI
Unsuccessful
$S_pO_2 \geq 90\%$?
No
Failed airway
Yes
Bronchoscopic method
I-LMA
Lighted stylet
Nasotracheal
Cricothyrotomy

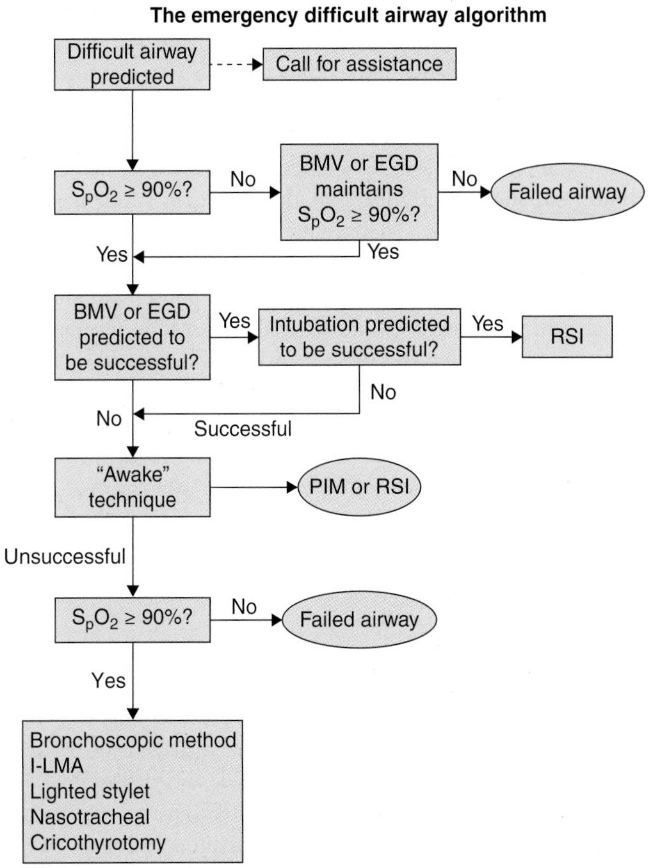

FIGURE 2-5. Emergency Difficult Airway Algorithm.

The failed airway algorithm

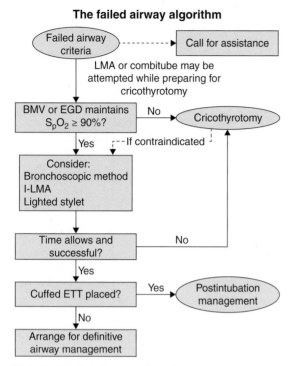

FIGURE 2-6. Failed Airway Algorithm.

below. The Emergency Airway Algorithms do not address the indications for intubation and do not deal with the decision to intubate. Therefore, the entry point for each one is immediately after the decision to intubate has been made.

These algorithms, though consistent with the thinking imbedded in the ASA algorithm, are tailored for urgent and emergency clinical situations and adhere to the principles fundamental to such clinical situations. They are meant to guide the development of response strategies to high threat/low-frequency events for which one has not developed automatic responses. Importantly, the algorithms presented in this chapter are not meant to be memorized and followed slavishly, as with a recipe. They are the ways of rapidly thinking through urgent clinical situations and helping to make crucial decisions and actions.

The practitioner may fail to appreciate the failed airway and subsequently fail to move quickly to a salvage strategy or to secure a surgical airway. It must be emphasized that there ought to be no hesitation in performing a surgical airway or cricothyrotomy in the face of airway management failure.

2.5.2   The overview algorithm

The Overview Algorithm (Figure 2-3) presents the way most practitioners approach the issue of airway management. Most of the time, it is routine, elective, controlled, and deliberate. Most intubations are not crash or emergency situations. So the first real question faced in daily practice is, "Is this a difficult airway?" If not, it is handled in a routine fashion as preferred by the individual.

If it is deemed to be difficult (based on a nonreassuring airway examination, an awkward environment, poor patient

condition, etc), an awake intubation procedure may be indicated depending on the judgment of the airway practitioner. There are a number of considerations that will inform and influence this decision.

- If direct laryngoscopy is deemed likely to be difficult, is the airway practitioner skilled in an alternative technique that is likely to be effective in the situation, or is the skill set limited to direct laryngoscopy? If the latter statement most accurately describes the situation, then awake intubation is likely the most prudent course. If the former statement most accurately describes the case, consideration may be given to induction of anesthesia, with or without muscle paralysis, followed by tracheal intubation using an alternate strategy, provided there is no anticipated difficulty in ventilation using BMV or an EGD.

- Is there a need to protect the airway from gastric contents? If so, it should be recognized that the ability to protect the airway with cricoid pressure is limited;[44-51] and that multiple attempts at direct laryngoscopy over a prolonged period of time are associated with regurgitation and aspiration.[23] The combination of difficult laryngoscopy and a full stomach in a cooperative patient may best be managed with an awake intubation (see Chapters 3 and 5).

In the event the patient is unresponsive or near death, a crash intubation is indicated and the Crash Algorithm is employed. "Unresponsive" means that the patient does not respond adversely to oral laryngoscopy (the newly dead or nearly dead).

Failure to meet the criteria for a crash intubation does not mean that the intubation is not an emergency. Intubation is urgently indicated in the event when a patient is unable to:

- Maintain reasonable oxygenation
- Protect the airway
- Maintain the airway
- Is faced with intubation to manage some other condition, or neuromuscular blockade is to be instituted.

Once the decision is made that this is an urgent or emergency intubation, the next question is "Will this be a difficult intubation?" This decision must be made quickly, and Chapter 1 presents efficient strategies for assessing the airway quickly for difficulty. If the urgent/emergency intubation is not judged to be difficult, a Rapid Sequence Induction/Intubation (RSI) is indicated as the method most likely to rapidly and safely secure the airway.

In the event the airway is judged difficult, the Emergency Difficult Airway Algorithm should be employed. Should any of these approaches fail, the Failed Airway Algorithm is used to rapidly and definitively gain control of the airway.

Four algorithms emerge from this conceptual approach to the airway and its management:

- The Crash Airway Algorithm (Figure 2-4)
- The Emergency Difficult Airway Algorithm (Figure 2-5)
- The Failed Airway Algorithm (Figure 2-6)
- The Extubation Algorithm (Figure 2-7)

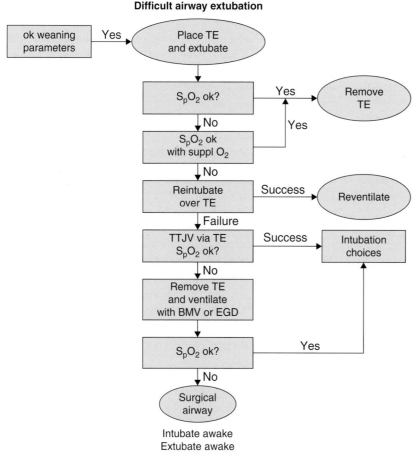

Difficult airway extubation

FIGURE 2-7. Difficult Airway Extubation Algorithm.

2.5.3   The crash airway algorithm

Entry at this point requires an unconscious, unresponsive patient with immediate need for airway management. The first step in the Crash Algorithm is to attempt oral intubation immediately by direct laryngoscopy without pharmacologic assist. If the oral intubation is successful, then the practitioner proceeds with postintubation management. If oral intubation is not initially successful with direct laryngoscopy, then a decision point is reached and several questions must be asked.

2.5.3.1   Is BMV Successful?

If BMV is successful, then one has time and further attempts at oral intubation are possible. If BMV is difficult and one is certain in this unresponsive patient that an EGD such as an LMA would resolve the issue, it may be reasonable to try it.

In the event that BMV is unsuccessful in the context of a *failed oral intubation* with a crash airway, then a *failed airway* is present. BMV should be optimized with the use of oral and nasal airways and include maneuvers such as jaw thrust, chin lift, or a head tilt if appropriate. A two-hand mask hold may improve mask seal. Additionally, if cricoid pressure is being applied, consideration should be given to relaxing the force being applied or temporarily discontinuing it and assessing airway patency in its absence. One further attempt at intubation may be indicated, but no more than one, because intubation

has failed and the failure of BMV places the patient in serious and immediate jeopardy. This is a CICV situation, and in such circumstances, the Failed Airway Algorithm (Figure 2-6) mandates immediate surgical airway management. If surgical airway management is not *immediately* possible, temporizing methods, such as the placement of an EGD (eg, LMA or Combitube™), should be attempted, but such attempts should not delay preparation for, and the creation of, a surgical airway. The successful use of an EGD in permitting adequate gas exchange may obviate the need for a surgical airway.

2.5.3.2   Is the Patient Completely Relaxed and Flaccid?

During the first attempt at orotracheal intubation in the unconscious, unresponsive patient, the patient is assessed for degree of relaxation to permit intubation. If the impression is one of absolute, complete skeletal muscle relaxation, then further intubation attempts are indicated. If the patient is felt to be exhibiting any resistance whatsoever to intubation, then a single dose of succinylcholine, 2.0 mg·kg⁻¹, should be given and oral intubation attempted again. Usually, only one dose is indicated. It should be noted that this dose of succinylcholine is higher than the 1.0 to 1.5 mg·kg⁻¹ recommended elsewhere. However, there is compelling evidence that excellent intubating conditions are achieved in virtually 100% of patients at 60 seconds with 2 mg·kg⁻¹ of succinylcholine.[19]

2.5.3.3   Have There Been Three Attempts at Intubation by an Experienced Airway Practitioner?

If the answer to this question is yes, then consistent with the definition above, the situation represents a "failed airway" (Figure 2-6). The futility of further attempts may be evident after the first attempt dictating an immediate move to a different device or technique. If fewer than three attempts have been made by an experienced airway practitioner, and it is the opinion of the practitioner that it is possible to be successful by this route, a repeat attempt at oral intubation is justified. No more than three attempts at direct laryngoscopy can be supported,[42] and some would say two.[1,23]

As detailed above, the evidence suggests that there is a low likelihood of success with persistent use of the direct laryngoscope after three failed attempts and an increased likelihood of patient morbidity and cardiac arrest. Between each intubation attempt, defined by a single laryngoscopy, the patient should receive ventilation and oxygenation through a bag-mask.

2.5.3.4   Is It Appropriate to Repeat Laryngoscopic Intubation Until Three Attempts Have Failed?

As stated above, it is often apparent after a single attempt that further attempts at orotracheal intubation will be futile. In such cases, move to Plan B if oxygenation can be maintained, the Failed Airway Algorithm if it cannot be maintained.

2.5.3.5   Were Repeated Efforts Successful?

If intubation is achieved, then proceed to postintubation management; if not, cycle back to make another attempt or to proceed to the Failed Airway Algorithm, depending on the number of attempts which have already been made. The failure of three attempts indicates a very low likelihood of ultimate success with oral intubation. There is a diminishing return with subsequent attempts and an increased risk of hypoxia, aspiration, and cardiac arrest. After three attempts, efforts to ensure oxygenation should be the priority while preparations are being made to perform a surgical airway.

2.5.3.6   Postintubation Management

This is undertaken in the event of a successful intubation.

2.5.4   The emergency difficult airway algorithm

This algorithm (Figure 2-5) is specifically designed to guide airway management in an emergency. Decisions are binary by design. It incorporates the notion of the failed airway. Though a fairly busy-appearing figure with 13 boxes, in reality it simply poses a series of four simple questions:

1. Is the airway difficult (MOANS, LEMON, RODS, and SHORT)? (See Sections 1.6.1-1.6.4.)

2. Do I have time (is the oxygen saturation within a normal range)? Or can I make time (with BMV)?

3. On reconsideration, is an RSI technique reasonable?

4. Failing that, what is my best option?

Bear in mind that patients presenting in an emergency should almost always be considered having a full stomach.

2.5.4.1   Is a Difficult Airway Predicted?

If, for whatever reason, airway management is predicted to be difficult, nothing should be taken from the patient that the airway practitioner cannot replace. This refers particularly to the administration of paralytic drugs. Furthermore, the ability to protect the airway with cricoid pressure is limited, and multiple attempts at laryngoscopy over a prolonged period of time have been associated with regurgitation and aspiration.[23] Therefore, careful consideration should be given to awake intubation in the setting of dual concerns of difficult airway and full stomach.

2.5.4.2   Is BMV or EGD Ventilation Predicted to Be Successful (MOANS and RODS)? (See Sections 1.6.1 and 1.6.3)

In other words, if intubation fails, will BMV or rescue with some other device (commonly an EGD) be possible? These are the only other airway methods possible aside from a surgical airway. So careful consideration is warranted and one must have a high degree

of certainty that this question is answered in the affirmative, particularly if the use of one of neuromuscular blocking (NMB) drugs is contemplated. Planning for and being prepared to undertake rescue maneuvers (Plans B and C) are crucial, as is the preemptive evaluation for difficulty. For example, if one is planning to perform a rapid cricothyrotomy (Plan B) should induction and paralysis (Plan A) fail, then an evaluation for difficult cricothyrotomy must be performed (SHORT, see Section 1.6.4) before embarking on Plan A.

2.5.4.3   Is Intubation Deemed Reasonably Likely?

The decision to proceed with an RSI technique in the patient with a predicted difficult airway must be associated with the likelihood that it will be successful. Airway practitioners must be confident in their abilities and must possess a broad array of equipment and skills to rescue the airway in the event that conventional direct vision orotracheal intubation fails.

2.5.4.4   Should an Awake Look Employing Topical Anesthesia and Sedation Be Attempted to Assist in Decision Making?

A variety of techniques are available to obtund the airway, the patient, or both, without burning any bridges. The condition of the patient and the clinical situation will dictate the aggression of this maneuver (ie, how much does one need to see?). It may be that the airway practitioner simply needs to verify that the epiglottis is in the midline to make the decision to back off and move to a rapid-sequence technique. At other times, it may indicate that an awake intubation is appropriate.

The value of the *awake look* as a maneuver to reassure oneself that oral intubation is likely to be possible following the administration of induction and NMB medications ought to be tempered by the findings of Sivarajan and Fink.[52] These authors measured the position of larynx in lateral radiographs of necks taken in human volunteers when they were awake, and after the induction of general anesthesia with muscle paralysis. They found that the hyoid bone and epiglottis shifted anteriorly and the vestibule of the larynx enlarged with the onset of general anesthesia and muscle paralysis. In addition, the larynx also stretched longitudinally with wide separation of the vestibular and vocal folds. The authors concluded that consciousness is associated with tonic muscular activity that folds the larynx and partially closes it and that onset of general anesthesia and muscle paralysis widens the larynx and shifts it anteriorly. This may make visualization of the larynx difficult during direct laryngoscopy in some patients. Remember: bad things sometime happen with induction after successful awake looks.

2.5.5   The failed airway algorithm

The failure to intubate is rarely accompanied by the failure to ventilate and oxygenate. This situation has variously been termed CICV or "can't intubate, can't oxygenate" (CICO), the latter being the more precise term. It is a clinical emergency of such magnitude that it leads to neurologic compromise and death if not rectified rapidly. Decisive action in selecting a technique most likely to lead to a secure airway (ie, an emergency surgical airway) is essential to success in such a situation. It cannot be overemphasized that a failing technique (eg, direct laryngoscopy) cannot be considered as an appropriate salvage technique and there is no defence for persistent attempts with a failing technique.

Most often the failure to intubate is associated with some degree of success with BMV oxygenation, giving the airway practitioner time to consider alternative techniques. This CICV/O situation is amenable to nonsurgical rescue techniques. In this scenario, practiced alternatives to the direct laryngoscope such as the lighted stylet, or a rigid or flexible endoscope, may be used or an EGD may be placed to provide a more secure, bridging airway. In the latter case, these EGDs may be used to facilitate intubation (eg, LMA-Fastrach™, Cook ILA) or provide time to prepare for a more definitive solution (surgical airway).

The Failed Airway Algorithm is presented in Figure 2-6. The essential message from this algorithm is that the decision to move to a surgical airway must be taken early once the failure to maintain oxygenation is recognized. Wasting valuable time attempting a variety of devices or techniques is to be avoided at all costs, unless it is while the practitioner is concurrently preparing to perform a surgical airway. There is little or no value at this time in making attempts with tools or techniques with which the practitioner has no experience.

2.5.5.1 Have Failed Airway Criteria Been Met?

This is the entry point to the Failed Airway Algorithm. The criteria are either three failed attempts at intubation via oral laryngoscopy by an experienced practitioner or a single failed attempt at oral intubation with inability to maintain S_PO_2 ≥90% using a bag-mask. A mandated intubation in a patient with a difficult or crash airway in whom BMV has failed represents a failed airway. As with the difficult airway, it is advisable to call for assistance when a failed airway has occurred.

2.5.5.2 Is BMV Possible and Adequate?

In the circumstance of a failed airway, if BMV is not adequate, then immediate cricothyrotomy is mandatory. Simultaneously with preparations for a cricothyrotomy, the immediate placement of an EGD is attempted. If successful in rescuing the airway, cricothyrotomy may be averted.

Further attempts at intubation or use of alternate devices will merely prolong the patient's hypoxemic state. If surgical airway management is itself *relatively* contraindicated (in a life and death situation all contraindications to cricothyrotomy are relative), then alternative methods may be tried first. For example, if the patient has known laryngeal pathology in the area of the anticipated surgical intervention, such as a tumor or hematoma, then alternative techniques may be preferred. However, if these methods are not immediately successful, cricothyrotomy should be performed, even in the presence of relative contraindications. SHORT (see Section 1.6.4) identifies conditions that present difficulty and should *not* be thought of as contraindications.

2.5.5.3 Consider Combitube™, Flexible Endoscopes, I-LMA, Lighted Stylet, Trans-tracheal Jet Ventilation, Retrograde, Rigid Video-optic Devices, or Some Other Method

If ventilation and oxygenation by bag-mask can maintain acceptable S_PO_2 values (≥90% or some acceptable number), then a number of different devices and procedures may be attempted to rescue the patient with the failed airway. At all times, the patient must be monitored for adequate oxygenation. If oxygenation becomes inadequate at any time and cannot be restored via BMV, then cricothyrotomy is mandatory. Likewise, if there is failure of each of the techniques considered appropriate, then cricothyrotomy should be undertaken. Videolaryngoscopic (eg, the Glidescope®, Storz C-MAC) and flexible endoscopic methods, and the rigid video laryngoscopes (eg, Shikani, Bonfils, Bullard) have all been shown to be effective and safe rescue techniques. The choice of the tool should be governed primarily by the practitioner's experience and expertise. The application of a tool with which the practitioner has little experience is difficult to defend as a prudent intervention.

2.5.5.4 Enough Time for Successful Airway Rescue?

If there is sufficient time to achieve oxygenation and ventilation using one of these devices or techniques, proceed down the main path of the algorithm. If not, cricothyrotomy is mandated.

2.5.5.5 Was an Endotracheal Tube Placed?

If an endotracheal tube is successfully placed at any time, postintubation management may be undertaken. If another method of gas exchange (eg, EGD) has been employed successfully, then the airway should be considered to be temporary at best and arrangements for a definitive airway be made. If the airway placed is unable to provide adequate ventilation and oxygenation, then immediate cricothyrotomy is indicated.

2.5.6 The extubation algorithm

The Extubation Algorithm (Figure 2-7) is specifically intended to be employed in those situations in which reintubation, if needed, is judged to be difficult or impossible (eg, the patient was initially intubated awake because intubation was judged to be impossible).[53,54] At the core of the algorithm is a trial of extubation over a *tube exchanger* (TE) (eg, Cook Endotracheal Tube Exchange Catheter). It needs to be emphasized that the airway practitioner needs to be absolutely certain that patient is awake and *cognitively responsive* before removing tube in a difficult extubation setting! Agitation is not responsiveness.

It is important to note that a failure to reintubate should be immediately followed by an assessment of the ability to maintain oxygen saturations. If oxygen saturation can be maintained by some form of ventilation through the catheter or by BMV, there is likely some time to use alternative methods of intubation, such as lightwands and flexible bronchoscopes. On the other hand, the failure to maintain oxygen saturation should be immediately followed by attempts to employ rescue devices such as a Combitube™, intubating laryngeal mask, and trans-tracheal ventilation while preparations are undertaken to perform a surgical airway.

2.6   SUMMARY

The failure to adequately manage the airway is a major contributor to poor outcomes in anesthesia, emergency medicine, emergency medical services, and critical care. Adverse respiratory events constitute the largest cause of injury in the ASA Closed Claims Project. The single most important factor leading to a failed airway is failure to predict the difficult airway.[37,38]

Emergency airway management is always stress provoking. Crucial decisions must be made in a timely manner, and the airway practitioner is expected to possess expertise in a variety of primary (Plan A) and backup (Plans B and C) maneuvers.

Well-designed algorithms based on the best available evidence are intended to improve the outcome of difficult and failed airway emergencies. However, it is incumbent on the airway practitioner to identify which algorithm to employ, particularly in the event that a *difficult airway* has progressed to a failed airway.

REFERENCES

1. Rose DK, Cohen MM. The airway: problems and predictions in 18,500 patients. *Can J Anaesth*. 1994;41:372-383.
2. Langeron O, Masso E, Huraux C, et al. Prediction of difficult mask ventilation. *Anesthesiology*. 2000;92:1229-1236.
3. Kheterpal S, Martin L, Shanks AM, Tremper KK. Prediction and outcomes of impossible mask ventilation: a review of 50,000 anesthetics. *Anesthesiology*. 2009;110:891-897.
4. Kheterpal S, Han R, Tremper KK, et al. Incidence and predictors of difficult and impossible mask ventilation. *Anesthesiology*. 2006;105:885-891.
5. Petito SP, Russell WJ. The prevention of gastric inflation—a neglected benefit of cricoid pressure. *Anaesth Intensive Care*. 1988;16:139-143.
6. Cass NM, James NR, Lines V. Difficult direct laryngoscopy complicating intubation for anaesthesia. *Br Med J*. 1956;1:488-489.
7. Mallampati SR. Clinical sign to predict difficult tracheal intubation (hypothesis). *Can Anaesth Soc J*. 1983;30:316-317.
8. Mallampati SR, Gatt SP, Gugino LD, et al. A clinical sign to predict difficult tracheal intubation: a prospective study. *Can Anaesth Soc J*. 1985;32:429-434.
9. Samsoon GL, Young JR. Difficult tracheal intubation: a retrospective study. *Anaesthesia*. 1987;42:487-490.
10. Shiga T, Wajima Z, Inoue T, Sakamoto A. Predicting difficult intubation in apparently normal patients: a meta-analysis of bedside screening test performance. *Anesthesiology*. 2005;103:429-437.
11. Karkouti K, Rose DK, Wigglesworth D, Cohen MM. Predicting difficult intubation: a multivariable analysis. *Can J Anaesth*. 2000;47:730-739.
12. Karkouti K, Rose K, Cohen M, Wigglesworth D. Models for difficult laryngoscopy. *Can J Anaesth*. 2000;47:94-95.
13. Yentis SM. Predicting difficult intubation—worthwhile exercise or pointless ritual? *Anaesthesia*. 2002;57:105-109.
14. Yentis SM. Predicting trouble in airway management. *Anesthesiology*. 2006;105:871-872.
15. Thiboutot F, Nicole PC, Trepanier CA, et al. Effect of manual in-line stabilization of the cervical spine in adults on the rate of difficult orotracheal intubation by direct laryngoscopy: a randomized controlled trial. *Can J Anaesth*. 2009;56:412-418.
16. Shorten GD, Alfille PH, Gliklich RE. Airway obstruction following application of cricoid pressure. *J Clin Anesth*. 1991;3:403-405.
17. Shorten GD. Airway obstruction from cricoid pressure. *Anesth Analg*. 1993;76:668.
18. Ho AM, Wong W, Ling E, Chung DC, Tay BA. Airway difficulties caused by improperly applied cricoid pressure. *J Emerg Med*. 2001;20:29-31.
19. Neilipovitz DT, Crosby ET. No evidence for decreased incidence of aspiration after rapid sequence induction. *Can J Anaesth*. 2007;54:748-764.
20. Smith CE, Boyer D. Cricoid pressure decreases ease of tracheal intubation using fibreoptic laryngoscopy (WuScope System™). *Can J Anaesth*. 2002;49:614-619.
21. Hodgson RE, Gopalan PD, Burrows RC, Zuma K. Effect of cricoid pressure on the success of endotracheal intubation with a lightwand. *Anesthesiology*. 2001;94:259-262.
22. Shulman GB, Connelly NR. A comparison of the Bullard laryngoscope versus the flexible fiberoptic bronchoscope during intubation in patients afforded inline stabilization. *J Clin Anesth*. 2001;13:182-185.
23. Mort TC. Emergency tracheal intubation: complications associated with repeated laryngoscopic attempts. *Anesth Analg*. 2004;99:607-613, table of contents.
24. Mort TC. Complications of emergency tracheal intubation: immediate airway-related consequences: part II. *J Intensive Care Med*. 2007;22:208-215.
25. Mort TC. Complications of emergency tracheal intubation: hemodynamic alterations—part I. *J Intensive Care Med*. 2007;22:157-165.
26. Hung OR, Pytka S, Morris I, Murphy M, Steward RD. Lightwand intubation: II—clinical trial of a new lightwand for tracheal intubation in patients with difficult airways. *Can J Anaesth*. 1995;42: 826-830.
27. Heidegger T, Gerig HJ, Ulrich B, Kreienbuhl G. Validation of a simple algorithm for tracheal intubation: daily practice is the key to success in emergencies—an analysis of 13,248 intubations. *Anesth Analg*. 2001;92:517-522.
28. Combes X, Le Roux B, Suen P, et al. Unanticipated difficult airway in anesthetized patients: prospective validation of a management algorithm. *Anesthesiology*. 2004;100:1146-1150.
29. Mort TC. The incidence and risk factors for cardiac arrest during emergency tracheal intubation: a justification for incorporating the ASA Guidelines in the remote location. *J Clin Anesth*. 2004;16:508-516.
30. Connelly NR, Ghandour K, Robbins L, Dunn S, Gibson C. Management of unexpected difficult airway at a teaching institution over a 7-year period. *J Clin Anesth*. 2006;18:198-204.
31. Crosby ET, Cooper RM, Douglas MJ, et al. The unanticipated difficult airway with recommendations for management. *Can J Anaesth*. 1998;45:757-776.
32. Rosenblatt WH, Wagner PJ, Ovassapian A, Kain ZN. Practice patterns in managing the difficult airway by anesthesiologists in the United States. *Anesth Analg*. 1998;87:153-157.
33. Jenkins K, Wong DT, Correa R. Management choices for the difficult airway by anesthesiologists in Canada. *Can J Anaesth*. 2002;49:850-856.
34. Wong DT, Lai K, Chung FF, Ho RY. Cannot intubate-cannot ventilate and difficult intubation strategies: results of a Canadian national survey. *Anesth Analg*. 2005;100:1439-1446, table of contents.
35. Kristensen MS, Moller J. Airway management behaviour, experience and knowledge among Danish anaesthesiologists—room for improvement. *Acta Anaesthesiol Scand*. 2001;45:1181-1185.
36. Ezri T, Szmuk P, Warters RD, et al. Difficult airway management practice patterns among anesthesiologists practicing in the United States: have we made any progress? *J Clin Anesth*. 2003;15:418-422.
37. Caplan RA, Posner KL, Ward RJ, Cheney FW. Adverse respiratory events in anesthesia: a closed claims analysis. *Anesthesiology*. 1990;72:828-833.
38. Cheney FW, Posner KL, Caplan RA. Adverse respiratory events infrequently leading to malpractice suits. A closed claims analysis. *Anesthesiology*. 1991;75:932-939.
39. Miller CG. Management of the difficult intubation in closed malpractice claims. ASA Newsletter 200:64 2000. Available at: www.asahq.org/Newsletters/2000.
40. Cook TM, Bland L, Mihai R, Scott S. Litigation related to anaesthesia: an analysis of claims against the NHS in England 1995-2007. *Anaesthesia*. 2009;64:706-718.
41. A report by the American Society of Anesthesiologists Task Force on Management of the Difficult Airway. Practice guidelines for management of the difficult airway. *Anesthesiology*. 1993;78:597-602.
42. Practice guidelines for management of the difficult airway: an updated report by the American Society of Anesthesiologists Task Force on Management of the Difficult Airway. *Anesthesiology*. 2003;98:1269-1277.
43. Henderson JJ, Popat MT, Latto IP, Pearce AC. Difficult Airway Society guidelines for management of the unanticipated difficult intubation. *Anaesthesia*. 2004;59:675-694.
44. Brimacombe JR, Berry AM. Cricoid pressure. *Can J Anaesth*. 1997;44:414-425.
45. Timmermann A, Byhahn C. Cricoid pressure. Protective manoeuvre or established nonsense? *Anaesthesist*. 2009;58:663-664.

46. Rice MJ, Mancuso AA, Gibbs C, et al. Cricoid pressure results in compression of the postcricoid hypopharynx: the esophageal position is irrelevant. *Anesth Analg.* 2009;109:1546-1552.

47. Priebe HJ. Cricoid pressure: an expert's opinion. *Minerva Anestesiol.* 2009;75:710-714.

48. Lerman J. On cricoid pressure: "may the force be with you". *Anesth Analg.* 2009;109:1363-1366.

49. Fenton PM, Reynolds F. Life-saving or ineffective? An observational study of the use of cricoid pressure and maternal outcome in an African setting. *Int J Obstet Anesth.* 2009;18:106-110.

50. Benkhadra M, Lenfant F, Bry J, et al. Cricoid cartilage and esophagus: CT scan study of the dynamic variability of their relative positions. *Surg Radiol Anat.* 2009;31:537-543.

51. Gobindram A, Clarke S. Cricoid pressure: should we lay off the pressure? *Anaesthesia.* 2008;63:1258-1259.

52. Sivarajan M, Fink BR. The position and the state of the larynx during general anesthesia and muscle paralysis. *Anesthesiology.* 1990;72:439-442.

53. Peterson GN, Domino KB, Caplan RA, Posner KL, Lee LA, Cheney FW. Management of the difficult airway: a closed claims analysis. *Anesthesiology.* 2005;103:33-39.

54. Miller KA, Harkin CP, Bailey PL. Postoperative tracheal extubation. *Anesth Analg.* 1995;80:149-172.

SELF-EVALUATION QUESTIONS

2.1. All of the following are features of well-designed, clinically useful algorithms **EXCEPT**

   A. They are designed by reputable organizations.

   B. They have clear entry and exit points.

   C. Decision points are binary.

   D. They are easily remembered in crisis.

   E. They are easy to represent graphically.

2.2. All of the following are true of the ASA Difficult Airway Algorithm **EXCEPT**

   A. It is evidence based.

   B. It has likely helped to reduce the rate of airway management failure in anesthesia practice.

   C. It is meant to represent the "standard of care" in medicolegal proceedings.

   D. It has two sections: one for the difficult airway and one for the failed airway.

   E. The use of the LMA is a discrete step.

2.3. All of the following are identified weaknesses of the ASA Difficult Airway Algorithm **EXCEPT**

   A. The algorithm actually addresses both difficult and failed airway management, but does not explicitly identify the two pathways.

   B. The nonbinary nature of the decision matrices and the multiplicity of pathways have limited the clinical usefulness of the algorithm in guiding day-to-day practice.

   C. The algorithm does not provide for uncooperative patients (children, mentally challenged, and patients who refuse to cooperate with the planned airway management) and different patient populations (eg, obstetrical and pediatric patients).

   D. The algorithm is silent with respect to whether or not they ought to apply outside the operating room.

   E. The algorithm is clear that awakening the patient is not always possible.

CHAPTER (3)

Preparation for Awake Intubation

Ian R. Morris

3.1   INTRODUCTION

3.1.1   What are the fundamentals of an *awake, bronchoscopically facilitated* intubation?

Awake bronchoscopic intubation, if it is to be performed rapidly and with minimal patient discomfort, requires an in-depth knowledge of the anatomy of the airway, adequate regional anesthesia, and dexterity with bronchoscopic manipulation. In order to achieve optimal regional anesthesia of the airway and avoid complications, a thorough knowledge of the local anesthetics employed and techniques of administration is necessary. The primary requirement for successful awake intubation is effective regional anesthesia of the airway.[1]

3.2   AIRWAY ANATOMY

3.2.1   Why is knowledge of upper airway anatomy beneficial in airway management?

Knowledge of the structure, function, and pathophysiology of the upper airway permits the practitioner to anticipate potential life-threatening problems and better utilize the full spectrum of airway management techniques.[2] Functionally, the upper airway can be considered to consist of the nasal cavities, pharynx, larynx, and trachea (see Figure 3-1).[3] The oral cavity provides an alternate access route to the pharynx.

3.2.2   The nose

Anatomically, the nose can be divided into an external component and the nasal cavity.[4] The external nose consists of a bony vault posterior superiorly, a cartilaginous vault anteriorly, and the lobule at the inferior-anterior aspect (see Figure 3-2).[3] The cavity of the nose is divided into bilateral compartments by the nasal septum and continues posteriorly from the nostrils (nares), to communicate with the nasopharynx at the posterior aspect of the septum (the choanae) (see Figures 3-3 to 3-5).[3] The nasal vestibule is a small dilatation located immediately inside the nostrils.[3,4] Each nasal cavity is bounded by a floor, a roof, and medial and lateral walls.[3-5] The roof of the nasal cavity extends posteriorly from the bridge of the nose, and consists of the lateral nasal cartilages, the nasal bones and spine of the frontal bone, the cribriform plate of the ethmoid, and the inferior aspect of the sphenoid (see Figure 3-2).[3,4,6] The nasal septum forms the medial wall, and is formed by the quadrilateral cartilage, the perpendicular plate of the ethmoid, and the vomer (see Figure 3-5).[3] The lateral wall is formed anterior-inferiorly by the frontal process of the maxilla, the nasal bones anterior-superiorly, the nasal aspect of the ethmoid superiorly, and the perpendicular plate of the palatine and medial pterygoid plate posteriorly.[3,7] A series of three horizontal scroll-like ridges (conchae or turbinates) project medially from the lateral walls of the nasal cavities, each of which overhangs a corresponding groove or meatus (see Figures 3-2 to 3-4).[3,8] Septal deviation is common, may be associated with compensatory hypertrophy of the turbinates, and can produce nasal obstruction.[3,4] The paranasal sinuses and the nasolacrimal duct empty into the nasal cavity through ostia in the lateral wall.[3] Obstruction of the ostia of the paranasal sinuses can occur with prolonged nasal intubation and can cause sinusitis.[2,3] The floor of each nasal cavity is concave and is formed by the palatine process of the maxilla and the horizontal

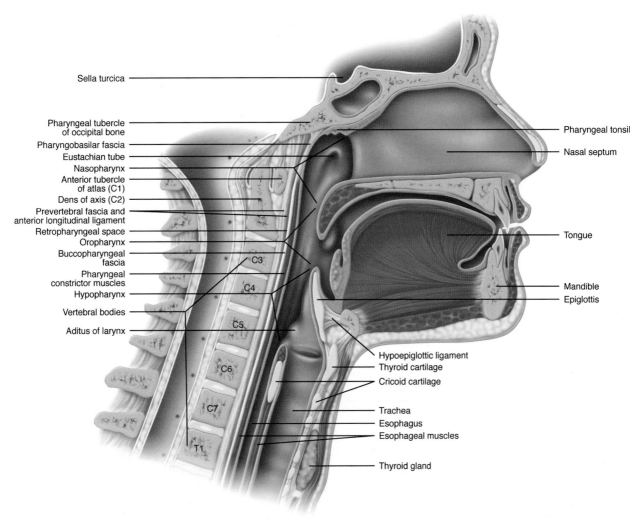

FIGURE 3-1. Sagittal view of the upper airway.

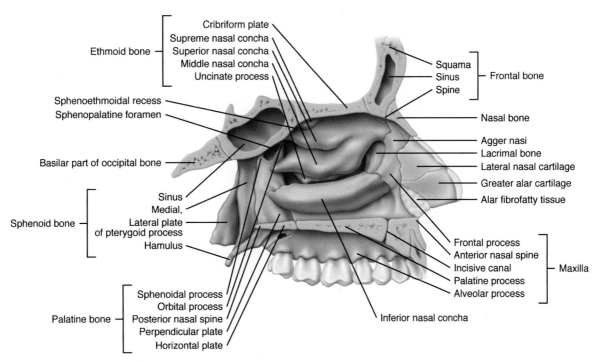

FIGURE 3-2. Bony components of lateral nasal wall.

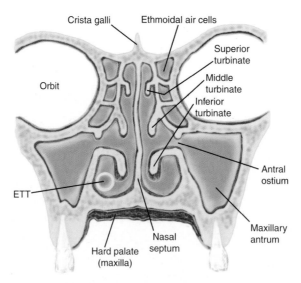

FIGURE 3-3. Coronal section of the maxillary sinus. The position of a nasotracheal tube (ETT) is shown in the right nasal cavity.

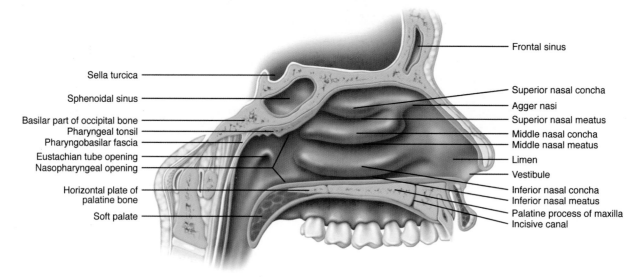

FIGURE 3-4. Lateral nasal wall.

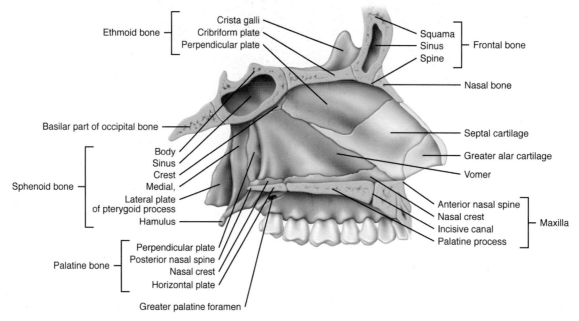

FIGURE 3-5. Medial nasal wall.

plate of the palatine bone.[3,4] The floor extends posteriorly in a transverse plane from the vestibule.

The major nasal airway is located below the inferior turbinate, declines slightly front to back (approximately 20 degrees), and a nasotracheal tube or flexible endoscope should be directed backward and slightly inferiorly along the floor of the nose.[2-4] Occasionally, the posterior aspect of the inferior turbinate may be hypertrophied and resistance to the passage of a nasotracheal tube may be encountered at this location.[4] Alternating counter-clockwise/clockwise rotation of the tube changes the orientation of the bevel and may facilitate negotiation of the nasal cavity (see Chapter 11).

The anterior and posterior ethmoidal branches of the internal carotid artery supply the anterior-superior aspect of the nasal cavity and the sphenopalatine branch of the external carotid supplies the posterior-inferior aspect.[3,9] The vestibule receives blood supply from both the anterior ethmoidal and sphenopalatine arteries as well as from nasal branches of the superior labial branch of the facial artery (see Figures 3-6 A and B).[3,9] Anastomoses between vessels from these three different sources occur particularly at the anterior-inferior aspect of the septum (Little's area or Kiesselbach's plexus), and this is a common site of epistaxis.[3,4,9] Tintinalli reported moderate to severe epistaxis in 7% of 71 attempted emergency nasotracheal intubations.[10] The single case of severe epistaxis in this series occurred in a patient with cirrhosis. Minimal epistaxis has been reported in 11% to 40% of nasal intubations.[10,11] In a series of 99 patients undergoing nasotracheal intubation for oromaxillofacial surgery, epistaxis occurred in 6 patients but was sufficient to result in a visible accumulation of blood in the pharynx in only 1 patient.[12] Of 175 anesthetists who underwent

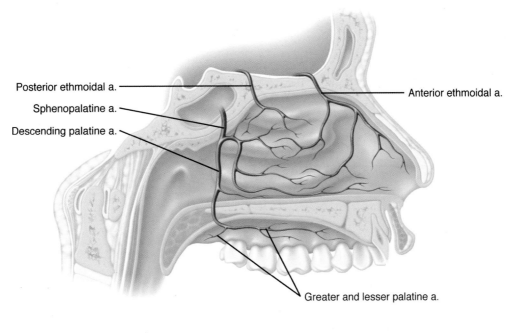

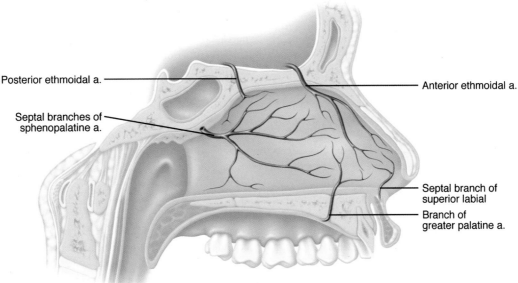

FIGURE 3-6. (A and B.) Blood supply to mucosa of lateral nasal wall and septum.

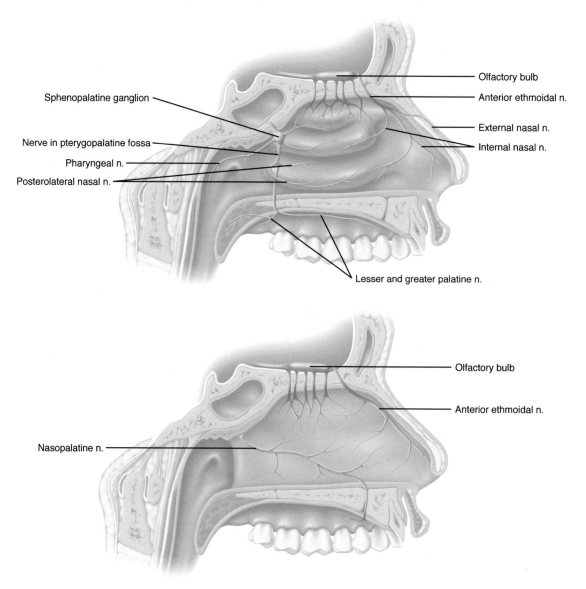

FIGURE 3-7. (A and B.) Nerve supply to mucosa of the lateral nasal wall and nasal septum.

nasotracheal intubation at a training course, minor nasal bleeding was seen in 20 during endoscopy or after extubation.[13] None of the 20 subjects required suction to control bleeding or clear the airway, and the bleeding did not interfere with endoscopy. During nasal intubation passing the tube with the bevel at the tip facing the septum directs the leading edge away from the vascular septum; however, the optimum orientation of the tube is controversial (see Blind Nasal Intubation section in Chapter 11).[14] Perforation into the submucosal space can occur and lead to hematoma and abscess formation in the retropharyngeal space.[2,3] Excessive force must be avoided.[3]

Common sensation to the nasal cavities is supplied by the ophthalmic and maxillary divisions of the trigeminal nerve.[2,3] The posterior aspect of the septum is innervated by the short and long sphenopalatine branches of the maxillary nerve.[3,4] Anteriorly the septum and the lateral wall is supplied by the anterior ethmoidal branch of the ophthalmic nerve (see Figures 3-7A and B).[7] The posterior-superior aspect of the lateral wall is innervated by the short sphenopalatine nerve and the inferior aspect by the posterolateral nasal branches of the sphenopalatine nerve.[3,4,9] Anteriorly, the floor of the nose is supplied by the anterior-superior dental branch of the infraorbital nerve and posteriorly by the greater palatine.[3,4] Rootlets of the olfactory nerve located in the roof of the nose adjacent to the cribriform plate transmit the sense of smell.[3]

In addition to being a respiratory pathway, the nose humidifies and warms inspired air, houses the olfactory receptors, removes bacteria, dust, and other particles from inspired air, and acts as a voice resonator.[3,4,8]

3.2.3   The mouth

Anatomically, the mouth consists of (1) the vestibule which is bounded externally by the lips and cheeks and internally by the gums and teeth and (2) the mouth cavity.[3,4] The mouth cavity is bounded by the alveolar arches and the teeth anteriorly and laterally, the hard palate and the anterior aspect of the soft palate above, and the anterior two-thirds of the tongue and the reflection of its mucosa onto the floor of the mouth and mandible below.[3,4] Posteriorly, the oral cavity opens into the oropharynx at the oropharyngeal isthmus.[3-5] The anterior two-thirds of the palate (hard palate) is composed of the palatine plates of the maxillae and the horizontal plates of the palatine bones (see Figure 3-2).[3,4,15] Posteriorly the hard palate is continuous with the soft palate, which is composed of a tough, fibrous sheath and extends to a free posterior border. In the midline, the soft palate ends in the uvula[3,4,15] then curves laterally to blend into the lateral pharyngeal wall at the palatoglossal and palatopharyngeal folds (anterior and posterior tonsillar pillars), respectively.[3,4,15] The anterior and inferior aspect of the soft palate faces the mouth cavity and oropharynx, whereas the posterior and superior aspect is part of the nasopharynx.[3,4,15] The uvula is a valuable midline landmark during bronchoscopic intubation through the mouth. Movement of the soft palate is controlled by five paired muscles including palatoglossus and palatopharyngeus, which descend in their respective folds to blend with the side of the tongue (palatoglossus) and the side wall of the pharynx (palatopharyngeus) and serve to approximate the folds.[3,4] These folds can be used as landmarks for transmucosal glossopharyngeal nerve blocks. The palatine muscles help to isolate the nasopharynx from the mouth during swallowing and phonation.[3,4] Paralysis permits regurgitation of food into the nasopharynx and results in nasal speech.[3,4] Sensation to the palate is primarily supplied by the trigeminal nerve; however the glossopharyngeal nerve supplies the most posterior aspect (see Figure 3-8).[3,4]

The anterior two-thirds of the body of the tongue occupies most of the floor of the mouth.[2,4,6] The posterior third of the tongue lies in the oropharynx and is separated from the anterior two-thirds by a V-shaped groove on the dorsal aspect of

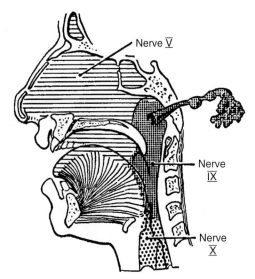

FIGURE 3-8. The sensory distribution of the glossopharyngeal nerve. (Reproduced with permission from Basmajian JV: Grant's Method of Anatomy, 8th edn. Baltimore: Williams and Wilkins (after Edwards), 1981.)

the tongue, the sulcus terminalis.[3] The posterior third of the tongue has abundant lymphoid nodules, the lingual tonsil,[6] and hypertrophy of this lymphoid tissue can make intubation by direct laryngoscopy difficult or impossible.[16] The tongue is also subdivided by a median vertical fibrous septum represented on the dorsum of the tongue by a shallow midline groove,[15] another useful landmark during bronchoscopic intubation (see Figure 3-9). The tongue musculature is divided into intrinsic

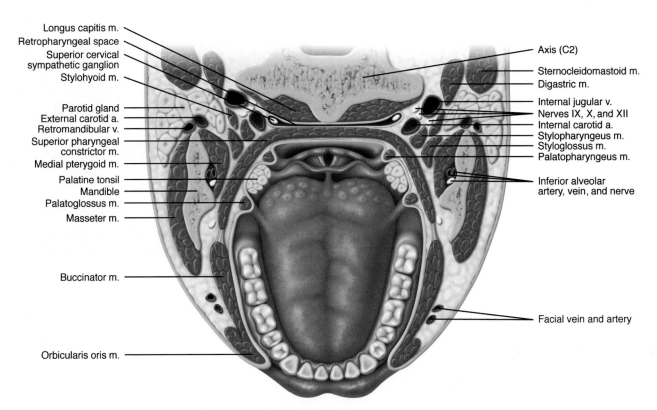

FIGURE 3-9. Horizontal section below lingua of mandible: superior view.

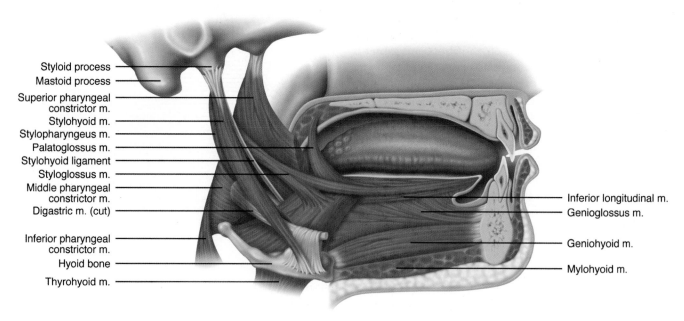

Styloid process
Mastoid process
Superior pharyngeal constrictor m.
Stylohyoid m.
Stylopharyngeus m.
Palatoglossus m.
Stylohyoid ligament
Styloglossus m.
Middle pharyngeal constrictor m.
Digastric m. (cut)
Inferior pharyngeal constrictor m.
Hyoid bone
Thyrohyoid m.

Inferior longitudinal m.
Genioglossus m.
Geniohyoid m.
Mylohyoid m.

FIGURE 3-10. Extrinsic muscles of the tongue.

muscles that alter the shape of the tongue[14] and extrinsic muscles that move the tongue as a whole (see Figure 3-10).[2,3,15] The extrinsic muscles connect the tongue to the symphysis of the mandible (genioglossus), hyoid (hyoglossus), styloid process (styloglossus), and the soft palate (palatoglossus).[14,15] In the supine unconscious individual, a decrease in genioglossal tone allows the tongue to move posteriorly and airway obstruction can occur. Sensation to the anterior two-thirds of the tongue is supplied by the lingual branch of the mandibular nerve,[3,15] whereas sensation to the posterior third is supplied by the glossopharyngeal and superior laryngeal branches of the vagus.[6,15] Stimulation of the posterior third of the tongue during awake intubation typically provokes the gag reflex and reflex secretions, and can be particularly problematic during bronchoscopic intubation. The tongue receives its blood supply from the lingual branch of the external carotid[15] and is a very vascular structure.[6] At the lateral aspect of the tongue, the mucous membrane is reflected onto the floor of the mouth and extends laterally to reach the gingiva, the "lingual sulcus."[3] The "buccal sulcus" lies between the teeth and the cheek. Deep to the mucous membrane in the floor of the mouth on either side of the tongue anteriorly lie the sublingual glands, and deep to these structures lies the mylohyoid muscle which forms a sling to support the floor of the mouth (see Figure 3-11).[3,6,7,15] The submandibular gland straddles the mylohyoid muscle posteriorly.[3] Both the lingual and the hypoglossal nerves travel in the floor of the mouth lateral to the tongue in the lingual sulcus.[3] Lingual branches of the glossopharyngeal nerve lie deep to the mucosa of the palatoglossal arch (anterior tonsillar pillar) at the lateral aspect of the tongue and can be blocked in this location (see Figure 3-12). The mylohyoid muscle divides the floor of the mouth into two potential spaces: the submandibular space below the muscle and the sublingual space above.[2] Hematoma formation or infection in either of these fascial spaces can displace the tongue superiorly and posteriorly to produce airway

compromise and can make intubation difficult (eg, Ludwig's angina).

The mandible consists of a horseshoe-shaped body anteriorly and two rami posteriorly, which extend superiorly to end in a condylar head and a coronoid process with an intervening mandibular notch (see Figure 3-13).[3] The condylar head articulates with the mandibular fossa of the temporal bone at

Submandibular gland, deep part

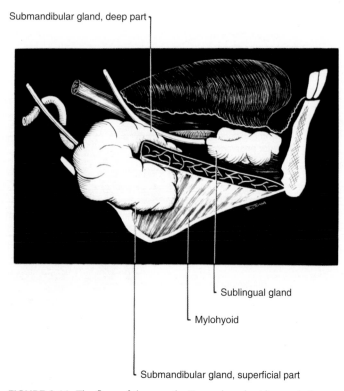

Sublingual gland

Mylohyoid

Submandibular gland, superficial part

FIGURE 3-11. The floor of the mouth. (Reproduced, with permission, from Friedman SM. *Visual Anatomy.* Vol. 1. *Head and Neck.* New York: Harper & Row; 1970.)

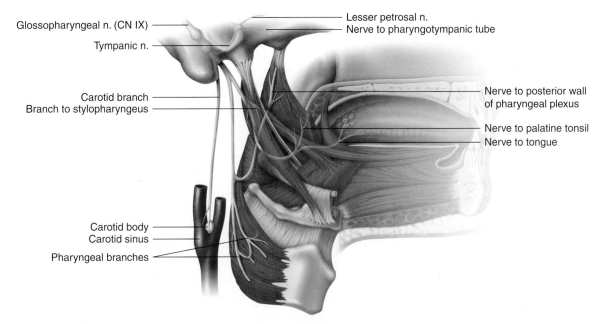

FIGURE 3-12. Distribution of the glossopharyngeal nerve (CN IX). (Reproduced, with permission, from Moore KL, Dalley AF. *Clinically Oriented Anatomy.* 4th ed. Philadelphia, PA: Lippincott, Williams & Wilkins; 1999.)

the temporomandibular joint (TMJ).[3] Two types of movement occur at the TMJ—rotation and a forward gliding or forward *translation*—thereby opening the mouth (see Figure 3-14).[3,6] Normal mandibular opening in the adult is about 4 cm, or at least two finger breadths, between the upper and lower incisors.[3,8] Decreased mandibular mobility and anatomic variants, in particular micrognathia, can make intubation by direct laryngoscopy difficult or impossible.

FIGURE 3-13. Lateral view of mandible. (Reproduced, with permission, from Basmajian JV. *Grant's Method of Anatomy.* 8th ed. Baltimore, MA: Lippincott, Williams & Wilkins; 1981.)

3.2.4   The pharynx

The pharynx is a U-shaped musculofascial tube which extends from the base of the skull to the lower border of the cricoid cartilage where at the level of the sixth cervical vertebrae it is continuous with the esophagus (see Figure 3-1).[2,3,6] Posteriorly, it rests against the prevertebral fascia. Anteriorly, it communicates with the nasal cavity, mouth, and the larynx at the *naso-*, *oro-*, and *laryngo*pharynx, respectively (see Figure 3-15).[3,4] From the inner aspect outward, the pharynx consists of mucosa, submucosa, muscle, and a loose areolar sheath, the buccopharyngeal fascia. This buccopharyngeal fascia is the thin fibrous capsule of the pharynx, contains the plexi of pharyngeal veins and nerves, and is continuous with the areolar sheath of the buccinator muscles and the

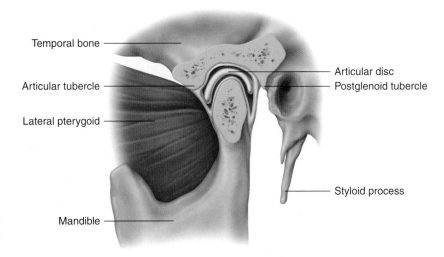

FIGURE 3-14. The temporomandibular joint, on saggital section. (Reproduced, with permission, from Basmajian JV. *Grant's Method of Anatomy.* 8th ed. Baltimore, MA: Lippincott, Williams & Wilkins; 1981.)

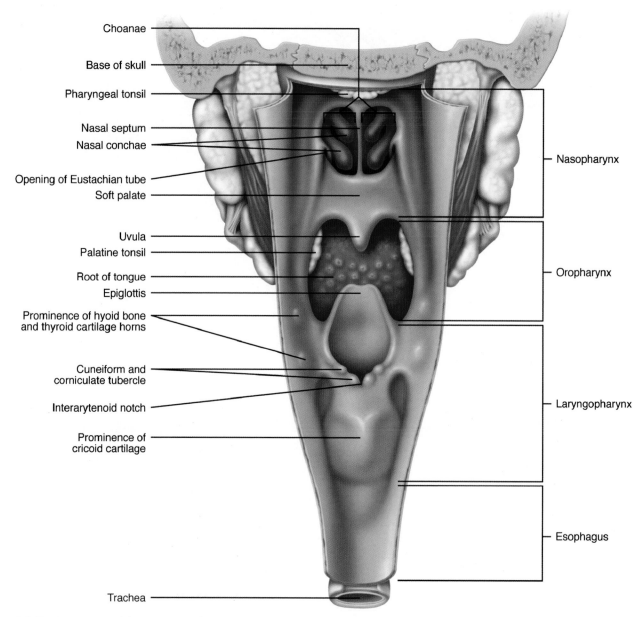

Choanae

Base of skull

Pharyngeal tonsil

Nasal septum

Nasal conchae

Opening of Eustachian tube

Soft palate

Uvula

Palatine tonsil

Root of tongue

Epiglottis

Prominence of hyoid bone
and thyroid cartilage horns

Cuneiform and
corniculate tubercle

Interarytenoid notch

Prominence of
cricoid cartilage

Trachea

Nasopharynx

Oropharynx

Laryngopharynx

Esophagus

FIGURE 3-15. Opened posterior view of the pharynx.

adventitia of esophagus.[2,3,6] Superiorly, it is attached to the base of the skull.[2] Edema associated with infection in the floor of the mouth, such as Ludwig's angina, is limited by the buccopharyngeal fascia, can spread into the pharynx and larynx, and may lead to airway obstruction.[3,4] The muscular layer of the pharynx is made up primarily of three paired constrictor muscles that curve around the pharyngeal lumen and telescope into one another (see Figure 3-16). The inferior constrictor consists of an upper oblique part and a lower transverse part (the cricopharyngeus) that is continuous with the esophagus and functions as an upper esophageal sphincter.[3,6] The junction of the pharynx with the esophagus is the narrowest part of the gastrointestinal tract and is a common place for foreign bodies to impact.[3,6]

The *naso*pharynx extends from the posterior choanae to the tip of the uvula[3,9] and forms a backward extension of the nasal cavities (see Figure 3-17).[3,6] It is bounded inferiorly by the soft palate.[3,4,6]

It communicates with the oropharynx at the pharyngeal isthmus, which is closed during swallowing by the soft palate, the palatopharyngeus, and a ridge of the superior pharyngeal constrictor at the level of the second cervical vertebra, the ridge of Passavant.[3,4,6] The roof of the nasopharynx is formed by the sphenoid bone and curves into the posterior pharyngeal wall at the level of the atlas and axis.[3,6,9] The nasopharyngeal tonsils (adenoids) are located in the roof of the nasopharynx and can extend laterally.[3,6] The Eustachian tube enters the nasopharynx through the lateral wall.[3,4] A prominent arch of the atlas vertebra (C1) may protrude anteriorly into the nasopharynx and during nasal intubation, the endotracheal tube can impact the mucosa and resist advancement at this level.[17] Rotation of the tube will facilitate passage around this prominence. However, on occasion, digital manipulation through the mouth may be required, or it may be necessary to first pass a soft nasal trumpet into the pharynx beyond the anterior tubercle of the atlas.

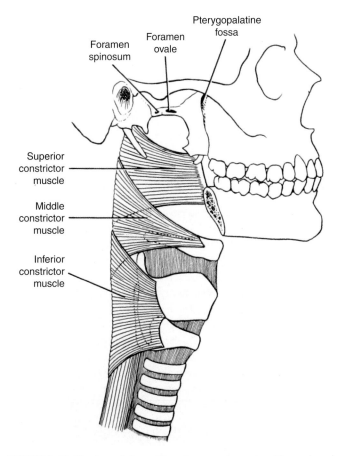

Foramen
spinosum
Foramen
ovale
Pterygopalatine
fossa

Superior
constrictor
muscle

Middle
constrictor
muscle

Inferior
constrictor
muscle

FIGURE 3-16. The lateral view of the pharyngeal muscles. (Reproduced, with permission, from Graney DO, Baker SR. Basic science: anatomy. In: Cummings CW, et al, eds. *Otolaryngology Head and Neck Surgery.* 3rd ed. St. Louis: Mosby; 1998.)

A nasogastric tube cut off at its proximal end can then be passed into the pharynx through the trumpet and the trumpet removed. A nasal endotracheal tube can then be passed over the nasogastric tube beyond the tubercle of the atlas. The NG tube can then be removed and the endotracheal tube passed into the trachea.

The *oro*pharynx extends from the soft palate to the epiglottis[3,4,9] and lies behind the mouth cavity and posterior third of the tongue. The palatoglossal folds arch downward from the soft palate to the junction of the anterior two-thirds and posterior third of the tongue and provide the dividing line between the mouth and oropharynx (see Figure 3-9).[3,6] This oropharyngeal isthmus is completed by the soft palate and the sulcus terminalis of the tongue.[3,6] The palatine tonsils lie on either side of the oropharynx in the triangle formed by the tongue and the palatoglossal and palatopharyngeal arches.[3,4,6] The glossopharyngeal nerve can be blocked as it runs deep to the mucosa posterior to the palatopharyngeal fold.

The *laryngo*pharynx (also referred to as the hypopharynx) extends from the epiglottis to the lower border of the cricoid cartilage, and is continuous with the esophagus (see Figures 3-15 and 3-17).[3,4,15] The upper border of the laryngopharynx has been located at the tip of the epiglottis by some authors[3,15] and the base of the epiglottis by others.[9,18] The oblique inlet of the larynx bounded by the epiglottis, aryepiglottic folds, arytenoid cartilages, and the posterior commissure lies anteriorly.[3,6] The cylindrical larynx itself bulges posteriorly into the center of the laryngopharynx creating a deep recess, the piriform fossa

(or sinus), on either side leading into the esophagus.[3,4] As seen during direct laryngoscopy, the larynx can be conceptualized to be a smaller cylinder eccentrically placed within and at the anterior aspect of the larger cylindrical pharynx. Laterally, the piriform fossae are bounded by the thyroid cartilage and the thyrohyoid membrane.[3,6] Superior to the piriform fossae, the median glossoepiglottic fold connects the epiglottis to the tongue in the midline and the lateral glossoepiglottic folds connect it to the pharyngeal wall.[3,6] The depressions formed between these folds are termed the valleculae[6] and are considered to be within the oropharynx.[9] During direct laryngoscopy, the Macintosh blade is inserted into the base of the vallecula to engage the hyoepiglottic ligament (beneath the glossoepiglottic fold) and thereby move the epiglottis anteriorly to expose the glottis.

Sensation to the nasopharynx and oropharynx is supplied primarily by the glossopharyngeal nerve.[3,6] The glossopharyngeal nerve enters the neck in company with the internal carotid artery and the internal jugular vein.[19] At the level of the styloid process, it leaves this position and winds anteriorly and inferiorly lateral to stylopharyngeus which it supplies (see Figure 3-18).[7] The nerve then passes forward between the superior and middle constrictors and gives off pharyngeal branches as well as lingual branches to the posterior third of the tongue (see Figure 3-12). Glossopharyngeal nerve blocks can be performed posterior to the midpoint of the palatopharyngeal fold or at the base of the palatoglossal fold in the mouth. The maxillary branch of the trigeminal nerve supplies sensation to the roof of the nasopharynx and contributes to the sensory supply of the soft palate and the adjacent part of the tonsil.[3,6] The laryngopharynx receives sensory innervation from the internal branch of the superior laryngeal branch of the vagus nerve, which pierces the thyrohyoid membrane and runs in the submucosa of the piriform fossae.[3] This nerve also supplies sensation to the larynx above the level of the false or true cords.[6,7,20-22] Cotton pledgets soaked in local anesthetic can be held against the mucosa of the piriform fossa using Kraus or Jackson forceps to produce a block of the internal branch of the superior laryngeal, or the nerve can be approached percutaneously. It has been said that the superior aspect (pharyngeal surface) of the epiglottis is innervated by the glossopharyngeal nerve, whereas the inferior aspect (laryngeal surface) receives sensory innervation from the superior laryngeal nerve.[21,23] Others have stated that both the surfaces of the epiglottis are innervated by the superior laryngeal branch of the vagus.[20]

3.2.5   The larynx

The larynx is a complex structure made up of a framework of cartilages and fibroelastic membranes covered by a layer of muscles and lined by mucous membrane.[3,4] It functions as an open valve during respiration, a partially closed valve during phonation, a closed value during swallowing, and to produce increased intrathoracic pressure when effort is required (Valsalva maneuver).[2,3,9,15] It extends from its oblique entrance or aditus to the lower border of the cricoid cartilage and bulges posteriorly into the laryngopharynx (see Figure 3-15).[3,6] It is suspended from the hyoid bone which is itself attached to the mandible, tongue, and the base of the skull.[15]

The laryngeal cartilages include the thyroid, cricoid, epiglottic and the paired arytenoid, corniculate, and cuneiform cartilages (see Figure 3-19). The quadrilateral laminae of the thyroid cartilage

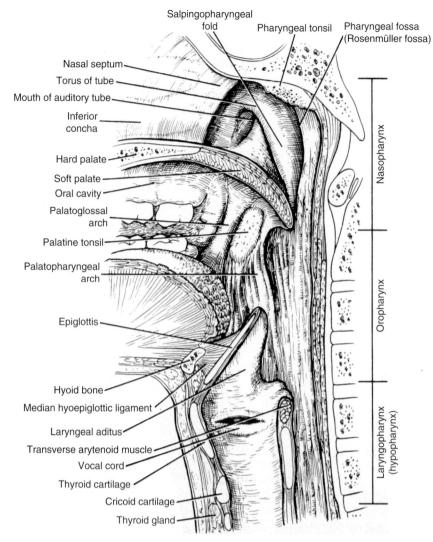

FIGURE 3-17. The medial view of the pharyngeal mucosa. (Reproduced, with permission, from Graney DO, Baker SR. Basic science: anatomy. In: Cummings CW, et al, eds. *Otolaryngology Head and Neck Surgery*. 3rd ed. St. Louis: Mosby; 1998.)

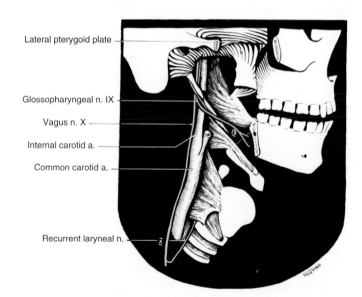

FIGURE 3-18. The glossopharyngeal nerve. (Reproduced, with permission, from Friedman SM. *Visual Anatomy*. Vol. 1. *Head and Neck*. New York: Harper & Row; 1970.)

meet in the midline anteriorly to form the thyroid prominence (Adam's apple). Superiorly, the thyroid cartilage is attached to the hyoid by the thyrohyoid membrane.[3] Posteriorly the lower horns of the thyroid cartilage articulate with the posteriorly oriented signet ring-shaped cricoid cartilage. Anteriorly, the thyroid cartilage is attached to the cricoid by the cricothyroid membrane, a suitable site for emergency surgical airway access in the adult. The cricoid cartilage is the only complete skeletal ring of the airway and can be used to provide cricoid pressure (Sellick maneuver) during rapid sequence induction/intubation. The paired arytenoid cartilages articulate with the superior aspect of the cricoid cartilage posteriorly. The corniculate cartilages in turn articulate with the apices of the pyramidal shaped arytenoids.[3] The shallow depression between the two corniculate cartilages (the posterior commissure) is a useful landmark during laryngoscopy.[3,9] The cuneiform cartilages are located lateral to the corniculate cartilages and lie within the aryepiglottic folds. The leaf-shaped epiglottis is attached directly to the thyroid cartilage inferiorly and the hyoid bone superiorly by the hyoepiglottic ligament.[3] The remaining framework of the larynx consists of two paired fibroelastic folds, the quadrangular and triangular membranes (see Figure 3-20).[3,9] The quadrangular membrane spans the space between the lateral border of the epiglottis and the arytenoid cartilages.[3,9] Its free upper edge forms the aryepiglottic ligament at the laryngeal aditus, and its thickened lower border forms the vestibular ligament (false vocal cord).[3,6] The triangular ligament is attached in the midline anteriorly to the thyroid and cricoid cartilage and extends posteriorly to attach to the arytenoid cartilage. The inferior border of the triangular ligament is attached obliquely to the cricoid cartilage whereas the upper border is free and thickened to form the vocal ligament (true vocal cord).[3,9] In coronal section, the relationship of the true vocal cords to the false vocal cords and the laryngeal ventricle or sinus (between the true and false cords) can be readily appreciated (see Figure 3-21).[3,9] The aryepiglottic, the vestibular (false cords), and the vocal folds (true cords) form a trilevel sphincter mechanism that regulates and protects the airway.[3,9] The folds also divide the larynx into three spaces: the supraglottic compartment or *vestibule* above the false cords, the *glottic* compartment between the false and true cords, and the *infraglottic* compartment between the true cords and the lower border of the cricoid.[3,6,15] The absence of a submucosal layer at the vocal ligament causes the cords to appear white and limits the extent to which they can swell in edematous conditions.[15] The average distance from the incisors to the vocal cords is 12 to 16 cm.[24,25]

A complex arrangement of intrinsic muscles alters the configuration of the laryngeal folds. The cricothyroid muscle is classified by itself as the only extrinsic muscle of the larynx; muscles that

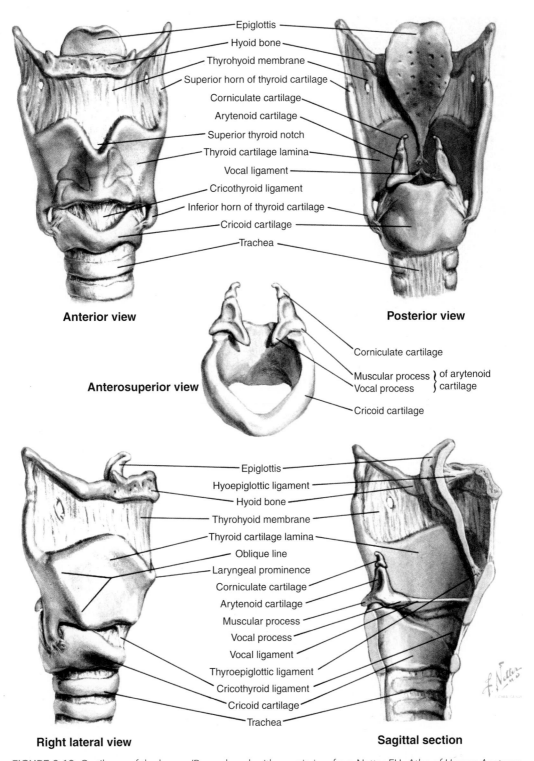

Epiglottis
Hyoid bone
Thyrohyoid membrane
Superior horn of thyroid cartilage
Corniculate cartilage
Arytenoid cartilage
Superior thyroid notch
Thyroid cartilage lamina
Vocal ligament
Cricothyroid ligament
Inferior horn of thyroid cartilage
Cricoid cartilage
Trachea

Anterior view

Posterior view

Anterosuperior view

Corniculate cartilage
Muscular process } of arytenoid
Vocal process } cartilage
Cricoid cartilage

Epiglottis
Hyoepiglottic ligament
Hyoid bone
Thyrohyoid membrane
Thyroid cartilage lamina
Oblique line
Laryngeal prominence
Corniculate cartilage
Arytenoid cartilage
Muscular process
Vocal process
Vocal ligament
Thyroepiglottic ligament
Cricothyroid ligament
Cricoid cartilage
Trachea

Right lateral view

Sagittal section

FIGURE 3-19. Cartilages of the larynx. (Reproduced, with permission, from Netter FH. *Atlas of Human Anatomy.* Summit. New Jersey: CIBA-GEIGY Corporation; 1989.)

elevate or depress the larynx as a whole (eg, during swallowing) are considered to be accessory laryngeal muscles.[3,9]

The larynx receives its nerve supply from the superior and recurrent laryngeal nerves.[3,4] The superior laryngeal nerve arises from the vagus just below the pharyngeal plexus, passes medial to both the internal and external carotids, and then divides into a large sensory internal and a small motor external branch which supplies the cricothyroid muscle (see Figure 3-22).[3,4,7] The internal branch pierces the thyrohyoid membrane to provide sensation to the laryngeal mucosa above the level of the false cords[3,9,21,22] or true cords.[6,7,20]

On the right side, the recurrent laryngeal nerve leaves the vagus as it crosses the subclavian artery, loops posteriorly under the artery, and ascends to the larynx in the groove between the esophagus and

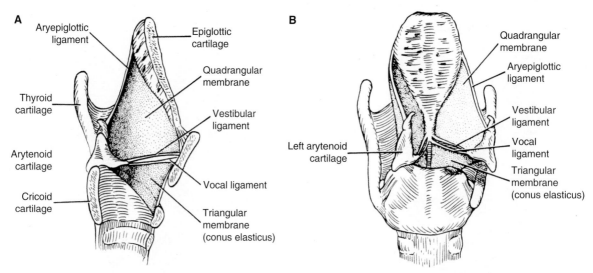

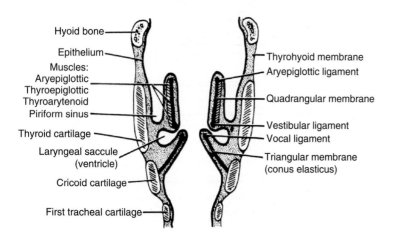

FIGURE 3-20. (A) Saggital section of laryngeal membranes. (B) Posterior view of laryngeal membranes (right arytenoid cartilage moved laterally). (Reproduced, with permission, from Graney DO, Baker SR. Basic science: anatomy. In: Cummings CW, et al, eds. *Otolaryngology Head and Neck Surgery*. 3rd ed. St. Louis: Mosby; 1998.)

trachea. On the left, the nerve leaves the vagus as it crosses the aortic arch and similarly loops posteriorly under the arch and then runs superiorly between the esophagus and the trachea to reach the larynx.[3,4] The recurrent laryngeal nerves supply all the intrinsic muscles of the larynx and provide sensation below the level of the false[3,9,21,22] or true cords.[6,7,20] Hoarseness produced by damage to the superior laryngeal nerve is usually temporary as the contralateral cord exerts a compensatory action.[3,4] Damage to the recurrent laryngeal nerve also produces hoarseness, and if both nerves are affected, severe airway obstruction can occur.[3,15]

The cricothyroid membrane or ligament can be identified in the anterior neck as a concavity between the convex inferior border of the thyroid cartilage and the superior portion of the cricoid cartilage (see Figures 3-19 and 3-23). The space is trapezoidal in shape with a cross-sectional area of 2.9 cm² and a mean height of 9 mm (range 5-12 mm).[26,27] The average vertical distance between the true cords and the midpoint of the cricothyroid membrane is 13 mm in the adult.[26] The vertical distance from the lower border of the thyroid cartilage to the vocal cords is 5 to 11 mm.[27,28]

The cricothyroid branches of the superior thyroid arteries run transversely across the membrane, usually the upper third,[27,28] and tributaries of the anterior jugular veins occasionally run anterior to the membrane, although considerable variation exists in the vascular pattern.[27] During cricothyrotomy or membrane puncture, the cricothyroid membrane should be traversed at its inferior third to minimize vascular injury.[27,28]

3.2.6   The trachea

The trachea extends inferiorly from its junction with the larynx at the lower border of the cricoid cartilage to the carina (see Figure 3-24).[3,4,29] It is approximately 10 to 15 cm in length in the adult and about 13 to 20 mm in diameter.[3,4,6,22,24] The inferior half of the trachea lies within the superior mediastinum.[6] The cervical trachea is in the midline; however the intrathoracic portion is deviated to the right by the aortic arch.[4] The patency of the trachea is maintained by 16 to 20 U-shaped rings of hyaline cartilage[6] joined by fibroelastic tissue and closed posteriorly by the trachealis muscle.[3,4] Longitudinal mucosal markings can be seen posteriorly when the trachea is viewed through the bronchoscope, and these can be used for spatial orientation. The average distance from the central incisors to the carina is 27 cm in the adult male and 23 cm in the adult female.[17] The distance from the nostrils to the carina is an additional 4 cm.[17] Tracheotomy is usually performed between the second and third or third and fourth tracheal rings.[4,27,30]

3.2.7   How is the anatomy of the pediatric airway different from that of the adult?

Awake intubation is most often performed in the adult population, and this chapter on preparation for awake intubation is directed to this age group. Management of the pediatric airway does require consideration of anatomic differences in children. The reader is directed to the pediatric sections of the text for further information (see Chapter 42 and Figure 42-5).

FIGURE 3-21. Coronal section of larynx. (Reproduced, with permission, from Graney DO, Baker SR. Basic science: anatomy. In: Cummings CW, et al, ed. *Otolaryngology Head and Neck Surgery*. 3rd ed. St. Louis: Mosby; 1998.)

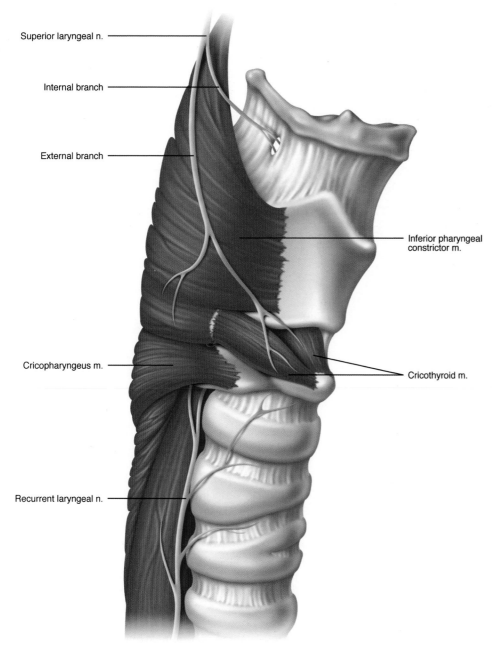

Superior laryngeal n.

Internal branch

External branch

Inferior pharyngeal constrictor m.

Cricopharyngeus m.

Cricothyroid m.

Recurrent laryngeal n.

FIGURE 3-22. Nerves innervating the larynx.

3.3   LOCAL ANESTHESIA OF THE AIRWAY

3.3.1   What drugs are useful for airway anesthesia? What are their toxicities and associated complications?

Lidocaine, tetracaine, cocaine, benzocaine, and dyclonine have all been used to produce topical anesthesia of the airway, and lidocaine is commonly used to perform glossopharyngeal and superior laryngeal nerve blocks.

3.3.2   Lidocaine

Introduced in 1948, lidocaine is the prototypical member of the amide class of local anesthetics and is metabolized in the liver by mixed function oxidases.[31] The principle metabolite is monoethylglycinexylidide (MEGX) which has a local anesthetic effect and side effect profile similar to lidocaine.[32] Hepatic metabolism of lidocaine appears to be limited by liver perfusion[33] as well as parenchymal disease such as cirrhosis[34] and the clearance of lidocaine is reduced in the presence of cardiac and hepatic insufficiency.[32] Orally ingested lidocaine undergoes first pass metabolism in the liver[35] and about 35% of an oral dose reaches the systemic circulation.[36] Lidocaine is probably the local anesthetic most commonly used for regional anesthesia of the airway and has also been used extensively in the past for the treatment of ventricular arrhythmias.[31,37,38]

Following application to the mucous membranes of the airway, lidocaine produces an anesthetic effect which is limited to the mucous membrane in 1 to 2 minutes.[24,39] The peak anesthetic effect occurs within 2 to 5 minutes,[31] and the duration of the airway anesthesia is said to be 30 to 40 minutes,[31] 20 to 40 minutes,[40] or 15 to 30 minutes.[41] Watanabe et al found the duration of anesthesia following the application of lidocaine to the oral mucosa to be 40 minutes with glycopyrrolate pretreatment, and 20 minutes without it.[42] Schonemann et al sprayed 10% (100 mg·mL^{-1}) lidocaine onto the oral mucosa of the lower lip and demonstrated a hypoalgesic effect that lasted 14 mintues.[43] Maximum hypoalgesia was observed after 4 to 5 minutes.[43] Adriani et al found that the maximum effective concentration of topical lidocaine applied to the tongue was 4% (40 mg·mL^{-1}), and that this concentration had a latent period of 2 minutes, and a duration of effect of 15.2 minutes.[39] The latent period has a profound significance when bronchoscopic intubation is performed using a spray-as-you-go technique and suggests that a significant risk of insufficient anesthesia may exist.[43] Concentrations of lidocaine of 1% (10 mg·mL^{-1}) to 10% (100 mg·mL^{-1}) have been used for topical anesthesia of the airway. Excellent topical anesthesia of the airway in the adult can be produced by 4% lidocaine, but at 2% (20 mg·mL^{-1}) concentration, topical anesthesia may be inadequate, and 1% lidocaine has been found to be insufficient for airway instrumentation.[44] Increasing the concentration beyond the optimum level does not affect the latent period or duration of action,[39] and increasing the

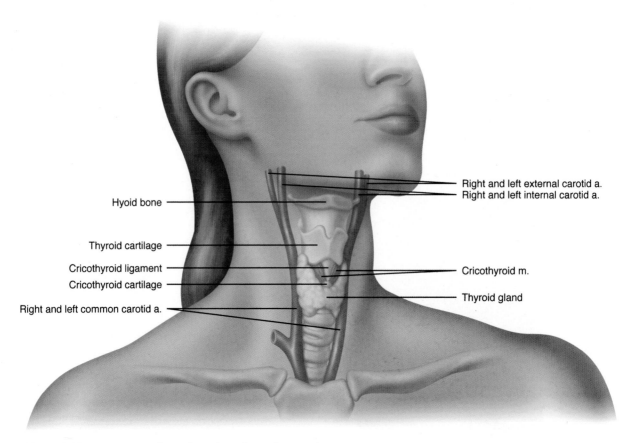

FIGURE 3-23. Anterior view of cricothyroid membrane (ligament).

dose to a given area of mucosa beyond 15 mg of lidocaine per square centimeter does not increase the anesthetic effect.[43] Importantly, topical epinephrine penetrates mucous membranes poorly, has no significant local effect, does not prolong the duration of topical local anesthesia,[31] and will not slow the rate of anesthetic absorption.[45]

Local anesthetics applied to the mucous membranes of the airway are rapidly absorbed into the circulation.[31] The extent of

FIGURE 3-24. The trachea and extrapulmonary bronchi, and their relations. (Reproduced, with permission, from Basmajian JV. *Grant's Method of Anatomy*. 8th ed. Baltimore: Lippincott, Williams & Wilkins; 1981.)

systemic absorption depends on the site and technique of application, tissue vascularity, the total dose administered,[46,47] the state of the mucosa, the concomitant use of drying agents,[42,48] the amount of mucous present, the rate and depth of respiration, the state of the circulation, the patient's disease state,[49,50] and individual variation.[49,50] Slower uptake occurs from the more proximal parts of the respiratory tract.[49,50] Absorption is particularly rapid when local anesthetics are applied to the tracheobronchial tree,[31] whereas decreased rates of absorption occur in the upper airway secondary to decreased vascularity and surface area.[47] Absorption from alveoli may approximate IV administration[51] due to osmotic relationships in the pulmonary vascular bed designed to prevent the collection of fluid in the alveolar spaces.[39,52] The therapeutic serum concentration of lidocaine when the drug is used as an antiarrhythmic is usually considered to be 1.5 to 4.0 μg·mL^{-1},[49] or 1.5 to 5 μg·mL^{-1}.[53] As serum lidocaine concentrations increase however, systemic toxicity is produced. The commonly accepted toxic plasma concentration of lidocaine has been said to be 5 μg·mL^{-1}.[54] At the upper limit of the antiarrhythmic therapeutic range, lightheadedness, tinnitus, and circumoral and tongue numbness can occur.[55] As serum concentrations continue to rise, visual disturbances and muscle twitching occur and can be followed by generalized seizure activity.[55] Seizures are most frequently seen at plasma concentrations more than 8 to 10 μg·mL^{-1},[51,56] although they have occurred at plasma concentrations as low as 6 μg·mL^{-1}.[47] Cardiorespiratory arrest can occur at plasma lidocaine concentrations of 20 to 25 μg·mL^{-1}.[47,55] Levels in arterial blood have been shown to be 20% to 30% higher than those in venous samples[48,56,57] and more closely correlate with CNS effects.[58] However, most clinicians consider venous blood levels to be reliable indicators of clinical toxicity.[47] Hypersensitivity reactions to lidocaine, although exceedingly rare, can also occur and can be catastrophic.[40] Clinically significant methemoglobinemia has been reported in association with lidocaine administration, although these occurrences have been extremely rare.[59-63] A 2007 review of the literature found 12 episodes of methemoglobinemia related to lidocaine without associated prilocaine or benzocaine use.[64] In seven of these cases an oxidative drug had been administered concomitantly. In one case the episode occurred within 24 hours of exposure to benzocaine, and one case occurred after the chronic abuse of lidocaine gel. Of the remaining three cases, one developed cyanosis about 21 hours after lidocaine injection.[60] Methemoglobin levels were not reported but the patient responded to methylene blue.[60]

The maximum safe dose of topical lidocaine has been stated to be 4 mg·kg^{-1},[3,4,65-70] mg·kg^{-1},[37] and 6 mg·kg^{-1}.[17] However, when topically applied to the mucous membranes of the airway, these maximal doses can only be interpreted when the method of topical administration is known. The exact dose of lidocaine delivered to the airway when an inhalational technique is used is difficult to measure,[58] and the dose administered may bear little relation to the dose actually absorbed.[71] Lidocaine administered to the airway by nebulization has been reported to produce low peak plasma concentrations as compared to other techniques.[47,48,58,72] This has been attributed to the loss of up to 50% of the nebulized solution to the environment with continuous nebulization.[58,73] Absorption of local anesthetics administered by aerosols is also dependent on droplet size. Typical nebulizers produce droplets that range from 1 to 20 μm in diameter.[74] The peak deposition of aerosol droplets occurs in the peripheral airway for droplets of about 2 μm, in bronchioles for droplets of about 8 μm, in bronchi for droplets of about 15 μm, and in the upper airway for droplets larger than 40 μm.[75] Higher oxygen flow rates through nebulizers create smaller droplets (<30 μm) that travel further distally into the bronchial tree and increase the rate of absorption.[41]

Droplets larger than 60 μm are preferred for airway anesthesia during awake intubation because they *rain out* in the proximal airway where the topical anesthesia is required.[41] The droplet size produced by manually squeezing the bulb of the hand-held DeVilbiss #40 nebulizer tends to be much larger than that produced by conventional aerosol delivery systems and is dependent on the pressure generated in the atomizer.[76] The mean bulb pressure produced by a firm squeeze is 250 to 340 mm Hg (4.86-6.01 psi). The mass median diameter (MMD) of the droplets thus produced was found to be 6.2 to 12.0 μm with 28% to 50% of the particles being less than 6.2 μm in diameter, small enough to penetrate the tracheobronchial tree.[76] With increasing firmness of the manual squeeze and increased bulb pressure, these nebulizers increase output and decrease MMD. When an oxygen flow through the RD 15 DeVilbiss atomizer of 5.0 L·min^{-1} was utilized, pressures at the inlet of the device of 3.8 to 4.0 psi were generated, and at 8 L.min^{-1} oxygen flow pressure was 11.2 to 11.4 psi. This technique may produce smaller droplets leading to increased systemic absorption, although it has been shown that only about 7% to 12% of the nebulized dose of a drug actually reaches the lung.[77,78] Furthermore, the anesthetic expectorated after gargle and atomizer administration must be subtracted from the total dose administered.

Many investigators have endeavored to link route of administration and dosage of lidocaine used for airway anesthesia to plasma levels and toxicity:

- In a study performed by Melby et al, 1.5 mg.kg^{-1} of 4% lidocaine was injected into the endotracheal tube of six patients under general anesthesia. Peak serum lidocaine concentrations of 1.4 to 3.3 μg·mL^{-1} occurred at 11.7 ± 5.2 minutes following administration. Three of the six patients experienced almost instantaneous absorption.[79]

- Chu et al measured plasma lidocaine concentrations produced by tracheal spraying using 3.3 mg.kg^{-1} of 4% lidocaine and IV injection of 1 mg.kg^{-1} of 2% lidocaine. After tracheal spraying, maximum plasma lidocaine levels of 2.0 to 5.6 μg·mL^{-1} were recorded at 15 to 20 minutes. Following IV administration, peak concentrations of 5.0 to 6.85 μg·mL^{-1} were reached within 12 minutes.[75]

- Curran et al measured the concentration of lidocaine in venous blood following tracheal as compared to laryngeal spraying in 10 patients under general anesthesia. Each group received 3 mL of 10% lidocaine. The peak lidocaine concentration in the tracheal group ranged from 1.9 to 8.2 μg·mL,$^{-1}$ whereas in the laryngeal group the range was 0.4 to 2.5 μg·mL^{-1}. Lidocaine levels in the tracheal group tended to rise more rapidly and reach a peak earlier than in the laryngeal group.[80]

- Eyres et al administered 4 mg.kg^{-1} of 4% lidocaine into the larynx and immediate subglottic area of 96 children under general anesthesia and measured plasma lidocaine levels at 2, 4, 6, 10, 15, 20, and 30 minutes after administration. Mean peak lidocaine levels measured were 4.3 ± 1.9 μg·mL^{-1} for those less than 1 year of age, 5.7 ± 2.0 for those 1 to 3 years of age, 5.3 ± 1.4 for those 3 to 5 years of age, and 5.3 ± 2.0 for those more than 5 years of age. Plasma lidocaine levels exceeded 8.0 μg·mL^{-1} in 13 patients. The time to peak concentration varied from 8.5 ± 2.5 minutes in those less than 1 year of age to 11.7 ± 4.3 minutes in those more than 5 years of age.[81]

- Parks et al administered 6 mg.kg^{-1} of 10% lidocaine to 10 ASA I volunteers via a *nebulizer* connected to a *facemask* powered by an oxygen flow of 6 L·min^{-1}. The mean peak serum concentration of lidocaine produced was 0.29 μg·mL^{-1}, and the highest measurement was 0.45 μg·mL^{-1}. The peak concentration occurred 30 minutes after nebulization was commenced.[48]

- Chinn et al administered 10 mL of 4% lidocaine to five healthy subjects using a DeVilbiss 35B ultrasonic *nebulizer* connected to a Hudson *oxygen mask*.[73] Plasma lidocaine levels were measured at the start of nebulization, at 5-minute intervals for 30 minutes and then at 45, 60, 90, and 120 minutes after the start of nebulization. The mean peak plasma level occurred at 10 minutes and, as measured from the published graph, was 0.95 ug.mL^{-1}.[73]

- Mostafa et al similarly administered 6 mg.kg^{-1} of 10% lidocaine to 14 ASA I and II patients scheduled for head and neck surgery using a *nebulizer* system with a *mouthpiece* and an oxygen flow of 7 L·min⁻¹.[78] The mean plasma lidocaine level 10 minutes after nebulization was 0.95 ± 0.62 µg·mL⁻¹, and at 20 minutes it was 0.68 ± 0.32 µg·mL⁻¹.[72]

- Sutherland and Williams administered 5 mL of 4% lidocaine to 20 adult patients using a standard *nebulizer* connected to a *mouthpiece* and an oxygen flow of 8 L·min⁻¹. The mouthpiece was connected to an oral airway intubator that was advanced into the oropharynx during the latter part of the nebulization process. The subjects also gargled 5 mL of 2% lidocaine gel for 1 minute, and 2 mL of 2% lidocaine was injected through the bronchoscope onto the vocal cords, as well as 2 mL into the trachea. The dosage range was 2.5 to 11 mg·kg⁻¹ (mean dose, 5.3 ± 2.1 mg·kg⁻¹). The mean peak plasma concentration was 0.7 ± 0.4 µg·mL⁻¹, and the highest plasma concentration was 1.6 µg·mL⁻¹. The mean peak concentration occurred 23 minutes following intubation.[82]

- Kirkpatrick et al administered 10 mL of nebulized 4% lidocaine to 10 normal volunteers using a DeVilbiss 646 *nebulizer*, an oxygen flow of 6 L·min⁻¹, and a *mouthpiece* during tidal breathing.[83] Blood was sampled at 10, 20, 30, 40, and 50 minutes after the start of nebulization. In three subjects additional samples were obtained at 60, 80, and 120 minutes. The mean peak serum lidocaine level was 0.52 ug·mL⁻¹ and occurred 20 minutes after beginning nebulization. The highest single measurement was 1.05 ug·mL⁻¹.[83]

- Wieczorek et al administered topical lidocaine to a group of 27 obese patients prior to bronchoscopic intubation.[84] Forty milliliters of either 2% lidocaine (14 patients) or 4% lidocaine (13 patients) was administered using a DV-15-RD *atomizer* and an oxygen flow of 10 L·min⁻¹. Plasma lidocaine concentrations were measured at intervals from before atomization to 120 minutes following the completion of atomization. Peak plasma concentrations were recorded in the 10 minute samples in both groups. The mean peak level in the 4% group was 6.5 ug·mL⁻¹ (standard error of the mean, 1.0 ug·mL⁻¹). In the 2% group, the peak level was 2.8 (0.8) ug·mL⁻¹. No clinical signs of lidocaine toxicity were detected.[84]

- Woodruff et al subsequently reported a prospective randomized blinded study from the same center which compared 1% lidocaine with 2% lidocaine using the same *atomization* technique.[85] Forty milliliters of either 1% or 2% lidocaine was administered. Mean peak plasma lidocaine levels were measured 5 minutes after completion of topicalization and were 3.8 (0.5) ug·mL⁻¹ in the 2% group and 1.4 (0.3) ug·mL⁻¹ in the 1% group. No signs of lidocaine toxicity were detected.[85]

- Gomez et al measured serum lidocaine levels in 29 patients who underwent bronchoscopy and who had between 180 and 400 mg of lidocaine *instilled* onto the tracheobronchial muscosa.[86] Blood was sampled at intervals between 10 minutes and 2 hours after administration in 9 patients, and from 45 minutes to 2 hours in 20 patients. In the group who had the whole serum concentration curve determined, the average maximum serum concentration was 1.21 ± 0.64 ug·mL⁻¹. The peak concentration occurred at 34.02 ± 10.74 minutes. The average serum level 2 hours after administration was 0.69 ± 0.29 ug·mL⁻¹ and

the average serum half-life of lidocaine was 1.35 ± 0.41 hours. The percentage of lidocaine absorbed was calculated to be between 60.88% and 20.89% with an average value of 36.55 ± 13.95%.[86]

- Patterson et al reported the administration of up to 380 mg of lidocaine almost entirely delivered as a 1% solution *through the bronchoscope* to 21 adult patients. With the exception of one patient, the maximum blood levels of lidocaine recorded were less than 2.48 µg·mL⁻¹. The peak concentration occurred between 5 and 75 minutes following lidocaine administration, usually between 5 and 30 minutes. Considerable individual variation in the maximum concentration measured was noted. One patient with abnormal liver function was found to have a plasma concentration of 18.2 µg·mL⁻¹ but developed no signs of toxicity.[87]

- Xue et al performed a randomized double-blind study which compared 2% and 4% lidocaine administered via the bronchoscope using a *spray-as-you-go* technique in a group of 52 sedated patients prior to bronchoscopic intubation.[35] The mean dose of lidocaine administered was 3.4 ± 0.6 mg·kg⁻¹ (range 3.2-4 mg·kg⁻¹) in the 2% group, and 7.1 ± 2.1 mg·kg⁻¹ in the 4% group (range 6.1-8.1 mg·kg⁻¹). The highest lidocaine concentration measured in the 2% group was 2.0 ug·mL⁻¹, and in the 4% group the highest concentration measured was 3.6 ug·mL. Concentrations above 3 ug·mL⁻¹ occurred in only three patients, all in the 4% group. In most patients the peak lidocaine concentration was observed at 20 to 30 minutes after lidocaine administration. Again, significant individual variation in plasma levels was noted.[35]

- Boye and Bredesen administered about 7 mL of 4% lidocaine to nine adult patients prior to bronchoscopy utilizing nebulization, a topical applicator, instillation, and injection through the bronchoscope.[88] Blood was sampled about 8 minutes after the start of anesthesia and after bronchoscopy, about 38 minutes after the start of anesthesia. The mean maximum plasma concentration of lidocaine was 2.7 ug·mL⁻¹. No clinical signs of lidocaine toxicity occurred.[88]

- Bigeleisen et al administered a total of 7 mg·kg⁻¹ of lidocaine to a group of 20 patients who underwent bronchoscopic intubation. Four mg·kg⁻¹ of atomized 4% lidocaine was applied to the nose and nasopharynx, and percutaneous superior laryngeal nerve blocks were performed using 0.5 mg·kg⁻¹ of 1% lidocaine.[89] The patients were then randomized into two groups. Group 1 underwent transtracheal injection of 2 mg·kg⁻¹ of 4% lidocaine, whereas Group 2 received an additional equivalent dose of 4% lidocaine applied to the nasopharynx. Plasma lidocaine levels were measured every 2.5 minutes for 10 minutes after the last dose of lidocaine and then every 5 minutes for an additional 20 minutes. The mean peak lidocaine level in the transtracheal group was 4.06 ug·mL⁻¹ and occurred at 10 minutes. The highest level recorded was 6.04 ug·mL⁻¹. In the nasotracheal group, the mean peak level was 3.16 ug·mL⁻¹ and occurred at 7.5 minutes. The highest level was 6.57 ug·mL⁻¹. No signs of systemic toxicity were detected.[89]

- Loukides et al measured plasma lidocaine levels for up to 2 hours after the start of topicalization in 12 patients who underwent fiberoptic bronchoscopy.[53] The lidocaine was administered as a 2% gel to the nose and a 2% solution injected through a laryngeal syringe or the bronchoscope. The mean total dose administered was 622 ± 20 mg (range 500-720 mg). Peak plasma concentrations were observed at 20 minutes in eight patients, at 30 minutes in three patients, and at 60 minutes in one patient. The highest value measured was 2.25 ug·mL^{-1}.[53]

- Efthimiou et al measured plasma concentrations of lidocaine in a group of 41 patients who underwent topical airway anesthesia before fiberoptic bronchoscopy. In 32 patients, 14 sprays of 10% lidocaine were administered to the nose and oropharynx followed by 8 mL of 4% lidocaine solution administered via the bronchoscope to the pharynx and vocal cords, and 14 mL of 1% lidocaine to the bronchial tree. In nine patients, 8 mL of 2% lidocaine gel was applied to the nose and the use of the 10% spray was omitted. The average dose of lidocaine administered was 9.3 ± 0.5 mg·kg^{-1}. The average peak plasma concentration was 2.9 ± 0.5 μg·mL^{-1} and correlated with dose per unit body weight. Two patients had plasma levels above 5 μg·mL^{-1} but demonstrated no clinical evidence of toxicity. The average time to peak concentration was 42.6 minutes in the aerosol group and 48.4 minutes in the gel group. In a second study of 10 volunteers, plasma concentrations following 4% lidocaine gargle and swallow was compared with 10% oropharyngeal spray. The dose in each group was 6.8 mg·kg^{-1}. The gargle produced a peak concentration of 2.4 μg·mL^{-1}, whereas the spray produced a peak concentration of 1.9 μg·mL^{-1} at 50 minutes.[46]

- Reasoner et al randomized 40 adult patients undergoing awake fiberoptic intubation and surgery for cervical spine instability into topical and nerve block groups. Up to 20 mL of 4% lidocaine was administered to the topical group via a nebulizer attached to a facemask using a flow rate of 10 L·min^{-1}. Nebulization required about 10 minutes and was followed by cricothyroid puncture and injection of an additional 3 mL of 4% lidocaine. In the nerve block group, airway anesthesia was achieved with 50 mg of 10% lidocaine spray applied to the tongue, bilateral glossopharyngeal nerve block at the palatoglossal fold using 0.5 to 1.0 mL 2% lidocaine, superior laryngeal nerve block using 1 to 2 mL 2% lidocaine, and 3 mL 4% lidocaine injected through the cricothyroid membrane. Arterial blood was sampled for the plasma lidocaine level following administration of local anesthesia, 2 minutes prior to intubation (time zero), and again 10 minutes later. The topical group received 815 ± 208 mg of lidocaine whereas the nerve block group received 349 ± 44 mg. Mean plasma lidocaine levels at time zero were 2.16 ± 1.48 μg·mL^{-1} in the topical group, and 4.23 ± 1.12 μg·mL^{-1} in the nerve block group. Ten minutes later, the levels were 3.34 ± 1.87 μg·mL^{-1} and 4.02 ± 1.02 μg·mL^{-1}, respectively. No plasma sampling was performed after the 10-minute recording. The quality of anesthesia achieved was similar with both the techniques, and intubation was achieved in 3.2 minutes on average. No complications were identified.[90]

- Langmack et al administered topical lidocaine to 51 asthmatic volunteers who underwent research bronchoscopy.[91] Atomized 4% lidocaine was sprayed into the nose and throat, 2 mL of vicous lidocaine was applied to the nose, and 1% lidocaine was administered to the tracheobronchial tree via the bronchoscope.

The 2% viscous was excluded from the total dose calculation and the authors considered absorption of intranasal lidocaine to be less than 50%. The mean *calculated* total dose administered was 8.2 ± 2.0 mg·kg^{-1} (range 4.3-14.3 mg·kg^{-1}). The venous serum lidocaine concentration was measured at 30 minutes after topical anesthesia was completed (T1) and 30 minutes after the bronchoscopy was completed (T2). The serum lidocaine concentration ranged between 0.1 and 2.90 ug·mL^{-1} at T1 and between 0.5 and 3.2 ug·mL^{-1} at T2. The serum lidocaine concentration correlated with the total dose administered, although considerable individual variability among subjects who received the same dose was noted. No signs or symptoms of lidocaine toxicity were detected.[91]

- Williams et al measured serum concentrations of lidocaine in 25 participants in a bronchoscopy training course.[54] Five milliliters of 4% lidocaine was administered by nebulizer, 2 mL of 5% lidocaine with 0.5% phenylephrine was sprayed into the nose and 4 mL of 10% lidocaine was sprayed into the oropharynx. Four percent lidocaine was also administered via the endoscope. *Seventy five percent of the nebulizer dose was excluded from the total dose calculation.* The average *calculated* dose administered was 8.8 mg·kg^{-1} (range 7.3-9.2 mg·kg^{-1}). Serum lidocaine concentrations were measured before topicalization (T0), 20 minutes after topicalization (T20), and then at 10 minutes intervals until 60 minutes after the last dose of lidocaine. The duration of sampling ranged from 100-120 minutes. The highest recorded lidocaine concentration was 4.5 ug·mL^{-1} and only two subjects experienced peak levels above 3 ug·mL^{-1}. In 8 of the 25 subjects, the highest lidocaine concentration was observed in the final sample, 60 minutes after the last dose of lidocaine was administered. Multiple symptoms of lidocaine toxicity were reported by the subjects including lightheadedness, dysphoria, nausea, and shivering.[54]

- Berger et al performed transnasal fiberoptic bronchoscopy on 21 normal volunteers and 18 patients under topical lidocaine anesthesia administered using a combination of gargle, atomization (spraying), nebulization, gel, and in the 18 patients, endobronchial instillation.[92] The total mean dose of lidocaine administered to the 18 patients was 2086 mg and to the volunteers 1534 mg. Plasma lidocaine levels were measured in eight patients and six volunteers after gargling, after spraying, after nebulization, and then at 5, 10, 15, 30, and 60 minutes. The mean peak level in the patients was about 3.1 ug·mL^{-1} and in the volunteers about 1.0 ug·mL^{-1} as measured from the published graphs. In the patient group the peak concentration occurred at 30 minutes. In the volunteers, the peak occurred after nebulization and this level was sustained until the 30-minute sample.[92]

- Ameer et al administered topical lidocaine for bronchoscopy to 19 adults using a combination of lidocaine gargle, atomized lidocaine, lidocaine jelly, and lidocaine solution injected through the bronchoscope. The time over which lidocaine was administered was 0.79 ± 0.31 hours in 5 young patients and 0.69 ± 0.22 hours in 14 elderly subjects. The total dosage administered was 19.01 ± 1.67 mg·kg^{-1} in the young adults, and 17.15 ± 2.28 mg·kg^{-1} in the elderly. The mean maximum plasma concentrations achieved were 3.04 ± 1.27 ug·mL^{-1} in the young and 2.40 ± 0.92 μg·mL^{-1} in the elderly. The times required to reach peak levels were 0.77 ± 0.28 hours in the young and 1.21 ± 0.55 hours in the elderly. No serious drug toxicity occurred.[93]

Reference has also been made to peak blood levels not occurring until 90 minutes after completion of bronchoscopy[94] and occurring 30 to 90 minutes from the start of airway local anesthesia.[53]

Toxicity associated with lidocaine topically applied to the airway can however occur.

- Martin et al administered 7.14 to 14.77 mg·kg^{-1} of topical lidocaine (median dose 9.6 mg·kg^{-1}) to 39 volunteers participating in a bronchoscopy training study.[95] The airway topicalization included 2% viscous lidocaine gargle, 10% spray, and 2% lidocaine administered through the bronchoscope. Thirty-six of the 39 subjects reported side effects associated with lidocaine topicalization including drowsiness, disorientation, hyperacusis, disinhibition, lightheadedness, visual disturbance, and dysphoria. Tremulousness was clinically evident in three subjects who received 9.7, 10.2, and 13.4 mg·kg^{-1}, respectively, two of whom had a single involuntary limb movement. No serum lidocaine concentrations were measured. No major adverse events occurred.[95]

- Wu et al reported a grand mal seizure which occurred following the topical application of 300 to 320 mg of lidocaine applied as a 4% spray to the larynx and 10 to 12 mL of 1% viscous lidocaine to the oropharynx and trachea of a 30-year-old, 48-kg woman with renal failure, congestive heart failure, cardiomyopathy, and abnormal liver function tests. The plasma lidocaine level shortly after the seizure was 12 µg·mL^{-1}. They also reviewed seven cases of seizure after the administration of topical lidocaine to mucous membranes of the airway. In each of these seven cases, the topical lidocaine was administered as 2% viscous or 2% to 4% solution.[47]

- Kotaki et al in 1996 reported a seizure following the application of up to 800 mg of lidocaine as a 2% viscous preparation and 4% solution to the oropharynx. The serum lidocaine concentrations were found to be 11.6 µg·mL^{-1} and 9.0 µg·mL^{-1} after 30 and 150 minutes postseizure, respectively. The authors reviewed three cases of seizure in addition to those reviewed by Wu et al associated with topical application of lidocaine to the mucous membranes of the oral cavity and pharynx. In each of these three cases, the lidocaine had been administered as a 4% solution or 2% viscous preparation.[56]

- In 1996 a healthy 19-year-old female volunteer died as a result of lidocaine toxicity following a bronchoscopy performed as part of a research project.[94] The amount of lidocaine administered was not documented in the record of the procedure. Details of the technique of administration, as determined from the references reviewed, were limited to *as a spray into the throat*, and that 4% lidocaine was administered in the upper airway and 2% in the lower airway. No reference to the use of atomized or nebulized lidocaine or documentation of the subject's body weight was found in the references reviewed.[94,96] The subject was left alone after release from the Medical Center and then found apparently having a seizure about an hour later. Emergency 911 was called and mouth-to-mouth breathing was initiated for apparent apnea. On arrival in the emergency department the subject was in cardiac arrest. The blood lidocaine level measured about 3 hours after the research procedure was 12.9 ug·mL^{-1}. Based on this blood level of lidocaine it was reported that it was "likely that she had received in excess of 1200 mg of lidocaine." The Medical Examiner's Office found no evidence of any impairment in the subject's ability to metabolize or detoxify lidocaine.[94]

- In 2001 the British Thoracic Society recommended that the dose of lidocaine used for bronchoscopy be limited to 8.2 mg·kg^{-1} and that extra care be used in the elderly or those with liver or cardiac impairment.[97] This maximum dosage recommendation appears to apply to all techniques, and the method of topicalization does not seem to have been taken into consideration. The Thoracic Society of Australia and New Zealand, also in 2001, recommended that the total dose of lidocaine used for bronchoscopy not exceed 4 to 5 mg·kg^{-1}.[98]

In summary, the maximum safe dose of lidocaine that can be topically applied to the mucous membrane of the airway is difficult to determine and must take into account the method of topicalization employed as well as the time course of administration. Traditional dosage guidelines may be excessively conservative when some or the entire dose is administered by aerosol, based on the available evidence with respect to serum levels and toxicity occurrences. Caution must be exercised however and a precalculated dose should not be exceeded. In clinical practice, the smallest amount of anesthetic sufficient to achieve the desired effect should be used,[92] and in general, for awake bronchoscopic intubation, the use of large doses is unnecessary. As always, clinical judgment is required and meticulous attention to detail should be employed when lidocaine is applied to the airway such that effective anesthesia is achieved without producing toxicity.

3.3.2.1   Can Topical Lidocaine Anesthesia of the Upper Airway Cause Airway Obstruction?

Several studies have looked at this issue:

- In a study of seven normal subjects, Gal administered 4% lidocaine by ultrasonic aerosol and measured airway responses. After the inhalation of lidocaine, the subjects noted an impaired ability to swallow, and a husky voice suggesting vocal cord paresis. Three of the seven subjects described a sensation of obstruction during deep inspiration, although this was not reflected by significant changes in peak inspiratory flow as recorded in maximum effort flow volume loops. Peak expiratory flow rates were also unchanged. Interestingly, statistically significant *increases* in maximum inspiratory flow were observed at 60%, 50%, and 40% of forced vital capacity (FVC) following the lidocaine aerosol. The author concluded that the administration of 4% lidocaine by ultrasonic nebulization produced mild bronchodilation and did not adversely affect airway function in normal subjects.[99]

- Gove et al administered 10 mL of 4% lidocaine by means of an ultrasonic nebulizer attached to a mouthpiece to 33 patients prior to bronchoscopy. Five of the 33 patients required additional boluses of lidocaine to the bronchial tree during the procedure. Spirometry was recorded in 32 patients. A wide variation in individual response to the nebulized lidocaine was observed. Forced expiratory volume in 1 second (FEV1) varied between −18% and +45%, FVC between −27% and +18%, and peak expiratory flow rate (PEFR) between −41% and +34%. However, no overall effect on airflow was demonstrated. The bronchoconstriction that did occur was not clinically significant and bronchodilator therapy was not required.[100]

- Kuna et al performed pulmonary function tests (PFTs) on 11 normal subjects before and after topical anesthesia of the airway. The topical anesthesia was achieved using 4% lidocaine spray to the soft palate and posterior oropharynx, an internal approach superior laryngeal nerve block using cotton pledgets soaked in 4% lidocaine, and 1.5 mL of 10% cocaine applied by means of a cannula to the epiglottis and vocal cords by direct laryngoscopy. The PFTs consisted of flow volume loops, body box determinations of functional residual capacity (FRC), and airway resistance. The area under the inspiratory curve, peak inspiratory flow (PIF), and forced inspiratory flow (FIF) at 25%, 50%, and 75% of FRC were decreased after airway anesthesia, as was peak expiratory flow. However, the area under the expiratory curve and forced expiratory flow at 25%, 50%, and 75% FVC were unchanged. The authors noted that the configuration of the flow volume envelope following topical anesthesia in most subjects demonstrated a plateau or sudden reversible reduction in airflow on inspiration but a relative preservation of gas flow on expiration, and concluded that laryngeal anesthesia can compromise upper airway patency.[101]

- Listro et al measured specific airway conductance and maximum inspiratory and expiratory flow rates before and 15, 35, and 45 minutes after topical anesthesia of the upper airway. Anesthesia was achieved using four 10% lidocaine sprays to the oropharynx and hypopharynx, and 2 mL of 4% lidocaine solution instilled twice onto the vocal cords using a laryngeal syringe. Average values of maximum inspiratory flow rate (MIFR) decreased 15 minutes after upper airway anesthesia, but returned to control levels or nearly so at 45 minutes. Transient decreases in flow rates reaching zero flow on some occasions were observed in 13 of 16 subjects during forced inspiratory vital capacity (FIVC) and in 7 of 16 during forced expiratory vital capacity (FEVC) maneuvers. The site of obstruction to air flow was determined in 13 patients using simultaneous measurements of supraglottic pressure, flow rates, and lung volume. In 12 of these 13 patients, the site of obstruction was localized to the glottis, and in one, both supraglottic and glottic obstruction occurred. However, upper airway anesthesia in the absence of maximum forced respiratory maneuvers did not result in a decrease in flow rates. The authors concluded that topical anesthesia of the upper airway induces a glottic obstruction that produces a profound but transient decrease in maximum inspiratory and expiratory gas flow consistent with reflex regulation of upper airway caliber.[102]

- Beydon et al measured airway flow resistance in nine healthy volunteers using a random noise forced oscillation technique before and after the application of topical anesthesia to the upper airway.[103] On two separate occasions, either 100 mg of 5% lidocaine liquid was sprayed into one nostril and onto the mucosa of the pharynx and larynx and then gargled, or 100 mg of lidocaine paste was gargled. Airway flow resistance increased in all but one subject. On average the increase was 81% after lidocaine spray and 68% after lidocaine paste. The increased resistance lasted for 13 ± 3 minutes in the spray group and 12 ± 3 minutes in the paste group. At a separate session no change in resistance was detected 3 minutes after spraying normal saline into the upper airway. The two volunteers who experienced the greatest increase in airway flow resistance subsequently underwent transnasal fiberlaryngoscopy under aqueous topical lidocaine anesthesia. Dramatic changes were observed at the larynx. The vocal cords appeared slack and remained in a semi-closed position. During quiet inspiration, the vocal cords moved medially, producing incomplete obstruction at the glottis. During maximal inspiratory efforts the epiglottis moved toward the vocal cords to produce complete airway obstruction similar to that which occurs during swallowing. The authors concluded that topical lidocaine produces an increase in airway resistance in most normal subjects and that the larynx and epiglottis appeared to be main site of obstruction.[103]

- Weiss and Patwardhan administered lidocaine aerosols to 22 patients with stable asthma and demonstrated an initial decrease of expiratory gas flow of approximately 20% within 5 minutes of aerosol administration. Following this initial response, 12 of 22 patients continued to demonstrate a reduction in measured expiratory gas flow that persisted up to 60 minutes, whereas the remaining 10 patients revealed a significant improvement in expiratory gas flow above baseline.[104]

- McAlpine and Thomson similarly measured FEV1 in 20 asthmatic patients following the administration of 6 mL of 4% nebulized lidocaine. The maximum percentage change in FEV1 following lidocaine inhalation varied from −42.1% to +28.2%, with a mean of −8.2%. Five of the 20 patients experienced a decrease in FEV1 greater than 15%.[105]

- Groben et al measured changes in FEV1 in 10 volunteers with mild asthma after topical airway anesthesia with either lidocaine or dyclonine and awake bronchoscopic intubation. The local anesthetic was initially administered by nebulizer and supplemented with a gargle and administration of the anesthetic solution onto the epiglottis via the bronchoscope. Following baseline measurements, FEV1 was measured after saline or salbutamol inhalation, local anesthetic inhalation, intubation, and extubation. No significant difference was found in FEV1 following lidocaine or dyclonine inhalation. Salbutamol inhalation significantly increased FEV1. Following awake bronchoscopic intubation under lidocaine anesthesia, FEV1 decreased 35% and 51% after dyclonine. This decrease in FEV1 was significantly attenuated by salbutamol pretreatment in both groups. Two to five minutes after extubation, FEV1 returned to values close to those obtained following saline or salbutamol administration. No significant difference was found between FEV1 values after extubation as compared to the respective FEV1 baseline.[106]

- In 2006 Ho et al reported a prospective observational study of the effect of upper airway topical anesthesia on dynamic airflow.[107] Six healthy volunteers, all authors of the study, underwent a series of spirometric measurements before and after topical anesthesia of the upper airway produced by topical lidocaine using an aspiration technique (see Section 3.4.4). Peak inspiratory flow rate (PIFR), forced inspiratory flow (FIF) between 25% and 75% of maximum inhaled volume, FEV1, and FVC were measured before the administration of lidocaine, immediately afterward, and at 10, 20, and 30 minutes afterward. A significant reduction in PIFR and FIF_{25-75} was demonstrated at all time points following the administration of lidocaine. Expiratory flow parameters were not affected. The authors concluded that maximum inspiratory flow is impeded by topical anesthesia of the upper airway and they suggested that caution be exercised in the setting of preexisting airway obstruction.[107]

- Thomson also reported a fall in specific conductance of the airway following bupivacaine aerosol administration to asthmatics.[108]

Case reports of airway obstruction following topical anesthesia and instrumentation of the airway have also been published:

- Shaw et al reported a case of respiratory distress following the administration of 10% lidocaine spray to the tongue and oropharynx in the presence of a compromised airway associated with goiter.[109] Air entry could not be maintained despite repositioning the patient onto her left side, jaw thrust, chin lift, and placement of an oral airway. The authors felt that a combination of laryngospasm due to irritation caused by the lidocaine spray, and loss of muscle tone as a result of the local anesthetic action, contributed to the airway obstruction.[109]

- McGuire and El-Beheiry reported complete airway obstruction during attempted awake bronchoscopic intubation under local anesthesia in two patients with unstable cervical spine fractures. Both required surgical airways. Both patients also received sedative agents. One patient developed stridor then complete airway obstruction following introduction of the endoscope after topicalization using 1% lidocaine spray and cricothyroid puncture. The second patient was topicalized using swabs soaked in 4% lidocaine. Insertion of the endoscope was associated with gagging and coughing followed by complete airway obstruction.[110]

- Ho et al reported a case of complete airway obstruction which occurred following the topical administration of 2% lidocaine onto the tongue and pharynx and suctioning in a patient with recurrent neck carcinoma following radiotherapy, who had hoarseness and stridor preoperatively.[111]

Extensive clinical experience with lidocaine has shown it to be an effective topical agent for airway anesthesia and to have a wide margin of safety.[78,87] However, in the presence of preexisting airway compromise, topical anesthesia and instrumentation of the airway can be associated with complete airway obstruction and in this setting, due consideration must be given to the performance of an awake tracheotomy under local anesthesia.[111-113]

3.3.3 Tetracaine

Tetracaine (pontocaine), a long-acting amino ester derivative of para-aminobenzoic acid was introduced in 1932, and is still used extensively for spinal anesthesia and topical anesthesia of the eye.[31,45] Although once widely used for topical anesthesia of the airway,[114] its use for this indication fell into disfavor after reports of toxic reactions including fatalities were published in the 1950s.[52,114] Of the local anesthetics possessing topical action, dibucaine and tetracaine are the most potent as well as the most toxic.[52] The maximal effective concentration of topical tetracaine is 1%. This concentration has a latent period of 0.6 to 1.1 minutes and a duration of 50.2 to 55.5 minutes.[39] When applied to the tongue, 0.5% tetracaine has a latent period of 1.6 minutes and a duration of action of 18.1 minutes.[39] The latent period for 0.4% tetracaine is 3.8 minutes and the duration of action is 35.8 minutes; for 2% tetracaine, these are 1.1 and 48.6 minutes, respectively.[39] The duration of action on the conjunctiva is approximately twice than that at the tip of the tongue, whereas the duration of action on the lip and palate is intermediate. Tetracaine appears to be superior to other topical anesthetics and this may be due to its ability to anesthetize structures deep to the mucous membrane.[52,115]

Tetracaine applied to the mucous membranes of the pharynx and trachea is rapidly absorbed into the circulation such that blood levels are almost comparable to those obtained after IV injection.[115,116] Epinephrine added to the tetracaine does not retard its absorption.[115] In 1951, Weisel and Tella reported a series of 1000 bronchoscopies performed with topical tetracaine.[114] There were 12 minor and 7 severe toxic reactions, including 6 seizures and 1 severe bronchospasm. Loss of consciousness preceded convulsions in two of the cases. Cotton pledgets were dipped into a solution of 2% tetracaine and placed successively between the faucial pillars and in each piriform fossa for about 1 minute at each location. Then 1 mL of 2% tetracaine was injected into the trachea using a syringe and a laryngeal cannula.[114] The dose administered was estimated to be ≤40 mg in most cases, although measurement was inexact. The toxic reaction occurred following application of the fourth pledget in two patients, and tracheal instillation in five patients, and was heralded by syncope or presyncope.[114] Adriani and Campbell noted 10 fatalities at their institution over a 15-year period caused by topical tetracaine.[52] The maximum safe dosage of tetracaine has never been clearly defined.[115] However, maximum safe doses cited in the literature are said to be 50 mg,[31] 80 mg,[24] or 100 mg[117,118] in the adults. A maximum dose of 20 mg of tetracaine hydrochloride has also been recommended.[119] Again, when maximum safe doses are considered, the method of administration must also be taken into account. In a 1995 review, topical tetracaine was said to be no longer recommended for topical airway anesthesia because of its narrow margin of safety.[68] Tetracaine (0.45%) administered by atomizer produces excellent intubating conditions; however, the potential for toxicity must be appreciated. Allergic reaction, although rare, is more likely with the ester group of local anesthetics as compared to the amides. As of 2007, a single case of methemoglobinemia had been reported associated with tetracaine.[64] In general, metabolism of local anesthetics with an ester linkage occurs by hydrolysis in plasma and requires plasma cholinesterase. The presence of an atypical pseudocholinesterase is associated with decreased metabolism.[34]

3.3.4   Does cocaine have a role in providing topical airway anesthesia in current anesthesia practice?

Cocaine, an ester of benzoic acid and a nitrogen base, was first isolated in 1860 and serendipitously discovered to have anesthetic properties.[31,45] It is the only local anesthetic that inhibits reuptake of norepinephrine and thereby produces vasoconstriction, hence its continued popularity for nasal procedures.[37,38,120] The maximum effective concentration of topical cocaine is 20%, and this solution produces an anesthetic effect within 0.3 minutes and has a duration of action of 54.5 minutes.[39] Topical anesthesia produced with 10% cocaine has a latent period of 2 minutes and a duration of action of 31.5 minutes, whereas 4% cocaine has a latent period of 4 minutes and a duration of action of 10.2 minutes.[39] The same degree of blockade is produced with 20% cocaine as with 1% tetracaine.[39] Typically 1% to 10% cocaine is used clinically.[31,69] The vasoconstriction produced by cocaine occurs after a latent period of 5 to 10 minutes.[66] The maximum recommended dose for topical nasal application has been said to be from 1.5 $mg \cdot kg^{-1}$,[121] to 3.0 $mg \cdot kg^{-1}$,[41] and 1-3 $mg \cdot kg^{-1}$;[122] however, toxic reactions have occurred after nasal administration of as little as 20 to 30 mg.[122,123] The use of cocaine has been associated with coronary artery vasoconstriction, increased myocardial demand,[68] and hypertension.[121] Doses as small as 0.4 $mg \cdot kg^{-1}$ may cause ventricular fibrillation,[121] and fatalities have been reported.[45] Cocaine should be avoided or used cautiously in the presence of hypertension, hyperthyroidism, angina, or in patients taking monoaminoxidase inhibitors (MAOIs).[41] Blood levels of cocaine after topical application to the piriform fossae were similar to levels produced after IV injection.[45,116] Oxymetazoline has been shown to be as effective as cocaine in the prevention of epistaxis caused by nasotracheal intubation[124,125] as has normal saline,[125] phenylephrine/lidocaine,[12,123] and phenylephrine alone.[123]

From the available evidence, the disadvantages associated with the use of cocaine to produce nasal anesthesia for awake intubation appear to outweigh the advantages.

3.3.5   How safe and effective is benzocaine?

Benzocaine, an ethyl ester of para-aminobenzoic acid,[126] is a water-soluble ester type local anesthetic that is widely used for topicalization of the airway.[118] It is available as a 20% spray which can deliver between 60 mg[117] and 200 to 295 mg per 1 second spray.[126] Benzocaine is also a component of cetacaine which consists of 14% benzocaine, 2% tetracaine, and 2% butyl aminobenzoate (butamben).[127] The maximum effective concentration of topical benzocaine is 20%, has a latent period of 0.17 minutes, and a duration of action of 4.3 minutes.[39] An onset time of 15 to 30 seconds and a duration of action of 5 to 10 minutes have also been cited.[68] The maximum dose recommended for upper airway anesthesia has been quoted to be 1.5 $mg \cdot kg^{-1}$,[41] although a dose of 100 mg in the adult has also been cited to be toxic.[118] Benzocaine

can produce methemoglobinemia following the administration of as little as 150 to 300 mg in the adult.[128] In a 2007 literature review, 159 episodes of methemoglobinemia associated with the use of benzocaine were identified.[64] Of these, benzocaine had been used alone in 105 episodes. Additional cases have occurred since that time.[129,130] A letter of warning has been issued by the Federal Drug Administration (FDA) in the USA. Methemoglobinemia is potentially fatal[127,131] and treatment with a 1% solution of methylene blue 1 to 2 $mg \cdot kg^{-1}$ is recommended for methemoglobin levels greater than or equal to 30% or at lower levels if symptoms of hypoxia are present.[132] Normal levels of methemoglobin should be achieved within 20 minutes to 1 hour.[133] However, repeat doses of methylene blue may be necessary.[133] The maximum total dose recommended is 4 $mg \cdot kg^{-1}$ to 7 $mg \cdot kg^{-1}$.[133,134] Rebound methemoglobinemia has been reported 2.5 to 20 hours after methylene blue administration.[64,135] In a 2009 review of methhemoglobinemia related to local anesthetics, it was recommended that benzocaine should no longer be used.[64] Benzocaine is metabolized by plasma cholinesterase[126] to para-aminobenzoic acid, a highly allergenic molecule[68] and allergic reactions to benzocaine can occur. Given its short duration of action, and its potential for toxicity, the use of benzocaine as a topical anesthetic for airway management seems difficult to justify.

3.3.6   Cetacaine

Cetacaine is a topical anesthetic spray that contains benzocaine 14%, butamben 2%, and tetracaine hydrochloride 2%. According to the manufacturer, the onset time of local anesthesia is 30 to 60 seconds and the duration is typically 30 to 60 minutes. (Cetylite Industries, Inc. Cetacaine Spray product sheet. Cited 2009 Dec 15. Available from: http://www.cetylite.com/cetacaine_spray.html). The manufacturer recommends that cetacaine be applied for approximately 1 second or less for normal anesthesia. A spray in excess of 2 seconds is considered to be contraindicated. The manufacturer states that "dosages should be reduced in the debilitated elderly, acutely ill, and very young patients." The average expulsion rate from the spray is 200 $mg \cdot s^{-1}$ at normal temperatures. Each 200 mg of cetacaine contains 28 mg of benzocaine, 4 mg of butamben, and 4 mg of tetracaine. Hypersensitivity reactions can occur and there have been multiple case reports of methemoglobinemia associated with the use of cetacaine.[131,133,136-142]

3.3.7   Dyclonine hydrochloride

Dyclonine, a ketone, is a unique local anesthetic agent that was introduced in 1952 and is structurally distinct from the aminoesters and aminoamides.[143] It can be used as a 0.5% to 1% solution for topical anesthesia.[31,143] When applied to mucous membranes, the onset time is 2 to 10 minutes and the duration of action is 20 to 30 minutes. Adriani et al noted that dyclonine had limited systemic toxicity but a saturated solution may cause residual numbness that persists for many hours suggesting local injury.[39] One percent dyclonine administered by aerosol has been shown to produce topical airway anesthesia as effective as, and longer lasting than, 4% lidocaine.[106] In a study of 10 volunteers with mild asthma, 4 of the 10 subjects reported much more intense topical anesthesia following 1% dyclonine inhalation as compared to 4% lidocaine.[106] However, FEV1 decreased to a greater extent in the dyclonine group and the authors concluded that dyclonine must be considered relatively contraindicated in the setting of bronchial hyperreactivity.

Bacon et al reported the use of dyclonine for awake bronchoscopic intubation in a patient with apparent allergy to local anesthetics.[143] The patient gargled and then swallowed 25 mL of 1% dyclonine solution, and 5 mL of 1% dyclonine was then administered by nebulizer. Adequate anesthesia was achieved.[143] Dyclonine has not been widely used, however, for airway anesthesia and is no longer marketed for this purpose in the USA or Canada.

3.4   AIRWAY ANESTHESIA TECHNIQUES

3.4.1   What techniques are available for upper airway anesthesia?

Regional anesthesia of the airway can be achieved using a wide variety of techniques. Each technique requires a meticulous approach, attention to detail, and knowledge of relevant anatomy as well as the pharmacology of the agents employed if an adequate block is to be achieved. The most important prerequisite for a successful awake intubation is adequate regional anesthesia of the airway.

3.4.2   Spray/ointment/gel/EMLA

The posterior third of the tongue, the soft palate, the tonsillar pillars, and the adjacent pharynx can be sequentially anesthetized using commercially available 10% lidocaine spray,[37,38,120] simply by directing the spray onto the relevant structures. A tongue depressor can be used to gently retract the tongue. The commercially available 10% lidocaine aerosol is fitted with a metered valve that delivers 10 mg of lidocaine as an aerosol with each depression of the pump mechanism.[51] This simple pump mechanism uses manually compressed air as the driving force. Adequate regional anesthesia for awake intubation by direct laryngoscopy can readily be achieved in this manner, and in the emergency setting, time may not permit additional regional techniques. The 10% lidocaine aerosol is marketed in Canada by Odan Laboratories Limited but is not currently available in the USA (see Figure 3-25). Alternatively, 4% lidocaine administered using a mucosal atomization device can be used (Wolf Tory Medical Incorporated, Salt Lake City, Utah). A curved metal cannula can also be used to inject lidocaine solution into the laryngopharynx and larynx as time and circumstances permit; however, this is not necessary for awake intubation by direct laryngoscopy, and blood levels of lidocaine produced with this technique will probably be higher than those produced by aerosol techniques.[48] Cooperative patients can also gargle 2% to 4% lidocaine in order to achieve topical anesthesia of the posterior tongue and adjacent oropharynx. Residual anesthetic should be expectorated to avoid excessive drug exposure and potential nausea and vomiting.[38,120,144] Lidocaine ointment (5%) can be very useful to anesthetize the posterior third of the tongue especially when patients are unable to gargle. Lidocaine gel

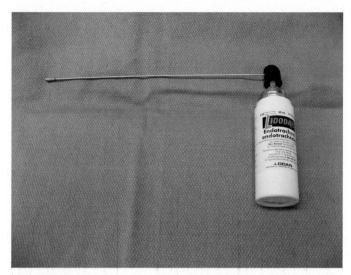

FIGURE 3-25. Lidocaine aerosol fitted with a malleable stainless steel nozzle. (Available from Odon Laboratories, Montreal, Canada).

2% can also be used. With any of these techniques, time (at least 1 minute[24] to 2 minutes[39] and perhaps as long as 5 minutes[31]) must be allowed for the anesthetic effect to occur.

EMLA cream, a 1:1 eutectic mixture of 2.5% lidocaine and 2.5% prilocaine, has also been used to produce airway anesthesia. Larijani et al applied up to 4 g of EMLA cream to the tongue and pharynx in a series of 20 patients who underwent awake bronchoscopic intubation.[145] The intubation was performed via a Williams airway. The mean time from the application of the EMLA cream to placement of the oral airway was 11 ± 6 minutes. All patients were successfully intubated but all coughed when the scope was passed into the trachea. No toxic plasma levels of lidocaine or prilocaine occurred. A statistically significant increase in methemoglobin levels occurred within 6 hours; however, these levels did not exceed normal values (1.5%).[145] Sohmer et al used 4 mL of EMLA cream applied to the tongue and gargled before performing awake bronchoscopy in 57 patients.[146] In addition, 79.05 ± 14.39 mg of lidocaine was administered through the flexible bronchoscope (FB) for laryngeal anesthesia. Fifty-six of the cases did not require supplemental anesthesia. Bronchoscopic conditions were excellent in 55 cases and good in the remaining 2 cases.[146] The mean time from EMLA application to insertion of the bronchoscope was 5.10 ± 0.45 minutes. EMLA cream applied to the nostril prior to the passage of a flexible bronchoscope provoked rhinorrhea and sneezing that persisted for several hours in 21 of 31 individuals, although the endoscopy was well tolerated.[147] EMLA cream may be an alternative for oropharyngeal topical anesthesia, although experience is limited.

3.4.3   Aerosols

Excellent anesthesia of the airway can be produced by the administration of aerosolized local anesthetic delivered by an atomizer, such as the DeVilbiss RD 15 (see Figure 3-26). The device consists of a glass reservoir, which holds the anesthetic solution, and a nozzle assembly, which can be connected to a high-pressure oxygen source by means of standard oxygen tubing. A small bleed hole

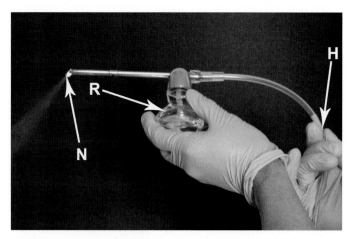

FIGURE 3-26. DeVilbiss atomizer. The device consists of a glass reservoir (R), which holds the anesthetic solution, and a nozzle assembly, which can be connected to standard oxygen tubing. A small bleed hole (H) is cut in the oxygen tubing. When oxygen flow is delivered into the tubing at about 6.0 to 8.0 L·min^{-1}, occlusion of the bleed hole with a finger produces a fine spray of local anesthetic from the atomizer nozzle (N).

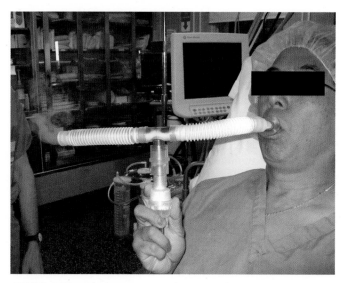

FIGURE 3-27. Nebulizer connected to a mouthpiece and airway intubator.

is cut in the oxygen tubing at a convenient location near its connection to the atomizer. When oxygen flow is delivered into the tubing at about 6 to 8 L·min^{-1}, occlusion of the bleed hole with a fingertip produces a fine spray of local anesthetic from the atomizer nozzle. When held at the nostril, and coordinated with deep breaths on command ("in through the nose and out through the mouth"), the device can produce profound anesthesia of the airway from the nose to the trachea and beyond in about 5 minutes.[38,120] The atomized local anesthetic can also be administered through the mouth, although superior gas flow characteristics through the nose may deliver the anesthetic more efficiently to the pharynx, larynx, and trachea.[38,120] Obstruction of the nasal cavity of course precludes nasal administration. At the author's institution, the DeVilbiss atomizer has been used routinely for awake intubation for more than two decades with excellent results and no toxic reactions. An excellent block can be achieved with 10 to 12 mL of 3% or 4 % lidocaine. Others have recommended up to 20 mL of 0.5% tetracaine or 10 mL of 4% lidocaine with this technique.[118]

In the study by Wieczorek et al in which either 2% or 4% lidocaine was administered by atomizer to a group of obese patients, the authors concluded that atomized lidocaine for awake intubation was efficacious, rapid, and safe.[84] A subsequent study from the same center compared 2% and 1% lidocaine using the same atomization technique and volume of anesthetic.[85] The authors concluded that 1% lidocaine provided measurably inferior airway anesthesia.

Atomization can also be used as a part of a combined technique of airway anesthesia.

Aerosolized local anesthetic can also be administered through the mouth using a standard nebulizer attached to a mouthpiece.[148] An oral airway intubation device can be attached to the nebulizer and advanced into the oropharynx as tolerated to deliver the anesthetic to the more distal airway (see Figure 3-27).[148] The authors of the noted report used 4 mL of 4% lidocaine at 8 L·min^{-1} oxygen flow with this technique and the nebulization required

8 minutes.[148] Additionally, 4 mL of 2% lidocaine was administered through the FB during intubation.[148]

Kirkpatrick et al reported that the gag reflex was abolished for a mean time of 32±5.9 minutes in 10 healthy volunteers following the administration of 10 mL of 4% lidocaine using a DeVilbiss 646 nebulizer and mouthpiece. No bronchoscopy or intubation was performed.[83]

Nebulized local anesthetic has also been administered by facemask using 4 to 20 mL of 4% lidocaine[58,72,74,90] or 6 mg·kg^{-1} of 10% lidocaine.[44] Nebulization by this technique required 10 to 22 minutes.[48,58,72,74,90] In a study reported by Kundra et al, 7 of 24 patients required supplemental lidocaine through the fiberoptic bronchoscope after nebulization of 4 mL of 4% lidocaine and administration by mask.[72] This study compared nebulization with a combined regional block (CRB) technique consisting of nasal lidocaine-soaked swabs, superior laryngeal nerve block, and transtracheal injection of lidocaine for awake nasotracheal bronchoscopic intubation. The authors reported that the patients in the CRB group were more comfortable during the procedure. Four of five other reports of awake intubation or bronchoscopy using nebulization by mask also used supplemental anesthesia.[58,74,90,149,150]

Chinn et al reported that only one of five healthy subjects lost the gag reflex following administration of 10 mL of 4% lidocaine by means of a DeVilbiss 35B nebulizer and Hudson oxygen mask.[73] No bronchoscopy or intubation was performed.

Nebulization has also been used by others as part of a combined technique of airway anesthesia.[13,54,88,92,95,151]

3.4.4   Local anesthetic aspiration

Local anesthesia of the airway can also be achieved using an aspiration technique.[152] In this technique, lidocaine solution is simply dripped onto the dorsum of the tongue of a supine patient during tongue traction.[152] The swallowing reflex is initially stimulated, but lidocaine subsequently pools in the posterior pharynx and is aspirated into the trachea.[152] Gargling with two consecutive 5-mL aliquots of 2% lidocaine can decrease the intensity of this swallowing reflex.[152] Chung et al instilled the lesser of 0.2 mL·kg⁻¹ or 20 mL of 1.5% lidocaine following the gargle as described above and reported satisfactory bronchoscopic intubating conditions in 39 patients, although mild coughing or gagging did occur with the scope in the trachea in 10 patients, and with the tube in the trachea in another 21 patients. Supplemental local anesthesia was not required. Eighteen patients were intubated orally, using a Williams airway intubator, whereas 21 were intubated nasally. Gauze packing soaked in 1.5 mL of 5% lidocaine was used for nasal anesthesia. The time required for intubation varied from 1 to 10 minutes (median time 3.25 minutes).[152] By comparison, intubation after a DeVilbiss technique can usually be accomplished in about 30 seconds.

3.4.5 Nasal anesthesia

Local anesthesia of the nasal cavity can be achieved by a variety of methods. Nebulized lidocaine can be administered by facemask and the patient instructed to breathe through the nose.[72,74] Lidocaine or tetracaine administered with a DeVilbiss atomizer can also be very effective in achieving topical anesthesia of the nasal cavity. Alternatively, long cotton-tipped applicators or pledgets, held in bayonet forceps and soaked in 4% lidocaine or 4% cocaine, can be introduced into the selected nostril.[118] One applicator can be inserted parallel to the anterior border of the nasal cavity along the septum until it reaches the anterior end of the cribriform plate at a depth of about 5 cm (see Figure 3-28).[153] The local anesthetic-soaked applicator can then be left in place for 5 to 15 minutes to produce a transmucosal block of the anterior ethmoidal nerve.[118,153] A second applicator can be inserted at an angle of about 20 to 45 degrees to the floor of the nose until bony resistance is felt at a depth of about 6 to 7 cm.[153] In this location, the tip of the applicator is adjacent to the sphenopalatine ganglion located deep to the nasal mucosa and similarly can be left in contact with the mucosa for 5 to 15 minutes to produce a transmucosal block of the sphenopalatine nerves.[118,153] Nasal anesthesia has also been produced using sprays from a multiorificed cannula,[123] a 20-gauge angiocatheter,[118] an epidural catheter,[154] 10% lidocaine aerosol, and lidocaine gel.

A vasoconstrictor is frequently applied topically to the nasal mucosa in an effort to prevent the epistaxis that can occur with nasotracheal intubation.[124] In a prospective, randomized, double-blind study of 36 patients, Rector et al found no difference in the incidence of epistaxis associated with nasotracheal intubation following nasal spraying with 0.05% oxymetazoline, 10% cocaine, or normal saline.[125] Similarly, Gross et al found no significant difference among groups pretreated with 4% cocaine, 3% lidocaine with 0.25% phenylephrine, or 0.25% phenylephrine.[123] Mitchell et al compared 5% cocaine, 4% lidocaine/0.5% phenylephrine, and normal saline and again found no significant difference in the prevention of epistaxis.[155] Latorre et al compared 10% cocaine with 3% lidocaine/0.25% phenylephrine and found no difference.[12] Katz et al found lidocaine 4% with epinephrine 1:100000 to be less effective than 0.05% oxymetazoline but no difference between 10% cocaine and oxymetazoline, or cocaine and lidocaine with epinephrine.[124]

Thus, the efficacy of the practice of administering vasoconstrictors to prevent epistaxis associated with nasotracheal intubation is doubtful and cocaine would appear to offer no significant advantage over oxymetazoline or phenylephrine.

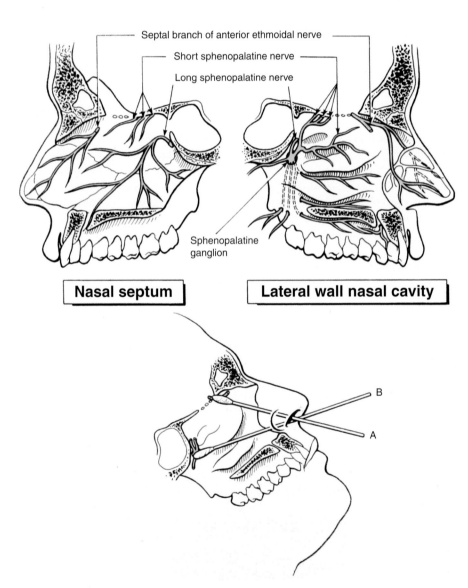

FIGURE 3-28. Placement of cotton-tipped applicators to contact the anterior ethmoidal nerve (A) and the sphenopalatine ganglion and nerves (B). (Reproduced, with permission, from Murphy TM. Somatic blockade of the head and neck. In: Cousins MJ, Bridenbaugh PO, eds. *Neural Blockade in Clinical Anesthesia and Management of Pain.* 3rd ed. Philadelphia, PA: Lippincott-Raven Publishers; 1998:489-574.)

3.4.6 Translaryngeal anesthesia

Injection of local anesthetic through the cricothyroid membrane was described in the 1920s, and use of this technique to facilitate endotracheal intubation was described in 1949.[26,156] A 21- to 23-gauge needle can be passed posteriorly in the midline immediately cephalad to the cricoid cartilage to enter the larynx (see Figure 3-29).[26,38,157] Alternatively, a 20-gauge angiocatheter can be used.[118] Directing the needle caudally will direct it away from the vocal cords which are located 1.3 cm cephalad from the transverse plane at the midpoint of the cricothyroid membrane.[26] The correct intraluminal position of the needle can be confirmed by the aspiration of air.[26,118] Then, 0.5 to 2.0 mL of 4% lidocaine,[157,158] 3 mL of 4% lidocaine,[90] 4 mL of 2% to 4% lidocaine,[118] or 2 to 3 mL of 2% lidocaine[159] can be injected either at end exhalation[160] or inhalation.[118] Translaryngeal injection predominantly produces anesthesia of the infraglottic mucosa.[72] The cough precipitated by the injection facilitates the spread of the anesthetic which has been shown to reach the superior aspect of the true cords in 95% of cases.[161] The sensory blockade above the glottis is dependent on the magnitude of the cough response.[72] If the goal is to spread anesthetic into the larynx and pharynx then injection at end inspiration seems most logical. Four milliliter of 2.5% cocaine[149] or 3 mL of 4% cocaine[158] have also been used for translaryngeal anesthesia. Tetracaine has also been used in the past[26]; however, severe reactions have been reported with the injection of tetracaine solution into the larynx.[114] Serum lidocaine levels following injection of 5 mg·kg⁻¹ of a 10% solution into the larynx via cricothyroid puncture have been found to be in the antiarrhythmic therapeutic range at a mean time of 5.1 ± 3.2 minutes.[162]

Contraindications to cricothyroid puncture include coagulopathy, local pathology, and an inability to clearly identify the cricothyroid membrane due to obscured landmarks as in the morbidly obese.[26,158] Relative contraindications include those circumstances in which vigorous cough could be deleterious, such as raised intracranial pressure or intraocular pressure, open eye injury, or unstable cervical spine injuries.[118] The use of translaryngeal anesthesia in the presence of a full stomach is controversial.[68] Complications of laryngeal anesthesia including laryngospasm and soft tissue infection have been rarely reported.[26,157] Potential complications

include bleeding, subcutaneous emphysema, pneumomediastinum, pneumothorax, vocal cord damage, and esophageal perforation.[118] A review of 17,500 cricothyroid punctures revealed only 8 complications: 2 laryngospasms, 2 broken needles, and 4 soft tissues infections of the neck.[26] In a series of 286 emergency department nasal intubations using translaryngeal anesthesia, Danzl and Thomas reported only 1 complication due to the cricothyroid membrane puncture, a case of superficial cellulitis.[157]

Bigeleisen et al compared the local anesthesia achieved with and without a transtracheal component in a group of 20 patients who underwent bronchoscopic intubation.[89] Atomized lidocaine was administered to all patients and superior laryngeal nerve blocks were performed prior to randomization into a transtracheal and nasopharyngeal groups. Transtracheal injection of 2 mg·kg⁻¹ of 4% lidocaine was performed in group 1 and in group 2 the same dose of lidocaine was applied topically to the nasopharynx. The authors reported that the patients appeared equally comfortable in both groups and that there was no qualitative difference in the ease of intubation between the groups.[89]

3.4.7 Spray-as-you-go

Lidocaine administered through the bronchoscope is commonly used during diagnostic bronchoscopy.[163] This technique can also be used for awake bronchoscopic intubation and can be combined with other methods of local anesthetic administration.[13,32,54,72,91,92,95,149] However, the time required to produce maximal local anesthesia after bronchoscopic instillation may be as long as 5 minutes, and this technique may provoke unnecessary reflex glottic closure and cough.

In the study reported by Xue et al the safety and efficacy of 2% and 4% lidocaine administered by a spray-as-you-go technique for bronchoscopic intubation were compared.[35] The patients were sedated and an oral airway and a jaw lift were used. Nineteen of 26 patients in the 2% group and 17 of 26 in the 4% group exhibited a change in facial expression or grimace when the endotracheal tube was advanced into the trachea. The tube impinged at the level of the glottis in 5 of 26 patients in the 2% group and 7 of 26 in the 4% group and required tube rotation. Slight and moderate coughing occurred in 54% and 15%, respectively, of those in the 2% group, as compared to 50% and 12%, respectively in the 4% group. Intubation times were 30.2 ± 9.8 seconds in the 2% group and 29.3 ± 10.1 seconds in the 4% group. Overall 61.5% to 73.1% of patients displayed grimacing or coughing responses during intubation. The authors reported intubating conditions to be excellent or acceptable in all patients, although a lack of complete anesthesia was reported in both groups.[35]

Webb et al compared transcricoid injection of lidocaine with the spray-as-you-go technique in a group of 62 patients who underwent transnasal diagnostic bronchoscopy.[164] The authors concluded that the transcricoid method was more effective than the spray-as-you-go technique in that, despite a lower dose of lidocaine, the bronchoscopy required less time to complete, the cough rate was lower, and the procedure was at least as acceptable to the patients in the transcricoid group.[164]

Graham et al compared transtracheal injection of cocaine, cocaine injected through the bronchoscope, and lidocaine administered by

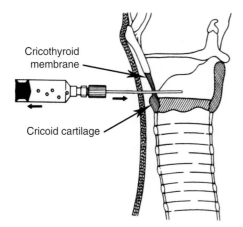

FIGURE 3-29. Anatomical relationships in translaryngeal anesthesia (lateral view). The needle punctures the cricothyroid membrane immediately cephalad to the cricoid cartilage to enter the larynx.

Cricothyroid membrane

Cricoid cartilage

nebulizer in a group of 53 patients who underwent flexible bronchoscopy.[149] The patients in the transtracheal group coughed less, experienced less stridor, and required less supplemental lidocaine. The authors concluded that transtracheal injection was the superior technique.

Sethi et al compared the spray-as-you-go technique, transtracheal injection, and nebulization in a group of 60 patients who underwent bronchoscopic transnasal intubation prior to elective surgery.[150] The nasal passages of all patients were lubricated with 2 mL of 2% lidocaine jelly, four sprays of 4% lidocaine were applied to the posterior pharynx and the patients gargled the excess solution. The patients were then randomized into a transtracheal group (A) who were given 4 mL of 4% lidocaine, a spray-as-you-go group (B) who were given 2 mL of 4% lidocaine into the larynx and 2 mL into the trachea through the bronchoscope, and a nebulization group (C) who were given 4 mL of 4% lidocaine starting 20 minutes before the procedure. Additional aliquots of 2% lidocaine were administered as required. The patients' VAS for symptoms and the endoscopist's unblinded assessment showed a preference for the spray-as-you-go technique. The cough count in Group B was 12, as compared to 18 in Group A, and 20 in Group C. Stridor occurred in 2 of 20 patients in Group B, as compared to 3 of 20 in Group A, and 10 of 20 in Group C. The best intubating conditions occurred in 16 patients in Group B, 10 in Group A, and 6 in Group C. Eight patients in Group B required a mean extra lidocaine dose of 60 mg, as compared to 2 patients (20 mg) in Group A and 12 patients (120 mg) in Group C. The data suggests that all three groups in this study had incomplete anesthesia.[150]

Spray as you go can also be used as part of a combined technique.

3.4.8 Glossopharyngeal nerve block

In the majority of individuals, the application of topical anesthesia to the mucosa of the oropharynx is sufficient to abolish the gag reflex. However, in the presence of a very pronounced gag reflex or excess secretions, glossopharyngeal nerve block may be a reasonable alternative approach. Submucosal pressure receptors in the posterior third of the tongue may also be involved in the gag reflex[70,118,165-168] and are not felt to be susceptible to topically applied local anesthetics.[118,168]

The glossopharyngeal nerve can be blocked using a posterior approach as it runs about 1 cm deep to the mucosa behind the midpoint of the palatopharyngeal fold (see Figure 3-30).[37,118,120,165,167-169] A 23-gauge angled tonsillar needle with 1 cm exposed shaft at the tip can be inserted 0.5 cm behind the midpoint of the palatopharyngeal fold, directed laterally and slightly posteriorly to a depth of about 1 cm.[165,169] Following a negative aspiration test, 2 mL of 2% lidocaine[127] or 3 to 5 mL of 1% lidocaine[167,169] can be injected. Mouth opening must be sufficient to permit visualization of the palatopharyngeal fold (posterior tonsillar pillar),[70] and adequate topical anesthesia of the tongue and adjacent pharyngeal mucosa is necessary to permit exposure of the tonsillar pillar with a tongue blade or laryngoscope.[70,118] Barton and Williams reported a series of 130 patients who underwent glossopharyngeal nerve block for bronchoscopic procedures or tonsillectomy with no complications,

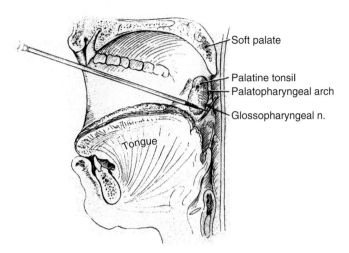

FIGURE 3-30. Glossopharyngeal nerve block, posterior to palatopharyngeal fold. (Reproduced, with permission, from Barton S, Williams JD. Glossopharyngeal nerve block. *Arch Otolaryng.* 1971;93:186-188.)

and elimination of the gag reflex in all but three patients.[165,127] Cooper and Watson similarly reported a series of 893 patients who underwent bronchoscopy or tonsillectomy using glossopharyngeal block.[169] Again no complications were reported. Onset time of the block has been noted to be about 1 minute[169] and the duration of the block to be 45 to 60 minutes.[167] Demeester and Skinner performed glossopharyngeal nerve block on 500 patients who underwent bronchoscopic procedures.[167] Superior laryngeal nerve blocks were also performed and supplemental anesthetic was administered through the bronchoscope. An inadequate block occurred in 10 patients. Blood was aspirated in six patients requiring needle repositioning and four additional patients complained of headache thought to have been due to partial intra-arterial injection of the local anesthetic. Two patients had a seizure during the endoscopy and five developed an arrhythmia following the block. The overall complication rate secondary to the glossopharyngeal nerve block was reported to be 2%.[167] Complications in addition to those noted above include local infection and hematoma formation.[118] Contraindications include coagulopathy and local pathology. This posterior approach, glossopharyngeal nerve block, is not widely used and may be impractical in the setting of difficult intubation.

Alternatively, the lingual branch of the glossopharyngeal nerve can be blocked as it runs deep to the mucosa of the palatoglossal fold (anterior tonsillar pillar) (see Figure 3-31).[118,166,168,170] Although the lingual branch of the nerve supplying the posterior third of the tongue is blocked primarily, in some cases retrograde submucosal tracking of the local anesthetic has been shown to occur, with blockade of the pharyngeal and tonsillar branches.[118,171] A 22- to 27-gauge needle is inserted in the floor of the mouth, 0.5 cm lateral to the lateral aspect of the base of the tongue at the palatoglossal fold (see Figure 3-31).[118,168,170] The needle is inserted to a depth of about 0.5 cm,[168,170] and following a negative aspiration test, 2 mL of 2% lidocaine[166,168] or 2 to 5 mL of 1% lidocaine[118,170] can be injected. If blood is aspirated, the needle should be redirected medially.[118] If air is aspirated, the needle has passed through the palatoglossal fold to enter the oropharynx and should be withdrawn until no air is aspirated.[118] Woods and Landers reported

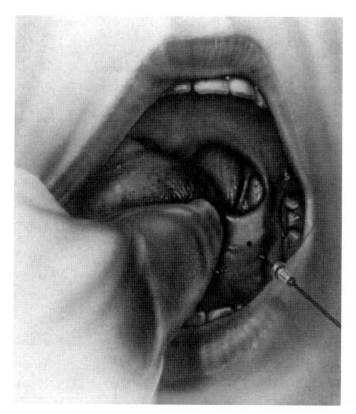

FIGURE 3-31. Glossopharyngeal nerve block at the palatoglossal fold. (Reproduced, with permission, from Bogdonoff DL, Stone DJ. Emergency management of the airway outside the operating room. *Can J Anaesth.* 1992;39(10):1069-1089.)

34 anterior approach glossopharyngeal nerve blocks and noted a duration of action of 15 to 20 minutes with plain lidocaine and 60 minutes with lidocaine and epinephrine.[168,130] The blocks were performed with a minimum of patient discomfort.[168] The gag reflex was not completely obliterated in "a number of patients."[168] Sitzman et al reported a prospective, randomized, single-blinded crossover study of airway anesthesia for direct laryngoscopy on 11 anesthesiologist volunteers which compared 2% viscous lidocaine swish and gargle (S&G), S&G combined with 10% lidocaine spray, and S&G combined with bilateral anterior glossopharyngeal nerve blocks.[170] There was no significant difference between the S&G/spray and S&G/block groups with respect to discomfort during direct laryngoscopy; however, the S&G group did experience significantly more discomfort than the other two groups. A trend toward less coughing and gagging with S&G/spray compared with S&G/block was noted, although the difference was not significant. Oropharyngeal discomfort lasting 24 hours or more occurred in 91% of the participants in the block group, and four participants had discomfort lasting more than 3 days. The study was stopped due to this oropharyngeal discomfort. The study used 5 mL of 1% plain lidocaine bilaterally, and the authors suggest that the discomfort may have been related to the volume of solution injected.[170,132] Contraindications include coagulopathy and local pathology. Potential complications include intra-arterial injection, patient discomfort, hematoma formation, and anatomic distortion. In addition, local anesthetic injected into the floor of the mouth *anterior* to the palatoglossal fold may produce

bilateral hypoglossal nerve block and impair the ability to swallow.[168] The block is considered to be acceptable in the presence of a full stomach.[157]

3.4.9   Superior laryngeal nerve block

The internal branch of the superior laryngeal nerve can be blocked as it runs just deep to the mucosa of the piriform fossa using Kraus or Jackson forceps to hold a cotton pledget soaked in 4% lidocaine against the mucosa for about 1 minute (see Figure 3-32).[22,38,65,69,120] Keeping the lidocaine-soaked pledget in contact with the mucosa of the piriform fossa for 5 minutes has also been recommended[68,69,118] but in the author's experience, this is not necessary.

Alternatively, this block can be performed using an external approach to the superior laryngeal nerve as it penetrates the thyrohyoid membrane just below the greater cornu of the hyoid bone.[22,38,68,69,118,120,160,172] With the patient supine and the head extended, the hyoid can be palpated as a freely mobile bony structure cephalad from the thyroid cartilage (see Figures 3-33 and 3-34).[160,172] The hyoid can be fixed between the operator's index finger and thumb[157] and displaced manually toward the side to be blocked.[70] A 21- to 25-gauge needle[69,70,160] can be passed medially in the frontal plane through the skin to contact the hyoid at or

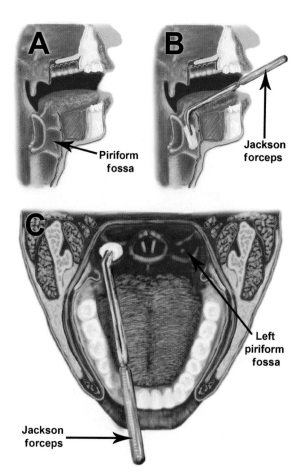

FIGURE 3-32. Schematic illustration of transmucosal superior laryngeal nerve block using Jackson forceps and a cotton pledget soaked in 4% lidocaine. A and B show the lateral view of the block and C shows the superior view of the block.

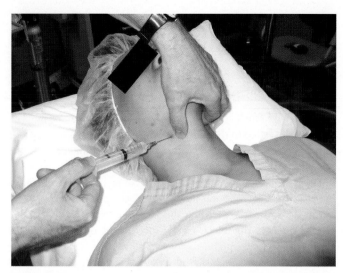

FIGURE 3-33. Percutaneous superior laryngeal nerve block. The hyoid can be fixed between the operator's index finger and thumb and displaced manually toward the side to be blocked. A 22-gauge needle is passed medially in the frontal plane through the skin to contact the hyoid at or near the greater cornu.

near the greater cornu[160,172] and then walked caudad until it slips off the bone.[160] The needle is then advanced 2 to 3 mm.[70,118] In this location, the needle tip has entered a closed space bounded by the thyrohyoid membrane laterally and the mucosa of the piriform fossa medially. A slight resistance may be appreciated as the needle is advanced through the ligament,[118] and a definite give as the needle passes through the deep aspect of the membrane.[159]

Following a negative aspiration, 2 to 3 mL of 2% lidocaine[68,69,160] can then be injected. If blood is aspirated, the needle may have entered the superior laryngeal artery or vein or the carotid artery, and in this circumstance it should be withdrawn and redirected anteriorly.[118] If air is aspirated, the pharyngeal lumen has been entered and the needle must be withdrawn until no air is aspirated prior to injection.[118] Entry into the laryngopharynx has been used as an integral part of the technique,[167,173] although this is not necessary. If the hyoid bone cannot be identified by palpation or if palpation produces undue patient discomfort, the thyroid cartilage can be used as a landmark.[37,38,68-70,118,120,160,173] The thyroid cartilage can be displaced toward the side to be blocked and the needle passed medially in the frontal plane to contact the cartilage at a point at or near the greater cornu[68,118,120] or at a point one-third of the distance from the midline to the superior cornu.[108] The needle is then walked cephalad to reach and perforate the thyrohyoid membrane.[31,68-70,160,172] Alternatively, the thyrohyoid membrane itself can be identified by palpation with the index finger immediately cephalad to the lateral aspect of the thyroid cartilage.[70,167,173] The carotid pulse can be felt posteriorly (see Figure 3-35).[167] The needle can then be passed medially anterior to the fingertip.[167,173] The feeling of resistance changes as the needle punctures the membrane and is relied on to indicate proper depth.[70] The needle may also be advanced to contact the thyroid cartilage as a depth guide and then walked cephalad.[173]

The onset time for the block is 5 to 10 minutes[41,68,69] and the duration of action is at least 90 minutes[171] and may be as long as 4 to 6 hours when 2% lidocaine is used.[68,172] Complications include intra-arterial injection, hematoma (reported incidence 1.4%),[9] unintended pharyngeal perforation,[41,68,160,167] hypotension, and bradycardia.[118] Contraindications include local pathology, coagulopathy, and poor anatomic landmarks.[41,68,160,167] The block has also been said to be contraindicated in patients at risk of aspiration.[22,118,160,171]

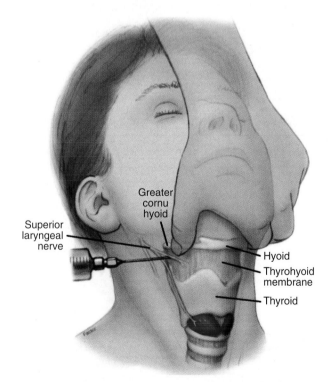

Superior laryngeal nerve
Greater cornu hyoid
Hyoid
Thyrohyoid membrane
Thyroid

FIGURE 3-34. Schematic illustrations of superior laryngeal nerve block. (Reproduced, with permission, from Brown D, ed. *Atlas of Regional Anesthesia.* 2nd ed. Philadelphia, PA: Saunders; 1999:205-208.)

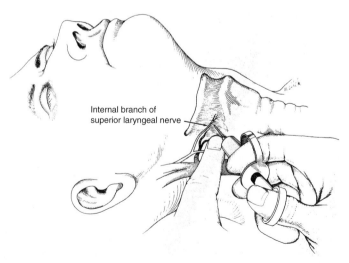

Internal branch of superior laryngeal nerve

FIGURE 3-35. Alternative technique of superior laryngeal nerve block. (Reproduced, with permission, from DeMeester TR, Skinner DB, Evans RH, et al. Local nerve block anesthesia for peroral endoscopy. *Ann Thoracic Surg.* 1977;24(3):278-282.)

3.5   OTHER CONSIDERATIONS

3.5.1   Is regional anesthesia of the airway contraindicated in the presence of a full stomach?

Local anesthesia of the larynx and trachea obtunds protective airway reflexes and may predispose to aspiration.[37,38,158,174] However, local anesthesia of the airway has been used in circumstances associated with increased risk for aspiration without aspiration actually occurring.[26,157-159,174-177] Thomas reported a series of 25 patients who were intubated awake, 21 of whom had a full stomach.[159] Topical anesthesia was administered to all 25 and bilateral superior laryngeal nerve blocks were performed on 21 patients. Nine patients were given translaryngeal injections. No incident of aspiration occurred.[159] Duncan reported 12 patients who underwent awake intubation for emergency surgery under regional anesthesia of the airway including transtracheal injection and recorded no incident of aspiration.[158] Kopman et al reported 55 awake intubations in patients with full stomachs under topical anesthesia to the nose, mouth, pharynx, and larynx. There was no evidence of aspiration in any of the patients.[175] Danzl and Thomas performed 286 emergency nasotracheal intubations under transtracheal anesthesia and reported no aspirations.[157] Meschino et al reported a series of 165 patients with cervical spine fracture who underwent awake intubation.[176] Sixty-four patients required emergent endotracheal intubation, and "a regional block or local anesthesia of the larynx" was administered in 137 patients. No evidence of aspiration of gastric contents was documented during intubation.[176] Ovassapian et al performed 114 awake bronchoscopic intubations on patients with a full stomach risk under regional anesthesia of the airway including translaryngeal injection or injection into the larynx and trachea through the flexible bronchoscope.[177] Again no aspirations occurred.[175,177] Gold and Buechel reviewed 17,500 cases of translaryngeal anesthesia reported in the literature.[26] They recorded eight complications, but no aspirations.[26]

The risk of aspiration during awake intubation under regional anesthesia of the airway must be weighed against the risks associated with other airway management modalities.[37,38] As always, good clinical judgment and a common sense approach are mandatory.[37,38]

3.5.2   Are antisialagogues helpful or even essential in awake bronchoscopic intubation?

Secretions in the airway interpose a mechanical barrier between the mucosa and topically applied local anesthetics, dilute the anesthetic solution, and wash it away from the intended site of action.[37,38,40,68,69,120,178,179] Additionally, the view through the bronchoscope can also be impaired by the presence of secretions.[41] Antisialagogues are therefore invaluable adjuncts to facilitate awake bronchoscopic intubation.[33,34,47,97] Atropine and glycopyrrolate are both effective, although glycopyrrolate is the more

potent drying agent.[33,97,142] Scopolamine has also been used as an antisialagogue; however, it produces sedation as well as amnesia and can produce delirium.[69]

These antimuscarinic drugs dry the airway by decreasing the *production* of secretions.[41,68,69] They must therefore be administered far enough in advance of planned airway manipulation to allow eradication of secretions that have already accumulated, as well as to permit the drug to exert its antisialagogic effect.[41,69] Following IV administration of glycopyrrolate to volunteers, dryness of the mouth was noted 7 minutes after injection and a significant drying effect was observed after 15 minutes.[42] Following IM administration, glycopyrrolate has an onset of action of 20 to 40 minutes[69,180] and the peak effect occurs at 30 to 45 minutes.[180] Inhibition of salivary secretions persists for up to 7 hours after parenteral administration of glycopyrrolate[181] and is dose related.[182] The appropriate dose of IM glycopyrrolate when used as a drying agent is 0.2 to 0.4 mg in the adult.[182] The corresponding dose in children is about 10 $\mu g \cdot kg^{-1}$.[182] Glycopyrrolate can also be given subcutaneously.[68,69,181] After IM administration, doses of glycopyrrolate sufficient to produce a 75% inhibition of salivation produced only minimal heart rate changes,[182] although an increase in heart rate can occur after IV administration.[182] Glycopyrrolate is a quaternary ammonium compound and does not cross the normal blood–brain barrier.[41,118]

Following the IM administration of atropine, inhibition of salivation is seen within 30 minutes,[180] the peak effect is seen at 1.0 to 1.6 hours,[180] and the duration of action is 4 hours.[69] The heart rate increases 5 to 40 minutes after the IM administration of atropine and peaks within 20 to 60 minutes.[180] At doses necessary to produce a 75% inhibition of salivation, atropine increases the heart rate by more than 15%.[182] When used as an antisialagogue, 0.2 to 0.8 mg of atropine can be given IM or subcutaneously 30 to 60 minutes before airway manipulation.[69,180] Rarely at low doses, atropine can exert a parasympathomimetic effect and produce a bradycardia.[180] Atropine readily crosses the blood–brain barrier and can produce a CNS effect.[183]

In a prospective, randomized, double-blind study of 37 surgical patients, the drying effect of glycopyrrolate 0.2 mg IM administered 90 minutes preoperatively was compared to 0.2 mg IV given 10 minutes preoperatively,[184] to 2 mg given by mouth 90 minutes preoperatively, and to placebo. No significant difference was found in the patient's sensation of mouth dryness 10 minutes after IV injection of glycopyrrolate or placebo, and no difference between groups in the anesthetist's perception of dryness of the airway following intubation by direct laryngoscopy. Ten minutes may not be sufficient time to permit significant drying to occur after IV injection as the effect has been shown to increase for up to 15 minutes.[42] The peak effect of IM glycopyrrolate occurs at 30 to 45 minutes following injection[180] and 90 minutes following injection may not have been the optimal time for observation. Furthermore, the inhibition of salivation is dose related and 0.2 mg is at the low end of the dose range recommended in the adult.[182] Direct laryngoscopy is also a different stimulus as compared to awake bronchoscopic intubation under local anesthesia. Cowl et al reported a double-blind, placebo-controlled study of 217 patients who underwent bronchoscopy and intubation under local anesthesia and sedation.[185] Patients were randomly allocated to receive atropine 0.01 mg·kg⁻¹ IM, glycopyrrolate 0.005 mg·kg⁻¹ IM, or saline placebo 2 mL IM, 15 to 45 minutes preoperatively. The time of administration in each patient was not recorded however, and the number of patients who received glycopyrrolate 15 minutes before the procedure is unknown. The operators noted no significant difference in antisialagogic effect or cough suppression for either atropine or glycopyrrolate as compared to placebo. However, the patients reported significantly higher visual analog scores for secretion control with glycopyrrolate.[185] Roffe et al randomly allocated 190 consecutive patients undergoing bronchoscopy employing local anesthesia and sedation to receive either IM atropine 0.6 mg, IM glycopyrrolate 0.3 mg, or no antisialagogue 30 minutes preoperatively.[186] Troublesome coughing was less frequent in the glycopyrrolate group as was patient movement. Mouth dryness was most common with glycopyrrolate but overall assessment of discomfort was similar in all three groups. In 2009, Malik et al reported a double-blind, placebo-controlled study of 1000 patients who underwent diagnostic bronchoscopy under local anesthesia and sedation.[187] Patients were randomly assigned to receive atropine 0.01 mg·kg⁻¹, glycopyrrolate 0.005 mg·kg⁻¹, or 2 mL normal saline IM 20 to 40 minutes before the procedure. The time of administration in each patient was not reported. Nebulized 4% lidocaine was administered and 5 mL of 2% lidocaine was instilled into the trachea via the bronchoscope. Additional boluses were administered via the bronchoscope as required. Neither the total dose of lidocaine administered nor any differences in doses among the groups were reported. The nasotracheal approach was used in approximately 95% of patients but any differences in approach among the groups were not reported. The authors reported that the patient and bronchoscopist's visual analogue scores for airway secretions, cough, and discomfort were lower in the patients treated with antimuscarinics compared with placebo, but only reached statistical significance in the bronchoscopist's score for secretions. In the atropine group changes in the blood pressure and heart rate were statistically significant as compared to glycopyrrolate and placebo. These changes were however clinically modest. There was no significant difference in the occurrence of major adverse events among the groups.[187] Brookman et al randomized 80 adult patients undergoing elective dental extraction to receive 0.4 mg hyoscine hydrobromide PO, 0.4 mg hyoscine hydrobromide IM, 0.4 mg glycopyrrolate IM, or placebo 60 minutes preoperatively.[188] All patients underwent nasal bronchoscopic intubation. The clarity of the visual field was noted to be significantly improved in all three antimuscarinic groups.[188]

The results of these studies are somewhat difficult to extrapolate to the awake bronchoscopic intubation setting. In the author's experience, drying agents are immensely helpful in facilitating awake bronchoscopic intubation. Glycopyrrolate 0.4 mg IM given to the adult 30 minutes before airway manipulation will provide optimum conditions for topical anesthesia of the airway in the vast majority of patients. Inflammatory conditions of the airway can be associated with excess secretion production and antisialagogues may be less effective in this setting. In the absence of pathology at the site of injection, superior laryngeal nerve block, or glossopharyngeal nerve blocks may be more effective in this circumstance; however, intubation under topical anesthesia alone can usually be achieved. The nasal approach requires less suppression of the gag reflex and may be the more appropriate route in the presence of excess secretions.

3.5.3   Is sedation useful in facilitating awake intubation?

If adequate local anesthesia of the airway can be achieved, awake intubation can be rapidly and easily accomplished without the use of sedation. Regional anesthesia of the airway can be achieved with minimal patient discomfort, although stimulation of the gag and cough reflexes can be unpleasant.[146] The emphasis should however be placed on the development of regional anesthesia skills, rather than on the use of sedation in an attempt to compensate for poor airway anesthesia.[37] As time and circumstances permit, sedation can be used to further minimize discomfort, produce anxiolysis, and attenuate recall,[37] although the need for anxiolysis or amnesia is reduced or eliminated if airway anesthesia can be rapidly and skillfully achieved. In the presence of airway compromise or respiratory distress, any additional impairment of the level of consciousness can lead to deterioration in the clinical situation. The goal of sedation during awake intubation is a calm and cooperative patient who remains crisply responsive to command.[37,38] During awake bronchoscopic intubation, the ability of the patient to breathe deeply on command improves visualization of the airway structures, moves the epiglottis anteriorly out of the path of the advancing bronchoscope and endotracheal tube, and by producing maximum abduction of the vocal cords facilitates glottic cannulation. Sedation can therefore make bronchoscopic intubation more difficult.

Sedation to facilitate awake intubation can be achieved using a variety of drugs. In general, the minimum amount of sedation required for anxiolysis should be used and the dose carefully titrated to effect.[118]

Midazolam administered in increments of 0.25 to 0.5 mg to the adult produces anxiolysis and amnesia,[189] and titration to a suitable end point without losing patient cooperation is usually achievable,[37] although the ability of the patient to briskly respond to command may be impaired. The onset time is 1 to 3 minutes and the duration of action is about 2 hours.[37,68] Fentanyl can provide sedation, analgesia, and euphoria, can attenuate laryngeal reflexes, and has an antitussive effect.[34,37,64] Respiratory depression can also occur,[37] as can bradycardia.[150] When used in combination, a synergism between fentanyl and midazolam occurs which potentiates the effects of both drugs.[34,64] Hypotension and apnea can occur. However, when administered in low doses and titrated carefully to affect, midazolam and fentanyl in combination can be used to produce satisfactory sedation, and side effects can be avoided.[37] Diazepam, lorazepam, and long-acting opioids do not appear to provide any advantage during awake intubation and may be more difficult to titrate. Overdose with benzodiazepines or opioids can be reversed with flumazenil and naloxone, respectively.

Droperidol, a butyrophenone that produces a state of quiescence with reduced motor activity and indifference to one's surroundings,[189] also has been used to facilitate awake intubation. However, about 10% of individuals exposed to droperidol experience a feeling of mental restlessness and agitation, so-called dysphoria,[24,41] and prolongation of the QT interval can occur even at low doses.[190] Ketamine can produce excessive secretions, disorientation,[191] hallucinations, and mild respiratory depression and is not commonly used to facilitate awake intubation.[68]

In the emergency situation, when judicious chemical restraint is required to permit airway management of combative and intoxicated patients, haloperidol, also a butyrophenone, can be immensely helpful.[38] Intravenous doses of 2 to 10 mg in the adult can be carefully titrated to effect.[33] Ketamine may be particularly useful in the uncooperative patient without IV access who requires chemical restraint.[191]

Recently, the use of remifentanil for awake bronchoscopic intubation as a single agent and in combination with propofol or midazolam has been reported.[192-197]

- Reusche and Egan reported a case of Ludwig's angina in which awake nasotracheal intubation was performed using a remifentanil infusion at 0.05 to 0.175 µg·kg⁻¹·min⁻¹.[197] The patient was also given glycopyrrolate 0.2 mg, droperidol 0.625 mg, and midazolam 2.0 mg IV. Four milliliter of 4% lidocaine was administered by nebulizer, the right naris was swabbed with 4% cocaine, and 2 mL of 4% lidocaine was sprayed on the vocal cords through the bronchoscope. The patient was intubated without gagging, bucking, or coughing.[197]

- Johnson et al reported the use of a remifentanil bolus of 3.2 µg·kg⁻¹ in addition to 26 µg·kg⁻¹ of midazolam to perform direct laryngoscopy on a patient who was predicted to be a difficult intubation on physical examination.[193] The patient remained conscious and followed commands throughout the direct laryngoscopy and subsequent intubation, appeared to tolerate the procedure well, and had no recall of the event. No local anesthetic was used.

- Puchner et al reported the use of a remifentanil infusion to facilitate awake nasotracheal intubation of a patient with odontogenic, facial, and cervical infection.[196] The nose was anesthetized with 4% lidocaine spray, and 2 mL of 4% lidocaine was sprayed through the bronchoscope onto the vocal cords and subglottic area. The patient remained conscious, calm, and cooperative. No reflex glottic closure was observed.[196] Remifentanil infusion was subsequently compared to a combination of fentanyl and midazolam during awake bronchoscopic intubation in 74 patients.[155] Remifentanil was administered in dosages of 0.1 to 0.5 µg·kg⁻¹·min⁻¹. Both groups received PO midazolam 1 hour preoperatively. Four percent lidocaine spray was administered to the nose, and 4 mL of 4% lidocaine was sprayed through the bronchoscope onto supraglottic and subglottic areas. Patients in the remifentanil group had a significantly reduced response to the nasal passage of the tube and less cough as the larynx was intubated. The investigators felt that remifentanil suppressed laryngeal reflexes significantly better than fentanyl and midazolam and improved intubating conditions.[195]

- Machata et al compared a remifentanil 0.75 µg·kg⁻¹ bolus, followed by 0.075 µg·kg⁻¹·min⁻¹ with a 1.5 µg·kg⁻¹ bolus followed by 0.15 µg·kg⁻¹·min⁻¹ for awake intubation in 24 patients.[194,154] All patients were premedicated with midazolam 0.05 mg·kg⁻¹ and glycopyrrolate 0.2 mg IV. The nostril was anesthetized using 2% lidocaine gel coating on nasopharyngeal tubes. The

supraglottic region was sprayed with 5 mL of 2% lidocaine and 2 mL was instilled onto the vocal cords through the working channel of the bronchoscope. No respiratory rate less than eight breaths per minute occurred, no patient recalled pain, and all patients remained cooperative. Intubating conditions were adequate in all patients and comparable between the groups.[194] Both regimens blunted airway reflexes sufficiently.

- Xu et al determined that when combined with midazolam 0.1 mg·kg⁻¹ IV and topical anesthesia of the airway, the ED_{50} of remifentanil for successful awake direct laryngoscopy and intubation was a bolus of 0.62 ug·kg⁻¹ followed by an infusion of 0.062 ug·kg⁻¹·min⁻¹.[198]

- Mingo et al reported the use of remifentinil for awake bronchoscopic nasotracheal intubation in a group of 24 patients scheduled for elective surgery.[199] Topical anesthesia was limited to the nasal mucosa. The remifentinil infusion was started at 0.3 ug·kg⁻¹·min⁻¹ and titrated between 0.2 and 0.5 ug·kg⁻¹·min⁻¹ to produce adequate sedation defined as "falling asleep if unstimulated but immediately responsive to command." Intubation difficulty as rated by the endoscopist and an observing anesthetist was reported, respectively, to be easy in 17 and 15 of 24 patients, and moderate in 5/24 and 7/24. Both raters reported the intubation as difficult in two patients. Coughing during intubation occurred in six patients and grimacing in six. Ten patients recalled the procedure but only one would not repeat it if it were considered necessary. The authors concluded that intubation had most likely been made possible by the suppression of airway reflexes and the intense analgesia produced by remifentinil. Although the results of this study cannot be readily extrapolated to the setting of acute airway compromise, attenuation of airway reflexes by remifentinil in this emergency setting may be beneficial.[199]

- Rai et al compared remifentinil and propofol administered as target-controlled infusions in a group of 24 patients who underwent bronchoscopic intubation under topical anesthesia.[200] All patients received 1 to 2 mg of IV midazolam based on weight, and IV glycopyrrolate. They were then randomized into remifentinil and propofol groups and topical anesthesia was administered. Sedation scores were similar in each group. Endoscopy and intubation were more difficult in the propofol group and required more time to complete. Twenty three patients were intubated on the first attempt. One patient in the propofol group requited two attempts. The patients in the remifentinil group tolerated the procedure much better as determined by discomfort and postintubation scores. Despite a higher level of recall in the remifentinil group, patient satisfaction was the same in both groups. No adverse events were recorded.[200]

- Remifentanil has also been administered by infusion in combination with low-dose propofol during awake intubation.[192]

The ester structure of remifentanil is unique among fentanyl congeners and results in very rapid metabolism. The peak effect-site concentration of remifentanil occurs within 1 to 2 minutes of bolus injection,[193] and the offset is also rapid. The time necessary to reach a 50% decrease in serum concentration after stopping a continuous infusion at steady state is 4 minutes.[195] The median dose of remifentanil administered over 2 minutes, required to produce loss of consciousness, has been found to be 12 $\mu g \cdot kg^{-1}$, and at doses ≤5 $\mu g \cdot kg^{-1}$ no subjects lost consciousness.[193,201] It has been recommended that dosing should be calculated on lean body mass and reduced by as much as 50%-70% in the elderly.[193] Remifentanil therefore appears to be very easily titrated. Jhaveri et al noted mild muscle rigidity in 40% and moderate rigidity in an additional 40% of a group of elective surgical patients following the administration of 2 $\mu g \cdot kg^{-1}$ of remifentanil over 2 minutes.[201] No severe muscle rigidity was observed at doses less than or equal to 4 $\mu g \cdot kg^{-1}$. Wilhelm et al administered remifentanil by infusion to a group of patients undergoing oocyte removal and did not observe muscle rigidity at doses up to 0.4 $\mu g \cdot kg^{-1} \cdot min^{-1}$.[202]

Anecdotally, in the author's experience remifentanil infusion appears to attenuate the gag reflex as well as laryngeal reflexes, and can facilitate airway anesthesia. It may be particularly useful in patients with hyperactive gag reflexes, and in the presence of excess secretions. Remifentanil may prove to be an exception to the general rule that sedatives cannot or should not be used to compensate for poor regional anesthesia of the airway.

Dexmedetomidine (DEX) is a centrally acting alpha-2-adrenoceptor agonist, which produces sedation, analgesia, anxiolysis, xerostomia, and some degree of amnesia.[203-208] The sedation produced by DEX is unique in that patients appear to be asleep but are readily aroused.[204] The term "cooperative sedation" has been used[191,205] as DEX appears to maintain[191,209] or enhance[210] patient cooperation, and the ability to follow commands.[209] DEX produces minimal[204,206,209,211] or no respiratory depression[191,203,210] but can produce hypotension, hypertension, tachycardia, and bradycardia.[191,203-206] When administered as a continuous IV infusion, however, it is associated with a predictable and stable hemodynamic response.[203] Caution is necessary when DEX is administered to patients who are volume depleted, vasoconstricted, or who have *severe* heart block.[203] Contraindications to DEX as listed by Unger include hypovolemia, hypotension, aortic stenosis, idiopathic hypertrophic subaortic stenosis, pulmonary hypertension, and heart block in the absence of a pacemaker.[191] The recommended loading dose of DEX is 0.5 to 1.0 $ug \cdot kg^{-1}$ over 10 to 20 minutes, which can then be followed by a continuous infusion of 0.2 to 0.7 $ug \cdot kg^{-1} \cdot h^{-1}$.[191,205,206,209-211] The elimination half-life is 2 hours.[203]

Avitsian et al performed a retrospective review of 19 patients who underwent awake bronchoscopic intubation using DEX for sedation.[211] Midazolam and/or fentanyl was also given to all but two patients, and topical anesthesia was utilized. A dose of 1 $ug \cdot kg^{-1}$ of DEX was administered over 10 to 15 minutes and this was followed by a continuous infusion of 0.2 to 0.7 $ug \cdot kg^{-1} \cdot h^{-1}$ if required. The intubation was "smooth" in all cases with good patient tolerance and no airway obstruction. Thirteen patients developed hypotension after induction of general anesthesia that was managed with ephedrine or phenylephrine.[211]

Grant et al reported three cases of awake bronchoscopic intubation in which DEX was used for sedation.[206] Local anesthesia was utilized but no other sedatives were administered. Intubating conditions were acceptable in all three patients. No clinically important hypotension or bradycardia was reported. One patient recalled the intubation but was not distressed by that recollection.

Abdulmalak et al reported five cases in which DEX was used as the sole sedative for awake bronchoscopic intubation.[209] Topical lidocaine was also utilized. The patients remained responsive to

command and were all intubated on the first attempt. Four of the five patients had no recall of the intubation. Hypotension required treatment in two cases. The lowest heart rate reported was 48 bpm.

Bergese et al reported the use of dexmedetomidine sedation in four patients with difficult airways who underwent successful awake bronchoscopic intubation.[210] Two patients also received midazolam. Local anesthesia was used in three patients. Two patients were initially uncooperative, but following the administration of DEX were able to follow command, and excellent intubating conditions were achieved. Hemodynamics remained stable during the procedure in all four cases.

Neumann et al and Maroof et al have also reported successful awake bronchoscopic intubations in patients with difficult airways under topical anesthesia and DEX sedation.[212,213]

Dexmedetomidine infusion in combination with ketamine infusion has also been used for awake bronchoscopic intubation.[214] Scher and Gitlin administered a bolus of 1 $\mu g \cdot kg^{-1}$ of dexmedetomidine over 10 minutes and followed this with an infusion of 0.7 $\mu g \cdot kg^{-1} \cdot h^{-1}$.[160] Upon completion of the dexmedetomidine bolus, 15 mg of ketamine was administered as a bolus, and then followed by an infusion of 20 $mg \cdot h^{-1}$. The patient remained responsive to command and calm. Regional anesthesia of the airway was then performed "in the usual manner," and bronchoscopic intubation via a bronchoscopic oral airway was performed.[214] Intubating conditions were reported to be excellent and included a secretion-free airway. The patient had no recall of the procedure.

Hagberg et al performed a randomized double-blind comparison of remifentinil (R) and dexmedetomidine (DEX) for sedation during awake bronchoscopic intubation in a group of 30 patients.[207] All patients were given glycopyrrolate and midazolam and their airways were topicalized with 4% lidocaine. Patients in the remifentinil group were given a bolus of 0.75 $ug \cdot kg^{-1}$, followed by an infusion of 0.075 $ug \cdot kg^{-1} \cdot min^{-1}$. Patients in the DEX group received a bolus of 0.4 $ug \cdot kg^{-1}$ over 10 minutes followed by an infusion of 0.7 $ug \cdot kg^{-1} \cdot h^{-1}$. All patients were successfully intubated. Thirteen of 17 patients in the R group were intubated on the first attempt, 3 required 2 attempts, and 1 required 3 attempts. In the DEX group, 5 of 13 patients were intubated on the first attempt, 4 required 2 attempts, and 4 required 3 attempts. Minimal hemodynamic instability was observed in both groups. Intraoperative recall was significantly lower in the DEX group.

Dexmedetomidine appears to be very useful as a sedative to facilitate awake bronchoscopic intubation. It is however not available in Canada and the author has no personal experience with this drug. The reports of its use in uncooperate patients, who following the administration of DEX were able to follow command, are particularly intriguing, as is its use in the absence of local anesthesia.

3.5.4 How should a patient be prepared psychologically to undergo awake intubation?

Undergoing any medical procedure can be intimidating, anxiety provoking, even frightening, and the practitioner must make every effort to minimize patient anxiety. As time permits in the emergency setting, and routinely in the elective situation, a full explanation of the circumstances requiring awake intubation should be given to the patient.[37] This explanation of the procedure and its necessity should be provided in as controlled a manner as possible, again as time and circumstances permit. The explanation should be delivered in a calm, unhurried, sincere, methodical manner[40,69] and should emphasize the margin of safety maintained as well as the dangers associated with intubation under general anesthesia in the presence of a difficult airway.[37,68] The explanation should be frank and straightforward, yet sufficiently detailed that the patient understands the necessity for the procedure as well as what to expect during the procedure itself.[41,69] Possible adverse consequences can be discussed as appropriate.[69] The patient must be able to develop a sense of trust in the operator's judgment and expertise if cooperation is to be established.[68] Perhaps in no other procedure is a good bedside manner more important than in awake bronchoscopic intubation.

Following the preoperative interview, the patient should be brought into the procedure room (eg, operating room) only after all the equipment has been made ready. The room should be calm and quiet. Only those who are working in the room should be present. One learner is appropriate, but spectators should be minimized or disallowed. The operator and an assistant should perform the awake intubation in a controlled methodical manner, should remain in verbal contact with the patient, and should calmly explain each step of the procedure to further allay anxiety. Nervous behavior by individuals in the room should be avoided. Local anesthesia of the airway should be achieved in 15 minutes or less and the intubation itself in about 30 seconds.

3.5.5   What technique works well for the average patient?

In the emergency setting, regional anesthesia of the airway for awake intubation by direct laryngoscopy can be readily achieved using 10% lidocaine spray. The spray can be directed onto the posterior third of the tongue, the uvula, and the tonsillar pillars using the malleable, stainless steel nozzle, and a tongue depressor to retract the tongue. Sprays can also be delivered into the piriform fossae; however, spraying into the larynx should be avoided as laryngospasm, cough, and a loss of patient cooperation may be precipitated. An explanation of the procedure should be provided to the patient as time and circumstances permit. In general, the use of sedation should be avoided in the emergency awake intubation and the time required for antisialagogues to provide mucosal drying is not available. If neck movement is permissible, then awake intubation by direct laryngoscopy is most easily performed with the patient in the sitting position.

In the setting of an anticipated difficult intubation in which awake bronchoscopic intubation is planned, profound regional anesthesia of the airway can be achieved using the following technique:

- A full explanation of the procedure should be provided to the patient.

- Glycopyrrolate should be administered IM about 20 to 30 minutes or IV at least 15 minutes prior to planned airway manipulation. The tongue should appear dry prior to airway manipulation.

- If neck movement is allowed, the patient should be in the sitting or semi-sitting position.

- A remifentinil infusion can be initiated at 0.1 to 0.2 ug·kg^{-1}·min^{-1}.

- Five percent lidocaine ointment can be gently applied to the posterior third of the tongue using a tongue depressor. Alternatively, the patient can be asked to gargle 40 to 50 mL of 4% lidocaine solution and expectorate the residual or 10% lidocaine spray can also be directed onto the posterior third of the tongue, uvula, and fauces.

- About 12 mL of aerosolized 3% lidocaine can then be administered optimally via the nose using a DeVilbiss atomizer attached to a high-pressure oxygen source. The spray delivered by the atomizer should be coordinated with respiration, with inhalation through the nose, and exhalation through the mouth. Alternatively, the aerosol can be administered via the mouth.

- Cotton pledgets held securely by Jackson forceps can be soaked in 4% lidocaine and then gently advanced over the tongue into the piriform fossa on each side to ensure or supplement laryngeal anesthesia. As the pledget is removed, the mucosa of the oropharynx can be swabbed to confirm the absence of the gag reflex.

Bronchoscopic intubation can then be rapidly achieved as described in Chapter 9.

Awake intubation under topical anesthesia with and without sedation has also been described using various rigid bronchoscopic devices.[215-219]

3.6   SUMMARY

Awake intubation can be achieved rapidly with minimal patient discomfort. Knowledge of airway anatomy, the medications that can be employed, and techniques of regional anesthesia of the airway are necessary. Manual dexterity, gentleness, and an appropriate bedside manner are also essential.

REFERENCES

1. Mongan PD, Culling RD. Rapid oral anesthesia for awake intubation. *J Clin Anesth*. 1992;4:101-105.
2. Redden RJ. Anatomic airway considerations in anesthesia. In: Hagberg CA, ed. *Handbook of Difficult Airway Management*. Philadelphia, PA: Churchill Livingstone; 2000:1-13.
3. Morris IR. Functional anatomy of the upper airway. *Emerg Med Clin North Am*. 1988;6:639-669.
4. Ellis H, Feldman S. *Anatomy for Anesthetists*. 4th ed. Oxford: Blackwell Scientific Publications; 1983.
5. Morris IR. Airway management. In: Rosen P, ed. *Emergency Medicine: Concepts and Clinical Practice*. St. Louis: Mosby Yearbook; 1992:79-105.
6. Basmajian JV. *Grant's Method of Anatomy*. 8th ed. Baltimore: Williams & Wilkins; 1981.
7. Friedman SM. *Head and Neck*. New York: Harper & Harper; 1970.
8. Hall IS. *Diseases of the Nose, Throat and Ear: A Handbook for Students and Practitioners*. 11th ed. Edinburgh: Churchill Livingstone; 1985.
9. Graney DO. *Basic Science: Anatomy*. St. Louis: Mosby; 1986.
10. Tintinalli JE, Claffey J. Complications of nasotracheal intubation. *Ann Emerg Med*. 1981;10:142-144.
11. Iserson KV. Blind nasotracheal intubation. *Ann Emerg Med*. 1981;10:468-471.
12. Latorre F, Otter W, Kleemann PP, Dick W, Jage J. Cocaine or phenylephrine/ lignocaine for nasal fibreoptic intubation? *Eur J Anaesthesiol*. 1996;13:577-581.

13. Woodall NM, Harwood RJ, Barker GL. Complications of awake fibreoptic intubation without sedation in 200 healthy anaesthetists attending a training course. *Br J Anaesth*. 2008;100:850-855.

14. Smith JE, Reid AP. Identifying the more patent nostril before nasotracheal intubation. *Anaesthesia*. 2001;56:258-262.

15. Ellis H. *Clinical Anatomy: A Revision and Applied Anatomy for Clinical Students*. 6th ed. Oxford: Blackwell Scientific Publications; 1977.

16. Ovassapian A, Glassenberg R, Randel GI, Klock A, Mesnick PS, Klafta JM. The unexpected difficult airway and lingual tonsil hyperplasia: a case series and a review of the literature. *Anesthesiology*. 2002;97:124-132.

17. Atkinson RS, Rushman GB, Lee JA. *A Synopsis of Anaesthesia*. 8th ed. Bristol: John Wright & Sons; 1977.

18. Netter FH. *Atlas of Human Anatomy*. Summit: CIBA–Geigy; 1989.

19. Snell RS. *Clinical Neuroanatomy for Medical Students*. 5th ed. Philadelphia: Lippincott, Williams & Wilkins; 2001.

20. Williams PL, Warwick R, Dyson M, Bannister LH. *Gray's Anatomy*. 37th ed. New York: Churchill Livingstone; 1989.

21. Donlon JVJ. Anesthetic and airway management of laryngoscopy and bronchoscopy. In: Benumof JL, ed. *Airway Management Principles and Practice*. St. Louis: Mosby, Inc.; 1996:666-685.

22. Stone DJ, Gal TJ. Airway management. In: Miller RD, ed. *Anesthesia*. 5th ed. Philadelphia, PA: Churchill Livingstone; 2000:1414-1451.

23. Stoelting RK. Endotracheal intubation. In: Miller RD, ed. *Anesthesia*. New York: Churchill Livingstone; 1981:233-255.

24. Dripps RD, Eckenhoff JE, VanDam LD. *Introduction to Anesthesia: The Principles of Safe Practice*. 6th ed. Philadelphia, PA: WB Saunders Co.; 1982.

25. Ovassapian A, Wheeler M. Flexible fiberoptic tracheal intubation. In: Hagberg C, ed. *Handbook of Difficult Airway Management*. Philadelphia, PA: Churchill Livingstone; 2000:83-114.

26. Gold MI, Buechel DR. Translaryngeal anesthesia: a review. *Anesthesiology*. 1959;20:181-185.

27. Melker RJ, Florete OGJ. Percutaneous dilatational cricothyrotomy and tracheostomy. In: *Airway Management Principles and Practice*. Benumof JL, ed. St. Louis: Mosby, Inc.; 1996:448-572.

28. Wong MEK, Bradick JP. Surgical approaches to airway management of anesthesia practitioners. In: Hagberg CA, ed. *Handbook of Difficult Airway Management*. 1st ed. Philadelphia, PA: Churchill Livingstone; 2000:185-218.

29. Kastendiek JG. Airway management. In: Rosen P, ed. *Emergency Medicine Concepts and Clinical Practice*. 2nd ed. St. Louis: Mosby, Inc.; 1988:26-53.

30. Davidson TM, Mogit AE. Surgical airway. In: Benumof JL, ed. *Airway Management Principles and Practice*. St. Louis: Mosby, Inc.; 1996:513-530.

31. Catterall W, Mackie K. Local anesthetics. In: Hardman JG, Limbird LE, Gilman AG, eds. *Goodman and Gilman's The Pharmacological Basis of Therapeutics*. 10th ed. New York: McGraw-Hill; 2001:367-384.

32. Milman N, Laub M, Munch EP, Angelo HR. Serum concentrations of lignocaine and its metabolite monoethylglycinexylidide during fibre-optic bronchoscopy in local anaesthesia. *Respir Med*. 1998;92:40-43.

33. Benowitz NL, Meister W. Clinical pharmacokinetics of lignocaine. *Clin Pharmacokinet*. 1978;3:177-1201

34. DiFazio CA. Local anesthetics: action, metabolism, and toxicity. *Otolaryngol Clin North Am*. 1981;14:515-519.

35. Xue FS, Liu HP, He N, et al. Spray-as-you-go airway topical anesthesia in patients with a difficult airway: a randomized, double-blind comparison of 2% and 4% lidocaine. *Anesth Analg*. 2009;108:536-543.

36. Boyes RN, Scott DB, Jebson PJ, et al. Pharmacokinetics of lidocaine in man. *Clin Pharmacol Ther*. 1971;12:105-116.

37. Morris IR. Airway anesthesia, sedation and awake intubation. *The Difficult Airway Course: Anesthesia Airway Course Manual*. 64-81.

38. Morris IR. Fibreoptic intubation. *Can J Anaesth*. 1994;41:996-1007; discussion 1007-1008.

39. Adriani J, Zepernick R, Arens J, Authement E. The comparative potency and effectiveness of topical anesthetics in man. *Clin Pharmacol Ther*. 1964;45:49-62.

40. Kirkpatrick MB. Lidocaine topical anesthesia for flexible bronchoscopy. *Chest*. 1989;96:965-967.

41. Walsh ME, Shorten GD. Preparing to perform an awake fiberoptic intubation. *Yale J Biol Med*. 1998;71:537-549.

42. Watanabe H, Lindgren L, Rosenberg P, Randell T. Glycopyrronium prolongs topical anaesthesia of oral mucosa and enhances absorption of lignocaine. *Br J Anaesth*. 1993;70:94-95.

43. Schonemann NK, van der Burght M, Arendt-Nielsen L, Bjerring P. Onset and duration of hypoalgesia of lidocaine spray applied to oral mucosa—a dose response study. *Acta Anaesthesiol Scand*. 1992;36:733-735.

44. Ovassapian A. The flexible bronchoscope. A tool for anesthesiologists. *Clin Chest Med*. 2001;22:281-299.

45. Schenck NL. Local anesthesia in otolaryngology. A re-evaluation. *Ann Otol Rhinol Laryngol*. 1975;84:65-72.

46. Efthimiou J, Higenbottam T, Holt D, Cochrane GM. Plasma concentrations of lignocaine during fibreoptic bronchoscopy. *Thorax*. 1982;37:68-71.

47. Wu FL, Razzaghi A, Souney PF. Seizure after lidocaine for bronchoscopy: case report and review of the use of lidocaine in airway anesthesia. *Pharmacotherapy*. 1993;13:72-78.

48. Parkes SB, Butler CS, Muller R. Plasma lignocaine concentration following nebulization for awake intubation. *Anaesth Intensive Care*. 1997;25:369-371.

49. Pelton DA, Daly M, Cooper PD, Conn AW. Plasma lidocaine concentrations following topical aerosol application to the trachea and bronchi. *Can Anaesth Soc J*. 1970;17:250-255.

50. Rosenberg PH, Heinonen J, Takasaki M. Lidocaine concentration in blood after topical anaesthesia of the upper respiratory tract. *Acta Anaesthesiol Scand*. 1980;24:125-128.

51. Scott DB, Littlewood DG, Covino BG, Drummond GB. Plasma lignocaine concentrations following endotracheal spraying with an aerosol. *Br J Anaesth*. 1976;48:899-902.

52. Adriani J, Campbell D. Fatalities following topical application of local anesthetics to mucous membranes. *JAMA*. 1956;162:1527-1530.

53. Loukides S, Katsoulis K, Tsarpalis K, et al. Serum concentrations of lignocaine before, during and after fiberoptic bronchoscopy. *Respiration*. 2000;67:13-17.

54. Williams KA, Barker GL, Harwood RJ, Woodall NM. Combined nebulization and spray-as-you-go topical local anaesthesia of the airway. *Br J Anaesth*. 2005;95:549-553.

55. Berde CB, Strichartz GR. Local anesthetics. In: Miller RD, ed. *Anesthesia*. 5th ed. Philadelphia, PA: Churchill Livingstone; 2000:494-521.

56. Kotaki H, Tayama N, Ito K, et al. Safe and effective topical application dose of lidocaine for surgery with laryngomicroscopy. *Clin Pharmacol Ther*. 1996;60:229-235.

57. Karvonen S, Jokinen K, Karvonen P, Hollmen A. Arterial and venous blood lidocaine concentrations after local anaesthesia of the respiratory tract using an ultrasonic nebulizer. *Acta Anaesthesiol Scand*. 1976;20:156-159.

58. Korttila K, Tarkkanen J, Tarkkanen L. Comparison of laryngotracheal and ultrasonic nebulizer administration of lidocaine in local anaesthesia for bronchoscopy. *Acta Anaesthesiol Scand*. 1981;25:161-165.

59. Burne D, Doughty A. Methaemoglobinaemia following lignocaine. *Lancet*. 1964;67:971.

60. Deas TC. Severe methemoglobinemia following dental extractions under lidocaine anesthesia. *Anesthesiology*. 1956;17:204.

61. Karim A, Ahmed S, Siddiqui R, Mattana J. Methemoglobinemia complicating topical lidocaine used during endoscopic procedures. *Am J Med*. 2001;111:150-153.

62. O'Donohue WJ, Jr., Moss LM, Angelillo VA. Acute methemoglobinemia induced by topical benzocaine and lidocaine. *Arch Intern Med*. 1980;140:1508-1509.

63. Rothrock SG, Green SM. Methemoglobinemia resulting from an unusual treatment for costochondritis. *J Emerg Med*. 1992;10:494-495.

64. Guay J. Methemoglobinemia related to local anesthetics: a summary of 242 episodes. *Anesth Analg*. 2009;108:837-845.

65. Donlon JVJ. Anesthetic management of patients with compromised airways. *Anesth Rev*. 1980;7:22-31.

66. Donlon JVJ. Anesthetic for eye, ear, nose and throat surgery. In: Miller RD, ed. *Anesthesia*. New York: Churchill Livingstone; 1981:1265-1321.

67. Donlon JVJ. Anesthesia for eye, ear, nose and throat surgery. In: Miller RD, ed. *Anesthesia*. 2nd ed. New York: Churchill Livingstone; 1986:1837-1894.

68. Reed AP. Preparation for intubation of the awake patient. *Mt Sinai J Med*. 1995;62:10-20.

69. Reed AP, Han DG. Preparation of the patient for awake fiberoptic intubation. *Anesth Clin North Am*. 1991;9:69-81.

70. Simmons ST, Schleich AR. Airway regional anesthesia for awake fiberoptic intubation. *Reg Anesth Pain Med*. 2002;27:180-192.

71. Jenkins SA, Marshall CF. Awake intubation made easy and acceptable. *Anaesth Intensive Care*. 2000;28:556-561.

72. Kundra P, Kutralam S, Ravishankar M. Local anaesthesia for awake fibreoptic nasotracheal intubation. *Acta Anaesthesiol Scand*. 2000;44:511-516.

73. Chinn WM, Zavala DC, Ambre J. Plasma levels of lidocaine following nebulized aerosol administration. *Chest*. 1977;71:346-348.

74. Bourke DL, Katz J, Tonneson A. Nebulized anesthesia for awake endotracheal intubation. *Anesthesiology*. 1985;63:690-692.

75. Chu SS, Rah KH, Brannan MD, Cohen JL. Plasma concentration of lidocaine after endotracheal spray. *Anesth Analg*. 1975;54:438-441.

76. Chan KN, Clay MM, Silverman M. Output characteristics of DeVilbiss No. 40 hand-held jet nebulizers. *Eur Respir J*. 1990;3:1197-1201.

77. Clay MM, Clarke SW. Wastage of drug from nebulisers: a review. *J R Soc Med*. 1987;80:38-39.

78. Mostafa SM, Murthy BV, Hodgson CA, Beese E. Nebulized 10% lignocaine for awake fibreoptic intubation. *Anaesth Intensive Care*. 1998;26:222-223.

79. Melby MJ, Raehl CL, Kruel JK. Pharmacokinetic evaluation of endotracheally administered lidocaine. *Clin Pharm*. 1986;5:228-231.

80. Curran J, Hamilton C, Taylor T. Topical analgesia before tracheal intubation. *Anaesthesia*. 1975;30:765-768.

81. Eyres RL, Bishop W, Oppenheim RC, Brown TC. Plasma lignocaine concentrations following topical laryngeal application. *Anaesth Intensive Care*. 1983;11:23-26.

82. Sutherland AD, Williams RT. Cardiovascular responses and lidocaine absorption in fiberoptic-assisted awake intubation. *Anesth Analg*. 1986;65:389-391.

83. Kirkpatrick MB, Sanders RV, Bass JB, Jr. Physiologic effects and serum lidocaine concentrations after inhalation of lidocaine from a compressed gas-powered jet nebulizer. *Am Rev Respir Dis*. 1987;136:447-449.

84. Wieczorek PM, Schricker T, Vinet B, Backman SB. Airway topicalisation in morbidly obese patients using atomised lidocaine: 2% compared with 4%. *Anaesthesia*. 2007;62:984-988.

85. Woodruff C, Wieczorek PM, Schricker T, et al. Atomised lidocaine for airway topical anaesthesia in the morbidly obese: 1% compared with 2% *Anaesthesia*. 2009.

86. Gomez F, Barrueco M, Lanao JM, et al. Serum lidocaine levels in patients undergoing fibrobronchoscopy. *Ther Drug Monit*. 1983;5:201-203.

87. Patterson JR, Blaschke TF, Hunt KK, Meffin PJ. Lidocaine blood concentrations during fiberoptic bronchoscopy. *Am Rev Respir Dis*. 1975;112:53-57.

88. Boye NP, Bredesen JE. Plasma concentrations of lidocaine during inhalation anaesthesia for fiberoptic bronchoscopy. *Scand J Respir Dis*. 1979;60:105-108.

89. Bigeleisen PE, Schisler JQ, Finucane BT. Plasma lidocaine levels following transtracheal injection during topical anesthesia of the upper airway. *Can J Anesth*. 1988;35:S95.

90. Reasoner DK, Warner DS, Todd MM, et al. A comparison of anesthetic techniques for awake intubation in neurosurgical patients. *J Neurosurg Anesthesiol*. 1995;7:94-99.

91. Langmack EL, Martin RJ, Pak J, Kraft M. Serum lidocaine concentrations in asthmatics undergoing research bronchoscopy. *Chest*. 2000;117:1055-1060.

92. Berger R, McConnell JW, Phillips B, Overman TL. Safety and efficacy of using high-dose topical and nebulized anesthesia to obtain endobronchial cultures. *Chest*. 1989;95:299-303.

93. Ameer B, Burlingame MB, Harman EM. Systemic absorption of topical lidocaine in elderly and young adults undergoing bronchoscopy. *Pharmacotherapy*. 1989;9:74-81.

94. Wentzel M. Death of a healthy college student volunteer in a research study. *Clin Trial Adv Newslet*. 1996;Supplement:1-26.

95. Martin KM, Larsen PD, Segal R, Marsland CP. Effective nonanatomical endoscopy training produces clinical airway endoscopy proficiency. *Anesth Analg*. 2004;99:938-944, table of contents.

96. Day RO, Chalmers DR, Williams KM, Campbell TJ. The death of a healthy volunteer in a human research project: implications for Australian clinical research. *Med J Aust*. 1998;168:449-451.

97. British Thoracic Society guidelines on diagnostic flexible bronchoscopy. *Thorax*. 2001;56(Suppl 1):i1-i21.

98. Wood-Baker R, Burdon J, McGregor A, et al. Fibre-optic bronchoscopy in adults: a position paper of The Thoracic Society of Australia and New Zealand. *Intern Med J*. 2001;31:479-487.

99. Gal TJ. Airway responses in normal subjects following topical anesthesia with ultrasonic aerosols of 4% lidocaine. *Anesth Analg*. 1980;59:123-129.

100. Grove RI, Wiggins J, Stableforth DE. A study of the use of ultrasonically nebulized lignocaine for local anaesthesia during fibreoptic bronchoscopy. *Br J Dis Chest*. 1985;79:49-59.

101. Kuna ST, Woodson GE, Sant'Ambrogio G. Effect of laryngeal anesthesia on pulmonary function testing in normal subjects. *Am Rev Respir Dis*. 1988;137:656-661.

102. Liistro G, Stanescu DC, Veriter C, et al. Upper airway anesthesia induces airflow limitation in awake humans. *Am Rev Respir Dis*. 1992;146:581-585.

103. Beydon L, Lorino AM, Verra F, et al. Topical upper airway anaesthesia with lidocaine increases airway resistance by impairing glottic function. *Intens Care Med*. 1995;21:920-926.

104. Weiss EB, Patwardhan AV. The response to lidocaine in bronchial asthma. *Chest*. 1977;72:429-438.

105. McAlpine LG, Thomson NC. Lidocaine-induced bronchoconstriction in asthmatic patients. Relation to histamine airway responsiveness and effect of preservative. *Chest*. 1989;96:1012-1015.

106. Groeben H, Schlicht M, Stieglitz S, et al. Both local anesthetics and salbutamol pretreatment affect reflex bronchoconstriction in volunteers with asthma undergoing awake fiberoptic intubation. Anesthesiology. 2002;97:1445-1450.

107. Ho AM, Chung DC, Karmakar MK, et al. Dynamic airflow limitation after topical anaesthesia of the upper airway. *Anaesth Intensive Care*. 2006;34:211-215.

108. Thomson NC. The effect of different pharmacological agents on respiratory reflexes in normal and asthmatic subjects. *Clin Sci (Lond)*. 1979;56:235-241.

109. Shaw IC, Welchew EA, Harrison BJ, Michael S. Complete airway obstruction during awake fibreoptic intubation. *Anaesthesia*. 1997;52:582-585.

110. McGuire G, el-Beheiry H. Complete upper airway obstruction during awake fibreoptic intubation in patients with unstable cervical spine fractures. *Can J Anaesth*. 1999;46:176-178.

111. Ho AM, Chung DC, To EW, Karmakar MK. Total airway obstruction during local anesthesia in a non-sedated patient with a compromised airway. *Can J Anaesth*. 2004;51:838-841.

112. Mason RA, Fielder CP. The obstructed airway in head and neck surgery. *Anaesthesia*. 1999;54:625-658.

113. Wong DT, McGuire GP. Management choices for the difficult airway (author reply). *Can J Anaesth*. 2003;50:624.

114. Weisel W, Tella RA. Reaction to tetracaine (pontocaine) used as topical anesthetic in bronchoscopy: study of 1,000 cases. *JAMA*. 1951;147:218-222.

115. Noorily AD, Noorily SH, Otto RA. Cocaine, lidocaine, tetracaine: which is best for topical nasal anesthesia? *Anesth Analg*. 1995;81:724-727.

116. Campbell D, Adriani J. Absorption of local anesthetics. *JAMA*. 1958;168:873-877.

117. Benumof JL. *Anesthesia for Thoracic Surgery*. Philadelphia, PA: WB Saunders Company; 1995.

118. Sanchez AF, Morrison DE. Preparation of the patient for awake intubation. In: Hagberg CA, ed. *Handbook of Difficult Airway Management*. Philadelphia, PA: Churchill Livingstone; 2000.

119. Drugdex System, Thompson Micromedex. Edited by Klesco RK. Colorado Healthcare Services, Volume 109. http://www.thompsonhc.com. Accessed December 9, 2009.

120. Morris IR. Pharmacologic aids to intubation and the rapid sequence induction. *Emerg Med Clin North Am*. 1988;6:753-768.

121. Donlon JVJ. Anesthesia for eye, ear, nose and throat surgery. In: Miller RD, ed. *Anesthesia*. 5th ed. Philadelphia, PA: Churchill Livingstone; 2000:2173-2298.

122. Lewin NA, Goldfrank LR, Hoffman RS. Cocaine. In: Goldfrank LR, Weisman RS, Flomenbaum NE, et al, eds. *Toxicologic Emergencies*. 5th ed. Norwalk: Appleton and Lange; 1994:847-862.

123. Gross JB, Hartigan ML, Schaffer DW. A suitable substitute for 4% cocaine before blind nasotracheal intubation: 3% lidocaine-0.25% phenylephrine nasal spray. *Anesth Analg*. 1984;63:15-18.

124. Katz RI, Hovagim AR, Finkelstein HS, et al. A comparison of cocaine, lidocaine with epinephrine, and oxymetazoline for prevention of epistaxis on nasotracheal intubation. *J Clin Anesth*. 1990;2:16-20.

125. Rector FT, DeNuccio DJ, Alden MA. A comparison of cocaine, oxymetazoline, and saline for nasotracheal intubation. *Aana J*. 1987;55:49-54.

126. Klesco RK. Drugdex System, Thompson Micromedex Expires 9/2001; Volume 109.

127. Nguyen ST, Cabrales RE, Bashour CA, et al. Benzocaine-induced methemoglobinemia. *Anesth Analg*. 2000;90:369-371.

128. Rinehart RS, Norman D. Suspected methemoglobinemia following awake intubation: one possible effect of benzocaine topical anesthesia—a case report. *AANA Journal*. 2003;71:117-118.

129. Kwok S, Fischer JL, Rogers JD. Benzocaine and lidocaine induced methemoglobinemia after bronchoscopy: a case report. *J Med Case Reports*. 2008;2:16.

130. Lin SK, Wu JL, Lee YL, Tsao SL. Methemoglobinemia induced by exposure to topical benzocaine for an awake nasal intubation—a case report. *Acta Anaesthesiol Taiwan*. 2007;45:111-116.

131. Gutta R, Louis PJ. Methemoglobinemia—an unusual cause of intraoperative hypoxia. *Oral Surg Oral Med Oral Pathol Oral Radiol Endod*. 2007;103:197-202.

132. White CD, Weiss LD. Varying presentations of methemoglobinemia: two cases. *J Emerg Med*. 1991;9(Suppl 1):45-49.

133. Byrne MF, Mitchell RM, Gerke H, et al. The need for caution with topical anesthesia during endoscopic procedures, as liberal use may result in methemoglobinemia. *J Clin Gastroenterol.* 2004;38:225-229.

134. Fitzsimons MG, Gaudette RR, Hurford WE. Critical rebound methemoglobinemia after methylene blue treatment: case report. *Pharmacotherapy.* 2004;24:538-540.

135. Rodriguez LF, Smolik LM, Zbehlik AJ. Benzocaine-induced methemoglobinemia: report of a severe reaction and review of the literature. *Ann Pharmacother.* 1994;28:643-649.

136. Basra SK, Vives MJ, Reilly MC, et al. Methemoglobinemia after fiberoptic intubation in a patient with an unstable cervical fracture: a case report. *J Spinal Disord Tech.* 2006;19:302-304.

137. Lunenfeld E, Kane GC. Methemoglobinemia: sudden dyspnea and oxyhemoglobin desaturation after esophagoduodenoscopy. *Respir Care.* 2004;49:940-942.

138. Mogos M, Thangathurai D, Roffey P, Tay C. Cetacaine-induced complication during transesophageal echocardiography placement. *J Cardiothorac Vasc Anesth.* Epub 2009 Aug 31.

139. Sandza JG, Jr., Roberts RW, Shaw RC, Connors JP. Symptomatic methemoglobinemia with a commonly used topical anesthetic, cetacaine. *Ann Thorac Surg.* 1980;30:187-190.

140. Ferraro L, Zeichner S, Greenblott G, Groeger JS. Cetacaine-induced acute methemoglobinemia. *Anesthesiology.* 1988;69:614-615.

141. Khan NA, Kruse JA. Methemoglobinemia induced by topical anesthesia: a case report and review. *Am J Med Sci.* 1999;318:415-418.

142. Seibert RW, Seibert JJ. Infantile methemoglobinemia induced by a topical anesthetic, Cetacaine. *Laryngoscope.* 1984;94:816-817.

143. Bacon GS, Lyons TR, Wood SH. Dyclonine hydrochloride for airway anesthesia: awake endotracheal intubation in a patient with suspected local anesthetic allergy. *Anesthesiology.* 1997;86:1206-1207.

144. Benumof JL. Upper airway obstruction. *Can J Anaesth.* 1999;46:906-907.

145. Larijani GE, Cypel D, Gratz I, et al. The efficacy and safety of EMLA cream for awake fiberoptic endotracheal intubation. *Anesth Analg.* 2000;91:1024-1026.

146. Sohmer B, Bryson GL, Bencze S, Scharf MM. EMLA cream is an effective topical anesthetic for bronchoscopy. *Can Respir J.* 2004;11:587-588.

147. Randell T, Yli-Hankala A, Valli H, Lindgren L. Topical anaesthesia of the nasal mucosa for fibreoptic airway endoscopy. *Br J Anaesth.* 1992;68:164-167.

148. Sutherland AD, Sale JP. Fibreoptic awake intubation—a method of topical anaesthesia and orotracheal intubation. *Can Anaesth Soc J.* 1986;33:502-504.

149. Graham DR, Hay JG, Clague J, et al. Comparison of three different methods used to achieve local anesthesia for fiberoptic bronchoscopy. *Chest.* 1992;102:704-707.

150. Sethi N, Tarneja VK, Houche S, Madhusudanan TP. Local anaesthesia for fiberoptic intubation: a comparison of three techniques. *MJAFI.* 2005;61:22-25.

151. Patil V, Barker GL, Harwood RJ, Woodall NM. Training course in local anaesthesia of the airway and fibreoptic intubation using course delegates as subjects. *Br J Anaesth.* 2002;89:586-593.

152. Chung DC, Mainland PA, Kong AS. Anesthesia of the airway by aspiration of lidocaine. *Can J Anaesth.* 1999;46:215-219.

153. Murphy TM. Somatic blockade of the head and neck. In: Cousins MJ, Bridenbaugh P, eds. *Nerual Blockade in Clinical Anesthesia and Management of Pain.* 3rd ed. Philadelphia, PA: Lippincott Raven; 1998:489-574.

154. Hannenberg AA. An atraumatic method for topical application of local anesthetics to the nasal mucosa. *Anesthesiology.* 1983;59:596-597.

155. Mitchell RL, DeNuccio DJ, Alden MA. A comparison of nasal spray with cocaine, lidocaine/phenylephrine and saline for nasal intubation. *Anesthesiology.* 1984;61:A217.

156. Bonica JJ. Transtracheal anesthesia for endotracheal intubation. *Anesthesiology.* 1949;10:736-738.

157. Danzl DF, Thomas DM. Nasotracheal intubations in the emergency department. *Crit Care Med.* 1980;8:677-682.

158. Duncan JA. Intubation of the trachea in the conscious patient. *Br J Anaesth.* 1977;49:619-623.

159. Thomas JL. Awake intubation. Indications, techniques and a review of 25 patients. *Anaesthesia.* 1969;24:28-35.

160. Gotta AW, Sullivan CA. Superior laryngeal nerve block: an aid to intubating the patient with fractured mandible. *J Trauma.* 1984;24:83-85.

161. Walts LF, Kassity KJ. Spread of local anesthesia after upper airway block. *Arch Otolaryngol.* 1965;81:77-79.

162. Boster SR, Danzl DF, Madden RJ, Jarboe CH. Translaryngeal absorption of lidocaine. *Ann Emerg Med.* 1982;11:461-465.

163. Antoniades N, Worsnop C. Topical lidocaine through the bronchoscope reduces cough rate during bronchoscopy. *Respirology.* 2009;14:873-876.

164. Webb AR, Fernando SS, Dalton HR, et al. Local anaesthesia for fibreoptic bronchoscopy: transcricoid injection or the "spray as you go" technique? *Thorax.* 1990;45:474-477.

165. Barton S, Williams JD. Glossopharyngeal nerve block. *Arch Otolaryngol.* 1971;93:186-188.

166. Bogdonoff DL, Stone DJ. Emergency management of the airway outside the operating room. *Can J Anaesth.* 1992;39:1069-1089.

167. DeMeester TR, Skinner DB, Evans RH, Benson DW. Local nerve block anesthesia for peroral endoscopy. *Ann Thorac Surg.* 1977;24:278-283.

168. Woods AM, Lander CJ. Abolition of gagging and the hemodynamic response to laryngoscopy. *Anesthesiology.* 1987;67:A220.

169. Cooper M, Watson RL. An improved regional anesthetic technique for peroral endoscopy. *Anesthesiology.* 1975;43:372-374.

170. Sitzman BT, Rich GF, Rockwell JJ, Leisure GS, Durieux ME, DiFazio CA. Local anesthetic administration for awake direct laryngoscopy. Are glossopharyngeal nerve blocks superior? *Anesthesiology.* 1997;86:34-40.

171. Benumof JL. Management of the difficult adult airway. With special emphasis on awake tracheal intubation. *Anesthesiology.* 1991;75:1087-1110.

172. Gotta AW, Sullivan CA. Anaesthesia of the upper airway using topical anaesthetic and superior laryngeal nerve block. *Br J Anaesth.* 1981;53:1055-1058.

173. Gaskill JR, Gillies DR. Local anesthesia for peroral endoscopy. Using superior laryngeal nerve block with topical application. *Arch Otolaryngol.* 1966;84:654-657.

174. Walts LF. Anesthesia of the larynx in the patient with a full stomach. *JAMA.* 1965;192:705-706.

175. Kopman AF, Wollman SB, Ross K, Surks SN. Awake endotracheal intubation: a review of 267 cases. *Anesth Analg.* 1975;54:323-327.

176. Meschino A, Devitt JH, Koch JP, Szalai JP, Schwartz ML. The safety of awake tracheal intubation in cervical spine injury. *Can J Anaesth.* 1992;39:114-117.

177. Ovassapian A, Krejcie TC, Yelich SJ, Dykes MH. Awake fibreoptic intubation in the patient at high risk of aspiration. *Br J Anaesth.* 1989;62:13-16.

178. Derbyshire DR, Smith G, Achola KJ. Effect of topical lignocaine on the sympathoadrenal responses to tracheal intubation. *Br J Anaesth.* 1987;59:300-304.

179. Telford RJ, Liban JB. Awake fibreoptic intubation. *Br J Hosp Med.* 1991;46:182-184.

180. Repchinsky C, ed. *Compendium of Pharmaceuticals and Specialties: The Canadian Drug Reference for Health Professionals.* Ottawa: Canadian Pharmacists Association; 2004:868-869.

181. McEvoy GK, Litvak K, Welsh OH, et al. Glycopyrrolate. In: *AHFS Drug Information.* Bethesda, MD: American Society of Health System Pharmacists Inc.; 2005:1243-1244.

182. Mirakhur RK, Dundee JW. Glycopyrrolate: pharmacology and clinical use. *Anaesthesia.* 1983;38:1195-1204.

183. Stoelting RK. *Pharmacology and Physiology in Anesthetic Practice.* Philadelphia, PA: JB Lippincott Company; 1991.

184. Bernstein CA, Waters JH, Torjman MC, Ritter D. Preoperative glycopyrrolate: oral, intramuscular, or intravenous administration. *J Clin Anesth.* 1996;8:515-518.

185. Cowl CT, Prakash UB, Kruger BR. The role of anticholinergics in bronchoscopy. A randomized clinical trial. *Chest.* 2000;118:188-192.

186. Roffe C, Smith MJ, Basran GS. Anticholinergic premedication for fibreoptic bronchoscopy. *Monaldi Arch Chest Dis.* 1994;49:101-106.

187. Malik JA, Gupta D, Agarwal AN, Jindal SK. Anticholinergic premedication for flexible bronchoscopy: a randomized, double-blind, placebo-controlled study of atropine and glycopyrrolate. *Chest.* 2009;136:347-354.

188. Brookman CA, Teh HP, Morrison LM. Anticholinergics improve fibreoptic intubating conditions during general anaesthesia. *Can J Anaesth.* 1997;44:165-167.

189. Marshall BE, Wollman H. General anesthetics. In: Goodman LS, Gilman A, eds. *The Pharmacological Basis of Therapeutics.* 6th ed. New York: MacMillan Publishing Company; 1980.

190. Merchant RN. Droperidol. *Canadian Anesthesiol Society Newslet.* 2002;4.

191. Unger RJ. Dexmedetomidine sedation for awake fiberoptic intubation. *Sem Anesth Periop Med Pain.* 2006;25:65-70.

192. Donaldson AB, Meyer-Witting M, Roux A. Awake fibreoptic intubation under remifentanil and propofol target-controlled infusion. *Anaesth Intens Care.* 2002;30:93-95.

193. Johnson KB, Swenson JD, Egan TD, Jarrett R, Johnson M. Midazolam and remifentanil by bolus injection for intensely stimulating procedures of brief duration: experience with awake laryngoscopy. *Anesth Analg.* 2002;94:1241-1243.

194. Machata AM, Gonano C, Holzer A, et al. Awake nasotracheal fiberoptic intubation: patient comfort, intubating conditions, and hemodynamic stability during conscious sedation with remifentanil. *Anesth Analg.* 2003;97:904-908.

195. Puchner W, Egger P, Puhringer F, Lökinger A, Obwegeser J, Gombotz H. Evaluation of remifentanil as single drug for awake fiberoptic intubation. *Acta Anaesthesiol Scand.* 2002;46:350-354.

196. Puchner W, Obwegeser J, Puhringer FK. Use of remifentanil for awake fiberoptic intubation in a morbidly obese patient with severe inflammation of the neck. *Acta Anaesthesiol Scand.* 2002;46:473-476.

197. Reusche MD, Egan TD. Remifentanil for conscious sedation and analgesia during awake fiberoptic tracheal intubation: a case report with pharmacokinetic simulations. *J Clin Anesth.* 1999; 11:64-68.

198. Xu Y, Xue F, Luo M, et al. Median effective dose of remifentanil for awake laryngoscopy and intubation. *Chinese Med J.* 2009;122:1507-1512.

199. Mingo OH, Ashpole KJ, Irving CJ, Rucklidge MW. Remifentanil sedation for awake fibreoptic intubation with limited application of local anaesthetic in patients for elective head and neck surgery. *Anaesthesia.* 2008;63:1065-1069.

200. Rai MR, Parry TM, Dombrovskis A, Warner OJ. Remifentanil target-controlled infusion vs propofol target-controlled infusion for conscious sedation for awake fibreoptic intubation: a double-blinded randomized controlled trial. *Br J Anaesth.* 2008;100:125-130.

201. Jhaveri R, Joshi P, Batenhorst R, et al. Dose comparison of remifentanil and alfentanil for loss of consciousness. *Anesthesiology.* 1997;87:253-259.

202. Wilhelm W, Biedler A, Hammadeh ME, et al. Remifentanil for oocyte retrieval: a new single-agent monitored anaesthesia care technique. *Anaesthesist.* 1999;48:698-704.

203. Carollo DS, Nossaman BD, Ramadhyani U. Dexmedetomidine: a review of clinical applications. *Curr Opin Anaesthesiol.* 2008;21:457-461.

204. Coursin DB, Maccioli GA. Dexmedetomidine. *Curr Opin Crit Care.* 2001;7:221-226.

205. Gerlach AT, Dasta JF. Dexmedetomidine: an updated review. *Ann Pharmacother.* 2007;41:245-252.

206. Grant SA, Breslin DS, MacLeod DB, et al. Dexmedetomidine infusion for sedation during fiberoptic intubation: a report of three cases. *J Clin Anesth.* 2004;16:124-126.

207. Hagberg CA, Abramson SI. A randomized, double-blind comparison of dexmedetomine and remifentanil for sedation during awake fiberoptic intubations. *J Clin Anesth.* 2007; 77-78, abstract.

208. Hall JE, Uhrich TD, Barney JA, et al. Sedative, amnestic, and analgesic properties of small-dose dexmedetomidine infusions. *Anesth Analg.* 2000;90:699-705.

209. Abdelmalak B, Makary L, Hoban J, Doyle DJ. Dexmedetomidine as sole sedative for awake intubation in management of the critical airway. *J Clin Anesth.* 2007;19:370-373.

210. Bergese SD, Khabiri B, Roberts WD, et al. Dexmedetomidine for conscious sedation in difficult awake fiberoptic intubation cases. *J Clin Anesth.* 2007;19:141-144.

211. Avitsian R, Lin J, Lotto M, Ebrahim Z. Dexmedetomidine and awake fiberoptic intubation for possible cervical spine myelopathy: a clinical series. *J Neurosurg Anesthesiol.* 2005;17:97-99.

212. Maroof M, Khan RM, Jain D, Ashraf M. Dexmedetomidine is a useful adjunct for awake intubation. *Can J Anaesth.* 2005;52:776-777.

213. Neumann MM, Davio MB, Macknet MR, Applegate RL, 2nd. Dexmedetomidine for awake fiberoptic intubation in a parturient with spinal muscular atrophy type III for cesarean delivery. *Int J Obstet Anesth.* 2009;18:403-407.

214. Scher CS, Gitlin MC. Dexmedetomidine and low-dose ketamine provide adequate sedation for awake fiberoptic intubation. *Can J Anaesth.* 2003;50:607-610.

215. Abramson SI, Holmes AA, Hagberg CA. Awake insertion of the Bonfils Retromolar Intubation Fiberscope in five patients with anticipated difficult airways. *Anesth Analg.* 2008;106:1215-1217, table of contents.

216. Dimitriou VK, Zogogiannis ID, Liotiri DG. Awake tracheal intubation using the Airtraq® laryngoscope: a case series. *Acta Anaesthesiol Scand.* 2009;53:964-967.

217. Lopez AM, Valero R, Pons M, Anglada T. Awake intubation using the LMA-CTrach in patients with difficult airways. *Anaesthesia.* 2009;64:387-391.

218. McGuire BE. Use of the McGrath® video laryngoscope in awake patients. *Anaesthesia.* 2009;64:912-914.

219. Suzuki A, Kunisawa T, Takahata O, Iwasaki H, Nozaki K, Henderson JJ. Pentax-AWS (airway scope) for awake tracheal intubation. *J Clin Anesth.* 2007;19:642-643.

SELF-EVALUATION QUESTIONS

3.1. The lower border of the quadrangular ligament forms

   A. the true vocal cord

   B. the false vocal cord

   C. the aryepiglottic ligament

   D. the triangular ligament

   E. the hyoepiglottic ligament

3.2. The maximum effective concentration of topical lidocaine applied to the tongue is

   A. 1%

   B. 2%

   C. 4%

   D. 10%

   E. 15%

3.3. Benzocaine

   A. is an ester

   B. is metabolized to para-aminobenzoic acid

   C. can produce methemoglobinemia

   D. is an effective topical anesthetic

   E. all of the above

CHAPTER (4)

Pharmacology of Intubation

Ronald B. George and Orlando R. Hung

4.1 PHYSIOLOGY OF TRACHEAL INTUBATION

4.1.1 What are the physiological responses to tracheal intubation?

The goal of tracheal intubation is to provide a secure, definitive airway. Unfortunately, laryngoscopy and intubation can result in a cascade of physiological and pathophysiological reflex responses. These responses are initiated by stimulation of afferent receptors in the posterior pharynx supplied by the glossopharyngeal and vagus nerves. The central nervous system (CNS), cardiovascular system, and respiratory system all respond predictably to these afferent stimuli, and in selected patients the resultant physiologic manifestations may adversely affect the patients' outcome. Though no data exist to suggest that patient outcomes are altered by attenuating the increases in intracranial pressure (ICP), stimulation of the autonomic nervous system with increases in the heart rate and blood pressure, and stimulation of the upper and lower respiratory tract resulting in increases in airway resistance, in light of the possible adverse effects in a compromised patient, it seems both reasonable and logical to attempt to attenuate these responses.

The CNS responds to airway manipulation by increasing cerebral metabolic oxygen demand ($CMRO_2$) and cerebral blood flow (CBF). If the intracranial compliance is decreased (tight brain), the increase in CBF may increase the ICP further. This response is important in situations in which there is a loss of autoregulation such that blood flow to the brain, or regions of the brain, becomes pressure-passive (ie, increases in blood pressure result in increases in ICP).

Laryngoscopy stimulates protective reflexes and predictably leads to cardiovascular and respiratory system responses mediated by the sympathetic nervous system. In children, this process is believed to be primarily a monosynaptic reflex promoting vagal stimulation of the sinoatrial node, resulting in bradycardia. In adults, a polysynaptic event predominates whereby impulses travel afferently via the 9th and 10th cranial nerves to the brain stem and spinal cord. An efferent sympathetic response results in norepinephrine release from adrenergic nerve terminals, epinephrine release from the adrenal glands, and activation of the renin–angiotensin system leading to tachycardia and hypertension. These responses may be detrimental in patients with myocardial ischemia (tight heart), known intracerebral or aortic aneurysms, major vessel dissection, or those with major vascular injuries. Hypertension may also lead to significant increases in ICP if autoregulation has been lost (eg, acute severe head injury or intracranial hemorrhage).

The respiratory system may respond in three important ways to laryngoscopy and intubation: activation of the upper airway reflexes leading to laryngospasm; coughing; and bronchospasm (tight lungs). Laryngospasm, a forceful involuntary spasm of the laryngeal musculature, may produce difficulty with intubation as well as ventilation. Persistent and life-threatening laryngospasm is treated with a gentle continuous positive airway pressure with 100% oxygen, intravenous lidocaine (1.5 mg·kg^{-1}), or if persistent, neuromuscular blockade (eg, succinylcholine at 10% of the intubating dose). Negative intrathoracic pressure created by inspiration attempts against a closed glottis (laryngospasm) may result in negative pressure pulmonary edema (see Chapter 58).

Coughing may produce significant adverse effects in patients with increased ICP, unstable cervical spine injury, or penetrating eye injuries.

Activation of the lower airway reflexes leads to an increase in airway resistance. This reaction is most often manifested by bronchospasm brought about by reflexes, irritants, or antigens, and may be mitigated in adults by the intravenous administration of lidocaine 1.5 mg·kg⁻¹.

Whether mitigation of these reflexes improves patient outcome is not known. However, it is known that specific prelaryngoscopy therapy is capable of mitigating these potentially harmful physiologic effects. The useful agents are most easily remembered by the mnemonic *LOAD*, which stands for *L*idocaine, *O*pioid, *A*tropine, and *D*efasciculating agent. Current evidence is most compelling for the use of lidocaine and opioids, and much less so for atropine and defasciculating doses of nondepolarizing agents.

This chapter provides a general discussion of the appropriate pharmacological agents used in airway management and their relevant properties. It should be emphasized that the goal of this chapter is not to discuss the rationale of using a specific sedative or muscle relaxant in an anticipated difficult airway. Rather, this discussion will center on the use of drugs to facilitate tracheal intubation and mitigate adverse physiological consequences.

4.2   PRETREATMENT AGENTS USING THE *LOAD* APPROACH

4.2.1   What is the LOAD approach and why do we use it?

Prelaryngoscopy agents, also known as "pretreatment agents," are used to attenuate the adverse physiologic responses to laryngoscopy and intubation. LOAD is a mnemonic that might be used to enhance recall of the commonly used pretreatment medications: *L*idocaine, *O*pioids, *A*tropine, and *D*efasciculating agents. Ideally, all pretreatment agents should be administered shortly before (typically about 3 minutes) induction to synchronize the onset of peak drug effects of all drugs administered in the airway management sequence.

While short-acting beta blockers, such as esmolol, have been shown to be beneficial in attenuating the sympathetic response to laryngoscopy,[1] they are not effective in attenuating to any extent a rise in ICP. They potentially increase airway resistance, especially in patients with reactive airways disease. Furthermore, beta blockers are also negative inotropes and in some clinical situations, particularly emergencies in which maximum cardiac reserve should be preserved, the combination of beta blockers and the negative cardiovascular effects of most induction agents could be catastrophic.

4.2.2   What is the rationale of using lidocaine for tracheal intubation?

Local anesthetics bind to closed, inactivated sodium channels and prevent subsequent channel activation. Sodium channels in the closed inactivated state are not permeable to sodium and therefore action potentials cannot be generated. Local anesthetic agents are a combination of a lipophilic benzene ring and a hydrophilic amine either linked by an amide or an ester bridge. Lidocaine is a low-potency, rapid-onset, and intermediate-acting amide local anesthetic. The literature is replete with articles that offer varying conclusions as to the efficacy of lidocaine when used in the pretreatment phase of tracheal intubation to attenuate various adverse effects of laryngoscopy and intubation.

Attenuation of the elevation of ICP related to airway manipulation is ascribed to lidocaine's ability to increase the depth of anesthesia, decrease $CMRO_2$ demand globally, decrease CBF, and increase cerebrovascular resistance. Patients with intracranial pathology may have an abnormal intracranial pressure–volume relationship which can predispose them to abrupt, extreme, and prolonged elevations of ICP. Such increases can contribute to secondary injury of the brain, such as herniation of the brain and impaired perfusion leading to ischemia. Indirect evidence exists that lidocaine can attenuate the intracranial hypertensive response to laryngoscopy and intubation. For instance, intracranial hypertension associated with endotracheal suctioning is suppressed by intravenous lidocaine.[2-5] Intratracheal lidocaine is equally effective.[4] Lidocaine (1.5 mg·kg⁻¹) administered 3 minutes before intubation suppresses the cough reflex and attenuates the increase in airway resistance resulting from laryngoscopy and endotracheal intubation.

Lidocaine's effect on antigenic-mediated bronchospasm is more controversial. Lidocaine and other local anesthetics may lead to bronchoconstriction in patients with reactive airway disease when given via the inhalational route[6] (see Chapter 3 for a full discussion of this evidence). In normal individuals, lidocaine does not alter airways resistance, and has been shown to produce mild bronchodilation.[7] Groeben et al[8-10] in three similar trials showed that intravenous lidocaine attenuated the response to an inhalational histamine challenge in patients with mild asthma. The inhalational administration of lidocaine to such patients, however, was met with short-lived initial increases in airway resistance.[10] Intravenous lidocaine but not inhalational lidocaine seems appropriate for the attenuation of the bronchoconstrictive response to upper airway manipulation and tracheal intubation. Lidocaine (1.5 mg·kg⁻¹) 3 minutes before induction is advocated for patients with reactive airway disease (ie, tight lungs) or elevated ICP (ie, tight brains). Lidocaine has a wide safety margin, particularly at a dose of 1.5 mg·kg⁻¹. The primary toxic effect is the development of seizures, which usually occurs at much higher doses.

4.2.3   Why do we use opioids prior to tracheal intubation?

Opium, derived from the seeds of the poppy (*Papaver somniferum*), is composed of more than 20 alkaloids, some of which serve as the foundation molecules for modern opioids. A German pharmacist isolated the first alkaloid from opium in 1806 and named it morphine after the Greek god of dreams, Morpheus.[11] A broad definition of the term "opioid" includes all drugs, synthetic and natural, which interact with opioid receptors, whether endogenous, exogenous, agonist, or antagonists. Opioids are routinely employed during an anesthetic induction and with the advent of newer, more rapid-acting agents, such as remifentanil, they continue to play a role in airway management.

TABLE 4-1

Pharmacokinetics of Opioids in Clinical Use[11]

	MORPHINE	FENTANYL	SUFENTANIL	REMIFENTANIL
pK_a	7.9	8.4	8	7.2
% Ionization	23	8.5	20	58
% Protein bound	35	84	90	66
Rapid Redistribution-$t_{\frac{1}{2}\pi}$ (min)		1.2-1.9	1.4	0.4-0.5
Redistribution-$t_{\frac{1}{2}\alpha}$ (min)	1.5-4.4	9.2-19	17	2-3.7
Elimination-$t_{\frac{1}{2}\beta}$ (h)	1.7-3.3	3.6-6.6	2.2-4.1	0.17-0.33

Opioids act throughout the nervous system, including the dorsal horn of the spinal cord (substantia gelatinosa), periaqueductal gray matter, and in the periphery. They inhibit presynaptic release and postsynaptic response to excitatory neurotransmitters such as acetylcholine (ACh) and substance P by altering the potassium and calcium conductance.[11] As such, they are useful in attenuating adverse responses to airway manipulation in patients with *tight brains* and *tight hearts*.

Although highly selective, opioid effects typically involve complex interactions among various receptor sites. The list of opioid receptors continues to expand. Mu (μ), kappa (κ), and delta (δ) receptor classes and their subtypes have been firmly established.[12] Most clinically useful opioids are highly selective μ agonists, which are responsible for the bulk of supraspinal and spinal analgesia.

Opioids are typically of low molecular weight but vary widely in their lipid solubility, percent of ionization, and degree of binding to proteins (Table 4-1). Commonly used opioids for induction (fentanyl, sufentanil, and remifentanil) are more lipid soluble, which accounts for their speed of onset of action. Redistribution is responsible for the termination of their CNS drug action. Metabolism of most opioids occurs through a two-stage hepatic process that generally results in an inactive metabolite. The exception is remifentanil, which contains an ester linkage and is rapidly hydrolyzed by nonspecific esterases in the blood and tissue.

Physiologically, opioids exert their effect on all organ systems. Venodilation and depressed sympathetic reflexes typically result in a decrease in heart rate and blood pressure. Unlike some opioids (most notably morphine) fentanyl, sufentanil, and remifentanil do not release histamine. This is partly why they cause less hypotension than morphine. All opioids depress ventilation by blunting the carbon dioxide response at the respiratory center, raising the apneic threshold and depressing the slope of the CO_2 response curve.

The primary reason to include an opioid in the intubation sequence is their ability to significantly attenuate the sympathetic response that occurs with manipulation of the airway. Unfortunately, the rapid administration of fentanyl and its derivatives has been associated with brief episodes of coughing and chest wall rigidity.[13-15] Large induction doses of an opioid can decrease pulmonary compliance in 50% to 86% of patients and potentially induce glottic closure interfering with ventilation of the patient.[13-16] Doses of this magnitude are seldom if ever employed in emergency airway management, in or out of the operating room (OR).

4.2.4   What types of opioids are commonly used for tracheal intubation?

The hemodynamic and intracranial responses to tracheal intubation are usually short lived. Therefore, the *ideal* choice of an opioid for tracheal intubation should be based on its pharmacokinetic and pharmacodynamic characteristics, namely, a rapid onset and a brief duration of drug effect. While there are currently many opioids available, the following discussion will be restricted to only those opioids with a rapid onset and short duration of drug effect.

4.2.4.1   Fentanyl

Like meperidine, fentanyl is a phenylpiperidine-derived synthetic opioid agonist. It is roughly 100 times more potent than morphine. Fentanyl in large doses (10-30 $\mu g \cdot kg^{-1}$) causes chest wall rigidity in 35% to 85% of patients.[13,15,17] This side effect is present in all age groups.[18] Rigidity is a unique and idiosyncratic response to opioids and is probably related to the dose and speed of administration. Although the exact mechanism is unknown, an animal study demonstrated opioid-induced muscle rigidity coincident with activation of central μ-receptors.[19] Others have suggested mechanisms involving the cerulospinal noradrenergic system[20,21] and the neurochemical system affected in Parkinson disease.[22]

Tagaito et al[23] found that increasing doses of fentanyl reduced the incidence of respiratory and laryngeal responses to laryngeal irritation under propofol anesthesia. Fentanyl is a short-acting opioid owing to redistribution of the drug, although accumulation with repeated dosing can limit its use. Peak drug effect occurs 3 to 5 minutes following intravenous administration with an equilibration half-time between the plasma and brain of 5 minutes.[24] Doses recommended for attenuating the adverse effects of airway manipulation range from 1 to 4 $\mu g \cdot kg^{-1}$. One must be prepared to treat dose-related hypotension and respiratory depression that may occur with fentanyl administration.

4.2.4.2   Sufentanil

A thienyl derivative of fentanyl, sufentanil is 10 to 15 times more potent than fentanyl. Sufentanil is a highly specific μ agonist with similar pharmacokinetic properties as fentanyl. It is extremely lipophilic, permitting rapid penetration of the blood–brain barrier and onset of CNS effects. Sufentanil 0.3 to 1 $\mu g \cdot kg^{-1}$, administered 1 to 3 minutes prior to intubation, will blunt the response to laryngoscopy. Rigidity has been reported with larger doses.[17] The difficult ventilation associated with opioid rigidity may be due in part to vocal cord closure.[14,16]

4.2.4.3   Remifentanil

Remifentanil is a structurally unique opioid. It is a piperdine analog with a methyl ester side chain. The ester linkage renders it susceptible to cleavage by nonspecific plasma and tissue esterases.[25] The rapid metabolism of remifentanil, rather than redistribution, is responsible for its ultrashort duration of action; and with limited redistribution, there is no accumulation. It is rapidly cleared from the plasma (3 L·min^{-1}).[17] Remifentanil is not, however, a substrate for pseudocholinesterase and therefore it is unaffected by pseudocholinesterase deficiency.

Remifentanil is a potent μ receptor agonist with a similar potency to fentanyl. Doses of 0.25 to 3 μg·kg^{-1} have successfully attenuated the response to laryngoscopy.[26-31] At higher doses, centrally mediated depression of sympathetic tone and vagally induced bradycardia may occur. This bradycardia can be attenuated by the prior administration of glycopyrrolate or other antimuscarinics.[11] Peak respiratory depression occurs 5 minutes after bolus dosing, and lasts 10 minutes after 1.5 μg·kg^{-1} and 20 minutes after 2 μg·kg^{-1}.[32] Remifentanil, like other opioids, may cause chest wall rigidity depending on the dose and speed of administration.[33]

The clinical utility of remifentanil is reflected in its distinctive pharmacokinetic characteristics. Its rapid onset, brief duration, and easily titratable nature have enhanced its profile for airway management, particularly in emergency settings, and for short surgical procedures. A small dose of remifentanil (0.25 μg·kg^{-1}) can provide excellent conditions for laryngeal mask airway insertion with minimal hemodynamic disturbance.[34] The trachea may be successfully intubated without muscle relaxants with the combination of remifentanil and an induction agent. Remifentanil, 2 to 4 μg·kg^{-1}, in this setting, provides good to excellent intubating conditions.[28,35-37]

Suppression of airway reflexes while maintaining patient comfort without compromising spontaneous ventilation for awake tracheal intubation is possible with remifentanil via continuous infusion (0.07-0.25 μg·kg^{-1}·min^{-1}).[38-40] Puchner et al[41] successfully used remifentanil, 0.07 μg·kg^{-1}·min^{-1}, for procedural sedation in a case of severe neck swelling in a morbidly obese patient with no alternative to awake bronchoscopic intubation. Similarly, in cases of head and neck surgery where a tenuous airway needs to be maintained, remifentanil allows a high degree of titratability with high rates of success.[42]

4.2.5   What is the role of atropine (or other antimuscarinic) administration prior to tracheal intubation?

Vagally mediated, succinylcholine-induced bradycardia may be seen in children. Bradycardia can be attenuated or abolished by administering atropine 0.02 mg·kg^{-1} or glycopyrrolate 0.01 mg·kg^{-1} [43] as pretreatment before administering succinylcholine. However, there is no evidence that pretreatment with an antimuscarinic in children is any more effective than responsive therapy in the event bradycardia occurs. The age after which this response to succinylcholine

disappears is unknown. Regardless of the age, *repeated doses* of succinylcholine may produce vagally mediated bradycardia, necessitating the administration of an antimuscarinic.

Unlike the natural derivatives of *Atropa belladonna*, atropine and scopolamine, glycopyrrolate is a synthetic, quaternary ammonium antimuscarinic agent. Because of its polar nature, glycopyrrolate is unable to cross the blood–brain barrier, and so is devoid of CNS activity. It is a potent antisialagogue with minimal sedating properties, which makes glycopyrrolate a useful pretreatment medication. Glycopyrrolate increases the heart rate in a manner similar to atropine with an onset of effect in 2 minutes, lasting 30 to 60 minutes.[44] Typically, increases in the heart rate following glycopyrrolate administration are more gradual than those with atropine, thereby avoiding a rapid tachycardia that may be a particular concern in patients with cardiovascular disease.

4.2.6   Why do we use defasciculating agents for tracheal intubation?

Fasciculations are involuntary muscle contractions. Practically, all patients who receive succinylcholine will experience fasciculations. Fasciculations have been associated with an increase in catecholamine release and elevations of ICP. Small doses of nondepolarizing muscle relaxants (NDMRs), such as vecuronium, rocuronium, and pancuronium, when administered prior to succinylcholine have been clearly shown to decrease the incidence of succinylcholine-induced fasciculations.[45-50]

Arguably, their greatest benefit is in mitigating the increase in ICP caused by succinylcholine. The appropriate defasciculating dose for any of the NDMRs is 10% of their ED$_{95}$. Typically, the suggested intubating dose is twice the ED$_{95}$. Therefore, the defasciculating dose would be approximately 5% of the intubating dose of the NDMRs. The use of higher doses will increase the incidence of muscle weakness and apnea prior to the induction of anesthesia. When used as a defasciculating agent, rocuronium 0.06 mg·kg^{-1} should be administered 1.5 to 3 minutes prior to succinylcholine.[51]

4.3   INDUCTION AGENTS

The ideal induction agent would quickly render the patient unconscious, unresponsive, and amnesic in one arm/heart/brain circulation time. Such an agent would also provide analgesia, maintain stable cerebral perfusion pressure (CPP) and cardiovascular hemodynamics, be immediately reversible, and have few, if any, adverse side effects. Unfortunately, such an induction agent does not exist.

Most induction agents are highly lipophilic, and therefore have a rapid onset of effect within 30 to 45 seconds of intravenous administration. Their clinical effect is likewise terminated quickly as the drug rapidly redistributes from the CNS to less well-perfused tissues. All induction agents have the potential to cause myocardial depression and hypotension. These effects depend on the particular drug and the patient's underlying physiologic condition. The faster the drug is administered, the larger the amount of the drug that will be delivered to those organs with the greatest blood flow (such as the brain and heart) and the more pronounced the effect. The choice of drug and the dose must be individualized to each patient to capitalize on desired effects, while minimizing adverse effects.

Anesthetic induction is intended to rapidly render the patient unable to appreciate, respond to, or recall noxious stimuli. It is at one end of a spectrum that runs from awake, alert, and oriented at one end to deep anesthesia and death on the other.

The induction agents include short-acting barbiturates: thiopental and methohexital; benzodiazepines: principally midazolam; and miscellaneous agents: etomidate, ketamine, and propofol. Opioids can function as anesthetic induction agents when used in very large doses (eg, fentanyl 30 $\mu g \cdot kg^{-1}$) but are rarely, if ever, used for that purpose during routine or emergency intubation, so will not be discussed in this chapter.

All of the induction agents discussed in this chapter share similar pharmacokinetic characteristics. As mentioned previously, they are highly lipophilic, and therefore a standard induction dose of an induction agent administered to a euvolemic, normotensive patient will take effect within 30 seconds. The duration of observed clinical effect of each drug is measured in minutes and is due to the redistribution of the drug from the central circulation (brain) to larger, but less well-perfused tissues, for example, fat and muscle. The elimination half-life ($t_{1/2\beta}$, usually measured in hours) is characterized by each drug's reentry from fat and lean muscle into plasma down a concentration gradient followed by hepatic metabolism which precedes renal excretion. Generally it requires four to five elimination half-lives to clear the drug completely from the body.

Because the target organ is the brain, and the desired effect is produced rapidly following bolus injection of the drug, dosing of induction agents in normal-sized and obese adults should be based on ideal body weight in kilograms. Hypovolemia results in the patient having a contracted central compartment; therefore, lower doses of induction agents are necessary to achieve adequate levels at the target organ (brain). Aging affects the pharmacokinetics of induction agents. In older adults, lean body mass and total body water decrease while total body fat increases, resulting in an increased volume of distribution, an increase in $t_{1/2\beta}$, and an increased duration of drug effect. Older adults are also much more sensitive to the hemodynamic and respiratory depressant effects of these agents, and consequently, most induction doses should be reduced.

4.3.1　Barbiturates

4.3.1.1　Discuss the Different Types of Barbiturate Induction Agents

Barbiturates are derived from barbituric acid, a cyclic compound obtained by the combination of urea and malonic acid. They are prepared as water-soluble, alkaline (2.5% solution with pH >10) sodium salts that are dissolved in isotonic saline or water. These agents act at the barbiturate receptor, which forms part of the GABA-receptor complex to enhance and mimic the action of GABA. Thiopental decreases GABA dissociation from its receptor, which enhances GABA's neuroinhibitory activity, directly opens the chloride channel, and, at higher drug concentrations, causes hyper-polarization of this chloride channel resulting in

global depression of neuronal excitation and subsequent unconsciousness. The most commonly used barbiturates are thiopental and methohexital.

Thiopental is the prototypical barbiturate. It is highly lipid soluble and highly protein bound. Thiopental undergoes hepatic oxidation to hydroxythiopental and carboxylic acid derivatives, which are water soluble and excreted via the kidney. Methohexital shares similar clinical pharmacologic properties with thiopental although it is significantly less lipid soluble and is two to three times more potent than thiopental. The elimination of methohexital is three to four times faster than thiopental.[52]

4.3.1.2　What Are the Indications and Contraindications of Barbiturate Induction Agents?

Barbiturates are primarily used as an induction agent for patients suspected of having increased ICP. Their ability to decrease ICP stems from the cerebral vasoconstriction and subsequent decrease in CBF. The decreased systemic vascular resistance is not matched by the decreased CBF and so cerebral perfusion pressure (CPP) is maintained and possibly increased.[53] Barbiturates remain a mainstay of intravenous cerebroprotective measures despite limited outcome data.[54-57]

Barbiturates have significant anticonvulsant activities in addition to their cerebroprotective properties.[58] Methohexital is often used in those patients undergoing electroconvulsive therapy (ECT) because of its desirable rapid onset of amnesia and short duration of action. While methohexital is often preferred over thiopental for ECT because of longer seizure activities, the clinical efficacy of ECT does not appear to correlate with the duration of seizure activity.[59] Thiopental and other barbiturates are absolutely contraindicated in patients with acute intermittent porphyria, or variegate porphyria, as they can activate the enzyme responsible for precipitating an acute attack, which can be life threatening.

4.3.1.3　What Are the Clinical Doses of Barbiturate Induction Agents?

The dosing of thiopental depends on the hemodynamic status of the patient and the concomitant use of other agents. Apart from stimulating the release of histamine from mast cells, thiopental is a potent venodilator and myocardial depressant.[60,61] Consequently, the dose must be decreased in patients with decreased intravascular volume, those with compromised myocardial function, elderly adults, and whenever thiopental is used with other drugs that affect sympathetic tone or cardiovascular function. In euvolemic, normotensive adults, a recommended induction dose of thiopental is 3 to 5 $mg \cdot kg^{-1}$. For most emergency intubations, the lower dose of this range (3 $mg \cdot kg^{-1}$) achieves excellent sedation and intubating conditions with fewer tendencies to cause hypotension that often occurs with the 5 $mg \cdot kg^{-1}$ dose. Thiopental should be avoided entirely in severely hypotensive patients for whom other drugs, especially etomidate or ketamine, may preserve greater hemodynamic stability. The onset of methohexital is more rapid and the duration of action shorter than it is with thiopental. The recommended induction dose of methohexital in the euvolemic, normotensive patient is 1.5 $mg \cdot kg^{-1}$.

4.3.1.4   What Are the Common Side Effects of Barbiturates?

The chief side effects of thiopental include central respiratory depression, venodilation, and myocardial depression. These last two may produce hypotension that tends to be greater in treated, and untreated, hypertensive patients compared with normotensive patients. Both of these effects may be detrimental in patients where optimal preload is required to maintain cardiac output and prevent organ ischemia. Thiopental causes a dose-related release of histamine (anaphylactoid response) which in most situations is not clinically significant, but may exacerbate hypotension or bronchospasm in patients with reactive airways disease.[61] Although barbiturates produce dose-dependent depression of ventilation centers, they do not completely blunt airway reflexes.[62]

There is a 10% to 20% incidence of nausea and vomiting that occurs during recovery from a barbiturate induction. Two to five percent of patients will experience pain on injection of thiopental or methohexital, especially if small veins are used. Inadvertent intra-arterial injection or subcutaneous extravasation of thiopental can result in chemical endarteritis and distal thrombosis, ischemia, and tissue necrosis. Methohexital has a greater incidence than thiopental of twitching and hiccups (excitatory phenomena) that may be misdiagnosed as seizures.[63]

4.3.2   Benzodiazepines

4.3.2.1   Discuss the Clinical Pharmacology of Benzodiazepines

Although chemically distinct from the barbiturates, the benzodiazepines also exert their effects via the GABA-receptor complex. Benzodiazepines specifically facilitate the binding of GABA to the benzodiazepine receptor, which in turn modulates chloride conduction, inhibiting neuronal function. The benzodiazepines provide amnesia, anxiolysis, sedation, anticonvulsant effects, and hypnosis (sleep). This potent, dose-related amnesic property is perhaps their greatest asset.

Benzodiazepines generally contain a benzene and diazepine ring. All have similar pharmacologic profiles, though various substitutions in the ring structures make each agent pharmacologically unique and their clinical usefulness variable. The lipophilicity of the benzodiazepines varies widely. Greater lipid solubility confers a more rapid onset of action because of the brain's high lipid content. The two benzodiazepines most clinically used during airway manipulation are midazolam and diazepam. Of the two, midazolam is the most lipid soluble. Although midazolam is prepared as a water-soluble agent in acidic aqueous medium, the imdazole ring structure closes at physiological pH greatly increasing the lipid solubility. Many studies have shown that the onset of effect is slower for midazolam than diazepam.[64] Regardless, the time to clinical effectiveness of benzodiazepines is longer than any of the other induction agents, which hinders their role in emergency airway management. The termination of action of midazolam and diazepam is due to redistribution and subsequent hepatic metabolism via cytochrome P450 to 3A4 microsomal oxidation. The innate structure of each parent compound determines the precise mechanism of hepatic degradation, and the production of active or inactive metabolites, both of which will dictate the eventual elimination half-life ($t_{1/2\beta}$) of each drug. Midazolam has one insignificant active metabolite and a $t_{1/2elim}$ of 2 to 4 hours. Diazepam has two active metabolites, both of which can prolong its sedative effect but more importantly are metabolized and excreted more slowly than diazepam and account for its prolonged $t_{1/2\beta}$ of 20 to 40 hours. The benzodiazepines do not release histamine, and allergic reactions are very rare.

4.3.2.2   What Are the Clinical Uses and Adverse Effects of Benzodiazepines?

The primary indications for benzodiazepines are anxiolysis, amnesia, and sedation. In this regard, the benzodiazepines are unparalleled. Midazolam is primarily used for procedural sedation, anxiolysis, and seizure management. Because of their dose-related reduction in systemic vascular resistance and direct myocardial depression, dosage must be adjusted in volume-depleted or hemodynamically compromised patients. Unlike the other induction agents, including those that cause hypotension, midazolam is generally underdosed during emergency induction. It is postulated that this is due to the clinicians' familiarity with sedating doses of midazolam employed during procedural sedation and lack of familiarity with the dosing and pharmacokinetics of midazolam as an induction agent.

The dose of midazolam for induction of anesthesia is 0.1 to 0.3 mg·kg^{-1}. Berggren and Eriksson[65] prospectively demonstrated that midazolam 0.4 mg·kg^{-1} provided anesthetic depth similar to that of thiopental 6 mg·kg^{-1} in 60 female patients undergoing induction for elective abortion. Driessen et al[66] found that 0.2 mg·kg^{-1} midazolam and 5 mg·kg^{-1} thiopental provided similar depth of anesthesia in 40 women undergoing outpatient anesthesia. Jensen et al[67] found similar results using 0.2 mg·kg^{-1} midazolam versus 3 mg·kg^{-1} of thiopental for 40 orthopedic surgeries and Izuora et al[68] found 0.15 to 0.2 mg·kg^{-1} midazolam comparable to thiopental 4 to 6 mg·kg^{-1} in 145 patients undergoing surgical procedures. Interestingly, Sagarin et al[69] recently demonstrated that most emergency intubations are performed using midazolam doses in the range of 0.03 to 0.04 mg·kg^{-1}. The lower dosing appears to be due to the inexperience with the larger doses of midazolam used for induction or the concern that hypotension may ensue. Other induction agents, including thiopental and etomidate, were used in recommended doses.[69]

Except for midazolam, the benzodiazepines are insoluble in water and are usually supplied in a propylene glycol solution. Unless injected into a large vein, pain and venous irritation on injection can be significant.

4.3.3   Etomidate

4.3.3.1   Discuss the Clinical Pharmacology of Etomidate

Etomidate is a carboxylated imidazole derivative that is primarily an intravenous hypnotic agent used for the rapid induction of anesthesia. It is available in a 0.2% solution dissolved in 35%

propylene glycol. It inhibits the reticular activating system, mimicking GABA at the GABA-receptor complex. Etomidate owes its rapid onset to its high lipid solubility and large nonionized portion at physiological pH (pK_a = 4.2).[17] Its rapid redistribution leads to prompt awaking following administration. The elimination half-life of etomidate is 2 to 5 hours. It is rapidly hydrolyzed by hepatic metabolism and plasma esterases to water-soluble inactive metabolites excreted primarily by the kidneys.

Etomidate is a potent direct cerebral vasoconstrictor.[70] It attenuates underlying elevated ICP by decreasing CBF and $CMRO_2$. Its hemodynamic stability preserves CPP. The use of etomidate in patients with seizure disorders ought to be limited to the induction of anesthesia and not its maintenance. Etomidate has been shown to increase electroencephalographic activity in certain leads[71] and is less effective than other agents in attenuating the motor activity associated with seizures.[72]

The respiratory system may be centrally stimulated by etomidate, so administration is not usually associated with apnea unless opioids are coadministered.[17,73] Etomidate lacks any direct bronchodilatory properties. Eames et al[62] prospectively demonstrated that 2.5 mg·kg⁻¹ of propofol was superior to either 0.4 mg·kg⁻¹ etomidate or 5 mg·kg⁻¹ thiopental in decreasing mean airway pressure during bronchoscopy in 75 patients.

Etomidate is touted as *the* most hemodynamically stable induction agent.[74-76] It mildly decreases the systemic vascular resistance but appears to have no direct effect on cardiac output or contractility. Gauss et al[77] conducted an echocardiographic assessment of the hemodynamics of various induction agents and showed that etomidate produced no changes in the hemodynamic variables measured.

4.3.3.2   What Is the Role of Etomidate as an Induction Agent for Tracheal Intubation?

Etomidate is becoming the induction agent of choice for most emergency rapid-sequence inductions (RSI) because of its rapid onset, its profound hemodynamic stability, its positive CNS profile, and its rapid recovery. As with any induction agent, dosage must be adjusted in hemodynamically compromised patients. The use of etomidate to facilitate airway management in the patient with status epilepticus is not contraindicated, as it does depress the level of consciousness, and long-term medication with benzodiazepines or propofol ordinarily follows the intubation.

In euvolemic and hemodynamically stable patients, the normal induction dose of etomidate is 0.2 to 0.4 mg·kg⁻¹. In compromised patients, the induction dose should be reduced commensurate with the patient's clinical status. Etomidate has no analgesic properties.

4.3.3.3   What Are the Adverse Effects of Etomidate?

Etomidate is associated with nausea and vomiting during recovery in 30% to 40% of patients undergoing general anesthesia. Pain on injection is common because of the propylene glycol solvent. The incidence can be as high as 80%.[78] Myoclonic movements due to an imbalance of inhibition and excitation in the thalamocortical

tract are common and have been confused with seizure activity.[71] It is of no clinical consequence and generally terminates promptly. The occurrence of hiccups, usually during awakening, is highly variable, ranging between 0% and 70%.[79]

The most significant and controversial side effect of etomidate is its reversible blockade of 11-beta-hydroxylase. Etomidate causes reversible adrenocortical suppression by interfering with 11-beta-hydroxylation of 11-deoxycortisol, which prevents its conversion to cortisol. It decreases both serum cortisol and aldosterone levels. Single bolus induction doses of etomidate have transiently inhibited cortisol and aldosterone synthesis.[80-82] The possible long-term adrenocortical suppression has limited the use of etomidate as a sedative for intensive care management and total intravenous anesthesia.

4.3.4   Ketamine

4.3.4.1   Discuss the Clinical Pharmacology of Ketamine

Ketamine, an arylcyclohexylamine, is a structural analog of phencyclidine, which may account for the psychomimetic side effects such as hallucinations and nightmares. The compound has a chiral center producing stereoisomers and is commercially available as a racemic mixture. It is fairly lipid soluble and minimally protein bound accounting for its rapid onset (45-60 second). Ketamine is extensively taken up by the liver and metabolized by the cytochrome P-450 biotransformation system. The primary metabolite, norketamine, has roughly one-fifth the potency of the parent molecule. Its high lipid solubility produces rapid redistribution and short duration of effect. Rapid hepatic metabolism is responsible for the short elimination half-life of 2 to 3 hours. Ketamine has been touted as a "complete" anesthetic by many, as it provides analgesia, amnesia, and hypnosis (unconsciousness). Besides blocking polysynaptic spinal cord reflexes, ketamine is a noncompetitive antagonist of *N*-methyl-D-aspartate (NMDA) receptors at the GABA-receptor complex, promoting the inhibition of excitatory neurotransmitters in selected areas of the brain. An interaction between ketamine and a number of the opioid receptors may be partially responsible for its analgesic properties. Ketamine produces dissociative anesthesia by electrophysiologically separating the thalamus from the limbic system. Patients may appear conscious but are unable to respond to stimuli. Ketamine centrally stimulates the sympathetic nervous system, which in turn releases catecholamines, augmenting the heart rate and blood pressure in those patients who are not catecholamine depleted secondary to the demands of their underlying disease. Similar to most other anesthetics, however, ketamine in the face of catecholamine depletion causes dose-dependent myocardial depression.

Traditionally, ketamine's direct stimulation of the CNS is thought to increase cerebral metabolism, $CMRO_2$, and CBF, thus potentially increasing ICP in patients with CNS injury. These generalizations may not be valid. Pfenninger et al[83] investigated the effect of 2 mg·kg⁻¹ of ketamine on the ICP and CPP of ventilated pigs. There was no increase in ICP in normal pigs with induced intracranial hypertension. Likewise, in ventilated goats, ketamine significantly decreased the $CMRO_2$, while the ICP did not increase.[84] Albanese et al[85] studied the effects of ketamine (5 mg·kg^{-1}) in eight patients with traumatic brain injury who were ventilated and sedated with propofol. There was a significant decrease in the ICP, while the CPP and middle cerebral artery blood flow velocity were unchanged. Mayberg et al[86] found similar results with a cohort of patients presenting for a craniotomy anesthetized with isoflurane and nitrous oxide who received 1 mg·kg^{-1} of ketamine. The mean arterial blood pressure, CPP, and arterial carbon dioxide did not change, while the ICP significantly decreased. There is emerging evidence that the antagonist behavior of ketamine at NMDA receptors may have a neuroprotective benefit.[87] Unfortunately, the evidence with respect to the use of ketamine for induction of anesthesia specifically in the patient with intracranial hypertension is lacking. However, it can be said that ketamine may be used in the sedated, mechanically ventilated patient with little concern for worsening intracranial hypertension. Ketamine's long-term exclusion from the induction of patients with decreased intracranial compliance may be an overgeneralization.

A key feature of ketamine is its effects on the respiratory system. Despite inducing a profound anesthesia, upper airway reflexes and central respiratory drive are preserved to a degree following ketamine administration, although with high doses, hypoventilation and apnea will occur. In addition, ketamine directly relaxes bronchial smooth muscle, producing bronchodilation. Ketamine has been successfully used to treat status asthmaticus and less severe bronchospasm.[88-92] Hemmingsen et al[89] in a placebo-controlled trial showed that ketamine (1 mg·kg^{-1}) successfully relieved bronchospasm in ventilated subjects.

4.3.4.2 With Its Unique Characteristics, What Is the Role of Ketamine as an Induction Agent in Management of the Airway?

Ketamine is the traditional induction agent for patients with reactive airways disease who require tracheal intubation. Because of its unique pharmacologic profile, ketamine may also be considered for induction in patients who are hypovolemic and for patients with hemodynamic instability due to cardiac tamponade or distributive shock. In normotensive or hypertensive patients with ischemic heart disease, catecholamine release may adversely increase myocardial oxygen demand, but it is not known whether this effect is clinically significant. Ketamine's preservation of central respiratory drive makes it appealing for awake upper airway evaluation in the difficult airway patient. On the basis of the previous discussion, the use of ketamine in patients with elevated ICP remains controversial. Traditional teaching would have us avoid ketamine despite there being little to no evidence to support such a practice.

4.3.4.3 Discuss the Clinical Use and Adverse Effects of Ketamine

The induction dose of ketamine is 1 to 2 mg·kg^{-1}. This dose needs to be adjusted for hypovolemic and/or hypotensive patients.

Ketamine may be mixed with propofol as a 50:50 mixture (5 mg·mL^{-1} of each), "ketofol," a combination that produces less hypotension and respiratory depression than propofol alone. Because of its stimulating effects, ketamine enhances laryngeal reflexes and increases pharyngeal and bronchial secretions. These secretions may precipitate laryngospasm and be bothersome during upper airway examination in the difficult airway patient or during procedural sedation. An antimuscarinic agent, such as glycopyrrolate, may be administered in conjunction with ketamine to promote a drying effect. The maintenance of airway reflexes does not negate the need for intubation and airway protection when faced with patients at risk for aspiration.

Five to thirty percent of patients will experience hallucinations or dreams on emergence from ketamine. They are more common in the adult than in the child and can be eliminated by the concomitant or subsequent administration of a benzodiazepine.[93] This is less of an issue in emergency airway management, in which often the patient is sedated with benzodiazepines for prolonged periods.

4.3.5 Propofol

4.3.5.1 Discuss the Clinical Pharmacology of Propofol

Propofol (2,6-diisopropylphenol) is an alkylphenol derivative with hypnotic properties. Propofol is supplied in an emulsion of 10% soybean oil, 2.25% glycerol, and 1.2% egg lecithin.[94] It is highly lipid soluble and hence rapidly acting. The initial redistribution half-life is 2 to 8 minutes. It is rapidly metabolized to inactive, water-soluble metabolites.

Propofol enhances GABA activity at the GABA-receptor complex. It decreases $CMRO_2$ and ICP.[95-97] Propofol causes a direct reduction in blood pressure through vasodilation and direct myocardial depression, resulting in a decrease in CPP, which may be detrimental in a compromised patient.[98] Propofol has profound anticonvulsant properties.[99] It is a potent depressor of ventilation inhibiting hypoxic and hypercarbic ventilatory drive.

4.3.5.2 What Is the Role of Propofol as an Induction Agent for Tracheal Intubation?

Propofol is an excellent induction agent in hemodynamically stable patients. Its potential for hypotension and reduction in CPP may reduce its role as an induction agent for rapid-sequence intubation/induction (RSI). However, it remains a commonly used agent in this setting as the adverse hemodynamic changes and other pharmacological effects of propofol are very predictable. Altered dosing for the unstable patients or using it in conjunction with ketamine, *ketofol*, helps to attenuate the undesirable hemodynamic effects. Apart from avoiding the use of propofol in patients with known egg allergy (egg lecithin emulsion), there are no absolute contraindications to the use of propofol.

The induction dose of propofol is 1 to 2 mg·kg^{-1} in a euvolemic, normotensive patient. Because of its predictable tendency to reduce mean arterial blood pressure, smaller doses are generally used when propofol is given as an induction agent for emergency induction. Young adults and children may require 2 to 3 mg·kg^{-1}.

The pain associated with the injection of propofol is comparable to that of methohexital, less than etomidate, and more than thiopental.[11] This effect can be attenuated by injecting the medication through a rapidly running intravenous infusion in a large vein. Alternatively, pretreatment with a small dose of 1% lidocaine (4 mL)[100] or mixing the propofol with a small amount of 1% lidocaine (2-4 mL) prior to injection[101] have both been shown to minimize the discomfort. Propofol can cause mild clonus but to a lesser degree than thiopental, etomidate, or methohexital.[71]

4.3.6   Inhalational agents

4.3.6.1   What Is the Role of Inhalational Anesthetics as Sedating/Induction Agents in Management of the Airway?

From the beginnings of anesthesia, volatile anesthetics have been an integral part of anesthesia induction. This technique is more commonly used in pediatrics than in adults. In the early days of ether anesthesia, inductions were stormy affairs. With the advent of newer volatile agents that are potent, less pungent, and poorly soluble (leading to rapid onset), a smooth inhalational induction can be easily accomplished.[102]

The major advantage of an inhalational induction is that spontaneous ventilation can be preserved and patients can regulate their own depth of anesthesia. The technique of inhalational induction in pediatric epiglottitis is well established. The safety of extending this practice to other causes of upper airway obstruction, and in adults with upper airway obstruction of any cause, has yet to be conclusively established. However, some have reported that tracheal intubation can be successfully carried out using this technique while maintaining spontaneous ventilation in an uncooperative patient with a difficult airway.[103-105] While halothane mask induction had played a major role in inducing pediatric patients in the past, most practitioners currently favor sevoflurane. Theoretically, the addition of nitrous oxide may speed the onset of anesthesia. However, unconsciousness can be accomplished in less than 60 seconds with sevoflurane and oxygen when using a primed circuit with 8% sevoflurane and fresh gas flow of 8 L·min^{-1}.[105,106] Although, intravenous induction seems to be the preferred induction technique, inhalational means of induction will remain a core anesthetic skill for the foreseeable future.

4.4   NEUROMUSCULAR BLOCKING AGENTS

Neuromuscular blocking agents are the cornerstone of emergency airway management and are used to obtain total control of the patient to facilitate rapid endotracheal intubation while minimizing the risks of aspiration or other adverse physiologic events. Neuromuscular blocking agents do not provide analgesia, sedation, or amnesia, and an induction or sedative agent must be used during RSI in patients who are not completely unresponsive. Similarly, appropriate sedation is essential when neuromuscular blockade is maintained for controlled mechanical ventilation following intubation.

4.4.1   Discuss the clinical pharmacology of neuromuscular blocking agents

In order to understand the pharmacology of neuromuscular blocking agents, it is important to understand their effects at the postjunctional, cholinergic, nicotinic receptors at the neuromuscular junction. Under normal circumstances, the neuron synthesizes acetylcholine (ACh) from choline and acetate and packages it in vesicles. Each vesicle contains 5,000 to 10,000 ACh molecules. Calcium enters the nerve through channels that open in response to the action potential propagating the length of the nerve. Calcium permits the binding of specific proteins to the vesicles necessary for them to bind to the nerve end membrane. Binding produces fusion and the release of ACh. The ACh migrates across the synaptic cleft and attaches to nicotinic ACh receptors, promoting muscle fiber depolarization producing muscle contraction. ACh then detaches from the receptor to be eligible for reuptake into the nerve terminal or hydrolysis by acetylcholinesterase, which also resides in the cleft.

Neuromuscular blocking agents are either ACh agonists (depolarizers of the motor end plate) or antagonists (nondepolarizers of the motor end plate). The antagonists attach to the receptors and competitively block ACh from accessing ACh receptors. Because they are in competition with ACh for the motor end plate, they can be displaced from the end plate by increasing concentrations of ACh, the end result of reversal agents (the cholinesterase inhibitors), such as neostigmine and edrophonium, which inhibit acetylcholinesterase and allow ACh accumulation and the return of neuromuscular function.

In clinical practice, there are two classes of neuromuscular blocking agents: the noncompetitive or depolarizing neuromuscular blocking agents, of which succinylcholine is the prototype and the only one in common clinical use. The competitive or nondepolarizing agents are divided into two main classes: the benzylisoquinolinium compounds and the aminosteroid compounds. The benzylisoquinolines, *d*-tubocurarine, metocurine, atracurium, cisatracurium, and mivacurium share common properties. The aminosteroids, vecuronium, pancuronium, rapacuronium, and rocuronium also share common attributes that are distinct from those of the benzylisoquinolines.

The ideal muscle relaxant to facilitate tracheal intubation would have a rapid onset, a short duration of action, no significant adverse side effects, and metabolism and excretion independent of liver and kidney function. Unfortunately, such an agent does not exist. Succinylcholine comes closest to meeting all these desirable goals. Despite the historic and well-known adverse effects of succinylcholine and the continuous advent of new competitive neuromuscular blocking agents, succinylcholine remains an essential drug in facilitating tracheal intubation.

4.4.2   Depolarizing neuromuscular blocking agent

4.4.2.1   What Are the Clinical Pharmacological Characteristics of Succinylcholine that Make it a Unique Neuromuscular Blocking Agent?

Succinylcholine is chemically similar to ACh. It consists of two molecules of ACh linked by an ester bridge and, as does ACh, succinylcholine stimulates the nicotinic and muscarinic cholinergic receptors of the sympathetic and parasympathetic nervous systems. Once succinylcholine reaches the neuromuscular junction, it binds tightly to the ACh receptors. ACh receptors related to neuromuscular transmission are located in three areas:

- The presynaptic receptors, responsible for regulation of ACh vesicles release, generate an action potential along the neuron.

- The postsynaptic receptors: the principle paralyzing component of succinylcholine occurs at the postsynaptic receptor. The resultant depolarization and subsequent desensitization to further stimulation produced by succinylcholine occurs because unlike ACh, succinylcholine is not rapidly hydrolyzed by acetylcholinesterase. Succinylcholine is resistant to degradation by cleft acetylcholinesterase and is susceptible to rapid hydrolysis by pseudocholinesterase, an enzyme of the liver and plasma not present at the neuromuscular junction. Therefore, diffusion away from the neuromuscular junction motor end plate and back into the vascular compartment is ultimately responsible for succinylcholine metabolism. This also explains why only a fraction of the initial intravenous dose of succinylcholine ever reaches the motor end plate to promote paralysis.

- Extrajunctional receptors, although numerous, are generally not of clinical significance. In pathological states such as denervation injuries or severe muscle crush injury, these receptors become unregulated and proliferate. The depolarization of the extrajunctional receptors in large numbers can result in clinically significant hyperkalemia.

Succinylmonocholine, the initial metabolite of succinylcholine, sensitizes the cardiac muscarinic receptors in the sinus node to repeat doses of succinylcholine, which may then lead to atropine responsive bradycardia.

4.4.2.2   What Are the Indications and Contraindications for Succinylcholine?

Succinylcholine remains the neuromuscular blocking agent of choice for emergency RSI because of its rapid onset and relatively brief duration of action. A personal or family history of malignant hyperthermia (MH) is an absolute contraindication to the use of succinylcholine. Patients judged to be at risk for succinylcholine-related hyperkalemia also represent absolute contraindications to its use. Under these circumstances, to facilitate tracheal intubation rapidly, a large dose of a competitive, nondepolarizing neuromuscular blocking agent should be used.[107] Relative contraindications to the use of succinylcholine are dependent on the skill and proficiency of the airway practitioner and individual patient's clinical circumstance (ie, "context sensitive"; see Chapter 6). A patient who is felt to represent a difficult intubation, and in whom bag-mask-ventilation is also felt to be difficult or impossible, should not receive any neuromuscular blocking agents except as part of a planned approach to the difficult airway.

4.4.2.3   How Can Succinylcholine Be Used Safely?

In the normal-sized adult patient, the recommended dose of succinylcholine for intubation is 1 to 2 mg·kg^{-1}. In a rare, life-threatening circumstance when succinylcholine must be given IM because of inability to secure venous access, a dose of 3 to 4 mg·kg^{-1} IM may be used.

The intubating dose is typically felt to be two to three times the dose that produces on average 95% decrease in twitch height of the adductor pollicis muscle (effective dose or ED$_{95}$). The ED$_{95}$ of succinylcholine is 0.3 to 0.6 mg·kg^{-1} in adults,[108,109] 0.5 mg·kg^{-1} in children, and 0.7 mg·kg^{-1} in infants and neonates.[110] Therefore, an appropriate intubating dose of succinylcholine for a normal-sized adult is 1 mg·kg^{-1}. For obese patients dosing would appear to be more successful if the total body weight is used rather than ideal body weight.[111] The average onset time is 1 to 1.5 minutes. Defasciculation with a nondepolarizing muscle relaxant will decrease the potency of succinylcholine by half. Therefore, if one intends to pretreat the fasciculations with a nondepolarizing agent, a succinylcholine dose of 1.5 to 2 mg·kg^{-1} is required for intubation.[109]

Succinylcholine is rapidly cleared by plasma pseudocholinesterase which is an enzyme manufactured in the liver. Once succinylcholine diffuses out of the synaptic cleft it is hydrolyzed to succinylmonocholine and then to succinic acid. The mean elimination half-life of succinylcholine is 43 seconds.[112] The rate of metabolism determines the duration of action. A normal adult has a theoretical 8-minute apneic reserve of oxygen. The mean time to return of spontaneous ventilation after an intubating dose of succinylcholine (1 mg·kg^{-1}) is approximately 5 to 8 minutes.[113] Hayes et al[113] did however have 10% of their patients desaturate before the return of spontaneous ventilation. The airway practitioner still has to provide mechanical ventilation until the function of the respiratory muscles returns. Doses less than 1 mg·kg^{-1} may not compromise the intubation nor do they shorten the apneic period.[114]

4.4.2.4   What Are the Adverse Effects of Succinylcholine and How Can We Minimize These Side Effects?

The recognized side effects of succinylcholine include fasciculations, hyperkalemia, bradycardia, asystole, prolonged neuromuscular blockade, MH, and masseter muscle spasm. Each of these will be discussed separately.

Fasciculations. Fasciculations are involuntary, unsynchronized muscle contractions caused by depolarization of ACh receptors. Fasciculations cause muscle damage that manifests itself as myalgias, increased creatinine kinase, myoglobinemia, and an increase in catecholamines leading to increases in heart rate and blood pressure. These uncontrolled muscle contractions increase oxygen consumption and carbon dioxide production, and can lead to increased cardiac output, and potentially CBF and ICP. In an animal study, the increase in ICP was found to be secondary to the increase in muscle spindle activation caused by succinylcholine-induced spindle depolarization.[115] Lastly, fasciculations tend to increase intragastric pressure, though this is not clinically significant as it is offset by an increase in lower esophageal sphincter tone.

Virtually all patients receiving succinylcholine will experience fasciculations. The same cannot be said for postoperative myalgias which occur following the administration of succinylcholine at a rate 1.5% to 89%.[116] However, 15% to 20% subjects undergoing surgery without being exposed to succinylcholine will suffer from postoperative myalgias.[117] Not only is the link between fasciculations and myalgias controversial, there is no evidence that the severity of fasciculations corresponds with more severe myalgias[116], nor does it appear to be a dose-related side effect. In fact, McLoughlin et al[118] suggest that increasing the dose of succinylcholine may decrease the incidence of myalgias, suggesting that the larger dose leads to a more synchronous contraction and a reduction in shearing forces.

Small doses of NDMRs given prior to succinylcholine have clearly been shown to decrease the incidence and intensity of fasciculations[45-50], but their ability to effectively relieve postoperative myalgias is not quite as clear.[46-48] A meta-analysis did determine that atracurium, d-tubocurarine, galamine, and pancuronium can decrease the frequency of fasciculations and myalgias.[50] Traditionally, 10% of the intubating dose of an NDMR has been given to pretreat for fasciculations. However, at this dose, a significant number of patients experience weakness. While a dose of 0.06 mg·kg^{-1} of rocuronium has been shown to decrease the incidence of fasciculations, it does not decrease the incidence of myalgias.[47-49,119] Harvey et al[46] showed that rocuronium at doses 0.03 and 0.05 mg·kg^{-1} was equally effective in decreasing the incidence of fasciculations. The timing of rocuronium administration (3 vs 1.5 minutes) prior to the succinylcholine does not seem to affect it effectiveness.[49]

Lidocaine is an alternative to nondepolarizing muscle relaxants for defasciculation. At doses of 1.5 mg·kg^{-1}, lidocaine effectively decreases the incidence of fasciculation and myalgias following the administration of succinylcholine.[50,116] Lidocaine appears to work by preventing ionic exchange across the sodium channels.

Hyperkalemia. Under normal circumstances, serum potassium increases minimally when succinylcholine is administered (0-0.5 mEq·L^{-1}) due to depolarization of the myocytes. A pathological response to succinylcholine can occur, however, resulting in rapid and dramatic increases in serum potassium. These pathologic hyperkalemic responses occur by two distinct mechanisms: receptor upregulation and rhabdomyolysis. In either situation, potassium increase may approach four times the normal efflux of potassium, resulting in hyperkalemic dysrhythmias, or cardiac arrest.[120] Two forms of postjunctional ACh receptors exist, mature (junctional) and immature (extrajunctional). Each ACh receptor is composed of five proteins arranged in circular fashion around a common channel. Both types of receptors contain two alpha subunits. ACh must attach to both alpha subunits to open the

channel and effect depolarization and muscle contraction. When receptor upregulation occurs, the mature receptors at and around the motor end plate are gradually converted over a 4 to 5-day period to immature receptors that propagate throughout the entire muscle membrane. Upregulated receptors are characterized by low conductance and prolonged channel-opening times, resulting in increasing levels of potassium, clinically significant dysrhythmias, and cardiac arrest.[119] Most of the entities associated with hyperkalemia during emergency RSI are the result of receptor upregulation. Interestingly, these same extrajunctional nicotinic receptors are relatively refractory to nondepolarizing agents, so larger doses of vecuronium, pancuronium, or rocuronium will be required to produce paralysis.

Rhabdomyolysis is the other mechanism by which hyperkalemia may occur. It is most often associated with myopathies. In cardiac arrest situations related to rhabdomyolysis and continued loss of potassium, resuscitation seems to be less successful than in receptor upregulation. Gronert[120] reviewed 129 cases of cardiac arrest from hyperkalemia; 57 were due to rhabdomyolysis and 78 due to upregulation. The mortality was higher in those cases of rhabdomyolysis (30%) compared to cases of upregulation (11%). Succinylcholine is a toxin to unstable membranes in any patient with a myopathy and should be avoided.

Receptor upregulation occurs in burn victims, patients that suffer denervation injury, and in patients with sepsis or widespread inflammation. In burn victims, extrajunctional receptor sensitization becomes clinically significant at 4 to 5 days postburn. It lasts an indefinite period of time, although the *at risk* period is deemed to have passed at the point healing of the burned area is complete. It is prudent not to administer succinylcholine to postburn patients if any question exists regarding the status of their burn. The percent of body surface area burned does not determine the magnitude of hyperkalemia; significant hyperkalemia has been reported in patients with as little as 8% total body surface area burn.[121] Most emergency intubations for burns are performed well within the safe 4-day window after the burn occurs. There have been no reports of hyperkalemia in the first 24 hours postburn. It seems rational to avoid the administration of succinylcholine until the burn has completely healed.

The patient who suffers a denervation event secondary to a lower motor neuron or upper motor neuron injury is at risk for hyperkalemia. Following lower motor neuron denervation injuries, patients exhibit a sensitivity to succinylcholine, which begins 3 to 4 days postinjury[119] and patients suffering from severe polyneuropathies display increased potassium release following the administration of succinylcholine.[122,123] Upper motor neuron lesions, such as stroke and traumatic closed head injuries, display a similar sensitivity to succinylcholine, usually 3 to 5 days after the event.[119] As long as any neuromuscular disease is active, one ought to expect that there will be augmentation of the extrajunctional receptors and risk for hyperkalemia with the use of succinylcholine. Congenital upper motor neuron and lower motor neuron lesions, such as cerebral palsy and myelomeningocele, do not exhibit an altered response to succinylcholine.[124,125] The duration of the upregulation and altered response to succinylcholine in neuromuscular disorders is not clear. Upregulation has been observed 3 years following an injury and may last even longer in progressive disease types.[119] Unlike fasciculations, the hyperkalemic response cannot be attenuated by administering defasciculating doses of NDMRs, and therefore, these specific clinical situations should be considered absolute contraindications to succinylcholine during the specified time periods.

Infection or inflammation can alter the neuromuscular junction response to muscle relaxants.[119] This situation is complicated by the intensive care unit environment where total body disuse atrophy and chemical denervation of the ACh receptors can occur if muscle relaxants are chronically infused. Exaggerated hyperkalemic responses to succinylcholine have been observed in patients with life-threatening infections.[126,127] The at-risk time period appears to be 5 days after the illness has begun and continues indefinitely as long as the disease process is present.

Succinylcholine is absolutely contraindicated in patients with inherited myopathies such as Duschene and Becker muscular dystrophies. The combination of the succinylcholine-induced contractures and the fragile muscle membrane of the myopathic patients predisposes them to rhabdomyolysis.[51] In children up to 10 years of age, an elevated creatine kinase is a highly sensitive indicator of muscular dystrophy.[128] Myopathic rhabdomyolysis and hyperkalemia-induced cardiac arrest is associated with a significant degree of mortality. The hyperkalemic efflux can be four times the expected normal response. Any inappropriate response by young males following the use of succinylcholine should alert the practitioner to the possibility of undiagnosed Duschene muscular dystrophy.[129]

There is a paucity of evidence supporting the notion that chronic renal failure patients with normal levels of serum potassium present a risk of an exaggerated hyperkalemic response with the administration of succinylcholine. Indeed, the majority of renal failure patients are successfully intubated using succinylcholine without adverse cardiovascular complications. A review of the literature by Thapa et al[130] concluded that there was insufficient evidence to support a recommendation to avoid succinylcholine in patients with renal failure.

Patients with hyperkalemia may be different. Despite succinylcholine being used successfully in patients with hyperkalemia[131] without any adverse events, succinylcholine still cannot be recommended for such patients. Even the normal 0.5 mEq.L^{-1} efflux of potassium could be lethal in a patient with preexisting significant hyperkalemia and acidosis.

Bradycardia. Bradycardia following the administration of succinylcholine is seen most commonly in children because of their heightened vagotonic state. This is especially so as the sympathetic nervous system does not mature until 4 to 6 months of age. Bradycardia is attenuated or abolished by administering atropine 0.02 mg·kg^{-1} or glycopyrrolate 0.01 mg·kg^{-1} [43] as pretreatment before administering succinylcholine. The age above which prophylactic atropine is no longer needed is unknown. McAuliffe et al[132] have shown that the incidence of bradycardia following succinylcholine in children 1 to 12 years of age is lower than previously thought, stating that atropine pretreatment may not be necessary. Expert opinion has gravitated to this same recommendation: treat bradycardia if it preexists or occurs following succinylcholine administration rather than employing routine pretreatment. Regardless of the age, repeated doses of succinylcholine

may produce the profound vagally mediated bradycardia requiring the administration of antimuscarinics.

Prolonged Neuromuscular Blockade. Prolonged neuromuscular blockade may result from an acquired reduction in pseudocholinesterase concentration, a congenital absence of pseudocholinesterase, or the presence of an atypical form of pseudocholinesterase, all of which will delay the degradation of succinylcholine and prolong paralysis. Reduced concentrations of pseudocholinesterase may be a result of liver disease, pregnancy, burns, oral contraceptives, uremia, drug abuse, or plasmapheresis. This quantitative loss of pseudocholinesterase is rarely clinically significant. Atypical or abnormal genetic variants of pseudocholinesterase can be uncovered by testing. The patient who is a homozygous for atypical pseudocholinesterase (1:1500) may have paralysis for 3 to 6 hours after a single dose of succinylcholine.

Increase in Intraocular Pressure. Elevated intraocular pressure results from muscle contractures of the orbital muscles that occur following stimulation of the postsynaptic ACh receptors. Although succinylcholine can increase the intraocular pressure by 6 to 8 mm Hg,[133] there have been no reported cases of vitreous extrusion in the presence of an opened globe injury related to the administration of succinylcholine or during intubation. The use of succinylcholine has been advocated in patients for whom the prompt securing of the airway is indicated in the face of open globe injuries.[134] The more pressing concern should be protection and the prevention of the deleterious side effects of intubation, such as hypoxia and coughing.

Malignant Hyperthermia. A personal or family history of MH is an absolute contraindication to the use of succinylcholine. MH is an acute hypermetabolic disorder of skeletal muscle. The incidence of MH ranges from 1:50000 to 1:4000.[135] It is an inherited syndrome typified by alteration of the Ry1 ryanodine receptor which modulates calcium release from the sarcoplasmic reticulum. It can be triggered by halogenated anesthetics and succinylcholine. Following the initiating event, its onset can be acute and progressive or delayed for hours. Generalized awareness of MH, earlier diagnosis, and the availability of dantrolene have decreased the mortality to approximately 10%.[136]

MH is characterized by an acute loss of intracellular calcium control. This results in a cascade of rapidly progressive events manifested primarily by increased metabolism (increased oxygen consumption and carbon dioxide production) as well as muscular rigidity, autonomic instability, hypoxia, hypotension, severe lactic acidosis, hyperkalemia, and myoglobinemia. An elevation in temperature is a highly variable manifestation. The treatment for MH consists of discontinuing the known or suspected precipitant and the immediate administration of dantrolene. Dantrolene is essential to successful resuscitation and should be given as soon as the diagnosis is seriously entertained. Dantrolene is a hydantoin derivative that acts directly on skeletal muscle to prevent calcium release from the sarcoplasmic reticulum without affecting calcium reuptake. The initial dose is 2.5 mg·kg^{-1} and is repeated every 5 minutes until muscle relaxation occurs or the maximum dose of 10 mg·kg^{-1} is administered. Dantrolene is free of any serious side effects. Additionally, measures to control body temperature, manage hyperkalemia, maintain acid–base balance, and enhance urinary output to preserve renal function must be instituted as soon as possible.

All cases of MH require constant monitoring of pH, arterial blood gases, and serum potassium. Immediate and aggressive management of hyperkalemia with the administration of calcium gluconate, glucose, insulin, and sodium bicarbonate may be necessary. Following an acute MH crisis, intensive care monitoring is recommended for 24 to 36 hours. Arterial pH, myoglobinemia, and creatine kinase should be serially monitored. Recrudescence occurs in 25% of MH cases.[135] Patients should be maintained on dantrolene (1 mg·kg[-1] every 6-8 hours) for the first 24 hours after a crisis.

Masseter Muscle Rigidity. Masseter muscle rigidity (MMR) is defined as the transient inability to distract the mandible from the maxilla such that the mouth cannot be opened or opened only with force.[137] The incidence of MMR following succinylcholine is 0.3% to 1%.[138] Pretreatment with defasciculating doses of nondepolarizing NMBAs will not prevent masseter rigidity. MMR typically subsides in 2 to 3 minutes. More than 50% of patients with MMR are susceptible to MH based on caffeine–halothane contracture studies.[139] In the setting of the OR where an operation is contemplated, continuance of a nontriggering anesthetic following tracheal intubation is reasonable if proper monitoring is available (end-tidal carbon dioxide, temperature, creatine kinase, and myoglobin) and the anesthesia practitioner is comfortable treating MH,[138] otherwise the anesthetic should be discontinued and patient monitored for signs of MH.

4.4.3   Nondepolarizing (competitive) neuromuscular blocking agents

4.4.3.1   Discuss the Clinical Pharmacology of Nondepolarizing Neuromuscular Blocking Agents

Nondepolarizing muscle relaxants (NDMRs) competitively antagonize the action of ACh transmission at the postjunctional, cholinergic, nicotinic receptors at the neuromuscular junction. They are incapable of inducing the conformational change necessary to initiate the depolarization of the neuromuscular junction. NDMRs prevent ACh access to both alpha subunits of the nicotinic receptor, which is required for muscle contraction. This competitive blockade is characterized by the absence of fasciculations and the reversal of paralysis by acetylcholinesterase inhibitors that prevent

metabolism of ACh to allow its reaccumulation and the potential for retransmission at the motor end plate, promoting a muscle contraction. Metabolism and elimination of NDMRs occur through a variety of biochemical pathways involving the liver, kidney, and Hofmann degradation. Hofmann degradation, a nonenzymatic degradation, is largely responsible for the metabolism of cisatracurium and atracurium.

Mivacurium is a benzylisoquinoline derivative that unlike the rest of the NDMRs is metabolized by pseudocholinesterase. Intubating doses range from 0.15 to 0.2 mg·kg[-1] with a short onset time and brief duration. Mivacurium duration will be prolonged in patients with atypical pseudocholinesterase. As well, mivacurium releases histamine that can induce hypotension.

Cisatracurium, as previously mentioned, undergoes Hofmann degradation and elimination, rendering it virtually independent of liver and renal function. It is devoid of autonomic side effects. Cisatracurium has a relatively long onset time and intermediate duration.

Rocuronium, an aminosteroid, is eliminated primarily by the liver. It has an ED_{95} of 0.3 mg·kg[-1]. A dose of 0.6 mg·kg[-1] can provide good intubating conditions in 90 seconds. In order to provide good intubating conditions in 60 seconds, similar to that of succinylcholine, a larger dose (1-1.2 mg·kg[-1]) is commonly required for an RSI.[107] However, it has an intermediate duration of action.

Rapacuronium, a newer rapid-onset aminosteroid NDMR, provides good intubating conditions in doses of 1.5 mg·kg[-1] and has a short duration of action (17 minutes).[140] Unfortunately, rapacuronium has caused life-threatening bronchospasm and as a result its sale has been suspended.[141]

4.4.3.2   What Are the Indications and Contraindications of NDMRs?

The NDMRs serve a multipurpose role in emergency airway management (Table 4-2). They can be used as pretreatment agents to attenuate the many undesirable side effects associated with muscle fasciculations (eg, myalgia and the increase in ICP, IOP, etc) following the use of succinylcholine. They can also serve as the muscle relaxant of choice if succinylcholine is contraindicated or unavailable, or to maintain postintubation paralysis. NDMRs are contraindicated in the face of difficult ventilation/intubation and/or an inexperienced airway practitioner.

▶ TABLE 4-2

Commonly Used NDMRs, Their Therapeutic Intubating Doses, Pretreatment Doses for Preventing Fasciculation and Myalgias, and Their Basic Pharmacokinetics[11]

	INTUBATING DOSE (mg·kg[-1])	PRETREATMENT (mg·kg[-1])	ONSET (s)	DURATION (min)
Rocuronium	0.6-1.2	0.03-.06	60-90	45
Vecuronium	0.15	0.005-.01	300	45
Cisatracurium	0.15	0.005	300	45
Mivacurium	0.2	0.01	120-180	30

4.4.3.3   How Can We Use NDMRs Effectively?

Defasciculation prior to the administration of succinylcholine is used in patients to minimize myalgias and the elevation of ICP secondary to the increased CBF associated with the increase of carbon dioxide production from the fasciculations and muscle spindle activation. The appropriate dose is 10% of the ED_{95} of any of the nondepolarizing agents. Presently, rocuronium appears to be the most commonly used NDMR to abate fasciculations[51] and it can be given 1.5 to 3 minutes prior to the induction of anesthesia.[49]

NDMRs are the only option for rapid-sequence induction when succinylcholine is contraindicated or not available. In these situations, NDMRs can be used for emergency RSI. The drug of choice is rocuronium 1 to 1.2 mg·kg⁻¹ based on its time to onset. If rocuronium is not available, vecuronium 0.15 mg·kg⁻¹ is a reasonable alternative (Table 4-2).

4.4.4   How do we decide when to use a nondepolarizing muscle relaxant versus succinylcholine for tracheal intubation?

The use of neuromuscular blocking agents to facilitate endotracheal intubation results in an increased success rate and fewer complications.[107,142-144] Whether succinylcholine or an NDMR is used to accomplish the task is a hotly debated topic. Succinylcholine is superior to the slower onset NDMRs such as pancuronium, atracurium, and vecuronium.[145] The most commonly used muscle relaxants in a rapid-sequence induction/intubation are succinylcholine and rocuronium based on their pharmacokinetic and pharmacodynamic profiles. For each drug, the dosage is critical to their success of intubation. The most appropriate dose of succinylcholine is 1 to 2 mg·kg⁻¹.[108,109,114] Doses of 1 to 1.2 mg·kg⁻¹ of rocuronium provide better intubating conditions within 60 to 90 seconds than the lower dose of 0.6 mg·kg⁻¹.[107,146,147] In the emergency department and the OR, succinylcholine (1-2 mg·kg⁻¹) and rocuronium (1-1.2 mg·kg⁻¹) in the appropriate doses have been used safely and efficaciously with unparalleled success.[143,144,147,148] However, one must always be wary of the potentially difficult intubation, and in those cases, the selection of rocuronium would be unwise.

4.4.5   Are there any new muscle relaxants or adjuncts with a better pharmacodynamic profile?

The next generation of neuromuscular blocking drugs aims for a rapid onset with a short duration of action, mimicking succinylcholine, but with minimal side effects. The ideal NDMR was thought to be rapacuronium, a newer rapid-onset aminosteroid NDMR. It provided good intubating conditions with a short duration of action.[140] However, after widespread usage of rapacuronium, it became evident that it can cause severe bronchospasm associated with arterial desaturation and difficult ventilation.[140,141,146] As a result of its life-threatening bronchospasm, rapacuronium was withdrawn from the market in 2001.

Another new generation muscle relaxant candidate is an asymmetrical mixed tetrahydroisoquinolinium chlorofumarate, Gantacurium (GW280430A). It is an NDMR with an ultrashort duration of action, developed to replace succinylcholine. Belmont[149] has estimated the ED_{95} to be 0.19 mg·kg⁻¹. The onset of action at doses 2.5 to 3 times the ED_{95} was within 90 seconds with transient cardiovascular adverse effects suggestive of histamine release.[149] Spontaneous recovery to a train-of-four of 0.9 was evident 12 to 15 minutes after large doses $(3 \times ED_{95})$.[150] Gantacurium's metabolism is nonenzymatic; partially due to rapid formation of an inactive cysteine product; the other portion undergoes ester hydrolysis to inactive metabolites.[150] The early studies indicate no significant adverse cardiovascular or respiratory side effects in humans.[141] A phase-2 trial in adults has been completed (http://clinicaltrials.gov/show/NCT00235976), but no results have yet been published.

The most promising new agent is not a muscle relaxant but a new reversal agent for muscle relaxants. Sugammadex is a modified γ-cyclodextrin. Cyclodextrins are cyclic oligosaccharides, whose 3D structures resemble a hollow, truncated cone or doughnut.[151] They have a hydrophobic interior and hydrophilic exterior, the hydrophobic portion traps drugs within the cyclodextrin cavity. Sugammadex is a muscle relaxant-binding agent; it does not interact with nicotinic receptors or with acetylcholinesterases, and acts independently of the degree of neuromuscular blockade. Sugammadex encapsulates and inactivates rocuronium and vecuronium; the resultant complex is excreted in the urine.[152] Sugammadex does not appear to have any significant hemodynamic or respiratory consequences.

Sugammadex may enable the rapid reversal of a profound nondepolarizing block in cases of difficult laryngoscopy and potentially eliminate succinylcholine from the standard anesthetic drug cart, cost notwithstanding. Reversal of profound rocuronium blockade (1.2 mg·kg⁻¹) with sugammadex (16 mg·kg⁻¹) was significantly faster than spontaneous recovery from succinylcholine (1 mg·kg⁻¹).[153] Jones et al[154] administered either sugammadex (4 mg·kg⁻¹) or neostigmine and glycopyrrolate to reverse a profound rocuronium neuromuscular block. The drugs were administered at the reappearance of 1 to 2 post-tetanic counts; sugammadex reversed the neuromuscular block significantly faster than the traditional reversal agents.

Rocuronium binds tightly to sugammadex rendering recurarisation as unlikely. However, if an inadequate dose of sugammadex is administered, unbound rocuronium redistributed from peripheral compartments may hinder the efficacy of sugammadex.[155] Because of its renal clearance, more study is required on its use in individuals with renal disease and other comorbidities. Although sugammadex is a useful addition to the armamentarium of airway practitioners, the intelligent use of muscle relaxants ought to limit the need for such an agent in difficult and failed airway management.

4.5   SUMMARY

Tracheal intubation and manipulation of the airway are associated with significant physiological changes. Although it is unknown if pharmacological attenuation of these responses improves outcomes, it seems both reasonable and logical to minimize these responses, particularly in compromised patients: *tight heart*, *tight brain*, and *tight lungs*. This chapter provides a general discussion of the appropriate pharmacological agents and their relevant properties. Successful and safe use of these drugs requires a clear understanding of patient's physiology, the pharmacokinetic and pharmacodynamic properties of the drugs, as well as the associated side effects.

REFERENCES

1. Figueredo E, Garcia-Fuentes EM. Assessment of the efficacy of esmolol on the haemodynamic changes induced by laryngoscopy and tracheal intubation: a meta-analysis. *Acta Anaesthesiol Scand*. 2001;45:1011-1022.

2. Donegan MF, Bedford RF. Intravenously administered lidocaine prevents intracranial hypertension during endotracheal suctioning. *Anesthesiology*. 1980;52:516-518.

3. Robinson N, Clancy M. In patients with head injury undergoing rapid sequence intubation, does pretreatment with intravenous lignocaine/lidocaine lead to an improved neurological outcome? A review of the literature. *Emerg Med J*. 2001;18:453-457.

4. White PF, Schlobohm RM, Pitts LH, Lindauer JM. A randomized study of drugs for preventing increases in intracranial pressure during endotracheal suctioning. *Anesthesiology*. 1982;57:242-244.

5. Yano M, Nishiyama H, Yokota H, et al. Effect of lidocaine on ICP response to endotracheal suctioning. *Anesthesiology*. 1986;64:651-653.

6. McAlpine LG, Thomson NC. Lidocaine-induced bronchoconstriction in asthmatic patients. Relation to histamine airway responsiveness and effect of preservative. *Chest*. 1989;96:1012-1015.

7. Kirkpatrick MB, Sanders RV, Bass JB, Jr. Physiologic effects and serum lidocaine concentrations after inhalation of lidocaine from a compressed gas-powered jet nebulizer. *Am Rev Respir Dis*. 1987;136:447-449.

8. Groeben H, Foster WM, Brown RH. Intravenous lidocaine and oral mexiletine block reflex bronchoconstriction in asthmatic subjects. *Am J Respir Crit Care Med*. 1996;154:885-888.

9. Groeben H, Silvanus MT, Beste M, Peters J. Combined intravenous lidocaine and inhaled salbutamol protect against bronchial hyperreactivity more effectively than lidocaine or salbutamol alone. *Anesthesiology*. 1998;89:862-868.

10. Groeben H, Silvanus MT, Beste M, Peters J. Both intravenous and inhaled lidocaine attenuate reflex bronchoconstriction but at different plasma concentrations. *Am J Respir Crit Care Med*. 1999;159:530-535.

11. Barash PG, Cullen BF, Stoelting RK. *Clinical Anesthesia*. 4th ed. Philadelphia, PA: Lippincott Williams & Wilkins; 2001.

12. Atcheson R, Lambert DG. Update on opioid receptors. *Br J Anaesth*. 1994;73:132-134.

13. Bailey PL, Wilbrink J, Zwanikken P, et al. Anesthetic induction with fentanyl. *Anesth Analg*. 1985;64:48-53.

14. Bennett JA, Abrams JT, Van Riper DF, Horrow JC. Difficult or impossible ventilation after sufentanil-induced anesthesia is caused primarily by vocal cord closure. *Anesthesiology*. 1997;87:1070-1074.

15. Streisand JB, Bailey PL, LeMaire L, et al. Fentanyl-induced rigidity and unconsciousness in human volunteers. Incidence, duration, and plasma concentrations. *Anesthesiology*. 1993;78:629-634.

16. Abrams JT, Horrow JC, Bennett JA, et al. Upper airway closure: a primary source of difficult ventilation with sufentanil induction of anesthesia. *Anesth Analg*. 1996;83:629-632.

17. Stoelting RK. *Pharmacology and Physiology in Anesthetic Practice*. 3rd ed. Philadelphia, PA: Lippincott-Raven; 1999.

18. Muller P, Vogtmann C. Three cases with different presentation of fentanyl-induced muscle rigidity—a rare problem in intensive care of neonates. *Am J Perinatol*. 2000;17: 23-26.

19. Vankova ME, Weinger MB, Chen DY, et al. Role of central mu, delta-1, and kappa-1 opioid receptors in opioid-induced muscle rigidity in the rat. *Anesthesiology*. 1996;85:574-583.

20. Liu RH, Fung SJ, Reddy VK, Barnes CD. Localization of glutamatergic neurons in the dorsolateral pontine tegmentum projecting to the spinal cord of the cat with a proposed role of glutamate on lumbar motoneuron activity. *Neuroscience*. 1995;64:193-208.

21. Lui PW, Lee TY, Chan SH. Involvement of locus coeruleus and noradrenergic neurotransmission in fentanyl-induced muscular rigidity in the rat. *Neurosci Lett*. 1989;96:114-119.

22. Mets B. Acute dystonia after alfentanil in untreated Parkinson's disease. *Anesth Analg*. 1991;72:557-558.

23. Tagaito Y, Isono S, Nishino T. Upper airway reflexes during a combination of propofol and fentanyl anesthesia. *Anesthesiology*. 1998;88:1459-1466.

24. Shafer SL, Varvel JR. Pharmacokinetics, pharmacodynamics, and rational opioid selection. *Anesthesiology*. 1991;74:53-63.

25. Egan TD, Lemmens HJ, Fiset P, et al. The pharmacokinetics of the new short-acting opioid remifentanil (GI87084B) in healthy adult male volunteers. *Anesthesiology*. 1993;79:881-892.

26. Batra YK, Al Qattan AR, Ali SS, et al. Assessment of tracheal intubating conditions in children using remifentanil and propofol without muscle relaxant. *Paediatr Anaesth*. 2004;14:452-456.

27. Blair JM, Hill DA, Wilson CM, Fee JP. Assessment of tracheal intubation in children after induction with propofol and different doses of remifentanil. *Anaesthesia*. 2004;59:27-33.

28. Grant S, Noble S, Woods A, et al. Assessment of intubating conditions in adults after induction with propofol and varying doses of remifentanil. *Br J Anaesth*. 1998;81:540-543.

29. Habib AS, Parker JL, Maguire AM, et al. Effects of remifentanil and alfentanil on the cardiovascular responses to induction of anaesthesia and tracheal intubation in the elderly. *Br J Anaesth*. 2002;88:430-433.

30. Maguire AM, Kumar N, Parker JL, et al. Comparison of effects of remifentanil and alfentanil on cardiovascular response to tracheal intubation in hypertensive patients. *Br J Anaesth*. 2001;86:90-93.

31. McAtamney D, O'Hare R, Hughes D, et al. Evaluation of remifentanil for control of haemodynamic response to tracheal intubation. *Anaesthesia*. 1998;53:1223-1227.

32. Glass PS, Hardman D, Kamiyama Y, et al. Preliminary pharmacokinetics and pharmacodynamics of an ultra-short-acting opioid: remifentanil (GI87084B). *Anesth Analg*. 1993;77:1031-1040.

33. Joshi GP, Warner DS, Twersky RS, Fleisher LA. A comparison of the remifentanil and fentanyl adverse effect profile in a multicenter phase IV study. *J Clin Anesth*. 2002;14:494-499.

34. Lee MP, Kua JS, Chiu WK. The use of remifentanil to facilitate the insertion of the laryngeal mask airway. *Anesth Analg*. 2001;93:359-362.

35. Alexander R, Olufolabi AJ, Booth J, et al. Dosing study of remifentanil and propofol for tracheal intubation without the use of muscle relaxants. *Anaesthesia*. 1999;54:1037-1040.

36. Erhan E, Ugur G, Alper I, et al. Tracheal intubation without muscle relaxants: remifentanil or alfentanil in combination with propofol. *Eur J Anaesthesiol*. 2003;20:37-43.

37. Klemola UM, Mennander S, Saarnivaara L. Tracheal intubation without the use of muscle relaxants: remifentanil or alfentanil in combination with propofol. *Acta Anaesthesiol Scand*. 2000;44:465-469.

38. Donaldson AB, Meyer-Witting M, Roux A. Awake fibreoptic intubation under remifentanil and propofol target-controlled infusion. *Anaesth Intensive Care*. 2002;30:93-95.

39. Machata AM, Gonano C, Holzer A, et al. Awake nasotracheal fiberoptic intubation: patient comfort, intubating conditions, and hemodynamic stability during conscious sedation with remifentanil. *Anesth Analg*. 2003;97:904-908.

40. Puchner W, Egger P, Puhringer F, et al. Evaluation of remifentanil as single drug for awake fiberoptic intubation. *Acta Anaesthesiol Scand*. 2002;46:350-354.

41. Puchner W, Obwegeser J, Puhringer FK. Use of remifentanil for awake fiberoptic intubation in a morbidly obese patient with severe inflammation of the neck. *Acta Anaesthesiol Scand*. 2002;46:473-476.

42. Mingo OH, Ashpole KJ, Irving CJ, Rucklidge MW. Remifentanil sedation for awake fibreoptic intubation with limited application of local anaesthetic in patients for elective head and neck surgery. *Anaesthesia*. 2008;63:1065-1069.

43. Lerman J, Chinyanga HM. The heart rate response to succinylcholine in children: a comparison of atropine and glycopyrrolate. *Can Anaesth Soc J*. 1983;30:377-381.

44. Bevan DR, Donati F, Kopman AF. Reversal of neuromuscular blockade. *Anesthesiology*. 1992;77:785-805.

45. D'Honneur G, Gall O, Gerard A, et al. Priming doses of atracurium and vecuronium depress swallowing in humans. *Anesthesiology*. 1992;77:1070-1073.

46. Harvey SC, Roland P, Bailey MK, et al. A randomized, double-blind comparison of rocuronium, d-tubocurarine, and "mini-dose" succinylcholine for preventing succinylcholine-induced muscle fasciculations. *Anesth Analg*. 1998;87:719-722.

47. Martin R, Carrier J, Pirlet M, et al. Rocuronium is the best non-depolarizing relaxant to prevent succinylcholine fasciculations and myalgia. *Can J Anaesth.* 1998;45:521-525.

48. Mencke T, Schreiber JU, Becker C, et al. Pretreatment before succinylcholine for outpatient anesthesia? *Anesth Analg.* 2002;94:573-576.

49. Motamed C, Choquette R, Donati F. Rocuronium prevents succinylcholine-induced fasciculations. *Can J Anaesth.* 1997;44:1262-1268.

50. Pace NL. Prevention of succinylcholine myalgias: a meta-analysis. *Anesth Analg.* 1990;70:477-483.

51. Donati F. Succinylcholine in modern anesthesia. *Anesthesiol Round.* 2002;1.

52. Beskow A, Werner O, Westrin P. Faster recovery after anesthesia in infants after intravenous induction with methohexital instead of thiopental. *Anesthesiology.* 1995;83:976-979.

53. Bedford RF, Persing JA, Pobereskin L, Butler A. Lidocaine or thiopental for rapid control of intracranial hypertension? *Anesth Analg.* 1980;59:435-437.

54. Brain Resuscitation Clinical Trial I Study Group. Randomized clinical study of thiopental loading in comatose survivors of cardiac arrest. *N Engl J Med.* 1986;314:397-403.

55. Gunaydin B, Babacan A. Cerebral hypoperfusion after cardiac surgery and anesthetic strategies: a comparative study with high dose fentanyl and barbiturate anesthesia. *Ann Thorac Cardiovasc Surg.* 1998;4:12-17.

56. Nussmeier NA, Arlund C, Slogoff S. Neuropsychiatric complications after cardiopulmonary bypass: cerebral protection by a barbiturate. *Anesthesiology.* 1986;64:165-170.

57. Ward JD, Becker DP, Miller JD, et al. Failure of prophylactic barbiturate coma in the treatment of severe head injury. *J Neurosurg.* 1985;62:383-388.

58. Modica PA, Tempelhoff R, White PF. Pro- and anticonvulsant effects of anesthetics (Part II). *Anesth Analg.* 1990;70:433-444.

59. Dew RE, Kimball JN, Rosenquist PB, McCall WV. Seizure length and clinical outcome in electroconvulsive therapy using methohexital or thiopental. *J ECT.* 2005;21:16-18.

60. Filner BE, Karliner JS. Alterations of normal left ventricular performance by general anesthesia. *Anesthesiology.* 1976;45:610-621.

61. Hirshman CA, Edelstein RA, Ebertz JM, Hanifin JM. Thiobarbiturate-induced histamine release in human skin mast cells. *Anesthesiology.* 1985;63:353-356.

62. Eames WO, Rooke GA, Wu RS, Bishop MJ. Comparison of the effects of etomidate, propofol, and thiopental on respiratory resistance after tracheal intubation. *Anesthesiology.* 1996;84:1307-1311.

63. Todd MM, Drummond JC, Hoi Sang U. The hemodynamic consequences of high-dose methohexital anesthesia in humans. *Anesthesiology.* 1984;61:495-501.

64. Mould DR, DeFeo TM, Reele S, et al. Simultaneous modeling of the pharmacokinetics and pharmacodynamics of midazolam and diazepam. *Clin Pharmacol Ther.* 1995;58:35-43.

65. Berggren L, Eriksson I. Midazolam for induction of anaesthesia in outpatients: a comparison with thiopentone. *Acta Anaesthesiol Scand.* 1981;25:492-496.

66. Driessen JJ, Booij LH, Crul JF, Vree TB. Comparative study of thiopental and midazolam for induction of anesthesia. *Anaesthesist.* 1983;32:478-482.

67. Jensen S, Schou-Olesen A, Huttel MS. Use of midazolam as an induction agent: comparison with thiopentone. *Br J Anaesth.* 1982;54:605-607.

68. Izuora KL, Ffoulkes-Crabbe DJ, Kushimo OT, et al. Open comparative study of the efficacy, safety and tolerability of midazolam versus thiopental in induction and maintenance of anaesthesia. *West Afr J Med.* 1994;13:73-80.

69. Sagarin MJ, Barton ED, Sakles JC, et al. Underdosing of midazolam in emergency endotracheal intubation. *Acad Emerg Med.* 2003;10:329-338.

70. Milde LN, Milde JH, Michenfelder JD. Cerebral functional, metabolic, and hemodynamic effects of etomidate in dogs. *Anesthesiology.* 1985;63:371-377.

71. Reddy RV, Moorthy SS, Dierdorf SF, et al. Excitatory effects and electroencephalographic correlation of etomidate, thiopental, methohexital, and propofol. *Anesth Analg.* 1993;77:1008-1011.

72. Avramov MN, Husain MM, White PF. The comparative effects of methohexital, propofol, and etomidate for electroconvulsive therapy. *Anesth Analg.* 1995;81:596-602.

73. Choi SD, Spaulding BC, Gross JB, Apfelbaum JL. Comparison of the ventilatory effects of etomidate and methohexital. *Anesthesiology.* 1985;62:442-447.

74. Choi YF, Wong TW, Lau CC. Midazolam is more likely to cause hypotension than etomidate in emergency department rapid sequence intubation. *Emerg Med J.* 2004;21:700-702.

75. Guldner G, Schultz J, Sexton P, et al. Etomidate for rapid-sequence intubation in young children: hemodynamic effects and adverse events. *Acad Emerg Med.* 2003;10:134-139.

76. Jellish WS, Riche H, Salord F, et al. Etomidate and thiopental-based anesthetic induction: comparisons between different titrated levels of electrophysiologic cortical depression and response to laryngoscopy. *J Clin Anesth.* 1997;9:36-41.

77. Gauss A, Heinrich H, Wilder-Smith OH. Echocardiographic assessment of the haemodynamic effects of propofol: a comparison with etomidate and thiopentone. *Anaesthesia.* 1991;46:99-105.

78. Holdcroft A, Morgan M, Whitwam JG, Lumley J. Effect of dose and premedication on induction complications with etomidate. *Br J Anaesth.* 1976;48:199-205.

79. Ghoneim MM, Yamada T. Etomidate: a clinical and electroencephalographic comparison with thiopental. *Anesth Analg.* 1977;56:479-485.

80. Duthie DJ, Fraser R, Nimmo WS. Effect of induction of anaesthesia with etomidate on corticosteroid synthesis in man. *Br J Anaesth.* 1985;57:156-159.

81. Wagner RL, White PF. Etomidate inhibits adrenocortical function in surgical patients. *Anesthesiology.* 1984;61:647-651.

82. Wagner RL, White PF, Kan PB, et al. Inhibition of adrenal steroidogenesis by the anesthetic etomidate. *N Engl J Med.* 1984;310:1415-1421.

83. Pfenninger E, Dick W, Ahnefeld FW. The influence of ketamine on both normal and raised intracranial pressure of artificially ventilated animals. *Eur J Anaesthesiol.* 1985;2:297-307.

84. Schwedler M, Miletich DJ, Albrecht RF. Cerebral blood flow and metabolism following ketamine administration. *Can Anaesth Soc J.* 1982;29:222-226.

85. Albanese J, Arnaud S, Rey M, et al. Ketamine decreases intracranial pressure and electroencephalographic activity in traumatic brain injury patients during propofol sedation. *Anesthesiology.* 1997;87:1328-1334.

86. Mayberg TS, Lam AM, Matta BF, et al. Ketamine does not increase cerebral blood flow velocity or intracranial pressure during isoflurane/nitrous oxide anesthesia in patients undergoing craniotomy. *Anesth Analg.* 1995;81:84-89.

87. Hirota K, Lambert DG. Ketamine: its mechanism(s) of action and unusual clinical uses. *Br J Anaesth.* 1996;77:441-444.

88. Hemming A, MacKenzie I, Finfer S. Response to ketamine in status asthmaticus resistant to maximal medical treatment. *Thorax.* 1994;49:90-91.

89. Hemmingsen C, Nielsen PK, Odorico J. Ketamine in the treatment of bronchospasm during mechanical ventilation. *Am J Emerg Med.* 1994;12:417-420.

90. Hirshman CA, Downes H, Farbood A, Bergman NA. Ketamine block of bronchospasm in experimental canine asthma. *Br J Anaesth.* 1979;51:713-718.

91. L'Hommedieu CS, Arens JJ. The use of ketamine for the emergency intubation of patients with status asthmaticus. *Ann Emerg Med.* 1987;16:568-571.

92. Sarma VJ. Use of ketamine in acute severe asthma. *Acta Anaesthesiol Scand.* 1992;36:106-107.

93. Cartwright PD, Pingel SM. Midazolam and diazepam in ketamine anaesthesia. *Anaesthesia.* 1984;39:439-442.

94. Bryson HM, Fulton BR, Faulds D. Propofol. An update of its use in anaesthesia and conscious sedation. *Drugs.* 1995;50:513-559.

95. Cavazzuti M, Porro CA, Barbieri A, Galetti A. Brain and spinal cord metabolic activity during propofol anaesthesia. *Br J Anaesth.* 1991;66:490-495.

96. Lagerkranser M, Stange K, Sollevi A. Effects of propofol on cerebral blood flow, metabolism, and cerebral autoregulation in the anesthetized pig. *J Neurosurg Anesthesiol.* 1997;9:188-193.

97. Pinaud M, Lelausque JN, Chetanneau A, et al. Effects of propofol on cerebral hemodynamics and metabolism in patients with brain trauma. *Anesthesiology.* 1990;73:404-409.

98. Searle NR, Sahab P. Propofol in patients with cardiac disease. *Can J Anaesth.* 1993;40:730-747.

99. Ebrahim ZY, Schubert A, Van Ness P, et al. The effect of propofol on the electroencephalogram of patients with epilepsy. *Anesth Analg.* 1994;78:275-279.

100. King SY, Davis FM, Wells JE, et al. Lidocaine for the prevention of pain due to injection of propofol. *Anesth Analg.* 1992;74:246-249.

101. Johnson RA, Harper NJ, Chadwick S, Vohra A. Pain on injection of propofol. Methods of alleviation. *Anaesthesia.* 1990;45:439-442.

102. Doi M, Ikeda K. Airway irritation produced by volatile anaesthetics during brief inhalation: comparison of halothane, enflurane, isoflurane and sevoflurane. *Can J Anaesth.* 1993;40:122-126.

103. Mostafa SM, Atherton AM. Sevoflurane for difficult tracheal intubation. *Br J Anaesth.* 1997;79:392-393.

104. Muzi M, Robinson BJ, Ebert TJ, O'Brien TJ. Induction of anesthesia and tracheal intubation with sevoflurane in adults. *Anesthesiology.* 1996;85:536-543.

105. Thwaites A, Edmends S, Smith I. Inhalation induction with sevoflurane: a double-blind comparison with propofol. *Br J Anaesth.* 1997;78:356-361.

106. Yogendran S, Prabhu A, Hendy A, et al. Vital capacity and patient controlled sevoflurane inhalation result in similar induction characteristics. *Can J Anaesth.* 2005;52:45-49.

107. Andrews JI, Kumar N, van den Brom RH, et al. A large simple randomized trial of rocuronium versus succinylcholine in rapid-sequence induction of anaesthesia along with propofol. *Acta Anaesthesiol Scand.* 1999;43:4-8.

108. Kopman AF, Klewicka MM, Neuman GG. An alternate method for estimating the dose-response relationships of neuromuscular blocking drugs. *Anesth Analg.* 2000;90:1191-1197.

109. Szalados JE, Donati F, Bevan DR. Effect of d-tubocurarine pretreatment on succinylcholine twitch augmentation and neuromuscular blockade. *Anesth Analg.* 1990;71:55-59.

110. Meakin G, McKiernan EP, Morris P, Baker RD. Dose-response curves for suxamethonium in neonates, infants and children. *Br J Anaesth.* 1989;62:655-658.

111. Lemmens HJ, Brodsky JB. The dose of succinylcholine in morbid obesity. *Anesth Analg.* 2006;102:438-442.

112. Roy JJ, Donati F, Boismenu D, Varin F. Concentration-effect relation of succinylcholine chloride during propofol anesthesia. *Anesthesiology.* 2002;97:1082-1092.

113. Hayes AH, Breslin DS, Mirakhur RK, et al. Frequency of haemoglobin desaturation with the use of succinylcholine during rapid sequence induction of anaesthesia. *Acta Anaesthesiol Scand.* 2001;45:746-749.

114. Donati F. The right dose of succinylcholine. *Anesthesiology.* 2003;99:1037-1078.

115. Lanier WL, Milde JH, Michenfelder JD. Cerebral stimulation following succinylcholine in dogs. *Anesthesiology.* 1986;64:551-559.

116. Wong SF, Chung F. Succinylcholine-associated postoperative myalgia. *Anaesthesia.* 2000;55:144-152.

117. Mikat-Stevens M, Sukhani R, Pappas AL, et al. Is succinylcholine after pretreatment with d-tubocurarine and lidocaine contraindicated for outpatient anesthesia? *Anesth Analg.* 2000;91:312-316.

118. McLoughlin C, Leslie K, Caldwell JE. Influence of dose on suxamethonium-induced muscle damage. *Br J Anaesth.* 1994;73:194-198.

119. Martyn JA, White DA, Gronert GA, et al. Up-and-down regulation of skeletal muscle acetylcholine receptors. Effects on neuromuscular blockers. *Anesthesiology.* 1992;76:822-843.

120. Gronert GA. Cardiac arrest after succinylcholine: mortality greater with rhabdomyolysis than receptor upregulation. *Anesthesiology.* 2001;94:523-529.

121. Viby-Mogensen J, Hanel HK, Hansen E, Graae J. Serum cholinesterase activity in burned patients. II: anaesthesia, suxamethonium and hyperkalaemia. *Acta Anaesthesiol Scand.* 1975;19:169-179.

122. Feldman JM. Cardiac arrest after succinylcholine administration in a pregnant patient recovered from Guillain-Barre syndrome. *Anesthesiology.* 1990;72:942-944.

123. Fergusson RJ, Wright DJ, Willey RF, et al. Suxamethonium is dangerous in polyneuropathy. *Br Med J (Clin Res Ed).* 1981;282:298-299.

124. Dierdorf SF, McNiece WL, Rao CC, et al. Effect of succinylcholine on plasma potassium in children with cerebral palsy. *Anesthesiology.* 1985;62:88-90.

125. Dierdorf SF, McNiece WL, Rao CC, et al. Failure of succinylcholine to alter plasma potassium in children with myelomeningocoele. *Anesthesiology.* 1986;64:272-273.

126. Khan TZ, Khan RM. Changes in serum potassium following succinylcholine in patients with infections. *Anesth Analg.* 1983;62:327-331.

127. Kohlschutter B, Baur H, Roth F. Suxamethonium-induced hyperkalaemia in patients with severe intra-abdominal infections. *Br J Anaesth.* 1976;48:557-562.

128. Larach MG, Rosenberg H, Gronert GA, Allen GC. Hyperkalemic cardiac arrest during anesthesia in infants and children with occult myopathies. *Clin Pediatr (Phila).* 1997;36:9-16.

129. Smith CL, Bush GH. Anaesthesia and progressive muscular dystrophy. *Br J Anaesth.* 1985;57:1113-1118.

130. Thapa S, Brull SJ. Succinylcholine-induced hyperkalemia in patients with renal failure: an old question revisited. *Anesth Analg.* 2000;91:237-241.

131. Schow AJ, Lubarsky DA, Olson RP, Gan TJ. Can succinylcholine be used safely in hyperkalemic patients? *Anesth Analg.* 2002;95:119-122.

132. McAuliffe G, Bissonnette B, Boutin C. Should the routine use of atropine before succinylcholine in children be reconsidered? *Can J Anaesth.* 1995;42:724-729.

133. Cunningham AJ, Barry P. Intraocular pressure—physiology and implications for anaesthetic management. *Can Anaesth Soc J.* 1986;33:195-208.

134. Vachon CA, Warner DO, Bacon DR. Succinylcholine and the open globe. Tracing the teaching. *Anesthesiology.* 2003;99:220-223.

135. Rosenbaum HK, Miller JD. Malignant hyperthermia and myotonic disorders. *Anesthesiol Clin North America.* 2002;20:623-664.

136. Rosenberg H FJ, Brandom BW: Malignant hyperthermia and other pharmaco-genetic disorders. In: Barash PG, Cullen BF, Stoelting RK, eds. *Clinical Anesthesia.* 4th ed. Philadelphia, PA: Lippincott Williams & Wilkins; 2001:521-549.

137. Rosenberg H. Trismus is not trivial. *Anesthesiology.* 1987;67:453-445.

138. Littleford JA, Patel LR, Bose D, et al. Masseter muscle spasm in children: implications of continuing the triggering anesthetic. *Anesth Analg.* 1991;72:151-160.

139. O'Flynn RP, Shutack JG, Rosenberg H, Fletcher JE. Masseter muscle rigidity and malignant hyperthermia susceptibility in pediatric patients. An update on management and diagnosis. *Anesthesiology.* 1994;80:1228-1233.

140. Sparr HJ, Mellinghoff H, Blobner M, Noldge-Schomburg G. Comparison of intubating conditions after rapacuronium (Org 9487) and succinylcholine following rapid sequence induction in adult patients. *Br J Anaesth.* 1999;82:537-541.

141. Moore EW, Hunter JM. The new neuromuscular blocking agents: do they offer any advantages? *Br J Anaesth.* 2001;87:912-925.

142. Kovacs G, Law JA, Ross J, et al. Acute airway management in the emergency department by non-anesthesiologists. *Can J Anaesth.* 2004;51:174-180.

143. Laurin EG, Sakles JC, Panacek EA, et al. A comparison of succinylcholine and rocuronium for rapid-sequence intubation of emergency department patients. *Acad Emerg Med.* 2000;7:1362-1369.

144. Mazurek AJ, Rae B, Hann S, et al. Rocuronium versus succinylcholine: are they equally effective during rapid-sequence induction of anesthesia? *Anesth Analg.* 1998;87:1259-1262.

145. Mehta MP, Sokoll MD, Gergis SD. Accelerated onset of non-depolarizing neuromuscular blocking drugs: pancuronium, atracurium and vecuronium. A comparison with succinylcholine. *Eur J Anaesthesiol.* 1988;5:15-21.

146. McCourt KC, Salmela L, Mirakhur RK, et al. Comparison of rocuronium and suxamethonium for use during rapid sequence induction of anaesthesia. *Anaesthesia.* 1998;53:867-871.

147. Perry JJ, Lee J, Wells G. Are intubation conditions using rocuronium equivalent to those using succinylcholine? *Acad Emerg Med.* 2002;9:813-823.

148. Cheng CA, Aun CS, Gin T. Comparison of rocuronium and suxamethonium for rapid tracheal intubation in children. *Paediatr Anaesth.* 2002;12:140-145.

149. Belmont MR, Lien CA, Tjan J, et al. Clinical pharmacology of GW280430A in humans. *Anesthesiology.* 2004;100:768-773.

150. Naguib M, Brull SJ. Update on neuromuscular pharmacology. *Curr Opin Anaesthesiol.* 2009;22:483-490.

151. Brull SJ, Naguib M. Selective reversal of muscle relaxation in general anesthesia: focus on sugammadex. *Drug Des Devel Ther.* 2009;3:119-129.

152. Yang LP, Keam SJ. Sugammadex: a review of its use in anaesthetic practice. *Drugs.* 2009;69:919-942.

153. Lee C, Jahr JS, Candiotti KA, et al. Reversal of profound neuromuscular block by sugammadex administered three minutes after rocuronium: a comparison with spontaneous recovery from succinylcholine. *Anesthesiology.* 2009;110:1020-1025.

154. Jones RK, Caldwell JE, Brull SJ, Soto RG. Reversal of profound rocuronium-induced blockade with sugammadex: a randomized comparison with neostigmine. *Anesthesiology.* 2008;109:816-824.

155. Craig RG, Hunter JM. Neuromuscular blocking drugs and their antagonists in patients with organ disease. *Anaesthesia.* 2009;64(Suppl 1):55-65.

SELF-EVALUATION QUESTIONS

4.1. Which of the following is a true statement about the elimination of remifentanil?

    A. It is metabolized by hepatic enzymes.

    B. It is primarily removed from the body unchanged by the kidneys.

    C. It is metabolized primarily by plasma and tissue esterases.

    D. It is primarily removed from the body by Hofmann degradation.

    E. It is metabolized primarily by plasma pseudocholinesterases.

4.2. To avoid serious hyperkalemia, which of the following is **NOT** considered a safe period to administer succinylcholine to a burned patient?

    A. immediately after the burn

    B. more than 1 day after the burn

    C. more than 2 days after the burn

    D. more than 3 days after the burn

    E. more than 4 days after the burn

4.3. Which of the following statements is **NOT** true about Sugammadex?

    A. Sugammadex is a modified γ-cyclodextrin.

    B. Sugammadex selectively binds and inactivates vecuronium, enhancing neuromuscular recovery.

    C. Sugammadex selectively binds and inactivates rocuronium, enhancing neuromuscular recovery.

    D. Sugammadex interacts with nicotinic receptors by displacing rocuronium and vecuronium.

    E. Sugammadex does not appear to have any significant hemodynamic or respiratory effects.

CHAPTER 5

Aspiration: Risks and Prevention

Saul Pytka, Edward Crosby, and Idena Carroll

5.1   INTRODUCTION

Pulmonary aspiration, an uncommon occurrence in nonemergency airway management, may lead to a spectrum of sequelae, from no discernable effects to significant morbidity and mortality. In this chapter, we will outline the known factors that increase the risks of aspiration and how airway management may be optimized to reduce the risks to the patient.

Although reported in the literature as a relatively uncommon complication of nonemergency airway management, a majority of airway practitioners will acknowledge that the risk of aspiration is a major concern to them in daily practice. Most would acknowledge that if they have not had an episode of aspiration in one of their patients, they know a colleague who has had to deal with the complication. Kluger and Willemsen[1] reported in 1998 that over 71% of all anesthesiologists responding to a national mail-in survey in New Zealand had had at least one case of aspiration in their careers.

5.2   HISTORICAL PERSPECTIVE

5.2.1   When was gastric aspiration first described?

Mendelson was the first to describe the occurrence of aspiration in conjunction with the delivery of obstetrical anesthesia.[2] Since that time, a plethora of publications have followed, outlining the risks and ways of preventing the problem. Unfortunately, much of the information is conflicting, and conclusions have been derived from studies with surrogate endpoints that may have very little to do with actual clinical risks. For example, the often-quoted study by Roberts and Shirley[3] suggested a gastric volume of greater than 25 mL and pH of less than 2.5, as a specific risk factor for aspiration. This postulation was accepted by subsequent investigators who directed their efforts for prevention of aspiration to the assumption that these specific values were critical factors in predicting the outcome of aspiration.

5.2.2   What was Sellick's approach to minimize the risk of gastric aspiration?

In the discussion section of his 1961 paper advocating the use of cricoid pressure during the induction of anesthesia to prevent the aspiration of gastric contents, Sellick examined alternatives available at the time.[4] He identified inhalational induction in the supine or lateral position (with head-down tilt) and rapid IV induction of anesthesia in the sitting position. He commented that, with inhalational induction, vomiting usually occurred in lighter stages of anesthesia when protective reflexes were hopefully still present and noted that any difficulty during induction predisposed to regurgitation and anoxia. Rapid IV induction in the sitting position often led to cardiovascular collapse in critically ill patients, and pulmonary aspiration was made more likely by the sitting position, if gastric reflux occurred. Sellick advocated the use of cricoid pressure during induction of anesthesia as a third option.

Sellick suggested that the stomach should be emptied before induction and the nasogastric tube then be removed. He was of the opinion that the nasogastric tube would prevent esophageal occlusion with cricoid pressure. The patient was positioned with the head and neck fully extended and, following denitrogenation, induction ideally occurred with an IV barbiturate-muscle relaxant combination. Cricoid pressure was instituted before induction, moderate pressure was applied during induction, and this was increased to firm pressure once consciousness was lost. Sellick suggested that the lungs may be ventilated without risk of gastric regurgitation. Once intubation was completed and the cuff inflated, cricoid pressure could be safely released.

In his description of cricoid pressure, Sellick reported its application in 23 high-risk cases. He noted no instance of pulmonary aspiration in any patient but did report that, in three cases, release of cricoid pressure after intubation was followed immediately by reflux into the pharynx of gastric or esophageal contents, suggesting that cricoid pressure had indeed been effective.

5.3   INCIDENCE AND RISK

5.3.1   What is the incidence of aspiration in anesthesia practice?

The difficulty in determining the actual incidence of aspiration relates to a number of factors. Firstly, because it occurs rarely, studies addressing the topic need to be very large. Most, if not all, of the better studies to date have been derived from large computerized databases. Secondly, aspiration is not always easy to recognize and, as will be illustrated below, rarely leads to clinical findings, let alone serious sequelae. Hence, it is an event likely to be missed and therefore underreported.

The recognition of gastric material in the pharynx does not alone support a diagnosis of aspiration. Despite the evident regurgitation, pulmonary aspiration may not have occurred. Even if foreign material is seen below the level of the true vocal cords, there may be a wide spectrum of clinical consequences. Silent aspiration may occur, wherein the patient exhibits no signs or symptoms of aspiration and there are no disruptions of physiological parameters. Indeed, it has been reported that asymptomatic aspiration may occur in up to 45% of normal subjects during sleep, and as many as 70% of people who have a blunted level of consciousness and responsiveness.[5]

Aspiration may become symptomatic, with cough and audible wheeze. Acute lung injury may be associated with tachypnea, increase in alveolar-arterial (A-a) gradient, hypoxemia, and radiological evidence of lung injury—with infiltrates and/or atelectasis. Frank respiratory failure may ensue, with the development of acute respiratory distress syndrome (ARDS), the need for ventilatory support, and (rarely) death.

Although many papers have reviewed the topic of aspiration, there has been a notable absence of consistent end points. In 1993, Warner[6] published a retrospective review of 215,488 general anesthetics over a period of 6 years. Aspiration was defined as:

> …either the presence of bilious secretions, or particulate matter, in the tracheobronchial tree; or, in patients who did not have their tracheobronchial airways directly examined after regurgitation, the presence of an infiltrate on postoperative chest roentgenogram that was not identified by preoperative roentgenogram, or physical examination.

Of the anesthetics included, 202,061 were elective and the remaining 13,427 were emergency cases. There were 52 and 15 aspirations in these two groups, respectively. The overall incidence of aspiration was 1:3216. Aspiration occurred in 1:3886 of elective surgeries and 1:895 of emergency procedures. Sixty-seven cases of significant aspiration were recognized; one patient died from surgical causes intraoperatively. Of the remaining 66 patients, 42 (64%) experienced no obvious sequelae from the aspiration. Of the remaining 24 patients, 13 required mechanical ventilation with 6 needing prolonged (>24 hours) mechanical support. Half of these (three) died of complications from their aspiration, giving a death rate of 1:71,829.

Mellin-Olsen,[7] in 1996, reported a prospective review of 85,594 cases over a 5-year period. They defined aspiration as "what the anesthetist has interpreted as such during, or immediately after the anesthetic procedures, based on clinical signs like gastric content, in the pharynx/larynx/trachea and a drop in O_2 saturation." In their study, a total 25 cases of aspiration were recorded; 52,650 patients had received a general anesthetic, with the remainder undergoing either regional or IV sedation. All cases of aspiration occurred in the general anesthetic population, giving an incidence of 1:2106. The incidence of aspiration was 1:3303 in elective procedures under general anesthetic and 1:809 for emergency procedures, both rates similar in magnitude to those reported by Warner. In the patients who had aspirated, there were similar complications to those described by Warner.[6] No deaths occurred and 22/25 patients had either no or minimal sequelae; three experienced more serious consequences. One patient required ventilation for 7 days, but made a complete recovery from his lung injury.

Olsson et al[8] reported a similar retrospective review, with an incidence of aspiration of 1:2131 and a mortality rate of 1:46,000. Finally, Sakai et al[9] conducted a 4-year retrospective review of 99,441 anesthetics at a single American university hospital. There were 14 cases of confirmed pulmonary aspiration for an incidence of 0.014% or 1:7103 overall. Seven cases of aspiration occurred in gastroesophageal procedures and patients in whom aspiration occurred had one or more identifiable risk factors. Six patients developed pulmonary complications related to the aspiration and one died. All these studies reaffirm that aspiration is a relatively uncommon occurrence and the mortality due to aspiration in the perioperative period is rare.

Kluger and Short[10] reported, in 1999, the analysis of data from the Australian Anaesthetic Incident Monitoring Study (AIMS). AIMS is a voluntary, anonymous reporting system of anesthesia-related incidents, collected in a central database. Unfortunately, the nature of this type of study does not allow for a denominator (ie, the total number of anesthetics performed by all reporting clinicians) and the incidence is unavailable. Of the 5000 reported events, 133 dealt with aspiration. Aspiration was deemed to have occurred if "any obvious nonrespiratory secretions were suctioned via a tracheal tube, there was chest X-ray evidence of new pathology after an incident, and/or there were signs of new wheeze or crackles after an episode of regurgitation or vomiting." In this group of 133 aspirations, 5 deaths were recorded. Of interest, aspiration did occur in a number of patients undergoing regional anesthesia in the AIMS study (7 out of the 133), whereas none were reported to have occurred in almost 31,000 regional and sedation cases in the paper by Mellin-Olsen et al.[7]

The American Society of Anesthesiologists (ASA) Closed Claims Database reviewed the incidence of aspiration as a cause of liability to anesthesiologists. In 2000, Cheney[11] reported that aspiration represented 3.5% of all claims as a primary or secondary event, and in half of those it was the offending event leading to a claim. Seven percent of the aspiration claims were during regional anesthesia.

In conclusion, the incidence of aspiration in a population is consistently estimated at between 1:2000 and 1:4000, depending on the population studied, and when the data had been reported. Emergency surgery increases the risk of aspiration fourfold, or more, yet overall mortality remains low.

5.3.2   What are the risk factors that contribute to aspiration? What about nonanesthesia settings?

In published studies measuring the incidence of aspiration, the most common association was with emergency surgery.[6-8,10,11] Olsson[8] reported that the timing of surgery also correlated with an increased incidence of aspiration, with a sixfold increase in the rate of aspiration between 18:00 and 06:00 hours. The causative factors that relate to the increased risk of aspiration with emergency surgery are not outlined in the studies, but numerous issues such as lack of fasting, stress, depression of GI motility, less staff availability, higher dependence upon less-experienced anesthesia staff, and fatigue may all play contributing roles. A preponderance of the cases of aspiration reported by Olsson[8] occurred in patients who had abdominal surgery performed, with esophageal and upper abdominal procedures predominating. The incidence of aspiration in cesarean section was 1:661. Interestingly, Warner,[6] roughly 10 years later, had no cases of aspiration during cesarean section. In another paper reviewing the incidence of aspiration in children, Warner[12] reviewed 63,180 anesthetics in children under the age of 18 and also found the incidence of aspiration in the emergency patient (1:373) to be significantly higher than that in the elective situation (1:4544).

There is a paucity of well-controlled, clinical trials that examine the incidence of aspiration in the prehospital and emergency department (ED) settings. In the prehospital setting, the rates of occurrence of aspiration vary from 6% to 90%, depending on the study populations and facilities, and whether the study considered survivors, nonsurvivors, or postmortem examinations.[13,14] Often, aspiration had already occurred prior to attempted intervention and provision of care. In some papers, the incidence of failure to intubate the trachea is as high as 47%.[14,15,16] In the study by Gausche,[15] patients were randomized into intubation group versus transport by bag-mask. There was an intubation success rate by the paramedics of only 57% and the only aspirations occurred in the intubation group. The outcomes between the two groups, in terms of survival, were similar. In the prehospital literature, the source of aspirate in trauma patients differs from that of the emergency surgical population. In the study by Lockey,[13] 34%, or a total of 18 of the trauma patients, had evidence suggestive of aspiration. Of these, 15 had blood contaminating their airway, while only 3

had evidence of gastric contents. All had significant head injuries, with a Glasgow Coma Scale of 8 or less.[13]

Taryle reviewed 43 consecutive intubations in the ED in a major teaching institution and reported a total of 38 complications in half of the patients (22/43). Aspiration occurring prior to airway manipulation was not included as an aspiration within their data. There were eight aspirations; the second most common complication after prolonged intubating time.[17] Sakles[18] reported a 1-year review of all intubations in an ED that had a census of 60,000 patients per year. In 610 consecutive intubations, 49 patients had a total of 57 immediate complications. Although there were 10 cases of vomiting, they did not report any occurrences of aspiration. Mort,[19] while reporting on airway complications during emergency intubation occurring outside of the operating room, noted that fewer aspirations occurred in the ED than on the wards or the medical ICU. The obstetrical population will be discussed later in this chapter.

5.3.3   What happens during an aspiration that determines its severity?

The consequences of aspiration can occur as a result of a chemical injury to the airway mucosa from either acid or bile. Injury may occur from particulate material in the aspirate causing either airway obstruction, or an inflammatory response. Finally, there may be pneumonia secondary to contamination from bacteria in the stomach or upper airway.

Injury resulting from aspiration is often that of an acute chemical burn and is a function of both volume and pH of the aspirate. Subsequent release of inflammatory substances, such as cytokines and interleukins from injured tissue, provokes neutrophil migration to the affected areas and further airway reaction. Airway edema, as well as capillary leak in the alveoli, can increase airway resistance and worsen lung compliance. The end result is ventilation–perfusion mismatching and hypoxemia, as well as inflammatory infiltration and/or atelectasis.

The initial chemical burn effect occurs within seconds, followed by neutralization of the acid within 15 seconds. The sudden onset of bronchospasm and laryngospasm may occur. Full evolution of injury can take several days. Repair of the injury is of the order of 3 to 7 days. Particulate materials can induce a local reaction themselves and lead to a pneumonia. Indeed, attempts to neutralize the gastric pH with particulate antacids may aggravate reaction in the lung due to the particles rather than from the acid itself. Particulate materials of sufficient size or number can produce substantive airway obstruction in their own right.

Pneumonia may follow, related to organisms from the upper airway, esophagus, and stomach. This is usually of a mixed flora, with anaerobes and aerobes present. Depending on the organism and the premorbid condition of the patient, this may progress to lung abscess. This is unlikely in the healthy patient. Differentiating between inflammatory pneumonitis and pneumonia may be difficult. The clinical and radiological picture may be similar. Pneumonitis is usually acute, resolving in hours to a day. If the presentation is one of progression without resolution, lasting days, with fever and purulent sputum, a diagnosis of pneumonia is more likely.[20-24]

5.4   PATIENT POPULATIONS AT RISK

5.4.1   What is the relevance of the issues of gastric volume, pH, and constituency of the gastric contents?

Roberts and Shirley[3] concluded that a pH of less than 2.5 and a gastric volume of 25 mL (or 0.4 mL·kg^{-1}) correlated with aspiration and resultant pneumonitis. In their study, an acid solution was injected directly into the bronchus of a monkey and extrapolations were made in regard to the volume and pH that would place humans at risk. These conclusions have been challenged by numerous investigators.[25,26] Schreiner[26] in 1998 pointed out that over 30% to 60% of patients have a gastric fluid volume of greater than 0.4 mL·kg^{-1} (median 0.3, but as high as 4.5 mL·kg^{-1}), yet the incidence of aspiration is quite rare. Indeed, it has been demonstrated that the incidence of gastroesophageal reflux (GER) is not associated with residual gastric volume (RGV).[27] Rather, it has been shown that GER during anesthesia is related to episodes of straining on an endotracheal tube when inadequate anesthesia has been provided.[28]

Maltby[25] argues that the risk of aspiration is due to loss of the barrier pressure at the gastroesophageal sphincter (GES), also referred to as the lower esophageal sphincter (LES). Normally, stomach contents are prevented from refluxing into the esophagus by the pressure exerted by the LES. The difference between LES pressure and intragastric pressure is the barrier pressure. The stomach is a very compliant structure and intragastric pressure can remain stable until volumes greater than 1000 mL are present.[29] Indeed, as intragastric pressure rises, because of its anatomical design, so does LES pressure, maintaining the barrier pressure. In one study, measurements of the intragastric pressure and LES pressure during laparoscopy demonstrated that a rise in mean gastric pressure from 5.2 to 15.7 was matched by a rise in LES tone from 31.2 to 47.0 cm H$_2$O.[30]

There is a clear association between aspiration and vomiting or gagging.[1,6-8,10] With active vomiting, or gagging, the sudden onset of high intragastric pressure is associated with relaxation of both the lower and upper esophageal sphincter mechanisms. This combination enhances the risk of pulmonary aspiration.

The higher the baseline intragastric pressure, the greater the tendency for GER and pulmonary aspiration. With an intestinal obstruction, for example, the intragastric pressure is high in association with the large RGV. This accounts for the high incidence of aspiration in this patient population and the finding that it is one of the most common factors associated with aspiration in most publications. By the same reasoning, patients with a documented hiatal hernia, or a history of GER disease (GERD), are also exposed to a higher risk of regurgitation and aspiration.

Active vomiting, in association with an unprotected airway, is most likely to occur during induction of anesthesia, with airway manipulation prior to placement of the endotracheal tube, and at the end of a procedure as the patient is awakening and the airway is no longer protected. Inadequate levels of anesthesia at these times, as well as difficulty securing an airway, are the essential elements favoring the occurrence of aspiration. Two-thirds of aspiration events are reported during induction and extubation, equally divided between the two periods.[6]

5.4.2   How important is a history of heartburn? Acid taste or burping? A history of GERD? How much reflux is significant?

Reflux occurs when the barrier pressure fails to prevent gastric contents moving from the stomach into the esophagus. Intuitively, those with a clear history of reflux should be at greater risk of aspiration. Kluger[10] found that a history of reflux and hiatal hernia were the ninth and tenth most common predisposing factors for aspiration, representing 7 and 6 cases, respectively, in the database of 133 total cases of aspiration. The patient with a history of acid reflux, with complaints of acid taste or choking at night, represents a more significant risk than one with only complaints of heartburn. The latter may simply suggest gastric mucosal pathology. However, no specific data are available to indicate that one symptom is more helpful than another in identifying who is at greater risk. Again the larger the volume of reflux, the more significant is likely to be the risk of aspiration.

5.4.3   What clinical situations and characteristics predispose to aspiration?

5.4.3.1   Emergency Surgery

Emergency surgery is the most significant risk factor associated with aspiration in the studies outlined earlier, increasing the incidence of aspiration by four- to sixfold.[6]

5.4.3.2   ASA Physical Status

When Warner[6] compared the ASA status to the risk of aspiration in elective situations, the risk or aspiration increased by almost sevenfold as ASA status rose from I to IV or V. In emergency situations, the occurrence of aspiration increased from 1:2949 for ASA I patients to 1:343 for ASA IV and V patients, or almost a ninefold increment (Table 5-1). Olsson[8] also reported an increased risk of aspiration and increased morbidity with increasing ASA status. Most, if not all, of the reported aspiration-associated deaths occur in ASA IV and V patients.

5.4.3.3   Airway and Intubation Difficulties

Difficult intubation is associated with an increased risk of aspiration. Vomiting during airway interventions is frequently associated with aspiration, far more so than passive regurgitation. In Olsson's paper,[8] out of 15 cases of aspiration in elective patients in which no risk factors predisposing to aspiration could be identified from the chart review, 10 (67%) had difficulty with intubation preceding the vomiting and aspiration. In total, 58 out of the 87 patients who aspirated did so due to difficulty with intubation or,

TABLE 5-1

Risk of Pulmonary Aspiration in Elective and Emergency General Anesthetics by ASA Physical Status Classification[6]

ASA PHYSICAL STATUS	ELECTIVE	EMERGENCY	P
I	4/36,916 (1:9,229)	1/2,949 (1:2,949)	.319
II	11/82,436 (1:7,494)	3/5,036 (1:1,679)	.043
III	31/74,301 (1:2,397)	8/4,413 (1:552)	Less than .001
IV and V	6/8,409 (1:1,401)	3/1,029 (1:343)	.066
Total	52/202,061 (1:3,886)	15/13,427 (1:895)	Less than .001

with airway manipulation. Warner[6] described aspiration in 69% of his patients in whom active vomiting or gagging occurred during intubation or extubation. Mort demonstrated that when the number of intubation attempts went from ≤2 to greater than 2, a significant increase in complications occurred. The incidence of regurgitation rose from 1.9% to 22% and aspiration from 0.8% to 13%, directly correlated with an increase in the number of intubation attempts.[19] Sakai et al[9] reported that 5 of 16 reported aspirations occurred during laryngoscopy or airway interventions including the exchange of airway devices in at-risk patients.

In summary, there are multiple studies describing morbidity and mortality associated with airway interventions and difficulties.[19,31-33]

5.4.3.4   Obesity

There was no correlation between obesity and aspiration in the studies by Warner et al[6] or Mellin-Olson et al.[7] Olsson,[8] however, did find obesity to be a contributing factor for aspiration risk. Obesity is frequently listed as an aspiration-associated factor in many other references. The association of obesity with an elevated risk of aspiration may relate to a high incidence of pertinent comorbidities. For example, delayed gastric emptying is known to be associated with diabetes, which is a more frequent finding in the obese. Other factors related to the obese include GER, difficult intubation, and inadequate anesthesia at the time of induction. This may account for the larger number of obese patients reported in aspiration populations.[10]

Obese patients have the same gastric emptying rate for liquids as nonobese patients. Depending on the meal content, the gastric emptying in obese patients for solids may be faster, slower, or the same as in the nonobese patients.[25,34-37] Maltby[25] reported that obesity did not slow gastric emptying in the absence of other predisposing comorbid conditions and suggested that fasting guidelines should be applied to obese patients using the same criterion as for the nonobese. In their paper, obese patients, with no comorbid conditions, were randomized into fasting and nonfasting groups. The later received a 300-mL clear-fluid challenge preoperatively, with no difference in RGV demonstrated postintubation between the two groups. A study reviewing anesthesia for electroconvulsive therapy in 50 obese patients reported no cases of aspiration in 660 procedures.[38]

5.4.3.5   Pregnancy

It has been well accepted that the obstetrical population is at increased risk of aspiration. This has been felt to be secondary to a number of factors. Hormones, particularly progesterone, cause relaxation of the LES and impair gastric emptying. Mechanical effects of the gravid uterus alter the position of the stomach and, as term approaches, create a gastric *pinchcock* partially obstructing the gastroduodenal junction. The gravid uterus also increases intra-abdominal pressure, which then increases intragastric pressure. It has been demonstrated that the intragastric pressure in pregnancy is increased to 17.2 cm H_2O from the nonpregnant level of 7.3 cm H_2O. Women experiencing heartburn in pregnancy have a drop in the LES tone from the normal in pregnancy of 44 cm H_2O to 24 cm H_2O. Heartburn in pregnancy is reported in some series to be between 45% and 70%, with 27% of these patients having hiatal hernias. The onset of labor with pain and stress, coupled with the presence of opioid analgesics, are independent factors associated with a reduction in gastric emptying. Increased difficulty with intubation occurs in the parturient related to hormonally induced mucosal edema and increased breast mass. For many reasons, the parturient is at an increased risk for aspiration.[3,39-41]

Interestingly, however, this risk has significantly decreased since Mendelson reported a maternal death rate from aspiration during C-section of 1:667.[2,5] This may well be due to the increased use of regional anesthesia, as well as the application of rapid-sequence induction (RSI) techniques, with cricoid pressure and cuffed endotracheal tubes. The use of pharmacologic interventions, although not proven to alter the incidence, may also be a contributing factor. The adoption of difficult airway practices that discourage persistent failing attempts at intubation may be an important factor, as is the increased use of regional anesthesia.

A number of recent publications support the contention that the risk of aspiration has become a much smaller contributor to maternal morbidity and mortality. Mhyre et al[42] reviewed all reported maternal deaths in the state of Michigan, USA, between 1985 and 2003. Of the recorded 855 deaths over that time, 15 were felt to be associated with anesthesia in either a related or contributing form. Of the 15 cases, only 1 was felt to be due to aspiration. This occurred in the PACU following caesarian delivery of a stillbirth. The rest of the deaths had no association with aspiration. Interestingly, all anesthesia-related deaths from airway issues occurred during emergence from general anesthesia or in the recovery room. None occurred during induction.

In a recent prospective observational study, McDonnell et al[43] reported on the incidence of problems associated with airway management in the parturient, during the period 2005 to 2006, in 13 hospitals with just under 50,000 deliveries per year. During that period, 1095 general anesthetics were performed. In that series, eight cases reported regurgitation (0.7%), with one case of aspiration confirmed (0.1%). Two of the regurgitation cases occurred in elective caesarian sections. Of the eight regurgitation cases, four occurred during induction, and five at emergence (one patient regurgitated at both times). Interestingly, the incidence of difficult intubation was 3.3%, with failed intubation of 0.36%. The later were managed with laryngeal mask airway (LMA).

The low incidence of aspiration is supported by the Closed Claims Analysis of the ASA[44]. From 1990 onward, only two cases of aspiration were implicated in a maternal death or permanent brain damage, with one of these being in association with general, the other with regional anesthesia.

In conclusion, the incidence of aspiration in obstetrics continues to decline as a source of morbidity and mortality. Increased use of regional anesthesia, a larger number of skilled practitioners comfortable with airway management options, better monitoring, and the use of prophylaxis may all be contributing factors.

5.4.3.6   Age

According to Warner,[6] age was not found to be an independent risk factor for aspiration. Olsson,[8] however, did find that extremes of age increased the risk of aspiration. Warner[12] reviewed 63,180 anesthetics in children under the age of 18. The incidence of aspiration in that population was not dissimilar to adults, except that there was an increased incidence of aspiration in patients less than 3 years of age. Over 91% of the aspirations in this population had either a bowel obstruction or ileus perhaps skewing the incidence in young children, although there is some uncertainty as to the effectiveness of the LES in this population. Distended stomachs from both fluids and air entrained during crying or using a pacifier predisposes to gastric reflux when these infants cry or gag. The efficacy and method of application of cricoid pressure during RSI in small children has not been defined.

Borland found that the incidence of aspiration in the pediatric population was 10.2:10,000 higher than Warner's reported 3.8:10,000.[12,45]

5.4.3.7   Decreased Levels of Consciousness and Neurological Disease

It is recognized that the incidence of aspiration of extraglottic (eg, blood) and lower GI tract (eg, stomach contents) contaminants is increased in patients with a reduced level of consciousness.[8,13] In these patient populations, loss of function of the LES and upper esophageal sphincter and delayed gastric emptying combine with a reduction of upper airway protective reflexes to promote both regurgitation and aspiration.[46,47] This has relevance for the postanesthetic period as well, as it has been shown that patients left in the supine position with a reduced level of consciousness have an increased incidence of aspiration.

Patients with other underlying neurological diseases, such as Parkinson disease and multiple sclerosis, are also at increased risk of aspiration due to impairment of their protective airway reflexes.[48] The diabetic with autonomic neuropathy has been demonstrated to have delayed gastric emptying, sometimes manifested by early postprandial satiety, but it is usually asymptomatic. Diabetics have a theoretically increased incidence of difficult laryngoscopy and intubation due to glycosylation of collagen in the cervical vertebrae. Inspite of speculation that diabetics ought to be at increased risk of regurgitation and aspiration,[49,50] no studies have found diabetes to be an independent risk factor for aspiration.[1,6-8,10-12,45]

5.4.3.8   Bowel Obstruction or Other Gastrointestinal Pathology

As discussed in Section 5.4.1 in this chapter, increased gastric volume predisposes patients to an increased risk of aspiration. Gastric obstruction, and or ileus, is one of the commonest associations with aspiration.[8,10,12] The incidence of aspiration in esophageal endoscopy is 1:188, and appendectomy is 1:751.

5.4.3.9   Full Stomach

Even in the absence of bowel pathology, recent ingestion of a meal has been documented to be a risk factor for aspiration.[6,12] Guidelines for fasting have been developed for the elective population. However, fasting does not guarantee an empty stomach and RGVs can be quite variable.

5.4.4   Is there a difference in gastric emptying in emergency patients or those who have received opioids?

Trauma patients have been shown to have delayed gastric emptying up to a week after injury. Patients who are critically ill, in ICU, also have significantly delayed gastric emptying.[51] Neurological injury, either head or spinal cord, is associated with significant delays in gastric emptying related, in part, to catecholamine surge.[52]

Opioids, irrespective of the manner of administration, have been shown to decrease gastric emptying significantly.[53-55]

5.5   STRATEGIES AIMED AT MINIMIZING ASPIRATION RISK

5.5.1   What are the current fasting guidelines? What evidence supports their use?

The American Society of Anesthesiologists has published a set of fasting guidelines, generated from a review of the available literature and expert opinion.[56] These guidelines were developed with the healthy patient in mind, booked for elective surgery. They are not intended to be applied to patients with comorbidities that would increase the risk of aspiration. There is a striking paucity of evidence around the relationships between fasting times, gastric volume, pH, and the risk of pulmonary aspiration. The consensus guidelines recommended the following:

For clear fluids, the Task Force recommended a minimum 2-hour period of preoperative abstinence. Clear fluids consist of water, black tea or coffee, pulp-free juices, fat-and protein-free drinks, and carbonated drinks. There is controversy as to the benefits of ingestion of carbohydrate-containing beverages. Some investigators feel that they may reduce gastric volume and raise pH, although this difference is not of clinical significance. There is some evidence to suggest that fasting itself may have detrimental effects, particularly in the pediatric population, resulting in greater anxiety and hunger.

For breast milk, the Task Force recommended a fasting period, for both infants and neonates, of 4 hours. Commercial milk and infant formula have a recommended fasting period of 6 hours.

A minimum period of 6 hours is recommended from the last ingestion of solids until the provision of anesthesia for elective surgery following a light meal. Indeed, some studies have noted that solids, particularly fats, can be found in the stomach for periods of over 8 hours after a meal. The Task Force recommended that consideration should be taken into account of the amount and type of food prior to the provision of anesthetic care after consumption of meals other that what is considered "light" (ie, clear liquids and toast).[57,58]

There is growing controversy as to the application of these guidelines in the parturient,[59] a complex group, as there is always a potential need for emergency surgery. It would seem reasonable to allow the moderate intake of clear fluids or ice chips for the low-risk parturient. However, the high-risk parturient, either due to comorbidities or at increased risk of requiring an operative delivery, should be fasted.[60] For elective cesarean sections, a fast of 8 hours following solids is recommended.

5.5.2   What role do pharmacological agents play at minimizing aspiration risk?

Although evidence exists to support the contention that pharmacological agents reduce gastric acid production, gastric volume, or both, no evidence exists to support their use in preventing or reducing the incidence of aspiration or improving outcome if aspiration was to occur. Furthermore, the administration of many of the pharmacological agents could not be justified on the basis of cost-benefit analysis. Subsequently, the ASA Task Force has not recommended the routine use of any pharmacological interventions for the prevention of aspiration.

Similarly, there are no recommendations regarding the *at-risk* patient, other than the use of nonparticulate antacids in the obstetrical population. The majority of studies looking at the efficacy of these drugs have been carried out in the healthy, low-risk populations.

H-2 antagonists, such as ranitidine, famotidine, and nizatidine, act by binding competitively to the histamine receptors on the gastric parietal cell. They are effective in increasing gastric pH and reducing gastric volume within 2 to 3 hours of administration. Unfortunately, the effect of the drug diminishes after a few days as tolerance develops.[61]

Proton pump inhibitors interfere with the H^+/K^+ ATPase pump on the parietal cells. They are less effective than H-2 antagonists if the intent is to use them for a single dose as they require at least two doses to be effective, both the night before and the morning of surgery. Tachyphylaxis does not develop with these agents.

Although reductions in gastric acid and volume have been shown with these agents, they do not reduce the harm from biliary fluid or particulate matter aspiration. Evidence from the animal literature suggests that pulmonary injury from bile is as significant, if not more so, than acid alone.[62] Bile, with a pH of 7.19, caused severe chemical pneumonitis and edema in one animal study.[62]

Prokinetic agents are used to accelerate emptying of the stomach, thereby reducing RGV. The most commonly used of these is metoclopramide. It has multiple effects, including prokinetic properties, antiemetic properties, and finally, an effect on increasing the tone of the LES. It acts by antagonizing dopamine and serotonin receptors. Depending on the receptor subtype, it may also act as an agonist. Its antiemetic effects are largely due to the 5HT3 antagonism and the prokinetic effects from the 5HT4 agonism. Its prokinetic properties, however, are quickly inhibited by the presence of opioids and anticholinergic agents.

Of interest, the antibiotic erythromycin has been shown to be an effective agent in stimulating gastric motility, thereby increasing the rate of gastric emptying. It exerts its effect via the motilin receptor. Unlike metoclopramide, it has no extrapyramidal side effects and its prokinetic properties are not inhibited by opioids or anticholinergics. Doses of 1 to 2 $mg \cdot kg^{-1}$ have been reported to be effective in reducing gastric fluid volume.[63,64]

The use of antacids has been demonstrated to reduce the pH of gastric contents for variable lengths of time. As discussed earlier in this chapter, the administration of particulate antacids can be problematic. The use of clear nonparticulate antacids has been in wide use for more than two decades, primarily in the obstetrical population. Sodium citrate is in routine use, prior to elective or emergency obstetrical procedures. Bicitra is a commercially available form of sodium citrate. The mechanism of action is by conversion to sodium bicarbonate. Rebound acidity will occur with prolonged use, increasing the volume of acid production.[65]

5.5.3   What is the role of rapid-sequence induction?

Rapid-sequence induction with cricoid pressure has been described as the standard of care in anesthesia for patients at risk for gastric regurgitation.[66] As well, it is cited to be the most common method of airway management by emergency physicians for critically ill and injured emergency patients. It is characterized by a high success rate and a low rate of serious complications.[18,67,68] RSI is also the principal salvage technique when other oral or nasal intubation methods fail in the emergency department.[8]

The use of a rapid-sequence technique results in fewer attempts, more rapid intubations, and higher success rates when compared to intubation with no sedation or sedation alone, both in hospital and in the prehospital setting.[69-71] Concerns about the role of rapid-sequence techniques in the prehospital setting for the care of severely head-injured patients relate to the potential for hypoxemia under some circumstances. The major issues seem to be the occurrence of severe hypoxia during induction in patients who were not hypoxic before induction and the excess morbidity and mortality in those patients. An effective strategy for maintenance of oxygenation is needed before it can be concluded that rapid-sequence intubation is of value in the out-of-hospital care of patients with serious closed head injury.[72,73]

5.5.4   Describe the technique of RSI

The patient should be placed at a height that is most convenient for the airway practitioner performing laryngoscopy. The head should be placed in the "sniffing" position with a firm pillow under the occiput. Although the benefit of the sniffing position compared to simple extension was recently challenged by Adnet, it did provide an advantage in patients who were obese or in whom there was at least one factor predictive of difficult intubation.[74]

5.5.4.1   Denitrogenation

The usual method for denitrogenating patients involves having the patient breathe 100% oxygen at tidal volumes through a snug-fitting facemask for 3 to 5 minutes. An alternative strategy is to have patients take four vital capacity breaths, but there is evidence that the former methodology is preferable.[75] Having said that, a recent review has concluded that having the patient take eight deep breaths (8DB) in 60 seconds provides a similar duration of safe apnea as does 3 to 5 minutes of tidal volume ventilation.[76] For this reason, whenever possible, it is recommended that either the tidal-volume breathing or the 8DB technique be employed. The same review concluded that denitrogenation of obese patients in the head-up compared to supine position also provided a longer period of safe apnea after the induction of anesthesia.

5.5.4.2   Cricoid Pressure

The cricoid cartilage should be identified by the assistant during denitrogenation, before induction of anesthesia, and the accuracy of the landmark should be confirmed by the airway practitioner. Cricoid pressure may be gently applied at the start of the induction sequence and the pressure increased to the amount recommended concurrent with the induction of anesthesia. The pressure should not be released until the cuff is inflated and the intratracheal position of the tube has been confirmed.

5.5.4.3   Nasogastric Tubes and Gastric Evacuation

Sellick recommended evacuating the stomach with a gastric tube and then removing the tube before induction of anesthesia.[4] Stept[77] argued that there was little evidence to support an effect of the tube on esophageal sphincter competence and suggested that the risk would be outweighed by the advantage of continuous gastric decompression when the tube was left in situ. Satiani et al[78] demonstrated no difference in the incidence of regurgitation with or without a nasogastric tube. Salem and colleagues demonstrated the effectiveness of cricoid pressure in preventing reflux in both infant and adult cadavers with nasogastric tubes in place.[79] It is recommended that a nasogastric tube be used to empty the stomach and then be left open to atmosphere to limit increases in intra-gastric pressure during induction of anesthesia.

5.5.4.4   Sedatives/Hypnotics during RSI

Despite wide acceptance and use of RSI, no single agent has emerged as the drug of choice for sedation and hypnosis during RSI. A deeper plane of anesthesia may improve intubating conditions in emergency patients undergoing RSI by complementing incomplete muscle paralysis.[80]

The use of etomidate, ketamine, a benzodiazepine, or no sedative agent prior to neuromuscular blockade is associated with a lower likelihood of successful intubation on the first attempt, as compared with thiopental, methohexital, or propofol.[80] The use of the benzodiazepine midazolam alone is associated with a prolonged delay to time of laryngoscopy, and doses greater than 0.1 mg·kg^{-1} are associated with a dose-related incidence of hypotension.[80-83]

Etomidate, thiopental, and propofol have a favorable effect on intraocular pressure (IOP) and intracranial pressure (ICP).[84-86] Barbiturates provide cerebral protective qualities against ischemia caused by elevated ICP. However, barbiturates may significantly lower mean arterial blood pressure and thereby lower cerebral perfusion pressure, potentially compromising collateral blood flow to ischemic regions of the brain.[84] Although propofol also reduces ICP, it reduces mean arterial pressure (MAP) more than barbiturates and can thus cause a significant reduction of cerebral perfusion pressure.[87] Etomidate, in contrast to barbiturates and propofol, reduces ICP to a similar degree while maintaining or increasing MAP and cerebral perfusion pressure, but there is evidence of neurotoxicity in experimental models.[88,89]

Ketamine, when used in the presence of hypovolemic shock, can be unpredictable in its effect on the hemodynamic profile. It possesses both indirect sympathomimetic stimulation and direct myocardial depressant properties, which support or raise systemic blood pressure in the acutely injured and hypovolemic patient. However, a patient who has been physiologically stressed for an extended period may be depleted of endogenous catecholamines, thereby rendering indirect autonomic stimulation ineffective and allowing the direct myocardial depressant effects to dominate.

Although it clearly has some advantages in a compromised patient, a significant disadvantage of etomidate is that it does not blunt the sympathetic response to endotracheal intubation.[90] This may result in hypertension and tachycardia during endotracheal intubation secondary to sympathetic stimulation. This response may raise ICP and increase myocardial work. Mitigation of this effect is achieved with the use of 1.5 to 5 µg·kg^{-1} of fentanyl in conjunction with etomidate.[91]

Lidocaine is widely used as a pretreatment agent to decrease the magnitude of increase of ICP in patients with closed head injury (with or without increased ICP). In fact, the evidence that IV lidocaine reduces the magnitude of the increase in ICP with elective tracheal intubation or suctioning in patients with increased ICP is indirect, and there is no evidence that it renders this effect in head-injured patients undergoing RSI.[92]

5.5.4.5   The Choice of Muscle Relaxant during Rapid-Sequence Techniques

Succinylcholine is widely used in anesthesia and emergency medicine during rapid-sequence techniques. Doses approximating 1 mg·kg⁻¹ have been conventionally used for intubation; the average time to return to 50% of twitch height following this dose is 8 to 9 minutes, and 10 to 11 minutes for a return to 90% twitch height. A number of authors have explored the use of smaller doses to decrease the time to recovery and to limit the dose-dependent sequelae. El-Orbany[93] assessed onset times and time to twitch recovery for succinylcholine in doses of 0.3, 0.4, 0.5, 0.6, and 1 mg·kg⁻¹ after anesthesia was induced with fentanyl and propofol. Onset times ranged between 82 and 52 seconds, decreasing with increasing doses of succinylcholine but not differing between 0.6 and 1 mg·kg⁻¹. Intubation conditions were often unacceptable after 0.3 and 0.4 mg·kg⁻¹ doses, but acceptable conditions were achieved in all patients receiving more than 0.5 mg·kg⁻¹; intubation conditions in patients receiving 0.6 and 1.0 mg·kg⁻¹ were identical. The times to twitch recovery and to regular spontaneous reservoir bag movements were significantly shorter in the 0.6 mg·kg⁻¹ dose group compared with patients receiving 1 mg·kg⁻¹. Naguib[94] carried out a similar study administering succinylcholine 0.3 to 1.0 mg·kg⁻¹ after anesthesia was induced with fentanyl and propofol. Intubating conditions were acceptable (excellent plus good grade combined) in 30%, 92%, 94%, and 98% of patients after 0.0, 0.3, 0.5, and 1.0 mg·kg⁻¹ succinylcholine, respectively. The calculated doses of succinylcholine that were required to achieve acceptable intubating conditions in 90% and 95% of patients at 60 seconds were 0.24 mg·kg⁻¹ and 0.56 mg·kg⁻¹, respectively.

While these results may have significant clinical implications, more studies are needed to examine the effectiveness of these smaller doses of succinylcholine in different patient populations, including obese, pregnant, pediatric, trauma, and critically ill patients. It must also be emphasized that the goal is "100% acceptable intubating conditions," particularly in an emergency.

There is considerable enthusiasm in anesthesia practice to replace succinylcholine with a nondepolarizing muscle relaxant. At this time, rocuronium has emerged as the most likely nondepolarizer to fill this role. Rocuronium 1 mg·kg⁻¹ given after induction in a rapid-sequence technique is clinically equivalent to succinylcholine 1 mg·kg⁻¹.[95] The incidences of clinically acceptable intubating conditions with rocuronium and succinylcholine were 93.2% and 97.1%, respectively. Clinically acceptable conditions occurred less frequently when rocuronium 0.6 mg·kg⁻¹ was used. The use of propofol 2.5 mg·kg⁻¹ combined with rocuronium 0.6 mg·kg⁻¹ results in satisfactory intubating conditions in 90% of patients within 61 seconds (range 50-81 seconds).[96] The use of either thiopental (5.0 mg·kg⁻¹) or etomidate (0.3 mg·kg⁻¹) combined with rocuronium 0.6 mg·kg⁻¹ results in a longer time to achieve, as well as a lower incidence of satisfactory intubating conditions than that achieved with propofol/rocuronium combinations.[97] The addition of alfentanil 10 μg·kg⁻¹ to these doses of etomidate and thiopental results in an increased likelihood of acceptable intubation conditions at 60 seconds following rocuronium administration.[98]

A recent review has concluded that a dose of succinylcholine of greater than 1 mg·kg⁻¹ is required to ensure *excellent* intubating conditions and that smaller doses may not consistently provide such conditions.[76] Rocuronium 1 mg·kg⁻¹ is a suitable alternative to succinylcholine during RSI, and although it will provide *acceptable* intubation conditions as often as equivalent doses of succinylcholine, it will provide *excellent* conditions less often. The time to full twitch recovery following paralyzing doses of rocuronium may be in excess of 1 hour, a factor that may exceed the comfort level of some practitioners. The availability and use of *Sugammadex* would be a potential solution in the situation where rocuronium is required for rapid-sequence induction, rather than succinylcholine as concern exists due to the prolonged neuromuscular block from the dose of rocuronium required.[99]

5.5.4.6   Positive Pressure Ventilation during RSI

In the 18th century, application of pressure in the cricoid area was advocated to allow for ventilation of the lungs without causing gastric distention.[100] Sellick,[4] in his description of cricoid pressure, also recommended ventilating the lungs while awaiting onset of muscle paralysis. On the other hand, Stept et al recommended against the use of ventilation after application of cricoid pressure[77] and conventional practice has favored this recommendation. However, there is now evidence that not only is there a benefit to ventilating the patient's lungs during the period of apnea but also that it can be done safely.

The average time to return to 90% of twitch height following an intubating dose of succinylcholine is considerably longer than it will take most patients to desaturate, even under ideal circumstances.[101] Using a simulator model, Hardman et al have identified the factors that shorten the time to desaturate with apnea.[102] The factors that have a moderate effect are a reduced ventilatory minute volume preceding apnea and a reduced duration of denitrogenation. Those that have a large effect are increased oxygen consumption and reduced functional residual capacity. All of those factors are likely to be relevant in many instances of RSI.

There is a relationship between airway pressure and gastric inflation.[103,104] In subjects ventilated by bag-mask without cricoid pressure, airway pressures below 15 cm H_2O rarely cause stomach inflation. Pressures between 15 and 25 cm H_2O will result in gastric insufflation in some patients, and pressures greater than 25 cm H_2O do so in most patients.[103] Application of cricoid pressure during BMV increases the maximum pressure that may be generated during mask-ventilation, without air entering the stomach, to about 45 cm H_2O.[104]

Petito and Russell measured the ability of cricoid pressure to prevent gastric inflation during BMV of the lungs.[105] Fifty patients were randomized to either have or not have cricoid pressure applied during a 3-minute period of standardized mask-ventilation. Patients who had cricoid pressure applied had less gas in the stomach after mask-ventilation. However, more patients who had cricoid pressure applied (36% vs 12%) were considered more difficult to ventilate and these patients tended to have more air in the stomach than those patients considered easy to ventilate with applied cricoid pressure.

In summary, the application of cricoid pressure significantly reduces the volume of air entering the stomach at low to moderate ventilation pressures. It allows for continued ventilation of the lungs even in situations where past convention would have discouraged it, such as in RSI. Ventilating the lungs while awaiting the onset of muscle block would clearly be a useful maneuver to prevent oxygen desaturation, and there is an evidence base that supports this intervention. In order to prevent gastric insufflation, every effort should be made to ventilate the lungs at the lowest pressure possible.

5.6   CRICOID PRESSURE

5.6.1   Discuss the applied anatomy of cricoid pressure

The cricoid cartilage is shaped like a signet ring with the narrow part of the ring being oriented anteriorly. The anterior arch of the cricoid cartilage is attached to the thyroid cartilage by the cricothyroid membrane. Laterally the cricothyroid muscles are situated in the cricothyroid gap (see Figure 3-23). The inferior horns of the thyroid cartilage articulate with the lateral surfaces of the cricoid cartilage. The cricoid cartilage is attached to the first tracheal ring by the cricotracheal ligament. The esophagus begins at the lower border of the posterior aspect of the cricoid cartilage. Sellick proposed the application of cricoid pressure during induction of anesthesia, to prevent regurgitation of gastric or esophageal contents by compressing the esophagus between the cricoid and the cervical spine, obliterating the esophageal lumen.[4] To perform the maneuver, the neck was extended, increasing the anterior convexity of the cervical spine and stretching the esophagus. Sellick hypothesized that this prevented lateral displacement of the esophagus when cricoid pressure was applied. However, Vanner[106] reported that contrast CT scanning in one patient revealed that when cricoid pressure was applied, although the cricoid cartilage and cervical vertebrae were approximated, only part of the esophageal lumen was obliterated. There was also slight lateral movement of the cricoid cartilage, which allowed the nonobliterated lumen to be pressed against the body of the longus colli muscle adjacent to the vertebral body. Smith[107] reviewed 51 cervical CT scans of normal patients to assess the anatomic relationships between the cricoid cartilage and the esophagus. Lateral esophageal displacement relative to the cricoid cartilage was evident in half (25 of 51) of the patients; 64% of those with lateral displacement had esophageal displacement beyond the lateral border of the cricoid cartilage. Smith subsequently reported on MRI taken of 22 volunteers with and without cricoid pressure applied. The esophagus was again seen to be displaced laterally relative to the cricoid cartilage in 52.6% of the subjects; this increased to 90.5% with the application of cricoid pressure. Lateral laryngeal displacement and airway compression were observed in 66.7% and 81% of the necks, respectively, with the application of cricoid pressure.[108] In neither study by Smith were the patients placed in the tonsillectomy position as recommended by Sellick. However, there is no evidence that doing so would have resulted in different findings than those reported.

The potential for lateral positioning and displacement of the esophagus relative to the cricoid cartilage possibly explains a number of case reports where, despite seemingly appropriate application of cricoid pressure during RSI, regurgitation and aspiration occurred.

5.6.2   What is the Sellick technique?

Sellick[109] outlined a number of steps in his original description of cricoid pressure applied concurrent with anesthetic induction. The patient was placed in the tonsillectomy position with the cervical spine in extension. Before induction of anesthesia, the cricoid was palpated and lightly held between the thumb and index finger; as induction commenced, pressure was exerted on the cricoid cartilage mainly by the index finger. As the patient lost consciousness, Sellick recommended firm pressure sufficient to seal the esophagus. Cricoid pressure was initially felt to be contraindicated by Sellick in the setting of active vomiting, in the belief that the esophagus may be damaged by vomit under high pressure. He later modified this stand, stating that he felt the risk of rupture to be almost nonexistent.[109] Since his original description, the technique has been exposed to much study and critique. Data have now accumulated to provide evidence to support many of Sellick recommendations.

5.6.3   Does cricoid pressure reliably protect against regurgitation and aspiration?

There are no outcome studies confirming the clinical benefit of cricoid pressure when used either in anesthesia or resuscitation. Brimacombe cites numerous case reports documenting the occurrence of aspiration despite the application of cricoid pressure.[66] There are also multiple studies documenting a negative impact of cricoid pressure on patient interventions, usually relating to airway management. There is also a single case report in the literature attributing rupture of the esophagus to cricoid pressure.[110] It involved an elderly female subjected to laparotomy after repeated episodes of hematemesis. The patient, who vomited on induction, was positioned laterally, cricoid pressure was released, and the trachea was intubated after pharyngeal suctioning. At surgery, a longitudinal split was found in the lower esophagus. It was concluded, by the reporting authors, that the esophageal rupture represented an esophageal injury attributable to the cricoid pressure. However, the diagnosis of rupture of the esophagus as a result of the repeated episodes of hematemesis represents as likely a diagnosis, as the stomach adjacent to the area of esophageal injury was noted to be bruised and swollen during the surgery, suggesting a temporally more remote injury.

There are a number of factors that would explain why cricoid pressure cannot provide absolute protection against aspiration, in addition to the anatomic factors already outlined. The landmarks on the patient's neck may not be identified properly and, as a result, pressure not exerted on the cricoid cartilage itself. Cricoid pressure may not have been commenced prior to induction, allowing for an interval between loss of consciousness and application of pressure, during which the patient is at risk for aspiration. Personnel may be inadequately trained. Cricoid pressure may be released inadvertently before the trachea is intubated and the cuff inflated. Finally, it may be difficult to maintain occlusive pressures for prolonged periods and the maneuver may become less effective in preventing aspiration during instances of difficult intubation.

There is a paucity of data to evaluate the role of cricoid pressure in preventing patient complications. Despite the lack of conclusive evidence supporting the role of cricoid pressure in the emergency management of the airway in the setting of a full stomach, the absence of evidence of an effect does not prove that there is no benefit to the intervention. It is likely to continue to be encouraged as a pattern of practice.

5.6.4   How much cricoid pressure is needed to prevent gastric regurgitation?

Twenty newtons of applied cricoid pressure is probably adequate in many instances and 30 N is more than enough to prevent regurgitation into the pharynx in most patients. Pressures of greater than 30 N (approximately 3 kg, or 7 lb) are unlikely to be necessary.[37,111-113] The originally described forces (40 N) would rarely be necessary to prevent gastric regurgitation.

5.6.5   How do you measure the performance of cricoid pressure?

Meek investigated the cricoid pressure technique of anesthetic assistants.[114] A large variation in the force applied (from <10 N to >90 N) was observed. Performance was improved markedly by providing simple instruction and further improved by practical training in the application of target force on a simulator. Meek also studied six operating room assistants performing simulated cricoid pressure (on a model of the larynx) to determine how long and under what conditions cricoid pressure could be sustained.[115] Subjects were asked to maintain forces of 20, 30, and 40 N for a target time of 20 minutes, with the arm either extended or flexed; most could not do so. Mean times to release of cricoid pressure varied from 3.7 minutes (flexed) to 7.6 minutes (extended) at 40 N, to 6.4 to 10.2 minutes at 30 N, and 13.2 to 14.6 minutes at 20 N, respectively. These findings suggest that the ability to generate forces sufficient to provide esophageal occlusion and airway protection is limited.

5.6.6   Is bimanual cricoid pressure better than a one-handed technique?

Flexion of the head on the neck may occur as a result of cricoid pressure and this may impede laryngoscopy. Bimanual (two-handed) cricoid pressure with the free hand of the assistant placed behind and supporting the neck or alternatively, with the use of a small support placed behind the patient's neck, has been recommended to overcome the tendency to neck flexion.[116] However, Vanner found no benefit for laryngoscopy when a cushion was placed behind the neck to prevent neck flexion during the application of cricoid pressure.[117] Cook compared the view of the larynx at laryngoscopy in 121 patients with one- or two-handed cricoid pressure applied.[118] In 28 cases the laryngeal view was better with one-handed cricoid pressure, and in 11 cases the laryngeal view was better with two-handed cricoid pressure. In 81 cases, the view was unaffected by the type of cricoid pressure applied. Two-handed cricoid pressure was not demonstrated to routinely provide an advantage over the one-handed technique.

Yentis[119] also studied the effect of the two different methods of cricoid pressure on laryngoscopic view in 94 patients and reached contrary conclusions to those of Cook. In 21 cases, a better laryngoscopic view was obtained with the bimanual technique; in 8 cases it was better with the single-handed technique; and in 65 cases the method of cricoid pressure made no difference. The force applied may have some impact on both the amount of neck flexion and the balancing potential of a bimanual technique. In the study by Yentis, considerably larger forces were applied (50-55 N) than in either Vanner's (30 N) or Cook's (40 N) studies. It is possible that more neck flexion occurred with the larger applied force and more benefit was thus realized when a bimanual technique was employed.

In summary, the technique of cricoid pressure which produces the best laryngoscopic view in an individual patient cannot be predicted. However, an alternative technique should be considered if it is suspected that the technique of cricoid pressure application is having a deleterious effect on direct laryngoscopy.

5.6.7   Does it matter which hand is used to apply cricoid pressure?

Cook assessed the cricoid force applied by trained anesthesia assistants, as well as the ability to maintain the applied force, and compared the two hands.[120] Overall, the assistants applied a lower force than is classically taught but were able to maintain the force with either hand for a sustained period. The use of the left hand resulted in slightly lower applied forces but the differences were not felt to be clinically relevant. Thus, no recommendation can be made regarding position of the assistants as it relates to the handedness of the cricoid pressure.

5.6.8   How does cricoid pressure affect ventilation and airway interventions?

A concern about cricoid pressure in general, and at higher applied pressures in particular, has been the potential for compromise of either the quality of the airway or the effectiveness of airway interventions.[121-123] In a recent report of 23 failed intubations over a 17-year period in one maternity unit, cricoid pressure was maintained during the failed intubation drill.[124] In 14 patients (60%), ventilation via a facemask was not difficult, indicating that cricoid pressure was at least not harmful in these patients. In the remaining nine patients, ventilation was difficult in seven patients (30%) and impossible in two (9%). Although some patients had laryngeal edema, it is possible that cricoid pressure contributed to the difficult ventilation in these patients.[121]

Vanner[123] reported that difficulty in breathing occurred in about half of awake patients with 40 N forces applied, and Lawes[125] reported that airway obstruction occurred in about 10%. Hartsilver and Vanner investigated whether airway obstruction is related strictly to the force applied or whether the technique of application was also relevant.[126] They recorded expired tidal volumes and inflation pressures during mask-ventilation in anesthetized patients. Airway obstruction occurred in 2% of patients with pressure applied at 30 N, and in 35% with 44 N. If the force is applied in an upward and backward direction, obstruction at 30 N occurs in 56%.

Aoyama assessed the effect of cricoid pressure (prior to insertion) on the positioning of and ventilation through the laryngeal mask airway (LMA).[127] Ventilation was considered adequate in all patients in the group with no cricoid pressure applied but in only 25% of those with pressure applied. The glottis was visible fiberoptically below the mask aperture in all patients when no pressure was applied, suggesting correct placement. Correct placement was evident in only 15% of patients who had the LMA placed with cricoid pressure applied. Fiberoptic evaluation showed that the mask was not inserted far enough in the remaining 85% of patients. Radiographs taken showed that the tip of the mask in the no-cricoid-pressure group was located below the level of the cricoid cartilage (C6 or C7 vertebra), whereas the mask tip in the cricoid pressure group was above this level (C4 or C5).

Asai[128] studied 50 patients to assess if the cricoid pressure applied after placement of the laryngeal mask prevented gastric insufflation, without affecting ventilation. Cricoid pressure significantly decreased mean expiratory volume delivered through an LMA. This inhibitory effect was greater when the pressure was applied without support of the neck. Cricoid pressure also reduced the incidence of gastric insufflation. In no patient was the mask dislodged. The inhibitory effect of cricoid pressure on ventilation without support of the neck was greater than cricoid pressure with support of the neck.

MacG Palmer and Ball[129] studied the effect of cricoid pressure on airway anatomy in 30 anesthetized patients examined fiberoptically through an LMA. They assessed the effect of 20, 30, and 44 N on the internal appearance of the cricoid and vocal cords. At 44 N, cricoid deformation occurred in 90% of patients and 50% had cricoid occlusion; 43% had cricoid occlusion at 30 N and 23% at 20 N. Associated difficulty in ventilation was present in 50% of patients and 60% had vocal cord closure with associated difficult ventilation, at forces up to 44 N.[130-132]

Smith and Boyer evaluated the ease of rigid fiberoptic (WuScope System™) intubation in anesthetized adults receiving cricoid pressure.[133] Each patient had their trachea intubated under two conditions: with and without cricoid pressure. An easy intubation occurred in 91% of patients without cricoid pressure and in 66% of patients with cricoid pressure applied. Cricoid pressure compressed the vocal cords in 27% of patients and impeded tracheal tube placement in 15%. In three patients (9%), pressure had to be released in order to successfully intubate their tracheas.

Hodgson[134] assessed the effect of application of cricoid pressure on the success of lightwand intubation in 60 adult female patients presenting for abdominal hysterectomy. All 30 patients allocated to intubation without cricoid pressure were intubated successfully, at the first attempt, within a median time of 28 seconds. Lightwand intubation with cricoid pressure was successful in 26 of 30 patients at the first attempt, but the median time to successful intubation was significantly longer at 48.5 seconds. Three patients required two attempts for successful intubation and one

could not be intubated with the lightwand while cricoid pressure was applied.

Shulman compared the Bullard laryngoscope (BL) with the flexible bronchoscope (FB) in a cervical spine injury model. Using in-line stabilization with or without cricoid pressure, he concluded that BL is more reliable when used in the setting of in-line stabilization with cricoid pressure applied. He determined as well that BL is also quicker and more resistant to the effect of cricoid pressure than is FB.[135]

In summary, properly applied cricoid pressure has a limited impact on the ability to ventilate the lungs, the quality of the airway realized, and the effectiveness of airway interventions. However, as applied pressures are increased, the potential for compromise of both the airway and airway interventions is also increased.

5.6.9 What is the impact of cricoid pressure on cervical spine movement?

In the setting of potential or actual cervical injury, concerns have been expressed that the application of cricoid pressure may result in cervical spine displacement, causing or worsening cord injury. Although cricoid pressure is widely used during airway management in trauma settings, there are no data either affirming its safety or implying that it actually poses a risk. Gabbott[136] assessed the impact of single-handed cricoid pressure applied concurrent with manual in-line stabilization of the neck in a neutral position in 30 healthy patients undergoing general anesthesia with neuromuscular paralysis. Vertical displacement was measured from the midpoint of the neck (directly below the cricoid cartilage), and mean neck displacement (vertebral) was 4.6 mm with a range of 0 to 8 mm.

Gabbott then measured the effect of single-handed cricoid pressure on cervical spine movement after applying manual in-line stabilization in cadavers.[137] The median vertical displacement measured from the body of C5 was 0.5 mm (range 0 to 1.5 mm). There was no disruption of the lines formed by the anterior or posterior borders of the cervical bodies. In this second study, Gabbott was unable to demonstrate that single-handed cricoid pressure caused clinically significant displacement of the cervical spine in a cadaver model.[136]

Wood[138] studied the effect of cricoid pressure on the view obtained at laryngoscopy with concurrent cervical stabilization maneuvers. Laryngoscopic view was best in the unrestrained position, with 77.4% of these views being Grade 1. More frequently, Grade 3 views were obtained in the presence of cervical stabilization with or without cricoid pressure. When in the stabilized position, application of cricoid pressure improved the view in 26% of patients. Wood concluded that cricoid pressure may actually improve the view of the larynx when the neck is stabilized even though it is often detrimental to the view in the absence of stabilization.

In summary, there is no evidence which would either encourage or discourage the use of cricoid pressure in the setting of real or potential cervical injury. However, its use in this setting is common and there is no evidence of harm caused. Cricoid pressure may actually facilitate laryngoscopy when cervical immobilization is employed, in much the same fashion that anterior laryngeal pressure does.

5.7   OTHER CONSIDERATIONS

5.7.1   What is the aspiration risk associated with the use of extraglottic devices?

When discussing extraglottic devices, the focus is generally on the LMA and its various forms. Other devices are available such as the laryngeal tube. However, the vast majority of the literature relates to the LMA.

The LMA has enjoyed over a decade of widespread use in anesthesia worldwide and has been hailed for its ease of use, efficacy, and low incidence of complications. As its use expanded, so did the nature of its application and it began to be employed for positive pressure ventilation, prolonged anesthesia (more than 2 hours duration), laparoscopic and nonlaparoscopic abdominopelvic surgery, and for surgery in the prone position. These applications have been labeled nonconventional applications and as these patterns of practice have become more common, increasing concerns about aspiration are being expressed.

Authors have addressed these concerns in three ways:

(1) Esophageal pH probes have been employed to determine the incidence and extent of GER during anesthesia with LMAs in place.

(2) Deliberate pharyngeal soiling has been used to measure the protection afforded to the respiratory tract by the LMA. Clinical studies have compared the incidence of reflux when the LMA was employed relative to endotracheal tubes or alternate airways.

(3) Finally, retrospective series and case reports have been presented to both estimate the incidence of aspiration associated with LMA and detail the clinical events and sequelae when aspiration occurred. The bulk of the published literature refers to the LMA Classic™ but more recently, literature relating to the newer iterations of the LMA, including the LMA ProSeal™ (PLMA) and the intubating LMA, has appeared.

Roux et al[139] studied esophageal reflux, using esophageal pH probes, in 60 patients administered anesthesia with either a face-mask or an LMA. They concluded that the use of the LMA was associated with an increased incidence of gastric reflux in the lower esophagus, but not mid-esophagus, and that reflux was not influenced by either volume of air or pressure inside the LMA cuff. Joshi et al[140] found no evidence of hypopharyngeal aspiration using pH probes in a study that compared the LMA with the endotracheal tube in spontaneously breathing patients. Ho et al[141] reported that the use of positive pressure ventilation in a similar setting did not increase the risk of reflux. Hagberg et al[142] studied both reflux and tracheal aspiration using pH electrodes measuring in both the proximal and distal esophagus, as well as the trachea. The patients were managed with either an LMA or a Combitube™. No changes in esophageal or pharyngeal pH were observed, but 12% of the LMA group and 4% of the Combitube™ group had pH changes at the tracheal level. No patient demonstrated clinical signs or symptoms of aspiration.

Using pH probes, McCrory and McShane[143] determined the incidence and level of reflux during spontaneous respiration with the LMA and compared the supine and lithotomy positions. The pH was measured in both the esophagus and the bowl of the LMA. Esophageal reflux occurred in 38% of the patients in the supine position and 100% of the patients in the lithotomy position. A change in pH was also measured in the bowl of the LMA in 57% of patients in the lithotomy position, but was not seen in the supine position.

Cheong et al[144] compared the incidence of reflux and regurgitation in adults associated with LMA removal and compared the incidence when two strategies were employed for removal. In one group, the LMA was removed when signs of rejection were observed (swallowing, struggling, restlessness) and in the second, when the patients could open their mouth to command. A pH probe was used to assess reflux and a gelatin capsule containing methylene blue, swallowed before anesthesia induction, was employed to identify regurgitation. Instances of reflux measured with the pH probe were more common in the late-removal group. There were no regurgitation events observed in either group.

Evans et al[145] assessed the ability of the LMA ProSeal™ to isolate the respiratory tract from the digestive tract. Methylene blue-dyed saline was instilled into the hypopharynx via the drainage tube once the mask was in place in 102 patients. A flexible bronchoscope was used to view the bowl of the mask to assess for evidence of methylene blue. Although an effective barrier was observed in all patients initially, mask displacement occurred in two patients (2%) and dye leaked into the bowl of the mask.

Verghese and Brimacombe[146] surveyed the use of the LMA in 11,910 patients, with special emphasis on nonconventional use of the LMA, and the occurrence of airway-related complications. Of the 11,910 uses recorded, 2222 were considered to be nonconventional. Eighteen of the 44 documented critical incidents related to the airway including laryngospasm (8), regurgitation (4), bronchospasm (3), vomiting (2), and aspiration (1). There was no difference between the rates of occurrence of critical incidents in conventional (0.16%) versus nonconventional (0.14%) use of the LMA. Brimacombe and Berry[147] performed a meta-analysis of the published literature relevant to the association of LMA use and aspiration. In the reviewed papers, there were three cases of aspiration in 12,901 patients, with no death or permanent disabilities recorded.

Keller et al[148] described three cases of aspiration: the first death and the first case of severe permanent neurological injury was associated with aspiration and the use of the LMA. All three patients were considered by the authors to be at increased risk of aspiration; two had previous gastric surgery and the third had a hiatus hernia. Keller also reported a literature review designed to assess risk factors for LMA-associated aspiration. Twenty case reports were identified in the literature. In 14 cases, there were factors that could increase the risk of aspiration, including inadequate depth of anesthesia (7), intra-abdominal surgery (3), upper GI tract disease (2), lithotomy position (2), exchanging the LMA (2), a full stomach (1), multiple trauma (1), multiple insertion attempts (1), obesity (1), opioid use (1), and cuff deflation (1).

In summary, there is evidence that gastric reflux into the lower esophagus occurs with some frequency during anesthesia provided with an LMA even in healthy patients without obvious risk factors. Reflux to higher levels of the esophagus or into the pharynx appears to be less common but does occur. It may be increased by patient positioning, such as the lithotomy and lateral decubitus positions. Although the LMA cuff may provide somewhat a protective barrier to refluxing materials, the barrier is not absolute and aspiration may occur even with a PLMA in place. The incidence of aspiration associated with LMA use seems low and not significantly altered when the LMA is used in an unconventional manner. However, it is likely that many cases of LMA-associated aspirations have occurred and gone unreported. When aspirations are reported, it is common that factors traditionally associated with a higher risk of aspiration are present.

In the opinion of the authors, in situations suggesting that the patient is at an increased or high risk of aspiration, it would seem prudent to electively employ alternate methods to the LMA when managing the airway.

5.7.2 Is it safe to use a lightwand intubation technique (eg, Trachlight™) in patients at risk of aspiration?

The Trachlight™ represents an alternate airway device that has proven its efficacy in many clinical situations. Studies have shown that it is both safe and effective, with minimal trauma and its ability to secure the airway in clinical situations where anatomical features make the use of the laryngoscope less likely to be successful. Indeed, features that predict difficult laryngoscopy have little or no correlation with the ease or difficulty of Trachlight™ intubation.[149]

The question of the safety of the Trachlight™ in the patient at risk of aspiration is one not well addressed in the literature. Only one paper[134] exists which reviews the use of the Trachlight™ in the presence of cricoid pressure and RSI in a randomized trial and it suggests that the use of the Trachlight™ is hampered by the presence of cricoid pressure. Sixty healthy patients were randomized into a cricoid pressure group and a noncricoid pressure group. Of the noncricoid pressure group, there was a 100% success rate on the first attempt. In the cricoid pressure group of 30 patients, only 26 were intubated on the first attempt, three on the second, and one failed with the Trachlight™. The conclusion was that the Trachlight™ should not be used as a first-line choice for RSI.

As discussed earlier, a failed or difficult intubation increases the risk of aspiration. Under circumstances where a difficult laryngoscopic intubation is predicted, one could argue that the use of the Trachlight™ might represent a safer choice. Hung et al[149] documented that the success of the Trachlight™ was at least as good, if not better than, as the laryngoscope in a series of 950 patients randomized into Trachlight™ and laryngoscope intubation. In another study, Hung et al[150] studied 265 patients deemed to be difficult laryngoscopic intubations. Of these, 206 were felt to be difficult either because of previously documented problems or anatomical factors predicting difficulty, such as cervical fusion, small mandibles, and impaired mouth opening. The remaining 59 were unanticipated failed laryngoscopic intubations whose airways were secured with the Trachlight™. A total of two failures occurred, both of which could have been predicted due to anatomical abnormalities that made the transillumination difficult.

Clearly, clinical judgment is required. The patient with a full stomach from a recent meal does not have the same risk of aspirating as the patient with an acute bowel obstruction. In addition, coughing and gagging in relation to prolonged attempts at laryngoscopy are as likely, if not more so, to expose the patient to the potential of aspirating than if the assistant releases cricoid pressure momentarily to facilitate insertion of a Trachlight™.

Unfortunately, apart from the solitary paper cited above, there is not enough evidence to draw a firm conclusion.

5.7.3 Is awake intubation with an anesthetized airway associated with a lower risk of aspiration than under anesthesia?

Airway anesthesia is routinely used for awake intubation. Many sources caution against these airway anesthesia techniques in the patient with a *full stomach*, fearing that anesthetizing the upper airway impairs the cough reflex, leaving the patient at risk should regurgitation occur.[151-154] The question then arises how should one proceed in a patient who has an anticipated difficult airway in the presence of elevated risk of regurgitation? Only one relevant study[152] has been published in 1989. The tracheas of 123 patients at high risk for aspiration were intubated awake, but sedated, with an FB. In 114 cases, the vocal cords were anesthetized by either injection of 4% lidocaine through the working channel of the bronchoscope or by transtracheal injection of lidocaine. No local anesthetics were used on 15 occasions. Topical anesthesia was applied to the oropharynx by benzocaine–amethocaine (Cetacaine) spray and benzocaine ointment for oral intubations. Patients having nasal intubations received topical 4% cocaine to the nasal mucosa. No incidences of aspiration were identified in this study.

While many use propofol boluses for *awake* intubation, this technique must be used with great caution. Propofol and other sedatives decrease LES tone, predisposing to aspiration. In addition, the patient with airway compromise may depend on voluntary muscle tone for airway patency.[154]

Clearly, each situation is unique. An anesthetized airway in an awake patient can prevent gagging, retching, and coughing during intubation. In addition, the awake, cooperative patient maintains the LES tone and can anticipate vomiting and assist in maneuvers to prevent aspiration—turning their head to the side, opening their mouth for suctioning, etc.[152] On the other hand, sedation can produce an uncooperative patient with depressed airway reflexes.

In the patient at high risk for aspiration, one must weigh each technique carefully in securing an airway while minimizing the risks of aspiration.

5.7.4 What is the appropriate management for aspiration?

When aspiration is suspected prompt measures should be taken to prevent further aspiration. The head of the bed should immediately be adjusted to a 30-degree head down position and the patient's head turned to the left side to facilitate drainage of secretions. The upper airway should be suctioned thoroughly. If the patient aspirates on induction, intubation should follow immediately with aggressive tracheal suctioning before ventilation, if possible.

If intubation was not intended (as in procedural sedation) and the patient is spontaneously breathing, then supplemental oxygen by face mask should be applied after suctioning as one prepares for further assessment.[5,155,156]

As was mentioned earlier, damage to the lungs after the aspiration of gastric contents occurs within seconds, with subsequent neutralization of acid in 15 seconds. Consequently, bronchoscopy is not indicated except to remove large particulate matter. The decision to proceed with or cancel the surgery should depend on the severity of the aspiration, the patient's clinical status, and the urgency of the procedure. The patient should be notified that aspiration has occurred, when it is appropriate to do so and observed for signs of pneumonitis initially and pneumonia over the ensuing days.

Since gastric acid normally prevents the growth of bacteria, antibiotics are not indicated following aspiration alone. The incidence of progression to bacterial pneumonia following chemical lung injury is unknown. Symptoms of pneumonitis include wheezing, coughing, dyspnea, and cyanosis. Further complications may include pulmonary edema, hypotension, hypoxemia, and severe ARDS.[23] Treatment of pneumonitis largely consists of supportive therapy, varying from simple oxygen supplementation to full ventilatory support.

5.7.5   Should corticosteroids be administered following the aspiration of gastric contents?

The use of steroids following aspiration has been historically based on theoretical considerations, which remain unproven. These relate to anti-inflammatory properties, stabilizing effects on lysosomal membranes, ability to reduce platelet aggregation, and improvement of peripheral release of oxygen from erythrocytes.[157] Studies conducted in the 1960s, 1970s, and 1980s consistently failed to prove a benefit of high-dose steroids after aspiration.[158-160] Nevertheless, the practice continues[23] despite a significantly higher death rate from secondary infections in the group receiving steroids.[161]

The use of high-dose steroids has not been proven effective and can adversely affect mortality in the critically ill population.[5,161] Therefore, its use in episodes of aspiration is not recommended.

5.7.6   Should antibiotics be administered to prevent pneumonia following the aspiration of gastric contents?

The majority of literature on the treatment of aspiration pneumonia is related to aspiration of colonized oropharyngeal secretions,[23] not gastric contents. Treatment should focus on supportive care to maintain oxygenation followed by organism-specific antibiotic therapy should bacterial pneumonia develop. The incidence of post aspiration pneumonia is more common in debilitated patients with comorbid conditions, and patients who have been on ventilatory support, due to leakage around the tracheal tube cuff that occurs in these patients.

The proplylactic use of antibiotics after aspiration has not been demonstrated to prevent infectious pneumonia and is not recommended.[162] Some exceptions may include patients with bowel obstruction[23] and elderly or debilitated patients.[162] The choice of antibiotics varies according to the syndrome and the clinical situation. For example, institutionalized elderly patients with aspiration pneumonia more commonly have anaerobic microorganisms cultured[163] than other populations.

The recommendations for antibiotic selection change frequently and current guidelines for antibiotic therapy should be consulted. Such guidelines have been published by the following medical societies: American Thoracic Society,[164] Infectious Diseases Society of America,[165] Canadian Infectious Disease Society,[166] and the Canadian Thoracic Society.[166] Most commonly, it is recommended that antibiotic selection be guided by culture and sensitivity determinations.[23]

5.7.7   How long should the patient be observed following the aspiration of gastric contents?

In a retrospective study of the perioperative course of 172,334 patients receiving general anesthesia, Warner et al[6] reviewed 67 cases of aspiration. Forty-two of these patients, who were asymptomatic at 2 hours postaspiration or procedure, never manifested any symptoms, acute or delayed. Eighteen of these were day surgeries, and 12 were discharged home on the day of surgery. Twenty-four developed symptoms within 2 hours including cough or wheeze (17), decrease in arterial oxygen saturation of greater than 10% on room air (10), an increase in the A-a gradient greater than 300 (1), or radiographic changes (12). Of the 24 with symptoms, 18 required respiratory support or ICU admission, with 6 being ventilated for more than 24 hours because of the development of ARDS. Only one patient developed pneumonia and required antibiotics.

Patients who have been discharged home after suspected episodes of aspiration should be informed of the symptoms of pulmonary complications and instructed to report them promptly.

5.8   SUMMARY

The prevention of aspiration is a significant focus of the airway practitioner. Certain factors markedly increase the risk of this event occurring. Some are inherent to the patients themselves, primarily premorbid conditions known to predispose to aspiration, some related to the patients' pathology and planned intervention, such as emergency surgery, bowel pathology, high ASA risk scores, pregnancy, difficult airway, and decreased level of consciousness. Airway management in the semiconscious patient may lead to coughing and gagging during attempts to secure the airway, accounting for over two-thirds of the perioperative aspirations.

Recognition of high-risk patients is important. Maneuvers to reduce gastric acid and volume, both pharmacologically and with drainage, may have their role but need to be targeted to specific situations. Bile and particulate materials are potentially as harmful to the lung as is the acid that tends to be the primary focus. Thus use of particulate antacids has been abandoned in the perioperative setting should they be aspirated.

Although the efficacy of the Sellick maneuver has come under recent criticism, it is still a standard of care in the protection of the airway at risk. A well-trained assistant is crucial. Under certain conditions when it hampers intubation or ventilation, the reduction or even release of cricoid pressure momentarily may be appropriate. The wisdom of the use of extraglottic devices in the high aspiration-risk patient, when other options are available, should be critically analyzed.

Finally, in the unlikely event that aspiration does occur, guidelines that are evidence based should be used in the assessment and management of these patients.

REFERENCES

1. Kluger MT, Willemsen G. Anti-aspiration prophylaxis in New Zealand: a national survey. *Anaesth Intensive Care.* 1998;26:70-77.
2. Mendelson C. The aspiration of stomach contents into the lungs during obstetric anesthesia. *Am J Obstet Gynecol.* 1946;52:191-205.
3. Roberts RB, Shirley MA. Reducing the risk of acid aspiration during cesarean section. *Anesth Analg.* 1974;53:859-868.
4. Sellick BA. Cricoid pressure to control regurgitation of stomach contents during induction of anaesthesia. *Lancet.* 1961;2:404-406.
5. Engelhardt T, Webster NR. Pulmonary aspiration of gastric contents in anaesthesia. *Br J Anaesth.* 1999;83:453-460.
6. Warner MA, Warner ME, Weber JG. Clinical significance of pulmonary aspiration during the perioperative period. *Anesthesiology.* 1993;78:56-62.
7. Mellin-Olsen J, Fasting S, Gisvold SE. Routine preoperative gastric emptying is seldom indicated. A study of 85,594 anaesthetics with special focus on aspiration pneumonia. *Acta Anaesthesiol Scand.* 1996;40:1184-1188.
8. Olsson GL, Hallen B, Hambraeus-Jonzon K. Aspiration during anaesthesia: a computer-aided study of 185,358 anaesthetics. *Acta Anaesthesiol Scand.* 1986;30:84-92.
9. Sakai T, Planinsic RM, Quinlan JJ, Handley LJ, Kim TY, Hilmi IA. The incidence and outcome of perioperative pulmonary aspiration in a university hospital: a 4-year retrospective analysis. *Anesth Analg.* 2006;103:941-947.
10. Kluger MT, Short TG. Aspiration during anaesthesia: a review of 133 cases from the Australian Anaesthetic Incident Monitoring Study (AIMS). *Anaesthesia.* 1999;54:19-26.
11. Cheney FW. *Aspiration: A Liability Hazard for the Anesthesiologist? ASA Newslet.* 2000;Sect. N6.
12. Warner MA, Warner ME, Warner DO, Warner LO, Warner EJ. Perioperative pulmonary aspiration in infants and children. *Anesthesiology.* 1999;90:66-71.
13. Lockey DJ, Coats T, Parr MJ. Aspiration in severe trauma: a prospective study. *Anaesthesia.* 1999;54:1097-1098.
14. McNicholl BP. The golden hour and prehospital trauma care. *Injury.* 1994;25:251-254.
15. Gausche M, Lewis RJ, Stratton SJ, et al. Effect of out-of-hospital pediatric endotracheal intubation on survival and neurological outcome: a controlled clinical trial. *JAMA.* 2000;283:783-790.
16. Nolan JD. Prehospital and resuscitative airway care: should the gold standard be reassessed? *Curr Opin Crit Care.* 2001;7:413-421.
17. Taryle DA, Chandler JE, Good JT, Jr., Potts DE, Sahn SA. Emergency room intubations—complications and survival. *Chest.* 1979;75:541-543.
18. Sakles JC, Laurin EG, Rantapaa AA, Panacek EA. Airway management in the emergency department: a one-year study of 610 tracheal intubations. *Ann Emerg Med.* 1998;31:325-332.
19. Mort TC. Emergency tracheal intubation: complications associated with repeated laryngoscopic attempts. *Anesth Analg.* 2004;99:607-613, table of contents.
20. Coriat P, Labrousse J, Vilde F, Tenaillon A, Lissac J. Diffuse interstitial pneumonitis due to aspiration of gastric contents. *Anaesthesia.* 1984;39:703-705.
21. Knight PR, Druskovich G, Tait AR, Johnson KJ. The role of neutrophils, oxidants, and proteases in the pathogenesis of acid pulmonary injury. *Anesthesiology.* 1992;77:772-778.
22. Knight PR, Rutter T, Tait AR, Coleman E, Johnson K. Pathogenesis of gastric particulate lung injury: a comparison and interaction with acidic pneumonitis. *Anesth Analg.* 1993;77:754-760.
23. Marik PE. Aspiration pneumonitis and aspiration pneumonia. *N Engl J Med.* 2001;344:665-671.
24. Smith G, Ng A. Gastric reflux and pulmonary aspiration in anaesthesia. *Minerva Anestesiol.* 2003;69:402-406.
25. Maltby JR, Pytka S, Watson NC, Cowan RA, Fick GH. Drinking 300 mL of clear fluid two hours before surgery has no effect on gastric fluid volume and pH in fasting and non-fasting obese patients. *Can J Anaesth.* 2004;51:111-115.
26. Schreiner MS. Gastric fluid volume: is it really a risk factor for pulmonary aspiration? *Anesth Analg.* 1998;87:754-756.
27. Hardy JF, Lepage Y, Bonneville-Chouinard N. Occurrence of gastroesophageal reflux on induction of anaesthesia does not correlate with the volume of gastric contents. *Can J Anaesth.* 1990;37:502-508.
28. Illing L, Duncan PG, Yip R. Gastroesophageal reflux during anaesthesia. *Can J Anaesth.* 1992;39:466-470.
29. Guyton AD, Hall JE. *Textbook of Medical Physiology.* 10th ed. Philadelphia, PA: WB Saunders Company; 2000:728-733.
30. Jones MJ, Mitchell RW, Hindocha N. Effect of increased intra-abdominal pressure during laparoscopy on the lower esophageal sphincter. *Anesth Analg.* 1989;68:63-65.
31. Mort TC. The incidence and risk factors for cardiac arrest during emergency tracheal intubation: a justification for incorporating the ASA Guidelines in the remote location. *J Clin Anesth.* 2004;16:508-516.
32. Rose DK, Cohen MM. The airway: problems and predictions in 18,500 patients. *Can J Anaesth.* 1994;41:372-383.
33. Schwartz DE, Matthay MA, Cohen NH. Death and other complications of emergency airway management in critically ill adults. A prospective investigation of 297 tracheal intubations. *Anesthesiology.* 1995;82:367-376.
34. Dubois A. Obesity and gastric emptying. *Gastroenterology.* 1983;84:875-876.
35. Horowitz M, Collins PJ, Cook DJ, Harding PE, Shearman DJ. Abnormalities of gastric emptying in obese patients. *Int J Obes.* 1983;7:415-421.
36. Maddox A, Horowitz M, Wishart J, Collins P. Gastric and oesophageal emptying in obesity. *Scand J Gastroenterol.* 1989;24:593-598.
37. Wright RA, Krinsky S, Fleeman C, Trujillo J, Teague E. Gastric emptying and obesity. *Gastroenterology.* 1983;84:747-751.
38. Kadar AG, Ing CH, White PF, Wakefield CA, Kramer BA, Clark K. Anesthesia for electroconvulsive therapy in obese patients. *Anesth Analg.* 2002;94:360-361, table of contents.
39. Ewah B, Yau K, King M, Reynolds F, Carson RJ, Morgan B. Effect of epidural opioids on gastric emptying in labour. *Int J Obstet Anesth.* 1993;2:125-128.
40. Macfie AG, Magides AD, Richmond MN, Reilly CS. Gastric emptying in pregnancy. *Br J Anaesth.* 1991;67:54-57.
41. Shinder SM, Levinson G. *Anesthesia for Obstetrics.* 2nd ed. Philadelphia, PA: Lippincott Williams & Wilkins; 1987:300-315.
42. Mhyre JM, Riesner MN, Polley LS, Naughton NN. A series of anesthesia-related maternal deaths in Michigan, 1985-2003. *Anesthesiology.* 2007;106:1096-1104.
43. McDonnell NJ, Paech MJ, Clavisi OM, Scott KL. Difficult and failed intubation in obstetric anaesthesia: an observational study of airway management and complications associated with general anaesthesia for caesarean section. *Int J Obstet Anesth.* 2008;17:292-297.
44. Davies JM, Posner KL, Lee LA, Cheney FW, Domino KB. Liability associated with obstetric anesthesia: a closed claims analysis. *Anesthesiology.* 2009;110:131-139.
45. Borland LM, Sereika SM, Woelfel SK, et al. Pulmonary aspiration in pediatric patients during general anesthesia: incidence and outcome. *J Clin Anesth.* 1998;10:95-102.
46. Kao CH, ChangLai SP, Chieng PU, Yen TC. Gastric emptying in head-injured patients. *Am J Gastroenterol.* 1998;93:1108-1112.
47. Saxe JM, Ledgerwood AM, Lucas CE, Lucas WF. Lower esophageal sphincter dysfunction precludes safe gastric feeding after head injury. *J Trauma.* 1994;37:581-584; discussion 4-6.
48. Hardoff R, Sula M, Tamir A, et al. Gastric emptying time and gastric motility in patients with Parkinson's disease. *Mov Disord.* 2001;16:1041-1047.
49. Kalinowski CP, Kirsch JR. Strategies for prophylaxis and treatment for aspiration. *Best Pract Res Clin Anaesthesiol.* 2004;18:719-737.
50. McAnulty GR, Robertshaw HJ, Hall GM. Anaesthetic management of patients with diabetes mellitus. *Br J Anaesth.* 2000;85:80-90.
51. Heyland DK, Tougas G, King D, Cook DJ. Impaired gastric emptying in mechanically ventilated, critically ill patients. *Intensive Care Med.* 1996;22:1339-1344.
52. Kao CH, Ho YJ, Changlai SP, Ding HJ. Gastric emptying in spinal cord injury patients. *Dig Dis Sci.* 1999;44:1512-1515.
53. Kelly MC, Carabine UA, Hill DA, Mirakhur RK. A comparison of the effect of intrathecal and extradural fentanyl on gastric emptying in laboring women. *Anesth Analg.* 1997;85:834-838.

54. Murphy DB, Sutton JA, Prescott LF, Murphy MB. Opioid-induced delay in gastric emptying: a peripheral mechanism in humans. *Anesthesiology.* 1997;87:765-770.

55. Porter JS, Bonello E, Reynolds F. The influence of epidural administration of fentanyl infusion on gastric emptying in labour. *Anaesthesia.* 1997;52:1151-1156.

56. ASA Task Force. Practice guidelines for preoperative fasting and the use of pharmacologic agents to reduce the risk of pulmonary aspiration: application to healthy patients undergoing elective procedures: a report by the American Society of Anesthesiologist Task Force on Preoperative Fasting. *Anesthesiology.* 1999;90:896-905.

57. Brady M, Kinn S, Stuart P. Preoperative fasting for adults to prevent perioperative complications. *Cochrane Database Syst Rev.* 2003:CD004423.

58. Soreide E, Eriksson LI, Hirlekar G, et al. Pre-operative fasting guidelines: an update. *Acta Anaesthesiol Scand.* 2005;49:1041-1047.

59. O'Sullivan G, Scrutton M. NPO during labor. Is there any scientific validation? *Anesthesiol Clin North America.* 2003;21:87-98.

60. Practice guidelines for obstetric anesthesia: an updated report by the American Society of Anesthesiologists Task Force on Obstetric Anesthesia. *Anesthesiology.* 2007;106:843-863.

61. Hatlebakk JG, Berstad A. Pharmacokinetic optimisation in the treatment of gastro-oesophageal reflux disease. *Clin Pharmacokinet.* 1996;31:386-406.

62. Porembka DT, Kier A, Sehlhorst S, Boyce S, Orlowski JP, Davis K, Jr. The pathophysiologic changes following bile aspiration in a porcine lung model. *Chest.* 1993;104:919-924.

63. Sturm A, Holtmann G, Goebell H, Gerken G. Prokinetics in patients with gastroparesis: a systematic analysis. *Digestion.* 1999;60:422-427.

64. Zatman TF, Hall JE, Harmer M. Gastric residual volume in children: a study comparing efficiency of erythromycin and metoclopramide as prokinetic agents. *Br J Anaesth.* 2001;86:869-871.

65. Gibbs CP, Schwartz DJ, Wynne JW, Hodd CI, Kuck EJ. Antacid pulmonary aspiration in the dog. *Anesthesiology.* 1979;51:380-385.

66. Brimacombe JR, Berry AM. Cricoid pressure. *Can J Anaesth.* 1997;44:414-425.

67. Bair AE, Filbin MR, Kulkarni RG, Walls RM. The failed intubation attempt in the emergency department: analysis of prevalence, rescue techniques, and personnel. *J Emerg Med.* 2002;23:131-140.

68. Sloane C, Vilke GM, Chan TC, Hayden SR, Hoyt DB, Rosen P. Rapid sequence intubation in the field versus hospital in trauma patients. *J Emerg Med.* 2000;19:259-264.

69. Pearson S. Comparison of intubation attempts and completion times before and after the initiation of a rapid sequence intubation protocol in an air medical transport program. *Air Med J.* 2003;22:28-33.

70. Ricard-Hibon A, Chollet C, Leroy C, Marty J. Succinylcholine improves the time of performance of a tracheal intubation in prehospital critical care medicine. *Eur J Anaesthesiol.* 2002;19:361-367.

71. Rocca B, Crosby E, Maloney J, Bryson G. An assessment of paramedic performance during invasive airway management. *Prehosp Emerg Care.* 2000;4:164-167.

72. Davis DP, Dunford JV, Poste JC, et al. The impact of hypoxia and hyperventilation on outcome after paramedic rapid sequence intubation of severely head-injured patients. *J Trauma.* 2004;57:1-8.

73. Dunford JV, Davis DP, Ochs M, Doney M, Hoyt DB. Incidence of transient hypoxia and pulse rate reactivity during paramedic rapid sequence intubation. *Ann Emerg Med.* 2003;42:721-728.

74. Adnet F, Baillard C, Borron SW, et al. Randomized study comparing the "sniffing position" with simple head extension for laryngoscopic view in elective surgery patients. *Anesthesiology.* 2001;95:836-841.

75. Gambee AM, Hertzka RE, Fisher DM. Preoxygenation techniques: comparison of three minutes and four breaths. *Anesth Analg.* 1987;66:468-470.

76. Neilipovitz DT, Crosby ET. No evidence for decreased incidence of aspiration after rapid sequence induction. *Can J Anaesth.* 2007;54:748-764.

77. Stept WJ, Safar P. Rapid induction-intubation for prevention of gastric-content aspiration. *Anesth Analg.* 1970;49:633-636.

78. Satiani B, Bonner JT, Stone HH. Factors influencing intraoperative gastric regurgitation: a prospective random study of nasogastric tube drainage. *Arch Surg.* 1978;113:721-723.

79. Salem MR, Wong AY, Fizzotti GF. Efficacy of cricoid pressure in preventing aspiration of gastric contents in paediatric patients. *Br J Anaesth.* 1972;44:401-404.

80. Sivilotti ML, Filbin MR, Murray HE, Slasor P, Walls RM. Does the sedative agent facilitate emergency rapid sequence intubation? *Acad Emerg Med.* 2003;10:612-620.

81. Adams P, Gelman S, Reves JG, Greenblatt DJ, Alvis JM, Bradley E. Midazolam pharmacodynamics and pharmacokinetics during acute hypovolemia. *Anesthesiology.* 1985;63:140-146.

82. Davis DP, Kimbro TA, Vilke GM. The use of midazolam for prehospital rapid-sequence intubation may be associated with a dose-related increase in hypotension. *Prehosp Emerg Care.* 2001;5:163-168.

83. Sivilotti ML, Ducharme J. Randomized, double-blind study on sedatives and hemodynamics during rapid-sequence intubation in the emergency department: the SHRED Study. *Ann Emerg Med.* 1998;31:313-324.

84. Michenfelder JD, Milde JH, Sundt TM, Jr. Cerebral protection by barbiturate anesthesia. Use after middle cerebral artery occlusion in Java monkeys. *Arch Neurol.* 1976;33:345-350.

85. Mirakhur RK, Elliott P, Shepherd WF, Archer DB. Intra-ocular pressure changes during induction of anaesthesia and tracheal intubation. A comparison of thiopentone and propofol followed by vecuronium. *Anaesthesia.* 1988;43 Suppl:54-57.

86. Thomson MF, Brock-Utne JG, Bean P, Welsh N, Downing JW. Anaesthesia and intra-ocular pressure: a comparative of total intravenous anaesthesia using etomidate with conventional inhalation anaesthesia. *Anaesthesia.* 1982;37:758-761.

87. Hartung HJ. Intracranial pressure in patients with craniocerebral trauma after administration of propofol and thiopental. *Anaesthesist.* 1987;36:285-287.

88. McCollum JS, Dundee JW. Comparison of induction characteristics of four intravenous anaesthetic agents. *Anaesthesia.* 1986;41:995-1000.

89. Moss E, Powell D, Gibson RM, McDowall DG. Effect of etomidate on intracranial pressure and cerebral perfusion pressure. *Br J Anaesth.* 1979;51:347-352.

90. Giese JL, Stockham RJ, Stanley TH, Pace NL, Nelissen RH. Etomidate versus thiopental for induction of anesthesia. *Anesth Analg.* 1985;64:871-876.

91. Weiss-Bloom LJ, Reich DL. Haemodynamic responses to tracheal intubation following etomidate and fentanyl for anaesthetic induction. *Can J Anaesth.* 1992;39:780-785.

92. Robinson N, Clancy M. In patients with head injury undergoing rapid sequence intubation, does pretreatment with intravenous lignocaine/lidocaine lead to an improved neurological outcome? A review of the literature. *Emerg Med J.* 2001;18:453-457.

93. El-Orbany MI, Joseph NJ, Salem MR, Klowden AJ. The neuromuscular effects and tracheal intubation conditions after small doses of succinylcholine. *Anesth Analg.* 2004;98:1680-1685, table of contents.

94. Naguib M, Samarkandi A, Riad W, Alharby SW. Optimal dose of succinylcholine revisited. *Anesthesiology.* 2003;99:1045-1049.

95. Andrews JI, Kumar N, van den Brom RH, Olkkola KT, Roest GJ, Wright PM. A large simple randomized trial of rocuronium versus succinylcholine in rapid-sequence induction of anaesthesia along with propofol. *Acta Anaesthesiol Scand.* 1999;43:4-8.

96. Dobson AP, McCluskey A, Meakin G, Baker RD. Effective time to satisfactory intubation conditions after administration of rocuronium in adults. Comparison of propofol and thiopentone for rapid sequence induction of anaesthesia. *Anaesthesia.* 1999;54:172-176.

97. Skinner HJ, Biswas A, Mahajan RP. Evaluation of intubating conditions with rocuronium and either propofol or etomidate for rapid sequence induction. *Anaesthesia.* 1998;53:702-706.

98. Fuchs-Buder T, Sparr HJ, Ziegenfuss T. Thiopental or etomidate for rapid sequence induction with rocuronium. *Br J Anaesth.* 1998;80:504-506.

99. Naguib M. Sugammadex: another milestone in clinical neuromuscular pharmacology. *Anesth Analg.* 2007;104:575-581.

100. Salem MR, Sellick BA, Elam JO. The historical background of cricoid pressure in anesthesia and resuscitation. *Anesth Analg.* 1974;53:230-232.

101. Farmery AD, Roe PG. A model to describe the rate of oxyhaemoglobin desaturation during apnoea. *Br J Anaesth.* 1996;76:284-291.

102. Hardman JG, Wills JS, Aitkenhead AR. Factors determining the onset and course of hypoxemia during apnea: an investigation using physiological modelling. *Anesth Analg.* 2000;90:619-624.

103. Lawes EG, Campbell I, Mercer D. Inflation pressure, gastric insufflation and rapid sequence induction. *Br J Anaesth.* 1987;59:315-318.

104. Ruben H, Knudsen EJ, Carugati G. Gastric inflation in relation to airway pressure. *Acta Anaesthesiol Scand.* 1961;5:107-114.

105. Petito SP, Russell WJ. The prevention of gastric inflation—a neglected benefit of cricoid pressure. *Anaesth Intensive Care.* 1988;16:139-143.

106. Vanner RG, Pryle BJ. Nasogastric tubes and cricoid pressure. *Anaesthesia.* 1993;48:1112-1113.

107. Smith KJ, Ladak S, Choi PT, Dobranowski J. The cricoid cartilage and the esophagus are not aligned in close to half of adult patients. *Can J Anaesth*. 2002;49:503-507.

108. Smith KJ, Dobranowski J, Yip G, Dauphin A, Choi PT. Cricoid pressure displaces the esophagus: an observational study using magnetic resonance imaging. *Anesthesiology*. 2003;99:60-64.

109. Sellick BA. Rupture of the oesophagus following cricoid pressure? *Anaesthesia*. 1982;37:213-214.

110. Ralph SJ, Wareham CA. Rupture of the oesophagus during cricoid pressure. *Anaesthesia*. 1991;46:40-41.

111. Hein C, Owen H. The effective application of Cricoid pressure. *J Emerg Prim Health Care*. 2005;3:1-2.

112. Vanner RG, O'Dwyer JP, Pryle BJ, Reynolds F. Upper oesophageal sphincter pressure and the effect of cricoid pressure. *Anaesthesia*. 1992;47:95-100.

113. Vanner RG, Pryle BJ. Regurgitation and oesophageal rupture with cricoid pressure: a cadaver study. *Anaesthesia*. 1992;47:732-735.

114. Meek T, Gittins N, Duggan JE. Cricoid pressure: knowledge and performance amongst anaesthetic assistants. *Anaesthesia*. 1999;54:59-62.

115. Meek T, Vincent A, Duggan JE. Cricoid pressure: can protective force be sustained? *Br J Anaesth*. 1998;80:672-674.

116. Crowley DS, Giesecke AH. Bimanual cricoid pressure. *Anaesthesia*. 1990;45:588-589.

117. Vanner RG, Clarke P, Moore WJ, Raftery S. The effect of cricoid pressure and neck support on the view at laryngoscopy. *Anaesthesia*. 1997;52:896-900.

118. Cook TM. Cricoid pressure: are two hands better than one? *Anaesthesia*. 1996;51:365-368.

119. Yentis SM. The effects of single-handed and bimanual cricoid pressure on the view at laryngoscopy. Anaesthesia 1997;52:332-335.

120. Cook TM, Godfrey I, Rockett M, Vanner RG. Cricoid pressure: which hand? *Anaesthesia*. 2000;55:648-653.

121. Allman KG. The effect of cricoid pressure application on airway patency. *J Clin Anesth*. 1995;7:197-199.

122. Moynihan RJ, Brock-Utne JG, Archer JH, Feld LH, Kreitzman TR. The effect of cricoid pressure on preventing gastric insufflation in infants and children. *Anesthesiology*. 1993;78:652-656.

123. Vanner RG. Tolerance of cricoid pressure by conscious volunteers. *Int J Obstet Anesth*. 1992;1:195-198.

124. Hawthorne L, Wilson R, Lyons G, Dresner M. Failed intubation revisited: 17-yr experience in a teaching maternity unit. *Br J Anaesth*. 1996;76:680-684.

125. Lawes EG, Duncan PW, Bland B, Gemmel L, Downing JW. The cricoid yoke—a device for providing consistent and reproducible cricoid pressure. *Br J Anaesth*. 1986;58:925-931.

126. Hartsilver EL, Vanner RG. Airway obstruction with cricoid pressure. *Anaesthesia*. 2000;55:208-211.

127. Aoyama K, Takenaka I, Sata T, Shigematsu A. Cricoid pressure impedes positioning and ventilation through the laryngeal mask airway. *Can J Anaesth*. 1996;43:1035-1040.

128. Asai T, Barclay K, McBeth C, Vaughan RS. Cricoid pressure applied after placement of the laryngeal mask prevents gastric insufflation but inhibits ventilation. *Br J Anaesth*. 1996;76:772-776.

129. Mac GPJH, Ball DR. The effect of cricoid pressure on the cricoid cartilage and vocal cords: an endoscopic study in anaesthetised patients. *Anaesthesia*. 2000;55:263-268.

130. Levitan RM, Kinkle WC, Levin WJ, Everett WW. Laryngeal view during laryngoscopy: a randomized trial comparing cricoid pressure, backward-upward-rightward pressure, and bimanual laryngoscopy. *Ann Emerg Med*. 2006;47:548-555.

131. McNelis U, Syndercombe A, Harper I, Duggan J. The effect of cricoid pressure on intubation facilitated by the gum elastic bougie. *Anaesthesia*. 2007;62:456-459.

132. Turgeon AF, Nicole PC, Trepanier CA, Marcoux S, Lessard MR. Cricoid pressure does not increase the rate of failed intubation by direct laryngoscopy in adults. *Anesthesiology*. 2005;102:315-319.

133. Smith CE, Boyer D. Cricoid pressure decreases ease of tracheal intubation using fibreoptic laryngoscopy (WuScope System™). *Can J Anaesth*. 2002;49:614-619.

134. Hodgson RE, Gopalan PD, Burrows RC, Zuma K. Effect of cricoid pressure on the success of endotracheal intubation with a lightwand. *Anesthesiology*. 2001;94:259-262.

135. Shulman GB, Connelly NR. A comparison of the Bullard laryngoscope versus the flexible fiberoptic bronchoscope during intubation in patients afforded inline stabilization. *J Clin Anesth*. 2001;13:182-185.

136. Gabbott DA. The effect of single-handed cricoid pressure on neck movement after applying manual in-line stabilisation. *Anaesthesia*. 1997;52:586-588.

137. Helliwell V, Gabbott DA. The effect of single-handed cricoid pressure on cervical spine movement after applying manual in-line stabilisation—a cadaver study. *Resuscitation*. 2001;49:53-57.

138. Wood PR. Direct laryngoscopy and cervical spine stabilisation. *Anaesthesia*. 1994;49:77-78.

139. Roux M, Drolet P, Girard M, Grenier Y, Petit B. Effect of the laryngeal mask airway on oesophageal pH: influence of the volume and pressure inside the cuff. *Br J Anaesth*. 1999;82:566-569.

140. Joshi GP, Morrison SG, Okonkwo NA, White PF. Continuous hypopharyngeal pH measurements in spontaneously breathing anesthetized outpatients: laryngeal mask airway versus tracheal intubation. *Anesth Analg*. 1996;82:254-257.

141. Ho BY, Skinner HJ, Mahajan RP. Gastro-oesophageal reflux during day case gynaecological laparoscopy under positive pressure ventilation: laryngeal mask vs. tracheal intubation. *Anaesthesia*. 1998;53:921-924.

142. Hagberg CA, Vartazarian TN, Chelly JE, Ovassapian A. The incidence of gastroesophageal reflux and tracheal aspiration detected with pH electrodes is similar with the Laryngeal Mask Airway and Esophageal Tracheal Combitube™—a pilot study. *Can J Anaesth*. 2004;51:243-249.

143. McCrory CR, McShane AJ. Gastroesophageal reflux during spontaneous respiration with the laryngeal mask airway. *Can J Anaesth*. 1999;46:268-270.

144. Cheong YP, Park SK, Son Y, et al. Comparison of incidence of gastroesophageal reflux and regurgitation associated with timing of removal of the laryngeal mask airway: on appearance of signs of rejection versus after recovery of consciousness. *J Clin Anesth*. 1999;11:657-662.

145. Evans NR, Gardner SV, James MF. ProSeal laryngeal mask protects against aspiration of fluid in the pharynx. *Br J Anaesth*. 2002;88:584-587.

146. Verghese C, Brimacombe JR. Survey of laryngeal mask airway usage in 11,910 patients: safety and efficacy for conventional and nonconventional usage. *Anesth Analg*. 1996;82:129-133.

147. Brimacombe JR, Berry A. The incidence of aspiration associated with the laryngeal mask airway: a meta-analysis of published literature. *J Clin Anesth*. 1995;7:297-305.

148. Keller C, Brimacombe J, Bittersohl J, Lirk P, von Goedecke A. Aspiration and the laryngeal mask airway: three cases and a review of the literature. *Br J Anaesth*. 2004;93:579-582.

149. Hung OR, Pytka S, Morris I, et al. Clinical trial of a new lightwand device (Trachlight™) to intubate the trachea. *Anesthesiology*. 1995;83:509-514.

150. Hung OR, Pytka S, Morris I, Murphy M, Stewart RD. Lightwand intubation: II—Clinical trial of a new lightwand for tracheal intubation in patients with difficult airways. *Can J Anaesth*. 1995;42:826-830.

151. Bourke DL, Katz J, Tonneson A. Nebulized anesthesia for awake endotracheal intubation. *Anesthesiology*. 1985;63:690-692.

152. Ovassapian A, Krejcie TC, Yelich SJ, Dykes MH. Awake fibreoptic intubation in the patient at high risk of aspiration. *Br J Anaesth*. 1989;62:13-16.

153. Simmons ST, Schleich AR. Airway regional anesthesia for awake fiberoptic intubation. *Reg Anesth Pain Med*. 2002;27:180-192.

154. Walsh ME, Shorten GD. Preparing to perform an awake fiberoptic intubation. *Yale J Biol Med*. 1998;71:537-549.

155. Benumof JL. Management of the difficult adult airway. With special emphasis on awake tracheal intubation. *Anesthesiology*. 1991;75:1087-1110.

156. McCormick PW. Immediate care after aspiration of vomit. *Anaesthesia*. 1975;30:658-665.

157. Wynne JW, Modell JH. Respiratory aspiration of stomach contents. *Ann Intern Med*. 1977;87:466-474.

158. Lee M, Sukumaran M, Berger HW, Reilly TA. Influence of corticosteroid treatment on pulmonary function after recovery from aspiration of gastric contents. *Mt Sinai J Med*. 1980;47:341-346.

159. Sukumaran M, Granada MJ, Berger HW, Lee M, Reilly TA. Evaluation of corticosteroid treatment in aspiration of gastric contents: a controlled clinical trial. *Mt Sinai J Med*. 1980;47:335-340.

160. Wolfe JE, Bone RC, Ruth WE. Effects of corticosteroids in the treatment of patients with gastric aspiration. *Am J Med*. 1977;63:719-722.

161. Bone RC, Fisher CJ, Jr., Clemmer TP, Slotman GJ, Metz CA, Balk RA. A controlled clinical trial of high-dose methylprednisolone in the treatment of severe sepsis and septic shock. *N Engl J Med*. 1987;317:653-658.

162. Johnson JL, Hirsch CS. Aspiration pneumonia. Recognizing and managing a potentially growing disorder. *Postgrad Med*. 2003;113:99-102,5-6,11-12.

163. El-Solh AA, Pietrantoni C, Bhat A, et al. Microbiology of severe aspiration pneumonia in institutionalized elderly. *Am J Respir Crit Care Med*. 2003;167:1650-1654.

164. Niederman MS, Bass JB, Jr., Campbell GD, et al. Guidelines for the initial management of adults with community-acquired pneumonia: diagnosis,

assessment of severity, and initial antimicrobial therapy. American Thoracic Society. Medical Section of the American Lung Association. *Am Rev Respir Dis.* 1993;148:1418-1426.

165. Bernstein JM. Treatment of community-acquired pneumonia—IDSA guidelines. Infectious Diseases Society of America. *Chest.* 1999;115:9S-13S.

166. Mandell LA, Marrie TJ, Grossman RF, Chow AW, Hyland RH. Canadian guidelines for the initial management of community-acquired pneumonia: an evidence-based update by the Canadian Infectious Diseases Society and the Canadian Thoracic Society. The Canadian Community-Acquired Pneumonia Working Group. *Clin Infect Dis.* 2000;31:383-421.

SELF-EVALUATION QUESTIONS

5.1. How much cricoid pressure has been shown to prevent gastric regurgitation?

A. 10 N

B. 20 N

C. 30 N

D. 40 N

E. 50 N

5.2. Which of the following is **NOT** true about cricoid pressure and airway techniques?

A. The difficulty in ventilation using the LMA is dependent on the amount of pressure applied.

B. Cricoid pressure reduces the incidence of gastric insufflation when using an LMA.

C. Improper LMA placement can occur when cricoid pressure is applied.

D. Ventilation via a facemask has not been shown to be affected by cricoid pressure.

E. Tracheal intubation using a rigid fiberoptic laryngoscope (eg, WuScope System™) is more difficult to perform when cricoid pressure is applied.

5.3. Which of the following is **NOT** a known factor that increases the risk of aspiration?

A. emergency surgery

B. timing of surgery

C. lack of fasting

D. pregnant patients

E. children

SECTION 2

Devices and Techniques for Difficult and Failed Airway Management

CHAPTER (6)

Context-Sensitive Airway Management

Steven Petrar, Orlando R. Hung, and Michael F. Murphy

6.1 CASE PRESENTATION

A 50-year-old man is in the waiting room of the emergency department (ED) awaiting evaluation for several days of hematuria. He has a remote history of prostate cancer. Suddenly, the man falls to the floor, becomes unresponsive, and has a generalized, tonic-clonic seizure. The emergency physician and paramedic on duty are summoned by the triage nurse. Intravenous (IV) access is established and the seizure is halted with multiple doses of intravenous lorazepam totaling 12 mg. Unfortunately, the patient is extremely somnolent and the emergency physician is concerned that he is at risk for airway obstruction, apnea, and aspiration. The decision to intubate the trachea is made.

The obtunded patient is positioned on a stretcher and monitors are applied. Evaluation of airway anatomy and ease of intubation reveal no significant predictors of difficulty. The physician elects to proceed with a rapid-sequence intubation (RSI). Direct laryngoscopy using a Macintosh #3 blade proves difficult, with two failed attempts by the physician. Bag-mask-ventilation (BMV) is performed between attempts and the patient's oxygen saturation never falls below 95%. On the third attempt, direct laryngoscopic intubation is successful with the aid of an Eschmann Tracheal Introducer (commonly known as the *gum-elastic bougie*) after establishing a partial (Cormack/Lehane Grade 2) view of the glottis.

The patient is sedated and transported to the CT scanner. CT scan is unremarkable. Collateral history reveals a history of heavy alcohol abuse, although the patient had recently decided to "quit drinking" and had been abstinent for 48 hours. A presumed diagnosis of alcohol withdrawal seizure is made and sedation is weaned. Three hours postintubation, the patient is noted to be awake, cooperative, and increasingly agitated by the tracheal tube.

Extubation is performed without incident and supplemental oxygen is applied by facemask. Several minutes later the bedside nurse summons the physician as the patient is having increasing difficulty in breathing with labored, noisy respirations. Moments later, the patient loses consciousness and becomes apneic and cyanotic.

The emergency physician immediately attempts tracheal intubation via direct laryngoscopy but fails due to a completely obstructed upper airway secondary to a massive tongue hematoma. The hematoma is presumed to be as a result of his earlier seizure. Help is summoned and a Code Blue is called.

6.2 INTRODUCTION

The fundamental goals of airway management are the maintenance of adequate ventilation, oxygenation, and protection from aspiration of foreign materials. In the majority of clinical settings, these three goals are achieved in tandem, usually via orotracheal intubation using a conventional laryngoscope. As the location, skill set of the practitioner, and the devices available (ie, the "context") change, the practitioner must be prepared to modify his or her approach and employ different techniques as appropriate. The provision of oxygenation, by whatever method possible, is ultimately the task that takes precedence over all others, particularly in emergency situations.

6.2.1 What is context-sensitive airway management?

The concept of "context-sensitive" airway management represents a paradigm shift in the approach to airway management. The skilled practitioner will be less focused on specific devices and techniques, and more aware of the *context* presented by each patient encounter—and how that context may influence the approach to the preservation of gas exchange.

The "context defining" questions can be conceptualized as the "who, what, where, when, why, and how" unique to each and every airway management encounter. These questions, or *situational modifiers*, influence the decision making of a skilled airway practitioner. In a more pragmatic sense, examples of these context defining factors might include: availability of equipment, the expertise of assistance, the skill set and personal experience of the practitioner, and the environment in which the patient encounter occurs. Additionally, individual patient factors, such as anatomy and physiology, acuity of the situation, and the distinction between cooperative and uncooperative patients all modify the context of the airway management encounter and must be considered in order to best approach the airway in a *context-sensitive* fashion.

6.2.2 Does the *context* of the case presented suggest which technique should be used to provide ventilation and oxygenation to an unconscious, apneic patient?

This case demonstrates how airway management by nature, is context-sensitive. "Who, what, when, where, why, and how" are all context-defining questions that affect the way the airway is best approached and managed. In this case, an airway successfully managed in one way, is unmanageable by the same team in a similar environment a short time later. This is owing to altered airway anatomy, that is, the context has changed and alternate methods of ventilation, oxygenation, and airway protection must be considered.

Traditionally, great emphasis has been placed on the provision of bag-mask-ventilation (BMV) as an initial approach to the unconscious and apneic patient. Indeed, among the four domains of airway management (BMV, extra-glottic devices, tracheal intubation, and surgical airway), BMV has been the most common initial maneuver employed by most airway practitioners. Unfortunately, mounting evidence and opinion suggests that BMV is a difficult skill to master, particularly in the hands of nonexpert practitioners.[1-4] In many cases, BMV is performed poorly with ineffective oxygenation and ventilation, and gastric insufflation the end result. As extraglottic devices (EGDs) continue to improve in quality and ease of use, many experts agree that the placement of an EGD ought to supplant BMV as the initial technique of choice for the airway management of an unconscious and apneic patient, particularly by nonexpert airway practitioners.[5]

Clearly, no single device or technique can be relied upon as the sole modality for airway management by *any* practitioner. The choice of device and technique depends on the context of the situation. The second airway management encounter in the case presented is likely to result in impossible BMV and failure of any oral intubation approach. The practitioner would be well advised to consider nasal route options (blind nasal intubation, nasal bronchoscopic intubation, and nasal intubation using a lightwand [Trachlight™]) while at the same time preparing for surgical options, such as cricothyrotomy.

6.2.3 How has increasing appreciation of the context-sensitive nature of airway management guided technological advances leading to improved airway management tools?

Technological advances over the past two decades have dramatically improved the quality and clinical utility of many airway management tools, including:

1. The manufacturing and marketing of newer and improved EGDs for use in a variety of situations.[6,7] Gone are the days where the LMA-Classic™ was the only, or even the *preferred*, EGD for use in difficult or failed airways. The airway practitioner now has to choose among devices that serve as tracheal intubation conduits in addition to those that have been shown to be effective rescue devices in situations where intubation is not possible.[8]

2. Advances in video resolution and LCD monitor technology, combined with high-quality color fidelity and optics have led to the development of several video-camera endoscopic-based devices. These include the Glidescope® (Verathon Medical, Bothell WA), the Video Macintosh Intubating Laryngoscope System (VMS, K. Storz Endoscopy Co., Culver City, CA), the LMA CTrach™, and the McGrath® Video Laryngoscope (Aircraft Medical, Edinburgh, UK). These devices remain subject to limitations due to fogging, and obscuration of glottic visualization in the presence of blood, vomitus, or secretions. Their utility is questionable in these contexts (see Chapter 10). Nonetheless, video laryngoscopy continues to be an evolving field with intriguing possibilities in the absence of bodily fluids that may obscure their optics.

3. Improved portability of sophisticated airway management devices, coupled with the introduction of disposable variants, has broadened their utility. Devices are becoming more lightweight, portable, and robust in construction. Battery-powered endoscopes and compact video laryngoscopes, such as the McGrath® and the Glidescope® Ranger Video Laryngoscopes, can be carried to the patient regardless of location and irrespective of external power sources or large video displays.

4. Enhanced light intensity of some airway instruments. The transillumination technique employed by lightwand devices, such as the Trachlight™, is substantially improved with the use of high-intensity bulbs.[9] Adequate transillumination is often possible under ambient lighting conditions, obviating the need to dim the lights or darken the room when these devices are being used. One study involving 950 patients demonstrated that nearly 88% of Trachlight™ intubations were effectively accomplished under ambient light with or without simple shading of the neck.[10]

6.2.4 In what contexts are blind intubating techniques indicated?

Over the years, direct laryngoscopic intubation has been shown to be an effective and safe technique that is relatively easy to perform. It has become the standard method of tracheal intubation in operating rooms, intensive care units, emergency departments, and in the field. Unfortunately, even in the hands of experienced laryngoscopists, the rapid and accurate placement of an endotracheal tube (ETT) remains a significant challenge in some patients. This is particularly true in *unprepared* patients, or those requiring emergency tracheal intubation. In these contexts, a blind or nonvisual technique *may* be more successful.

Alternative intubation techniques, such as flexible broncho-scopic intubation, have gained a measure of popularity over the past several decades. While effective and reliable, this technique requires expensive equipment, and special skill and training. Additionally, bronchoscopic intubation can be difficult in emergency situations in which *unprepared* or uncooperative patients may have copious secretions, blood or vomitus in the oropharynx, or airway. One large study involving more than 1600 fiberoptic intubations recorded a success rate of approximately 94%.[11]

Because of the difficulties posed by laryngoscopic intubation under direct vision, particularly under emergency conditions, the search for other techniques has led to the development of blind techniques using a variety of devices. During the last few decades, intubating guides and light-guided intubation using the principle of transillumination have proven to be effective, safe, and simple.

6.2.5 Would it not be safer to place a tracheal tube using a technique that is under direct vision?

One would anticipate that the placement of an endotracheal tube (ETT) into the trachea under direct vision using a laryngoscope ought to be safer and achieve higher success rates than nonvisual techniques. Such is not the case; success and complication rates are *not* substantially different with blind techniques performed by skilled practitioners,[10] as elaborated below. Furthermore, the technique of direct vision can be very difficult or even impossible because of distorted anatomy or the patient's disease—as illustrated in the preceding case study. However, several contextual factors *do* influence the success rates and safety of indirect laryngoscopic intubation including the inability to visualize the passage of the ETT through the glottic opening and the presence of blood, secretions, and vomitus.

Many practitioners fail to understand that after having placed the flexible bronchoscope into the trachea under indirect vision, the actual passage of the ETT over the bronchoscope is done blindly employing the scope as a guide. In other words, during bronchoscopic intubation, after advancing the tip of the broncho-scope into the trachea, the bronchoscope functions only as a stylet to guide the ETT into the trachea similar to that of an Eschmann Introducer. The use of advanced airway devices to enable continuous glottic visualization during endotracheal tube exchange has recently been reviewed.[12] This intriguing application of these devices may be applied to primary intubation to further increase the safety of *blind* intubation techniques, although further research is required.

Many other procedures performed in medicine are in fact *blind* techniques including the placement of pulmonary arterial catheters, arterial cannulae, epidural catheters, and femoral nerve sheath catheters. All of these procedures demand placement blindly under the guidance of anatomical landmarks, and physiological responses.

Blind intubating techniques have been shown to be effective and safe, and in the absence of abnormalities of the upper airway, these techniques are acceptable methods of airway management when employed in the appropriate contexts.

6.3 AIRWAY MANAGEMENT TOOLS

6.3.1 Which of the EGDs has been shown to provide better ventilation and oxygenation and in what contexts?

Implicit to any discussion about airway management tools and techniques is the realization that the *best* instrument for the situation depends entirely on the context, or the *situational modifiers*. Unfortunately, there is no 'one size fits all' device.

The context affects a variety of issues when one contemplates the use of an EGD. These include: patient anatomy and predicted ease of insertion, *full-stomach* precautions and the need for airway protection from aspiration, need for positive-pressure ventilation, and the presence or absence of airway-obstructing pathology. These are just a few of the *situational modifiers* which define the context of EGD use in airway management.

In general, EGDs are best reserved for fasted patients at low risk of aspiration, and those with acceptable airways resistance and pulmonary compliance should positive-pressure ventilation be desired. However, EGDs are invaluable *rescue* devices in the case of unexpected airway management difficulty or failure. They have proven to be valuable as primary airway management devices in EMS. In these situations, placement of an EGD with intubation capabilities and a parallel lumen for gastroesophageal venting may be advisable. In clinical practice, the actual device is less important than the thoughtful consideration of all contextual factors. In the opinion of the authors, the EGDs currently available which best fulfill these objectives are the LMA-Supreme™ (nonintubating EGD), the LMA-Fastrach™ (intubating EGD), and the King LTS-D™.

6.3.2 What extraglottic devices (EGDs) should I incorporate into my practice?

The most thoroughly studied EGDs currently in use are the Laryngeal Mask Airway and the Combitube™. Many competing designs and variations of these devices have been released to market and are in use worldwide. We now have the option of using intubating LMAs as well as alternatives to the Combitube™, such as the King Laryngeal Tube Airway (King LT™, King Systems) which are placed blindly into the oropharynx and seated in the hypopharynx, directing respiratory gases into the trachea. In addition, a new generation of disposable, single-use EGDs has entered the marketplace, including the Ambu LMA (Ambu USA), the Streamlined Liner of the Pharynx (SLIPA, SLIPA Medical Inc), and the i-Gel (Intersurgical Ltd).

Of particular use in the difficult or failed airway scenario are the various models of intubating LMAs such as the LMA-Fastrach™ and Cook Intubating LMA (ILMA). Intubating LMA systems are fundamentally designed to permit the practitioner to ventilate the patient and to provide a conduit for tracheal intubation. This may be accomplished using a flexible bronchoscope, a lightwand, or even by blind insertion. In the author's institution, an intubating LMA (LMA-Fastrach™) is kept in each anesthesia machine with the intention of immediate availability in the event of a failed airway or an airway emergency where other methods of preserving oxygenation have failed unexpectedly.

The final consideration of note when deciding on the best EGDs to purchase and implement in one's institution is the differentiation between disposable and reusable devices. Several high-quality disposable EGDs are now on the market. These were developed partially in response to concerns of potential transmission of prion-based infection disease, such as Creutzfeldt-Jakob disease. Disposable devices, such as the LMA-Supreme™, may be best suited to use in the pre-hospital context where a reusable device requiring sterilization may be discarded or lost. Environmental concerns with the routine use, disposable devices are worth noting.

6.3.3   What tracheal intubation techniques should I incorporate into my practice?

Recalling the principles of context-sensitive airway management, it is apparent that an expert practitioner should be comfortable with several techniques of tracheal intubation, including visual and nonvisual methods.

For most practitioners involved in airway management, tracheal intubation equates to direct laryngoscopy. It is true that the conventional laryngoscope, with interchangeable curved and straight blades, is likely the tool with the greatest recognition and use worldwide. Expertise with the use of this tool is an essential skill for any airway practitioner. In addition, all practitioners should become familiar with the use of an Eschmann introducer. This device should be kept readily at hand wherever airway management and direct laryngoscopy may be required. This includes: the operating room, emergency department, intensive care unit, and in crash-carts throughout the hospital.

Beyond direct laryngoscopy the best tracheal intubation tools for an individual's practice depends on the context of that practice. Specifically, what types of patients do you routinely expect to see? Does your institution deal with "difficult" airway situations on a regular basis? How will budgetary constraints dictate which tools may or may not be available for purchase?

While it is not possible to mandate a standard list of devices, it is reasonable to ensure access to a complementary armamentarium of tools to confront the challenges that might arise. This should include: laryngoscopes with curve and straight blades, the Eschmann Introducer, a flexible bronchoscope, a video laryngoscope, such as the Glidescope®, Storz VMAC or McGrath®, and a nonvisual technique, such as a lightwand (Trachlight™). The

remaining devices available should be considered on a case-by-case basis. Certainly a surgical airway kit, such as the Melker percutaneous cricothyrotomy kit (Cook Medical), is mandatory in all areas where airway management may occur.

6.4   CLINICAL APPLICATION OF AIRWAY MANAGEMENT TOOLS

There is a staggering array of airway management tools and techniques available today. For the average practitioner, it is unrealistic to expect to be proficient with all devices. However, to be an efficient and safe practitioner in a field where airway management is an expectation, one must be familiar with a number of airway management tools and techniques in order to be prepared for the inevitable challenges.

6.4.1   What is the most appropriate airway management tool for an unconscious patient?

The simple answer to this question is: Whichever device restores ventilation and oxygenation promptly! A subsidiary concern is that the device protects against gastric insufflation and aspiration. These goals suggest that tracheal intubation is the most-desired solution, most commonly achieved through direct laryngoscopy.

However, in reality, the context will define the 'best' way to manage an airway. In the example given at the beginning of this chapter, direct laryngoscopy, and indeed any *conventional* approach to tracheal intubation may be impossible. In this case, resorting to a surgical airway as the primary method of airway management may be the only viable option to establish oxygenation and ventilation.

Classically, individuals charged with emergency airway management have learned that BMV ought to be the initial airway management strategy in the unconscious patient. This paradigm may be shifting, particularly as evidence supporting the ease of use and effectiveness of EGDs in the hands of those who infrequently manage the airway mounts. EGDs and BMV have similar drawbacks in that they leave the patient with an *unprotected* airway in terms of aspiration risk, and the ability to administer effective positive-pressure ventilation is variable. Overall, it is the authors' opinion that EGDs should be taught to rescue personnel because the authors believe that they are *more* effective than BMV in most cases. EGDs should also be familiar to all other airway practitioners for primary use in appropriate patients, or as rescue devices in the setting of an intubation failure.

6.4.2   How would you manage this patient if this patient is awake, cyanotic, and uncooperative?

The situation (context) has changed. The management of the uncooperative patient will be covered in detail in Chapter 39. In this case, the practitioner is faced with the unenviable decision as to whether or not to induce anesthesia with or without muscle relaxation in the face of a potentially difficult airway. In other words, should a rapid-sequence induction/intubation (RSI) be preformed?

There is no simple answer to this question. In short, it is *always* desirable to have a controlled situation to permit examination and evaluation of the patient's anatomy prior to the induction of anesthesia or the start of an airway management procedure. Due to patient factors, this may not always be possible. In this context, one must judge whether maneuvers or interventions to correct the patient's cyanosis without invasive intervention are likely to succeed. These include administration of supplemental oxygen or simple airway maneuvers, such as a chin lift or jaw thrust. If these are *unlikely* to succeed, or are impossible due to the underlying pathology or the behavior of the patient, an RSI may be the only course of action while preparing for an immediate surgical airway in the event of failure (double setup). In this circumstance, calling for help, meticulous preparation for the primary plan, and preparation for several backup plans is critical.

6.4.3 What other factors influence the selection of an airway management tool?

Successful context-sensitive airway management depends on the interplay between three general categories of situational modifiers. Each modifier demands a *"who, what, where, when, why, and how"* analysis. Consider the following:

1. **Practitioner factors.** These are factors unique to each airway practitioner and include, but are not limited to: degree of expertise, past experiences, ability to rapidly assess the needs of the situation, and the ability to modify or adapt one's approach to a dynamic and variable situation. In general, the skilled practitioner will be able to quickly assess a given airway management situation and select the most appropriate technique from his or her personal arsenal of skills.

2. **Patient factors.** These factors are those unique to each individual patient including, but not limited to: degree of cooperation, anatomical features pertinent to airway management (eg, a parturient), size of the patient (children or morbidly obese patients), medical comorbidities and past medical/surgical history, full stomach considerations, presence of bodily fluids such as blood or vomitus in the airway, lung compliance, and the anticipated need for aggressive positive-pressure ventilation. In general, the patient factors are "what the patient brings to the table." They refer to things the practitioner *may* be able to modify. Patient factors must be considered for each individual for an airway management plan to be crafted that is best suited to that individual. There is no *one size fits all* in airway management!

3. **Situational factors.** This category refers to factors that are unique to the particular situation in which the airway must be managed. Situational factors include, but are not limited to: location of the encounter (pre-hospital vs emergency department vs intensive care unit vs operating room, etc), urgency (elective vs emergency situations), availability of skilled assistants, the airway management tools and equipment available, presence of confounding/complicating factors such as C-spine immobilization collars, and availability of expert backup in the event of difficulty. The situational factors present in the environment where one practices may be modifiable to some extent. For example, a practitioner can petition the hospital to purchase an airway management tool not currently available or advocate for higher standards of airway management training for pre-hospital care personnel.

6.5   SUMMARY

The aim of this chapter is to introduce the concept of *context-sensitive* airway management, and to serve as an introduction to a few of the general classes of airway management tools and techniques available. The most fundamental dilemma facing the practitioner wishing to improve their difficult or failed airway management skills is making logical, evidence-based, and clinically appropriate management decisions. The case at the beginning of this chapter is based on an encounter at the author's institution. It was used as an example of the principles involved in context-sensitive airway management.

This case presented an airway managed initially in a conventional way (direct laryngoscopy together with an Eschmann Introducer) that subsequently became unmanageable due to dynamic situational factors. In the case described, an emergency cricothyrotomy in the trauma bay was successful. The patient made an unremarkable recovery from this life-threatening episode.

Gaining familiarity and experience with a variety of airway management techniques and devices will best equip the practitioner for these inevitable and challenging situations. At the very least, a competent practitioner should be facile with the techniques of bag-mask-ventilation, direct laryngoscopy and tracheal intubation, placement of an extraglottic device, and performance of an emergency cricothyrotomy. In addition, all practitioners should have predetermined plans "A," "B," and "C" when approaching any airway situation. The rare but extremely important *can't intubate, can't ventilate* situation must be routinely considered. Under these circumstances, placement of a rescue device (eg, LMA, Intubating LMA, Combitube™, or King LT™) should be performed while concurrently preparing for a surgical airway.

REFERENCES

1. Augustine JA, Seidel DR, McCabe JB. Ventilation performance using a self-inflating anesthesia bag: effect of operator characteristics. *Am J Emerg Med.* 1987;5:267-270.

2. Lawrence PJ, Sivaneswaran N. Ventilation during cardiopulmonary resuscitation: which method? *Med J Aust.* 1985;143:443-446.

3. Lee HM, Cho KH, Choi YH, Yoon SY. Can you deliver accurate tidal volume by manual resuscitator? *Emerg Med J.* 2008;25:632-634.

4. Noordergraaf GJ, van Dun PJ, Kramer BP, et al. Airway management by first responders when using a bag-valve device and two oxygen-driven resuscitators in 104 patients. *Eur J Anaesthesiol.* 2004;21:361-366.

5. Petrar S, Murphy M, Hung O. Is a seismic shift in EMS airway management coming? A closer look at oxygenation, ventilation, intubation & alternative airways. *JEMS.* 2009;34:54-59.

6. Bogetz MS. Using the laryngeal mask airway to manage the difficult airway. *Anesthesiol Clin North America.* 2002;20:863-870, vii.

7. Cook TM. The classic laryngeal mask airway: a tried and tested airway. What now? *Br J Anaesth.* 2006;96:149-152.

8. Gerstein NS, Braude DA, Hung O, Sanders JC, Murphy MF. The Fastrach Intubating Laryngeal Mask Airway: an overview and update. *Can J Anaesth.* 2010;57:588-601.

9. Hung OR, Stewart RD. Lightwand intubation: I—a new lightwand device. *Can J Anaesth.* 1995;42:820-825.

10. Hung OR, Pytka S, Morris I, Murphy M, Launcelott G, Stevens S. Clinical trial of a new lightwand device (Trachlight™) to intubate the trachea. *Anesthesiology.* 1995;83:509-514.

11. Heidegger T, Gerig HJ, Ulrich B, Schnider TW. Structure and process quality illustrated by fibreoptic intubation: analysis of 1612 cases. *Anaesthesia.* 2003;58:734-739.

12. Mort TC. Tracheal tube exchange: feasibility of continuous glottic viewing with advanced laryngoscopy assistance. *Anesth Analg.* 2009;108:1228-1231.

SELF-EVALUATION QUESTIONS

6.1. A stridorous, mentally challenged patient was brought to the operating room for an urgent neck exploration because of a neck hematoma following a neck dissection 2 days prior. In the presence of hypoxemia with SaO_2 less than 80%, which of the following is a reasonable airway management option?

   A. bag-mask-ventilation

   B. the use of an extraglottic device

   C. tracheal intubation using a Macintosh laryngoscope

   D. surgical airway

   E. all of the above

6.2. For the same patient, and in the absence of hypoxemia (with SaO_2 >95%), which of the following is a reasonable intubating technique?

   A. direct laryngoscopy using a Macintosh blade

   B. tracheal intubation using the intubating LMA (Fastrach™)

   C. retrograde intubation

   D. intubation using a lightwand (Trachlight™)

   E. digital intubation

6.3. For the same patient, in the presence of severe hypoxemia with SaO_2 less than 70%, while setting up for a cricothyrotomy, which of the following is a reasonable intubating technique?

   A. direct laryngoscopy using a Macintosh blade

   B. tracheal intubation using the intubating LMA (Fastrach™)

   C. intubation using a lightwand (Trachlight™)

   D. intubation using a Glidescope®

   E. all of the above

CHAPTER 7

Manual Noninvasive Ventilation: Bag-Mask-Ventilation

George Kovacs and Michael F. Murphy

7.1 INTRODUCTION

Providing effective ventilation and oxygenation using a bag-mask is probably the single most important aspect of airway management. Bag-mask-ventilation (BMV) refers to the use of a bag-valve-mask (BVM) system/device to deliver gas rich in oxygen either passively or actively by manually ventilating the patient using a face-mask interface. Manual noninvasive ventilation also accurately describes the use of a BMV device to provide positive pressure ventilation (PPV). This should be differentiated from mechanical noninvasive ventilation which also uses a face-mask interface but provides respiratory effort assistance (PPV) delivered by specialized ventilator.

7.1.1 Is there still a role for bag-mask-ventilation in this advanced world of difficult airway devices?

Definitive airway management has traditionally been defined as the placement of an endotracheal tube in the trachea. Although few would argue that there has been a philosophical and evidence-based shift away from defining airway management by the method of gas exchange to focus on the goals of resuscitation namely, maintaining patient oxygenation and ventilation while preserving hemodynamic status. In other words, endotracheal tubes do not save lives; providing adequate perfusion and gas exchange does. Oxygenation and ventilation may be provided using endotracheal tubes, extraglottic devices, BMV devices, and surgical methods. Which method is most appropriately employed will depend on patient characteristics, the clinical situation, and practitioner's skill.

Bag-mask-ventilation particularly in the prehospital setting has been shown to be no less effective than endotracheal intubation (ETI) or extraglottic device (EGD) use.[1-3] With mounting evidence that prehospital ETI is of questionable benefit and in certain scenarios potentially harmful, alternative methods of maintaining oxygenation and ventilation, including BMV are being reaffirmed as an essential airway management skill.[4-10]

Bag-mask-ventilation has been compared to other ventilatory strategies in the prehospital, operating room, and simulation settings.[11-22] Extraglottic devices, such as the laryngeal mask airway (LMA) and Combitube™, have become accepted *intermediate* alternatives to BMV and *go to* options in failed intubation and failed BMV (or "can't intubate, can't ventilate") scenarios.

There is a theoretical advantage in using EGDs in patients suffering a of cardiac arrest where chest compressions can continue uninterrupted. In general, however, ventilation has been deemphasized in the early phase of adult nonasphyxia-related resuscitation, where oxygen delivery is more dependent on blood flow than on arterial oxygen content.

This is in keeping with the recent American Heart Association recommendation in which ventilation is de-emphasized in the early phase of adult non-asphyxia related resuscitation because oxygen delivery has been shown to be more dependent on blood flow than arterial oxygen content. Ultimately, however, the American Heart Association guidelines recommend BMV as an equivalent option compared to other advanced life support (ALS) options (ETI, LMA, or Combitube) stating that "there is no evidence that advanced airway measures improve survival rates in the setting of prehospital cardiac arrest."[11]

Bag-mask-ventilation is a challenging skill to learn and perform effectively.[23-25] Despite the advent of numerous alternative devices, just as direct laryngoscopy remains the current gold standard for endotracheal tube placement, BMV still remains the primary method of providing initial basic life support (BLS) oxygenation and ventilation in most resuscitation settings.[24,26] Although this may change, there currently is no compelling evidence of superiority of extraglottic devices over BMV.[11-22] Compared to BMV in the hands of inexperienced health-care providers, LMA insertion has been reported to be rapidly placed, *easy to use*, and effective as ventilation device.[1,27,28] Other reports of LMA field use have, however, demonstrated low success rates (64%) despite self-reported ease of use.[22] In the controlled setting of the operating room when compared to both LMA and Combitube use, it is reported that BMV performed favorably having no oxygenation failures and producing the smallest decline in oxygen saturation during placement.[1] Success and complications of any airway device are more often related to training and experience than the device itself.[1]

Despite its effectiveness in skilled hands, BMV is facing growing competition from EGDs that even in unskilled hands, are relatively easy to teach, learn, and ultimately deliver as a primary method for oxygenation and ventilation. While BMV remains a vital skill to master, it may be relegated to a subsidiary position to EGDs in the foreseeable future.

7.1.2   What are the key components of a bag-mask system?

Also referred to as manual resuscitators, these devices employ a bag and an integrated one-way valve to be connected to an endotracheal tube, an EGD, or a mask to manually provide positive-pressure ventilation. Despite there being various types of BMV systems, they share common features (Figure 7-1)[29]:

- A standard 22 mm connector which fits standard face masks, endotracheal tubes, EGDs, and surgical airway devices.
- A nonrebreathing valve.
- A self-inflating bag that is supplied in adult (1600 mL), child (500 mL), and infant (240 mL) sizes that when manually compressed deliver a tidal volume.
- An oxygen inlet valve that is used to provide unidirectional flow from the oxygen reservoir to the self-inflating bag.
- An oxygen reservoir bag that is inflated by receiving high oxygen flow through an adjacent connector.
- Other features of BMV systems may include a positive pressure relief or *pop-off* valve located on the patient end of the system with the intent of limiting peak inspiratory pressures to avoid barotrauma when the manual resuscitator is connected to an ETT.
- A flow-limiting valve that is located at the patient end of the self-inflating bag designed to limit inspiratory flow, decreasing the risk of both hyperventilation and excessive airway pressures (Smart Bag®).

The face masks used in conjunction with the manual resuscitator vary in material, size, seal type, and transparency. Traditionally, black/opaque rubber masks with an anatomically contoured seal were used in the operating room setting connected to an anesthetic circuit. These have been replaced to a large extent in most environments by transparent silicone, or plastic, latex-free, nondisposable, and single-use masks that provide the added benefit of being able to visualize the mouth/nose-mask interface and, therefore, react to the presence of vomitus and other secretions. Rather than anatomically conforming to the patient's face, the seals in these masks are either made of foam or an air-filled *cushion* that molds to the underlying facial anatomy.

7.2   BASIC PRINCIPLES

7.2.1   How do you accurately anticipate difficult mask-ventilation?

Perhaps the simple answer is you can never ensure 100% accuracy when you are trying to predict anything. The safest approach is *always anticipate the unexpected*. In the anticipated difficult airway, proceeding depends on context. In an elective operating room setting, predicted difficulty will often mean a very different course (including canceling the case) than in an emergency situation in which a choice of not proceeding is usually not an option. In trying to anticipate difficulty, the core two questions that all practitioners should ask themselves prior to proceeding are:

- Will I be able to maintain oxygenation and ventilation by BMV if intubation attempts fail?
- If not, will I be able to oxygenate and ventilate rapidly using a rescue device or technique, such as an extraglottic device or surgical airway?

Early literature on predicting the difficult airway focused on laryngoscopy and intubation.[30-32] Recognizing that maintenance of oxygenation and ventilation is the priority in airway management and that this is often best achieved rapidly and early by BMV, the identification of predictors of difficult mask-ventilation has been a focus of more recent research.[33-36] Most airway management

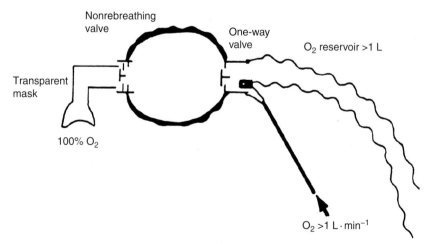

FIGURE 7-1. Bag-valve-mask schematic. (With permission from Mohamud D, Mariani R, Fernandes C. Basic life support. Dailey R, et al, eds. In: *The Airway: Emergency Management.* St. Louis: Mosby; 1992:47.)

decision algorithms require a *formal* patient assessment focused on identifying predictors of difficulty. This assessment is critically important in deciding whether neuromuscular blockade can be safely used to facilitate intubation. While it is important to assess all aspects of the difficult airway, BMV is perhaps most important as this intervention is the primary *go to* technique when tracheal intubation attempts fail. Despite numerous alternative rescue options available to the practitioner, BMV is universally available, familiar to most and almost always effective.

Earlier data estimated that *cannot intubate/cannot ventilate* clinical situations occurred at a rate between 0.01 and 2 in 10,000 general anesthetic cases.[30] More recent data have reported the incidence of difficult mask-ventilation (DMV) in the operating room setting as varying from a low of 0.9% to a high of 7.8%.[18,33-36] This variation likely relates to differences in definition, outcome criteria, and sample size. In the largest study of over 50,000 patients, DMV occurred in 2.2% of cases while "impossible" BMV defined as an inability to establish BMV using two-hand technique and multiple airway adjuvants, occurred in 0.15% of the study population.[34]

Langeron et al prospectively evaluated 1502 patients requiring routine general anesthesia to determine both the incidence and factors associated with DMV.[35] The reported incidence of DMV in this population was 5%. Five independent factors associated with DMV were identified: presence of a beard; age older than 55; body mass index greater than 26 kg·m⁻²; lack of teeth; and a history of snoring. The presence of two of these factors in a patient was 72% sensitive and 73% specific for DMV.[35]

Other studies involving large patient populations have validated the above findings and identified additional risk factors, including male gender, a history of neck radiation, high Mallampati grade (Grade III or IV), and limited jaw protrusion (Table 7-1).[33-36] In the study by Kheterpal et al[34] involving over 50,000 adult patients receiving a general anesthetic at a tertiary care hospital, there was a diverse group of practitioners (trainees, nurse, and physician anesthetists) however, being a *junior anesthesia practitioner* was not found to be an independent predictor for impossible mask-ventilation (IMV). The presence of three or more predictors (neck radiation, male, OSA, Mallampati Grade III or IV, beard) significantly increased the risk of IMV with an odds ratio of 8.9 compared to patients without these risk factors. In addition, this study also found that 25% of these IMV patients had difficult tracheal intubations.

These recent reports differentiating DMV from IMV.[18] A numeric representation this DMV continuum has been proposed; however, it has not been consistently used or accepted to date in the literature.[37] The difference between DMV and IMV is simply that difficult mask-ventilation is usually correctable (ie, two-hand and two-person technique) whereas impossible-mask ventilation represents a failure and the need to abandon BMV in favor of another intervention (DL if not attempted, EGD or a surgical airway).

It is important to appreciate the fact that these studies did not examine the incidence of DMV in patients requiring emergency airway management. Levitan et al examined the ability to assess for predictors of the difficult airway in emergency department

TABLE 7–1

Studies Reporting Independent Predictors of Difficult BMV

INVESTIGATORS	DESIGN	POPULATION	DMV INCIDENCE	RISK FACTORS	COMMENTS
Langeron et al, 2000	Prospective observational	1502, adult, routine GA[a] patients	5%	Age >55, BMI >26 kg·m⁻², beard, edentulous, snoring	First study evaluating independent risk factors
Yildiz et al, 2004	Prospective observational	576, adult, routine GA	7.8%, 15.5% of difficult intubations	Male, Mallampati IV, increasing age, snoring, increasing weight	Small sample size
Kheterpal et al, 2006	Prospective observational	22,660, adult, GA	1.4%	BMI >30 kg·m⁻², beard, Mallampati III IV, age >57, ↓ JP[c], snoring	Diverse clinician group
Kheterpal et al, 2009	Prospective observational	53,041, adult, GA	2.2%, 0.15% IMV[b]	IMV: neck radiation, male, OSA[d], Mallampati III IV, beard	Odds ratio 8.9 vs no risk factors

[a]*General anesthesia.*

[b]*Impossible BMV.*

[c]*Jaw protrusion.*

[d]*Obstructive sleep apnea.*

patients requiring intubation and found that only 32% of this population would have been able to be assessed adequately for difficulty because of limitations, such as an inability to follow commands or being immobilized for cervical spine (C-spine) precautions.[38]

The incidence of DMV is not known in this population. However, emergency department cricothyrotomy (as a marker for cannot intubate, cannot ventilate) rates between 0.5% and 1.0% have been reported, which are much higher than that reported in the controlled operating room setting.[39-41] Table 7-2 summarizes the likely pathophysiology behind the various predictors of DMV.

7.2.2   What anatomic factors need to be considered in providing safe and effective BMV?

In the unconscious or anesthetized patient with normal anatomy, it has been traditionally thought that obstruction to the easy to-and-fro movement of gas with BMV was primarily related to the effect of a *relaxed* tongue falling back against the posterior pharyngeal wall. Data gathered during fluoroscopy in studies of obstructive sleep apnea (OSA) patients has improved our understanding of the pathophysiology of upper airway dynamics in the sleeping patient. In addition to obstruction caused by the tongue, there is also a loss of velopharyngeal and hypopharyngeal muscle tone.[42,43] This results in soft tissue collapse leading to the posterior displacement of both the soft palate and epiglottis to oppose the posterior pharyngeal wall and contribute to obstruction (velopharyngeal and hypopharyngeal collapse).[42] The hypopharyngeal site of obstruction is clinically supported by the observation that placement of an OPA without performing an adequate jaw thrust may not alleviate obstruction caused by normal upper airway soft tissues.

When a patient is placed in the sniffing position, there is flexion in the cervicothoracic region with extension in occiptocervical region. This position has been traditionally thought to facilitate alignment of the axes necessary to visualize the glottic inlet during direct laryngoscopy. Although there has been some question as to whether this position provides any advantage over simple head extension, more recent data support the combination of neck flexion with head elevation in enabling glottic exposure during laryngoscopy.[44,45] It is less well understood, however, if this position improves upper airway patency for bag-mask-ventilation. There is some evidence that the retropalatal and retroglossal region is enlarged by placing anesthetized nonobese patients with OSA in the sniffing position.[46] In addition, it is well known that obese patients desaturate early, a clinical phenomena which can be delayed by denitrogenating in the sitting (as opposed to supine) position.[47] At this point, it is reasonable to state that head and neck repositioning from neutral to a position that involves a degree of neck flexion with head elevation may improve BMV and is appropriate in anticipation to perform direct laryngoscopy should it become necessary.

While head and neck positioning is considered vitally important for direct laryngoscopy, the key anatomic manipulation that facilitates BMV is performing a jaw thrust. This maneuver originally described over a century ago (Esmarch-Heiberg maneuver) has been demonstrated to be superior to *chin lift* and *head tilt* when performed alone, during observations made of anesthetized patients undergoing (preprocedure) head and neck fluoroscopy.[48,49] Recognizing that obstruction in the unconscious patient is related to more than the tongue falling posteriorly, the "triple airway" maneuver (open mouth, head tilt, jaw thrust) was

⬤ TABLE 7–2

DMV Pathophysiology and Response

DMV PREDICTOR	PATHOPHYSIOLOGY	RESPONSE
Obesity	Rapid desaturation, ↓ compliance, ↑ upper airway soft tissues	Positioning: sitting denitrogenation, ramp
Snoring (airway sounds)	Snoring: ↑ upper airway collapse; sounds: stridor, wheezing ↑ resistance	OPA, two-hand BMV, ↑ expiratory time
Age	↓ tissue elasticity, ↓ jaw and neck mobility, ↑ edentulous rate	Leave dentures in place[79]
Beard	Mask seal	Apply ointment
Edentulous	Mask size, fit	Leave dentures in, OPA
Neck radiation	Noncompliant, distorted tissues	OPA, two-hand BMV, early EGD
Mallampati III or IV	Excess soft tissues, upper airway collapse	OPA, two-hand BMV
Male	? associated comorbidities	
Diminished jaw protrusion	↓ ability to manage tongue, upper airway collapse	OPA, two-hand BMV, early EGD
Difficult intubation	As per above, secondary injury from difficult laryngoscopy	

suggested to be the best approach.[50,51] More recent evidence supports the jaw thrust alone as being equally effective to the triple airway maneuver in relieving obstruction.[49]

7.2.3   What is the role of BMV in difficult airway algorithms?

Numerous algorithms have been published to guide practitioners in the management of the difficult airway.[52-60] Most of these guidelines or recommendations are generated using available evidence and expert opinion by specialized working groups and/or anesthesiology societies. All algorithms have limitations, some are too complicated; and others impractical for application in emergency situations outside of the operating room, where awakening the patient or cancelling the case is not an option.

There are only a few difficult airway algorithms to guide the nonanesthesia practitioner responsible for airway management. ATLS guidelines have moved away from its early edition "can't intubate, cut the neck" approach to more recent versions defining the role of BMV and the use of extraglottic devices is more clearly defined.[61] Emergency medicine has also published airway algorithms which are presented in airway education programs such as *The Difficult Airway Courses* in the United States and *AIME (Airway Interventions and Management in Emergencies)* in Canada.[60,61]

A difficult airway may be any or all of the following difficult BMV, difficult laryngoscopy, difficult intubation, difficult extraglottic device use, or difficult surgical airway placement. Most algorithms or approaches separate the *anticipated* from the *unanticipated* (or encountered) difficult airway. In the former scenario, predicted difficulty leads a defined, usually more controlled path, whereas in the latter, whether predicted or not, real time difficulty *is* being experienced and demands an immediate and specific course of action, depending on the type of difficulty encountered.

When approaching the difficult airway, the ability to successfully perform BMV is a critical management junction in all algorithms. The most prominent place for BMV as part of any difficult airway algorithm is between failed intubation attempts. However, it is important to appreciate the role of BMV even before a first attempt at laryngoscopy and intubation. Assuming the patient can generate sufficient tidal volumes with an adequate respiratory rate, the bag portion of the BMV device does not have to be squeezed to deliver close to 100% oxygen. It is not uncommon (and in some situations is potentially hazardous) that when switching from a nonrebreathing mask (or another mask type) to BMV, positive pressure is often instinctively applied. If assisted BMV is applied without synchrony, gastric inflation is much more likely to occur.

In the preintubation phase of airway management, the use of a BMV device to denitrogenate should be encouraged. This approach offers several advantages:

1. Passive delivery of high-concentration (approaching 100%) oxygen

2. Opportunity to size the mask properly

3. Provides hands-on feel for predicting DMV

4. Provides opportunity to improve gas exchange with assisted BMV

Various methods of denitrogenation have been suggested in an attempt to minimize desaturation during laryngoscopy and intubation. This is relatively easy to accomplish in healthy adults with normal pulmonary mechanics and oxygen consumption rates. Mort examined the effects of PPV denitrogenation on critically ill patients using a manual resuscitator for both 4 and 8 minutes prior to performing an RSI and found only marginal benefit.[62,63] Traditionally, during RSI, it has been advised that BMV be halted after induction and neuromuscular blockade to avoid gastric insufflation. This teaching, however, was based more on theory than science. In fact, Sellick's original paper stated that manual PPV in combination with cricoid pressure could be done without gastric distention risk.[64] Data have since supported active denitrogenation using a manual resuscitator with or without the application of cricoid pressure as long as *good* technique is used (avoiding high airway pressures).[65] BMV is in fact clinically indicated during RSI in certain patients (obese, hypoxemic, or pediatric) who may have low baseline oxygen saturation, high oxygen consumption rates, and/or low functional residual capacity.[66] Finally, the knowledge of adequate BMV soon after the drugs are given is reassuring, particularly in situations where difficult intubation may be encountered.

7.3   TECHNIQUE

7.3.1   What defines optimal BMV technique and how do you assess the adequacy of ventilation?

There are three important components to proper BMV technique: mask seal, airway opening, and ventilation.

Mask Seal: An appropriately sized face mask is attached to the bag-mask device and applied to the patient's face. The lower border of the mask's cuff is first applied to the groove between the lower lip and the chin and then the mask can be placed down across the nasal bridge. The thumb and index finger of the airway practitioner's hand applies sufficient pressure on the face mask to achieve a good seal (Figure 7-2). Note, however, that sealing pressure must be achieved *without* excessive downward pressure on the patient's mandible, as this may worsen functional obstruction—rather, the mandible is *lifted* to meet the mask. Small adjustments to the position of the mask on the patient's face (eg, with small movements to left or right) are made as needed to achieve a seal.

Airway Opening: The ring and long fingers of the nondominant hand grasp the bony ridge of the patient's mandible, and, if practical, the fifth finger hooks under the angle of the mandible to provide a jaw thrust (Figure 7-2). In the event the airway practitioner has a small hand, the long finger is hooked under the mentum to provide a jaw pull. These three digits provide counter-pressure to the digits applying the mask to the face, but also apply an *upward lift* to the mandible to help perform an airway opening jaw thrust. Note that these three fingers should *not* be placed directly under the patient's chin unless lifting it forward, as midline pressure

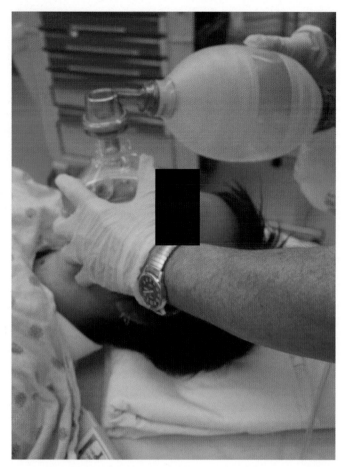

FIGURE 7-2. Proper bag-mask-ventilation technique: A good mask seal involves applying sufficient pressure on the face mask by the thumb and index finger of the practitioner's hand. The ring and long fingers of the nondominant hand grasp the bony ridge of the patient's mandible, and, if practical, the fifth finger hooks under the angle of the mandible to provide a jaw thrust.

under the chin can contribute to airway obstruction. This latter directive is particularly important in small children and infants. Concomitantly, the entire hand also attempts to keep the head extended (if no C-spine precautions).

Ventilation: The practitioner's dominant hand is free to gently squeeze the bag. Volumes should be delivered with attention to the inflating pressure as well as the patient's status: If apneic, the patient should be carefully ventilated (attached to high-flow oxygen) at a rate of 10 to 12 breaths per minute, at a tidal volume of 6 mL·kg^{-1}, or 500 to 600 mL in the average adult.[11] Smaller tidal volumes (eg, 300-400 mL in the adult) at increased rates (15-18 breaths per minute) may lead to less gastric insufflation. Although adult (1.6 L) manual resuscitators may deliver varied volumes, excessive and rapid compression of the bag must be avoided. The goal, as stated previously, is to produce *visible* chest rise.[11] In the patient still demonstrating respiratory effort, *assisted* bag-mask-ventilation should be performed, synchronizing the positive pressure breath to the patient's inspiratory effort. If the patient is tachypneic, it will be appropriate to simply deliver an assisted ventilation with every third or fourth breath.

7.3.2   What do you do if BMV is difficult?

With optimal technique, significant difficulty with BMV is rarely encountered in the absence of airway pathology.[33-36] In the acute setting, BMV is often delegated to non-physician health-care practitioner while the physician prepares for definitive airway management. While this may be appropriate, it is important to accept that BMV is a difficult skill for those who perform it infrequently, and vigilance rather than inattention is recommended. Abandoning BMV in the uncommon scenario of failing BMV should only occur after the most experienced *set of hands* have failed.

Difficult BMV (DMV) is often defined as the inability to maintain an acceptable oxygen saturation despite using good technique. Failure to maintain acceptable oxygen saturations or falling saturations demands a change in approach. Although one response to a DMV situation is to proceed to intubation, DMV may itself predict difficulty with laryngoscopy and/or intubation.[67]

In the setting of a failed airway in which one is not able to maintain acceptable saturations, immediate preparation for a cricothyrotomy is mandatory while one simultaneously attempts better BMV. Response to DMV requires a staged response that may include the following:

A. Reposition the head by performing an exaggerated head tilt/chin lift (if not contraindicated).

B. Open the mouth to permit anterior translation of the mandible and tongue in concert with an aggressive jaw thrust.

C. Insert an appropriate size oropharyngeal airway (Figure 7-3) and as many as two nasopharyngeal airways.

D. Perform two-person mask-ventilation technique.

E. If cricoid pressure is being applied, ease up on, or release it.

F. Consider a mask change (size or type) if seal is an issue.

G. Rule out foreign body in the airway.

H. Consider a rescue ventilation device, for example, an EGD, such as a laryngeal mask airway (LMA) or Combitube™.

I. Consider an early attempt at intubation.

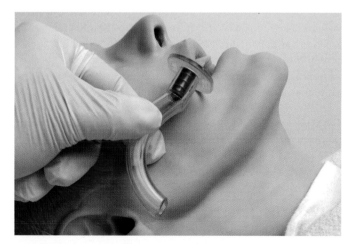

FIGURE 7-3. Insertion of an appropriate size oropharyngeal airway is necessary to alleviate airway obstruction.

Steps A, B, and C, as listed above, should occur almost simultaneously and very early in the DMV situation. DMV is often due simply to the failure to adequately open a functionally obstructed airway. Attempted ventilation against this obstruction results in a leak at the mask-face interface, often resulting in the practitioner's attempting to remedy the problem by pushing down harder on the mask to attain a seal.

This can worsen an already obstructed airway. Rather, what must occur is a more pronounced jaw *lift or thrust*, with resultant airway opening occurring as anterior movement of the mandible elevates the tongue, epiglottis, and soft palate away from the posterior pharyngeal wall. This is best performed with the aid of a second person. Two-person mask-ventilation is easy to perform and is often much more effective than one-person BMV. As shown in Figure 7-4, the two-person technique can be performed in a number of ways.[68]

Oropharyngeal airways (OPAs) help alleviate functional airway obstruction caused by relaxation of the tongue against the soft palate and to a lesser extent the posterior pharyngeal wall. They are most often used as an adjunct to bag-mask-ventilation of an obtunded or unconscious patient. Made of plastic, the component parts are a curved hollow lumen (in the Guedel version) (Figure 7-5) or side gutters (the Berman version), both with a proximal flange which

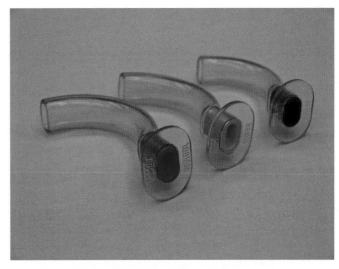

FIGURE 7-5. Different sizes of Guedel oropharyngeal airways.

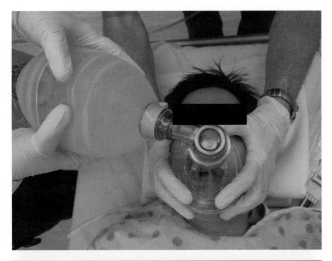

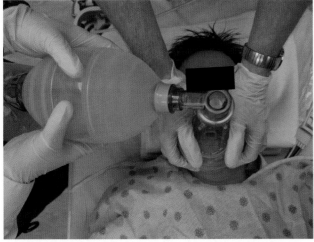

FIGURE 7-4. Two-hand, and two-person bag-mask-ventilation.

abuts the patient's lips, and a proximal bite block which may also be used as a color-coded size indicator.

OPAs are sized by length in centimeters, and are available in sizes for all ages. Choosing the appropriate size is important. If the OPA is too long, it may precipitate laryngospasm; if too small it may be ineffective. Although never formally validated, many airway practitioners approximate correct OPA length by placing it alongside the patient's cheek[69]: From the corner of the mouth, the tip of the OPA should reach the angle of the mandible or the tragus of the ear (Figure 7-3). A typical adult female will take an 8-cm OPA, and an adult male, 9 or 10 cm.

The OPA should be inserted inverted, (ie, with its concave surface directed cephalad) and advanced until the distal tip will proceed no further in the inverted position. At that point, the OPA is rotated 180 degrees, so that the concavity faces caudad. Advancement continues around the curve of the tongue until fully inserted. This technique prevents the tip of the OPA from impinging the tongue pushing it backwards and making the obstruction worse. Alternatively, it can be inserted noninverted with a tongue depressor to manage the tongue: This is the preferred technique in infants and younger children, to help avoid trauma to delicate tissues.

OPAs are not well tolerated in the awake or semiconscious patient with intact airway reflexes, where insertion may stimulate gagging, laryngospasm, or vomiting and aspiration. In addition, care must be taken to rule out a foreign body in the oropharynx prior to OPA insertion.

A nasopharyngeal airway (NPA) may be a useful option where trismus precludes OPA insertion, and may be better tolerated than an OPA in the awake or semiconscious patient with intact airway reflexes. While effective at alleviating functional airway obstruction, disadvantages of the NPA include transient patient discomfort during insertion and the potential for causing epistaxis. While the application of a vasoconstrictor (eg, oxymetazoline or phenylephrine) is frequently performed, there is no evidence that it reduces the incidence of epistaxis, nor may it be practical in an urgent situation. NPAs, also known as *nasal trumpets*, are made from soft material, for example, latex or silicon, have a hollow

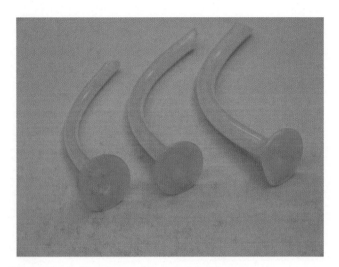

FIGURE 7-6. Different sizes of nasopharyngeal airways.

lumen and a bevelled leading edge, and a proximal flange to abut the patient's nostril (Figure 7-6).

Adult NPAs are generally sized by their internal diameter (ID) in millimeter. Typical adult sizes for small, medium, and large NPAs are 6, 7, and 8 mm ID respectively. One commonly used (but nonvalidated) sizing method is to use an NPA of a length corresponding to the distance from nose tip to the tragus of the ear. Sizing based on patient height makes more anatomic sense, resulting in a recommendation for a 6-mm ID NPA for an average adult female and 7 mm for an average male.

The NPA is lubricated and advanced into the patient's nostril, perpendicular to the face, resulting in passage along the floor of the major nasal airway. Authorities vary in their recommendation whether the bevel of the NPA should face toward or away from the nasal septum. A slight twisting motion can be used during insertion. If significant resistance is encountered, insertion should be attempted through the other nostril. Insertion continues until the flange of the NPA abuts the nasal ala.

NPA use is *relatively* contraindicated in known bleeding diathesis, including heparinized, warfarinized, or recently thrombolyzed patients, and in suspected cribriform plate fracture. In the head-injured patient, common sense dictates balancing the substantial risk of hypoxemia with the benefits of obtaining a patent nasopharyngeal airway, if an oral airway cannot be used.

Cricoid pressure can cause difficulty with both BMV and laryngoscopy as previously discussed. Excessive cricoid pressure (as may be applied during an RSI) may distort the airway and result in a partial or even complete obstruction. If significant difficulty with BMV is encountered during application of cricoid pressure, the assistant should momentarily ease (initially by 50%) or release the applied pressure.

It may become apparent once BMV is underway that the chosen mask size is incorrect. This is often the case where initial sizing occurred with the patient's dentures in place. Especially with encountered difficulty, the improved seal allowed by an appropriately sized mask makes the change worthwhile.

The decision to move to a rescue EGD, such as a laryngeal mask airway or laryngeal tube (King LT), will depend on the patient's clinical status and whether direct laryngoscopy (DL) has yet been attempted. If there has been no initial attempt at DL, it may be appropriate to proceed to an intubation attempt. If, on the other hand, DMV is encountered in the setting of an already failed attempt at intubation, placement of a rescue ventilation device, such as an LMA should be considered. Direct laryngoscopy is also the method of choice to rule out obstructing lesions, including foreign bodies and lingual tonsillar hypertrophy.

7.3.3   Is cricoid pressure appropriate to use with BMV?

Aspiration incidence rises with the number of attempts at intubation to a high of 22% in the emergency setting.[70] Mortality from aspiration has fallen but still remains relatively high at 4.6%.[18] Does the application of cricoid pressure prevent regurgitation and more importantly does it reduce morbidity and mortality?

Since Sellick's description in 1961, cricoid pressure has been recommended as a safe and necessary airway maneuver meant to reduce the risk of aspiration during airway management.[64] Supportive literature seemed to confirm its value during BMV in preventing gastric inflation, particularly in the pediatric population.[67,71-74] More recently, however, based on accumulating evidence, this standard use of Sellick's maneuver has been questioned.[71,72] In a review of the literature Ellis et al presented 10 studies reporting potential negative effects of cricoid pressure administered during BMV that include reduced tidal volumes, increased peak inspiratory pressure, and difficult ventilation.[71] It was concluded that there is little evidence to support the widespread use of cricoid pressure to prevent aspiration and that there is evidence of potential harm in certain situations.[71]

Anatomically, as studied by CT and MRI, the value of cricoid pressure has also been questioned based on observations that the cricoid cartilage moves laterally with compression and causes incomplete luminal esophageal opposition.[75] More recent literature has identified that the hypopharynx at the level of the glottis and not the esophagus is compressed by Sellick's maneuver because it moves in concert with the cricoid ring, making the position and degree of compression of the esophagus below it irrelevant.[26]

The question of whether cricoid pressure reduces morbidity and mortality by preventing aspiration has not, and likely will not be answered. Aspiration has been documented to occur in cases where cricoid pressure has been applied, however, it has been argued that this could have been from inadequate technique.[71,72] The clinical risk/benefit debate over the use of cricoid pressure will likely continue. At this point, it can be said that when performed correctly, by occluding the hypopharynx and in preventing gastric inflation during BMV, cricoid pressure may reduce the risk associated with aspiration during airway management. In addition, during BMV, care should be taken to employ good technique by opening the airway, paying attention to inspiratory time, inflation pressure, and delivering appropriate tidal volumes to avoid gastric inflation. If cricoid pressure is being applied, it should be done by an experienced assistant and if BMV becomes difficult, cricoid pressure should be released to assess whether it may be impeding ventilation.

7.4   COMPLICATIONS

7.4.1   How does one maximize gas exchange while minimizing the risk of gastric inflation and regurgitation BMV?

With an unprotected airway, the risks of gastric inflation and subsequent aspiration are a real risk during BMV. In autopsy patients of failed CPR attempts, the incidence of aspiration has been reported to be 29%.[74] Delivering an intended tidal volume and avoiding gastric inflation during BMV depends on various factors, such as lung compliance, airway resistance, and lower esophageal sphincter pressure (LESP).[76] In healthy adults, the LESP is 20 to 25 cm H_2O.[76] In the anesthetized patient, this pressure is likely lower and in cardiac arrest patients, it may be as low as 5 cm H_2O.[76] This information leads to the recommendation by the authors that airway practitioners performing BMV employ smaller tidal volumes at higher rates to minimize inflation pressures and the risk of gastric insufflation.

In order to minimize the risk of aspiration and its related potential morbidity, high airway pressure during BMV should be avoided. Underlying lung pathology and problems with pulmonary mechanics, such as obesity, will adversely affect lung compliance but are not always immediately modifiable. Airway resistance in the upper airway can be reduced during BMV by paying attention to technique, such as using an oral or nasal airway and applying a jaw thrust. Although most discussion around gastric inflation focuses around BMV use in the apneic patient, the breathing patient who is receiving assisted manual PPV using a BMV device is at particularly high risk. In this situation, if the airway practitioner is not paying close attention to timing, and delivery occurs during the patient's expiratory phase, higher airway pressures will more likely result in gastric inflation. This eventual gastric inflation cycle can result in increased intra-abdominal pressure causing reduced lung compliance, which in turn requires higher airway pressures and diverts more gas to the stomach.[76] In extreme circumstances this can lead to decreased cardiac output from increased intrathoracic pressure and a *can't ventilate* scenario.

Stress and an excited state may contribute to the overzealous ventilation with large tidal volume and rapid respiratory rates that have been documented in the acute prehospital setting.[27,77] This response often leads to further gastric inflation, breath stacking, and the cycle described above, resulting in worsening oxygenation and ventilation and a further decrease in cardiac output. The other consequence of increased minute ventilation is the development of respiratory alkalosis which is gaining recent attention as a contributor to poor patient outcomes in certain acute settings.[78]

Research related to the delivery of appropriate tidal volumes when using a BMV device has yielded different results depending on the clinical situation.[27] The American Heart Association recommendations for BMV is to deliver sufficient tidal volume to produce a *visible* chest rise.[11] This recommendation is based on evidence that in an unprotected airway, smaller tidal volumes (approximately 500 mL) result in less gastric inflation. Secondly, although in anesthetized patients with normal perfusion tidal volumes of 8 to 10 mL·kg^{-1} are used, during CPR perfusion is approximately 30% of normal with resultant delivery of oxygen and clearance of CO_2. Therefore, lower tidal volumes and respiratory rates are needed.

In patients with a sudden dysrhythmic cardiac arrest (ventricular fibrillation), hypoxemia and acidosis develop over several minutes.[27] In this very early phase of resuscitation, oxygen delivery is more dependent on tissue perfusion than arterial oxygen content.[11] These findings are in part behind the recommendations that prioritize early CPR in advance of ventilation in this subgroup of patients.[11] In the asphyxiated, respiratory arrest patient, maximal oxygen depletion has usually already developed (over time) in association with a lactic acidosis and CO_2 accumulation. In this situation, delay in oxygenation and ventilation should not occur during resuscitation efforts.

In a manikin study using a standard adult manual resuscitator, one-hand BMV provides tidal volumes between 450 mL and 600 mL. Squeezing the bag completely delivered volumes between 888 mL and 1192 mL.[79] When presented with the task of delivering 500-600 ml by 'half compression' of a 1.6 L bag with two hands subjects consistently delivered inadequate volumes.[80] Use of a pediatric self-inflating bag instead of the larger adult one, despite resulting in less gastric inflation provided inadequate tidal volumes.[16] Current recommendations are to deliver tidal volumes in the adult of 500 to 600 mL in both arrhythmia and asphyxia related cardiac arrest but emphasize that "the volume delivered should produce visible chest rise".[11]

7.5   SUMMARY

Bag-mask-ventilation remains an important potentially life-saving airway management skill. However, it can be a difficult skill to teach, learn, and perform adequately unless one does so on a regular basis. The advent of extraglottic devices that are easy to teach, learn and perform are likely to supplant BMV as a first-line airway management technique in certain settings in the future.

Difficult mask-ventilation will usually respond to corrective measures and impossible mask-ventilation is uncommon in experienced hands. Predicting difficult or impossible BMV is never fool-proof but is fundamental to the practice of advanced airway management, influencing subsequent decision making on how to proceed.

REFERENCES

1. Dorges V, Wenzel V, Knacke P, Gerlach K. Comparison of different airway management strategies to ventilate apneic, nonpreoxygenated patients. *Crit Care Med.* 2003;31:800-804.
2. Gausche M, Lewis RJ, Stratton SJ, et al. Effect of out-of-hospital pediatric endotracheal intubation on survival and neurological outcome: a controlled clinical trial. *JAMA.* 2000;283:783-790.
3. Stockinger ZT, McSwain NE, Jr. Prehospital endotracheal intubation for trauma does not improve survival over bag-valve-mask ventilation. *J Trauma.* 2004;56:531-536.
4. Denver Metro Airway Study Group. A prospective multicenter evaluation of prehospital airway management performance in a large metropolitan region. *Prehosp Emerg Care.* 2009;13:304-310.
5. Davis DP. Prehospital intubation of brain-injured patients. *Curr Opin Crit Care.* 2008;14:142-148.

6. Davis DP, Hwang JQ, Dunford JV. Rate of decline in oxygen saturation at various pulse oximetry values with prehospital rapid sequence intubation. *Prehosp Emerg Care.* 2008;12:46-51.

7. Lecky F, Bryden D, Little R, et al. Emergency intubation for acutely ill and injured patients. *Cochrane Database Syst Rev.* 2008:CD001429.

8. Stiell IG, Nesbitt LP, Pickett W, et al. The OPALS Major Trauma Study: impact of advanced life-support on survival and morbidity. *CMAJ.* 2008;178: 1141-1152.

9. Tam RK, Maloney J, Gaboury I, et al. Review of endotracheal intubations by Ottawa advanced care paramedics in Canada. *Prehosp Emerg Care.* 2009;13:311-315.

10. Warner KJ, Sharar SR, Copass MK, Bulger EM. Prehospital management of the difficult airway: a prospective cohort study. *J Emerg Med.* 2009;36:257-265.

11. ECC Committee, Subcommittees and Task Forces of the American Heart Association. 2005 American Heart Association Guidelines for Cardiopulmonary Resuscitation and Emergency Cardiovascular Care, Part 7.1: Adjuncts for Airway Control and Ventilation. *Circulation.* 2005;112 (Suppl IV):51-56.

12. Morimura N. Comparison of arterial blood gases of laryngeal mask airway and bag-valve-mask ventilation in out-of-hospital cardiac arrests. *Circ J.* 2009;73:490-496.

13. Alexander R, Hodgson P, Lomax D, Bullen C. A comparison of the laryngeal mask airway and Guedel airway, bag and facemask for manual ventilation following formal training. *Anaesthesia.* 1993;48:231-234.

14. Clayton TJ, Pittman JA, Gabbott DA. A comparison of two techniques for manual ventilation of the lungs by non-anaesthetists: the bag-valve-facemask and the cuffed oropharyngeal airway (COPA) apparatus. *Anaesthesia.* 2001;56:756-759.

15. Doerges V, Sauer C, Ocker H, Wenzel V, Schmucker P. Airway management during cardiopulmonary resuscitation—a comparative study of bag-valve-mask, laryngeal mask airway and combitube in a bench model. *Resuscitation.* 1999;41:63-69.

16. Dorges V, Ocker H, Wenzel V, Sauer C, Schmucker P. Emergency airway management by non-anaesthesia house officers—a comparison of three strategies. *Emerg Med J.* 2001;18:90-94.

17. Dorges V, Wenzel V, Schumann T, Neubert E, Ocker H, Gerlach K. Intubating laryngeal mask airway, laryngeal tube, 1100 mL self-inflating bag-alternatives for basic life support? *Resuscitation.* 2001;51:185-191.

18. El-Orbany M, Woehlck HJ. Difficult mask ventilation. *Anesth Analg.* 2009;109:1870-1880.

19. Grein AJ, Weiner GM. Laryngeal mask airway versus bag-mask ventilation or endotracheal intubation for neonatal resuscitation. *Cochrane Database Syst Rev.* 2005:CD003314.

20. Kurola J, Harve H, Kettunen T, et al. Airway management in cardiac arrest—comparison of the laryngeal tube, tracheal intubation and bag-valve mask ventilation in emergency medical training. *Resuscitation.* 2004;61:149-153.

21. Kurola JO, Turunen MJ, Laakso JP, Gorski JT, Paakkonen HJ, Silfvast TO. A comparison of the laryngeal tube and bag-valve mask ventilation by emergency medical technicians: a feasibility study in anesthetized patients. *Anesth Analg.* 2005;101:1477-1481.

22. Murray MJ, Vermeulen MJ, Morrison LJ, Waite T. Evaluation of prehospital insertion of the laryngeal mask airway by primary care paramedics with only classroom mannequin training. *CJEM.* 2002;4:338-343.

23. Cummins RO, Austin D, Graves JR, Litwin PE, Pierce J. Ventilation skills of emergency medical technicians: a teaching challenge for emergency medicine. *Ann Emerg Med.* 1986;15:1187-1192.

24. Elling R, Politis J. An evaluation of emergency medical technicians' ability to use manual ventilation devices. *Ann Emerg Med.* 1983;12:765-768.

25. Wynne G, Marteau TM, Johnston M, et al. Inability of trained nurses to perform basic life support. *Br Med J (Clin Res Ed).* 1987;294:1198-1199.

26. Rice MJ, Mancuso AA, Gibbs C, Morey TE, Gravenstein N, Deitte LA. Cricoid pressure results in compression of the postcricoid hypopharynx: the esophageal position is irrelevant. *Anesth Analg.* 2009;109:1546-1552.

27. Gabrielli A, Layon AJ, Wenzel V, Dorges V, Idris AH. Alternative ventilation strategies in cardiopulmonary resuscitation. *Curr Opin Crit Care.* 2002;8: 199-211.

28. Martin PD, Cyna AM, Hunter WA, et al. Training nursing staff in airway management for resuscitation. A clinical comparison of the facemask and laryngeal mask. *Anaesthesia.* 1993;48:33-37.

29. Mohamud D, Mariani R, Fernandes C. *Basic Life Support, The Airway: Emergency Management.* Dailey R, ed. St. Louis: Mosby; 1992:47.

30. Benumof JL. Management of the difficult adult airway. With special emphasis on awake tracheal intubation. *Anesthesiology.* 1991;75:1087-1110.

31. Cormack RS, Lehane J. Difficult tracheal intubation in obstetrics. *Anaesthesia.* 1984;39:1105-1111.

32. Mallampati SR, Gatt SP, Gugino LD, et al. A clinical sign to predict difficult tracheal intubation: a prospective study. *Can Anaesth Soc J.* 1985;32:429-434.

33. Kheterpal S, Han R, Tremper KK, et al. Incidence and predictors of difficult and impossible mask ventilation. *Anesthesiology.* 2006;105:885-891.

34. Kheterpal S, Martin L, Shanks AM, Tremper KK. Prediction and outcomes of impossible mask ventilation: a review of 50,000 anesthetics. *Anesthesiology.* 2009;110:891-897.

35. Langeron O, Masso E, Huraux C, et al. Prediction of difficult mask ventilation. *Anesthesiology.* 2000;92:1229-1236.

36. Yildiz TS, Solak M, Toker K. The incidence and risk factors of difficult mask ventilation. *J Anesth.* 2005;19:7-11.

37. Han R, Tremper KK, Kheterpal S, O'Reilly M. Grading scale for mask ventilation. *Anesthesiology.* 2004;101:267.

38. Levitan RM, Everett WW, Ochroch EA. Limitations of difficult airway prediction in patients intubated in the emergency department. *Ann Emerg Med.* 2004;44:307-313.

39. Sagarin MJ, Barton ED, Chng YM, Walls RM. Airway management by US and Canadian emergency medicine residents: a multicenter analysis of more than 6,000 endotracheal intubation attempts. *Ann Emerg Med.* 2005;46:328-336.

40. Sakles JC, Laurin EG, Rantapaa AA, Panacek EA. Airway management in the emergency department: a one-year study of 610 tracheal intubations. *Ann Emerg Med.* 1998;31:325-332.

41. Tayal VS, Riggs RW, Marx JA, Tomaszewski CA, Schneider RE. Rapid-sequence intubation at an emergency medicine residency: success rate and adverse events during a two-year period. *Acad Emerg Med.* 1999;6:31-37.

42. Hillman DR, Platt PR, Eastwood PR. The upper airway during anaesthesia. *Br J Anaesth.* 2003;91:31-39.

43. McGee J, Vender J. Nonintubation management of the airway. In: Hagberg C, ed. *Mask Ventilation, Benumof's Airway Management.* St. Louis: Mosby; 2007:345-370.

44. Adnet F, Baillard C, Borron SW, et al. Randomized study comparing the "sniffing position" with simple head extension for laryngoscopic view in elective surgery patients. *Anesthesiology.* 2001;95:836-841.

45. Levitan RM, Mechem CC, Ochroch EA, Shofer FS, Hollander JE. Head-elevated laryngoscopy position: improving laryngeal exposure during laryngoscopy by increasing head elevation. *Ann Emerg Med.* 2003;41:322-330.

46. Isono S, Tanaka A, Ishikawa T, Tagaito Y, Nishino T. Sniffing position improves pharyngeal airway patency in anesthetized patients with obstructive sleep apnea. *Anesthesiology.* 2005;103:489-494.

47. Altermatt FR, Munoz HR, Delfino AE, Cortinez LI. Pre-oxygenation in the obese patient: effects of position on tolerance to apnoea. *Br J Anaesth.* 2005;95: 706-709.

48. Kovacs G, Law J. Oxygen delivery and bag-mask ventilation in airway management. In: Kovacs G, Law J, eds. *Airway Management in Emergencies.* New York: McGraw-Hill Medical; 2007:33-52.

49. Uzun L, Ugur MB, Altunkaya H, Ozer Y, Ozkocak I, Demirel CB. Effectiveness of the jaw-thrust maneuver in opening the airway: a flexible fiberoptic endoscopic study. *ORL J Otorhinolaryngol Relat Spec.* 2005;67:39-44.

50. Boidin MP. Airway patency in the unconscious patient. *Br J Anaesth.* 1985;57: 306-310.

51. Morikawa S, Safar P, Decarlo J. Influence of the headjaw position upon upper airway patency. *Anesthesiology.* 1961;22:265-270.

52. Practice guidelines for management of the difficult airway: an updated report by the American Society of Anesthesiologists Task Force on Management of the Difficult Airway. *Anesthesiology.* 2003;98:1269-1277.

53. Crosby ET, Cooper RM, Douglas MJ, et al. The unanticipated difficult airway with recommendations for management. *Can J Anaesth.* 1998;45:757-776.

54. Heidegger T, Gerig HJ, Henderson JJ. Strategies and algorithms for management of the difficult airway. *Best Pract Res Clin Anaesthesiol.* 2005;19: 661-674.

55. Henderson JJ, Popat MT, Latto IP, Pearce AC. Difficult Airway Society guidelines for management of the unanticipated difficult intubation. *Anaesthesia.* 2004;59:675-694.

56. Law J, Kovacs G. Response to an encountered difficult airway. In: Kovacs G, Law J, eds. *Airway Management in Emergencies.* New York: McGraw-Hill Medical; 2007:199-210.

57. Lim MS, Hunt-Smith JJ. Difficult airway management in the intensive care unit: practical guidelines. *Crit Care Resusc.* 2003;5:43-52.

58. Petrini F, Accorsi A, Adrario E, et al. Recommendations for airway control and difficult airway management. *Minerva Anestesiol.* 2005;71:617-657.

59. Vaida SJ, Pott LM, Budde AO, Gaitini LA. Suggested algorithm for management of the unexpected difficult airway in obstetric anesthesia. *J Clin Anesth.* 2009;21:385-386.

60. Walls RM. The emergency airway algorithms. In: Walls RM, Murphy MF, eds. *Emergency Airway Management.* 3rd ed. Philadelphia, PA: Lippincott, Williams and Wilkins; 2008:8-22.

61. American College of Surgeons Committee on Trauma. *Advanced Trauma Life Support for Doctors.* 8th ed. 2002 Chicago: Americal College of Surgeons.

62. Mort TC. Preoxygenation in critically ill patients requiring emergency tracheal intubation. *Crit Care Med.* 2005;33:2672-2675.

63. Mort TC, Waberski BH, Clive J. Extending the preoxygenation period from 4 to 8 mins in critically ill patients undergoing emergency intubation. *Crit Care Med.* 2009;37:68-71.

64. Sellick BA. Cricoid pressure to control regurgitation of stomach contents during induction of anaesthesia. *Lancet.* 1961;2:404-406.

65. Lawes EG, Campbell I, Mercer D. Inflation pressure, gastric insufflation and rapid sequence induction. *Br J Anaesth.* 1987;59:315-318.

66. Brown JP, Werrett G. Bag-mask ventilation in rapid sequence induction. *Anaesthesia.* 2009;64:784-785.

67. Moynihan RJ, Brock-Utne JG, Archer JH, Feld LH, Kreitzman TR. The effect of cricoid pressure on preventing gastric insufflation in infants and children. *Anesthesiology.* 1993;78:652-656.

68. Davidovic L, LaCovey D, Pitetti RD. Comparison of 1- versus 2-person bag-valve-mask techniques for manikin ventilation of infants and children. *Ann Emerg Med.* 2005;46:37-42.

69. Levitan R, Ochroch EA. Airway management and direct laryngoscopy. A review and update. *Crit Care Clin.* 2000;16:373-388, v.

70. Mort TC. Emergency tracheal intubation: complications associated with repeated laryngoscopic attempts. *Anesth Analg.* 2004;99:607-613.

71. Ellis DY, Harris T, Zideman D. Cricoid pressure in emergency department rapid sequence tracheal intubations: a risk-benefit analysis. *Ann Emerg Med.* 2007;50:653-665.

72. Ovassapian A, Salem MR. Sellick's maneuver: to do or not do. *Anesth Analg.* 2009;109:1360-1362.

73. Salem MR, Wong AY, Mani M, Sellick BA. Efficacy of cricoid pressure in preventing gastric inflation during bag-mask ventilation in pediatric patients. *Anesthesiology.* 1974;40:96-98.

74. Lawes EG, Baskett PJ. Pulmonary aspiration during unsuccessful cardiopulmonary resuscitation. *Intensive Care Med.* 1987;13:379-382.

75. Smith KJ, Dobranowski J, Yip G, Dauphin A, Choi PT. Cricoid pressure displaces the esophagus: an observational study using magnetic resonance imaging. *Anesthesiology.* 2003;99:60-64.

76. Wenzel V, Idris AH, Dorges V, Nolan JP, Parr MJ, Gabrielli A. The respiratory system during resuscitation: a review of the history, risk of infection during assisted ventilation, respiratory mechanics, and ventilation strategies for patients with an unprotected airway. *Resuscitation.* 2001;49:123-134.

77. Davis DP, Heister R, Poste JC, Hoyt DB, Ochs M, Dunford JV. Ventilation patterns in patients with severe traumatic brain injury following paramedic rapid sequence intubation. *Neurocrit Care.* 2005;2:165-171.

78. Davis DP. Early ventilation in traumatic brain injury. *Resuscitation.* 2008;76:333-340.

79. Wolcke B, Schneider T, Mauer D, Dick W. Ventilation volumes with different self-inflating bags with reference to the ERC guidelines for airway management: comparison of two compression techniques. *Resuscitation.* 2000;47:175-178.

80. Lee HM, Cho KH, Choi YH, Yoon SY. Can you deliver accurate tidal volume by manual resuscitator? *Emerg Med J.* 2008;25:632-634.

SELF-EVALUATION QUESTIONS

7.1. Functional upper airway obstruction in the unconscious patient involves soft tissue collapse between:

A. the tongue and the posterior pharynx

B. the epiglottis and the posterior pharynx

C. the soft palate and the posterior pharynx

D. the tongue and the palate

E. all of the above

7.2. The most effective means of relieving a nonpathologic upper airway obstruction in the unconscious patient is:

A. placing the patient in sniffing position

B. placing a nasopharyngeal airway

C. simple extension of the neck

D. performing a jaw thrust

E. placing an extraglottic device

7.3. Difficult mask-ventilation is associated with:

A. increasing age

B. Mallampati II or III

C. difficult laryngoscopy

D. the presence of dentures

E. A and C

CHAPTER (8)

Direct Laryngoscopy

Richard M. Levitan and George Kovacs

8.1   HISTORY AND BACKGROUND

8.1.1   What is the history and evolution of direct laryngoscopy and tracheal intubation?

In the modern era, direct laryngoscopy is almost exclusively associated with tracheal intubation, even though the procedure was initially developed for diagnosing and treating laryngeal pathology. Following the development of mirror laryngoscopy in the 1800s (Czermark and others), Kirstein reported the first direct laryngoscopy in 1895.[1] Over the next 20 years the basic tenets of the procedure were refined by surgeons interested in laryngeal examination and surgical exposure.

A step-wise approach, the focus on epiglottoscopy, recognition of posterior laryngeal landmarks, optimal positioning for laryngeal exposure, and the benefits of external laryngeal manipulation and head elevation, etc are all detailed by Chevalier Jackson in his 1922 text, *Bronchoscopy and Esophagoscopy, A Manual for Peroral Endoscopy and Laryngeal Surgery.*[2]

With the evolution of modern anesthesia, the original straight laryngoscope designs by ENT surgeons gave way to instruments specifically designed for tracheal intubation, such as the straight Miller blade (1941)[3] and the curved Macintosh blade (1943).[4] It was also in this time period that the modern design of a detachable blade and battery handle became commonplace.

Between the 1930s and 1970s many different laryngoscope blades were designed to facilitate intubation (eg, Wisconsin, Phillips, Guedel, etc), but the Miller and Macintosh models (albeit with some modifications) remain universally used, and in most settings, are the only laryngoscope blades available.

The development of flexible fiberoptics, subsequent attachment of fiberoptics to rigid blades (Bullard laryngoscope, Wu Scope, etc), and more recently video laryngoscopes (Glidescope, McGrath, Video MAC, etc) have narrowed the clinical role of standard, line-of-sight, direct laryngoscopy, and now there is a wide array of indirect visual devices for both diagnostic imaging of the larynx and tracheal intubation. Direct laryngoscopy remains the predominant method of tracheal intubation. Alternative devices, however, are being increasingly deployed for both routine and anticipated difficult laryngoscopy.

8.2   EQUIPMENT

8.2.1   What are the principal design components of laryngoscopy blades and how do they work to facilitate endotracheal intubation?

Laryngoscope blade design, light, and battery systems affect procedural performance since they impact on illumination, laryngeal exposure, and endotracheal tube (ETT) delivery. This holds true for both straight and curved laryngoscope blade designs, but because these designs function differently, there are different considerations (see below).

The principal components of a laryngoscope blade are the spatula (that passes over the lingual surface of the tongue) and the flange that is used to direct the tongue (Figure 8-1), a fluid-filled noncompressible structure, to the side of the mouth and into the mandibular space (the space below the tongue). This concept of *mandibular space volume* is particularly important in clinical practice as the practitioner evaluates for difficult laryngoscopy and intubation (see Chapter 1).

Straight blades, such as the Magill blade (see Chapter 1, Figure 1-1), were originally designed to pick up the epiglottis and elevate it directly, while the curved Macintosh-type blades are intended to be advanced into vallecula and indirectly elevate the epiglottis by applying pressure to the hyoepiglottic ligament. These factors illustrate two distinguishing features of these blade designs: that straight blades are inserted more deeply than curved blades; and that curved blades have an atraumatic tip design to reduce the risk of vallecular injury.

Because laryngoscopy was originally an operative technique where the practitioner needed their dominant right hand (85% of the population is right-hand dominant) to be free to operate, the laryngoscope became by default a left-handed instrument.

Laryngoscopy and intubation are performed through the right side of the mouth. The left hand is used to insert the laryngoscope blade into the mouth to expose the glottis. The right hand is then free to perform a variety of tasks including the insertion of an intubation aid (eg, Eschmann Tracheal Introducer, [ETI]), manipulate the larynx, lift the head, suction the airway, and ultimately, pass the tube.

Early pioneers employing straight blades recognized that tongue displacement to one side facilitated laryngeal visualization, particularly if the blade of the laryngoscope was inserted in the corner of the mouth and along the paraglossal gutter. Importantly, it was recognized that this paraglossal or retromolar technique optimized the laryngeal view mostly because it shortened the distance between the teeth and the larynx (ie, the molars are closer to the larynx than the incisors). The other benefit of right paraglossal laryngoscopy is that the rigid laryngoscope blade impacts the molar teeth rather than the relatively more fragile central incisors. The flange of the laryngoscope remains a threat to dentition and should never be leveraged backward against the teeth.

Straight blade laryngoscopes tend to have smaller displacement volumes (defined by the dimensions of the spatula and flange) than curved designs. It is logical, therefore, that straight blades (and a paraglossal approach) are favored in patients who have a small mandibular volumes into which the tongue is displaced (or compressed) during direct laryngoscopy. Examples of such patients are small children (below the age of 8, but especially below age 5) and adults who have a receding chin.

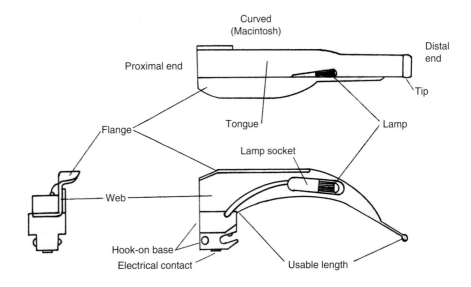

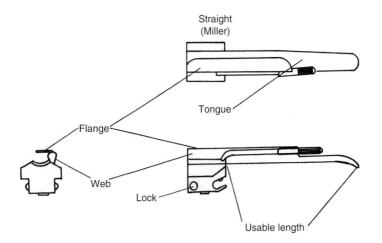

FIGURE 8-1. Design of the laryngoscope blades. (Modified with permission from Dorsch JA, Dorsch SE: Laryngoscopes. In: Dorsch JA, Dorsch SE (Eds). Understanding Anesthesia Equipment, 2nd ed. Williams & Wilkins; Baltimore, 1984)

8.2.2   What are the variables that determine the illumination created by a laryngoscope blade?

Illumination is critically important for direct laryngoscopy. Bright light is necessary for tissue edge and color discrimination, and the identification of tissues and structures. This is particularly important in preterm infants where the appreciation of subtle color differences is critical to intubation success.

Laryngoscope lighting systems can be divided into those with a light source mounted directly on the blade (bulb-on-blade), and those in which the light source is at the top of the handle (bulb-on-handle).

Bulb-on-blade designs (sometimes referred to as conventional blades) have a simple electrical connection between the bulb socket on the blade and the handle (with enclosed batteries). This connection is very robust and less subject to malfunction than the spring-loaded, on-off lights used with bulb-on-handle systems. These removable bulbs can usually be replaced if they fail. This feature confers the risk that should the bulb become loose it may flicker during operation, or worse yet, become dislodged and lost into the patient.[5,6] To eliminate this risk, some manufacturers fuse the bulb to the blade rendering the bulb nonreplaceable.

Laryngoscope bulbs for both designs are of several types: incandescent filament (tungsten with halogen gas), xenon gas, and light-emitting diodes (LED). The bulb itself can have either a frosted or clear lens, and may incorporate a reflector (common with bulb-on-handle designs).

Compared to other light-producing systems, LED bulbs use very little energy, operate with less heat, and have a much longer life span, thereby eliminating bulb replacement as a major concern. They now can be produced at less cost than other bulbs and produce brilliant light. The light from an LED tends to be whiter and bluer than traditional bulbs. All of the newer intubation devices (video laryngoscopes, mirror laryngoscopes, chip-on-stick CMOS-imaging devices, etc) use LED lights.

With bulb-on-handle systems, a light-conducting fiber, made of either glass or plastic, conveys the light from the top of the handle to the distal portion of the blade. Although such blades are often called fiber-optic, they have no optical fibers, per se, and a more appropriate term is fiber-lit. Glass fibers conduct light more efficiently, but cost significantly more. Disposable blades commonly use a light-conducting bundle made of plastic, whereas nondisposable fiber-lit blades use glass fiber bundles. In the United States, any blade or handle that uses fiber illumination has a green dot on the blade base and a green circle at the top of the handle (commonly referred to as a *green-line handle*). It is important for practitioners to appreciate that fiber-lit blades and handles and conventional blades and handles are not interchangeable.

A critical and essentially unexamined area of laryngoscope illumination involves batteries.[7]

Alkaline batteries have a gradually declining discharge curve. Failure to appreciate and rectify this declining illumination may compromise direct laryngoscopy by low light, heralded by a difficult or failed intubation.

Lithium batteries have a much flatter, higher discharge curve than alkaline batteries, but fail precipitously once the energy output falls below a certain threshold. Lithium batteries are much more expensive and generate more heat than alkaline batteries.

Some manufacturers, especially those producing high-quality fiber-lit blades, offer nickel-metal-hydride rechargeable battery systems, which produce very intense light when combined with a xenon bulb and glass fibers. While the light output from these high-end fiber-lit systems is impressive, they are very expensive.

Newer LED technology has the potential to rival the light output of these systems at a fraction of their cost, draw little energy, and are offered in a single-use, disposable, bulb-on-blade design.

Regardless of the type of light, the intensity of light reaching the distal end of a laryngoscope blade is dependent on the distance the light must travel. This phenomenon is governed by the inverse square law of physics, that is, if the distance from the light source to an object is doubled, the resultant amount of light energy reaching the object is reduced to one quarter of the original amount. So, generally, blade designs with shorter light-to-tip distances create more intense distal light. This produces substantial variability in the amount of light emitted by different combinations of blades

and handles used in clinical practice. In a study conducted in emergency departments, there was a 500-fold difference in light output between the best and worst blade-handle combinations.[8]

Few clinical settings monitor the light output with light meter testing. Lighting standards in dentistry or surgery recommend 5000 lux.[9] While there is no well-accepted light intensity standard for the laryngoscopes, the International Organization for Standardization has suggested 700 lux as a minimum light output for laryngoscopes.[10] In the presence of blood, secretions, and vomitus, common to emergency airways, more light is needed to discriminate landmarks.[10]

8.2.3 What are the distinguishing features of commonly used curved (Macintosh) blade designs?

The term "Macintosh blade" is generally used to mean any curved blade. However, since Macintosh's original description in 1943[4] several variations have been produced that are distinguishable by their flange height, flange shape, light position, and light type. These designs are commonly designated by their geographic manufacturing origins, that is, American (commonly known as "Standard"), English (commonly known as "Classic"), and German designs. The common features are a gently curved spatula and a large reverse Z-shaped flange (Figure 8-1).

American blades closely follow Macintosh's original description, that is, a large vertical, square-shaped, proximal flange that does not extend to the distal tip, coupled with a bulb-on-blade illumination system. The English design has a smaller, curvilinear proximal flange that runs all the way to the distal tip, and also uses a conventional light. Heine of Germany developed a fiber-lit blade that follows the English contour in terms of a short proximal flange. A large rectangular-shaped 5-mm glass fiber bundle is incorporated in the flange. The English and German designs have a much shorter light-to-tip distance than the American design (Figure 8-2). Most American designs use a frosted bulb, while most English designs have a clear lens. American and English designs now offer fiber illumination options. Numerous manufacturers

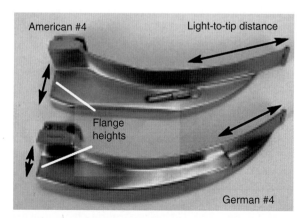

FIGURE 8-2. Design of the curved Macintosh laryngoscope blades. The German design has a much shorter light-to-tip distance than the American design.

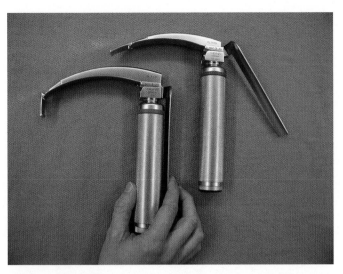

FIGURE 8-3. The McCoy (also known as Corazelli-London-McCoy [CLM]) levering laryngoscope blade.

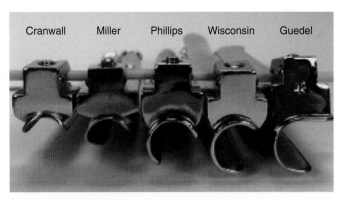

FIGURE 8-4. Different designs of the straight laryngoscope blades with different tubular shapes.

around the world now offer *American*, *English*, and *German* curved blades, and many blades have a mix of features.

It is interesting to note that Macintosh envisioned one adult size for his blade (corresponding to approximately a Macintosh size 3). Market demand lead to the current variety of pediatric and adult sizes available. Size selection is largely a matter of patient size and practitioner choice. No matter the size chosen, it should be noted that the most common error of the novice is inserting the blade too deeply and into the upper esophagus before visualization is performed. The shorter light-to-tip distance (and light source common to German or English designs) also provides better illumination relative to the American design.

A recent variation of the Macintosh design is the McCoy (also known as Corazelli-London-McCoy [CLM]) levering laryngoscope blade (Figure 8-3). This blade is a Macintosh design with an articulating distal tip that when activated is intended to elevate the tissue at the base of the tongue (improving epiglottis lift and laryngeal exposure). This blade has become quite popular in the United Kingdom (where it originated), but published clinical investigations have reported mixed results.[11-16]

8.2.4   What variations exist between Miller blade laryngoscope designs?

Robert Miller's straight blade design in 1941 adapted the straight shape of early laryngoscopes, in particular that of Magill (see Figure 1-1), but added a slightly upturned distal tip and narrower flange.[3] The flange had a compressed D-shape (when viewed longitudinally) with a height large enough to accept a 37 French Argyle tube. Compared to tubular shaped blades (eg, Jackson-Wisconsin) the much shallower proximal flange was intended to minimize dental injury (Figure 8-4). The light was situated at the distal tip on the right side of the spatula, opposite the flange side, and tilted toward midline (Figure 8-1).

Since Miller's original description various manufacturers have compressed the flange height, and some have changed the bulb location (to the left flange edge, or recessed within the flange).

Designs with light sources located on the exposed edge of the left flange are less preferred by some since a light at this location can become embedded in the tongue with resultant poor illumination. Most Miller designs currently made for adults cannot accommodate an adult-sized cuffed endotracheal tube down the barrel. In addition, tube passage down the barrel blocks the line-of-sight to the target. The very narrow design of modern Miller blades necessitates careful paraglossal placement (the small flange cannot sweep the tongue) and the extreme right corner of the mouth (which often requires manual retraction by an assistant) must be used for tube delivery. Alternatively, an ETI can be employed. Another challenge of the narrow-flange straight blades is that it makes landmark recognition down the barrel difficult.

8.2.5   What is the "straight blade paradox?"

Landmark recognition and ease of tube delivery improves as the flange height and spatula size of a straight blade is increased. Paradoxically, it gets harder to introduce the blade alongside the tongue, and reach the larynx, as the displacement volume of the blade increases. This was known to Miller, who shortened his flange height, but left the resulting D-shaped barrel large enough to accept an ETT.

Straight blade designs with larger flanges (and spatulas) than the Miller design include the Phillips (a two-third small C-shaped flange), Wisconsin (a higher, nearly full C-shaped flange), and the Guedel (a very large, sideways U-shaped flange and spatula) (Figure 8-4).

The Henderson straight blade has small incomplete two-third C-shaped flange that is large enough for tube delivery. It also has a uniquely visible distal tip (a knurled edge at the distal blade tip is visible when viewed down the barrel), and a large, recessed, fiber bundle light source (Figure 8-5).

8.2.6   Apart from the McCoy and Henderson blades already mentioned, are there other recent blade designs that might be of use?

The Dorges universal blade is intended to replace Macintosh size 2 to 4 blades with one blade for all patients from age 1 to adult.[17]

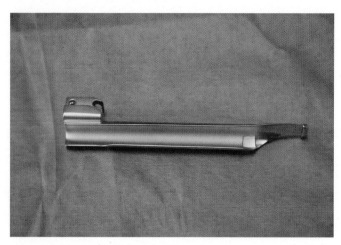

FIGURE 8-5. The Henderson laryngoscope blade.

The curve is much reduced, the spatula is tapered from proximal end to distal tip, and the proximal flange height is very short (15 mm), allowing it to be used with children and those with limited mouth opening, while at the same time permitting deeper insertion in larger adults owing to its length (Figure 8-6).

The Grandview blade is an emergency blade for adult patients that is available in two sizes.[18] It combines a very wide spatula with a slight overall curve and a narrow proximal flange (Figure 8-7). The resulting blade can be used to lift the epiglottis directly or indirectly.

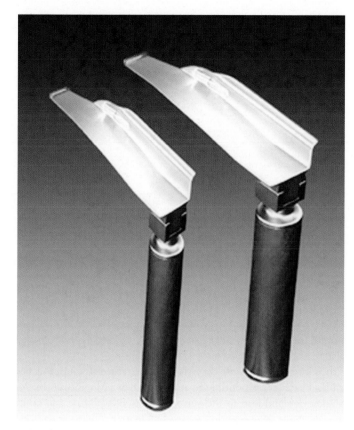

FIGURE 8-7. The Grandview universal laryngoscope blade.

8.3   BIOMECHANICS AND OPTICS

8.3.1   What optical and biomechanical considerations should practitioners appreciate when performing direct laryngoscopy?

Direct laryngoscopy is a procedure with inherent visual restrictions. Visual restrictions are created by the degree to which the mouth opens, the teeth, the tongue, the long-axis view down a laryngoscope blade, and the structures about the laryngeal inlet that surround the glottic opening. Laryngeal anatomy, which is exposed in piecemeal fashion initially, must be recognized when viewed down this restricted visual space. In many instances, only a small posterior portion of the glottic opening may be visible. Passage of the ETT further adds to the visual challenge. It is critical

for practitioners to know laryngeal anatomy in detail, to anticipate the sequence and appearance of structures as they come into view, and to be aware of how visual restrictions and biomechanics impact on laryngeal exposure and tube delivery.

8.3.2   What is the best way to maximize mouth opening and jaw distraction for laryngeal exposure and tube insertion?

As has been previously mentioned, employing the right corner of the mouth for laryngoscope blade insertion and tube passage is essential. A paraglossal approach is absolutely essential with straight blades. Even with curved blades, midline placement of the blade must be avoided because it will create *tongue flop* on each side of the blade, restricting glottic exposure and tube delivery.

The amount of mouth opening possible is a function of jaw distraction, and head and neck positioning. Positioning that facilitates jaw distraction and mouth opening is important in all patients, but most critical in the obese. Supine patients without cervical spine immobilization or known cervical pathology are optimally positioned for laryngoscopy when the external auditory meatus and sternal notch are horizontally aligned when viewed from the patient's side (see Chapter 18, Figures 18-1 and 18-2). This is called "ear-to-sternal notch" or "ramped position."

The traditional "sniffing position" is created by a combination of neck flexion and head extension at the atlanto-occipital joint. Ear-to-sternal notch positioning usually requires 8 to 10 cm of

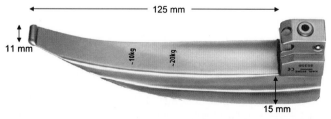

FIGURE 8-6. The Dorges universal laryngoscope blade.

elevation under the occiput, generally much more head elevation than that produced by the standard sniffing position. Furthermore, standard sniffing position posture fails to take into account size-related anatomical variations of the respiratory tract as it transitions from the thorax through the head and neck. On the other hand, ear-to-sternal notch positioning takes this variation into account permitting external landmark-based patient positioning to be individualized. These anatomical variations are most frequently appreciated in individuals who are obese and morbidly obese. In such patients, a ramp may be several feet high and incorporate support under the upper torso and shoulders as well as the head to achieve proper alignment. Head elevation and ramping in this manner optimizes laryngoscopy, while at the same time offering improved gas exchange mechanics.

When performing laryngoscopy with the patient supine, along with ear-to-sternal notch positioning, the face plane of the patient should be parallel to the ceiling (see Figure 18-2). A common error is to overextend or tilt the head backwards.[2] Atlanto-occipital extension may push the base of tongue and epiglottis against the posterior hypopharyngeal wall. Not only does this make recognition of the epiglottis more difficult upon blade insertion, this also narrows the space available to pass the laryngoscope and restricts laryngeal exposure. Extension alone may also create tension on the anterior neck muscles opposing simultaneous efforts to open the mouth and distract the jaw.

Successful laryngoscopy in this position requires that the patient's head be below the practitioner's xiphoid process, a position recommended by some texts. The reason for this is that increasing head elevation dynamically during laryngoscopy if laryngeal exposure is inadequate is made easier.[19] Dynamic head elevation cannot be done on the morbidly obese and these patients must be ramped into a proper position in advance (see Figure 18-2).

Mouth opening in the anesthetized or unresponsive patient usually occurs with head and neck positioning. In the event it does not, it can be achieved by simply pushing the chin in a caudad direction or by employing the cross-fingered or "scissors technique." This technique provides a more controlled and effective force than simply extending the head on the neck.

8.3.3 What is the optimal position for laryngoscopy in patients with known or suspected cervical spine injury? Is it safe to perform direct laryngoscopy?

Direct laryngoscopy has been shown to be safe in patients with known or suspected cervical spine injury, but it should be performed with manual in-line immobilization (MILI) (see Chapter 15). There has been considerable attention and controversy regarding airway management in the known or presumed C-spine-injured patient.[20-22] Some would argue that this concern has lead to unnecessary delay in managing the trauma airway, a decision which in some cases could result in increased morbidity and mortality (eg, hypoxemia and/or hypercarbia in head-injured patients). As a result, ATLS has backed away from an earlier recommendation that C-spine imaging precede airway management. Furthermore, there is little evidence to support secondary spinal cord injury directly attributable to airway management.[21-23]

Despite the fact that MILI does not completely prevent C-spine motion, it remains a recommendation. Care should be taken to ensure proper application of MILI in such a manner that mouth opening is not limited. Mouth opening is markedly limited with a collar in place where epiglottis only is visible (or worse). This can occur in more than 60% of cases.[24] Properly performed MILI will reduce the incidence of an epiglottis-only view to 22%.[25]

Research comparing intubation devices have revealed no convincing superiority of any device over well-performed DL in terms of limiting C-spine motion.[20] The major priority in managing suspected C-spine-injured patients is how to optimize view on laryngoscopy. Indicated airway management should not be delayed in fear of causing secondary spinal cord injury. The use of alternative devices, such as optical stylets or video laryngoscopy may help overcome a challenging view, although simple maneuvers, such as the application of optimal external laryngeal manipulation[26] (OELM or BURP [backwards upwards rightwards pressure][27]) and the use of an Eschmann tracheal introducer (commonly referred to as a *gum elastic bougie*) are equally effective in managing the trauma airway with suspected C-spine injury.[20]

Ear-to-sternal notch positioning cannot be used in such patients. The front of a cervical collar should be removed in order to permit jaw distraction. It is also helpful to drop the foot end of the stretcher while keeping the stretcher straight (ie, reverse Trendelunberg). This positions the airway higher than the stomach and may prevent passive regurgitation and improves pulmonary mechanics. An assistant must maintain MILI while laryngoscopy is carefully performed.

8.3.4 How should the laryngoscope be gripped to minimize the work of laryngoscopy while maintaining fine control of the blade tip?

The mechanics of laryngoscope lift are slightly different with curved versus straight blades. With the curved blade, the tip is guided into vallecula to depress the underlying hyoepiglottic ligament, lifting the epiglottis forward away from the glottic inlet. With straight blades, the tip of the blade lifts the epiglottis directly. Both curved and straight blade handles should be gripped with the tips of the fingers where the handle meets the proximal blade (Figure 8-8). The handle should be gripped low enough that the blade is essentially an extension of the forearm. Holding the handle higher increases the length of the lever arm requiring significantly more muscular effort. When properly gripped with the thumb pointing upward on the handle, fine control and effective mechanical advantage is achieved, and levering on the upper incisors is less likely to occur. Laryngoscopy is a delicate procedure, mostly dependent on gentle positioning of and correct vector forces at the blade tip. When properly positioned, the amount of force required for most patients is minimal and can be achieved by a light grip. When the blade tip is not correctly positioned, excessively forceful lifting will usually not correct the problem.

Another way to maximize lifting efficacy with minimal muscular effort is to keep the left elbow adducted to your side (roughly the anterior axillary line), not pointing outward. With the elbow in, the handle gripped down low, the forearm is kept straight and

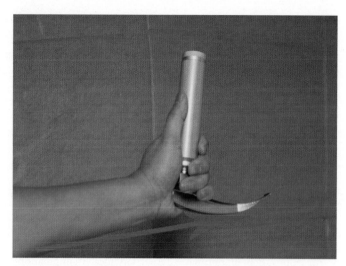

FIGURE 8-8. Laryngoscope grip. Both curved and straight blade handles should be gripped with the tips of the fingers where the handle meets the proximal blade. The handle should be gripped low enough that the blade is essentially an extension of the forearm.

body weight can be used to rock forward slightly so that minimal arm strain occurs. Force is efficiently transferred along the forearm and down the long axis of the blade.

8.3.5   How is the larynx sighted during direct laryngoscopy? Is performance improved by assuming a distance as far as possible from the target?

Contrary to popular belief and traditional instruction, even with an extended arm position, it is not possible to simultaneously see the larynx during laryngoscopy with both eyes.[28] This is due to the inherent visual restrictions of direct laryngoscopy, created by the opening of the mouth, the teeth, the tongue, the laryngoscope blade itself, and the structures of the laryngeal inlet. Visually, direct laryngoscopy is similar to looking down a narrow pipe at a target the size of a quarter, from a distance of 14 to 16 in.

Both eyes can be open during the procedure, but sighting of the larynx is with the dominant eye only; the brain subconsciously blocks out the nondominant image through a process called "binocular suppression." The same phenomenon occurs when looking through a peephole in a door, or when sighting during target sports. In situations without visual restriction, the right and left eyes have slightly different perspectives on an object, due to the distance separating the eyes in the skull. These slightly disparate views are fused into a single stereoscopic image. This cannot happen with the visual restrictions created during laryngoscopy; stereoscopic sight cannot be achieved. Because binocular suppression occurs subconsciously, even experienced laryngoscopists may not be aware of which eye they use to sight the larynx.

The monocularity of laryngeal sight during laryngoscopy is evident when viewing novice intubators attempting laryngoscopy for the first time by noting a subtle side-to-side head rotation, intermittently sighting the target with one eye and then the other.

The old adage that "experienced laryngoscopists maintain a distance from the target, while novices climb into the mouth" is due not to experience but rather restrictions on accommodation

that occur with age. By the mid-forties, the near visual accommodation point begins to move out approximately 2 to 3 cm·y^{-1}. By mid-fifties regardless of your underlying acuity, presbyopia results in the near focus point being at about arm's length. Younger practitioner's have the accommodation flexibility to focus on near objects. These changes are exacerbated in low light conditions. The amount of light needed for laryngoscopy by the same practitioner is different at age 40 versus age 50 and 60; more light improves the near focus ability significantly and is another reason for using laryngoscope systems with good light output.

8.3.6   Is it beneficial to identify ocular dominance, acuity, and accommodation distance in trainees and how is this done?

Ocular dominance, visual acuity, and accommodation should be assessed at the start of procedure training and in all practitioners on the steep curve of presbyopia (mid-forties).

Ocular dominance is tested by having the practitioner perform direct laryngoscopy on a training mannequin. After the practitioner confirms that the larynx is sighted, instruct him or her not to move their head. Selectively cover each eye, individually. When the nondominant eye is covered the laryngeal view is not compromised; when the dominant eye gets covered the larynx will no longer be sighted (or it will be seen partially, off angle). One cannot change one's natural ocular dominance. Eyedness tends to follow handedness assuming there is no unequal acuity, and since majority of the population is right-handed, most practitioners are also right-eyed. Persons who have a difference in visual acuity (wear lenses), or are left-handed, have a greater likelihood of being left-eyed when it comes to laryngoscopy.

Identification of ocular dominance, formal visual acuity, and accommodation testing is valuable to the trainee to proactively prevent procedural performance problems. Notwithstanding severe visual acuity problems, most accommodation issues can be addressed by corrective lenses. Unfortunately, many practitioners have lenses made for either driving, or reading, but not for the proper procedural distance of laryngoscopy. The proper procedural distance for a given practitioner is between their arm held at full extension, and the arm flexed at 90 degrees. For most practitioners this is about 14 to 16 in (35-40 cm). Corrective lenses become a valuable aid to direct laryngoscopy in most practitioners by their mid- to late forties.

8.4   DIFFICULT LARYNGOSCOPY— ASSESSMENT AND PREDICTION

8.4.1   What factors contribute to difficult laryngoscopy and how reliable is prediction?

Difficult laryngoscopy can result from two different issues: (1) problems with landmark recognition; and (2) mechanical problems that prevent laryngeal exposure.

Landmark recognition is much more difficult in the presence of blood, secretions, vomitus, or distorted anatomy from a myriad of causes, including burns, edema, and other pathology. Successful laryngoscopy hinges on recognizing the epiglottis and structures of the laryngeal inlet, in addition to the glottic opening and vocal cords. The epiglottis has a mucosal appearance that is very similar to the posterior hypopharynx even without the additional challenges of fluids, vomitus, or distorted anatomy. Fluids from the oropharynx and hypopharynx will collect above the epiglottis when a patient is positioned in a supine position with poor muscular tone (or after the use of muscle relaxants). This can easily cause epiglottis edge recognition failure as the blade is inserted. Elevation of the epiglottis out of the fluids by proper jaw distraction during the first phase of laryngoscopy, which is, in turn, a function of proper head and neck position, and avoidance of overextension may help. Because fluids are often present in the airway, it is appropriate to have a Yankauer suction immediately available.

Mechanical problems that can limit laryngeal exposure include limited mouth opening, prominent dentition and overbite, a large tongue-to-pharynx relationship (ie, the Mallampati score), short thyromental distance (a small displacement volume for the tongue), and limitations of neck mobility. Although great effort has been put into devising scoring systems for predicting difficult laryngoscopy, the clinical utility of such screening tests remains very limited, more so in emergency situations. Only about one in three emergency patients who undergo intubation can follow simple commands, permitting even a basic screening assessment. Emergency patients with poor muscular tone, lying in a supine position, will almost universally have a poor and different Mallampati score and a short thyromental distance. Compounding this are those with suspected C-spine injury because they cannot undergo neck mobility testing.

As reviewed by Yentis,[29] it is statistically challenging to devise an effective screening test, or combination of tests, for detecting a rare outcome (failed laryngoscopy). The trachea of a vast majority of patients can be successfully intubated with direct laryngoscopy, and unless a screening test has extremely high specificity and sensitivity, most predicted failures will be false positives. Conversely, some patients who would seem to be easy may be difficult or impossible because laryngoscopy primarily involves interaction with tissue not visible to oral inspection (the base of tongue and epiglottis, eg, lingual tonsillar hypertrophy).

While it is important to be aware of factors that can contribute to difficulty, screening performs poorly, and practitioners should always plan a means of rescue gas exchange and rescue technique should direct laryngoscopy and/or mask ventilation prove difficult or impossible.[30] Much of the historical concern about difficult laryngoscopy is no longer relevant, now that there are so many alternative effective options for intubation, and even more significant, an extraordinarily effective means of rescue ventilation should mask ventilation and intubation fail, namely, the laryngeal mask airway.

Given the effectiveness of rescue ventilation devices, and alternative intubation methods, direct laryngoscopy efforts should generally not exceed three attempts and in many settings (prehospital) be limited to one or two attempts depending on practitioner's experience. Poor outcomes, that is, hypoxemia, regurgitation, aspiration, cardiac arrest, etc, have been associated with three or more laryngoscopy attempts in emergency situations.[31]

8.4.2 How is direct laryngoscopy view articulated and how is this clinically relevant? Is difficult laryngoscopy synonymous with difficult intubation?

Laryngeal exposure is only one step in the sequence of steps leading to successful intubation employing direct laryngoscopy. It is possible to have an excellent laryngeal view and be unable to intubate, as can occur with tracheal stenosis, for example. Conversely, an epiglottis-only view can sometimes be easily intubated on first attempt using a blind technique (ETI).

For laryngoscopy research and for documentation purposes, different systems have been created for reporting the extent of laryngeal view. The original system of grading laryngeal view, developed by Cormack/Lehane (C/L), categorizes laryngeal exposure into four grades: Grade 1—all of the vocal cords/glottic opening; Grade 2—only the posterior aspect of the glottis is in view (depending on external laryngeal pressure, part of the vocal cords and/or arytenoids may be in view); Grade 3—epiglottis-only; and Grade 4—no landmarks (not even epiglottis).[32] Some researchers have subdivided the CL grading system to 3A and 3B. A 3A view is when the epiglottis is able to be lifted off the posterior hypopharynx, and 3B when it is touching the posterior wall (Figure 8-9).[33] This difference in the position of the epiglottis is important as a posteriorly directed epiglottis creates a relatively more anterior glottic inlet that will not be easily accessed using an adjunct such as an ETI. A moderate degree of interobserver and intraobserver variability with this scoring system is known to exist.

A more statistically useful method of reporting laryngeal view is the Percentage of Glottic Opening Score, which is a numerical value from 0% to 100%.[34,35] A full 100% POGO score would be a full view of the glottic opening from the anterior commissure of the vocal cords to the interarytenoid notch between the posterior cartilages. This system better distinguishes between CL Grades 1

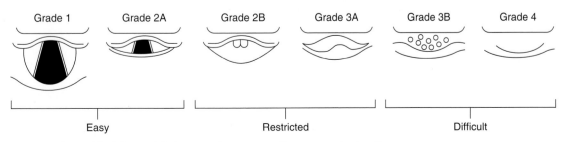

FIGURE 8-9. Modified Cormack/Lehane grading system of laryngoscopic view.[33]

and 2, which make up the vast majority of cases, but makes no distinction between CL 3 (including 3A vs 3B) and 4 (both would be POGO 0).

Adnet devised an Intubation Difficulty Scale, which incorporates laryngeal view as well as other aspects of intubation.[36] They proposed an Intubation Difficulty Scale (IDS) score that is a function of seven parameters, resulting in a progressive, quantitative determination of intubation complexity. The score was intended to be used to compare difficulty of intubation under varying circumstances by isolating variables of interest. The seven parameters include:

- The number of attempts
- The number of operators
- The number of techniques (or devices)
- Cormack/Lehane view grade
- Lifting force
- Need for external laryngeal manipulation
- Position of the vocal cords (abducted/adducted)

There are numerous challenges when applying grading systems of laryngoscopy or intubation to patients. Fundamentally, the effectiveness of the procedure is also about the skill and ability of the practitioner. A Grade 3 CL view or difficult intubation employing Adnet's scoring system may be a Grade 1 view and an easy intubation in a different practitioner's hands.

Direct laryngoscopy and intubation is not an objective, easily graded diagnostic test, such as coronary angiography, for example. Not only does practitioner's technique impact dramatically on the result, but the performance is not routinely graded from the practitioner's perspective, and therefore, cannot be objectively assessed by other persons. With angiography, the images of dye filling the coronaries are not likely to be different when performed by a different operator, and the results can be reviewed by others. Direct laryngoscopy is dynamic, with the larynx transiently visualized for 5 to 15 seconds, and sighted by only one eye of the practitioner. Even if it was possible to capture what the practitioner was actually seeing during direct laryngoscopy and evaluate the performance, it still captures the procedural performance of only one practitioner and one event.

8.5   PREPARING FOR LARYNGOSCOPY— OPTIMIZING CONDITIONS

8.5.1   What is optimal laryngoscopy and how should the practitioner prepare for direct laryngoscopy?

The "Optimum laryngoscopic attempt" was characterized by Benumof as possessing six factors[37]:

- Most skilled individual
- Best paralysis
- Best position

- Best laryngeal manipulation
- Best laryngoscope blade type
- Best laryngoscope blade length

"Optimal laryngoscopy" refers to a combination of the proper equipment, a preplanned laryngoscopy strategy, and ideal patient conditions that collectively create optimal conditions for laryngeal exposure and first-pass intubation success.

Equipment must include suction (Yankauer), functioning oxygen delivery devices, and well-functioning laryngoscopes with optimal illumination. Tube delivery requires appropriately sized tubes, and stylets, along with a means of managing an epiglottis-only view (ETI and/or optical stylet). It is critical to have oral and nasal airways and an appropriately sized rescue extraglottic device (eg, LMA) immediately available, should intubation fail and rescue ventilation be required. Given the wide variety of alternative intubation devices, it is also appropriate to have an alternative device for intubation immediately available.

The importance of proper positioning, for both ventilation and direct laryngoscopy, cannot be overstated. Not only will ventilation be more effective in the ear-to-sternal notch position, but it will lengthen the time to desaturation in the patient who has been rendered apneic from their underlying condition or RSI (apnea time).[38-40] Different methods of denitrogenation have been suggested to extend apnea time.[41] These include having the cooperative patient take eight vital capacity breaths. Tidal volume breathing for 3 to 4 minutes using high-flow oxygen via a bag-mask device yields the best results. However, in some patient populations, such as the young pediatric patients, and patients with morbid obesity and critical illness, oxygen utilization is increased while reserves may be diminished.[42] Desaturation will occur rapidly following apnea in these patients, requiring early mechanical ventilation, often before adequate intubation conditions (muscle relaxation) are achieved.[43] Assisted ventilation in patients with low baseline saturations may be indicated during the preintubation phase. The risk of aspiration in carefully applied BMV is much less than the risk of desaturation in the critically ill patient. Denitrogenation will allow sufficient time for laryngoscopy and intubation in most patients without pulmonary pathology before desaturation occurs (longer apnea times).

While there has been debate about the indications for muscle relaxants outside of the operating room, there is no doubt that laryngoscopy is easier, more successful and done more quickly, and with fewer attempts when relaxants are used. The use of muscle relaxants offers two other very significant advantages. It eliminates the risk of active vomiting during laryngoscopy, and it permits the use of rescue ventilation devices (ie, LMA) should laryngoscopy fail. In emergency patients with full stomachs and short apnea times, these advantages may be important.

8.5.2   Is there a role for decompression of the stomach prior to emergency laryngoscopy, and how should nasogastric tubes already in place be handled?

In patients with known bowel obstruction, significant GI bleeding, and perhaps in patients who have received prolonged assisted

BMV (long prehospital course) it may be helpful to decompress the bowel as much as possible prior to muscle relaxation and laryngoscopy. These patients are at significant risk of regurgitation with the onset of muscle relaxation (see Section 5.5.4). Sellick recommended evacuating the stomach with a gastric tube and then removing the tube before induction of anesthesia.[44] Others demonstrated no difference in the incidence of regurgitation with or without a nasogastric tube.[45] It is the opinion of the authors that the nasogastric tubes should, if placed, remain in situ for the intubation.

8.6 ANATOMIC CONSIDERATIONS AND LAYNGOSCOPY TECHNIQUE

8.6.1 What is epiglottoscopy and why is it important when performing laryngoscopy?

"Epiglottoscopy" emphasizes the importance of visualizing the epiglottis prior to exposing the larynx and was one of Chevalier Jackson's basic rules of laryngoscopy.[2] As an anatomic landmark the epiglottis has a unique importance to laryngoscopy for numerous reasons.

The epiglottis is the bridge between the starting anatomic landmark (the tongue) and the goal (the larynx). The relational anatomy, between the tongue, epiglottis, and larynx remains a constant despite person to person anatomic and pathologic variations. The epiglottis attaches to both the tongue and the larynx. It is connected to the base of the tongue at the vallecula. It is also the most superior aspect of the laryngeal inlet, a ring of structures that encircles the glottic opening. This ring is made up of the epiglottis, the paired aryepiglottic folds, the paired posterior cartilages, and the interarytenoid notch. Within the laryngeal inlet lies the glottic opening and vocal cords. The epiglottis is additionally a marker for the midline.

8.6.2 What is "epiglottis camouflage"?

As stated earlier, the mucosal appearance of the epiglottis is identical to that of the posterior pharyngeal wall. In a supine position, with poor muscular tone, or after the administration of muscle relaxants, the jaw and base of tongue fall backward and the epiglottis lies against the posterior pharynx. Depending upon head and neck position, and the manner in which the laryngoscope is directed, it is easy to advance past the epiglottis as it is camouflaged against the pharynx. Overextension of the head, at the atlanto-occipital joint, moves the base of the tongue and epiglottis backward, making the situation worse, as do secretions, blood, and vomitus.

To overcome epiglottis camouflage and make the epiglottis edge distinctly visible, it is necessary to distract the jaw effectively and lift the base of the tongue. Keeping the face plane horizontal to the floor and elevating the head to ear-to-sternal notch position (if possible) permits optimal jaw distraction.

8.6.3 What is the best method for controlling the tongue and how does tongue control integrate with epiglottoscopy?

Effective control of the tongue is critical for straight blade use, and important as well with curved blades. Any amount of tongue positioned to the right of a narrow-lumen straight blade will make target visualization and tube delivery very difficult. The small flange height, especially of some Miller designs, prevents any ability to sweep the tongue, and practitioners should not attempt to do so. Proper position is achieved with straight blades by deliberately directing the blade to the right paraglossal space.[23] When correctly positioned, the proximal portion of the blade is lateral to the right of the patient's right nostril and no tongue is present to the right of the blade. Insertion of the blade should occur through the right lateral mouth over the molar dentition. The distal blade may then be directed medially, although the proximal blade should never be brought back toward the midline upper incisors.

With a curved blade, the large reverse Z-shaped flange allows tongue sweeping. To avoid the thick chest or breasts, particularly in patients with a short neck, many practitioners prefer to insert the blade with the handle tilted sideways toward the right and insert the blade into the mouth at a slight right lateral position. A potential problem with this approach is that the epiglottis and the larynx are then approached *off angle* and depending upon the depth of insertion this can create landmark confusion. The aryepiglottic fold can be misinterpreted as the epiglottis edge, and if inserted too deeply the tip of the blade will pass under the posterior cartilages into the esophagus.

With the patient's face plane parallel to the ceiling, the author prefers to follow the curve of the blade down the curve of tongue, slightly to the right of midline, with early compression/lift of the tongue as necessary to visualize the epiglottis edge. In this first stage of laryngoscopy, only a gentle force is required to distract the jaw caudad, lifting the epiglottis edge off the posterior pharyngeal wall. The direction of the handle upon insertion and with initial jaw distraction is toward the patient's feet, and at a very shallow angle as the blade is advanced down the tongue (perhaps only approximately 20 degrees up from horizontal). Inexperienced users will commonly place the blade tip too far, before looking for landmarks. This is particularly common when using a longer blade (eg, #4 Macintosh blade). After the epiglottis has been recognized, and before the blade is engaged with greater force, the practitioner should check tongue position and move the blade rightward as necessary to effectively control the tongue. In practice, epiglottoscopy and tongue control happen simultaneously.

8.6.4 How can direct laryngoscopy be made more predictable and not a hit-or-miss procedure?

From insertion of the blade until visualization of the larynx, there is a predictable, sequential exposure of landmarks that results from progressive advancement of the line-of-sight (LOS). As a laryngoscope blade is advanced over and down the surface of the tongue, into the pharynx, and then the hypopharynx, the LOS moves from the uvula, to the posterior pharynx, and then at the base of the tongue, to the epiglottis.

With the curved blade, the epiglottis is indirectly elevated, while with the straight blade the epiglottis is directly lifted. Once the epiglottis is visualized, the practitioner knows where the larynx will be located. Effective epiglottis control (either indirectly with a curved blade or directly with a straight blade) will then permit progressive exposure of laryngeal landmarks.

The structures of the larynx become visible from the most posterior to the most anterior. The most posterior laryngeal structures and the first visible under the epiglottis edge are the interarytenoid notch and the accompanying right and left arytenoids cartilages. Above the interarytenoid notch, and just medial to the arytenoid cartilages, is the posterior aspect of the glottic opening. Moving more anteriorly, the aryepiglottic folds are visible laterally, and the true and false vocal cords medially. Finally, most anterior and farthest within the laryngeal inlet, is the anterior commissure of the vocal cords.

8.6.5 What are the subtleties of curved blade laryngoscopy, and what is bimanual laryngoscopy?

The effectiveness of indirect epiglottis elevation hinges on proper placement of the blade tip in the vallecula as well as correctly directing force down the blade. Following epiglottoscopy, the tip of the blade needs to be fully advanced into the vallecula and the lifting force increased compared to what was needed for distracting the jaw and visualizing the epiglottis. The force direction is along the forearm and down the blade, in a manner that the practitioner's arm and forearm are extended away from the torso. The handle should not be tilted backwards, otherwise the tip of the blade will come out of the vallecula and there will be inadequate pressure on the underlying hyoepiglottic ligament. With the force directed down the blade (ie, the force vector approximately perpendicular to the practitioner), the tip of the blade can be effectively driven into the vallecula and resulting pressure on the hyoepiglottic ligament will cause the epiglottis to indirectly elevate (Figure 8-10).

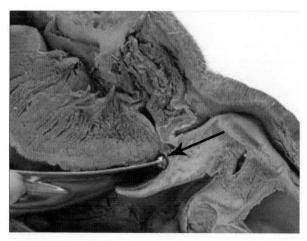

FIGURE 8-10. Direct laryngoscopy with a curved Macintosh laryngoscope in a cadaver. The tip of the blade should be placed into the vallecula and the resulting pressure on the hyoepiglottic ligament (arrow) will cause the epiglottis to indirectly elevate.

If the tip of the blade is not fully seated into the vallecula engaging the hyoepiglottic ligament, no amount of lifting force will correctly elevate the epiglottis. A difference in blade tip placement of millimeters will affect the degree of epiglottic control. This is likely one of the primary reasons for skill-/experience-based variations in the laryngoscopic views. One way to seat the blade tip correctly is by performing bimanual laryngoscopy.[46] The practitioner uses their free right hand to reach around to the anterior neck of the patient and apply external manipulation to the thyroid cartilage with a downward (backward, posterior) force.

The tip of the blade is like a key being inserted into the lock of the vallecula. Bimanual laryngoscopy serves to fully insert the key all the way into the lock, which only then will allow turning (elevating the epiglottis) and opening the larynx. In some cases, bimanual laryngoscopy may be best at the cricoid cartilage, or even the hyoid, although Benumof found that optimal manipulation was at the thyroid in almost 90% of cases.[26] The practitioner need not be concerned about the exact position of their right hand. There is instantaneous visual feedback about the effectiveness of epiglottis elevation, and it is easy to move the right hand slightly up or down on the patient's neck to optimize the view.

Bimanual laryngoscopy improves laryngeal view in two ways. First, it changes the mechanics as described, correctly sitting the blade tip where it needs to be. Second, it helps to move the larynx downward (backward) into the practitioner's LOS. The mobility of the larynx and the ability of the practitioner to move it backward into view during the procedure was something known even to Czermark in the mid-19th century, when mirror laryngoscopy was first developed. Early wood block prints of Czermark performing mirror laryngoscopy show one hand on the patient's neck while his other hand holds the mirror within the mouth.[2]

A critical component of bimanual laryngoscopy is the direct practitioner connection between neck manipulation and the immediately observed effect on laryngeal view. Cricoid pressure (discussed later) and backward upward rightward pressure (BURP[27]) involve an assistant applying pressure to the neck. Given the subtlety of laryngoscopy, and that minor changes in blade tip position or force can significantly alter exposure and epiglottis control, bimanual laryngoscopy performed by the practitioner (referred by some as optimal external laryngeal manipulation, OELM) is the most effective means of optimizing laryngeal view.[26] An assistant can be taught to maintain pressure at this location while the practitioner uses the right hand to pass the ETT.

The term "bimanual laryngoscopy" has also been used to describe a technique where the left hand manipulates the laryngoscope while the right hand is placed behind the occiput to manipulate the head and neck position to obtain the best view of the glottis.

8.6.6 How is OLEM different from cricoid pressure (the Sellick maneuver)? Can cricoid pressure and OELM be used together, or should they (see also Section 5.6)?

In 1961, Sellick described backward pressure on the cricoid ring by an assistant as a method of preventing passive regurgitation of stomach contents during elective anesthesia.[44] It has become a standard part of emergency laryngoscopy and rapid sequence intubation/induction (RSI). It seems logical that pressure on the cricoid could occlude the esophagus and that this is advantageous in full stomach or aspiration-risk patients.

It is critical for airway practitioners to evaluate recent evidence regarding cricoid pressure and whether it should be a standard part of emergency laryngoscopy for two reasons. First, imaging of the neck with CT and MRI by Smith has established that the mechanics are not what they seem.[47,48] Total occlusion of the esophagus does not occur in 91% of patients when cricoid pressure is applied because the esophagus is actually not midline, immediately behind the cricoid cartilage, but laterally displaced. However, Smith did find that the lumen of the esophagus was significantly compressed even if displaced laterally, and surmised that regurgitant fluid would be impeded by the maneuver, and recommended that there was no reason to suggest that traditional practice be abandoned.

The second reason why cricoid pressure should be examined critically is that the parameters of ventilation and positioning have changed dramatically from when Sellick conceived his technique. In Sellick's time, ventilation volumes averaged 10 to 15 mL·kg^{-1} and ventilation rates were 12 to 15 or more breaths per minute. Current practice is to use much smaller ventilation volumes, only 6 to 7 mL·kg^{-1}, and higher ventilation rates to reduce the risk of exceeding esophageal opening pressure (25-30 cm H_2O), yet again reducing the risk of gastric insufflation and regurgitation.

Sellick believed cricoid pressure would only work if the head and neck were placed in hyperextension in order to pin the esophagus between the cricoid and the vertebrae.[44] He further advocated that the head be in a head down position. Should any regurgitation recur, the material could drain out and not into the lungs.[44] This hyperextended head and neck position, and positioning the head down are antithetical to what we now know is optimal for effective ventilation and maximizing upper airway patency.

Laryngeal manipulation (BURP or bimanual laryngoscopy) should not be confused with cricoid pressure. Cricoid pressure is usually done by an assistant rather than the practitioner and it is not primarily intended to improve laryngeal exposure. It is also applied lower on the neck than laryngeal manipulation. If initiated upon induction (before blade insertion), cricoid pressure may prevent the blade tip from being correctly seated in the vallecula. Recent evidence has identified that the application of cricoid pressure may increase the incidence of a difficult emergency laryngoscopy (Grade 3 or 4 Cormack/Lehane view). A growing body of literature has highlighted the detrimental effects of cricoid pressure on laryngoscopy, mask-ventilation, and LMA placement although it has yet to demonstrate decreased gas exchange or increased intubation failure rates.[49,50]

In summary, it seems reasonable to continue with the practice of applying cricoid pressure (Sellick maneuver) at least until the evidence demonstrates that it is futile at preventing aspiration or leads to decreased gas exchange and increased intubation failure rates.

8.6.7 Apart from paraglossal placement, what are the specifics of correctly performing straight blade laryngoscopy?

Much of the specifics of straight blade laryngoscopy have already been discussed, that is, paraglossal placement, and use of the extreme

right corner of the mouth for blade positioning, tilting, and tube delivery. There is a critical aspect of straight blade laryngoscopy that needs to be addressed, however, and that is the direct lifting of the epiglottis.

After the epiglottis edge is identified, the handle must be tilted forward (eg, the tip backward, toward the posterior hypopharynx), the blade inserted slightly (approximately 1-2 cm), and the tip passed under the epiglottis. Once the epiglottis is *trapped* under the blade tip, the blade is rocked slightly backward (handle brought slightly more upright) and then the lifting force increased. Jackson described the lifting direction as suspending the patient's head with the flat section of the blade, at a point underneath the hyoid bone.[2]

Miller blades have an upturned distal tip that varies among manufacturers. This renders the distal blade tip invisible to the practitioner when viewed down the long axis of the blade. A potential problem with this design is that the practitioner does not know if the blade has been advanced far enough to trap the epiglottis until the blade is rocked backward; frequently the tip of the epiglottis is not trapped and the advancement and tilting maneuver needs to be repeated.

The Henderson blade is a novel straight blade design that has a deliberately visible distal tip. Underneath, within the barrel of the distal tip is a knurled edge that is easily seen when the practitioner looks down the blade (Figure 8-5). This allows the practitioner to place the tip under the epiglottis and know with certainty that the epiglottis is trapped.

OELM is helpful with straight blades because the posterior laryngeal pressure displaces the target into view.

8.6.8 In addition to OELM, what other maneuvers can be done during laryngoscopy to improve a poor laryngeal view?

Practitioners should understand and be ready to respond to poor laryngeal view within their first laryngoscopy attempt. There should be a specific planned approached to find the epiglottis and optimize blade tip position. In addition to OELM, and making sure the curved tip is driven fully into the vallecula, another technique for improving an epiglottis-only view is to dynamically lift the patient's head higher. This technique, which the author has called "head elevated laryngoscopy positioning" (HELP, and others have called "bimanual laryngoscopy"), was first described by Richard Johnston in 1909, and later adopted by Jackson and included in his subsequent textbooks.[1,2,51] As already noted, head elevation permits greater jaw distraction because of its mechanically favorable effect on mouth opening. It enlarges the area beneath the base of the tongue and epiglottis improving visualization. According to Jackson, exaggerated head elevation also better aligned the blade axis with the axis of the upper trachea and larynx.

The practitioner can perform head elevation by using their right hand to lift the patient's occiput. Some practitioners have used their abdomen to lean forward and prop up and elevate the patient's head. Alternatively, an assistant can easily help by using two hands to lift the head from the patient's side. In the morbidly obese, dynamic lifting is often not feasible given the weight involved. A large ramp is needed extending from under the occiput, to the upper shoulders which then tapers to the mid-low back, in order to provide proper positioning (see Figure 18-2). An inflatable ramp has been designed for this purpose for airway management in the morbidly obese, called the "Rapid Airway Management Positioner."[52] A noninflatable version is called the "Troop Pillow" (see Figure 49-2).

Regardless of which lifting technique is used, the patient's stretcher height must be kept low enough to permit head elevation and still provide a good perspective for the practitioner to look down the mouth into a patient whose face plane is parallel to the ceiling. For some practitioners, especially when dealing with larger patients, this may require a foot stool for the practitioner to be at proper height.

8.6.9 What are the most common errors of direct laryngoscopy by novices?

The three most common errors that novice practitioners make during laryngoscopy include:

1. Placing the blade too deep before looking (not performing epiglottoscopy)
2. Entering the vallecula and lifting without engaging the hyoepiglottic ligament
3. Not using their right hand (bimanual laryngoscopy, OELM, BURP, HELP) to optimize the view

Novice practitioners move right past the epiglottis, insert the blade tip too deep, and then cannot recognize any laryngeal structures. They typically try to transfer their practice experience from an intubation trainer to an actual patient and find recognition of structures very difficult. This occurs because of unrecognized visual restrictions, epiglottis camouflage, and little understanding of the nuances of laryngeal anatomy. They also do not appreciate how minor manipulative adjustments of the blade tip affects laryngeal exposure, instead resorting to extra lifting effort. Their response to a poor laryngeal view is to move the blade in and out with large movements, leading to edema, tissue trauma, bleeding, and possibly perforation of the upper esophagus or hypopharynx. The best way to avoid landmark confusion is to be meticulous about epiglottoscopy.

Novice practitioners should carefully study video imaging of direct laryngoscopy prior to practicing on real patients paying particular attention to the nuances of anatomy and technique. The visual restrictions inherent to laryngoscopy make targeted feedback and supervision during the procedure impossible. With intensive video training, novice intubators can achieve a 90% success rate on their first 10 attempts, while with standard mannequin-only training initial success rates are low (50%).[53] Following mannequin-only practice, a statistical modeling showed that the number of laryngoscopic intubations required to achieve a 90% success rate in anesthetized patients with a normal airway in an operating room environment was 47.[54]

8.6.10 Are there specific patients, apart from small children, in whom curved blades perform poorly or in whom a straight blade would be the first choice?

Patients who have lingual tonsillar hyperplasia have excess tissue at the base of the tongue and a small or nonexistent vallecula, making indirect epiglottis elevation very difficult. This is a rare condition, but can lead to unexpected failed laryngoscopy, since the base of tongue and epiglottis are not visible to oral examination during preprocedural assessment (see also Chapter 37). There are case reports of such patients being able to be intubated using a paraglossal straight blade technique.[55] If the condition was known in advance, it would be prudent to avoid direct laryngoscopy altogether since it could prevent laryngeal exposure with a laryngoscope and also lead to very difficult mask and LMA ventilation.

Patients with large central dental gaps may be more easily intubated using a straight blade, since the large flange on the curved blade may lock into the gap creating a very restricted space for tube delivery. In such instances, ETI can be very helpful, or alternatively, a straight blade can be used with a paraglossal approach.

8.7   ENDOTRACHEAL TUBE PLACEMENT

8.7.1 Tube delivery as a separate and distinct challenge from laryngeal exposure: role for stylets, tube introducers, and optical stylets

Polyvinyl chloride (PVC) ETTs have a gentle arcuate shape, as prescribed by American Society of Testing of Materials standards. The standard tube also has an asymmetric tip, with the bevel of the tube facing leftward when viewed from the practitioner's perspective ("Magill bevel"), down the long axis of the tube, as the tube is inserted into a patient.

The optical challenges of direct laryngoscopy have already been described. When there is favorable laryngeal exposure, tube delivery is rarely problematic. Conversely, when only a small portion of the glottic opening is visible, or even just the interarytenoid notch can be seen, tube delivery may obscure simultaneous visualization of the target.

All instruments designed to be passed into narrow body cavities have a narrow long-axis dimension and an upward distal turn. Instruments that adhere to this shape are alligator forceps, laryngeal mirrors, and ETI. The optical benefit of this shape is that the long straight section allows good maneuverability toward a target, while the upturned distal tip makes the tip of the device visible.

The large curvature of standard PVC ETTs (or those prepackaged with a matching arcuate-shaped stylet) is difficult to maneuver in the mouth and hypopharynx. They have a wide side-to-side dimension when viewed down the long axis, causing the tube to contact the sides of the mouth, tongue, and teeth. As efforts are made to direct the tip upward, for example, the midsection of the tube will contact the teeth when used with a stylet, causing bending of the midsection of the tube and stylet. The other problem with an arcuate-shaped tube (and stylet) is that minor rotational change will cause the distal tip to move substantially. When this occurs at the last moment of insertion toward the target, the midsection of the tube may visually block the target itself, leading to inadvertent and unseen passage of the tube into the esophagus.

A straight-to-cuff shaped tube and stylet has a narrow long axis and offers significant visual advantages than a tube alone, or a tube with an arcuate-shaped stylet.[56,57] When viewed down the long axis it has a very narrow dimension. It can be passed into the mouth and easily maneuvered without obscuring the target as it advanced toward the target. The ideal method of inserting an ETT is to always pass the tube from beneath the line-of-sight, and bring the distal tube tip up from below, passing over the interarytenoid notch under direct vision without obscuring the target itself. Many practitioners prefer using a styletted tube for all tracheal intubations because of this maneuverability and visualization advantage. When the tube is first inserted in the extreme right corner of the mouth, the tube is placed visually behind the maxilla, and the distal tip is not even seen. By rocking the proximal tube backward, the distal tip moves posteriorly from behind the maxilla, up into the line-of-sight, and anteriorly until it is placed above the posterior landmarks of the larynx and into the trachea.

8.7.2 Where exactly should the styletted tube be bent, and what is the appropriate angle to use to maximize tip visualization, but not mechanically affect insertion?

The historic approach to stylet shaping is to use a hockey stick. But this does not define the optimal bend point, or the proper angle. A more precise terminology is to use the term straight-to-cuff stylet shaping, followed by an angle not exceeding 35 degrees to the tube tip.[58] This narrow long-axis shape is ideal for tube delivery toward the glottis, without blocking the line-of-sight. It still provides enough of a bend upward allowing the distal tube tip to be easily seen. The bend point should be at the proximal end of the cuff and the stylet should stop at the distal end of the cuff. The stylet can be dangerous if it protrudes beyond the tube tip. It can cause the tip to be too stiff even if it extends just to the tip of the tube. By stopping the stylet tip at the distal cuff, it provides an effective bend without stiffening the tip of the tube.

Angles beyond 35 degrees confer no visual advantage and hinder maneuverability within the mouth and hypopharynx. After the tip has passed into the trachea, bend angles above 35 degrees cause the tip of the tube to impact on the anterior tracheal rings.[58] This phenomenon explains why it is possible to have a correctly sized tube between the vocal cords and be unable to pass the tube, even though the trachea itself is large enough to accept it.

8.7.3 What should the practitioner do if the tube tip catches in the cricothyroid space or on the tracheal rings after insertion?

One option is to withdraw the stylet without withdrawing the tube itself. An assistant is necessary to do this since the practitioner will be holding the laryngoscope in their left hand and the tube in their right hand. By reducing the stiffness of the distal tube it may then be able to advance into the trachea. This maneuver however can easily result in dislodgement of the tube with resultant esophageal intubation on advancement.

Another option to rectify this mechanical hang-up on the anterior tracheal wall is to rotate the tube clockwise if resistance is felt.

By turning the tube 90 degrees clockwise, the standard left-facing bevel of the ETT moves from facing leftward to facing upward. The leading edge of the tube rotates downward, away from the rings by this movement and it disengages.[57]

If time permits, Hung et al suggested the combination of softening of the ETT by immersing the ETT in warm saline solution, and reverse loading of the ETT onto the stylet may potentially overcome the problems with the hang up during intubation.[59] With the reverse loading, the tip of the ETT is more likely to be directed down the trajectory of the trachea during the retraction of the stylet, making it easier to advance.

8.7.4 What are the options for an epiglottis-only view?

Assuming every effort has been made to maximize laryngeal view with the laryngoscope, there are several options for intubation. The first of these is to hug the undersurface of the epiglottis with the straight-to-cuff styletted tube, and being mindful of the tip orientation (keeping it upright), to insert the tube blindly. In general, blind insertion should be avoided.

An ETI can be used for intubation in epiglottis-only views. Newer disposable tracheal tube introducers are inexpensive. When compared with the use of a stylet in simulated Cormack/Lehane Grade 3 views, the success rates using this device is as high as 96% with the ETI and 66% using a stylet.[60]

In the true epiglottis-only view, the tip of the ETI is directed upward, hugging the undersurface of the epiglottis. Practitioners should be aware that minor rotational change will cause the tip to move lateral to the aryepiglottic fold (missing the larynx). The Eschmann tracheal introducer (ETI) is approximately 60 cm long, straight over its entire length, except for its distal end, which has a slight upward bend (Coude tip). The original Portex product (made of resin-covered fiberglass) has a bend angle of 38 degrees and this angle has been copied in the many disposable tracheal introducers now produced. After the tracheal introducer has passed into the trachea, the anterior tracheal rings may be felt (clicks) as the rounded tip passes over them. This occurs in 60% to 95% of cases, but it is practitioner and situation dependent, and also a function of the orientation of the distal tip. If the tip rotates downward after insertion, the tip will ride along the posterior membranous portion of the trachea and not pass over the rings (ie, no tactile feedback of tracheal placement). In the trachea, as the tip passes beyond the main stem bronchus, the narrowing diameter will cause it to stop between 30 and 35 cm. This distinct endpoint is more reliable in assessing tracheal placement. On reaching this endpoint, the tracheal introducer should be pulled back by 2 to 3 cm. When the tracheal introducer is placed into the esophagus, no rings are felt, and there should be no limit to advancement.

After tracheal introducer placement, the ETT is placed over the proximally stabilized tracheal introducer (by an assistant) and slid down (*railroaded*) its length into the mouth and ultimately the trachea. The laryngoscope should be maintained in the same position as was achieved during the initial laryngoscopy attempt. This promotes a long-axis slide of the ETT over the tracheal introducer. Without the laryngoscope, the tracheal introducer will bend in the pharynx and be surrounded by adjacent soft tissues which can cause difficulties with tube advancement. The beveled leading edge of the larger diameter ETT can holdup at the laryngeal inlet (right aryepiglottic fold, right arytenoid cartilage, or right vocal cord) as the tube is advanced over the tracheal introducer. This can be avoided by using a smaller ETT. This holdup is easily managed by turning (quarter turn) the ETT counterclockwise as it approaches the laryngeal inlet. This maneuver positions the bevel facing inferiorly, allowing uninhibited passage into the trachea.

It is important to note that there is major difference between the Cormack/Lehane Grade 3A and 3B—the latter being the situation where the epiglottis is visible but lies against the posterior hypopharyngeal wall. In this situation the tracheal introducer is not stiff enough to lift the epiglottis and it becomes more difficult to direct it into the glottis. The true incidence of this view is not known, and as stated earlier, may relate to improper blade tip placement deflecting the epiglottis posteriorly.

A more effective means for approaching the epiglottis-only view for practitioners who have acquired the skill is to use a malleable optical stylet.[61] This permits target visualization either through an eyepiece or a monitor and the stylet tip can be advanced under indirect vision into the trachea. These devices require significant handling experience and recognition of fiberoptic landmarks and are addressed in Chapter 10.

8.8   SUMMARY

Placement of a tracheal tube under direct vision using a laryngoscope remains one of the most important skills to master for all airway practitioners. Many types of laryngoscopes with curve and straight blades have been developed over the years with the objectives to improve visualization of the glottis and easy passage of the tracheal tube. While these devices are highly effective and safe, they all have limitations. To improve outcome and minimize the risk of complications, basic principles and techniques must be applied when performing a laryngoscopic intubation.

REFERENCES

1. Zeitels SM. Universal modular glottiscope system: the evolution of a century of design and technique for direct laryngoscopy. *Ann Otol Rhinol Laryngol.* Suppl 1999;179:2-24.
2. Jackson C. *Bronchoscopy and Esophagoscopy. A Manual of Peroral Endoscopy and Laryngeal Surgery.* Philadelphia, PA: W. B. Saunders; 1922.
3. Miller RA. A new laryngoscope. *Anesthesiology.* 1941;2:318-320.
4. Macintosh RR. A new laryngoscope. *Lancet.* 1943;1:205.
5. Delport SD, Gibson BH. Ingestion of a laryngoscope light bulb during tracheal intubation. *S Afr Med J.* 1992;81:579.
6. Naumovski L, Schaffer K, Fleisher B. Ingestion of a laryngoscope light bulb during delivery room resuscitation. *Pediatrics.* 1991;87:581-582.
7. Cheung KW, Kovacs G, Law JA, Brousseau P, Hill W. Illumination of bulb-on-blade laryngoscopes in the out-of-hospital setting. *Acad Emerg Med.* 2007;14: 496-499.
8. Levitan RM, Kelly JJ, Kinkle WC, Fasano C. Light intensity of curved laryngoscope blades in Philadelphia emergency departments. *Ann Emerg Med.* 2007;50:253-257.
9. Illuminating Engineering Society of North America, Committee for Health Care Facilities. *Lighting for Hospitals and Health Care Facilities.* New York: Illuminating Engineering Society of North America; 2006.
10. International Organization for Standardization (ISO). *Standardization. of Anaesthetic and Respiratory Equipment—Laryngoscopes for Tracheal Intubation.* Geneva: ISO; 2005.
11. Chisholm DG, Calder I. Experience with the McCoy laryngoscope in difficult laryngoscopy. *Anaesthesia.* 1997;52:906-908.
12. Haridas RP. The McCoy levering laryngoscope blade. *Anaesthesia.* 1996;51:91.
13. Johnston HM, Rao U. The McCoy levering laryngoscope blade. *Anaesthesia.* 1994;49:358.
14. Laurent SC, de Melo AE, Alexander-Williams JM. The use of the McCoy laryngoscope in patients with simulated cervical spine injuries. *Anaesthesia.* 1996;51:74-75.
15. Uchida T, Hikawa Y, Saito Y, Yasuda K. The McCoy levering laryngoscope in patients with limited neck extension. *Can J Anaesth.* 1997;44:674-676.
16. Ward M. The McCoy levering laryngoscope blade. *Anaesthesia.* 1994;49: 357-358.
17. Gerlach K, Wenzel V, von Knobelsdorff G, Steinfath M, Dörges V. A new universal laryngoscope blade: a preliminary comparison with Macintosh laryngoscope blades. *Resuscitation.* 2003;57:63-67.
18. Kelley MA, Boskovich S, Allegretti PJ. Laryngoscope blade review. *Am J Emerg Med.* 2008;26:952-955.
19. Levitan RM, Mechem CC, Ochroch EA, Shofer FS, Hollander JE. Head-elevated laryngoscopy position: improving laryngeal exposure during laryngoscopy by increasing head elevation. *Ann Emerg Med.* 2003;41: 322-330.
20. Crosby ET. Airway management in adults after cervical spine trauma. *Anesthesiology.* 2006;104:1293-1318.
21. Manoach S, Paladino L. Manual in-line stabilization for acute airway management of suspected cervical spine injury: historical review and current questions. *Ann Emerg Med.* 2007;50:236-245.
22. Manoach S, Paladino L. Laryngoscopy force, visualization, and intubation failure in acute trauma: should we modify the practice of manual in-line stabilization? *Anesthesiology.* 2009;110:6-7.
23. Henderson JJ. The use of paraglossal straight blade laryngoscopy in difficult tracheal intubation. *Anaesthesia.* 1997;52:552-560.
24. Heath KJ. The effect of laryngoscopy of different cervical spine immobilisation techniques. *Anaesthesia.* 1994;49:843-845.
25. Robitaille A, Williams SR, Tremblay MH, Guilbert F, Thériault M, Drolet P. Cervical spine motion during tracheal intubation with manual in-line stabilization: direct laryngoscopy versus GlideScope videolaryngoscopy. *Anesth Analg.* 2008;106:935-941.
26. Benumof JL, Cooper SD. Quantitative improvement in laryngoscopic view by optimal external laryngeal manipulation. *J Clin Anesth.* 1996;8:136-140.
27. Knill RL. Difficult laryngoscopy made easy with a "BURP". *Can J Anaesth.* 1993;40:279-282.
28. Levitan RM, Higgins MS, Ochroch EA. Contrary to popular belief and traditional instruction, the larynx is sighted one eye at a time during direct laryngoscopy. *Acad Emerg Med.* 1998;5:844-846.
29. Yentis SM. Predicting difficult intubation—worthwhile exercise or pointless ritual? *Anaesthesia.* 2002;57:105-109.
30. Shiga T, Wajima Z, Inoue T, Sakamoto A. Predicting difficult intubation in apparently normal patients: a meta-analysis of bedside screening test performance. *Anesthesiology.* 2005;103:429-437.
31. Mort TC. Emergency tracheal intubation: complications associated with repeated laryngoscopic attempts. *Anesth Analg.* 2004;99:607-613.
32. Cormack RS, Lehane J. Difficult tracheal intubation in obstetrics. *Anaesthesia.* 1984;39:1105-1111.
33. Cook TM. A new practical classification of laryngeal view. *Anaesthesia.* 2000;55:274-279.
34. Levitan RM, Ochroch EA, Kush S, Shofer FS, Hollander JE. Assessment of airway visualization: validation of the percentage of glottic opening (POGO) scale. *Acad Emerg Med.* 1998;5:919-923.
35. Ochroch EA, Hollander JE, Kush S, Shofer FS, Levitan RM. Assessment of laryngeal view: percentage of glottic opening score vs Cormack and Lehane grading. *Can J Anaesth.* 1999;46:987-990.
36. Adnet F, Borron SW, Racine SX, et al. The intubation difficulty scale (IDS): proposal and evaluation of a new score characterizing the complexity of endotracheal intubation. *Anesthesiology.* 1997;87:1290-1297.
37. Benumof JL. Difficult laryngoscopy: obtaining the best view. *Can J Anaesth.* 1994;41:361-365.
38. Boyce JR, Ness T, Castroman P, Gleysteen JJ. A preliminary study of the optimal anesthesia positioning for the morbidly obese patient. *Obes Surg.* 2003;13:4-9.
39. Dixon BJ, Dixon JB, Carden JR, et al. Preoxygenation is more effective in the 25 degrees head-up position than in the supine position in severely obese patients: a randomized controlled study. *Anesthesiology.* 2005;102:1110-1115.

40. Lane S, Saunders D, Schofield A, Padmanabhan R, Hildreth A, Laws D. A prospective, randomised controlled trial comparing the efficacy of pre-oxygenation in the 20 degrees head-up vs supine position. *Anaesthesia.* 2005;60:1064-1067.

41. Benumof JL. Preoxygenation: best method for both efficacy and efficiency. *Anesthesiology.* 1999;91:603-605.

42. Benumof JL, Dagg R, Benumof R. Critical hemoglobin desaturation will occur before return to an unparalyzed state following 1 mg/kg intravenous succinylcholine. *Anesthesiology.* 1997;87:979-982.

43. Mort TC. Preoxygenation in critically ill patients requiring emergency tracheal intubation. *Crit Care Med.* 2005;33:2672-2675.

44. Sellick BA. Cricoid pressure to control regurgitation of stomach contents during induction of anaesthesia. *Lancet.* 1961;2:404-406.

45. Satiani B, Bonner JT, Stone HH. Factors influencing intraoperative gastric regurgitation: a prospective random study of nasogastric tube drainage. *Arch Surg.* 1978;113:721-723.

46. Levitan RM, Kinkle WC, Levin WJ, Everett WW. Laryngeal view during laryngoscopy: a randomized trial comparing cricoid pressure, backward-upward-rightward pressure, and bimanual laryngoscopy. *Ann Emerg Med.* 2006;47:548-555.

47. Smith KJ, Dobranowski J, Yip G, Daulphin A, Choi PTL. Cricoid pressure displaces the esophagus: an observational study using magnetic resonance imaging. *Anesthesiology.* 2003;99:60-64.

48. Smith KJ, Ladak S, Choi PT, Dobranowski J. The cricoid cartilage and the esophagus are not aligned in close to half of adult patients. *Can J Anaesth.* 2002;49:503-507.

49. Ellis DY, Harris T, Zideman D. Cricoid pressure in emergency department rapid sequence tracheal intubations: a risk-benefit analysis. *Ann Emerg Med.* 2007;50:653-665.

50. Neilipovitz DT, Crosby ET. No evidence for decreased incidence of aspiration after rapid sequence induction. *Can J Anaesth.* 2007;54:748-764.

51. Johnston RH. Extension and flexion in direct laryngoscopy: a comparative study. *Ann Oto Rhino Laryn.* 1910;19:19-24.

52. Cattano D, Melnikov V, Khalil Y, Sridhar S, Hagberg CA. An evaluation of the rapid airway management positioner in obese patients undergoing gastric bypass or laparoscopic gastric banding surgery. *Obes Surg.* 2010;20:1436-1441.

53. Levitan RM, Goldman TS, Bryan DA, et al. Training with video imaging improves the initial intubation success rates of paramedic trainees in an operating room setting. *Ann Emerg Med.* 2001;37:46-50.

54. Mulcaster JT, Mills J, Hung OR, et al. Laryngoscopic intubation: learning and performance. *Anesthesiology.* 2003;98:23-27.

55. Ovassapian A, Glassenberg R, Randel GI, Klock A, Mesnick PS, Klafta JM. The unexpected difficult airway and lingual tonsil hyperplasia: a case series and a review of the literature. *Anesthesiology.* 2002;97:124-132.

56. Levitan RM. *The Airway Cam Guide to Intubation and Practical Emergency Airway Management.* Wayne, PA: Airway Cam Technologies, Inc.; 2004.

57. Levitan RM, Kinkle WC. *The Airway Cam Pocket Guide to Intubation.* 2nd ed. Wayne, PA: Airway Cam Technologies, Inc.; 2007.

58. Levitan RM, Pisaturo JT, Kinkle WC, Butler K, Everett WW. Stylet bend angles and tracheal tube passage using a straight-to-cuff shape. *Acad Emerg Med.* 2006;13:1255-1258.

59. Hung OR, Tibbet JS, Cheng R, Law JA. Proper preparation of the Trachlight™ and endotracheal tube to facilitate intubation. *Can J Anaesth.* 2006;53:107-108.

60. Gataure PS, Vaughan RS, Latto IP. Simulated difficult intubation. Comparison of the gum elastic bougie and the stylet. *Anaesthesia.* 1996;51:935-938.

61. Levitan RM. Design rationale and intended use of a short optical stylet for routine fiberoptic augmentation of emergency laryngoscopy. *Am J Emerg Med.* 2006;24:490-495.

SELF-EVALUATION QUESTIONS

8.1. Regarding the mechanics of laryngoscopy, all are true **EXCEPT**

A. A fully extended arm position permits binocular sighting of the larynx for most operators.

B. A low grip, that is, where the blade meets the handle, provides greater control with less muscular effort.

C. Morbidly obese patients require proper ear-to-sternal notch positioning before laryngoscope insertion, since dynamic lifting of the head during the procedure is impossible.

D. The degree of lifting force applied during laryngoscopy is minimal when advancing the curved blade down the tongue and maximal after the blade is correctly positioned in the vallecula.

8.2. Bimanual laryngoscopy is

A. distinct from cricoid pressure because is applied by the laryngoscopist

B. distinct from cricoid pressure because it is done to improve laryngeal view

C. distinct from backward upward rightward pressure (BURP) because it is done by the operator, not an assistant

D. distinct from cricoid pressure because it is generally applied at the thyroid cartilage, not the cricoid ring

E. all of the above

8.3. The mechanical problem of railroading an endotracheal tube over a tube introducer (or a flexible bronchoscope)

A. can be overcome by rotating the tracheal tube counterclockwise (leftward) at 14 to 16 cm of insertion

B. is a consequence of the asymmetric left-facing bevel of a standard tracheal tube

C. is due to the gap between the outer diameter of the introducer (or scope) and the inner diameter of the tracheal tube

D. occurs at the laryngeal inlet, specifically at the right aryepiglottic fold and right posterior cartilages

E. all of the above

CHAPTER (9)

Flexible Bronchoscopic Intubation

Ian R. Morris

9.1 INTRODUCTION

9.1.1 How did bronchoscopic intubation develop?

The first recorded endoscopic tracheal intubation was reported by Murphy in 1967.[1] In that case report, the trachea of a patient with Still's disease was successfully intubated through the nose using a flexible choledochoscope.[1] The flexible fiberoptic bronchoscope was introduced into clinical practice in 1964, and although it was not developed for the purpose of airway management, its value as a device to facilitate endotracheal intubation was soon appreciated.[2,3] A series of 100 tracheal intubations using the flexible bronchoscope was reported in 1972, with a success rate of 96%.[4] However, utilization of flexible fiberoptic technology for endotracheal intubation remained limited among health-care providers throughout the 1970s and 1980s.[5] Seventy-five percent of those who completed questionnaires at a series of fiberoptic bronchoscope workshops between 1984 and 1989 had either no or minimal experience with the technique.[5] Following the publication of the ASA Guidelines on Difficult Airway Management in 1993,[6] the use of flexible bronchoscopic intubation among anesthesia practitioners greatly increased[7] and the technique has come to play a pivotal role in the management of the difficult airway.[8]

Although it has been advocated as the technique of choice in the management of the difficult intubation,[9-12] this view is not universally shared and a reluctance to perform awake bronchoscopic intubation continues to occur.[13,14] However, surveys from the United States, France, and Denmark published between 1998 and 2001 confirm the widespread use of flexible bronchoscopes particularly for management of the anticipated difficult airway.[15-18]

9.1.2 When is bronchoscopic intubation indicated?

The primary indication for bronchoscopic intubation is in the elective (or at least nonemergency) management of the anticipated difficult airway.

When endotracheal intubation is required and there has been a history of previous difficult intubation, or if difficult direct laryngoscopy is predicted on airway assessment, and in particular, when mask-ventilation is also predicted to be difficult, bronchoscopic intubation can be an invaluable alternative intubation technique. Although bronchoscopic intubation in this setting can be achieved under general anesthesia (GA), awake intubation maintains a wide margin of safety.[19-21] In general, if airway compromise or respiratory distress exists, awake intubation similarly maintains a wide margin of safety.[19] However, in this circumstance, the urgency with which airway control must be achieved and the extent of the airway compromise may limit the choice of technique, and bronchoscopic intubation may not be feasible or appropriate. In addition, incomplete local anesthesia of the upper airway makes bronchoscopic intubation more difficult, as does the presence of blood and secretions in the airway. Complete airway obstruction has been reported following the topical application of local anesthesia to the airway and suctioning in preparation for awake intubation in a stridorous patient with recurrent neck carcinoma and radiation therapy.[22] Complete airway obstruction after application of topical local anesthesia to the upper airway was also reported by Shaw et al in a patient with a compromised airway secondary to goiter.[23] Listro et al demonstrated a transitory but profound obstruction at the level of the glottis or supraglottis during forced inspiratory and expiratory vital capacity maneuvers that was produced in normal subjects with local anesthesia of the upper airway.[24] Kuna et al and Beydon et al also found a decrease in upper-airway caliber following local anesthesia of the airway in normal subjects.[25,26] Patients with severe airway obstruction due to edema or tumor must be approached with extreme caution if completion airway obstruction is to be avoided[3] (see Chapter 3).

In the presence of potential cervical spine instability, no intubation technique has been shown to be clearly superior.[19,20,27–31] However, movement of the cervical spine must be minimized during intubation if neurologic injury is to be avoided. Flexible bronchoscopic intubation (FBI) can be a valuable alternative in this setting and has been extensively used.[28,32] Complete airway obstruction has however been reported during attempted awake bronchoscopic intubation in this patient population.[32]

FBI can also be used as an alternative to direct laryngoscopy in any patient for whom intubation is indicated, and in particular when a high risk of dental injury exists.[3] In the setting of failed intubation by direct laryngoscopy or other techniques, FBI can be an invaluable option.

9.1.3   When is flexible bronchoscopic intubation best avoided?

Contraindications to FBI must be considered relative and weighed against the risks associated with alternative airway management techniques.[19] Some measure of patient cooperation is required for awake FBI, and the total absence of cooperation may preclude this technique, as can bleeding in the airway and massive tissue disruption.[3,19] Fixed laryngeal obstruction with stridor at rest implies a reduction in the caliber of the airway to 4.0 mm or less in diameter.[33] FBI is unlikely to be successful in this setting and at best will produce a higher grade of obstruction when the scope is passed through the involved area. In this setting, a surgical airway (eg, awake tracheotomy) performed under local anesthesia is a better alternative.[34] FBI is contraindicated when immediate airway control is necessary and the time required to complete the procedure is not available.[7]

Patient refusal in the adult population without psychiatric disease is exceedingly rare if an appropriate explanation of the procedure has been provided.

9.2   EQUIPMENT

9.2.1   How do flexible bronchoscopes work? What is the best instrument for flexible bronchoscopic intubation?

The standard adult flexible bronchoscope remains unsurpassed as an instrument for bronchoscopic intubation in the vast majority of circumstances in the adult population. These bronchoscopes have a sufficient length (about 60 cm) to accommodate an endotracheal tube (ETT) ensleeved proximally while leaving an adequate distal segment for maneuverability. Shorter bronchoscopes tend to make FBI more difficult. A bronchoscope with an outside diameter of 5.9 to 6.0 mm will readily accommodate a 7-mm inner diameter (ID) ETT and has adequate stiffness to function well as a stylet over which to advance the ETT (see Figure 9-1).[19,35]

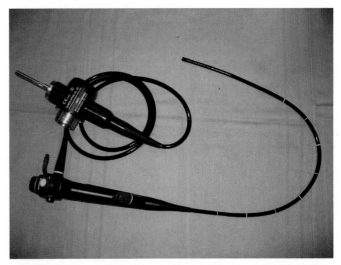

FIGURE 9-1. The adult flexible bronchoscope. An Olympus BF-XT160 is shown here with an insertion cord diameter of 6.3 mm and a length of 600 mm.

Bronchoscopes with thinner insertion cords tend to be more flexible and form a floppy stylet that is easily buckled away from the glottis as the ensleeved ETT is advanced into the airway (see Figure 9-2).[20]

The flexible bronchoscope consists of a proximal handle and a distal insertion cord or shaft. An umbilical or universal cord is attached to the side of the handle and connects the bronchoscope to an external light source (see Figure 9-3). Modern flexible bronchoscopes include fiberoptic bronchoscopes, video bronchoscopes, and hybrid designs. Flexible fiberoptic bronchoscopes are also available with a battery-operated light source, which greatly improves portability. The handle of the bronchoscope is fitted with a lever which controls flexion of the tip of the scope (the bending section)[11,36] in a single plane; the movement of the tip being produced by two wires which connect the control lever to

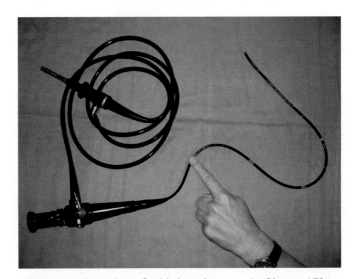

FIGURE 9-2. The pediatric flexible bronchoscope. An Olympus LF2 is shown here with an insertion cord diameter of 4 mm and a length of 600 mm. Note the increased flexibility of the thinner insertion cord.

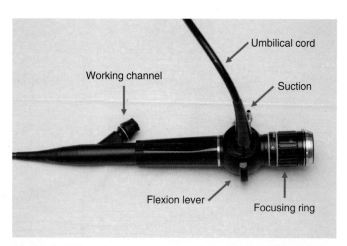

FIGURE 9-3. Features of the flexible bronchoscope: it consists of a proximal handle and a distal insertion cord or shaft. An umbilical or universal cord is attached to the side of the handle and connects the bronchoscope to an external light source. The handle also contains the proximal port of the working channel, a suction port, and the flexion lever.

the tip of the scope (see Figure 9-3).[11] The handle also contains the proximal port of the working channel which extends distally to the tip of the scope. This channel can be used to pass various instruments into the airway and can be used for irrigation, administration of medications, and suction. Oxygen insufflation has been used via the working channel; however gastric rupture has been reported with this technique.[37] Light is transmitted from the external light source to the tip of the insertion cord via a fiberoptic bundle made up of thin glass rods (see Figure 9-4).[11,36,38] In the flexible fiberoptic scope, light reflected from the object being viewed is focused by a lens located at the tip of the insertion cord onto the distal end of a second fiberoptic bundle which then

transmits the image to a second lens located in the eye piece.[11,36] The glass fibers in this image transmission bundle remain in the same relative location along the length of the bundle (coherent bundle) such that a mosaic image is accurately reconstructed at the eye piece.[11,36] The image seen through the scope is focused by means of a control located in the handle. In the video bronchoscope, a charged coupled device or silicone chip is located at the distal tip of the insertion cord and is used to sense and transmit the image (see Figure 9-5).[36] The image data are then transmitted electronically through the bronchoscope to an external video processing unit.[36] The image is then displayed on a screen and can be printed, stored electronically, or transmitted to a remote location.[36] A video camera can be coupled to the eye piece of a conventional fiberoptic bronchoscope. However, the image obtained is inferior to that provided by the video bronchoscope.[36]

Bronchoscopes are produced by a number of different manufacturers and are available with insertion cord diameters ranging from 2.2 to 6.3 mm.[36] In general, minimizing the discrepancy between the outside diameter (OD) of the bronchoscope and the internal diameter (ID) of the ensleeved ETT facilitates passage of the tube through the larynx over the scope.[2,3,20,39-45] Bronchoscopes with smaller diameter insertion cords have allowed FBI to be performed in the pediatric population, and very thin scopes such as the Olympus BF-N$_2$O with a shaft diameter of 2.2 mm can be used in infants. However, use of pediatric bronchoscopes to

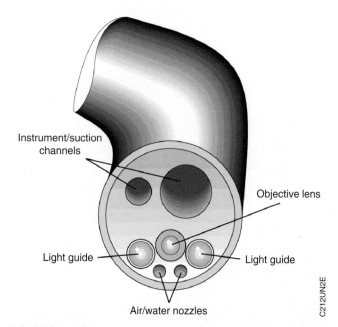

FIGURE 9-4. Schematic diagram of the cross section of the insertion cord of a flexible fiberoptic bronchoscope. (ECRI. Bronchoscopes. In: *Healthcare Product Comparison System.* Hospital ed. Plymouth Meeting, PA: ECRI; 2004.)

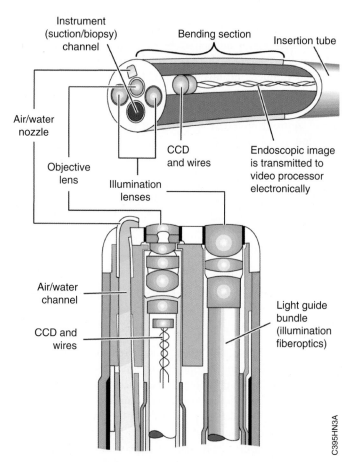

FIGURE 9-5. Schematic diagram of the insertion cord of a flexible videobronchoscope. (ECRI. Bronchoscopes. In: *Healthcare Product Comparison System.* Hospital ed. Plymouth Meeting, PA: ECRI; 2004.)

perform FBI of the adult in general makes the procedure more difficult.[20] The use of a pediatric bronchoscope to perform awake intubation in the adult with severe upper-airway obstruction may be complicated by complete obstruction and must be approached with great caution.[3,22,34,46,]

Bronchoscopes are delicate instruments and must be handled with care if damage to the instrument is to be avoided. Damage to the bronchoscope is not only costly to repair but it also means that the scope is unavailable for clinical use for a period of time.[11] Striking the distal tip of the insertion cord against a hard surface or excessive bending or twisting of the shaft of the scope can damage the lens and fiberoptic bundles, respectively.[36] If the external shaft of the insertion cord or the working channel wall is punctured, fluids can enter the inside of the scope and lead to a degradation or loss of the image transmitted.[36]

Flexible bronchoscopes with shaft diameters of 3.5 to 4.0 mm can readily be passed through the lumen of a #35-Fr or larger double-lumen tube and are invaluable for the precise tube placement required for lung isolation.

9.2.2   How are flexible bronchoscopes disinfected?

In general, the issue of sterilization of bronchoscopes is addressed by infection control and risk management personnel in each health-care facility.[36] Specific recommendations for sterilization are also provided by each manufacturer.[11,36] A typical sterilization process is as follows:

Immediately following a bronchoscopic procedure, a premixed enzymatic solution is suctioned through the working channel(s) of the bronchoscope and the instrument is wiped down with a lint-free cloth saturated with the premixed enzymatic solution. This is considered to be a "preclean setup" in the sterilization process and is performed at the bedside. The scope is then transferred to the sterile processing department where a leak tester is connected to the umbilical cord or handle and the inside of the scope is pressurized with air. The scope is then immersed in a water bath for 30 seconds and observed for escaping bubbles. The scope is removed from the water bath, the leak tester disconnected from the pressure source, and the scope allowed to vent at atmospheric pressure before the tester is disconnected from the self-sealing port. The scope is then placed in a predetermined concentration of an enzymatic solution and the working channels and external controls manually cleaned with appropriate brushes. The working channels are also flushed with the enzymatic solution followed by water and air. The scope is then immersed in a solution of peracetic acid using specially designed equipment that ensures flow through the working channels. These channels are subsequently irrigated with air and alcohol before the scope is dried manually and with an air flush. The sterilization process requires about 50 to 60 minutes to complete. If the scope is not reused within 1 week of the sterilization process, the sterilization is repeated. Glutaraldehyde, hydrogen peroxide, and ortho-phthalaldehyde (Cidex OPA) can also be used for disinfection of bronchoscopes.[36] Ethylene oxide (ETO) sterilization is also an effective agent for sterilization of bronchoscopes, although the process requires about 18 hours to complete. When the scope is *gassed*, an ETO cap must be attached to the leak tester port to permit the gas to enter the scope and thereby equalize internal and external pressures.[11]

Recently, it has been shown that routine cleaning and autoclaving do not remove protein material, including prions, from reusable airway devices,[47] and concern has been expressed with respect to the possible transmission of infection with subsequent usage.[48] Currently there is no information available with regard to the cleaning of bronchoscopes such that the absence of protein deposits can be ensured. Similarly, the risk of cross-contamination of patients following a standard cleaning procedure for the flexible bronchoscope is unknown.

9.3   TECHNIQUE

9.3.1   How is the bronchoscope maneuvered? What are the key aspects of technique for fast, successful bronchoscopic intubation?

The bronchoscope is most easily maneuvered by holding the handle of the scope in the palm of the dominant (usually right) hand with the **thumb** placed on the **flexion** lever (see Figure 9-6). The fingers should comfortably encircle the handle of the scope and the index finger can be used to activate the suction mechanism, although if antisialogogues are used, suction is rarely required during FBI. When the scope is held such that the flexion lever is in the 6 o'clock position, moving the lever downward (toward the shaft of the scope) flexes the tip of the scope upward toward the 12 o'clock position. Conversely, moving the lever up toward the proximal aspect of the handle flexes the tip downward toward the 6 o'clock position (see Figure 9-7). Movement of the flexion lever (**thumb flexion**) then flexes the tip of the scope *in a single plane*. To flex the tip in any other plane, *the entire instrument must be rotated* clockwise or counterclockwise using the wrist and hand holding the handle of

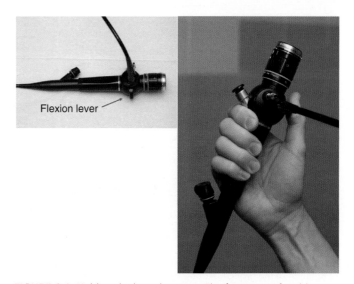

FIGURE 9-6. Holding the bronchoscope. The fingers comfortably encircle the handle. The thumb is placed on the flexion lever.

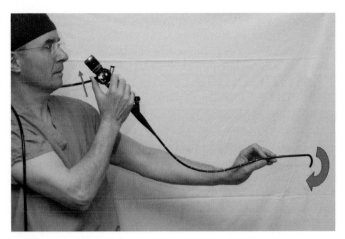

FIGURE 9-7. Movement of the flexion lever flexes the tip of the insertion cord in a single plane.

the scope. This **wrist rotation** is the second important and perhaps not intuitively obvious movement required when manipulating the bronchoscope during FBI (see Figures 9-8A and B). The tip of the bronchoscope can then be manipulated to view objects in any plane within the scope's field of vision by a combination of **wrist rotation and thumb flexion**. Many bronchoscopes have a triangular marker or divot[7,49] located at the 12 o'clock position at the periphery of the scope's field of vision (see Figure 9-9). This marker

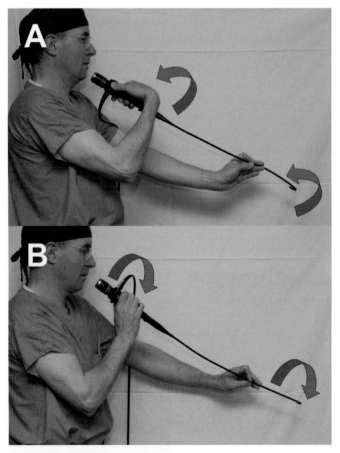

FIGURE 9-8. (A) Rotation of the bronchoscope counterclockwise. (B) Rotation of the bronchoscope clockwise. The entire instrument is rotated using the wrist at the handle of the scope. The hand holding the shaft allows the instrument to rotate.

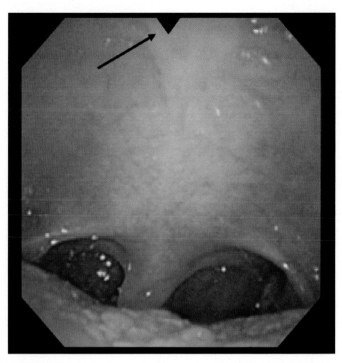

FIGURE 9-9. The marker or *divot* located at 12 o'clock (arrow) in the scope's field of vision.

helps the practitioner maintain spatial orientation as the tip of the scope always flexes in the diametrical plane of the marker. When a video camera is coupled to a fiberoptic bronchoscope, the divot must be adjusted to the 12 o'clock position (opposite the flexion lever on the handle) to maintain correct orientation.[49] The practitioner's nondominant (usually left) hand holds the shaft or insertion cord of the bronchoscope a few centimeters proximal to the tip with the forearm pronated (see Figure 9-10). The shaft should be held lightly between the thumb and index finger, and stabilized between the ring and middle finger or some other combination of digits. The hand that holds the distal shaft of the scope must feed the scope forward into the airway in a controlled manner without excessive (shaky) movement that can make visualization difficult.

Generally it is easier to rotate the bronchoscope using the dominant (usually right) hand positioned at the handle. The nondominant

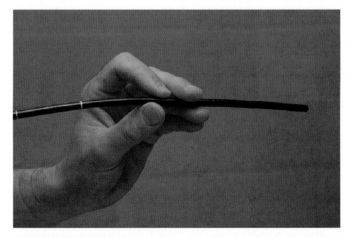

FIGURE 9-10. Holding the insertion cord of the bronchoscope. With the forearm pronated, the nondominant hand holds the insertion cord a few centimeters proximal to the tip of the bronchoscope.

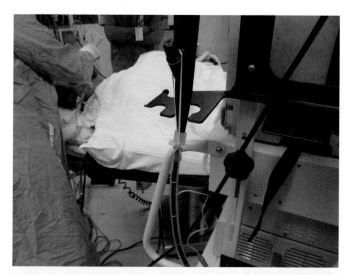

FIGURE 9-11. A 7.5-mm ID PVC ETT ensleeved over the adult bronchoscope and fixed to the handle with an elastic band.

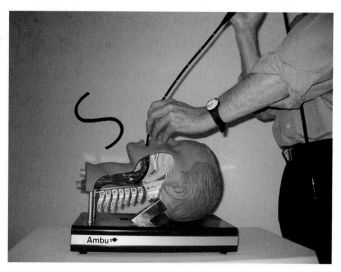

FIGURE 9-12. Flexible bronchoscopic intubation performed from the head of the bed requires the insertion cord to negotiate an S-shaped curve and the patient must be supine or nearly supine.

hand holding the distal aspect of the shaft **must however allow the shaft to rotate,** and therefore the shaft cannot be gripped tightly. If the distal aspect of the shaft is held tightly, rotation at the handle twists the insertion cord, the scope fails to go in the desired direction, and the components in the shaft can be damaged. Although rotation of the scope is usually more easily controlled by the hand positioned at the handle, the nondominant hand holding the distal shaft can also be used to rotate the instrument. In that maneuver, the hand at the handle **must follow the movement and allow the entire instrument to rotate as a single unit,** or again, twisting of the shaft will occur and the scope fails to go in the desired direction (see Figures 9-8A and B). As experience is gained in handling of the scope, the shaft does not need to be held taut to maneuver the tip. However, holding the shaft of the scope relatively straight can be useful to maintain orientation and control movement. The most important concepts to master are **thumb flexion** and **wrist rotation.** In addition, during FBI, movements of the scope (flexion, rotation, and forward feeding) should be small, slow, and deliberate. Oversteering of the scope is a common error.

The ETT can be precut to a desired length to maximize the length of the insertion cord beyond the tube and thereby optimize maneuverability.[19] The inside of the tube can be lubricated using lidocaine spray or sterile water. The tube is then ensleeved proximally and fixed to the handle with a single piece of easily removable tape or an elastic band (see Figure 9-11).[19] A lubricant jelly placed on the cuff of the tube may facilitate glottic entry. Lubricating the shaft of the scope is unnecessary and makes it difficult to handle.

9.3.2 Is bronchoscopic intubation more easily performed from the head of the bed or from the patient's right side? What instructions should be given to the patient during the procedure?

Awake FBI can be performed with the practitioner standing at the head of the bed, and for those who are most familiar with visualization of the airway by direct laryngoscopy, this position

preserves the spatial orientation of the airway structures as they are viewed through the scope.[19,20] However, this position requires the practitioner to negotiate an S-shaped curve to the trachea (see Figure 9-12) and the patient to be supine or nearly supine. Standing at the patient's right side facing cephalad facilitates negotiation of the natural C-shaped curve of the airway (see Figure 9-13) and permits easy visualization of patient monitors, and as eye contact can be readily maintained this position may be less intimidating for the patient.[19,20] The patient may be supine or in the semi-sitting or sitting position.[20] The semi-seated or sitting position may also be less intimidating for the awake patient and may better maintain the patency of the pharyngeal lumen.[20,50] Extension at the atlanto-occipital joint moves the epiglottis anteriorly away from the posterior pharyngeal wall and facilitates passage of the bronchoscope through the pharynx.[3,20,45,51,52] Neck flexion, however, tends to produce pharyngeal obstruction and can make FBI more difficult.[20,51-53]

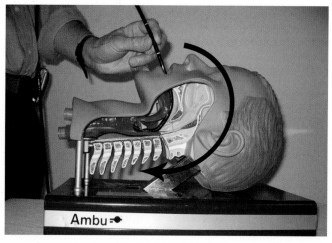

FIGURE 9-13. Flexible bronchoscopic intubation from the patient's right side requires the scope to negotiate a C-shaped curve.

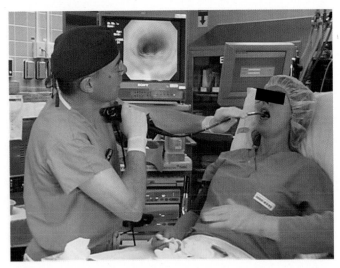

FIGURE 9-14. Flexible bronchoscopic intubation with the practitioner on the patient's right side facing the patient: the ETT is advanced in the midline during a deep inspiration while following the natural C-shaped curve of the airway.

For awake oral FBI, the author prefers to be positioned at the semi-sitting or sitting patient's right side (see Figure 9-14). The light source is to the practitioner's left, and the video screen is located in front of or slightly to the left of the practitioner. Oxygen can be administered by nasal prongs. An assistant is positioned at the patient's left side and provides gentle tongue traction using a piece of gauze.[20] The bronchoscope can be focused on printed material prior to insertion. Use of a bite block tends to push the tongue posteriorly and cephalad into the oropharyngeal isthmus, can make passage of the scope more difficult, and if adequate local anesthesia has been achieved, is not necessary.[20] The lens can be defogged using silicone solution or simply by holding the tip of the scope in warm water, or against the buccal mucosa for a few seconds to warm it and thereby prevent condensation.[19,20] The scope should be inserted into the oral cavity to the level of the dental arches in the midline, and then advanced a few centimeters posteriorly over the dorsum of the tongue following the midline groove toward **the first midline landmark, the uvula,** seen in the superior aspect of the scope's field of vision (see Figure 9-9).[20] Gently resting the hand holding the shaft of the scope on the patient's chin may help keep the scope in the midline.[20,45] If the uvula is in contact with the dorsal aspect of the tongue, the patient can be instructed to take a deep breath, thereby elevating the uvula and opening the oropharyngeal isthmus.[19,20] The scope is then advanced slowly forward just past the uvula and flexed caudally to visualize **the second midline landmark, the epiglottis,** seen inferiorly in the scope's field of vision (see Figure 9-15).[19,20] If the epiglottis is oriented posteriorly or is in contact with the posterior pharyngeal wall, the awake patient can again be instructed to take a deep breath and thereby move the epiglottis anteriorly to create an air space through which to pass the scope.[19,20] The scope is then passed, posterior to the epiglottis to visualize **the third midline landmark, the vocal cords** (see Figure 9-16).[19,20] If the bronchoscope is passed behind the epiglottis in the midline, then it is naturally lined up for the approach to the larynx. Conversely, if the bronchoscope is off midline at the level of the epiglottis, the

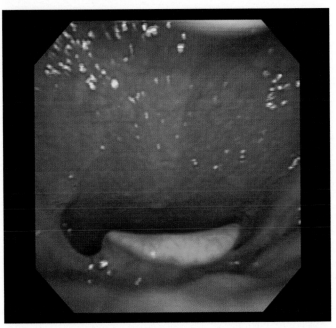

FIGURE 9-15. Bronchoscopic view of the second midline landmark (the epiglottis) during flexible bronchoscopic intubation with the practitioner on the patient's right side facing the patient.

approach to the larynx can be much more difficult. The scope is then advanced in the midline through the glottis and positioned proximal to the carina.[19,20] As the scope is advanced through the larynx, the patient is again instructed to take a deep breath to maximally abduct the vocal cords and thereby facilitate passage of the scope. As the bronchoscope is passed from the level of the dental arches to the trachea, flexion and rotation movements should be small and deliberate such that the scope can be kept in the midline

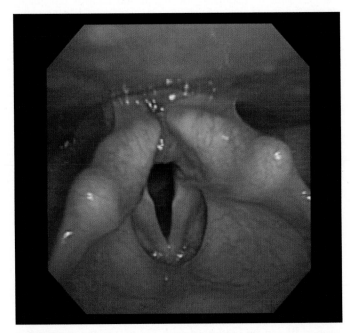

FIGURE 9-16. Bronchoscopic view of the third midline landmark (the vocal cords) during flexible bronchoscopic intubation with the practitioner on the patient's right side facing the patient.

and advanced along the C-shaped curve analogous to staying in a given lane during highway driving using small movements of the steering wheel. Unnecessary touching of the mucosa by the bronchoscope should be avoided. Having positioned the tip of the bronchoscope in the mid to distal trachea, the practitioner should then look directly at the patient and advance the ETT over the scope being careful to aim for the midline and to follow the natural curve of the airway (see Figure 9-14).[19,20] The bronchoscope must be kept stationary as the tube is advanced[9] in order to avoid inadvertent contact with the carina, cannulation of a main stem bronchus, or premature removal of the scope from the trachea. Again, as the tube is advanced, the patient should be instructed to take a deep breath to move the epiglottis anteriorly away from the advancing tube and to maximally abduct the vocal cords.[19,20] The correct intratracheal position of the ETT can be confirmed endoscopically before the scope is removed.[19,20] However, the presence of both the bronchoscope and ETT in the trachea produce a degree of airway obstruction that can be distressing for the awake patient, and the bronchoscope should be removed expeditiously once the ETT is in proper position. Correct position can be further confirmed by listening to and feeling gas exhaled via the ETT and by capnography.

9.3.3 How can difficulty in passing the ensleeved endotracheal tube into the trachea over the flexible bronchoscope be minimized?

Difficulty in passing the ensleeved ETT through the larynx has been variously reported to occur in 5% to 90% of FBIs,[42,54-58] and has occurred in awake patients, as well as those under GA, and with both the nasal and oral routes of tracheal intubation. During oral FBI, as the tube is advanced with the concave aspect of the tube facing anteriorly and the bevel facing toward the patient's left, the leading edge of the tube may meet resistance at the right arytenoid or aryepiglottic fold (see Figure 9-17).[56,59,60] Rotation of the tube

90 degrees counterclockwise orients the bevel posteriorly and the leading edge into the 12 o'clock position and has been advocated to improve passage of the ETT through the larynx.[60-63] Rotation of the tube counterclockwise may also keep the leading edge in closer contact with the bronchoscope and provide less of a gap between the two with which to catch a laryngeal structure.[64] During nasal FBI, it has been postulated that the tube tends to impinge on the epiglottis.[56,60,64] However the usual point of obstruction during nasal tracheal intubation may also be the right arytenoid.[64] Improved success rates have been reported for glottic cannulation during nasal FBI, using a 90-degree counterclockwise rotation of the tube.[56] Conversely, nasal FBI performed with the bevel up has also been advocated such that impingement on the epiglottis may be avoided.[63] In addition to the right arytenoid and epiglottis, impingement can occur at the posterior pharyngeal wall or other laryngeal structures.[58] The larger the discrepancy between the outside diameter of the bronchoscopic stylet and the internal diameter of the ensleeved ETT, the greater is the chance that the tube may impinge on laryngeal structures and resist entry into the trachea (see Figure 9-18).[2,3,20,41,42,59] Therefore this discrepancy should be minimized by choosing the largest bronchoscope which will easily fit into the ETT to be used.[20,44,45] In the adult, a bronchoscope with an outside diameter of 5.9 to 6.0 mm works well when used with a 7.5 to 8.5-mm ID ETT. When the combination of a relatively large bronchoscope and an ETT are both present in the trachea, the practitioner must be aware that a degree of airway obstruction has been produced[40] and the bronchoscope should be removed without delay following tube placement and confirmation. If the bronchoscope must remain inside the tube positioned in the trachea for a relatively long period as during diagnostic or therapeutic bronchoscopy, then the concentric airway remaining must be adequate to permit ventilation to occur.[20,40,65] Wire-reinforced spiral tubes are more flexible than polyvinyl chloride (PVC) tubes and may more easily follow the curve of the bronchoscope as it passes through the larynx.[20,59,65-68] Although flexible wire-reinforced tubes were reported to be associated with a lower rate of impingement in the larynx than a standard

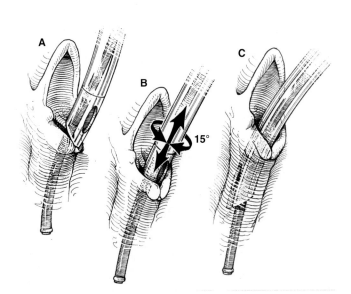

FIGURE 9-17. Impingement of ETT at the right arytenoid or right epiglottic fold. (*Crit Care Med.* 1990;18(8):883.)

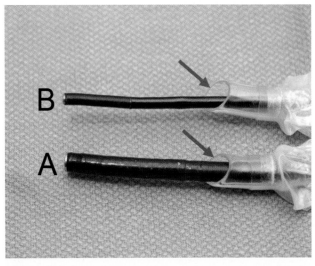

FIGURE 9-18. A 7.5-mm ID PVC ETT ensleeved over (A) a standard adult bronchoscope and (B) a pediatric bronchoscope. Note the discrepancy between the external diameters of the scopes and the IDs of the ETTs (arrows).

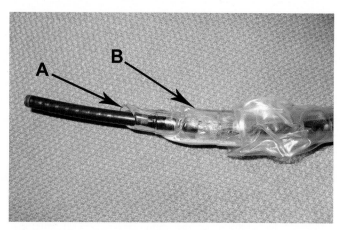

FIGURE 9-19. A smaller ETT (A) interpositioned between the broncho-scopic insertion cord and a larger ETT (B).

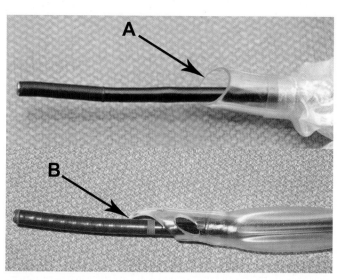

FIGURE 9-21. The Parker Flex-Tip tube: a 7-mm ID PVC endotracheal tube ensleeved over a standard pediatric bronchoscope (A) and a 7-mm ID Parker Flex-Tip tube ensleeved over a pediatric bronchoscope (B). Note the discrepancy between the leading edge of the two different types of endotracheal tubes (arrows).

tube,[66] subsequent studies reported frequent laryngeal impaction with spiral tubes.[54,55] Various methods to minimize the discrepancy between the outside diameter of the bronchoscope and the ID of the ETT have been proposed. These include the interposition of a smaller ETT between the scope and the larger ETT to be positioned in the trachea (see Figure 9-19),[39,68] or the use of a sleeve such as an airway exchange catheter,[68] split nasogastric tube,[69] or a custom-designed conical-shaped PVC sleeve.[70] The use of a Cook Airway Exchange Catheter passed alongside the bronchoscope through the ETT into the trachea to centralize the tube and facilitate glottic cannulation has also been reported.[71] Preformed PVC ETTs can also be warmed to increase flexibility.[11,19,20] Laryngeal cannulation with the ensleeved ETT may also be facilitated by using a tube with a modified tip design.[19,20,59,61] The silicone wire-reinforced tube for the intubating laryngeal mask airway (ILMA) is reusable and has a soft hemispherical bevel that has a leading edge in the midline (see Figure 9-20).[59] Greer et al found that the incidence of difficulty in passage of the ETT was significantly less using the IMLA tube as compared to the flexometallic tube during *oral* FBI under GA.[59] Barker et al found the Intravent Orthofix ILMA tube to be superior to both the reinforced and standard PVC tubes during *naso*tracheal intubation under GA.[54] All 15 Intravent tubes were easily passed through the larynx on the first attempt, whereas difficulty in passing

the ensleeved tube was encountered in 8/15 in the standard-tube group, and 6/15 in the flexible-tube group.[54] The Parker Flex-Tip tube shown in Figure 9-21 has a flexible tip that points toward the center of the distal lumen and the convex side of the tube.[42] Kristensen has reported a greater incidence of initial success with passage of the tube through the larynx as compared to a standard PVC ETT in a series of 76 patients who underwent oral FBI under GA.[42] A higher cuff pressure was required with this Parker Flex-Tip tube to establish a seal. However, in a recent randomized prospective study involving 111 patients with difficult airways or unstable cervical spines, Joo et al did not find any significant difference in the success rate between the Parker Flex-Tip tube and the PVC tube for awake oral FBI.[72] Difficulty in advancing the ETT through the larynx may be encountered as well in the awake patient without obtunded laryngeal reflexes.[3]

Difficulty with passage of the ETT through the larynx is exceedingly rare in the awake cooperative patient in the sitting position with adequate topical anesthesia of the airway, when an optimally sized bronchoscope is used relative to the ETT, and the tube is advanced during a deep inspiration.

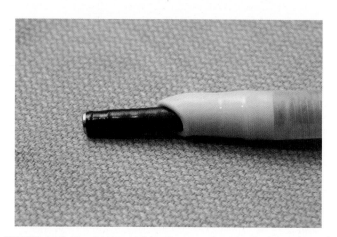

FIGURE 9-20. The ILMA reusable silicone endotracheal tube ensleeved over a standard adult bronchoscope; note the hemispherical bevel with a leading edge in the midline of the tube.

9.4   OTHER TECHNIQUES AND ADJUNCTS TO FACILITATE BRONCHOSCOPIC INTUBATION

9.4.1   Are oral intubating airways useful or necessary?

Various oral intubating airways are available and can be used during FBI. The purpose of these airways is to keep the bronchoscope in the midline and align it with the glottic opening, displace the tongue anteriorly and the soft palate superiorly thus opening the pharyngeal space, and to protect the scope from bite damage.[49,73]

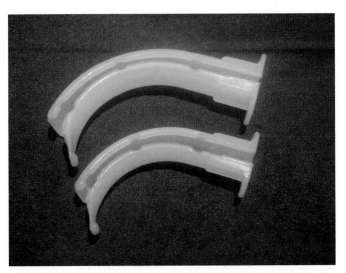

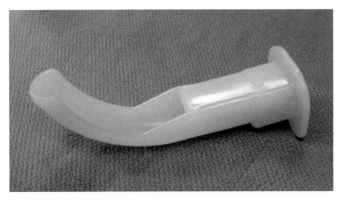

FIGURE 9-24. The Williams airway intubator: the Williams airway intubator has a cylindrical proximal half whereas the distal half of the device has an open lingual surface.

FIGURE 9-22. The Berman intubating pharyngeal airway: the Berman intubating pharyngeal airway is cylindrical and has a longitudinal opening along its side which permits its disengagement from the endotracheal tube following intubation. (From Ovassapian A, Wheeler M. Fiberoptic endoscopy-aided techniques. In: Benumof JL, ed. *Airway Management Principles and Practice*. St. Louis: Mosby, Inc.; 1996:289.)

The Berman intubating pharyngeal airway, also known as the Berman breakaway airway (see Figure 9-22), is cylindrical and has a longitudinal opening along its side which permits its disengagement (breakaway) from the ETT.[11] The maneuverability of the bronchoscope is limited when inside the airway, and if the airway is not in line with the glottis, visualization requires manipulation of the device.[11]

The Patil-Syracuse endoscopy airway (see Figure 9-23) is made of aluminum and is available in two sizes (adult and pediatric).

A central groove is located on the lingual surface for the bronchoscope, but manipulation of the bronchoscope is restricted.[47] An ETT will not pass through the airway.[11]

The Williams airway intubator has a cylindrical proximal half, whereas the distal half of the device has an open lingual surface (see Figure 9-24).[11,49] The airway is available in two sizes (90 and 100 mm ID) which admit 8.0 and 8.5 mm ID ETTs, respectively.[11,49] Manipulation of the bronchoscope inside the airway is limited.[11] If the distal aspect of the airway is not aligned with the glottis, visualization of the vocal cords can be difficult.[11,49]

The Ovassapian fiberoptic intubating airway has a flat lingual surface at the proximal half of the device which minimizes its movement (see Figure 9-25).[11,49] The distal half of the airway has a wide curve designed to prevent the tissues of the anterior pharyngeal wall from moving posteriorly. The posterior distal aspect of the airway is open.

A split Guedel airway has also been used for FBI.[10]

Randall et al found that the Berman airway was superior to the Ovassapian fiberoptic intubating airway during FBI.[74] However,

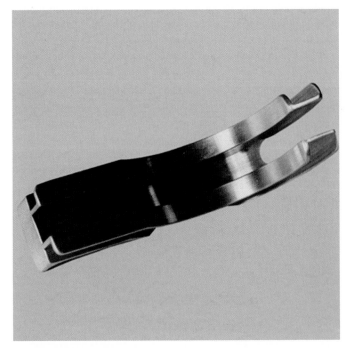

FIGURE 9-23. The Patil-Syracuse endoscopy airway: the airway is made of aluminum. A central groove is located on the lingual surface for the bronchoscope.

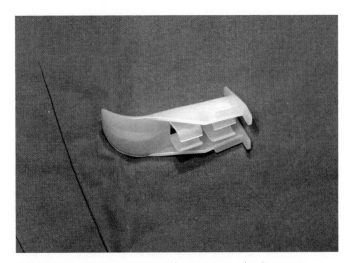

FIGURE 9-25. The Ovassapian intubating airway: the Ovassapian fiberoptic intubating airway has a flat lingual surface at the proximal half of the device which minimizes its movement. (Adapted from Ovassapian A, Wheeler M. Fiberoptic endoscopy-aided techniques. In: Benumof JL, ed. *Airway Management Principles and Practice*. St. Louis: Mosby, Inc.; 1996:289.)

only 1 of 63 bronchoscopies failed using the Ovassapian airway. Greenland et al compared the Williams airway intubator and the Ovassapian fiberoptic intubating airway in 60 Asian patients who underwent oral FBI under GA.[73] They reported that the Williams airway provided an unobstructed view of the glottis in 68.3% of cases, whereas the Ovassapian airway provided an unobstructed view in 25%. Four bronchoscopies failed using the Williams airway and 26 using the Ovassapian airway. Intubating conditions with either airway were similar when the glottis was visible.[73] Asai and Shingu suggest that it may be better to remove an airway intubator after the bronchoscope has been positioned in the trachea as it may interfere with the advancement of the ETT.[39]

Airway intubators can be used to facilitate FBI. However, FBI can be rapidly achieved without the use of these devices and the emphasis should be on the development of skill with bronchoscopic manipulation and regional anesthesia of the airway.

9.4.2   Is nasal bronchoscopic intubation easier? Which nostril is the more appropriate for intubation?

If the nasal route is chosen for FBI, an attempt to identify the more patent nostril can be made by asking the patient to assess airflow through each nasal cavity in turn during exhalation, and by palpating airflow from the nostril.[75] However, these simple diagnostic tests have been shown to have a failure rate of about 45%.[75] Some degree of nasal obstruction can be present in the absence of a history of nasal trauma, surgery, or obstruction and can interfere with the attempted passage of a nasal tube. The mucosa over the turbinates is easily traumatized.[75] Endoscopic examination of the nasal cavity may be helpful in identifying the more appropriate nostril for intubation.[75] Administration of a nasal vasoconstrictor may also increase the caliber of the nasal airway. In the absence of a history of nasal obstruction, it is controversial whether the left or right nostril should be used for nasal intubation as it is not known whether the bevel or the tip of the tube is more responsible for potential damage to the nasal mucosa (see also Blind Nasal Intubation section in Chapter 11).

During nasal FBI, either the ETT or the bronchoscope can be passed initially through the nasal cavity.[2,19,20,38] If the tube is passed first, it can be advanced along the floor of the nose using a gentle alternating clockwise-counterclockwise motion to facilitate its passage until the tip of the tube exits the choana to enter the nasopharynx.[2,20] The scope can then be passed through the lubricated tube and as it exits the distal aspect of the tube, the glottis is usually in view (see Figure 9-26). If on exiting the tip of the ETT the view is obstructed, the tube may be in contact with the pharyngeal mucosa or the tip of the scope may be covered with blood or debris. The scope can be removed, the tip cleaned and warmed, and then replaced into the tube. If on exiting the distal aspect of the tube still no recognizable structures are visualized, then the scope and tube should be slowly retracted together until pharyngeal or laryngeal landmarks (the uvula, epiglottis, or vocal cords) are identified.[19] If the epiglottis is oriented posteriorly against the posterior pharyngeal wall, the patient can be instructed to take a deep breath and thereby move the epiglottis anteriorly and create an adequate airspace for the scope to pass behind it without touching

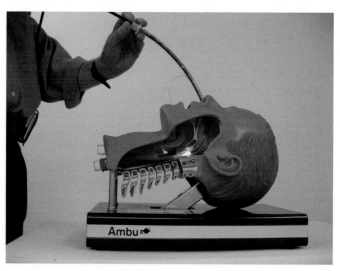

FIGURE 9-26. Nasal intubation using a flexible bronchoscope: the bronchoscope is passed through the endotracheal tube which was initially positioned in the pharynx.

mucosa and losing the visual field.[20] The flexible bronchoscope is then advanced into the trachea and the ETT advanced over the scope as for oral intubation during a deep inspiration, optimally with the patient in the semi-sitting or sitting position.[19,20] Alternatively, the flexible bronchoscope can be passed through the nasal cavity initially under endoscopic vision and then on into the trachea and the ensleeved ETT passed over the scope (see Figure 9-27). On advancing the ETT over the flexible bronchoscope, the leading edge of the tube may impact on the laryngeal structures and resist further advancement.[56] The most likely site of impingement during nasal FBI is controversial.[60,64] Rotating the tube such that the bevel faces anteriorly,[63] or posteriorly,[56] or advancing with a twisting motion[20,40,60] may facilitate glottic entry. A lubricated nasopharyngeal airway can be inserted temporarily into the nose before subsequent insertion of the ETT to explore the nasal cavity such that an appropriately sized ETT can be chosen.[20] Further decompression of the nasal mucosa may also be thereby

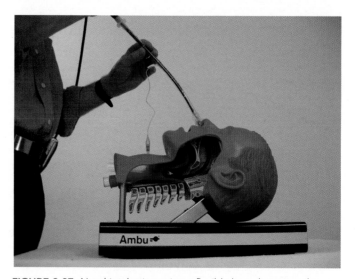

FIGURE 9-27. Nasal intubation using a flexible bronchoscope: the bronchoscope can be passed first into pharynx and trachea. The endotracheal tube is then advanced over the bronchoscope.

achieved[76] and trauma due to the more rigid ETT may be reduced. Alternatively, a nasopharyngeal airway split longitudinally can be inserted into the nasopharynx and used as a guide through which to pass the bronchoscope.[20,76] The split nasopharyngeal airway can then be removed before subsequent passage of the ETT. On occasion, the caliber of the nasal cavity may be such that it will permit passage of the ETT but not the bronchoscope through the tube due to external compression of the tube.[19,20] Conversely, the nasal cavity may permit initial passage of the scope but not the tube over the scope.[19,20] In this circumstance, it may be necessary to use a smaller scope, a smaller tube, the other nostril, oral intubation, or another means of airway management.

Nasotracheal intubation produces less stimulation of the gag reflex[3,7,57] and requires less patient cooperation, but is generally more uncomfortable for the awake patient. If the nasal cavity can be readily cannulated, it is technically somewhat easier than oral FBI.

Nasotracheal intubation has been considered to be contraindicated in the presence of a coagulopathy, intranasal abnormalities, paranasal sinusitis, extensive facial fractures, and basal skull fracture.[77-80] Conversely, basal skull fracture has been said not to be a contraindication to nasotracheal intubation.[77] Complications peculiar to nasotracheal intubation include epistaxis,[29,78,80-83] damage to the nasal or nasopharyngeal mucosa with creation of a false passage[3,81] and potential abscess formation,[78] bacteremia,[3,29,80] damage to nasal polyps or adenoidal tissue with possible dislodgement and aspiration, nasal necrosis,[3,29,78,80] sinusitis,[29,78,80] and otitis.[3,29,80] Minimal epistaxis has been reported in 11% to 40% of emergency nasotracheal intubations[81,83] and moderate to severe bleeding in 7%.[83] In a series of 99 patients undergoing maxillofacial surgery, nasotracheal intubation was associated with mild epistaxis in 5 patients and bleeding sufficient to produce a visible accumulation of blood in the pharynx in 1 patient.[82] Of 175 participants who underwent nasotracheal intubation at an awake bronchoscopic intubation training course, minor nasal bleeding was seen during endoscopy or after extubation in 20.[84] None of these 20 participants required suction to clear the airway and the bleeding did not interfere with endoscopy.[84]

9.4.3 When is bronchoscopic intubation under GA indicated? What are the problems with this technique?

FBI under GA can be performed as easily as intubation by direct laryngoscopy in patients with normal airway anatomy.[3] Oral FBI has also been successfully performed following simulated rapid sequence induction (RSI),[85] and FBI under GA has been used for training purposes.[86,87] FBI of the anticipated and unanticipated difficult intubation under GA has also been reported, although some intubation failures did occur.[10,88] This technique may be particularly useful in uncooperative patients.[89]

As consciousness is lost, loss of tone in the submandibular muscles allows the tongue and epiglottis to move posteriorly and potentially obstruct the airway at the level of the pharynx and larynx, respectively.[90,91] The soft palate also approximates the posterior pharyngeal wall.[90] The degree of airway obstruction produced is influenced by variations in airway anatomy, body habitus, and

depth of coma.[20,52] In the unconscious individual, this reduction in the caliber of the pharyngeal lumen can make endoscopic visualization more difficult.[3,20,92] Contact of the bronchoscope lens with the mucosa results in loss of the visual field, and the practitioner's ability to maneuver past an epiglottis in contact with the posterior pharyngeal wall is limited.[20,35,40,92] In the supine individual under GA, lingual traction with Duval forceps has been shown to move the tongue away from the uvula and soft palate better than the jaw thrust maneuver, whereas jaw thrust moved the epiglottis away from the posterior pharyngeal wall more effectively than tongue traction.[91] Jaw thrust and tongue traction applied simultaneously opened the airway at the soft palate and epiglottic level in all patients studied.[91] These combined maneuvers require two assistants.[91] Intubating airways such as the Berman or Ovassapian airway can also be used to keep the pharyngeal airway open as well as to direct the flexible bronchoscope toward the larynx; however multiple manipulations may be required, the intubation may be prolonged, and failure can occur.[91] Anterior displacement of the tongue base using the rigid laryngoscope may also improve visualization,[2,3,20,35] as can placing the patient in the semi-left lateral position with the head turned to the left.[93] If resistance is encountered in passing the ETT over the bronchoscope despite rotation of the tube, digital manipulation may be useful to facilitate glottic entry.[45] An endoscopy mask fitted with a diaphragm permits endoscopy during positive pressure mask-ventilation[94] and can be used in conjunction with an intubating airway.[3,7,11,94] The nasotracheal route can also be used in the unconscious individual.[2,92] In the presence of apnea or suboptimal ventilation, arterial desaturation imposes a time limit on bronchoscopic techniques.[3,19,20] FBI of a patient under GA can be difficult and arterial desaturation can occur,[95] although the technique has been used with high levels of success.[85,88]

9.5 UTILIZATION OF BRONCHOSCOPIC INTUBATION IN DIFFERENT SETTINGS

9.5.1 How useful is bronchoscopic intubation in the emergency setting?

Immediate airway control in the emergency setting can be difficult using bronchoscopic techniques due to the presence of blood, emesis, or secretions in the airway.[20,95-97] Poor preparation of the patient and lack of patient cooperation can also be problematic.[3,20,95,98] FBI can nevertheless be a valuable option in selected patients such as those with confirmed or suspected cervical spine injury,[97] those with anticipated difficult direct laryngoscopic intubation due to variant anatomy,[97] and in the presence of airway pathology such as Ludwig angina,[99] burn injury,[100] or angioedema.[96] Its use as part of a rapid sequence intubation technique has also been described.[101] Complete airway obstruction has however been reported during attempted FBI in the presence of upper-airway compromise.[22,32]

Awake FBI has been advocated in the management of penetrating neck injury (see Chapter 34).[101] However, this technique may only be feasible in cooperative stable patients who do not require immediate airway control.[101,102] The optimal initial airway management approach in the patient with penetrating neck injury remains controversial.[103,104] Mandavia et al reported a series of 58 patients with penetrating neck trauma who required emergency airway control.[103] Of the 58 patients, 39 underwent rapid-sequence orotracheal intubation with a 100% success rate, 5 unconscious patients underwent orotracheal intubation by direct laryngoscopy without paralysis, and 2 underwent successful emergency tracheostomy.[103] FBI was attempted in 12 patients. Three of these intubations failed, but all three were later successfully intubated orotracheally by direct laryngoscopy following RSI.[103] Of 107 patients with penetrating neck trauma reported by Shearer and Giesecke, 8 patients underwent oral FBI with a 100% success rate.[104] Eighty-nine patients underwent orotracheal intubation by direct laryngoscopy after RSI, six had a primary surgical airway, and four had blind nasotracheal intubation. Ninety-eight percent of the direct laryngoscopy RSI group was successfully intubated. The authors concluded that the technical and time constraints of FBI led them to prefer RSI and direct laryngoscopy, or a primary surgical airway, when an emergency airway was required.[104]

FBI has also been advocated for the emergency management of blunt injury to the airway, although reported experience is limited.[105,106] Awake nasal FBI of a patient with unstable bilateral mandibular fractures in the semi-prone position has been reported.[107] The patient was unable to tolerate the supine or sitting position due to airway obstruction.[107] Successful awake bronchoscopic orotracheal intubation has also been performed via an LMA in a patient with massive oropharyngeal bleeding following blunt trauma.[108] An attempt at FBI had failed due to blood in the airway, and an LMA was inserted to maintain gas exchange during a planned awake tracheotomy. Cuff inflation produced an unobstructed airway, resolution of respiratory distress, and permitted FBI through the LMA.[108] Emergency FBI has also been performed successfully in patients with respiratory failure, congestive heart failure, altered consciousness due to stroke, overdose, head trauma, status asthmaticus, hematemesis, and partial upper-airway obstruction.[95,97,98]

Success rates of emergency FBI have been reported by various authors to be 72%,[95] 87%, 83%,[97] and 75%.[109] Visualization can be improved by pharyngeal suctioning.[20,98] Insufflation of oxygen via the working channel of the flexible bronchoscope has been used to disperse secretions or vomitus and improve visualization.[98] However, gastric rupture has occurred with this technique,[37] and the potential for other barotrauma exists.[3,19]

In 1999, Levitan et al published a survey of devices used for difficult airway management in academic emergency departments in the United States.[110] Of 95 programs who responded, only 64% had a flexible bronchoscope, and although the most commonly used alternative to intubation by direct laryngoscopy was the flexible bronchoscope, it was in fact rarely used.[110] Only a small minority of patients requiring emergency endotracheal intubation need bronchoscopic techniques,[97] and as a result skill maintenance is problematic. However, Desjardins and Varon have reported the use of awake FBI in a large proportion of their trauma patients, as well as the use of the rapid sequence bronchoscopic technique.[101]

9.5.2   Can the flexible bronchoscope be combined with other intubation techniques?

FBI via the LMA has been described by a number of authors.[2,3,11,111-117] A 7-mm ID ETT can be passed through a #5 LMA, and a 6-mm ID ETT through a #3 or #4 LMA.[38,111] The LMA Classic Excel has a removable connector and an epiglottic elevating bar which facilitates intubation and permits the use of larger ETTs.[112] A #7.5 mm ID-cuffed ETT can be passed through a #5 LMA Classic Excel and a cuffed 7.0 mm ID ETT through a #3 and #4 Classic Excel.[112] An appropriately sized bronchoscope can then be passed through the ETT into the trachea and the tube advanced over the scope. The length of a #4 LMA is 20 cm from the proximal edge of the LMA adapter to the aperture bars,[113] and the distance from the aperture bars to the cords is about 3.5 to 4.0 cm.[11,114] A standard 6 mm ID ETT will therefore only be able to extend about 5 cm below the cords and will not provide an adequate length of ETT for satisfactory tracheal placement.[11] However, a 6 mm ID microlaryngoscopy tube (MLT, Mallinckrodt, Hospimetrix Sdn Bhd, Selangor, Malaysia) with a length of 40 cm can be used to overcome this problem.[115] Alternatively, a 6 or 7 mm ID nasal Ring-Adair-Elwyn (RAE) tube can be used, although the nasal RAE may need to be shortened by 2 cm to permit an adequate depth of intratracheal intubation by the flexible bronchoscope.[114] The LMA can be removed over the ETT using a second tube to exert counter pressure on the ETT in the trachea to prevent its inadvertent dislodgement during removal of the LMA.[116] The airway tube of the ILMA has a minimal ID of 13 mm and can accommodate any cuffed ETT size up to an 8-mm ID.[117] FBI through the LMA and ILMA has been performed with the patient awake or anesthetized.[3,11,118]

The reusable intubating laryngeal airway (ILA), (Mercury Medical, Clearwater FL, USA) is similar to the LMA both in its functionality and its insertion technique.[111] It has several advantages over the LMA Classic: the circuit connector is removable; the shaft is shorter; and there are no aperture bars.[111] A cuffed #7.5 mm ID ETT can be passed through a #3.5 ILA and a cuffed #8.5 mm ID ETT through a #4.5 ILA. Wong and McGuire reported successful intubation through the ILA using regular ETTs with and without bronchoscopic guidance.[111]

FBI can also be accomplished by passing a pediatric flexible bronchoscope with an ensleeved Aintree intubation catheter (AIC, Cook Medical Inc. Bloomington, IN) into the trachea through an in situ LMA Classic. The AIC is an ETT exchange catheter which has an internal diameter of 4.8 mm, an external diameter of 6.5 mm, and a length of 56 cm.[119] Introduced in 1996, it was designed to facilitate FBI through an LMA Classic.[120] The AIC can be ensleeved proximally over a 4.0 mm flexible bronchoscope such that the distal 3 cm of the shaft, the bending section, of the scope is free. The scope with the ensleeved catheter can then be passed through the LMA into the trachea. The scope can then be removed leaving the AIC in the trachea. The LMA can then be removed and an ETT ≥7.0 mm ID passed into the trachea over the AIC. The AIC is then removed. A Rapi-Fit adapter supplied with the AIC permits ventilation through the catheter if this becomes necessary[119,120] Ventilation can also continue through the LMA during the FBI.[120] Atherton et al reported that the experienced endoscopist could master the technique after four intubations and those inexperienced in FBI after six intubations.[120] Zura et al reported a case of failed intubation by direct laryngoscopy and GlideScope in which the trachea was successfully intubated bronchoscopically using a #5 LMA Unique, an ensleeved AIC, and a 7.5 mm ID Parker Flex-Tip ETT.[121] Avitsian et al reported a case of inadvertent tracheal extubation intraoperatively during cervical spine decompression.[122] Bronchoscopic reintubation was accomplished using an LMA Classic and an AIC while maintaining in-line stabilization.[122] Higgs et al reported a series of patients with difficult direct laryngoscopy who were successfully intubated bronchoscopically using an AIC and LMA.[123] In five of these cases attempted intubation by DL had failed. The authors also note that the consultant in charge of one of the cases anesthetizes "more than 50" cervical spine cases per year primarily using this technique. Zura et al subsequently reported that at their institution they had achieved a 100% success rate with this technique in "more than 50" cannot intubate, can ventilate cases without complications.[124] In a manikin study, FBI using the Aintree catheter through the LMA Proseal has been shown to be at least as easy and reliable as through an LMA Classic.[125]

In the Difficult Airway Society (DAS) guidelines for management of the unanticipated difficult intubation, FBI through the ILMA or the LMA Classic is included in Plan B (secondary intubation plan).[126] Plan B is implemented when tracheal intubation by DL or an alternate technique of proven value in experienced hands has failed. The ILMA has proven to be a useful device in the management of the unanticipated difficult intubation;[126] however blind intubation through the ILMA may require multiple attempts and esophageal intubation can occur.[126] FBI through the ILMA has a higher success rate than blind techniques.[126] However, techniques of insertion and intubation through the ILMA differ from those for the Classic LMA, and training and practice are essential if a high success rate is to be achieved while minimizing trauma in the unanticipated difficult intubation.[126] The DAS guidelines state that FBI through the Classic LMA should be considered if an ILMA is not available, and note that a two-stage technique with the AIC can be used.[126]

The revised American Society of Anesthesiologists Practice Guidelines for Management of the Difficult Airway in 2003 include the use of the LMA as an intubation conduit with or without bronchoscopic guidance in the alternative approaches to intubation.[127]

Higgs et al note that almost all international failed intubation guidelines include recourse to an LMA Classic to maintain airway patency.[123] The authors also note that the ILMA is a specialized piece of equipment that is not universally available in all areas where anesthetics are administered or airway management occurs, and that it requires a distinct skill with its own learning curve.[123] However, the LMA Classic is widely utilized, more likely to be immediately available, and easily inserted. The technique of FBI with an ensleeved Aintree catheter using the LMA as a conduit appears to be easy to learn and does not require a high level of bronchoscopic skill.[123]

In the unanticipated "cannot intubate, cannot ventilate" situation, an attempt to establish ventilation by insertion of an LMA Classic can be made while preparing to perform a cricothyrotomy. If ventilation can be established with the LMA Classic, it may be prudent to awaken the patient or proceed with a surgical airway as the clinical setting dictates. However, FBI can also be performed through the LMA Classic using an AIC.

FBI through the LMA Classic has been referred to as a "low skill bronchoscopic intubation"[123] and has been regarded as a core skill that should be within the ability of all anesthesia practitioners after minimal training.[123,128] The same can be said for all practitioners responsible for airway management.

The flexible bronchoscope can also be used to facilitate retrograde intubation (see Section 11.6.4).[2,3,129] During retrograde intubation, the tip of the ETT being advanced into the trachea over the guide wire may impinge on laryngeal structures and resist further advancement.[2,3] The flexible bronchoscope can be passed through the tube alongside the wire to visualize the glottis and then passed on into the trachea.[2,3] The wire can then be removed and the ETT advanced over the bronchoscope.[2,3] Alternatively, the wire can be passed in a retrograde direction through the working channel of the bronchoscope loaded with an ensleeved ETT.[2,129] The bronchoscope is then advanced over the wire into the trachea and the guidewire removed.[2,3] The ETT is then passed over the bronchoscope into the trachea.[2,3,129]

Blind nasotracheal intubation can also be assisted by the flexible bronchoscope.[2,3] The bronchoscope can be passed through the contralateral nostril to visualize and thereby facilitate manipulation of the ETT into the trachea.[2,3]

9.6   OTHER CONSIDERATIONS

9.6.1   What are the limitations and complications of bronchoscopic intubation?

FBI in the presence of secretions, emesis, or blood in the airway is difficult and the applicability of the technique in the emergency situation is limited. Some measure of patient cooperation is also necessary. When both the bronchoscope and the ensleeved ETT are in the larynx or trachea, significant airway obstruction can be produced[11,40] and can cause respiratory distress. Bronchoscopes are delicate, expensive instruments and require careful use if damage is to be avoided. The sterilization process is complex and requires time and resources.

Although they are rare, complications associated with FBI can occur. These include laryngospasm,[2,3] complete airway obstruction,[22,23,32] local anesthetic toxicity,[130] respiratory depression secondary to sedative overdose,[3] loss of the endoscopy mask diaphragm into the airway,[2,3] laryngeal trauma,[131] pyrexia and rigors,[132] and respiratory infection.[84] The ETT is advanced blindly over the bronchoscope and may impinge on laryngeal or pharyngeal structures. Supraglottic swelling, pharyngeal hematoma, and vocal cord immobility and bruising have been reported after

FBI.[131] The ETT should be advanced gently over the broncho-scope, the gap between the ETT and scope diameters minimized, and the use of tubes with modified bevels may be considered. Additional studies are required to determine the mechanism of pharyngeal or laryngeal injury during FBI as well as their inci-dence and severity.[131] In a series of 2031 FBIs, complications were limited to laryngospasm in 51, pain or hematoma secondary to cricothyroid injection in 33, gagging or vomiting in 8, and mild epistaxis in 70 who were nasally intubated.[3] None of the cases of epistaxis required packing.

9.6.2 How much training is required to develop proficiency in bronchoscopic intubation? How can the training be acquired?

FBI is not a difficult skill to master; however, it requires famil-iarity with the anatomy of the upper airway, and dexterity in bronchoscopic manipulation. Awake FBI requires skill in regional anesthesia of the airway and gentleness on the part of the practi-tioner. Each step of the procedure must be planned in advance and methodically carried out. The ability to quickly and reliably maneuver the bronchoscope in a given direction is an absolute requirement for fast, successful, and safe FBI.

Readily available intubation mannequins can be used to develop manual dexterity with the bronchoscope and with advancing the ETT over the scope. Nonanatomic models can also be used to develop bronchoscopic dexterity.

Naik et al reported that a group of 12 novice residents who underwent bronchoscopic training using a Choose-the-Hole model significantly outperformed a similar 12 subject didactic group, when performance was evaluated during FBI of an anesthe-tized paralyzed patient.[133] Marsland et al have described a nonana-tomical modular endoscopic training system called Dexter.[134] This system consists of a manikin, an image chart, a series of maps, and a structured training module. The objective is to endoscopi-cally explore the mannequin and find the images placed inside it. Novice endoscopists took about 3.5 hours to complete the Dexter training modules and were then able to perform clinical endoscopy on awake subjects from mouth to carina in a mean time of 32.5 seconds.[134] Marsland et al subsequently reported that 28 of 29 novice endoscopists were able to achieve bronchoscopic intuba-tion proficiency within 4 hours of bench training with the Dexter system.[135] Twenty seven of the 29 then demonstrated proficiency on clinical bronchoscopy to the carina.[135]

Martin et al compared the effectiveness of the Choose-the-Hole model with the Dexter system in the development of endo-scopic proficiency.[136] Members of the authors' Department of Anesthesia were given initial didactic teaching. Initial endoscopic performance on an anatomical manikin was then assessed. The participants then practiced in a self-directed manner on one of the two models for a 2-week period, following which endoscopy skills were again measured on the manikin and then during clinical bronchoscopy from mouth to carina on each other. Participants in the Dexter group significantly outperformed the Choose-the-Hole

group during clinical bronchoscopy. A positive correlation was also demonstrated between clinical and manikin performance scores. The authors concluded that Dexter is a more effective model for learning endoscopic dexterity than the Choose-the-Hole model, and that benchmark levels of endoscopic dexterity can be achieved without subjecting patients to novice learning curves.[136]

Smith et al studied the learning curve of a group of 12 anesthesia trainees who underwent a supervised, structured, video-controlled training session utilizing a bronchial tree model followed by 20 supervised and coached nasal FBIs on anesthetized patients.[137] The trainees were able to advance the scope to the carina within 2.5 minutes in 95% of the patients, and within an additional 2.5 minutes in the remaining 5%. The authors calculated that the half-life of the group learning curve was 9 endoscopies, and concluded that when using a videoscope under supervision, train-ees were beginning to develop a reasonable level of proficiency in fiberoptic nasotracheal intubation after performing, on average, 18 intubations. Extrapolation of the learning curve suggested that 45 endoscopies would be required to approach expert times of 35 seconds for the procedure. Speed was felt to be related to the development of hand-eye coordination or dexterity. The authors noted great individual variation in skill development.[137]

At the authors' institution a group of residents with no prior experience or training in FBI were given a brief slide show presen-tation on FBI, followed by expert demonstration on a manikin. Each resident was then coached by the instructor through a series of FBIs on the manikin. Each resident completed 50 supervised intubations within 1.5 hours. At the end of the session, all the participants had achieved a reasonable level of dexterity with the bronchoscope and were able to complete the intubation within about 30 seconds. Anecdotally, these skills were subsequently noted to be transferred to the clinical setting of awake intubation of the difficult airway.

Rowe et al reported the use of a virtual reality bronchoscopic simulator for FBI training.[138] Twenty pediatric residents who had no prior experience in bronchoscopy were randomized to a simula-tor or control group. All participants performed an initial FBI on a patient which was videotaped and graded. The simulator group (n=12) then underwent training on a virtual reality simulator. The residents in the simulator group practiced on an average of 17 virtual cases and spent 39 minutes on the simulator. They then performed a second awake intubation on a patient. The control group performed a second intubation without intervening train-ing. The simulator group significantly outperformed the control group in all the variables measured (intubation time, number of mucosal hits, time viewing mucosa, and airway). There were no complications. The authors concluded that the bronchoscopy simulator was very effective in teaching residents the psychomotor skills required for flexible bronchoscopy.[138]

FBI workshops can also be effective in improving skills.[139] Patil et al reported a training course in local anesthesia and FBI using course delegates as subjects.[140] Participants attended lectures, video demonstrations, and practical sessions using manikins and an arti-ficial throat endoscopy model. Endoscopy was also performed on an instructor. All fifteen course participants then underwent local airway anesthesia and endoscopy. Nasal FBI was completed in 10 subjects. Nasal obstruction precluded intubation in three cases. Nasal anesthesia was inadequate in one case and the procedure was abandoned in one case who developed paresthesia of the hands and feet that could have been due to local anesthetic toxicity. The course overall was rated as excellent by all delegates and no delegate found the procedure to be unacceptable.[140] In 2004 the same authors reported one subject who developed pyrexia and rigors about 6 hours after intubation and was treated with antibiotics.[132]

Woodall et al subsequently reported a training course at which 200 anesthetists underwent airway endoscopy and attempted FBI under local anesthesia.[84] One hundred and eighty delegates were intubated, 175 nasally and 5 orally, and 1336 endoscopies were performed. Intubation was abandoned due to nasal obstruction in 10 subjects, inadequate anesthesia in 8, symptoms suggestive of lidocaine toxicity in 1, and extreme agitation in 1. Minor nasal bleeding occurred in 20 subjects and symptoms that could be attributed to lidocaine in 71. Two subjects experienced rigors after the procedure and one developed a respiratory infection. Three delegates rated the intubation as distressing. The authors note that extreme caution is required when selecting subjects for a training course and concluded that the use of volunteers for this form of training carries risks and requires further evaluation.[84]

FBI has been advocated as an alternate technique that may be used whenever tracheal intubation is indicated,[3] and this FBI of normal airways under GA may be beneficial in learning to manipulate the bronchoscope and to advance the ETT over the scope.[3,87,141] However, the use of nonroutine techniques may require discussion with the patient beforehand.[142] Furthermore, the FBI of patients with normal airways under GA may not extrapolate well to the intubation of the difficult airway in the awake patient.[141,143]

Cole et al reported FBI training of eight novice anesthesia residents using anesthetized paralyzed patients.[86] The trainees were given two 1-hour lectures followed by a 20-minute hands-on workshop using a Choose-the-Hole model. Each trainee also performed one or two tracheal intubations in a manikin, and could practice using the manikin or model in their spare time. During the training period, each trainee performed 16 to 47 FBIs and 58 to 120 conventional rigid laryngoscopic intubations. Following the training period, bronchoscopic and laryngoscopic intubation skills were evaluated in a randomized single-blind prospective study. One hundred and thirty patients were randomized to either rigid laryngoscopic or bronchoscopic intubation. Each resident performed 5 to 10 rigid laryngoscopic intubations and 6 to 13 FBIs. There was one failed FBI and two failed rigid scope intubations. Successful FBI was achieved within 60 seconds of apnea in 52 of 71 cases. The average intubation time was less that 81 seconds for all residents and 5 of 8 residents achieved mean times of ≤60 seconds of apnea. There was no significant difference in the incidence of sore throat and hoarseness between the groups. There was no dental trauma.[86]

Schaeffer et al have also reported a study of bronchoscopic training in anesthetized paralyzed patients.[144] Five fourth-year anesthesia residents who had no prior experience in FBI performed tracheal intubation in 20 patients each in a random fashion either as an expert laryngoscopist or a bronchoscopic novice. The residents initially viewed two instructional videos and practiced on an intubation manikin until intubation times of ≤30 seconds were achieved. This required up to 20 supervised oral and nasal intubations. Each resident then performed nasal bronchoscopic intubations on 10 patients. The time to bronchoscopically identify the carina decreased from 64 seconds in each of the residents' first two intubations to 33 seconds in their last two intubations. The corresponding times to complete the intubation decreased from 96 seconds to 53 seconds. FBI was achieved on the first attempt in 98% of the patients. The incidence of sore throat, hoarseness, dysphagia, and hemodynamic change was similar between the groups.[144]

Ideally, FBI should be demonstrated by a knowledgeable and skilled instructor.[5] The learner should then be supervised until the principles of bronchoscopic manipulation are mastered. The availability of video bronchoscopes permit the instructor to easily coach the learner in the flexion and rotation movements required to properly steer the bronchoscope and appears to facilitate bronchoscopic skill acquisition.[145] Independent practice is then required to further develop and improve psychomotor skills. A reasonable level of dexterity in manipulating the bronchoscope can be achieved within 3 to 4 hours of independent mannequin practice.[5]

An acceptable level of technical expertise may be achievable after 10 FBIs in anesthetized patients[146] and 15 to 20 awake FBIs in patients with normal anatomy.[5] Smith and Jackson reported that trainees were "becoming reasonably proficient" after performing 20 FBIs in anesthetized patients in whom intubation was predicted to be difficult.[147] It has also been suggested that 30 FBIs in conscious and anesthetized patients be performed before a practitioner is ready to handle the difficult intubation.[148] The amount of experience and training required for safe and effective use of the flexible bronchoscope in the difficult airway is unknown;[11,20] however an experience of 100 or more bronchoscopic procedures may be necessary to acquire expertise in this setting.[5,11,20]

9.7   SUMMARY

Flexible bronchoscopic intubation is widely accepted as an invaluable alternate technique in the management of the difficult airway. It should be mastered by all anesthesia practitioners and other practitioners responsible for airway management.

REFERENCES

1. Murphy P. A fibre-optic endoscope used for nasal intubation. *Anaesthesia.* 1967;22:489-491.
2. Ovassapian A. The flexible bronchoscope. A tool for anesthesiologists. *Clin Chest Med.* 2001;22:281-299.
3. Ovassapian A, Wheeler M. Flexible fiberoptic tracheal intubation. In: *Handbook of Difficult Airway Management.* Hagberg CA, ed. Philadelphia, PA: Churchill Livingstone; 2000; 83-114.
4. Stiles CM, Stiles QR, Denson JS. A flexible fiber optic laryngoscope. *JAMA* 1972;221:1246-1247.
5. Ovassapian A, Yelich SJ. Learning fiberoptic intubation. *Anesth Clin N Am.* 1991;9:175-186.
6. ASA Task Force on Management of the Difficult Airway. Practice guidelines for management of the difficult airway. A report by the American Society of Anesthesiologists Task Force on Management of the Difficult Airway. *Anesthesiology.* 1993;78:597-602.
7. Stackhouse RA. Fiberoptic airway management. *Anesthesiol Clin North Am.* 2002;20:933-951.

8. Weiss YG, Deutschman CS. The role of fiberoptic bronchoscopy in airway management of the critically ill patient. *Crit Care Clin.* 2000;16:445-451.

9. Benumof JL. Management of the difficult adult airway. With special emphasis on awake tracheal intubation. *Anesthesiology.* 1991;75:1087-1110.

10. Heidegger T, Gerig HJ, Ulrich B, Kreienbuhl G. Validation of a simple algorithm for tracheal intubation: daily practice is the key to success in emergencies—an analysis of 13,248 intubations. *Anesth Analg.* 2001;92:517-522.

11. Ovassapian A, Wheeler M. Fiberoptic endoscopy-aided techniques. In: *Airway Management Principles and Practice.* Benumof JL, ed. St. Louis: Mosby, Inc.; 1996:282-319.

12. Sidhu VS, Whitehead EM, Ainsworth QP, et al. A technique of awake fibreoptic intubation. Experience in patients with cervical spine disease. *Anaesthesia.* 1993;48:910-913.

13. Allan AG. Reluctance of anaesthetists to perform awake intubation. *Anaesthesia.* 2004;59:413.

14. Basi SK, Cooper M, Ahmed FB, et al. Reluctance of anaesthetists to perform awake intubation. *Anaesthesia.* 2004;59:918.

15. Avargues P, Cros AM, Daucourt V, et al. Procedures used by French anesthetists in cases of difficult intubation and the impact of a conference of experts. *Ann Fr Anesth Reanim.* 1999;18:719-724.

16. Heidegger T, Gerig H. Anticipated difficult airway: the role of fiberoptics. *Anesth Analg.* 2002;95:1124; author reply 1125.

17. Kristensen MS, Moller J. Airway management behaviour, experience and knowledge among Danish anaesthesiologists—room for improvement. *Acta Anaesthesiol Scand.* 2001;45:1181-1185.

18. Rosenblatt WH, Wagner PJ, Ovassapian A, Kain ZN. Practice patterns in managing the difficult airway by anesthesiologists in the United States. *Anesth Analg.* 1998;87:153-157.

19. Morris IR. Airway anesthesia, sedation and awake intubation. *The Difficult Airway Course: Anesthesia Airway Course Manual.* 64-81.

20. Morris IR. Fibreoptic intubation. *Can J Anaesth.* 1994;41:996-1007; discussion 1007-1008.

21. Reed AP. Preparation for intubation of the awake patient. *Mt Sinai J Med.* 1995;62:10-20.

22. Ho AM, Chung DC, To EW, Karmakar MK. Total airway obstruction during local anesthesia in a non-sedated patient with a compromised airway. *Can J Anaesth.* 2004;51:838-841.

23. Shaw IC, Welchew EA, Harrison BJ, Michael S. Complete airway obstruction during awake fibreoptic intubation. *Anaesthesia.* 1997;52:582-585.

24. Liistro G, Stanescu DC, Veriter C, Rodenstein DO, D'Odemont JP. Upper airway anesthesia induces airflow limitation in awake humans. *Am Rev Respir Dis.* 1992;146:581-585.

25. Beydon L, Lorino AM, Verra F, et al. Topical upper airway anaesthesia with lidocaine increases airway resistance by impairing glottic function. *Intensive Care Med.* 1995;21:920-926.

26. Kuna ST, Woodson GE, Sant'Ambrogio G. Effect of laryngeal anesthesia on pulmonary function testing in normal subjects. *Am Rev Respir Dis.* 1988;137:656-661.

27. Crosby ET. Airway management in adults after cervical spine trauma. *Anesthesiology.* 2006;104:1293-1318.

28. Meschino A, Devitt JH, Koch JP, et al. The safety of awake tracheal intubation in cervical spine injury. *Can J Anaesth.* 1992;39:114-147.

29. Morris IR. Airway management. In: Rosen P, et al. *Emergency Medicine: Concepts and Clinical Practice.* St. Louis: Mosby Yearbook; 1992:79-105.

30. Suderman VS, Crosby ET, Lui A. Elective oral tracheal intubation in cervical spine-injured adults. *Can J Anaesth.* 1991;38:785-789.

31. Walls RM. Airway management. In: Rose P, ed. *Emergency Medicine: Concepts and Clinical Practice.* St. Louis: Mosby Yearbook; 1998:2-24.

32. McGuire G, el-Beheiry H. Complete upper airway obstruction during awake fibreoptic intubation in patients with unstable cervical spine fractures. *Can J Anaesth.* 1999;46:176-178.

33. Donlon JVJ. Anesthetic management of patients with compromised airways. *Anesth Rev.* 1980;7:22-31.

34. Wong DT, McGuire GP. Management choices for the difficult airway (Author reply). *Can J Anaesth.* 2003;50:624.

35. Edens ET, Sia RL. Flexible fiberoptic endoscopy in difficult intubations. *Ann Otol Rhinol Laryngol.* 1981;90:307-309.

36. ECRI. ECRI Healthcare Product Comparison System. https://www.ecri.org/Products/Pages/Hpcs.aspx?sub=Capital%20Equipmen. Accessed May, 2010.

37. Hershey MD, Hannenberg AA. Gastric distention and rupture from oxygen insufflation during fiberoptic intubation. *Anesthesiology.* 1996;85:1479-1480.

38. Fulling PD, Roberts JT. Fiberoptic intubation. *Int Anesthesiol Clin.* 2000;38:189-217.

39. Asai T, Shingu K. Difficulty in advancing a tracheal tube over a fibreoptic bronchoscope: incidence, causes and solutions. *Br J Anaesth.* 2004;92:870-881.

40. Dellinger RP. Fiberoptic bronchoscopy in adult airway management. *Crit Care Med.* 1990;18: 882-887.

41. El-Orbany MI, Salem MR, Joseph NJ. Tracheal tube advancement over the fiberoptic bronchoscope: size does matter. *Anesth Analg.* 2003;97:301; author reply 301.

42. Kristensen MS. The Parker Flex-Tip tube versus a standard tube for fiberoptic orotracheal intubation: a randomized double-blind study. *Anesthesiology.* 2003;98:354-358.

43. Marsh NJ. Easier fiberoptic intubations. *Anesthesiology.* 1992;76:860-861.

44. Sutherland AD, Williams RT. Cardiovascular responses and lidocaine absorption in fiberoptic-assisted awake intubation. *Anesth Analg.* 1986;65:389-391.

45. Witton TH. An introduction to the fiberoptic laryngoscope. *Can Anaesth Soc J.* 1981;28:475-478.

46. Deam R, McCutcheon C. Management choices for the difficult airway. *Can J Anaesth.* 2003;50:623-624; author reply 624.

47. Taylor DM, Brimacomb J, Stone T. Inactivation of prions by physical and chemical means. *J Hosp Infect.* 1999;43(Suppl):S69-S76.

48. Walsh EM. Reducing the risk of prion transmission in anaesthesia. *Anaesthesia.* 2006;61:64-65.

49. Walsh ME, Shorten GD. Preparing to perform an awake fiberoptic intubation. *Yale J Biol Med.* 1998;71:537-549.

50. Telford RJ, Liban JB. Awake fibreoptic intubation. *Br J Hosp Med.* 1991;46:182-184.

51. Morikawa S, Safar P, Decarlo J. Influence of the headjaw position upon upper airway patency. *Anesthesiology.* 1961;22:265-270.

52. Safar P. Ventilatory efficacy of mouth-to-mouth artificial respiration; airway obstruction during manual and mouth-to-mouth artificial respiration. *J Am Med Assoc.* 1958;167:335-341.

53. Boyson PG. Fiberoptic instrumentation for airway management. ASA Annual Refresher Course Lectures. 1993;266:1-5.

54. Barker KF, Bolton P, Cole S, Coe PA. Ease of laryngeal passage during fibreoptic intubation: a comparison of three endotracheal tubes. *Acta Anaesthesiol Scand.* 2001;45:624-626.

55. Hakala P, Randall T, Valli H. Comparison between tracheal tubes for orotracheal fibreoptic intubation. *Br J Anaesth.* 1999;82:135-136.

56. Hughes S, Smith JE. Nasotracheal tube placement over the fibreoptic laryngoscope. *Anaesthesia.* 1996;51:1026-1028.

57. Ovassapian A. Flexible bronchoscopic intubation of awake patients. *J Bronchology.* 1994;1:240-245.

58. Randell T. Fibreoptic orotracheal intubation—reply (correspondence). *Br J Anaesth.* 1999;83:683-684.

59. Greer JR, Smith SP, Strang T. A comparison of tracheal tube tip designs on the passage of an endotracheal tube during oral fibreoptic intubation. *Anesthesiology.* 2001;94:729-731; discussion 5A.

60. Katsnelson T, Frost EA, Farcon E, Goldiner PL. When the endotracheal tube will not pass over the flexible fiberoptic bronchoscope. *Anesthesiology.* 1992;76:151-152.

61. Jones HE, Pearce AC, Moore P. Fiberoptic intubation: influence of tracheal tube tip design. *Anaesthesia.* 1993;48:672-674.

62. Schwartz D, Johnson C, Roberts J. A maneuver to facilitate flexible fiberoptic intubation. *Anesthesiology.* 1989;71:470-471.

63. Wheeler M, Dsida RM. Fiberoptic intubation: troubles with the "Tube"? *Anesthesiology.* 2003;99:1236-1237; author reply 1237.

64. Nakayama M, Kataoka N, Usui Y, et al. Techniques of nasotracheal intubation with the fiberoptic bronchoscope. *J Emerg Med.* 1992;10:729-734.

65. Raj PP, Forestner J, Watson TD, et al. Technics for fiberoptic laryngoscopy in anesthesia. *Anesth Analg.* 1974;53:708-714.

66. Brull SJ, Wiklund R, Ferris C, et al. Facilitation of fiberoptic orotracheal intubation with a flexible tracheal tube. *Anesth Analg.* 1994;78: 746-748.

67. Calder I. When the endotracheal tube will not pass over the flexible fiberoptic bronchoscope. *Anesthesiology.* 1992;77:398.

68. Tan I. Easier fiberoptic intubation. *Anaesthesia.* 1994;49:830-831.

69. Aoyama K, Yasunaga E, Takenaka I. Another sleeve for fiberoptic tracheal intubation. *Anesth Analg.* 2003;97:1205; author reply 1205-1206.

70. Ayoub CM, Rizk MS, Yaacoub CI, Baraka AS, Lteif AM. Advancing the tracheal tube over a flexible fiberoptic bronchoscope by a sleeve mounted on the insertion cord. *Anesth Analg.* 2003;96:290-292, table of contents.

71. Ayoub CM, Lteif AM, Rizk MS, Abu Jalad NM, Hadi U, Baraka AS. Facilitation of passing the endotracheal tube over the flexible fiberoptic

bronchoscope using a Cook airway exchange catheter. *Anesthesiology.* 2002;96:1517-1518.

72. Joo HS, Naik VN, Savoldelli GL. Parker Flex-Tip are not superior to polyvinylchloride tracheal tubes for awake fibreoptic intubations. *Can J Anaesth.* 2005;52:297-301.

73. Greenland KB, Lam MC, Irwin MG. Comparison of the Williams airway intubator and Ovassapian fibreoptic intubating airway for fibreoptic orotracheal intubation. *Anaesthesia.* 2004;59:173-176.

74. Randell T, Valli H, Hakala P. Comparison between the Ovassapian intubating airway and the Berman intubating airway in fibreoptic intubation. *Eur J Anaesthesiol.* 1997;14:380-384.

75. Smith JE, Reid AP. Identifying the more patent nostril before nasotracheal intubation. *Anaesthesia.* 2001;56:258-262.

76. Lee AC, Wu CL, Feins RH, Ward DS. The use of fiberoptic endoscopy in anesthesia. *Chest Surg Clin N Am.* 1996;6:329-347.

77. Arrowsmith JE, Robertshaw HJ, Boyd JD. Nasotracheal intubation in the presence of frontobasal skull fracture. *Can J Anaesth.* 1998;45:71-75.

78. Bainton CR. Complications of managing the airway. In: Benumof JL, ed. *Airway Management Principles and Practice.* St. Louis: Mosby, Inc.; 1996: 886-899.

79. Dauphinee K. Nasotracheal intubation. *Emerg Med Clin North Am.* 1988;6:715-723.

80. Stone DJ, Gal TJ. Airway management. In: Miller RD, ed. *Anesthesia.* 5th ed. Philadelphia, PA: Churchill Livingstone; 2000:1414-1451.

81. Iserson KV. Blind nasotracheal intubation. *Ann Emerg Med.* 1981;10:468-471.

82. Latorre F, Otter W, Kleemann PP, Dick W, Jage J. Cocaine or phenylephrine/lignocaine for nasal fibreoptic intubation? *Eur J Anaesthesiol.* 1996;13: 577-581.

83. Tintinalli JE, Claffey J. Complications of nasotracheal intubation. *Ann Emerg Med.* 1981;10:142-144.

84. Woodall NM, Harwood RJ, Barker GL. Complications of awake fibreoptic intubation without sedation in 200 healthy anaesthetists attending a training course. *Br J Anaesth.* 2008;100:850-855.

85. Pandit JJ, Dravid RM, Iyer R, Popat MT. Orotracheal fibreoptic intubation for rapid sequence induction of anaesthesia. *Anaesthesia.* 2002;57: 123-127.

86. Cole AF, Mallon JS, Rolbin SH, Ananthanarayan C. Fiberoptic intubation using anesthetized, paralyzed, apneic patients. Results of a resident training program. *Anesthesiology.* 1996;84:1101-1106.

87. Hartley M, Morris S, Vaughan RS. Teaching fibreoptic intubation. Effect of alfentanil on the haemodynamic response. *Anaesthesia.* 1994;49:335-337.

88. Heidegger T, Gerig HJ, Ulrich B, Schnider TW. Structure and process quality illustrated by fibreoptic intubation: analysis of 1612 cases. *Anaesthesia.* 2003;58:734-739.

89. Nakazawa K, Ikeda D, Ishikawa S, Makita K. A case of difficult airway due to lingual tonsillar hypertrophy in a patient with Down's syndrome. *Anesth Analg.* 2003;97:704-705.

90. Albanon-Sofelo R, Atkins JM, Broom RS, et al. *Textbook of Advanced Cardiac Life Support.* American Heart Association, Dallas, TX; 1987.

91. Durga VK, Millns JP, Smith JE. Manoeuvres used to clear the airway during fibreoptic intubation. *Br J Anaesth.* 2001;87:207-211.

92. Coe PA, King TA, Towey RM. Teaching guided fibreoptic nasotracheal intubation. An assessment of an anaesthetic technique to aid training. *Anaesthesia.* 1988;43:410-413.

93. Yushi A, Satomoto M, Hiquchi H, et al. Fiberoptic orotracheal intubation in the left semi lateral position. *Anesth Analg.* 2002;94:477-478.

94. Patil V, Stehling LC, Zauder HL, Koch JP. Mechanical aids for fiberoptic endoscopy. *Anesthesiology.* 1982;57:69-70.

95. Afilalo M, Guttman A, Stern E, et al. Fiberoptic intubation in the emergency department: a case series. *J Emerg Med.* 1993;11:387-391.

96. Hamilton PH, Kang JJ. Emergency airway management. *Mt Sinai J Med.* 1997;64:292-301.

97. Mlinek EJ, Jr., Clinton JE, Plummer D, Ruiz E. Fiberoptic intubation in the emergency department. *Ann Emerg Med.* 1990;19:359-362.

98. Delaney KA, Hessler R. Emergency flexible fiberoptic nasotracheal intubation: a report of 60 cases. *Ann Emerg Med.* 1988;17:919-926.

99. Doyle DJ, Arellano R. Medical conditions affecting the airway: a synopsis. In: Hagberg CA, ed. *Handbook of Difficult Airway Management.* Philadelphia, PA: Churchill Livingstone; 2000:227-256.

100. Doyle DJ, Arellano R. Medical conditions affecting the airway: a synopsis. In: Hagberg CA, ed. *Handbook of Difficult Airway Management.* Philadelphia, PA: Churchill Livingstone; 2000:219-225.

101. Desjardins G, Varon AJ. Airway management for penetrating neck injuries: the Miami experience. *Resuscitation.* 2001;48:71-75.

102. Demetriades D, Velmahos GG, Asensio JA. Cervical pharyngoesophageal and laryngotracheal injuries. *World J Surg.* 2001;25:1044-1048.

103. Mandavia DP, Qualls S, Rokos I. Emergency airway management in penetrating neck injury. *Ann Emerg Med.* 2000;35:221-225.

104. Shearer VE, Giesecke AH. Airway management for patients with penetrating neck trauma: a retrospective study. *Anesth Analg.* 1993;77:1135-1138.

105. Morris IR. Anaesthesia and airway management of laryngoscopy and bronchoscopy. In: Hagberg CA, ed. *Benumof's Airway management Principles and Practice.* 2nd ed. Philadelphia, PA: Mosby Elsevier; 2006.

106. Walls RM, Vissers RJ. The traumatized airway. In: Hagberg C. *Benumof's Airway Management.* 2nd ed. Philadelphia, PA: Mosby Elsevier; 2007:939-960.

107. Neal MR, Groves J, Gell IR. Awake fibreoptic intubation in the semi-prone position following facial trauma. *Anaesthesia.* 1996;51:1053-1054.

108. Preis CA, Hartmann T, Zimpfer M. Laryngeal mask airway facilitates awake fiberoptic intubation in a patient with severe oropharyngeal bleeding. *Anesth Analg.* 1998;87:728-729.

109. Schafermeyer RW. Fiberoptic laryngoscopy in the emergency department. *Am J Emerg Med.* 1984;2:160-163.

110. Levitan RM, Kush S, Hollander JE. Devices for difficult airway management in academic emergency departments: results of a national survey. *Ann Emerg Med.* 1999;33:694-698.

111. Wong DT, McGuire GP. Endotracheal intubation through a laryngeal mask/supraglottic airway. *Can J Anaesth.* 2007;54:489-491; author reply 491.

112. The Laryngeal Mask Company Ltd. 2008 LMA North America, Inc. LMA/Classic Excel Product Brochure. www.LMANA.com. Accessed February 11, 2010.

113. Benumof JL. Laryngeal mask airway and the ASA difficult airway algorithm. *Anesthesiology.* 1996;84:686-699.

114. Benumof JL. A new technique of fiberoptic intubation through a standard LMA. *Anesthesiology.* 2001;95:1541.

115. Preis C, Preis I. Concept for easy fiberoptic intubation via a laryngeal airway mask. *Anesth Analg.* 1999;89:803-804.

116. Watson NC, Hokanson M, Maltby JR, Todesco JM. The intubating laryngeal mask airway in failed fibreoptic intubation. *Can J Anaesth.* 1999;46:376-378.

117. Brain AI, Verghese C, Addy EV, Kapila A. The intubating laryngeal mask. I: development of a new device for intubation of the trachea. *Br J Anaesth.* 1997;79:699-703.

118. Joo HS, Kapoor S, Rose DK, Naik VN. The intubating laryngeal mask airway after induction of general anesthesia versus awake fiberoptic intubation in patients with difficult airways. *Anesth Analg.* 2001;92:1342-1346.

119. Lin M, Hunt-Smith J. The Aintree Intubation Catheter. www.cookmedical.com. Accessed February 11, 2010.

120. Atherton DP, O'Sullivan E, Lowe D, Charters P. A ventilation-exchange bougie for fibreoptic intubations with the laryngeal mask airway. *Anaesthesia.* 1996;51:1123-1126.

121. Zura A, Doyle DJ, Orlandi M. Use of the Aintree intubation catheter in a patient with an unexpected difficult airway. *Can J Anaesth.* 2005;52:646-649.

122. Avitsian R, Doyle DJ, Helfand R, et al. Successful reintubation after cervical spine exposure using an Aintree intubation catheter and a Laryngeal Mask Airway. *J Clin Anesth.* 2006;18:224-225.

123. Higgs A, Clark E, Premraj K. Low-skill fibreoptic intubation: use of the Aintree catheter with the classic LMA. *Anaesthesia.* 2005;60:915-920.

124. Zura A, Doyle DJ, Avitsian R, DeUngria M. More on intubation using the Aintree catheter. *Anesth Analg.* 2006;103:785.

125. Blair EJ, Mihai R, Cook TM. Tracheal intubation via the Classic and Proseal laryngeal mask airways: a manikin study using the Aintree intubating catheter. *Anaesthesia.* 2007;62:385-387.

126. Henderson JJ, Popat MT, Latto IP, Pearce AC. Difficult Airway Society guidelines for management of the unanticipated difficult intubation. *Anaesthesia.* 2004;59:675-694.

127. ASA Task Force on Management of the Difficult Airway. Practice guidelines for management of the difficult airway: an updated report by the American Society of Anesthesiologists Task Force on Management of the Difficult Airway. *Anesthesiology.* 2003;98:1269-1277.

128. Pearce AC. Airway strategy. *Current Anaesth Crit Care.* 2001;12:207-212.

129. Sanchez AF, Morrison DE. Preparation of the patient for awake intubation. In: Hagberg CA, ed. *Handbook of Difficult Airway Management.* Philadelphia, PA: Churchill Livingstone; 2000.

130. Wu FL, Razzaghi A, Souney PF. Seizure after lidocaine for bronchoscopy: case report and review of the use of lidocaine in airway anesthesia. *Pharmacotherapy.* 1993;13:72-78.

131. Maktabi MA, Hoffman H, Funk G, From RP. Laryngeal trauma during awake fiberoptic intubation. *Anesth Analg.* 2002;95:1112-1114, table of contents.

132. Patil AA, Barker GL, Woodall NM, Harwood RJ. Pyrexia and rigors following fiberoptic intubation in a delegate attending an awake fiberoptic intubation training course. *Anaesthesia.* 2004;59:1045-1046.

133. Naik VN, Matsumoto ED, Houston PL, et al. Fiberoptic orotracheal intubation on anesthetized patients: do manipulation skills learned on a simple model transfer into the operating room? *Anesthesiology.* 2001;95:343-348.

134. Marsland CP, Robinson BJ, Chitty CH, Guy BJ. Acquisition and maintenance of endoscopic skills: developing an endoscopic dexterity training system for anesthesiologists. *J Clin Anesth.* 2002;14:615-619.

135. Marsland C, Larsen P, Segal R, et al. Proficient manipulation of fibreoptic bronchoscope to carina by novices on first clinical attempt after specialized bench practice. *Br J Anaesth.* 2010;104:375-381.

136. Martin KM, Larsen PD, Segal R, Marsland CP. Effective nonanatomical endoscopy training produces clinical airway endoscopy proficiency. *Anesth Analg.* 2004;99:938-944, table of contents.

137. Smith JE, Jackson AP, Hurdley J, Clifton PJ. Learning curves for fibreoptic nasotracheal intubation when using the endoscopic video camera. *Anaesthesia.* 1997;52:101-106.

138. Rowe R, Cohen RA. An evaluation of a virtual reality airway simulator. *Anesth Analg.* 2002;95:62-66, table of contents.

139. Dykes MH, Ovassapian A. Dissemination of fibreoptic airway endoscopy skills by means of a workshop utilizing models. *Br J Anaesth.* 1989;63:595-597.

140. Patil V, Barker GL, Harwood RJ, Woodall NM. Training course in local anaesthesia of the airway and fibreoptic intubation using course delegates as subjects. *Br J Anaesth.* 2002;89:586-593.

141. Ball DR. Awake versus asleep fibreoptic intubation. *Anaesthesia.* 1994;49:921.

142. Bray JK, Yentis SM. Attitudes of patients and anaesthetists to informed consent for specialist airway techniques. *Anaesthesia.* 2002;57:1012-1015.

143. Mason RA. Learning fibreoptic intubation: fundamental problems. *Anaesthesia.* 1992;47:729-731.

144. Schaefer HG, Marsch SC, Keller HL, Strebel S, Anselmi L, Drewe J. Teaching fibreoptic intubation in anaesthetised patients. *Anaesthesia.* 1994;49:331-334.

145. Smith JE, Fenner SG, King MJ. Teaching fibreoptic nasotracheal intubation with and without closed circuit television. *Br J Anaesth.* 1993;71:206-211.

146. Johnson C, Roberts JT. Clinical competence in the performance of fiberoptic laryngoscopy and endotracheal intubation: a study of resident instruction. *J Clin Anesth.* 1989;1:344-349.

147. Smith JE, Jackson AP. Learning fibreoptic endoscopy. Nasotracheal or orotracheal intubations first? *Anaesthesia.* 2000;55:1072-1075.

148. Sia RL, Edens ET. How to avoid problems when using the fibre-optic bronchoscope for difficult intubation. *Anaesthesia.* 1981;36:74-75.

SELF-EVALUATION QUESTIONS

9.1. Complications associated with bronchoscopic intubation include

A. laryngospasm

B. complete airway obstruction

C. local anesthesia toxicity

D. laryngeal trauma

E. all of the above

9.2. Which of the following is a reliable method of removing prions from the flexible bronchoscope following its use in a patient with Creutzfeldt-Jakob disease?

A. immersed in a solution of peracetic acid

B. disinfection of bronchoscopes using orthophthaldehyde

C. disinfection of bronchoscopes using ethylene oxide

D. disinfection of bronchoscopes using an autoclave

E. none of the above

9.3. During bronchoscopic intubation, which of the following can facilitate advancement of the ensleeved endotracheal tube to advance into the trachea over the bronchoscopic bronchoscope?

A. Profound regional anesthesia of the airway.

B. Rotation of the tube 90 degrees counterclockwise may be necessary to orient the bevel posteriorly.

C. Minimize the discrepancy between the outside diameter of the bronchoscope and the internal diameter of the endotracheal tube.

D. The use of the ILMA tube which has a soft hemispherical bevel and a leading edge in the midline.

E. All of the above.

CHAPTER (10)

Rigid and Semirigid Fiberoptic and Video Laryngoscopy and Intubation

Richard M. Cooper and J. Adam Law

10.1 INTRODUCTION

10.1.1 Why were rigid and semirigid fiberoptic and video laryngoscopes developed?

Macewan originally performed endotracheal intubation with his fingers.[1] In 1913 Janeway used a speculum very similar to the laryngoscopes introduced by Miller and Macintosh in 1941 and 1943.[2] And since that time, we've remained very much dependent upon the line-of-sight technique exemplified by direct laryngoscopy (DL). It was proposed that "the sniffing position" aligns the axes of the mouth, pharynx, and trachea, yet the incisors, the tongue, the epiglottis, and occasionally the position of the larynx itself, often conspire against a clear view. Studies on conscious adults with normal airway features, in neutral, sniffing, and simple extension demonstrate that positioning alone does not align the axes[3] and there was little difference between the sniffing position and simple extension in a large series of patients undergoing laryngoscopy.[4] If positioning does not align these axes, how do we accomplish intubation by DL? This is achieved by the application of force to displace and compress the tongue, mandible, and frequently the larynx itself. Yet even among adults with seemingly normal airways, it is not possible to view the larynx by direct means in approximately 6% to 10%[5,6] and studies suggest that when this method fails, all too often we try harder and more often[7] with dire consequences.[7,8]

Instruments that are more or less anatomically shaped can overcome restrictions in upper airway anatomy of most patients. Unfortunately, direct laryngoscopy using these instruments is difficult or impossible in some patients. Fiberoptic and video laryngoscopes are designed specifically for this purpose.

Another significant limitation of direct laryngoscopy is that the experience is difficult to share.[9,10] Only the laryngoscopist is able to view the procedure and this complicates the teaching and recording of laryngoscopy, limiting possibilities for quality improvement and the conduct of airway research. Video laryngoscopy circumvents many of these limitations but generally relies upon alternative devices. Viewing the anatomy and the procedure of intubation can be achieved using a conventional laryngoscope. The Airway Cam®, developed by Dr Richard Levitan, is a head-mounted camera which captures the laryngoscopist's view through an eye-level pentaprism and conveys the image to a video monitor and/or a recording device.[11,12] This device enables a student and mentor to simultaneously view the same object, record and replay the image at a time and pace conducive to and appropriate for teaching, clinical documentation, and research. While these achievements are clearly worthwhile, this technology does not improve laryngeal exposure.

Flexible bronchoscopes have greatly expanded our ability to diagnose and manage problems in previously inaccessible body parts. These devices are versatile but complex. For tracheal intubation, flexible bronchoscopes demand a different skill set than direct laryngoscopy. Nonetheless, practitioners must master these devices, since they are the best choice for some airway challenges. Their complexity and versatility also add to their cost and fragility. As well, blood, secretions, vomitus, or fogging may significantly interfere with the view. Although in some situations, flexible bronchoscopes are essential, other devices can do the job more easily, and quickly. Fiberoptic and video technologies have been incorporated into semirigid or rigid devices, designed specifically for intubation. These devices share the attributes of providing illumination and non-line-of-sight viewing. They may be in the form of a stylet (eg, the Shikani optical stylet, the Levitan FPS [first pass success]), a flat blade (eg, the Bullard laryngoscope), a hollow tube (eg, WuScope), or resemble a conventional laryngoscope (eg, Storz V-Mac, McGrath VL, or GlideScope® VL). As this is an evolving field, this chapter is not an exhaustive review of all the currently available devices.

(In discussing the features, costs, and cleaning of these devices, every effort has been made to obtain information from the manufacturer, current at the time of the writing. Prices and device configurations change and the authors strongly advise prospective users to consult further with the manufacturer and national and institutional authorities regarding acceptable methods of disinfection). All prices are in US dollars unless otherwise stated. All prices were accurate at the time of writing but may be subject to change.

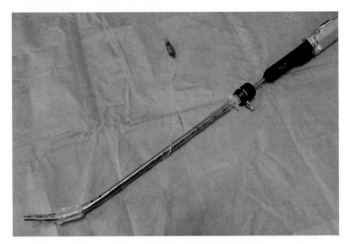

FIGURE 10-1. The Bonfils retromolar intubation fiberscope, shown here with a micro video module camera unit, enabling image display on an accompanying monitor.

10.2   FIBEROPTIC STYLETS

10.2.1   What are optical stylets?

Optical stylets ensleeve fiberoptic bundles within a metallic exterior and when inserted within an endotracheal tube (ETT) allow the practitioner to view ETT advancement through a proximal eyepiece or via a video monitor. The instruments vary in their external diameter, image resolution, source of illumination, and flexibility. At this point, the commercially available optical stylets with reasonable accompanying narrative in the literature include the Bonfils retromolar intubation fiberscope (Bonfils, Karl Storz Endoscopy, Culver City, CA), the Shikani optical stylet (SOS) and the Levitan FPS scope (both from Clarus Medical LLC, Minneapolis, MN), the fiberoptic StyletScope (FSS, Nihon Kohden Corp., Tokyo, Japan), and the video-optical intubation stylet (VOIS, Acutronic Medical Systems AG, Baar, Switzerland). The recently introduced Clarus video system (Clarus Medical LLC, Minneapolis, MN) is the first semirigid optical stylet to be entirely video based.

10.2.2   What are the unique characteristics of optical stylets?

Common to all optical stylets is a rigid or semirigid shaft, and a proximal tube holder compatible with a 15-mm ETT connector. Tube holders are generally movable on the stylet shaft, enabling appropriate positioning of the tip of the endoscope within the ETT. Most optical stylets transmit light distally and the image proximally to an eyepiece or camera through glass or plastic fibers of variable resolution. The distal viewing angle varies from 50 to 90 degrees. Light is generally powered from a battery source to enhance portability, although some scopes can be attached via a cable to a remote light source. None of the optical stylets have a hollow working channel of the type present on other classes of fiberoptic device.

10.2.3   Individual optical stylet description

10.2.3.1   What Are the Characteristics of the Bonfils Retromolar Intubation Fiberscope?

The Bonfils is the only scope in this class of instruments that is nonmalleable. The shaft of the adult scope is 40 cm long and has a fixed anterior bend of 40 degrees at the distal end. The adult version is 5.0 mm in diameter, so the instrument will accommodate ETTs of 5.5 mm internal diameter (ID) and larger (Figure 10-1). Two smaller versions are 3.5 mm and 2.0 mm in diameter. A movable tube holder permits ETT fixation on the stylet shaft as well as oxygen insufflation down the ETT. Light is provided by cable from a remote light source, or by attachable battery-powered LED. The image is transferred by glass fiber (12,000 pixels), and the distal viewing angle is 90 degrees. Two versions of each size of stylet are offered: one features a movable proximal eyepiece, while the other version accepts the direct-coupled interface (DCI™)—a quick connection on the proximal stylet that allows one-step attachment of a camera with a light/signal cable, compatible with Storz video towers or Telepack units.

10.2.3.2   What Are the Characteristics of the Shikani Optical Stylet?

The Shikani optical stylet (SOS) is an example of a semimalleable optical stylet (Figure 10-2). It is supplied with a bending tool and can accommodate an arc of up to 120 degrees. The stylet shaft is 27 cm long, and with a diameter of 5.0 mm, can accept ETTs greater than 5.5 mm ID. A pediatric version is compatible with ETTs in the 2.5 to 5.5 mm ID range. ETT fixation on the stylet shaft is achieved by a movable "Tube Stop" adapter. The adapter accepts an attachment through which oxygen can be delivered down the ETT. The distal viewing angle of the adult scope is 70 degrees. Glass fiberoptic bundles of 30,000 pixels are used to deliver the image to a fixed-focus, proximal eyepiece. Lighting is supplied from a standard Green specification fiberoptic laryngoscope

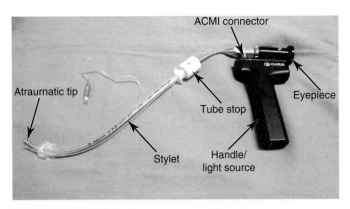

FIGURE 10-2. The Shikani optical stylet, adult version.

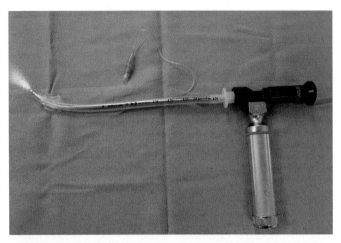

FIGURE 10-4. The Levitan FPS scope, shown here with a Greenline-compatible laryngoscope handle. It can also be used with a light-emitting diode (LED) battery pack.

handle or a small battery-powered LED source. The eyepiece is compatible with a proximally attached camera adapter, if desired. The company also supplies a passively flexible version of optical stylet called the Pocket Scope (Figure 10-3) designed for use with ETTs of 4 mm ID or larger. It can be used to confirm single- or double-lumen tube placement or patency.

10.2.3.3 What Are the Characteristics of the Levitan FPS Scope?

The Levitan first pass success (FPS) scope, developed by Dr Richard Levitan, has recently been introduced as a low-cost fiberoptic stylet (Figure 10-4). The light source is supplied via an adapter from a standard Greenline handle or a dedicated attached portable LED. The shaft of the instrument is malleable through 90 degrees. Unlike other fiberoptic stylets, the 15.0 mm ETT connector adapter is fixed proximally on the stylet's handle; so as to have the distal stylet tip appropriately placed just within the distal ETT, the ETT should be cut to 27.5 cm prior to loading. A proximal connector permits oxygen insufflation down the ETT once attached. The designer suggests shaping the Levitan FPS scope "straight to cuff" (ie, with an otherwise straight shaft bent anteriorly at an angle of no more than 25-35 degrees just proximal to the ETT cuff) and using it in conjunction with DL.[13]

10.2.3.4 What Are the Characteristics of the StyletScope?

The fiberoptic StyletScope (FSS) is unique among the optical stylets in incorporating a lever adjacent to the proximal handle, enabling manipulation of the distal stylet angle during the tracheal tube placement. When depressed toward the handle, the distal stylet tip, with loaded ETT, will flex anteriorly up to 75 degrees (Figure 10-5). The handle incorporates a holder that accepts the ETT's 15-mm connector, and stylet length is adjustable to conform to ETT length. Light supply is built in to the proximal battery handle, and is powered by two 1.5 V alkaline batteries.[14] Fiberoptic imaging occurs via plastic bundles (3500 pixels), and the obtainable field of view is 50 degrees. With an outer diameter of 6.0 mm, the FSS will accept a minimum ETT size of 7.0 mm ID. The scope can be sterilized in ethylene oxide.

10.2.3.5 What Are the Characteristics of the Video-Optical Intubating System?

The video-optical intubating stylet (VOIS) is a semirigid stylet malleable along its distal 40 cm (Figure 10-6). With an OD of 5.0 mm, glass fiberoptic bundles of 10,000 pixels transfer the image to a proximal ocular, which in turn is compatible with various CCD camera systems. Light is supplied from a remote source via a fiberoptic cable, and a 50-degree angle of view can be obtained.

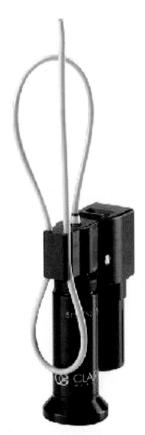

FIGURE 10-3. The Pocket Scope. (Courtesy Clarus Medical.)

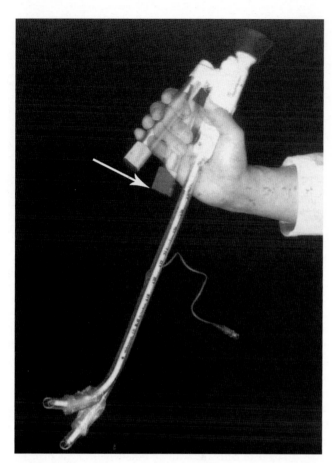

FIGURE 10-5. The Fiberoptic StyletScope (FSS). The photo shows the neutral and activated positions: as the proximal lever is depressed toward the device handle, the distal stylet and ensleeved tube flex anteriorly. (With permission from *Can J Anaesth.* 2001 Oct;48(9):919-923.)

10.2.3.6   What Are the Characteristics of the Clarus Video System?

The recently-introduced Clarus video system is a video-based optical stylet with a proximal handle-mounted video screen (Figure 10-7). The 3-in LCD screen can be variably angled using a thumb control.

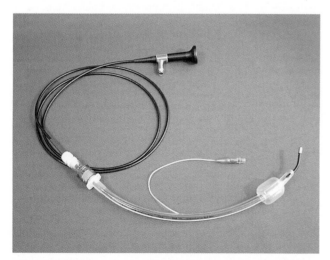

FIGURE 10-6. Video-optical intubating stylet (VOIS). (Courtesy Dr Marcus Weiss.)

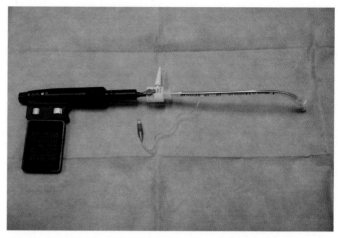

FIGURE 10-7. The Clarus video system is a video-based optical stylet with a proximal handle-mounted video screen which can be variably angled using a thumb control.

A CMOS image sensor is located at the distal end of the stylet, which is detachable from the handle, mainly for cleaning and sterilization purposes. The rechargeable scope features two light sources: two white light LEDs, and one red LED, which can be used for anterior neck transillumination, in similar fashion to lighted stylets. The stylet shaft is semimalleable, and as with other optical stylets, has a shaft-mounted Tube Stop adapter to enable optimal placement of the stylet tip just within the distal end of an ETT.

10.2.3.7   What Pediatric Optical Stylet Options Are Available?

The pediatric version of the Shikani optical stylet will accept a minimum tube size of 2.5-mm ID. An intermediate size of the Bonfils will accept a minimum tube size of 4.0-mm ID, while the smallest fiberoptic stylet in the Karl Storz family, named the Brambrink, will accept ETTs down to 2.5-mm ID.

10.2.4   Optical stylet use

Most of the optical stylets described above are similar in their structure, from which it follows that their function will also be similar. The following narrative describing the use of optical stylets, in general, can be applied to all.

10.2.4.1   How Are Optical Stylets Prepared for Tracheal Intubation?

An ETT should be loaded on the optical stylet, and the proximal ETT connector stabilized within the tube holder on the stylet's shaft. The tube holder and ETT are then positioned on the stylet's shaft such that the scope tip is located just proximal to the ETT bevel. The tube holder is then fixed to the stylet shaft by tightening a locking screw. As previously mentioned, with its fixed proximal ETT connector holder, the Levitan FPS requires the ETT be precut to 27.5 cm prior to loading. For semirigid devices, the desired degree of distal stylet angulation will depend on the technique of use: stand-alone use generally requires more angulation (eg, 40-90 degrees), while fiberoptic stylet used as adjunct to direct laryngoscopy should require a distal curvature of no more than 25 to 35 degrees.

As with all fiberoptic instruments, insertion of a cold instrument in a patient may result in an obscured view due to fogging. This can be avoided by prewarming the device with immersion of the stylet shaft in a container of warm water, or by applying a commercial antifog solution to the distal lens. As the presence of blood and secretions can interfere with viewing, the patient's pharynx should be suctioned prior to insertion of an optical stylet, or any fiberoptic device.

10.2.4.2 How Are Optical Stylets Used to Perform Tracheal Intubation?

Although optical stylets can also be used as an adjunct to DL, most clinicians opt for stand-alone use. A jaw lift, jaw thrust, tongue pull, or combination thereof[15] should be performed to enlarge the pharyngeal space[16] by elevating the tongue and epiglottis away from the posterior pharyngeal wall. The jaw thrust may also be beneficial by expanding the laryngeal aperture.[17] Following suctioning, the stylet/tube assembly is inserted from the side of the mouth (ie, advanced over or behind the molars) and slowly rotated upright and toward the midline during advancement,[15] or alternatively, it can be inserted and advanced via a midline approach. For the midline approach, the stylet should generally be bent at a more acute angle, and during advancement, identification of the uvula and epiglottis will help practitioner's orientation to the midline position of the tip of the device. Once at the laryngeal aperture, the ETT can be advanced off the stylet, through the glottis and into the trachea.

For optical stylet used as an adjunct to DL, the best laryngoscopic view is obtained. Faced with a poor view, for example, Cormack/Lehane (C/L) Grade 3, an optical stylet loaded with an ETT is carefully placed just beneath the epiglottis, under direct vision. With the ETT tip under, but no more than 0.5 cm beyond the tip of the epiglottis, the clinician then seeks a view through the stylet's eyepiece (or on-screen): the vocal cords should be immediately visible, facilitating advancement of the ETT up to and through the cords. If stand-alone use has failed, some practitioners elect to use the direct laryngoscope in this fashion to help control the tongue.[15,18,19] Concomitant use of DL with an optical stylet appears to be as effective as stand-alone use.[20]

Optical stylets have also been used in similar fashion to lighted stylets. Using only transillumination of the anterior neck to suggest successful tracheal access, secondary confirmation of correct placement can then follow by indirect visualization of the trachea through the eyepiece. This has been described with adult and pediatric optical stylets[21,22] with a success rate that rivals the traditional visual advancement techniques.

10.2.5 Clinical experience of optical stylets

10.2.5.1 What Is the Clinical Utility of Optical and Video-Optic Stylets?

Fiberoptic stylet use has been described to facilitate postinduction and awake[23-25] intubations of adult and pediatric patients, both with and without predicted difficult airway anatomy. Successful use has been reported with both single- and shortened double-lumened tubes.[26]

10.2.5.2 How Effective Are Optical Stylets for Intubation of Patient with a Difficult Airway?

Rudolph in 1996 reported on use of the Bonfils stylet in a series of 107 patients, of whom 18 presented C/L Grade 3 or 4 views at direct laryngoscopy. Tracheal intubation was successful in 16 of 18 of the difficult cases with the Bonfils, including all four C/L Grade 4 situations. Twenty-one percent of the total series required concomitant use of DL.[18] Shikani, in his initial study of the SOS,[19] looked at 120 patients, 74 of them children, including 7 patients with C/L Grade 3 or 4 views. All patients in the series, including five awake patients, were successfully intubated with the scope, 88% on the first attempt. Five of the seven C/L Grade 3 and 4 patients required concomitant use of DL. Later, Bein et al compared use of the Bonfils with the LMA Fastrach™ in 80 patients with predictors of difficult DL. Thirty-nine of 40 patients randomized to Bonfils use were intubated on the first attempt with a median time of 40 seconds, in contrast to a 70% first attempt success rate for the Fastrach.[27] A second study evaluated the Bonfils use after failed DL. In 25 patients recruited following two failed DL attempts, 88% were successfully intubated with the Bonfils at the first attempt, and all but one (96%) by the second attempt, with a median time of 47.5 seconds.[16]

10.2.5.3 How Effective Are Optical Stylets for Tracheal Intubation in the Simulated Difficult Airway?

Greenland and coworkers compared the Levitan FPS scope with the single-use Portex tracheal introducer in a randomized crossover study of 34 adult patients. They found equal success and a shorter time-to-intubation with the tracheal introducer under simulated C/L Grade 3A conditions.[28] This was consistent with one of two similar mannequin studies: Kovacs[29] found equivalent success and time-to-intubation with the tracheal introducer and Levitan FPS in a mannequin with fixed C/L Grade 3A conditions, while Evans, using the multiuse Eschmann tracheal introducer and an undifferentiated Grade 3 view, found the Levitan a better device with a significantly higher success rate.[30]

The Bonfils stylet was compared with Macintosh blade DL in a population of elective surgical patients in whom difficulty was simulated by application of a cervical collar. Tube placement was successful in 81.6% of patients randomized to the Bonfils stylet, versus 39.5% of the Macintosh DL patients.[31] A similar study in elective surgical patients undergoing only manual in-line neck stabilization compared the use of the StyletScope with attempted blind passage of an ETT styletted with a conventional metal stylet. In those patients presenting C/L Grade 3 or 4 views, StyletScope use required fewer attempts, and was successful more often than the conventional stylet.[32]

10.2.5.4   What Is the Role of the Optical Stylet for Intubation of the Patient with Known or Possible Cervical Spine Instability?

Two studies have compared Bonfils aided Macintosh blade (with attempted full exposure of vocal cords), one using intermittent direct laryngoscopy, one using intermittent still radiographs[33] and the other using external markers as a surrogate of cervical spine movement.[34] Subjects in the two studies started with the head and neck in a neutral position, but had no application of in-line neck stabilization. Both studies documented significantly less upper cervical spine movement with the Bonfils. Using the Shikani optical stylet with in-line neck stabilization and continuous fluoroscopy, another study similarly concluded that less movement occurred with the SOS than with Macintosh blade DL.[35] The clinical significance of such studies is unknown.

10.2.5.5   What Is the Learning Curve for Optical Stylet Use?

Using time to successful tracheal intubation as a marker for proficiency, published learning curve data on the Bonfils fiberoptic stylet suggest that 20 to 25 uses are needed to achieve expertise.[15,24] Other published reports of experience with optical stylets detail most of the failures at the beginning of their respective series (ie, within the first 10 uses).[19] In one series, the most commonly encountered preventable difficulties included secretions, fogging (both preventable by suctioning and antifogging, respectively), and difficulty getting under the epiglottis[15] (aided by jaw lift or concomitant direct laryngoscopy).

10.2.6   Optical stylets—other considerations

10.2.6.1   What Is the Pediatric Experience with Optical Stylet Use?

Case reports have been published documenting successful tracheal intubation using optical stylets in pediatric patients with actual or predicted difficulty due to Pierre Robin sequence[36,37], Hurler syndrome[38], Goldenhar syndrome[36], Treacher Collins syndrome[36], restricted mouth opening with popliteal pterygium syndrome[39], difficulty with these devices and small for gestational age conditions.[40] In all of these cases, either a Brambrink or Shikani stylet was used as a stand-alone technique. However, unlike the foregoing successes, Bein published a series of 55 uses of the Bonfils and Brambrink optical stylet in elective pediatric surgery patients without predictors of difficult airway anatomy. Although performed by an investigator experienced in adult use of the Bonfils, this study reported a relatively poor success rate with the device, with many of the failures due to secretions. In the series, the tracheas of only 40 of 55 (73%) patients were intubated on the first attempt, and after 3 attempts there was a failure rate of 9%.[41] Using the VOIS, prospective observational series of 50 pediatric patients with difficulty simulated by suboptimal DL (C/L Grade 3 view) showed successful tracheal intubation in 92% (46/50) of patients within 60 seconds.[42]

10.2.6.2   What Are the Potential Complications Associated with the Use of Optical Stylets?

To date, most complications reported in the literature due to optical stylets have been limited to failures to intubate[41]: reports of airway trauma are rare.[15] One case report has appeared documenting extensive facial and subcutaneous emphysema of the neck after an intubation attempt during which oxygen was insufflated at 10 L·min^{-1} via the tube holder adapter on a Bonfils stylet.[43] Otherwise, in many cases, failure to intubate has resulted from a view being obscured by fog or secretions, often a preventable complication.

10.2.6.3   What Are the Potential Advantages of Optical Stylets?

As a class, optical stylets are portable, and are, relative to their flexible counterparts, less expensive and more robust. Their rigidity may make them easier to navigate to the laryngeal inlet than flexible devices. As outlined above, published studies and case series suggest that at least in the hands of experienced users, optical stylets enable a high rate of successful tracheal intubation in patients presenting predicted or actual difficult direct laryngoscopy. Optical stylet use has also been associated with a lower incidence of adverse hemodynamic response than DL.[44,45]

10.2.6.4   What Are the Disadvantages of Optical Stylets?

Preparation for optical stylet use is needed by antifogging the stylet and ensuring the oropharynx has been suctioned prior to the tracheal intubation attempt. Some optical stylets require the ETT be cut to a specific length. During advancement toward the glottic opening, orientation within the upper airway can be difficult unless soft tissues are well controlled with a jaw lift or by concomitant use of a direct laryngoscope. It follows that poor jaw protrusion, as well as significant blood or secretions in the airway may predict difficulty with these devices. It should be noted that optical stylet use in mannequins, with their predictable, patent, and secretion-free upper airways, can seem deceptively easy. It is also probable that intubation using optical stylets will be more successful in the hands of practitioners already experienced in the use of flexible bronchoscopes.

10.2.6.5   How Are Optical Stylets Disinfected?[A]

Most optical stylets can be cleaned in similar fashion as flexible bronchoscopes (see Section 9.2.2), although individual recommendations should be sought from the manufacturer. After use, the stylet shaft should be washed with a detergent solution, while those stylets with a hollow working channel should have it cleaned with a brush supplied for the purpose. Most can be sterilized with ethylene oxide, Steris® or Sterrad® systems, or have high-level disinfection applied by cold-soak solutions (eg, Cidex).

[A]In all cases, please consult with the manufacturer for detailed cleaning instructions.

10.3   RIGID FIBEROPTIC LARYNGOSCOPES

10.3.1 What are rigid fiberoptic laryngoscopes?

These devices have in common a fiberoptic bundle and viewing channel within a rigid exoskeleton. The fibers are thereby protected from damage, making these devices more robust. Eliminating the angulation controller found on flexible scopes decreases their complexity, making rigid devices less expensive, also reducing their versatility. Rigid fiberoptic laryngoscopes were historically designed only to view the larynx and observe the insertion and advancement (or removal and exchange) of an ETT. However, this design feature is now being challenged by rigid optical and video-based devices such as the Airtraq® Optical Laryngoscope and Pentax AirwayScope, which will enable laryngeal visualization and act as a conduit for tube passage to and through the glottis.

During direct laryngoscopy using a laryngoscope, the view of the glottis is frequently obscured by the ETT. This is particularly true with the blade laryngoscope. During intubation using a flexible bronchoscope, typically the scope is directed into the distal trachea, after which the ETT is passed blindly over the scope into the trachea. The flexible scope essentially functions, in this setting, as a tracheal introducer (eg, Eschmann introducer). In contrast, the viewing element of the rigid fiberoptic laryngoscope is placed distally on the blade and to the side, providing an unobstructed view of the ETT as it advances through the larynx. This offers a superior degree of control, potentially reducing the danger of laryngeal injury caused by blind tube advancement.

The Bullard laryngoscope (BL) has been available for over two decades. Though clearly the device has its champions, despite its apparent utility in a wide variety of challenging settings, it does not enjoy widespread popularity.[46-48]

10.3.2 Specific devices

10.3.2.1 Bullard and Bullard Elite (Gyrus/ACMI) Laryngoscopes

10.3.2.1.1 What Are the Characteristics of the Bullard Laryngoscope?

The Bullard laryngoscope (BL, Gyrus ACMI, Inc., Southborough, MA) is an indirect rigid fiberoptic laryngoscope, developed by Roger Bullard (Figure 10-8). It is available in adult, pediatric, and neonatal sizes. The blade is anatomically shaped and has three channels: a 3.7-mm working channel, a light bundle, and an image bundle all close to the distal tip. The image bundle has 9500 pixels, producing an adequate although lower image resolution than other devices in its class. The unit is reasonably compact when field illumination is provided by an incandescent bulb powered by a battery handle. An external halogen light source provides more intense illumination and is better suited if a video camera is utilized. The working channel can be used for oxygen insufflation, suction, or the application of topical anesthesia using an epidural catheter. The eyepiece on the BL Elite has an integrated knob for

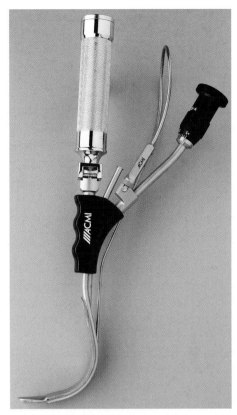

FIGURE 10-8. The Adult Bullard Elite™ Laryngoscope is shown with the dedicated stylet and battery handle. Note how the stylet is tucked tightly beneath the 6-mm spatula-like blade. An external fiberoptic light source is advised when a video camera is attached to the eyepiece. The working channel can be seen between the battery handle and the stylet. This can accommodate a suction catheter, oxygen, or an epidural catheter to apply topical anesthesia. (Photograph provided by ACMI.)

diopter adjustment. The eyepiece on both the BL and BL Elite can be connected to a standard 35-mm video attachment allowing the image to be displayed on a large monitor. This facilitates teaching and permits recording of the airway images.

The blade design resembles a spatula having a thickness of only 6.0 mm, allowing excellent glottic visualization even when mouth opening is very limited and cervical movement is restricted. The ETT can be introduced freehanded with a malleable stylet or with one of two types of dedicated stylets:

1. Bullard intubating stylet: This stylet anchors directly to the Bullard laryngoscope and fits snugly against the posterior and inferior aspect of the BL blade (Figure 10-8). The ETT is loaded onto the stylet and advanced through the Murphy eye. One of the authors recommends rotating the ETT 180 degrees so that the bevel points to the left. This reduces the tendency for the ETT to impact upon the right arytenoid during its insertion.

2. Straight-tipped "multifunctional stylet": This stylet also attaches to the BL and fits against its inferior aspect. In contrast to the intubating stylet, it is longer, straight at its distal end, and tubular in order to accommodate an intubation catheter over which the ETT is advanced.

A plastic blade extender can be attached to the distal tip of the laryngoscope for additional length.

10.3.2.1.2   How Is the BL Used?

To facilitate tracheal intubation using the Bullard laryngoscope, the authors suggest the following steps:

- Minimize secretions of the upper airway by using an antisialagogue prior to intubation and suctioning the pharynx prior to device insertion.

- Prepare the device with an antifogging spray or warm water immersion.

- Prepare free-handed, dedicated Bullard intubating stylet or multifunctional stylet with lubricant and an appropriately sized ETT.

- Place the head and neck of the patient in neutral position.

- Topical airway anesthesia should be used if laryngoscopy is to be done awake. This can be achieved by applying topical anesthesia to the tongue to suppress the gag reflex, lidocaine or EMLA ointment to the BL, and advancing an epidural catheter through the working channel. The epidural catheter is attached to a syringe containing local anesthetic. This allows topical airway anesthesia to be applied under visual control.

- The blade is inserted by rotation behind and around the tongue. With the scope handle now vertical, the blade is allowed to gently drop against the posterior pharyngeal wall. Manual elevation of the mandible with the right thumb will help to elevate the epiglottis and reduce contact with the posterior pharyngeal wall. The BL is then advanced caudally and elevated to view the glottic opening.

- When using either of the attached stylets, it is essential to grasp the stylet/ETT together with the handle such that they remain closely applied to the inferior aspect of the blade. This in turn will keep the tip of the stylet visible through the eyepiece.

- A clear view of the larynx should be obtained prior to advancing the ETT. If the dedicated intubating stylet is used, it should be pointed toward the posterior third of the left vocal fold or its arytenoid cartilage. As the laryngoscopist begins to advance the ETT, subtle adjustments of the scope are still possible, but if the tube fails to enter the glottis, it is often necessary to withdraw the scope and reload the ETT.

- If the multifunctional stylet is used, ETT advancement can be preceded by passage of an intubation catheter through the hollow lumen of the stylet into the trachea.

- Use of a "freehand" technique involves advancing an ETT off a well-lubricated stylet bent at an acute angle corresponding to that of the BL blade (90 degrees). To reduce the risk of hang up against the anterior tracheal wall, Hung et al have suggested reverse loading of the ETT onto the stylet.[49]

- After intubation, the BL should be removed from the patient by forward rotation of the scope out of the patient's mouth.

10.3.2.1.3   How Effective Is the BL for Tracheal Intubation in Patients with a History of Difficult Laryngoscopy?

MacQuarrie and coworkers compared the BL using a free-handed stylet and the dedicated multifunctional stylet in 80 adult patients lacking anatomical features predictive of a difficult laryngoscopy.[50]

A cervical collar was applied to simulate a difficult airway. This resulted in a C/L Grade 3 view in 65% of their patients when DL was performed using a Macintosh #3 blade. BL intubation however was unsuccessful in 12/80 patients (15%). Fogging or secretions were responsible for half of these failures. The cervical collar reduced mouth opening to 2.3 and 2.6 cm in the two groups making it difficult to manipulate the ETT. There was no significant difference between the two different stylets with respect to the number of attempts required, success rate, trauma, or time to tracheal intubation. Nasal tube insertion might have overcome the problems encountered in the patients in whom mouth opening did not permit manipulation of the ETT.

Use of the BL has been advocated in various conditions associated with difficult or failed DL, including microstomia, micrognathism, Pierre-Robin syndrome, and morbid obesity.[51-53]

Comparing the BL with the flexible bronchoscope in awake patients with cervical spine disease, the BL provided a better laryngeal view in less time.[51] Hastings and coworkers compared head and cervical spine movement and the laryngeal views obtained with the BL, Macintosh and Miller laryngoscopes in 35 unrestrained adult patients with normal cervical spine anatomy. Each patient underwent three laryngoscopies. Compared with DL, the BL resulted in a comparable or superior glottic view. DL failed to provide a view of the larynx in 10% of cases. Less head and cervical extension was required for BL.[54] On the other hand, Watts et al found that simulating emergency conditions by applying in-line stabilization and cricoid pressure resulted in longer intubation times using the BL compared with Macintosh DL.[55] More recently, Turner et al, using a series of cadaveric specimens with a surgically created unstable C4 to C5 segment, demonstrated that Macintosh blade DL caused more variance in subluxation at the unstable segment than the BL, with 3 of the 10 specimens exceeding physiologic limits. Median angulation and distraction, while significantly different, remained within physiologic limits for both laryngoscopes.[56]

Insertion of a double lumen tube in a patient with a difficult airway may be difficult since the tube is both larger, requiring more pharyngeal space, and longer with a complex preformed shape, making manipulation more difficult. The reduced inner diameter may not be compatible with available adult flexible bronchoscopes. Shulman and Connelly used the BL in 29 consecutive adult patients requiring lung separation.[57] This resulted in a C/L Grade 1 view in all patients and tracheal intubation was successful in 28 with a time to intubation of 28 ± 10 (14-55) seconds. Tracheal intubation was unsuccessful in the remaining patient who also had a failed intubation under DL owing to the selection of too large a DLT. (Two other patients had a failed DL but their tracheas were successfully intubated by BL.) Seven patients, however, had to have their DLTs exchanged because of a torn cuff (one patient) or inadequate size (six patients). This study was conducted using the standard dedicated stylet rather than the multifunctional stylet. The latter has greater length and will permit the use of a larger sized DLT.

10.3.2.1.4   What Is the Role of the BL for Unanticipated Difficult Laryngoscopy for Patients with Lingual Tonsillar Hyperplasia?

Although its prevalence is unknown, lingual tonsillar hyperplasia may be responsible for some situations where despite careful preoperative airway evaluation, mask ventilation or intubation by DL proves to be difficult or impossible (see also Chapter 37).[58] These patients may truly challenge our airway management skills. Even in the most expert hands, an LMA is not always successful in achieving adequate ventilation. Intubation using the flexible bronchoscope may also be difficult.[58] Crosby and Skene described a patient who on a previous occasion had been found to have LTH following an unexpected failed DL. On subsequent presentation to the operating room, laryngoscopy was performed using BL and intubation was achieved using glycopyrrolate, topical anesthesia, and sedation.[59] When using a BL in the patient with LTH, the practitioner may have difficulty elevating the epiglottis, particularly if the tonsillar tissue is markedly enlarged or when using the dedicated stylet.

10.3.2.1.5   What Is the Learning Curve of the BL?

Shulman and colleagues tested their impression that BL trainees acquire skill faster if their initial instruction is done with a video system rather than viewing through the eyepiece. They found the use of a video system did in fact reduce the laryngoscopy time and improved success; however the benefits were not discernible after 15 intubations.[60] They demonstrated significant skill acquisition after 5 laryngoscopies in the video group and after 10 in the standard (eyepiece) group.

10.3.2.1.6   What Are the Advantages of BL?

As indicated above, all of the rigid fiberoptic and video laryngoscopes allow visually-controlled ETT insertion and advancement. Compared with the blind approach employed with the flexible bronchoscope, this may be less stimulating and could avoid arytenoid or vocal fold injury.[61]

One distinct advantage of the BL is its flat spatula-like blade, permitting insertion and laryngoscopy in patients with a restricted mouth opening. Even with an inter-incisor distance of 6.0 mm, it may be possible to perform laryngoscopy, although in this instance nasal intubation would likely be necessary.

Although none of the above-mentioned optical stylets are appropriate when intubating nasally, some directional control can be achieved using an Endotrol® ETT (Mallinckrodt, Pleasanton, CA) or a Parker Flex-It™ stylet (Parker Medical, Englewood, CO). An alternative approach is to elevate the head or depress the larynx to influence the position of the ETT relative to the larynx in the anterior-posterior position and to apply torque to rotate the ETT from side to side. The relatively flat spatula-like blade also makes it relatively easy to pass the BL beneath the epiglottis, thereby exposing the glottic aperture. When this is difficult, pulling the mandible (or tongue) forward may elevate the epiglottis and facilitate passage of the BL.

The width and depth of the visual field enables the practitioner to easily discern anatomical landmarks. This is helpful, particularly in settings in which the structures may be altered by disease. Establishing reference landmarks, remaining in the midline, and advancing the BL toward a patent lumen will increase the likelihood of success. The working channel of the BL is a useful conduit for oxygen, suction, or topical anesthesia, all under visual control. The latter is best accomplished by advancing an epidural catheter through the working channel.

10.3.2.1.7   What Are the Disadvantages of the BL?

Like many of the rigid fiberoptic scopes, secretions,[50] fogging,[50] elevation of the epiglottis, and difficulty directing or advancing the

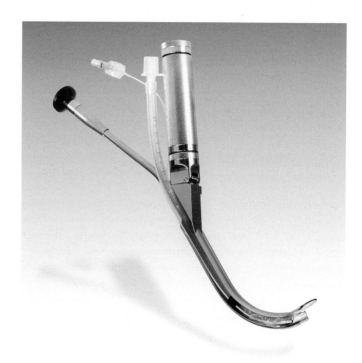

FIGURE 10-9. The UpsherScope Ultra™ is shown with a battery handle and an endotracheal tube residing in the tube slot.

ETT[50,52,62] through the vocal folds are the major obstacles to success.[62] Secretions can be dealt with using a Yankauer sucker or by attaching suction to the working channel. Fogging can be reduced by warming, or applying an antifogging agent to the optical bundle immediately prior to use. In addition, use of the working channel to insufflate oxygen (2.0-4.0 L·min⁻¹) may also reduce fogging and the effect of secretions on the view. Elevation of the epiglottis can frequently be further assisted by performing a mandibular thrust or pulling the tongue forward. Difficulties with tube passage may be lessened by using the LMA Fastrach-dedicated wire-reinforced ETT with its molded tip[63]; or similarly shaped Parker Flex-tip tube.[64] If the practitioner chooses to use a video attachment, an external fiberoptic light source is recommended, although this entire assembly becomes rather bulky.

The BL Elite adult and pediatric models sell for $5500 and $5700, respectively. The multifunctional and dedicated stylets are $600 and $400. The cost of the fiberoptic adapter, necessary if the device is to be connected to an external light source, is $495.

10.3.2.1.8   How Should the BL be Disinfected?[B]

After removing the light source (bulb or fiberoptic adapter) and blade extender (if used), the device and the working channel should be washed, brushed, and flushed with soap and water. The Bullard Elite can be disinfected with ethylene oxide or immersed in a high-level disinfectant.

10.3.2.2   UpsherScope (Mercury Medical)

The UpsherScope (Figure 10-9) and its successor, the UpsherScope Ultra (Mercury Medical, Clearwater FL) are no longer manufactured

---

[B]In all cases, please consult with the manufacturer for detailed cleaning instructions.

or sold. A brief description of the device will be provided for legacy purposes.

It was available in a single, adult-size and consisted of a J-shaped blade with a channel able to accommodate an ETT up to 8.5 mm ID. The light bundle and coherent fiberoptic channel ran along the left side of the blade. Light could be provided by a battery handle or an external halogen source. The eyepiece could be viewed directly or connected to a video system. The device was used much like the BL, requiring an antifogging solution or prewarming, placement of the head in a neutral position, midline blade insertion, and rotation around the base of the tongue attempting to pick up the epiglottis. An Eschmann introducer (Smiths Medical) or Frova intubating catheter (Cook Critical Care, Bloomington, IN) was advanced through the ETT and directed through the glottis. Although simple in design, the original version was not very effective.[65,66] Although the UpsherScope Ultra™ was an improved product, it was withdrawn from the market before establishing its clinical role.

10.3.2.3 WuScope System™ (Achi Corporation)

Like the UpsherScope™ and the UpsherScope Ultra™, the manufacturers of the WuScope System (WS) (Figure 10-10) have recently discontinued manufacturing or selling the device. It will be discussed briefly for legacy purposes.

In its final version, it consisted of dedicated battery-operated nasopharyngoscope (Achi FA-10WUBS), lacking an angulation controller, and two blades that fit together creating two internal channels, one for the ETT and the other for the endoscope. The blades were available in two adult sizes. A video camera could be attached to the eyepiece or the latter could be viewed directly.

Like the BL and the UL, the WS required antifogging preparation and was generally used with the head of the patient in a neutral position. It was introduced in the midline and positioned in the vallecula unless the epiglottis was obscuring the laryngeal view. Generally, an intubating catheter (eg, suction catheter, Eschmann introducer, Frova intubating catheter) was advanced through the

ETT into the glottis and the ETT was advanced over the guide. Then the blades were uncoupled and withdrawn while the ETT was held securely. Nasotracheal intubation was possible by introducing only one of the two blades into the mouth. Used in this manner, it provided glottic visualization and no longer functioned as a channeled device.

The WS was used in a variety of clinical settings where DL was often challenging. These included patients with a receding jaw, limited temporomandibular joint mobility, a reduced atlanto-occipital gap or a short mandibular ramus,[67-70] and lingual tonsillar hyperplasia.[71] The WS often succeeded when DL failed and was associated with a lower intubation difficulty score.[68]

10.3.2.4 What is the Acutronic Fiberoptic Laryngoscope (Acutronic Medical Systems, Switzerland)?

This device, developed by Swiss pediatric anesthesiologist Marcus Weiss, consists of a modified Macintosh laryngoscope (sizes 2, 3, 4, and 5) with a fiberoptic bundle 3.9 mm in diameter and 200 cm in length. (Figure 10-11). An eyepiece can be coupled to a video camera providing an image with 10,000 pixels. When approved for sale in North America, the estimated cost will be approximately $3400 for the laryngoscope and fiberoptic bundle.

10.3.2.5 What is the Angulated Video-Intubation Laryngoscope (Acutronic Medical Systems)?

This device is a modified plastic Macintosh laryngoscope (size #4), the distal 3 cm of which is angulated upward about 25 degrees, resembling a McCoy (CLM; levering tip) blade (Figure 10-12).

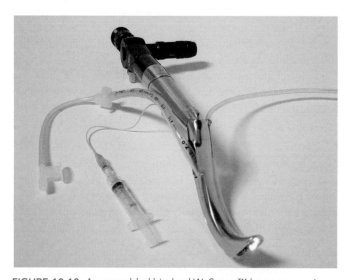

FIGURE 10-10. An assembled bivalved WuScope™ laryngoscope is shown with an attached battery-powered fiberscope, an endotracheal tube, and a suction catheter within the ETT. Intubation usually involves the passage of the suction catheter into the glottis and railroading of the ETT over the former. Oxygen is shown connected to a nipple on the right side of the device. (Photograph provided by Achi Corporation.)

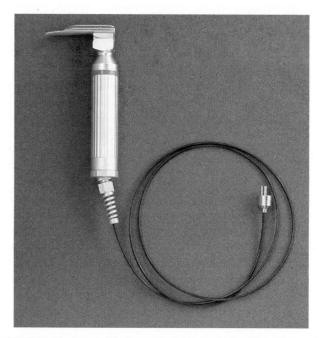

FIGURE 10-11. A pediatric Acutronic video intubating laryngoscope is shown. Various blades are available. The image can be viewed on an external monitor. The videocable is attached to an external monitor. (Photograph provided by Acutronic Medical Systems AG.)

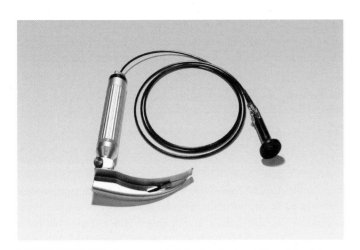

FIGURE 10-12. This shows an adult Acutronic angulating video intubating laryngoscope with a 25-degree anterior angulation of the distal tip. Note that the eyepiece can be viewed directly or connected to a videocamera. (Photograph provided by Dr Markus Weiss and is used with his permission.)

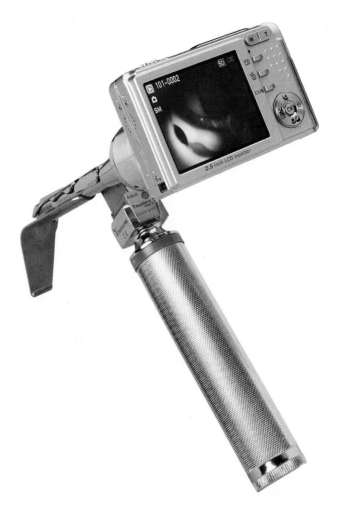

FIGURE 10-13. The new Truview EVO2 laryngoscope is shown connected to an optional, dedicated digital camera. The image is angulated upward approximately 45 degrees and enlarged on the camera's LCD. Alternatively, an existing operating room videocamera can also be attached to the eyepiece of the laryngoscope.

The vertical flange is also flattened, enabling it to be used in children. A thin fiberoptic bundle passes through the body of the laryngoscope, providing illumination and transmitting an image that can be viewed directly through an eyepiece or on a monitor via an attached video camera.

Use of the AVIL has been described in two children with Morquio's syndrome (hypoplasia of the odontoid process) in whom cervical extension posed a risk of spinal cord compression.[72] The device has been compared with the video-optical intubation stylet (VOIS).[10,73,74] In this study, head extension of an intubation manikin was modified so that only a C/L Grade 3 view could be obtained by DL. Thirty endoscopists, previously unfamiliar with both devices performed five intubations with each. Although the trachea was successfully intubated, in four early cases, AVIL intubation required multiple attempts and took longer than 60 seconds. Slightly less time was required for intubation using the VOIS (17.4 ± 6.8 seconds) compared with the AVIL (22.8 ± 13.4 seconds; $p = 0.027$) although greater improvement occurred with subsequent AVIL use compared with VOIS. Skill was easily achieved with both devices and they were highly rated by anesthesiologists and nurse anesthetists. The authors concluded that both techniques were well suited to high-risk situations, such as a rapid-sequence induction with cervical immobilization or as rescue of a failed conventional DL. Each device is estimated to cost €2000 (approximately $2700), although this does not include the video camera, light source, or monitor.

10.3.2.6 What Is the Viewmax® or Truview® or EVO (manufacturer: Truphatek; North American Distributor: Teleflex, Research Triangle Park, NC)

This device is neither a rigid fiberoptic nor a video laryngoscope and consists of an inexpensive proprietary lens inserted into the blade of a modified Macintosh laryngoscope. The blade is angled anteriorly approximately 45 degrees and the lens refracts the viewing angle approximately 42 degrees anteriorly (Figure 10-13), allegedly improving the laryngeal view. The view is observed through a small eyepiece, although with a specialized adapter, it can be displayed on a video monitor.

The product is analogous to a modern Huffman prism. The TruView (TV) is available in two sizes, corresponding to Macintosh 2.5 for children and 3.5 for adults. It was superceded by the TV EVO2 that includes an optional dedicated digital camera that both enlarges and captures the image. A new version, the TV PCD will soon be released which will include four different blade sizes and a magnetically coupled video camera that connects with an LCD monitor.[C]

After applying an antifogging solution, the laryngoscope is introduced into the midline to a depth indicated on the blade as "position 1." An Optiflex metal stylet, or Truphatek's dynamic TruFlex stylet can be used to deliver the ETT. The small image can be viewed directly through the eyepiece, on the digital camera (EVO2), or LCD monitor (PCD).

[C]Personal communication, Cynthia Yaakovi, Truphatek, January 2010.

In a manikin simulation of normal and difficult airways (tongue inflation or cervical rigidity), 20 anesthesiologists compared laryngoscopy and intubation using a Macintosh DL and TV EVO2. Better laryngeal views were obtained using the TV EVO2 when difficulty was simulated. Despite this, the anesthesiologists preferred DL.[75] A similar manikin study compared the TV with the Macintosh and McCoy laryngoscopes, observing better laryngeal views with the TV, but longer intubation times.[76] The time to intubation reached a plateau after six attempts. Barak and colleagues evaluated the TV EVO2 in 170 adult patients and found that laryngoscopy and intubation with the TV EVO2 resulted in better laryngeal views requiring less force but more time.[77] Li and coworkers randomized the sequence of DL or TV EVO2 laryngoscopy in 200 adults. Cormark-Lehane 1 or 2 views were obtained in 157 and 199 patients in the respective groups; however intubation took longer with the TV EVO2.[78]

Malik and coworkers compared the TV EVO2 with the Pentax AirwayScope (AWS), the GlideScope video laryngoscope (GVL), and the Macintosh in patients with cervical immobilization[79] and in manikins.[80] In the studies, the study operators were familiar with DL but had only 2 minutes of prior instruction with the alternative devices. In the simulated difficult airway, the TV EVO2 performed better than DL but not as well as the AWS or GVL.[79]

After use, the view tube is rinsed in clean water and gently scrubbed in soapy water. The TV tube and laryngoscope blade should be further disinfected by ethylene oxide, Steris or Sterrad systems cold soaks.

The price for the TV EVO2 adult blade is $750 ($1370 for the infant blade set). The new TV PCD system with four blade sizes, handles, stylets, and the 5-in LCD monitor with onboard dedicated camera module in a hard storage case costs US $6588. The TruFLEX dynamic stylets cost $279.

10.4 RIGID VIDEO LARYNGOSCOPES

10.4.1 What are the characteristic features of rigid video laryngoscopes?

The rigid fiberoptic laryngoscopes convey their image along a bundle of glass fibers to an eyepiece. If the eyepiece is connected to a video camera, the benefits of video laryngoscopy are achieved, albeit with greater complexity. The fiberoptic stylets, BL, UL, WS, and TV can all be connected to a video camera in this way. As previously mentioned, video laryngoscopy can also be achieved using a conventional laryngoscope and an AirwayCam™. An integrated video laryngoscope incorporates a video camera into its design. This has been achieved in various ways. The Storz V-Mac is a hybrid, combining a distal fiberoptic bundle and a video camera within the handle. The C-Mac, McGrath Video-Laryngoscope, and GlideScope® dispense with the fiberoptic bundle, relying exclusively on video technology.

At the moment, there are three video laryngoscopes that more-or-less resemble curved blades of conventional laryngoscopes. We will also discuss two-channeled devices which more closely resemble the UpsherScope. It is expected that a practitioner with

experience performing DL will find the operation of these devices easier than the rigid fiberoptic devices or flexible bronchoscopes but comparative studies in patients have not been conducted.

10.4.2 Specific devices

10.4.2.1 Pentax AirwayScope AWS-S100

10.4.2.1.1 What Are the Characteristics of the Pentax AirwayScope-S100?

The Pentax AirwayScope-S100 (Ambu Inc., Glen Burnie, MD) is a battery-powered, portable video laryngoscope. It has two components: a reusable handle and monitor and a disposable blade (PBlade). The handle features an integrated, proximal 2.4-in color LCD screen that can swivel for optimal viewing. A 12-cm video cable housing a CCD camera and an LED light source fits within the PBlade (Figure 10-14). The PBlade, available in only one adult size, is made of clear polycarbonate and has separate channels for introducing the CCD/LED cable, the ETT and a suction catheter if needed. It has a vertical profile of 2.5 cm, and will accommodate a 6.5 to 8.0 mm ID ETTs. A unique feature of the AWS is the presence of cross hairs that appear on the LCD screen to help line up the scope with the glottic opening to guide tube passage. The device is powered with two AA batteries, and is water resistant.

10.4.2.1.2 How Is the AWS Used?

For AWS use, a PBlade is attached, the device is turned on, and an appropriate size ETT is loaded in the blade's channel with its tip placed just beyond the end of the camera cable. With the patient's head and neck in the neutral position,[81] the mouth is opened and the scope is advanced into the oropharynx and rotated upright. The AWS is designed to directly elevate the epiglottis (Miller style). The scope is then lifted and adjusted to align the green target signal with the glottic inlet (Figure 10-15), whereupon the ETT is advanced between the cords into the trachea. Once placed,

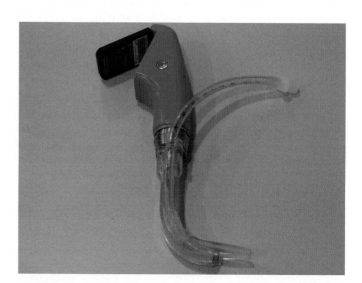

FIGURE 10-14. The Pentax AirwayScope-S100 has a reusable handle unit with a movable 2.4-in color LCD screen proximally and ends distally in a 12-cm cable that houses a CCD camera and an LED light source. It uses a disposable L-shaped introducer blade (the PBlade) which can accommodate 6.5 to 8.0 mm ID ETTs.

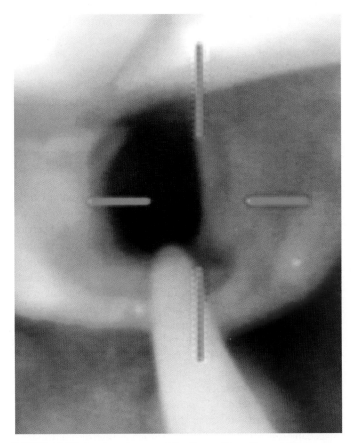

FIGURE 10-15. A unique feature of the Pentax AirwayScope is the presence of a target signal (crosshairs) that appears on the LCD screen to help line up the scope with the glottic opening, thus guiding tube passage.

the ETT is separated laterally from the tube channel and securely held while the AWS is withdrawn from the patient.

10.4.2.1.3 What Is the Clinical Utility of the AWS?

Initial published case series on the AWS have documented generally easy insertion, good glottic exposure, and nonproblematic tube passage.[82,83] Compared with Macintosh blade direct laryngoscopy (DL) in both routine elective surgical patients and those with predicted or encountered difficult DLs, AWS use has resulted in improved laryngeal exposure,[82-86] and lower intubation difficulty scores (IDS).[84,85,87]

In patients with restricted head and neck mobility, when compared with DL, the AWS provided a better laryngeal view,[79,88,89] resulted in a lower intubation difficulty score,[79,87,89] and facilitated improved success rates.[88] Under these same study conditions, faster intubation times have been reported when comparing the AWS to the GlideScope, StyletScope, or tracheal introducer-assisted Macintosh blade DL.[90-92] Radiographic studies have shown that AWS-aided intubation results in significantly less upper C-spine movement than DL with both attempted full exposure,[93,94] and minimal exposure[95] of the cords. One other radiographic study demonstrated a significant decrease in cervical spine movement when the AWS was used with prior passage of a tracheal introducer.[96]

Case reports have documented successful AWS-facilitated oral awake,[97-99] nasal,[100] and DLT[101,102] intubation (the latter with a modified blade or intermediary tracheal introducer or airway exchange catheter use); difficult tube changes;[103,104] and TEE probe

placement.[105,106] In the hands of inexperienced airway practitioners, compared to DL in patients, the AWS appears to have an advantage in terms of success, number of attempts, and time taken to successful intubation.[107] Infrequent reports of esophageal intubation[108] and damage to the soft palate[109] have occurred.

10.4.2.2 Airtraq (Prodol, Spain)

10.4.2.2.1 What Are the Characteristics of the Airtraq?

The Airtraq Optical Laryngoscope (Meditec S.A., Vizcaya, Spain) was developed by Dr Pedro Acha Gandarias. It is a single-use, anatomically shaped, battery-powered device (Figure 10-16). It has two channels, one that conveys the image by means of mirrors and prisms to a fog-resistant lens and viewer; the other directs the ETT. The airway is illuminated by a low-temperature, white LED. The optical viewer can be coupled to an optional camera and either connected by wire to a standard video monitor or wirelessly to a dedicated receiver. The Airtraq is available in a total of seven configurations suitable for small (6.0-7.5 mm ID) and regular (7.0-8.5) adult ETTs oral intubations, infant (2.5-3.5) and pediatric (4.0-5.5) oral intubations, adult and infant nasal

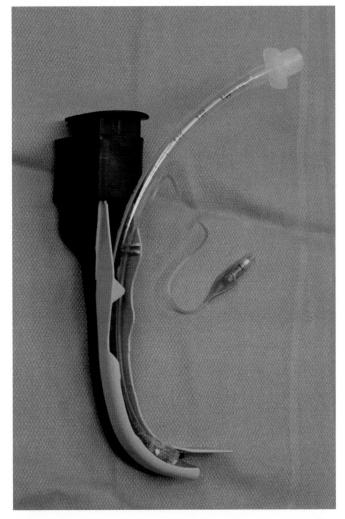

FIGURE 10-16. The Airtraq® Optical Laryngoscope is an anatomically shaped, battery-powered device. It has two channels, one which conveys the image by means of mirrors and prisms to a fog-resistant lens and viewer; the other directs the ETT.

intubations, and double lumen tube (DLT, sizes 35-41 Fr). The infant scopes require a mouth opening of 12.5 mm; the regular adult and DLT models require openings of 18 and 19 mm respectively. The image quality is surprisingly good for a disposable product. Laryngeal exposure, however, is often excellent and fogging is rarely a factor.

10.4.2.2.2   How Is the Airtraq Used?

The Airtraq is introduced in the midline and rotated around the base of the tongue. Space can be created by pulling the mandible forward and/or extending the head. The tip of the blade is preferentially introduced into the vallecula but if the epiglottis obstructs the view, it can be elevated directly by the blade. Like the VLs, insertion to an excessive depth reduces the visual field and demands greater precision when advancing the ETT. With channeled devices, ETT advancement is determined by the laryngoscope and cannot be manipulated independently. Thus it is important to advance the ETT slowly and adjust the Airtraq to optimize ETT delivery.[110,111]

10.4.2.2.3   What Is the Clinical Utility of the Airtraq?

Compared with Macintosh DL, the Airtraq provided comparable or superior conditions for intubation in patients with normal airways[112] as well as those at increased risk of a difficult DL.[113] In the latter study, the Airtraq reduced the duration of intubation attempts, the need for additional maneuvers, the Intubation Difficulty Score, and the hemodynamic changes associated with intubation.

Dhonneur and coworkers described two morbidly obese women undergoing emergency general anesthesia for cesarean section in whom DL and use of an Eschmann tracheal introducer (gum elastic bougie) failed. Using the Airtraq, an excellent glottic view and successful intubation were achieved promptly in both cases.[114] In another report, seven patients in whom multiple attempts at DL with optimization maneuvers, including the use of a Eschmann tracheal introducer proved unsuccessful, were easily intubated on the first attempt using the Airtraq.[115] In each case, the laryngeal view went from a C/L 4 to 1 and the Intubation Difficulty Score[87] went from 10 to 12 to 0 or 1.

As with nonchanneled devices,[116] a good view does not guarantee a successful intubation. Savoldelli described a patient in whom DL yielded a C/L 3 view. Airtraq laryngoscopy revealed the entire glottis but several corrective maneuvers, including partial withdrawal and a vertical lift, failed to redirect the ETT toward the glottis. Intubation was accomplished with a McGrath laryngoscope allowing independent manipulation of a styletted ETT.[111] In another report, the video recordings of 109 attempted Airtraq laryngoscopies were reviewed to determine the views associated with successful (50) and failed (59) intubations.[110] Dhonneur and coworkers found that intubation was most likely to occur when the glottic opening was in the vertical center with the interarytenoid cleft below the horizontal center of the visual field. Most of the initial failures resulted from an inappropriately high position of the glottic opening in the laryngoscopic view. Success generally followed a lowering of the position of the glottic opening (by tipping the blade downward, backward, and upward) and by reducing cervical extension. Although the blades of the AWS and Airtraq appear quite similar, the ETT emerges from the tube channel with different trajectories. Perhaps, because of the width of the Airtraq channel and the arcuate

shape of the ETT, the tube emerges more posteriorly with the Airtraq. This creates a space that may accommodate the epiglottis in a way not possible with the AWS.[85]

All indirect techniques, not requiring manual alignment of the airway axes, have potential value in patients with cervical spine injuries. Cervical spine movement was assessed during Airtraq and Macintosh DL in 20 patients with normal airway and cervical anatomy, each of whom underwent two laryngoscopies without restraint.[117] Although the radiographic images were static rather than continuous, the study found that significant cervical extension occurred with both groups; however it was 44% less with the Airtraq at C3/C4 while no difference was observed at C0/C1 or C1/C2. The reduction of movement from occiput to C4 was 29% with the Airtraq. Although patients with a suspected cervical spine injury are likely to be restrained during airway management, this study shows a potential role for this device in neck-injured patients. The Airtraq was compared with DL in 40 patients with normal airway anatomy, during the application of manual in-line stabilization (MILS).[118] The IDS, number of optimization maneuvers, the time to tracheal intubation and stimulation were less with the Airtraq. Turkstra and colleagues performed Airtraq and Macintosh laryngoscopies in 24 adults with normal airway and cervical anatomy, during the application of MILS with continuous fluoroscopic assessment.[119] Laryngoscopy, done by the same experienced anesthesiologist, performed to obtain a view adequate to allow visualized intubation showed a trend toward shorter laryngoscopy times with the Airtraq, defined as insertion of the ETT just past the vocal cords, but this did not achieve significance. Over three segments, there was an average reduction of C-spine motion by 66% less using the Airtraq. This difference was most apparent at the C0 to C1 and C5-thoracic segments. This study was conducted with patients in a neutral position with MILS, both of which may favor the Airtraq.[120,121]

Ndoko et al randomized 106 morbidly obese patients to Macintosh DL or Airtraq laryngoscopy and intubation.[122] DL failed in six patients, all of whom were successfully intubated with the Airtraq. The Intubation Difficulty Scores[87] were lower for the Airtraq (11 vs 0); times for tracheal intubation were faster (24 ± 16 seconds for Airtraq vs 56 ± 23 seconds for DL, p<0.001). Fewer patients assigned to Airtraq intubation experienced SpO$_2$ less than 92%. But this study was not blinded, patients may not have been optimally positioned for DL and finally, and they excluded patients with mouth opening less than 3 cm because of the thickness of the blade. Dhonneur et al have suggested an alternative means of inserting the Airtraq in obese patients. They described a "reverse maneuver," where the Airtraq is introduced into the mouth pointing upward and rotated 180 degrees. It is advanced into the pharnyx, like a Guedel airway.[120] In morbidly obese patients, this reduced the time to glottic exposure and increased first pass success. In the morbidly obese patients, significantly less pressure was required to insert the Airtraq, although this benefit was not observed among lean patients. In four patients, in whom difficulty was encountered with standard Airtraq insertion technique, superficial bleeding was observed at the base of the pharyngopalatine arch. The posterior hard palate was reddened in four patients in whom the reverse maneuver was employed. Review of their video clips demonstrated that all the injuries occurred in patients in whom pharyngeal insertion had been challenging, requiring considerable pressure to introduce and advance the blade. Clearly, a cautious or alternative approach would be appropriate. However in a single case report, Holst described a patient (BMI 32 kg·M^{-2}) in whom no difficulty was experienced using the standard insertion technique. Upon conclusion of the surgery, blood in the pharynx and a 2-cm laceration were noted in the midline of the posterior pharyngeal wall. A large coroner's clot was seen in the postnasal space that might easily have gone unnoticed. Direct pressure was applied and the subsequent extubation was uneventful.[123]

When doubt exists about the ability of a practitioner or device to successfully manage an airway, most would prefer to not sacrifice spontaneous ventilation. Suzuki describes a patient with a difficult airway and gastroesophageal reflux in whom awake Airtraq intubation was successfully performed.[98] Dimitriou describes successful tracheal intubation using the Airtraq in four patients with anticipated difficult intubation, one with severe ankylosing spondylitis. Spontaneous ventilation was preserved and topical anesthesia enabled awake intubation.[124]

The Airtraq is particularly well suited in remote settings where intubation is uncommonly performed or difficulties are infrequently encountered. There is no requirement for a large capital investment, and reprocessing time is eliminated. This may be useful in free-standing clinics, remote locations in a hospital, or on ambulances. In addition, it may be more useful in the hands of occasional intubators since the skill is more easily learned and retained compared with DL. Using a difficult airway manikin model, Woollard et al reported that tracheal intubation was more successful with the Airtraq than Macintosh DL in the hands of untrained paramedics,[125] as well as advanced paramedic students and experienced prehospital practitioners.[126] Maharaj confirmed that medical students, previously untrained in laryngoscopy, acquired and retained intubation skills better with the Airtraq than Macintosh DL although skill retention, in the absence of a refresher or interval practice, was poor with both techniques.[121]

Airtraq laryngoscopes are sold in cases of six, each case costing $474 ($79/use). The cost of NTSC Airtraq camera is $327 and the wireless monitor is for $1143.

In summary, the Airtraq is a single-use optical laryngoscope that provides excellent glottic exposure in routine as well as in challenging settings. It is available in a large range of sizes for multiple applications including nasal and double-lumen tube insertion. It is compatible with a video system using existing equipment or a wireless transmitter, receiver, and proprietary monitor. Although it requires no capital investment, the cost per case is high and may be a barrier to routine use.

10.4.3 DCI/V-MAC/C-MAC (Karl Storz Endoscope, VMS)

10.4.3.1 What Are the Unique Features of the Video-Macintosh?

The first version of the Storz Video-Macintosh laryngoscope was modified to accommodate a fiberoptic bundle that passes through a metal channel, terminating approximately 4.0 cm from the tip of the blade and was referred to as the DCI (Direct Coupled Interface model). The bundle passes through the heel of the blade

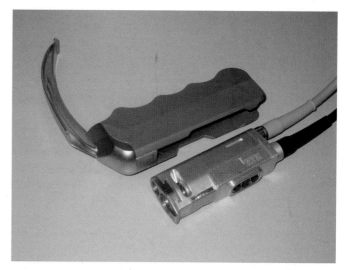

FIGURE 10-17. Three Storz Video-Macintosh (V-Mac) laryngoscope.

into the handle connecting to a video camera. A video cable and power supply passes to a proprietary video cart housing a light source, video processor, and monitor.[127]

The DCI has been replaced with the V-MAC, employing an American-style Macintosh blade with an integrated light source and video camera housed in a removable cassette (Figure 10-17). It provides intense illumination and a high-quality image, displayed on a proprietary monitor (Telepak™).

Recently, the V-MAC was updated to the C-MAC (Figure 10-18), replacing the fiberoptic components with a CMOS camera (complementary metal oxide semiconductor) and LED light source. It uses a conventionally shaped, German-style Macintosh laryngoscope blade with an optional suction channel. At present, the blades are available in sizes 2, 3, and 4, though additional blades are planned. The image is displayed on a Li-ion battery-powered, high-resolution (800 × 400) proprietary 7-in LCD monitor (Figure 10-18). This also enables still (jpeg) and video recordings

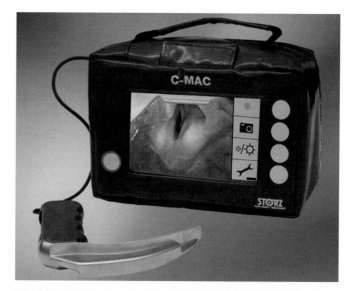

FIGURE 10-18. Tracheal intubation using the Storz C-MAC laryngoscope connected to a proprietary video display.

(M-PEG 4), stored on a removable Secure Digital (SD) memory card. The recording is activated and terminated by buttons located on both the handle and the monitor. No white balancing or focusing is required. Since there is no evidence that these devices are functionally different, for the purposes of this discussion, they will be considered together as the Video-Macintosh System (VMS).

10.4.3.2 What Is the Clinical Utility of the VMS?

Unlike the other video-laryngoscope (VL) devices, the VMS is introduced like the conventional Macintosh blade it resembles. The tongue is displaced leftward and compressed. The image can be viewed directly or indirectly on the monitor. A stylet is considered optional[128] and indeed, when no stylet was used—contrary to the recommendations of the manufacturers of the other devices—the VMS outperformed both the McGrath and GlideScope which frequently required second attempts after stylet insertion.[128] Kaplan and coworkers evaluated the DCI on 235 patients, 18 of whom had features suggesting a difficult conventional DL. In 22 of the 217 (10%) patients in whom no difficulties were anticipated, external laryngeal manipulation (ELM) was required and the video system enabled the assistant to evaluate its effect and make the appropriate adjustments. All but one of these intubations was successful. ELM was required in the patients predicted to be difficult and all these intubations were also successful.[127] The authors concluded that the VMS had a very short learning curve and provided a larger, brighter image that could be viewed by the practitioner and instructor. It was therefore a useful device for teaching. In this study, the direct and indirect views were not compared, making it difficult to know whether the advantage was primarily a larger brighter view. However, in another study, the DCI was evaluated in a multicenter study involving 867 adults.[129] All practitioners had performed at least 10 prior manikin intubations using the device. The patients were neither consecutive nor randomized and the airway characteristics differed from site to site. In this study, VL and DL views were compared, using the same laryngoscope. The indirect (VL) view was improved by at least one grade in 41.5% of patients (and worsened in only 2.7%). The larynx could not be exposed, despite ELM in 14.2% by DL and in 3.4% by VL (p<0/001). Fogging interfered with the view in 3% of cases.[129]

While it is useful for an assistant to be able to make adjustments to the location, direction, and force of ELM, the need to apply it in 40/238 (17%) cases suggests that the camera of the DCI (or V-MAC) does not provide better glottic exposure in challenging airways.

The DCI was used for DL and VL in 200 adult patients with modified Mallampati III or IV views, in an effort to identify patient at increased risk of difficult DL.[130] Two anesthesiologists performed all the laryngoscopies with patients in a neutral position, using the same device but comparing the glottic views seen directly and indirectly. The sequence was randomization and intubation was performed following the second assessment. The VL view was significantly better than direct viewing, although ELM and an Eschmann introducer was frequently required. Successful intubation was achieved in 99/100 and 92/100 with VL and DL respectively (p = 0.02) and when all patients were considered, intubation time was no different. When only patients with a C/L ≥3 view

were considered, intubation was faster by VL. While the observation that improved laryngeal exposure was achieved, more patients were successfully intubated—even though many required ELM and an Eschmann introducer—and in the most challenging cases, intubation was performed faster by VL, a laryngeal view could not be obtained in a significant number of patients by either VL (10) or DL (36). It is possible that the high failure rate was a consequence of the investigators' decision to perform laryngoscopy in the neutral position, but it is also possible that this outcome arises from the inherent shape of the Macintosh blade.

Serocki and colleagues performed laryngoscopies using three devices in random sequence.[131] Each of their 120 patients had at least one feature predictive of a difficult DL. The laryngoscopes included a conventional Macintosh DL, the Storz DCI, and the GlideScope (GVL). DL yielded a C/L ≥3 view in 30% of the patients, compared with the indirect view using the DCI (10.8%) and the GVL (1.6%). Clinically important improvements were more likely to result from use of the GVL than the DCI, but both outperformed the Macintosh DL with respect to the laryngeal view. Concerning intubation time, significantly more time was required to intubate with both DCI (27 seconds [17-94]) and GVL (33 seconds [8-68]) compared with DL (13 [5-33]). Finally, intubation could not be achieved within two attempts by DL in 4/40 cases compared with one in each of the 40 patients in whom it was attempted by DCI or GVL. Unfortunately, the sample size is too small to be conclusive.

To date, there has been only one study evaluating the C-MAC.[132] The optimal laryngeal view was assessed both directly and indirectly in 60 adults. ELM and an Eschmann introducer were permitted. Intubation was successful in all patients requiring 1, 2, or 3 attempts in 52, 6, and 2 patients respectively. An Eschmann introducer was required in 8 (13%) patients. A C/L grade 1, 2a, and 2b views were obtained in 30, 22, and 6 patients, respectively, which improved to 52, 6, and 2 when ELM was applied.

10.4.3.3 What Are the Advantages and Disadvantages of the Video-Macintosh?

The VMS results in a large, high-resolution color image. Since it is used like a conventional Macintosh DL and the view is likely identical, it is well suited to teaching this technique. Laryngoscopy can be recorded as still or video images. These features are desirable for teaching, documentation, and research. As previously mentioned, it enables an assistant to modify ELM, potentially improving the laryngeal view.

The cost of the components is a significant deterrent for a device that may not improve laryngeal exposure. The Video-Macintosh handle costs $8000 while each blade costs $220.[D] A video system and cart are also required to power, illuminate, and display the image. The cost of this additional equipment, sold by Karl Storz, is $25,000, although it can also be used with the Storz flexible fiberoptic scope or Bonfils fiberoptic stylet. The VMS can be used

---

[D]All prices are in US dollars unless otherwise stated. All prices were accurate at the time of publication but may be subject to change.

with most xenon light sources; however it requires a proprietary (Karl Storz) video camera to view the image.

The C-MAC pricing for the monitor and electronic module are $5200 and $750, respectively. The C-MAC blades are $4250 each. Additional accessories include a carrying case and mobile stand.

Although the DCI, V-MAC, and C-MAC blades are slightly different, it appears that their clinical performance will be very similar. This repackaged product has many compelling features, but it remains to be demonstrated that the C-MAC will outperform its predecessors. It appears to offer modest advantages in the management of the difficult airway, although it may be the best system currently available for teaching direct laryngoscopy. The technique is identical to DL and the laryngoscopist and mentor have very similar laryngeal views. Laryngoscopy can be recorded and replayed for feedback and the effects of either ELM or cricoid pressure can be assessed and modified as required.

10.4.3.4 How Is the VMS Disinfected?[E]

The C-MAC is disassembled by removing the electronic module from the laryngoscope housing. A reprocessing cap is affixed to the sockets on the laryngoscope and the electronic module and immediate surface cleaning is performed to remove heavy soiling. The laryngoscope and electronic module, once properly capped, can be immersed in an approved disinfectant and then rinsed and dried. A wide range of sterilization procedures are compatible but the C-MAC should not be subjected to temperatures greater than 60°C (The DCI and V-MAC blades should be washed immediately after use, to remove surface contamination and can then be autoclaved.). After processing, the optical surface of the C-MAC and its LED should be rewashed with 70% alcohol using a cotton tip applicator.

10.4.4 GlideScope® video laryngoscope (Verathon Medical, Bothell WA)[F]

10.4.4.1 What Are the Characteristics of the GlideScope® Video Laryngoscope?

This GVL was developed by a Canadian surgeon, John A. Pacey, and was introduced in late 2001. Since that time, it has undergone a number of modifications and is now available in a variety of sizes and formats. The reusable version consists of a plastic modified Macintosh-type laryngoscope blade, the distal half of which is angled upward approximately 60 degrees (Figure 10-19). The GVL® Cobalt is the single-use version and includes a video baton and a disposable plastic shell known as a STAT (Figure 10-20). The video batons are available in two sizes to be used with STATs sized 1 and 2 or 3 and 4 for neonates, infants, small- and large-size adults, respectively. The reusable GVLs are available in sizes 2 through 5 (Figure 10-19). A video chip (complementary metal oxide semiconductor or CMOS) captures an image that is

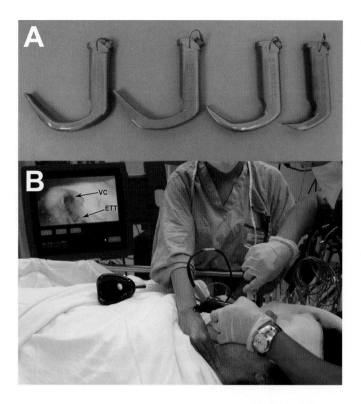

FIGURE 10-19. (A) The four GlideScope® video laryngoscopes. From left to right, these are the new adult Lo-Pro (14.5-mm profile), the discontinued Classic (monochrome, 18 mm), the pediatric, and the neonatal models. The integrated power supply/video cable and proprietary LCD videodisplay are not shown. (Provided by Saturn Medical Systems.) (B) Laryngoscopic intubation is displayed on the dedicated GlideScope® video monitor.

illuminated by adjustable light-emitting diodes. The image is displayed on a proprietary monitor—either a 3.4 in portable version known as the GVL® Ranger (Figure 10-21) or a 7-in display. Recently, the GVL® Advanced VL was released in the single-use format. This captures a higher resolution, time-annotated digital image, requiring a newly designed digital AVL display with an on-board image capturing feature. These saved video images can be transferred to a flash memory device via a USB port. The screen can also be

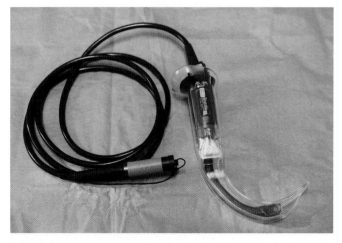

FIGURE 10-20. The GlideScope® Cobalt is the single-use version and includes a video baton and a disposable plastic shell known as a STAT.

[E]In all cases, please consult with the manufacturer for detailed cleaning instructions.

[F]Richard Cooper is an unpaid consultant to Verathon Medical Systems.

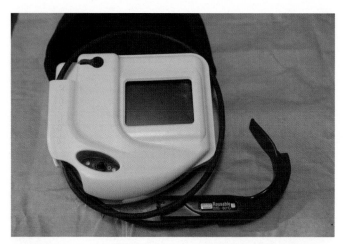

FIGURE 10-21. The GlideScope® Ranger is specifically developed for out of the operating room use. It is light-weight, compact, and was designed to demanding specifications including a rechargeable battery capable of 90 minutes of continuous use.

connected to an auxiliary display using an HDMI (High-Definition Multimedia Interface) port on the rear of the monitor.

Although the new AVL features are enticing, the monitor is not compatible with earlier GVL® laryngoscopes. Nonetheless, there are several ways that the images can be captured from earlier systems. Verathon has a digital video recorder (DVR) that when interposed between the laryngoscope and the monitor (Figure 10-22)

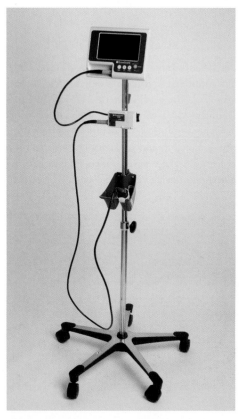

FIGURE 10-22. The GlideScope DVR is a digital video recorder when interposed between the laryngoscope and the monitor, is automatically activated to record a date and time-stamped video on a standard secure digital (SD) memory card.

is automatically activated to record a date and time-stamped video on a standard secure digital (SD) memory card. A lower cost alternative is a generic video capture system such as that offered by Pinnacle (www.pinnaclesys.com).

An important feature of all GVL® systems is a patented antifogging technology that automatically warms the glass covering the video chip, preventing condensation. To achieve this benefit, the device must be turned on at least 30 seconds prior to use.

All GVL® monitors—the Ranger, the GVL®, and the GlideScope AVL—use rechargeable batteries. The screen resolutions are 480 × 234, 440 × 234, and 640 × 480 pixels respectively.

The original GVL® employed a monochrome camera and had a vertical height of 18 mm. These are no longer produced. The distance of the camera from the laryngoscope tip as well as height, width, and length of the blade depend upon the specific size and model selected. The smaller and larger video batons have a height profile of 6 and 10.7 mm, respectively. With their corresponding STAT blades attached, they have a maximum height of 8.7 and 16 mm, slightly bulkier than their corresponding reusable equivalents. This dimension generally dictates the minimal inter-incisor distance required to accommodate the laryngoscope blade.

All GVLs employ a blade configuration that differs significantly from the standard Macintosh DL. With an upward camera orientation approximately 50 to 60 degrees from the line-of-sight, the image displayed on the monitor will be quite different from that seen when looking directly into the mouth. For example, with minimal lifting of the laryngoscope, the line-of-sight view may be limited to the uvula while complete laryngeal exposure is seen on the monitor.

10.4.4.2 How Is the GVL Used?

There are three components to GVL® use: (i) visualization, (ii) ETT delivery, and (iii) ETT advancement. With DL, visualization is the greatest challenge—generally, if you can see the glottis, you can place an ETT in it. With GVL® (and the McGrath VL), the larynx is not in the line-of-sight and it is necessary to have a means of delivering the ETT. Furthermore, because of the pronounced angle of the blade relative to the axis of the trachea, it is frequently necessary to redirect the ETT.

10.4.4.2.1 Laryngeal Visualization

The GVL® is introduced in the midline of the mouth and rotated around the base of the tongue. There is a tendency to introduce the blade to an excessive depth which has several disadvantages: (i) by reducing the distance of the camera from the larynx, it restricts the visual field; (ii) it requires greater precision when delivering the ETT to the larynx, and (iii) it increases the angle of incidence between the advancing ETT and the trachea. The practitioner should generally resist the temptation to maximize glottic exposure as this may make subsequent ETT delivery and advancement more difficult. Likewise, it is worth checking the orientation of the laryngoscope handle; the more vertical the handle, the less favorable the angle of incidence between the approaching ETT and the trachea. Nonetheless, if the epiglottis is obscuring laryngeal exposure, it can be elevated directly, as with a straight blade.

10.4.4.2.2 ETT Delivery

When DL is performed, the ETT insertion is directly observed as it passes through the oropharynx. When performing VL, there is a temptation to watch the monitor while the ETT is being introduced into the mouth. There have been several reports of perforations of the right palatopharyngeal pillar resulting from inadvertent penetration by the advancing ETT.[133-136] This complication is preventable and results from the unnecessary blind ETT insertion and advancement. This can and should be observed directly. Another approach, particularly helpful in patients with small mouths, is insertion of the ETT into the mouth prior to the GVL®.[137] This has the additional advantage of obligating the user to observe ETT insertion.

As previously mentioned, a stylet is highly desirable. Care must be taken to ensure that it does not protrude beyond the end of the tube. There are four ways that ETT can be delivered:

1. A malleable stylet, shaped like the distal aspect of the GVL® blade,[116] although various other configurations have been advocated.[138-140]

2. A rigid metal (GlideRite®) stylet is offered by Verathon, but this offers little advantage to the experienced user.[141]

3. A dynamic or directional stylet such as the Flex-It™[142,143] (Parker Medical, Highland Ranch, CO) or the TruFLEX (Truphatek, Israel). These permit the practitioner to modify the trajectory of the ETT during its delivery.

4. An Eschmann tracheal introducer or Frova Intubation Guide may prove helpful in redirecting the ETT and facilitating its advancement within the trachea.

It is helpful to introduce the ETT as close to the laryngoscope blade as possible. Essentially, the ETT is rotated about the base of the tongue, close to the midline. If this fails to direct the ETT to the larynx, the stylet can be reconfigured, flexed (if a dynamic stylet is used), an Eschmann or Frova introducer can be used, or external laryngeal manipulation can bring the larynx to the tube. A final strategy to deliver the ETT to a more anterior location is as follows: the orientation of the styletted ETT is changed from vertical (12 o'clock) to approximately 2 o'clock and the ETT is then rotated counterclockwise, thereby redirecting its tip (personal communication, Leonard Pott, September 2009).

10.4.4.2.3 ETT Advancement

The stylet is partially retracted after the tip passes through the laryngeal inlet. If the ETT cannot be advanced easily, there are several measures that can be helpful:

1. "Loss of resistance": A PVC ETT concaves upward. Advancing it may cause impaction on the anterior tracheal wall. Clockwise rotation of the ETT will generally result in a (satisfying) loss of resistance as the ETT descends into the airway.

2. Reverse loading[49,138]: This technique can be used with either a rigid GlideRite® or malleable stylet. The ETT is mounted on the stylet such that the imposed shape is opposite to its natural concavity. When the stylet is withdrawn, the ETT is oriented more posteriorly. To optimize the effectiveness of reverse loading, it is recommended that the bending of the ETT be employed immediately prior to intubation. Otherwise, the ETT will untwist itself around the well-lubricated stylet within a short period of time.

3. Force should never be applied in an effort to advance the ETT. If the above methods are unsuccessful and the ETT is within the trachea, the stylet can be fully withdrawn and replaced with either an Eschmann or Frova introducer. The latter permits oxygenation/ventilation and confirmation of intra-tracheal placement using capnography.

10.4.4.3 What Is the Clinical Utility of the GVL?

The clinical role of the GVL® is still being defined. All studies comparing DL with GVL® have confirmed equivalency in the case of easy airways or improved laryngeal views when more challenging conditions are encountered. Although laryngeal visualization is highly desirable and almost always achievable, it is not sufficient. Many of the studies have also been associated with a higher intubation failure rate or longer time to achieve tracheal intubation. These studies have been flawed by nonstandardized outcome definitions, inexperienced practitioners, clinical extrapolations from manikin simulations, and nonhomogenous patient mixing.[144,145] The challenge ahead is to define relevant outcomes for routine airway management and the role of this and similar devices for rescue of the unanticipated and anticipated difficult airways.

Use of the GVL® has been described in routine and difficult airways for oral, nasal, and double lumen tube insertions. It has also been described to perform visualized tube exchanges in patients in whom DL could not reveal the larynx (see Chapter 28).

Sun and colleagues compared laryngeal exposure and time to tracheal intubation in 200 adult patients, randomized to GVL or DL using a Macintosh 3.[146] All patients first underwent DL and the C/L view was scored. Subsequently, a second practitioner, unaware of the previous view, performed laryngoscopy and intubation. Among patients with a C/L greater than 1 view, use of the GVL significantly improved the view in 68% of patients (p < 0.001). Of the 15 patients with C/L 3, eight and six were converted to Grade 1 and 2 views, respectively, when the GVL was used. Time to tracheal intubation (TTI) was longer in the GVL group (30 seconds for DL vs 46 for GVL); however the time required increased as the laryngeal view deteriorated in the DL but not in the GVL group. There was no difference in the TTI between the two techniques in patients with DL-C/L 3. There was one failed intubation in the DL group (and the trachea of this patient was intubated after one attempt using the GVL). Multiple attempts were more frequently required in the DL group.

To date, the largest series reported the early experience by 133 users at five centers involving 728 consecutive uses.[116] Training was minimal and patient selection was at the discretion of the anesthesiologist. Failure was defined as abandonment of the device in favor of a more familiar alternative. In some cases, this occurred after a single unsuccessful attempt. During the evaluation period, the GVL came to be used in increasingly challenging settings, in an effort by some to define its limits. Despite minimal or no prior experience, C/L Grade 1 or 2 views were obtained in 92% and 7% of patients, respectively. A subset of 133 patients underwent both DL and GVL. A DL gave rise to a C/L ≥3 in 35 patients whereas GVL resulted in a C/L 1 or 2 view in 77% of these patients. Intubation could not be achieved in 3.7% of patients; over half (14/26) of these patients had a C/L 1 view. In contrast to DL, where intubation is frequently successful despite not seeing the larynx, the early experience with GVL showed that intubation occasionally failed *despite* good laryngeal exposure.[147] Clearly, as discussed in the section on ETT delivery and advancement, DL and VL require a different skill set—a good view is helpful but not enough.

VL not requiring tongue displacement and compression, anterior mandibular advancement, and tracheal depression should be less stressful to the patient;[116,121] however demonstrating this has been challenging,[148,149] in part because of variable hemodynamic responses to medications and interventions. Recent approaches are promising,[150,151] and comparisons of directly measured forces required to perform DL and VL intubations are currently under investigation.[152]

10.4.4.4 How Effective Is the GlideScope® for Tracheal Intubation in Patients with a Difficult Airway?

Agrò et al simulated a difficult airway by applying a cervical collar to the necks of 15 surgical patients.[153] Each patient was subjected to both direct laryngoscopy and GVL. The C/L view was improved by an average of one grade in 14 of 15 patients. One of 15 patients remained unchanged as a C/L 3 but tracheal intubation was successful using an Eschmann tracheal introducer under GVL visual control.

Turkstra et al compared the GVL, Macintosh 3 DL, and the Trachlight in 36 healthy adults with in-line cervical stabilization.[154] They evaluated tracheal intubation and assessed cervical spine movement under fluoroscopy. Compared with DL, cervical spine movement was reduced by 50% but only at the C2 to C5 segment. Elsewhere in the C-spine, there was no difference, and GVL prolonged intubation time. Robitaille and colleagues compared DL and GVL with manual in-line stabilization (MILS).[155] Although the GVL provided better laryngeal exposure, they failed to identify a difference between these devices with regard to cervical movement in four static views. In another study, laryngoscopy and intubation using the GVL was compared with the flexible bronchoscope.[156] Using continuous fluoroscopy in an unrestrained cervical spine, the authors found that the GVL resulted in greater cervical movement at all segments. However, the jaw thrust (more than a tongue pull) required to facilitate endoscopic intubation was associated with significant movement. It is noteworthy that there were significant differences between the interpreting neurosurgeon and neuroradiologist, pointing to the difficulty in evaluating such research. Furthermore, a patient with a compromised cervical spine is likely to be managed with MILS or some other cervical stabilization strategy.

Cooper has described a patient at risk of regurgitation who could not be intubated by DL on repeated presentations.[157] The patient had refused awake intubation using a flexible bronchoscope. The GVL was used with a rapid sequence induction and successful intubation was achieved on the first attempt (within 15 seconds); the patient presented on two subsequent occasions with the same outcome. It has been used in a wide variety of clinical settings where DL is challenging or has failed.[116,142,146,157-169]

In the preliminary report by Cooper et al,[116] BMI over 40 kg·m⁻² or body weight greater than 100 kg was not a significant impediment to either good laryngeal visualization or successful intubation. Despite the relative lack of experience on the part of the practitioners, a C/L 1 to 2 view was obtained in 102/104 patients and intubation was successful in 101 of these. A C/L 1 to 2 view was also achieved in 28/30 patients with a BMI more than 40 kg·m⁻² and 29 of these patients were successfully intubated. In a retrospective review from The Cleveland Clinic, 32 patients with a BMI more than 45 kg·m⁻² (average 54.1 ± 8.1; BW 155 kg ± 29) were identified.[170] A GVL had been used and the number of required intubation attempts was recorded on 29 charts. Intubation was accomplished on the first attempt in 27 of these. In one case, a second attempt was required to reduce the diameter of the ETT. Although several centers specializing in bariatric surgery are using the GVL routinely, the authors are unaware of any additional published reports.

The early neonatal blade was bulky and did not perform very well.[171] Subsequent iterations and increased clinical experience has been far more promising.[163,172-175]

The GVL Ranger (Figure 10-21) was specifically developed for prehospital and battlefield applications. It is light-weight, compact, and was designed to demanding specifications including a rechargeable battery capable of 90 minutes of continuous use, tolerance of temperatures from −4°F to 122°F and altitude to 22,000 ft. In a nonrandomized comparison of prehospital laryngoscopy and intubation performed by Advanced Life Support paramedics, Wayne and colleagues compared 300 DL and 315 GVL intubations.[176] The cohorts were similar. The care practitioners performed an average of only six intubations yearly. The average time to intubate was shorter (21 seconds, range 8-43 for GVL vs 42, 28-90 for DL, p = 0.05), and the average number of attempts required were fewer (1.2 vs 2.3, p = 0.05) with the GVL. There were fewer failures using the GVL Ranger but the difference was insignificant. It is known that the documentation of airway management in general is poor, but it may be especially so for prehospital care.[177] In one report, the authors had recently added the digital video recorder (DVR™) to their GVL Ranger™ allowing them to accurately quantify the number and duration of intubation attempts.[176] This could (and should) become mandatory for the quality control of prehospital airway management.

10.4.4.5 What Is the Learning Curve for the GlideScope®?

Numerous studies have evaluated skill acquisition with the GVL, but these must be evaluated cautiously. Some of the studies have involved students with no prior experience[178-180] or personnel not requiring these skills. Others involve very limited instruction or were conducted on manikins that may lack realism. Although manikins are obviously preferred as training objects, the validity of this model must be considered critically.[181] In a study comparing the performance of novices, trained on manikins but performed on patients, intubation was successful in 51% versus 93% when using Macintosh DL and GVL, respectively. Time to tracheal intubation was also significantly faster using GVL.[180]

Savoldelli and coworkers compared the learning curves of the GVL, McGrath, and the Airtraq in a manikin study involving nurses, residents, and staff anesthesiologists performing on a

Laerdal SimMan manikin.[182] In a normal simulation, performance with the Airtraq was best although they observed steep learning curves for the GVL and McGrath. The authors felt that this related to the added challenge of directing the ETT in the nonchanneled VLs.

In general, compared with DL, VL is an easier skill to acquire; however in nonchanneled devices with angled blades (such as the GVL and McGrath), ETT delivery and advancement require the acquisition of a separate set of skills.

10.4.4.6 What Is the Clinical Role of the GlideScope®?

Like the other VLs, the role of the GVL is still being defined for routine, anticipated, difficult DL and rescue airway management. Some argue that these devices have rendered line-of-sight techniques obsolete,[183] while others maintain that the evidence does not yet support such conclusions.[144,145] This technology is a compelling way to teach airway anatomy and for a mentor to provide more meaningful feedback to the learner. A legitimate question arises concerning the retention of skills required to perform DL. The same argument applies to the widespread adoption of extraglottic airways, the claim that ultrasound should be a standard of care for central line insertion (or that surgeons should continue to perform open cholecystectomies and appendectomies to retain their skill). What happens when such devices are not available? If and when VL is proven to surpass DL in relevant outcomes, should DL be abandoned?

10.4.4.7 What Are the Advantages and Disadvantages of the GVL?

The GVL is similar enough to DL that an experienced laryngoscopist can easily learn the technique. Even novice laryngoscopists have been able to obtain excellent glottic exposure. The device is portable and requires virtually no setup time, making it useful in the unanticipated difficult airway. The GVL Ranger is even more suitable for use outside of the operating room. The GVL is effectively resistant to fogging though rarely slight fogging may be observed.[184] Secretions or blood in the oropharynx do not significantly interfere with visualization. The high-resolution image can be displayed on an external video display and/or recorded as clinical documentation or for research or quality assurance purposes. It is constructed of an impact-resistant medical grade plastic and there are no fragile fiberoptic bundles. It provides non-line-of-sight laryngeal exposure even in circumstances where DL has proven unsuccessful. Like the other rigid fiberoptic and video laryngoscopes, it permits visualized control of endotracheal tube insertion and advancement.

The GVL is more expensive than DL and many of the rigid fiberoptic devices, although priced similarly to the other VLs. This cost differential is orders of magnitude greater than DL but less than flexible bronchoscopy. While the flexible bronchoscope has greater versatility, it is fragile, performs poorly in the presence of blood or secretions and in the setting of deteriorating oxygen saturation. Even more fundamentally, after its insertion in the trachea, intubation over the bronchoscope requires the blind manipulation of an endotracheal tube when advancement is arrested.

Verathon Medical did not wish to disclose a list price but encourages interested parties to contact the distributor at 1-800-331 2313.[G]

10.4.4.8 How Is the GVL Disinfected?[H]

Following tracheal intubation, the video/power cable should be detached from the laryngoscope, and the port is covered by a protective cap. The GVL should then be cleaned with a soapy solution to remove biological debris. The entire scope can then be disinfected by immersing in bleach, Cidex, Metricide, Steris, or Sterrad solutions.

10.4.5 McGrath Video Laryngoscope Series5 (Aircraft Medical)

10.4.5.1 Describe the Unique Features of the McGrath VL

The McGrath VL Series5® (MGL) was developed by industrial designer, Matt McGrath, and is manufactured by Aircraft Medical, Edinburgh Scotland. Introduced in Europe in January 2006, the MGL is compact and lightweight. It is ergonomically designed and powered by a single 1.5V AA NiMH or Li battery housed in its handle. It consists of an adjustable stainless steel CameraStick™ that can be advanced or retracted to three different lengths. The handle is a comfortable, medical grade hard rubber. A 1.7-in (diagonal, 3.3 × 2.25-cm) LCD screen is mounted atop the handle and can be tilted and swiveled for an optimal viewing angle (Figure 10-23). The power button is located on the top of the handle. When the button is depressed, an LED on the monitor flashes if the battery requires replacement.

The CameraStick contains two high-intensity light-emitting diodes and a CMOS video camera. The color image is displayed at 320 × 280 pixels. It has neither recording capability nor an antifogging system. A single-use, low-profile, polycarbonate blade cover with a maximal height of 13-mm covers the CameraStick and clicks securely into place. The system is designed to withstand high impact.

An antifogging solution can be applied to the external surface of the plastic blade but this is not specifically encouraged by the manufacturer. An ETT should be prepared with a stylet. Like the GVL, a malleable stylet, shaped like a hockey-stick or with a 60 to 70 degrees distal bend,[185,186] a dynamic stylet (like the Parker Flex-It™ or Truphatek TruFlex™), a rigid stylet (Verathon GlideRite), or an Eschmann or Frova introducer can be used (see Section 10.4.4.2 above). The blade is introduced into the mouth in the midline until the tip passes beyond the base of the tongue. An ETT is introduced into the mouth under direct vision, close to the laryngoscope blade. Keeping the ETT close to the tongue and laryngoscope blade, the tip is introduced into the glottis and the stylet is partially or fully withdrawn.

[G]All prices are in US dollars unless otherwise stated. All prices were accurate at the time of publication but may be subject to change.
[H]In all cases, please consult with the manufacturer for detailed cleaning instructions.

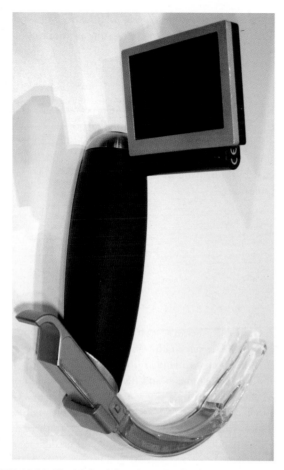

FIGURE 10-23. The McGrath® VL Series5 video laryngoscope consists of an adjustable stainless steel CameraStick that can be advanced or retracted to three different lengths. A 1.7-in (diagonal) LCD screen is mounted atop the handle and can be tilted and swiveled for an optimal viewing angle. A single-use, polycarbonate blade covers the CameraStick and clicks securely in place.

10.4.5.2 What Is the Clinical Utility of the MGL?

After a preliminary investigation in 75 adults, the device was tested in 75 additional consecutive patients. The combined success rate was 147/150 (98%); first pass success was 139/150 (92.7%) and C/L 1 and 2 views were seen in 95% and 4%.[185] The same investigators used the MGL successfully in three cases of failed DL[187] and a series of 35 rapid-sequence intubations.[188]

O'Leary described 30 patients in whom DL had failed and the MGL was used.[189] Most of the initial failures were a consequence of poor laryngeal exposure. Using a modified C/L classification,[190] the MGL resulted in marked improvements of the laryngeal views: C/L 1 and 2a views increased from 7 to 28/30. Failed laryngoscopy occurred in 2/30 (6.6%) rescue attempts; failed intubations occurred in a total of 5/30 attempted rescues (16.6%). Like the GVL, an adequate view of the larynx but inability to intubate was experienced in 3 of 28 patients. The authors concluded that with the MGL, an improved laryngeal view does not assure intubation. These authors believe that the failure rate described is more readily reducible than failed intubations associated with nonvisualization. Although little has been written about the MGL technique, the

similarities between the MGL and GVL would suggest that a very similar technique would enhance success.

O'Leary et al observed minor injuries (self-limiting, minor bleeding) associated with the MGL blade and the ETT.[189] Williams and Ball described a patient in whom, following failed DL, an MGL provided a full glottic view but the ETT was not seen on the monitor. Direct inspection showed a palatal perforation on the right side of the soft palate, likely very similar to the injury described with the GVL.[134,135,191,192] This is a preventable injury requiring direct observation of the ETT as it is introduced into the mouth (see below).

The MGL has been used as an airway assessment tool[193] and as a means of securing the airway in awake patients.[194] In the latter report, three patients with a difficult airway received topical anesthesia and a remifentanil infusion for sedation. In each case, laryngoscopy was well tolerated with good laryngeal visualization and successful tracheal cannulation.

10.4.5.3 What Is the Learning Curve Associated with the MGL?

Walker compared the performance of four anesthesiology residents in their first year of training, randomized to DL- or MGL-assisted endotracheal intubation of 120 elective, uncomplicated patients.[186] All had undergone manikin training and had completed 10 successful intubations. The primary outcome was time to tracheal intubation which they found to be significantly longer with the MGL (47.0 [25-202] seconds) compared with Macintosh DL 29.5 [15-121] seconds; p<0.001)). More C/L 1 views were obtained with the MGL; however all patients in the DL had C/L 1 or 2 views. While they had questioned whether the MGL should be provided for unsupervised, rapid sequence intubations to enhance success in patients with (unanticipated) difficult airways, they did not test this. These findings were consistent with most studies that have shown that among patients with normal airway anatomy, indirect techniques generally take longer.

Savoldelli and coworkers compared the learning curves of the GVL, MGL, and Airtraq in 60 subjects (20 staff anesthesiologists, 20 anesthesia residents, and 20 nurses) previously unfamiliar with these devices.[182] Standardized training was provided and they subsequently were instructed to swiftly intubate a Laerdal SimMan manikin five times with each device. The primary outcome was time to tracheal intubation (of a manikin), although this was divided into time to view and duration of intubation attempt. The time to view was less for DL and Airtraq although by the fifth intubation, the differences between the devices did not differ. The duration of intubation was shorter for DL and the Airtraq than the GVL and MGL, although these differences were of no clinical significance. Although all the laryngoscopes were judged easy to use, the McGrath was the favorite, followed closely by the familiar Macintosh DL. It is important to bear in mind that this study was conducted on new practitioners, performing a very limited number of laryngoscopies and intubations on a specific "normal" manikin. While the time to view and duration of intubation were comparable, additional attempts might have further reduced differences between devices. Furthermore, the manikin does not simulate the effect of fogging, secretions, or differences between simulators and humans that could favor certain devices.

Like the GVL, the curvature of the blade may cause the handle to abut on the patient's chest during insertion. The MGL blade can be disarticulated from the handle and inserted separately. Once the blade has been introduced, it can be reattached to the handle.[195]

10.4.5.4 What Are the Advantages and Disadvantages of the MGL?

The principal advantages of the MGL are its ergonomic design, portability, low-profile, ease of setup, lack of wires, excellent glottic views, and a high-quality image in the user's field of view. The disposable blade covers allow for a rapid turnaround between uses. The blade and handle can be disarticulated if the handle abuts on the chest during insertion. The disadvantages include the small screen size, the inability to record events or transmit the image, the lack of antifogging, and like the other indirect laryngoscopes, the need for a degree of hand-eye coordination not required for DL. Aircraft Medical advertises the advantages of not being tethered to a wire or cable. However the inability to charge the (single) battery between uses without its removal increases the likelihood that the battery will fail at the least opportune moment. Therefore, they recommend replacing the batteries between uses.

The price range for the MGL is between $10,000 and $15,000, depending on the purchased quantities. The list price for the disposable blade is about $15. Disposable blades and batteries add to the per case cost.

10.4.5.5 How Is the McGrath VL Disinfected?

There are two models of MGL. With the basic McGrath™ VL Series5, after the laryngoscope is used, the blade cover is removed, discarded, and the CameraStick is separated from the handle. Both are thoroughly wiped down with alcohol. Visible contamination may require a thorough wiping with a cloth containing an enzymatic detergent and brushing of contacts and crevices.

The Series5 HLDi (high-level disinfection) model can be cleaned as follows: immediately after use, the blade cover is removed and discarded. Surface soiling is removed with an enzymatic detergent and brush. The battery is removed and the cover reapplied. This unit is compatible with Ethylene Oxide, Steris®, or Sterrad® high-level disinfection.

10.5 SUMMARY

Traditionally, laryngoscopy has been dependent upon line-of-sight devices. Despite a variety of laryngoscope blades, it is not always possible to view the larynx even with our attempts to anatomically align the axes of the mouth, pharynx, and larynx. Fiberoptic and video technology now make it feasible to look around those corners that were concealed from our line-of-sight. Our predictors of a difficult intubation developed for direct laryngoscopy may have limited relevance to our success or failure with these alternative devices. This chapter reviewed some of the specific devices, and is not an exhaustive review of all devices now available.

Fiberoptic stylets (Bonfils retromolar intubation fiberscope, Shikani optical stylet, Levitan FPS scope, StyletScope, video-optical intubation system) require relatively limited space for insertion but provide a restricted visual field. Rigid fiberoptic laryngoscopes (Bullard Elite Laryngoscope, WuScope, Uspherscope Ultra, Acutronic Fiberoptic Laryngoscope, Angulated Video-Intubation Laryngoscope, Truview) and video laryngoscopes (Storz V-Mac or C-Mac, GlideScope, and McGrath) provide a wider visual field and space permitting, more readily identifiable anatomical identification. As the name suggests, the fiberoptic stylets are placed within the endotracheal tube and may be positioned at the laryngeal inlet or beyond, with the ETT being advanced over the stylet. The rigid fiberoptic and video laryngoscopes have a viewing channel adjacent to the ETT and remain outside the trachea. Advancement of the ETT toward and through the vocal folds is under visual control. The contrast between the latter technique and that of flexible bronchoscopic intubation is also worth emphasizing. The flexible bronchoscopes identify the larynx but ETT advancement is essentially a blind procedure.

This is a rapidly developing area. New products are added and older ones are modified or withdrawn. A user should not expect to reproduce the findings of experienced practitioners without some investment of time and effort. Although this may be associated with early failures, the authors are of the belief that this investment will ultimately pay dividends. Familiarity with a technique is best acquired when used electively, in patients with relatively normal airway features. Confidence is acquired and the benefits and limitations of specific devices are appreciated. It is not the device that intubates the trachea of a patient; it is the device in a particular practitioner's hands.

The role of these alternative techniques is evolving. Declarations that DL is obsolete[183] are provocative and perhaps premature. Calls for more compelling evidence[144,145] to justify the incremental cost will undoubtedly grow despite the enthusiasm of the video convicted. We need to critically examine the quality of the evidence and look for meaningful clinical outcomes. This will require carefully designed studies, adequately powered, involving those likely to use the device, properly trained to do so, and under conditions in which they are likely to be used. We look forward to seeing the evidence.

REFERENCES

1. James CD. Sir William Macewen and anaesthesia. *Anaesthesia*. 1974;29: 743-753.
2. Cooper RM. Laryngoscopy—its past and future. *Can J Anes*. 2004;51:R6.
3. Adnet F, Borron SW, Dumas JL, Lapostolle F, Cupa M, Lapandry C. Study of the "sniffing position" by magnetic resonance imaging. *Anesthesiology*. 2001;94:83-86.
4. Adnet F, Baillard C, Borron SW, et al. Randomized study comparing the "sniffing position" with simple head extension for laryngoscopic view in elective surgery patients. *Anesthesiology*. 2001;95:836-841.
5. Asai T, Enomoto Y, Shimizu K, Shingu K, Okuda Y. The Pentax-AWS video-laryngoscope: the first experience in one hundred patients. *Anesth Analg*. 2008;106:257-559, table of contents.
6. Rose DK, Cohen MM. The incidence of airway problems depends on the definition used. *Can J Anaesth*. 1996;43:30-34.
7. Rose DK, Cohen MM. The airway: problems and predictions in 18,500 patients. *Can J Anaesth*. 1994;41:372-383.
8. Mort TC. Emergency tracheal intubation: complications associated with repeated laryngoscopic attempts. *Anesth Analg*. 2004;99:607-613, table of contents.
9. Kaplan MB, Ward D, Hagberg CA, et al. Seeing is believing: the importance of video laryngoscopy in teaching and in managing the difficult airway. *Surg Endosc*. 2006;20(Suppl 2):S479-S483.

10. Weiss M, Schwarz U, Dillier CM, Gerber AC. Teaching and supervising tracheal intubation in paediatric patients using videolaryngoscopy. *Paediatr Anaesth*. 2001;11:343-348.

11. Levitan RM. A new tool for teaching and supervising direct laryngoscopy. *Acad Emerg Med*. 1996;3:79-81.

12. Levitan RM. *The Airway Cam Guide to Intubation and Practical Emergency Airway Management*. Wayne, PA: Airway Cam Technologies; 2004.

13. Levitan RM. Design rationale and intended use of a short optical stylet for routine fiberoptic augmentation of emergency laryngoscopy. *Am J Emerg Med*. 2006;24:490-495.

14. Kitamura T, Yamada Y, Du HL, Hanaoka K. Efficiency of a new fiberoptic Stylet Scope in tracheal intubation. *Anesthesiology*. 1999;91:1628-1632.

15. Halligan M, Charters P. A clinical evaluation of the Bonfils intubation fibrescope. *Anaesthesia*. 2003;58:1087-1091.

16. Bein B, Yan M, Tonner PH, Scholz J, Steinfath M, Dorges V. Tracheal intubation using the Bonfils intubation fibrescope after failed direct laryngoscopy. *Anaesthesia*. 2004;59:1207-1209.

17. Aoyama K, Takenaka I, Sata T, Shigematsu A. Use of the fibrescope-video camera system for difficult tracheal intubation. *Br J Anaesth*. 1996;77:662-664.

18. Rudolph C, Schlender M. Clinical experiences with fiber optic intubation with the Bonfils intubation fibrescope. *Anaesthesiol Reanim*. 1996;21:127-130.

19. Shikani AH. New "seeing" stylet-scope and method for the management of the difficult airway. *Otolaryngol Head Neck Surg*. 1999;120:113-116.

20. Young CF, Vadivelu N. Does the use of a laryngoscope facilitate orotracheal intubation with a Shikani Optical Stylet? *Br J Anaesth*. 2007;99:302-303.

21. Xue FS, Liu HP, Guo XL. Transillumination-assisted endotracheal intubation with the Bonfils fiberscope. *Eur J Anaesthesiol*. 2009;26:261-262.

22. Xue FS, Liu HP, Liao X, Zhang YM. Measures to facilitate smooth insertion of an endotracheal tube into the trachea with GlideScope videolaryngoscopy. *J Clin Anesth*. 2009;21:381-382.

23. Abramson SI, Holmes AA, Hagberg CA. Awake insertion of the Bonfils retromolar intubation fiberscope in five patients with anticipated difficult airways. *Anesth Analg*. 2008;106:1215-1217, table of contents.

24. Corbanese U, Possamai C. Awake intubation with the Bonfils fibrescope in patients with difficult airway. *Eur J Anaesthesiol*. 2009;26:837-841.

25. Kovacs G, Law AJ, Petrie D. Awake fiberoptic intubation using an optical stylet in an anticipated difficult airway. *Ann Emerg Med*. 2007;49:81-83.

26. Bein B, Caliebe D, Romer T, Scholz J, Dörges V. Using the Bonfils intubation fiberscope with a double-lumen tracheal tube. *Anesthesiology*. 2005;102:1290-1291.

27. Bein B, Worthmann F, Scholz J, et al. A comparison of the intubating laryngeal mask airway and the Bonfils intubation fibrescope in patients with predicted difficult airways. *Anaesthesia*. 2004;59:668-674.

28. Greenland KB, Liu G, Tan H, Edwards M, Irwin MG. Comparison of the Levitan FPS Scope and the single-use bougie for simulated difficult intubation in anaesthetised patients. *Anaesthesia*. 2007;62:509-515.

29. Kovacs G, Law JA, McCrossin C, et al. A comparison of a fiberoptic stylet and a bougie as adjuncts to direct laryngoscopy in a manikin-simulated difficult airway. *Ann Emerg Med*. 2007;50:676-685.

30. Evans A, Morris S, Petterson J, Hall JE. A comparison of the Seeing Optical Stylet and the gum elastic bougie in simulated difficult tracheal intubation: a manikin study. *Anaesthesia*. 2006;61:478-481.

31. Byhahn C, Nemetz S, Breitkreutz R, et al. Brief report: tracheal intubation using the Bonfils intubation fibrescope or direct laryngoscopy for patients with a simulated difficult airway. *Can J Anaesth*. 2008;55:232-237.

32. Kihara S, Yaguchi Y, Taguchi N, et al. The StyletScope is a better intubation tool than a conventional stylet during simulated cervical spine immobilization. *Can J Anaesth*. 2005;52:105-110.

33. Rudolph C, Schneider JP, Wallenborn J, Schaffranietz L. Movement of the upper cervical spine during laryngoscopy: a comparison of the Bonfils intubation fibrescope and the Macintosh laryngoscope. *Anaesthesia*. 2005;60:668-672.

34. Wahlen BM, Gercek E. Three-dimensional cervical spine movement during intubation using the Macintosh and Bullard laryngoscopes, the Bonfils fibrescope and the intubating laryngeal mask airway. *Eur J Anaesthesiol*. 2004;21:907-913.

35. Turkstra TP, Pelz DM, Shaikh AA, Craen RA. Cervical spine motion: a fluoroscopic comparison of Shikani Optical Stylet vs Macintosh laryngoscope. *Can J Anaesth*. 2007;54:441-447.

36. Shukry M, Hanson RD, Koveleskie JR, Ramadhyani U. Management of the difficult pediatric airway with Shikani Optical stylet. *Paediatr Anaesth*. 2005;15:342-345.

37. Stricker P, Fiadjoe JE, McGinnis S. Intubation of an infant with Pierre Robin sequence under dexmedetomidine sedation using the Shikani Optical Stylet. *Acta Anaesthesiol Scand*. 2008;52:866-867.

38. Aucoin S, Vlatten A, Hackmann T. Difficult airway management with the Bonfils fiberscope in a child with Hurler syndrome. *Paediatr Anaesth*. 2009;19:421-422.

39. Jansen AH, Johnston G. The Shikani Optical Stylet: a useful adjunct to airway management in a neonate with popliteal pterygium syndrome. *Paediatr Anaesth*. 2008;18:188-190.

40. Caruselli M, Zannini R, Giretti R, et al. Difficult intubation in a small for gestational age newborn by Bonfils fiberscope. *Paediatr Anaesth*. 2008;18:990-991.

41. Bein B, Wortmann F, Meybohm P, et al. Evaluation of the pediatric Bonfils fiberscope for elective endotracheal intubation. *Paediatr Anaesth*. 2008;18:1040-1044.

42. Weiss M, Hartmann K, Fischer J, Gerber AC. Video-intuboscopic assistance is a useful aid to tracheal intubation in pediatric patients. *Can J Anaesth*. 2001;48:691-696.

43. Hemmerling TM, Bracco D. Subcutaneous cervical and facial emphysema with the use of the Bonfils fiberscope and high-flow oxygen insufflation. *Anesth Analg*. 2008;106:260-262, table of contents.

44. Kimura A, Yamakage M, Chen X, Kamada Y, Namiki A. Use of the fibreoptic stylet scope (StyletScope) reduces the hemodynamic response to intubation in normotensive and hypertensive patients. *Can J Anaesth*. 2001;48:919-923.

45. Kitamura T, Yamada Y, Chinzei M, Du HL, Hanaoka K. Attenuation of haemodynamic responses to tracheal intubation by the StyletScope. *Br J Anaesth*. 2001;86:275-257.

46. Ezri T, Szmuk P, Warters RD, Katz J, Hagberg CA. Difficult airway management practice patterns among anesthesiologists practicing in the United States: have we made any progress? *J Clin Anesth*. 2003;15:418-422.

47. Jenkins K, Wong DT, Correa R. Management choices for the difficult airway by anesthesiologists in Canada. *Can J Anaesth*. 2002;49:850-856.

48. Rosenblatt WH, Wagner PJ, Ovassapian A, Kain ZN. Practice patterns in managing the difficult airway by anesthesiologists in the United States. *Anesth Analg*. 1998;87:153-157.

49. Hung OR, Tibbet JS, Cheng R, Law JA. Proper preparation of the Trachlight and endotracheal tube to facilitate intubation. *Can J Anaesth*. 2006;53:107-108.

50. MacQuarrie K, Hung OR, Law JA. Tracheal intubation using Bullard laryngoscope for patients with a simulated difficult airway. *Can J Anaesth*. 1999;46:760-765.

51. Cohn AI, Hart RT, McGraw SR, Blass NH. The Bullard laryngoscope for emergency airway management in a morbidly obese parturient. *Anesth Analg*. 1995;81:872-873.

52. Gorback MS. Management of the challenging airway with the Bullard laryngoscope. *J Clin Anes*. 1991;3:473-477.

53. Midttun M, Laerkholm Hansen C, Jensen K, Pedersen T. The Bullard laryngoscope. Reports of two cases of difficult intubation. *Acta Anaesthesiol Scand*. 1994;38:300-302.

54. Hastings RH, Vigil AC, Hanna R, et al. Cervical spine movement during laryngoscopy with the Bullard, Macintosh, and Miller laryngoscopes. *Anesthesiology*. 1995;82:859-869.

55. Watts AD, Gelb AW, Bach DB, Pelz DM. Comparison of the Bullard and Macintosh laryngoscopes for endotracheal intubation of patients with a potential cervical spine injury. *Anesthesiology*. 1997;87:1335-1342.

56. Turner CR, Block J, Shanks A, et al. Motion of a cadaver model of cervical injury during endotracheal intubation with a Bullard laryngoscope or a Macintosh blade with and without in-line stabilization. *J Trauma*. 2009;67:61-66.

57. Shulman GB, Connelly NR. Double lumen tube placement with the Bullard laryngoscope. *Can J Anaesth*. 1999;46:232-234.

58. Ovassapian A, Glassenberg R, Randel GI, et al. The unexpected difficult airway and lingual tonsil hyperplasia: a case series and a review of the literature. *Anesthesiology*. 2002;97:124-132.

59. Crosby E, Skene D. More on lingual tonsillar hypertrophy. *Can J Anaesth*. 2002;49:758.

60. Shulman GB, Nordin NG, Connelly NR. Teaching with a video system improves the training period but not subsequent success of tracheal intubation with the Bullard laryngoscope. *Anesthesiology*. 2003;98:615-620.

61. Maktabi MA, Hoffman H, Funk G, From RP. Laryngeal trauma during awake fiberoptic intubation. *Anesth Analg*. 2002;95:1112-1114, table of contents.

62. Katsnelson T, Farcon E, Schwalbe SS, Badola R. The Bullard Laryngoscope and the right arytenoid. *Can J Anaesth*. 1994;41:552-553.

63. Suzuki A, Tampo A, Abe N, et al. The LMA Fastrack endotracheal tube facilitates the use of the Bullard laryngoscope. *Anesth Analg*. 2007;104:1307.

64. Suzuki A, Tampo A, Abe N, et al. The Parker Flex-Tip tracheal tube makes endotracheal intubation with the Bullard laryngoscope easier and faster. *Eur J Anaesthesiol*. 2008;25:43-47.

65. Fridrich P, Frass M, Krenn CG, et al. The UpsherScope in routine and difficult airway management: a randomized, controlled clinical trial. *Anesth Analg*. 1997;85:1377-1381.

66. Pearce AC, Shaw S, Macklin S. Evaluation of the Upsherscope. A new rigid fibrescope. *Anaesthesia*. 1996;51:561-564.

67. Smith CE, Pinchak AB, Sidhu TS, et al. Evaluation of tracheal intubation difficulty in patients with cervical spine immobilization: fiberoptic (WuScope) versus conventional laryngoscopy. *Anesthesiology*. 1999;91:1253-1259.

68. Smith CE, Sidhu TS, Lever J, Pinchak AB. The complexity of tracheal intubation using rigid fiberoptic laryngoscopy (WuScope). *Anesth Analg*. 1999;89:236-239.

69. Sprung J, Weingarten T, Dilger J. The use of WuScope fiberoptic laryngoscopy for tracheal intubation in complex clinical situations. *Anesthesiology*. 2003;98:263-265.

70. Wu TL, Chou HC. A new laryngoscope: the combination intubating device. *Anesthesiology*. 1994;81:1085-1087.

71. Andrews SR, Mabey MF. Tubular fiberoptic laryngoscope (WuScope) and lingual tonsil airway obstruction. *Anesthesiology*. 2000;93:904-905.

72. Dullenkopf A, Holzmann D, Feurer R, Gerber A, Weiss M. Tracheal intubation in children with Morquio syndrome using the angulated video-intubation laryngoscope. *Can J Anaesth*. 2002;49:198-202.

73. Biro P, Weiss M. Comparison of two video-assisted techniques for the difficult intubation. *Acta Anaesthesiol Scand*. 2001;45:761-765.

74. Biro P, Weiss M, Gerber A, Pasch T. Comparison of a new video-optical intubation stylet versus the conventional malleable stylet in simulated difficult tracheal intubation. *Anaesthesia*. 2000;55:886-889.

75. Miceli L, Cecconi M, Tripi G, Zauli M, Della RG. Evaluation of new laryngoscope blade for tracheal intubation, Truview EVO2: a manikin study. *Eur J Anaesthesiol*. 2008;25:446-449.

76. Leung YY, Hung CT, Tan ST. Evaluation of the new Viewmax laryngoscope in a simulated difficult airway. *Acta Anaesthesiol Scand*. 2006;50:562-567.

77. Barak M, Philipchuck P, Abecassis P, Katz Y. A comparison of the Truview blade with the Macintosh blade in adult patients. *Anaesthesia*. 2007;62:827-831.

78. Li JB, Xiong YC, Wang XL, et al. An evaluation of the TruView EVO2 laryngoscope. *Anaesthesia*. 2007;62:940-943.

79. Malik MA, Maharaj CH, Harte BH, Laffey JG. Comparison of Macintosh, Truview EVO2, Glidescope, and Airwayscope laryngoscope use in patients with cervical spine immobilization. *Br J Anaesth*. 2008;101:723-730.

80. Malik MA, O'Donoghue C, Carney J, et al. Comparison of the Glidescope, the Pentax AWS, and the Truview EVO2 with the Macintosh laryngoscope in experienced anaesthetists: a manikin study. *Br J Anaesth*. 2009;102:128-134.

81. Hirabayashi Y. In-line head and neck positioning facilitates tracheal intubation with the Airway Scope. *Can J Anaesth*. 2007;54:774.

82. Asai T, Liu EH, Matsumoto S, et al. Use of the Pentax-AWS in 293 patients with difficult airways. *Anesthesiology*. 2009;110:898-904.

83. Hirabayashi Y, Seo N. Airway Scope: early clinical experience in 405 patients. *J Anesth*. 2008;22:81-85.

84. Malik MA, Subramaniam R, Maharaj CH, et al. Randomized controlled trial of the Pentax AWS, Glidescope, and Macintosh laryngoscopes in predicted difficult intubation. *Br J Anaesth*. 2009;103:761-768.

85. Suzuki A, Abe N, Sasakawa T, et al. Pentax-AWS (Airway Scope) and Airtraq: big difference between two similar devices. *J Anesth*. 2008;22:191-192.

86. Suzuki A, Toyama Y, Katsumi N, et al. Pentax-AWS improves laryngeal view compared with Macintosh blade during laryngoscopy and facilitates easier intubation. *Masui*. 2007;56:464-468.

87. Adnet F, Borron SW, Racine SX, et al. The intubation difficulty scale (IDS): proposal and evaluation of a new score characterizing the complexity of endotracheal intubation. *Anesthesiology*. 1997;87:1290-1297.

88. Enomoto Y, Asai T, Arai T, Kamishima K, Okuda Y. Pentax-AWS, a new videolaryngoscope, is more effective than the Macintosh laryngoscope for tracheal intubation in patients with restricted neck movements: a randomized comparative study. *Br J Anaesth*. 2008;100:544-558.

89. Malik MA, Subramaniam R, Churasia S, et al. Tracheal intubation in patients with cervical spine immobilization: a comparison of the Airwayscope, LMA CTrach, and the Macintosh laryngoscopes. *Br J Anaesth*. 2009;102:654-661.

90. Komatsu R, Kamata K, Hamada K, et al. Airway scope and StyletScope for tracheal intubation in a simulated difficult airway. *Anesth Analg*. 2009;108:273-279.

91. Komatsu R, Kamata K, Hoshi I, Sessler DI, Ozaki M. Airway scope and gum elastic bougie with Macintosh laryngoscope for tracheal intubation in patients with simulated restricted neck mobility. *Br J Anaesth*. 2008;101:863-869.

92. Liu EH, Goy RW, Tan BH, Asai T. Tracheal intubation with videolaryngoscopes in patients with cervical spine immobilization: a randomized trial of the Airway Scope and the GlideScope. *Br J Anaesth*. 2009;103:446-451.

93. Hirabayashi Y, Fujita A, Seo N, Sugimoto H. Cervical spine movement during laryngoscopy using the Airway Scope compared with the Macintosh laryngoscope. *Anaesthesia*. 2007;62:1050-1055.

94. Maruyama K, Yamada T, Kawakami R, et al. Upper cervical spine movement during intubation: fluoroscopic comparison of the AirWay Scope, McCoy laryngoscope, and Macintosh laryngoscope. *Br J Anaesth*. 2008;100:120-124.

95. Maruyama K, Yamada T, Kawakami R, Hara K. Randomized cross-over comparison of cervical-spine motion with the AirWay Scope or Macintosh laryngoscope with in-line stabilization: a video-fluoroscopic study. *Br J Anaesth*. 2008;101:563-567.

96. Takenaka I, Aoyama K, Iwagaki T, et al. Approach combining the airway scope and the bougie for minimizing movement of the cervical spine during endotracheal intubation. *Anesthesiology*. 2009;110:1335-1340.

97. Kato T, Kusunoki S, Kawamoto M, Yuge O. Usability of AirWay Scope for awake tracheal intubation in a burn patient with difficult airway. *Masui*. 2007;56:1179-1181.

98. Suzuki A, Kunisawa T, Takahata O, et al. Pentax-AWS (Airway Scope) for awake tracheal intubation. *J Clin Anesth*. 2007;19:642-643.

99. Suzuki A, Terao M, Aizawa K, et al. Pentax-AWS airway Scope as an alternative for awake flexible fiberoptic intubation of a morbidly obese patient in the semi-sitting position. *J Anesth*. 2009;23:162-163.

100. Kitagawa H, Sai Y, Tarui K, Imashuku Y, Yamazaki T, Nosaka S. Airway Scope-assisted nasotracheal intubation. *Anaesthesia*. 2009;64:229.

101. Nakamura R, Kusunoki S, Kawamoto M. Usability of modified INTLOCK for double-lumen endobronchial tube insertion with airway scope. *Masui*. 2007;56:817-819.

102. Poon KH, Liu EH. The Airway Scope for difficult double-lumen tube intubation. *J Clin Anesth*. 2008;20:319.

103. Asai T, Shingu K: Use of the Pentax-AWS videolaryngoscope and an exchange catheter for tube exchange. *Masui*. 2008;57:990-992.

104. Suzuki A, Kunisawa T, Aizawa K, et al. Stress-free tracheal tube exchange using the Pentax-AWS (airway scope). *J Cardiothorac Vasc Anesth*. 2009;23:133-134.

105. Kitagawa H, Imashuku Y, Yamazaki T. The airway scope: an aid also in transesophageal echocardiography probe placement. *J Cardiothorac Vasc Anesth*. 2009;23:275.

106. Tagawa T, Sakuraba S, Okuda M. Pentax-AWS-assisted insertion of a transesophageal echocardiography probe. *J Clin Anesth*. 2009;21:73-74.

107. Hirabayashi Y, Seo N. Tracheal intubation by non-anesthesia residents using the Pentax-AWS airway scope and Macintosh laryngoscope. *J Clin Anesth*. 2009;21:268-271.

108. Suzuki A, Yamagishi A, Sasakawa T, et al. Esophageal intubation: can it be avoided with the airway scope (Pentax-AWS)? *Masui*. 2008;57:1160-1163.

109. Ogino Y, Uchiyama K, Hasumi M, et al. A pitfall of AirWay Scope—an experience of distinctive airway edema after palatal laceration caused by irWay Scope. *Masui*. 2008;57:1245-1248.

110. Dhonneur G, Abdi W, Amathieu R, et al. Optimising tracheal intubation success rate using the Airtraq laryngoscope. *Anaesthesia*. 2009;64:315-319.

111. Savoldelli GL, Schiffer E. Videolaryngoscopy for tracheal intubation: the guide channel or steering techniques for endotracheal tube placement? *Can J Anaesth*. 2008;55:59-60.

112. Maharaj CH, O'Croinin D, Curley G, et al. A comparison of tracheal intubation using the Airtraq or the Macintosh laryngoscope in routine airway management: a randomised, controlled clinical trial. *Anaesthesia*. 2006;61:1093-1099.

113. Maharaj CH, Costello JF, Harte BH, Laffey JG. Evaluation of the Airtraq and Macintosh laryngoscopes in patients at increased risk for difficult tracheal intubation. *Anaesthesia*. 2008;63:182-188.

114. Dhonneur G, Ndoko S, Amathieu R, et al. Tracheal intubation using the Airtraq in morbid obese patients undergoing emergency cesarean delivery. *Anesthesiology.* 2007;106:629-630.

115. Maharaj CH, Costello JF, McDonnell JG, et al. The Airtraq as a rescue airway device following failed direct laryngoscopy: a case series. *Anaesthesia.* 2007;62:598-601.

116. Cooper RM, Pacey JA, Bishop MJ, McCluskey SA. Early clinical experience with a new videolaryngoscope (GlideScope) in 728 patients. *Can J Anaesth.* 2005;52:191-198.

117. Hirabayashi Y, Fujita A, Seo N, Sugimoto H. A comparison of cervical spine movement during laryngoscopy using the Airtraq or Macintosh laryngoscopes. *Anaesthesia.* 2008;63:635-640.

118. Maharaj CH, Buckley E, Harte BH, Laffey JG. Endotracheal intubation in patients with cervical spine immobilization: a comparison of Macintosh and Airtraq laryngoscopes. *Anesthesiology.* 2007;107:53-59.

119. Turkstra TP, Pelz DM, Jones PM. Cervical spine motion: a fluoroscopic comparison of the AirTraq Laryngoscope versus the Macintosh laryngoscope. *Anesthesiology.* 2009;111:97-101.

120. Dhonneur G, Ndoko SK, Amathieu R, et al. A comparison of two techniques for inserting the Airtraq laryngoscope in morbidly obese patients. *Anaesthesia.* 2007;62:774-777.

121. Maharaj CH, Costello J, Higgins BD, Harte BH, Laffey JG. Retention of tracheal intubation skills by novice personnel: a comparison of the Airtraq and Macintosh laryngoscopes. *Anaesthesia.* 2007;62:272-278.

122. Ndoko SK, Amathieu R, Tual L, et al. Tracheal intubation of morbidly obese patients: a randomized trial comparing performance of Macintosh and Airtraq laryngoscopes. *Br J Anaesth.* 2008;100:263-268.

123. Holst B, Hodzovic I, Francis V. Airway trauma caused by the Airtraq laryngoscope. *Anaesthesia.* 2008;63:889-890.

124. Dimitriou VK, Zogogiannis ID, Liotiri DG. Awake tracheal intubation using the Airtraq laryngoscope: a case series. *Acta Anaesthesiol Scand.* 2009;53:964-967.

125. Woollard M, Mannion W, Lighton D, et al. Use of the Airtraq laryngoscope in a model of difficult intubation by prehospital providers not previously trained in laryngoscopy. *Anaesthesia.* 2007;62:1061-1065.

126. Woollard M, Lighton D, Mannion W, et al. Airtraq vs standard laryngoscopy by student paramedics and experienced prehospital laryngoscopists managing a model of difficult intubation. *Anaesthesia.* 2008;63:26-31.

127. Kaplan MB, Ward DS, Berci G. A new video laryngoscope—an aid to intubation and teaching. *J Clin Anesth.* 2002;14:620-626.

128. Maassen R, Lee R, Hermans B, et al. A comparison of three videolaryngoscopes: the Macintosh laryngoscope blade reduces, but does not replace, routine stylet use for intubation in morbidly obese patients. *Anesth Analg.* 2009;109:1560-1565.

129. Kaplan MB, Hagberg CA, Ward DS, et al. Comparison of direct and video-assisted views of the larynx during routine intubation. *J Clin Anesth.* 2006;18:357-362.

130. Jungbauer A, Schumann M, Brunkhorst V, et al. Expected difficult tracheal intubation: a prospective comparison of direct laryngoscopy and video laryngoscopy in 200 patients. *Br J Anaesth.* 2009;102:546-550.

131. Serocki G, Bein B, Scholz J, Dorges V. Management of the predicted difficult airway: a comparison of conventional blade laryngoscopy with video-assisted blade laryngoscopy and the GlideScope. *Eur J Anaesthesiol.* 2010;27:24-30.

132. Cavus E, Kieckhaefer J, Doerges V, et al. The C-MAC videolaryngoscope: first experiences with a new device for videolaryngoscopy-guided intubation. *Anesth Analg.* 2009;110:473-477.

133. Cho JE, Kil HK. A maneuver to facilitate endotracheal intubation using the GlideScope. *Can J Anaesth.* 2008;55:56-57.

134. Choo MK, Yeo VS, See JJ. Another complication associated with videolaryngoscopy. *Can J Anaesth.* 2007;54:322-324.

135. Cooper RM. Complications associated with the use of the GlideScope videolaryngoscope. *Can J Anaesth.* 2007;54:54-57.

136. Malik AM, Frogel JK. Anterior tonsillar pillar perforation during GlideScope video laryngoscopy. *Anesth Analg.* 2007;104:1610-1611; discussion 1611.

137. Hirabayashi Y. Pharyngeal injury related to GlideScope videolaryngoscopy. *Otolaryngol Head Neck Surg.* 2007;137:175-176.

138. Dow WA, Parsons DG. 'Reverse loading' to facilitate GlideScope intubation. *Can J Anaesth.* 2007;54:161-162.

139. Doyle DJ, Zura A, Ramachandran M. Videolaryngoscopy in the management of the difficult airway. *Can J Anaesth.* 2004;51:95; author reply 95-96.

140. Jones PM, Turkstra TP, Armstrong KP, et al. Effect of stylet angulation and endotracheal tube camber on time to intubation with the GlideScope. *Can J Anaesth.* 2007;54:21-27.

141. Turkstra TP, Harle CC, Armstrong KP, et al. The GlideScope-specific rigid stylet and standard malleable stylet are equally effective for GlideScope use. *Can J Anaesth.* 2007;54:891-896.

142. Krasser K, Moser A, Missaghi SM, Lackner-Ausserhofer H, Zadrobilek E. Experiences with the Lo Pro Adult GlideScope Video Laryngoscope for Orotracheal Intubation. *Internet J Airway Manag.* 2007;4.

143. Turkstra TP, Jones PM, Ower KM, Gros ML. The Flex-It stylet is less effective than a malleable stylet for orotracheal intubation using the GlideScope. *Anesth Analg.* 2009;109:1856-1859.

144. Frerk CM, Lee G. Laryngoscopy: time to change our view. *Anaesthesia.* 2009;64:351-354.

145. Mihai R, Blair E, Kay H, Cook TM. A quantitative review and meta-analysis of performance of non-standard laryngoscopes and rigid fibreoptic intubation aids. *Anaesthesia.* 2008;63:745-760.

146. Sun DA, Warriner CB, Parsons DG, et al. The GlideScope Video Laryngoscope: randomized clinical trial in 200 patients. *Br J Anaesth.* 2005;94:381-384.

147. Cooper RM. The GlideScope videolaryngoscope. *Anaesthesia.* 2005;60:1042.

148. Ithnin F, Lim Y, Shah M, et al. Tracheal intubating conditions using propofol and remifentanil target-controlled infusion: a comparison of remifentanil EC50 for Glidescope and Macintosh. *Eur J Anaesthesiol.* 2009;26:223-228.

149. Siddiqui N, Katznelson R, Friedman Z. Heart rate/blood pressure response and airway morbidity following tracheal intubation with direct laryngoscopy, GlideScope and Trachlight: a randomized control trial. *Eur J Anaesthesiol.* 2009;26:740-745.

150. Maassen R, Lee R, van Zundert A, Cooper R. The videolaryngoscope is less traumatic than the classic laryngoscope for a difficult airway in an obese patient. *J Anesth.* 2009;23:445-448.

151. Santoni BG, Hindman BJ, Puttlitz CM, et al. Manual in-line stabilization increases pressures applied by the laryngoscope blade during direct laryngoscopy and orotracheal intubation. *Anesthesiology.* 2009;110:24-31.

152. Lee C, Katznelson R, Firat M, Cooper RM. Direct measurement of the force required for direct and Video Laryngoscopy in four commercial airway manikins, 2010. Abstract presented at the SAM meeting in Chicago, Sept, 2011.

153. Agro F, Barzoi G, Montecchia F. Tracheal intubation using a Macintosh laryngoscope or a GlideScope in 15 patients with cervical spine immobilization. *Br J Anaesth.* 2003;90:705-706.

154. Turkstra TP, Craen RA, Pelz DM, Gelb AW. Cervical spine motion: a fluoroscopic comparison during intubation with lighted stylet, GlideScope, and Macintosh laryngoscope. *Anesth Analg.* 2005;101:910-915, table of contents.

155. Robitaille A, Williams SR, Tremblay MH, et al. Cervical spine motion during tracheal intubation with manual in-line stabilization: direct laryngoscopy versus GlideScope videolaryngoscopy. *Anesth Analg.* 2008;106:935-941, table of contents.

156. Wong DM, Prabhu A, Chakraborty S, et al. Cervical spine motion during flexible bronchoscopy compared with the Lo-Pro GlideScope. *Br J Anaesth.* 2009;102:424-430.

157. Cooper RM. Use of a new videolaryngoscope (GlideScope) in the management of a difficult airway. *Can J Anaesth.* 2003;50:611-613.

158. Bishop S, Clements P, Kale K, Tremlett MR. Use of GlideScope Ranger in the management of a child with Treacher Collins syndrome in a developing world setting. *Paediatr Anaesth.* 2009;19:695-696.

159. Brar MS. Airway management in a bleeding adult following tonsillectomy: a case report. *AANA J.* 2009;77:428-430.

160. Cooper RM. Videolaryngoscopy in the management of the difficult airway: reply. *Can J Anaesth.* 2004;51:95-96.

161. Diaz-Gomez JL, Satyapriya A, Kolli Iv SV, et al. The usefulness of the GlideScope in the management of a "controlled" difficult airway. *J Clin Anesth.* 2009;21:79-80.

162. Doyle DJ. Awake intubation using the GlideScope video laryngoscope: initial experience in four cases. *Can J Anaesth.* 2004;51:520-521.

163. Eaton J, Atiles R, Tuchman JB. GlideScope for management of the difficult airway in a child with Beckwith-Wiedemann syndrome. *Paediatr Anaesth.* 2009;19:696-698.

164. Echeverri M, Tur A, Dese J, Marcelo S. GlideScope video laryngoscope intubation of a patient with ankylosing spondylitis. *Rev Esp Anestesiol Reanim.* 2007;54:576-577.

165. Gooden CK. Successful first time use of the portable GlideScope videolaryngoscope in a patient with severe ankylosing spondylitis. *Can J Anaesth.* 2005;52:777-778.

166. Gunaydin B, Gungor I, Yigit N, Celebi H. The Glidescope for tracheal intubation in patients with ankylosing spondylitis. *Br J Anaesth.* 2007;98:408-409.

167. Hirabayashi Y, Hakozaki T, Fujisawa K, et al. Use of a new video-laryngoscope (GlideScope) in patients with a difficult airway. *Masui.* 2007;56:854-857.

168. Jones PM, Harle CC. Avoiding awake intubation by performing awake GlideScope laryngoscopy in the preoperative holding area. *Can J Anaesth.* 2006;53:1264-1265.

169. Taub PJ, Silver L, Gooden CK. Use of the GlideScope for airway management in patients with craniofacial anomalies. *Plast Reconstr Surg.* 2008;121: 237e-238e.

170. Smith MP, Khodadadi O, Doyle DJ. Use of GlideScope Video Larynogoscope in morbidly obese patients (>45 BMI): a retrospective review. *Anesthesiology.* 2007;107:A926.

171. Trevisanuto D, Fornaro E, Verghese C. The GlideScope video laryngoscope: initial experience in five neonates. *Can J Anaesth.* 2006;53:423-424.

172. Hirabayashi Y, Otsuka Y. Early clinical experience with GlideScope video laryngoscope in 20 infants. *Paediatr Anaesth.* 2009;19:802-804.

173. Kim JT, Na HS, Bae JY, et al. GlideScope video laryngoscope: a randomized clinical trial in 203 paediatric patients. *Br J Anaesth.* 2008;101:531-534.

174. Redel A, Karademir F, Schlitterlau A, et al. Validation of the GlideScope video laryngoscope in pediatric patients. *Paediatr Anaesth.* 2009;19:667-671.

175. Xue FS, Liu HP, Liu JH, et al. Facilitating endotracheal intubation using the GlideScope video laryngoscope in children with difficult airways. *Paediatr Anaesth.* 2009;19:918-919.

176. Wayne MA, McDonnell M. Comparison of traditional versus video laryngoscopy in out-of-hospital tracheal intubation. *Prehosp Emerg Care.* 2010;14:278-282.

177. Dunford JV, Davis DP, Ochs M, Doney M, Hoyt DB. Incidence of transient hypoxia and pulse rate reactivity during paramedic rapid sequence intubation. *AnnEmergMed.* 2003;42:721-728.

178. Maharaj CH, Costello JF, Higgins BD, et al. Learning and performance of tracheal intubation by novice personnel: a comparison of the Airtraq and Macintosh laryngoscope. *Anaesthesia.* 2006;61:671-677.

179. Malik MA, Hassett P, Carney J, Higgins BD, Harte BH, Laffey JG. A comparison of the Glidescope, Pentax AWS, and Macintosh laryngoscopes when used by novice personnel: a manikin study. *Can J Anaesth.* 2009;56: 802-811.

180. Nouruzi-Sedeh P, Schumann M, Groeben H. Laryngoscopy via Macintosh blade versus GlideScope: success rate and time for endotracheal intubation in untrained medical personnel. *Anesthesiology.* 2009;110:32-37.

181. Cook TM, Green C, McGrath J, Srivastava R. Evaluation of four airway training manikins as patient simulators for the insertion of single use laryngeal mask airways. *Anaesthesia.* 2007;62:713-718.

182. Savoldelli GL, Schiffer E, Abegg C, et al. Learning curves of the Glidescope, the McGrath and the Airtraq laryngoscopes: a manikin study. *Eur J Anaesthesiol.* 2009;26:554-558.

183. Cooper RM. Is Direct Laryngoscopy Obsolete? http://www.adair.at/ijam/volume04/specialcomment01/default.htm. Accessed January 3, 2011.

184. Jones PM, Turkstra TP, Armstrong KP, et al. Comparison of a single-use GlideScope Cobalt videolaryngoscope with a conventional GlideScope for orotracheal intubation. *Can J Anaesth.* 2009;57:18-23.

185. Shippey B, Ray D, McKeown D. Case series: the McGrath videolaryngoscope—an initial clinical evaluation. *Can J Anaesth.* 2007;54:307-313.

186. Walker L, Brampton W, Halai M, et al. Randomized controlled trial of intubation with the McGrath Series 5 videolaryngoscope by inexperienced anaesthetists. *Br J Anaesth.* 2009;103:440-445.

187. Shippey B, Ray D, McKeown D. Use of the McGrath videolaryngoscope in the management of difficult and failed tracheal intubation. *Br J Anaesth.* 2008;100:116-119.

188. Shippey B, McKeown D, Ray D. Rapid sequence intubation using the McGrath videolaryngoscope. *Eur J Emerg Med.* 2006;13:A12-A13.

189. O'Leary AM, Sandison MR, Myneni N, et al. Preliminary evaluation of a novel videolaryngoscope, the McGrath series 5, in the management of difficult and challenging endotracheal intubation. *J Clin Anesth.* 2008;20:320-321.

190. Yentis SM, Lee DJ. Evaluation of an improved scoring system for the grading of direct laryngoscopy. *Anaesthesia.* 1998;53:1041-1044.

191. Cross P, Cytryn J, Cheng KK. Perforation of the soft palate using the GlideScope videolaryngoscope. *Can J Anaesth.* 2007;54:588-589.

192. Vincent RD, Jr, Wimberly MP, Brockwell RC, Magnuson JS. Soft palate perforation during orotracheal intubation facilitated by the GlideScope videolaryngoscope. *J Clin Anesth.* 2007;19:619-621.

193. Thong SY, Shridhar IU, Beevee S. Evaluation of the airway in awake subjects with the McGrath videolaryngoscope. *Anaesth Intensive Care.* 2009;37: 497-498.

194. McGuire BE. Use of the McGrath video laryngoscope in awake patients. *Anaesthesia.* 2009;64:912-914.

195. Osborn IP, Behringer EC, Kramer DC. Difficult airway management following supratentorial craniotomy: a useful maneuver with a new device. *Anesth Analg.* 2007;105:552-553.

SELF-EVALUATION QUESTIONS

10.1 Which of the following statements about video laryngoscopes is **TRUE**?

A. The video laryngoscopes facilitate the recording of the laryngoscopy.

B. The technique for using the GlideScope® makes it well suited for teaching direct laryngoscopy.

C. The laryngeal view obtained using the Storz Video-Macintosh makes it well suited for managing the difficult airway.

D. The laryngeal view is essentially the same as the line-of-sight view.

E. The images obtained using any of the video laryngoscopes is hampered by fogging.

10.2 Which of the following statements about optical/fiberoptic stylets (eg, the Bonfils, Shikani optical stylet, or Levitan FPS scope) is **TRUE**?

A. Fiberoptic stylets should generally be used as stand-alone tools.

B. Once the tube is loaded, fiberoptic stylets have the advantage of requiring no other preparation of patient or instrument.

C. Fiberoptic stylets have been proven to be effective in awake intubations.

D. Fiberoptic stylets can be used as an adjunct to direct laryngoscopy.

E. The learning curve of these devices is such that novices can be expected to have a good chance at a successful intubation using a fiberoptic stylet.

10.3 Which of the following regarding rigid fiberoptic laryngoscopes is **FALSE**?

A. The rigid fiberoptic laryngoscopes are delicate and are easily damaged.

B. The laryngeal view may be obscured by fogging or the presence of blood and secretions.

C. Advancement of the endotracheal tube can be observed.

D. All of these devices require wider mouth opening than is required for direct laryngoscopy.

E. These devices are well suited for managing difficult airways.

CHAPTER (11)

Nonvisual Intubation Techniques

Chris C. Christodoulou and Orlando R. Hung

11.1 INTRODUCTION

11.1.1 Do we still need nonvisual intubating techniques?

For many decades, tracheal intubation under direct vision using a laryngoscope has been considered the standard technique of intubation. Unfortunately, this approach to intubation has limitations. Difficult and failed intubation employing this technique can be as high as 21%, particularly in emergency situations.[1] Not surprisingly, studies have shown that considerable experience is required before a trainee becomes proficient in laryngoscopic intubation. Konrad and Mulcaster have constructed learning curves showing that a 90% probability of success requires between 47 and 57 laryngoscopic intubations.[2,3]

The high incidence of difficulty and failure, coupled with these kinds of learning curves for laryngoscopic intubation have driven the development of many alternative intubation devices and techniques such as rigid and flexible endoscopes, video laryngoscopes, and optical intubating stylets. All of these devices have gained a measure of popularity. Unfortunately, these devices are substantially more expensive than the laryngoscope. Furthermore, the cleaning and sterilization processes of some of these devices, such as the flexible bronchoscope, require an average of 50 to 60 minutes to complete, hindering their availability and practicality in emergency airway management and in prehospital care (ie, they may be context driven).

The challenge of visual techniques employing optical stylets and videoscopes is visualization of glottic structures and the passage of the Eschmann Tracheal Tube Introducer through the glottic opening in the face of fogging or the presence of blood, secretions, and vomitus in the upper airway. It is precisely these kinds of difficulties that have motivated the search for nonvisual techniques using a variety of devices such as intubating guides, light-guided intubation using the principle of transillumination, blind nasal intubation, digital intubation, and retrograde intubation, all of which have proven to be effective, safe, and simple techniques.

11.2 INTUBATING STYLETS OR GUIDES

11.2.1 What is the Eschmann tracheal tube introducer? How does it facilitate the placement of an endotracheal tube?

In 1949, Macintosh reported the use of an introducer (gum-elastic bougie) to facilitate orotracheal intubation under direct laryngoscopy.[4] Using the concept of the introducer, Venn designed the Eschmann Introducer (endotracheal tube [ETT], Portex Limited, Hythe, UK), a tubelike core woven from polyester threads and covered with a resin layer.[5] The Eschmann Introducer (EI) is 60 cm long, with a J (coudé) tip (a 35-degree angle bend) at the distal end to facilitate advancement anteriorly underneath the epiglottis into the trachea and to provide tactile tracheal confirmation (Figure 11-1). Centimeter markings designate the distance from the tip. The EI is often referred to as the "gum-elastic bougie" or "bougie." However, to avoid confusion, historically the "gum-elastic bougie" has been used to refer to a shorter urinary catheter made of different material and without a curved tip.[6]

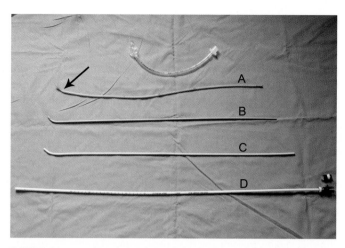

FIGURE 11-1. Intubating guides: (A) the Eschmann Introducer with a coudé tip (arrow) at the distal end; (B) Frova Intubation Introducer is an intubating catheter with a hollow lumen and a coudé tip at the distal end; (C) the endotracheal Tube Introducer is similar to the Eschmann Introducer in size and shape with a coudé tip, but it is 10 cm longer; and (D) the Cook Airway Exchange Catheter with an inner lumen, distal ports, and an adapter at the proximal end.

The EI is particularly useful when the glottic opening cannot be clearly seen using a laryngoscope (eg, Grade 3 laryngoscopic view as described by Cormack).[7] Under these circumstances, the EI can be hooked underneath the epiglottis and advanced into the trachea. If it is correctly placed in the trachea, a subtle tactile clicking sensation can be felt as the tip of the EI slides over the tracheal rings while advancing it into the trachea. Furthermore, if the EI correctly enters the trachea, as it is gently advanced it will eventually be lodged (or "holdup") in a distal airway and cannot advance beyond the 30 to 35 cm mark. In contrast, if it is placed in the esophagus, the entire EI can be advanced without encountering resistance. With the EI in place and positioned at 20 cm at the teeth, the ETT can then be advanced over the EI into the trachea. To facilitate the advancement of the ETT over the EI, the tongue and epiglottis must be elevated by a gentle jaw lift, a jaw thrust, or preferably, by the laryngoscope already in place. If difficulty persists while advancing the ETT, rotating the ETT 90 degrees counterclockwise will turn the ETT bevel posteriorly and minimize the risk of catching on glottic structures.[8] Following intubation, the position of the ETT is confirmed using conventional methods, such as end-tidal CO_2 and auscultation. The EI has also been used to facilitate retrograde intubation in a trauma patient,[9] and placement of a tracheostomy device during the performance of a difficult or emergency surgical airway (eg, cricothyrotomy).[10,11]

11.2.2 What other intubating guides or introducers are commercially available?

Since the introduction of the EI, many intubating guides of different sizes, shapes, lengths, and materials have been developed. All of the designs serve a function similar to the EI but many have some additional features.

a. The Flex-Guide ETT Introducer (Green Field Medical Sourcing, Inc., Northborough, MA) is a flexible plastic introducer with a distal tip that can be bent by means of a proximal handle.[12]

b. The Sheridan Tube Exchanger (Sheridan Catheter Corp., Oregon, NY) is a hollow flexible straight tube designed as a tube exchanger for patients with difficult airways. It can be used to ventilate patients under difficult circumstances through the inner lumen, distal ports, and an adapter at the proximal end.

c. The Cook Airway Exchange Catheter (Cook® Critical Care, Inc., Bloomington, IN) serves a similar function as the Sheridan Tube Exchanger (Figure 11-1).

d. Frova Intubation Introducer (Cook® Critical Care Inc., Bloomington, IN) is an intubating catheter with a coudé tip at the distal end (Figures 11-1 and 11-2).[13] It has a hollow lumen with side ports distally; Rapi-Fit® adapters (luer lock and standard 15/22 mm) come with the device to permit oxygen insufflation in the event intubation cannot be achieved. It also has a removable internal metal stylet to prevent kinking and damage during shipping and to increase stiffness, facilitating tracheal placement and ETT passage (Figure 11-2). The Frova Introducer has two sizes: the adult version for ETT with greater than 5.5 mm internal diameter (ID) and the pediatric version for ETTs 3 to 5 mm ID.

e. The Schroeder (Parker Flex-It™ Directional Stylet) Oral/Nasal Directional Stylet (Parker Medical, Englewood, CO) is a disposable articulating stylet that requires no bending prior to intubation (Figure 11-3). Inserting the stylet into an ETT allows the practitioner to elevate the tip of the ETT by wrapping the index and middle fingers around the proximal tracheal tube and using the thumb to depress the proximal end of the stylet. Although the stylet is suitable for both oral and nasal intubation, it has been reported to be somewhat awkward to use and the curvature created is not at the tip, but rather over the distal half of the tube.[14]

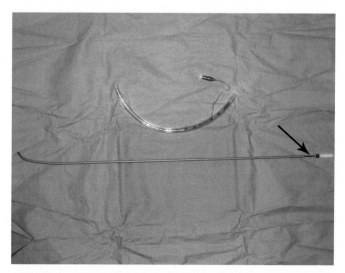

FIGURE 11-2. Frova Intubation Introducer is an intubating catheter with a hollow lumen and a coudé tip at the distal end. It also has a removable internal metal stylet (arrow) to increase stiffness to facilitate tracheal placement and ETT passage.

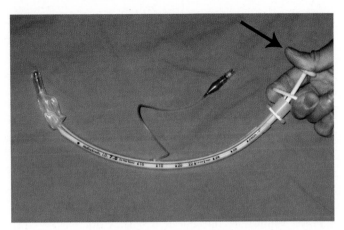

FIGURE 11-3. The Schroeder (Parker Flex-It Directional Stylet) Oral/Nasal Directional Stylet. Elevation of the tip of the ETT can be achieved by wrapping the index and middle fingers around the proximal tracheal tube and using the thumb to depress the proximal end of the stylet (arrow).

However, it has been reported to be effective for difficult as well as blind intubations.[15]

f. Endotracheal Tube Introducer (Sun Med, Largo, FL) is similar to the EI in size and shape, but it is 10 cm longer. This confers some advantage in employing the device as more of the device protrudes from the mouth, making it easier to thread a standard 30-cm adult-sized ETT and capture the proximal end of the introducer. It is stiffer than the EI, conferring an advantage in guiding the ETT, but at the same time serving to emphasize the importance of gentle maneuvers to prevent airway injury. There is a single marking at 20 cm on the device to indicate the depth of insertion. It is a single-use disposable device, though resterilization is possible (Figure 11-1).

g. Portex Intubation Stylet (SIMS Portex Ltd, Hythe, Kent, UK) is available in outer diameter sizes ranging from 2.2 mm to 5.0 mm. These stylets can be inserted into a variety of endotracheal tubes. Blind awake orotracheal intubation has been successfully performed utilizing a stylet loaded into an ETT, in a patient with a laryngeal carcinoma and ankylosing spondylitis.[16] Guided tactile probing is used to direct the ETT-stylet unit into the trachea.

11.2.3   Is there any clinical evidence to support the widespread use of these intubating introducers?

Over the last several decades, numerous studies have reported the effectiveness and safety of employing an EI to facilitate tracheal intubation in patients with difficult laryngoscopy.[17-20] The EI has been well accepted by most practitioners in the United Kingdom, and it continues to play an important role in the management of the difficult intubation. According to a recent survey in the United Kingdom, 100% of the respondents reported the use of the EI as their technique of choice when faced with an unanticipated difficult laryngoscopic intubation.[21] Though primarily a device used by anesthesia practitioners in the past, over the past decade this relatively inexpensive and simple device has found its way to the hands of emergency practitioners and prehospital health-care practitioners as a standard airway management adjunct.[22-24] A telephonic survey of emergency departments in England revealed that 99% of respondents stocked the EI on their difficult airway carts.[25]

Following a recent review of the evidence, the Difficult Airway Society Guidelines for Management of the Unanticipated Difficult Intubation in the United Kingdom recommend the use of the EI as the initial device to facilitate a difficult laryngoscopy.[26] Many authorities recommend that this device be a standard piece of equipment for every laryngoscopic intubation.

While the EI has been widely accepted as a useful tracheal intubation adjunct, other types of introducers bearing similar features do not share the same popularity. This may be due to a paucity of clinical evidence supporting their use compared to the EI. In addition, most of these new intubating guides and stylets are disposable devices intended for single use and perhaps less cost-effective than the reusable EI.

11.2.4   What are the potential limitations of these intubating guides and introducers?

The popularity of the EI rests on its simplicity, ease of use, high success rates, and relatively few complications. However, it does have limitations.

The much-anticipated clicks and the holdup as described by many may prove elusive. The appreciation of clicks is particularly subtle in many patients. In 1988, Kidd et al studied the reliability of these signs.[27] They found that holdup was observed in 100% of tracheal EI placement, whereas clicks were appreciated in only 90%. Importantly, however, neither were observed in any of the 22 esophageal placements. It is also possible that holdup might occur with esophageal placement of the EI in cases of esophageal stenosis, pharyngeal pouch or diverticulum, or with cricoid pressure, although one would anticipate these occurrences would be rare. Practitioners should be aware of these limitations, particularly where holdup can occur without the presence of clicks. It is the opinion of the author (ORH) that the probability of feeling the clicks with EI placement into the trachea depends largely on the angle of insertion of the EI relative to the trachea. It is unlikely that the tip of the EI will rub against the tracheal rings if the EI is advancing into the trachea from a more vertical position. It is also related to the degree to which the EI contacts other soft tissues in the airway (eg, tongue or lip), insulating against the transmission of the subtle tactile sensation.

Although complications are rare with these devices, they tend to occur when they are used improperly. Soft tissue lacerations, esophageal perforation, and tracheo-bronchial tree injuries have been reported with aggressive insertion of the EI and forceful railroading of the ETT over the EI.[28-30] The incidence of these complications can be minimized by employing a gentle advancement technique, and using the laryngoscope to move soft tissues out of the way to improve the angle of insertion of the ETT over the EI. Tip detachment has also been reported. Gardner et al reported a detachment of the tip of the EI following its withdrawal.[31] The tip was initially identified just above the bifurcation of the trachea, although it was later documented to have moved into the right middle lobe bronchus. Manually checking the integrity of the tip of the EI prior to use is recommended.

11.2.5 Are there any clinical differences between the EI and other introducers with identical features?

Inspired by the simplicity and effectiveness of the EI, many newer introducers (eg, the Frova Intubation Introducer, and the Endotracheal Tube Introducer) share similar characteristics such as the J (coudé) tip at the distal end. By and large, these newer devices are made of different materials and are designed for single use. The Frova Intubation Introducer and the Cook Airway Exchange Catheter are hollow intubating introducers that permit urgent oxygenation and ventilation, should the tracheal tube fail to advance into the trachea over the introducer. In addition to the tracheal clicks and holdup of the introducers during the insertion into the trachea, an aspiration test using a self-inflating bulb (SIB; also known as an Esophageal Detection Device [EDD]) can also be used with the hollow intubating introducers to further confirm tracheal placement. Tuzzo et al recently reported that a prompt and complete reinflation of the SIB failed to occur when the hollow intubating introducer was placed accidentally into the esophagus with 100% sensitivity and at a 3.5% false-positive rate.[32] While these newer devices appear to function similarly to the EI in facilitating tracheal intubation, they may not have comparable success rates. Using a simulated Grade 3 laryngoscopic view in a manikin, a recent comparative study showed that successful placement of the Frova Introducer (65%) and the EI (60%) was significantly higher than with the Portex Introducer (8%).[12] A separate experiment also revealed that the peak force exerted by the Frova and Portex introducers was two to three times greater than that which could be exerted by the EI, suggesting that placement of the single-use introducers may be more traumatic.

11.3 LIGHTWANDS

11.3.1 What is a lightwand? How does it help with the placement of an endotracheal tube?

The technique of transillumination using a lightwand (lighted-stylet) was first described by Yamamura et al in 1959 with nasotracheal intubation.[33] The lightwand employs the principle of transillumination of the soft tissues of the anterior neck to guide the tip of the lightwand, and the mounted ETT, into the trachea. It also takes advantage of the anterior (superficial) location of the trachea relative to the esophagus.

When the tip of the ETT/lightwand (ETT/LW) combination enters the glottic opening, a well-defined circumscribed glow can be readily seen slightly below the thyroid prominence (Figure 11-4A).

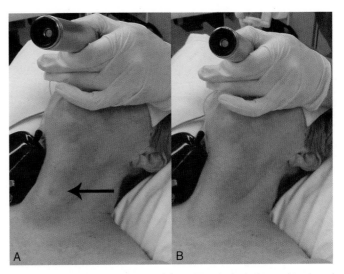

FIGURE 11-4. (A) When the tip of the ETT with the lightwand is placed at the glottic opening under direct laryngoscopy, a well-defined circumscribed glow (arrow) in the anterior neck just below the thyroid prominence can be readily seen. (B) When the tip of the endotracheal tube is placed in the esophagus under direct laryngoscopy, transillumination is poor and the transmitted glow is diffuse in the anterior neck and cannot be seen easily under ambient lighting condition.

However, if the tip of the ETT/LW is in the esophagus, the transmitted glow is diffuse and cannot be readily detected under ambient lighting conditions (Figure 11-4B). If the tip of the ETT/LW is placed in the vallecula, the light glow is diffuse and appears slightly above the thyroid prominence. Using these landmarks and principles, the practitioner can guide the tip of the ETT easily and safely into the trachea without the use of a laryngoscope.

11.3.2 Are all lightwands the same?

Through the 1970s and 1980s, many versions of a lighted stylet had been introduced, including the Fiberoptic Malleable Lighted Stylette (Metropolitan Medical Inc., Winchester, VA), Fiberoptic Lighted-Intubation Stylette (Anesthesia Medical Specialties, Santa Fe, CA), Lighted Intubation Stylet (Aaron Medical, St. Peterborough, FL), Flexilum™ (Concept Corporation, Clearwater, FL), Tubestat™ (Xomed, Jacksonville, FL) (Figure 11-5), and Imagica Fiberoptic Lighted Stylet (Fiberoptic Medical Products, Inc., Allentown, PA). Some of these devices have proven to be effective and safe in placing an ETT both orally and nasally.[34-36] Even though favorable results have been reported with these devices, substantial limitations have been identified: (1) poor light intensity; (2) short length, limiting the use of the lightwand device to a short or cut ETT; (3) absence of a connector to secure the ETT to the lightwand device; (4) rigidity of the lightwand, hampering use of the devices with other techniques, such as light-guided nasal intubation; and (5) most lightwands were designed for single use, increasing the cost per intubation. For these reasons and others, intubation using a lightwand did not receive widespread popularity until the Trachlight™ (Laerdal Medical, Wappingers Falls, NY) device became available.

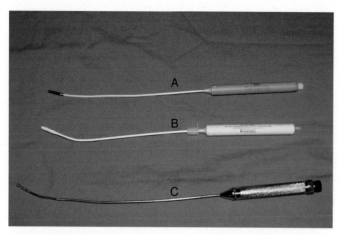

FIGURE 11-5. Commercially available lighted stylets: (A) Flexilum™, (B) Tubestat™, and (C) fiberoptic malleable lighted stylette.

11.3.3   What are some of the unique characteristics of the Trachlight™ compared to other lightwand devices?

The Trachlight™ (TL) consists of three parts: a reusable handle, a flexible wand, and a stiff retractable wire stylet (Figure 11-6). The power control circuitry and three triple A alkaline batteries are encased in the handle. A locking clamp located on the handle accepts and secures a standard 15-mm ETT connector. The stylet or wand consists of a durable, flexible plastic shaft with a bright light bulb affixed at the distal end, permitting intubation under ambient lighting conditions. After 30 seconds of illumination, the light bulb blinks to minimize heat production and provide a convenient reminder of elapsed time. Ensuring that the tip of the stylet is inside the distal tip of ETT enhances its heat safety profile. A recent animal study confirmed an absence of heat-related tissue

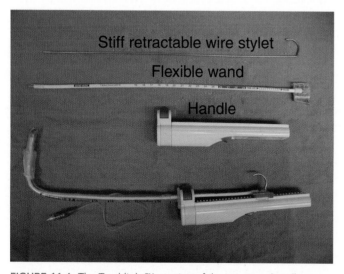

FIGURE 11-6. The Trachlight™ consists of three parts: a handle, a flexible wand, and a stiff retractable stylet wire. With the TL in place, the ETT-TL unit is bent at a 90-degree angle just proximal to the cuff of the tube in the shape of a field hockey stick.

histopathological changes, suggesting that thermal injury following the use of the TL is unlikely.[37]

A rigid plastic connector with a release arm at the proximal end of the TL handle allows adjustment of the wand along the handle and into the ETT when the release arm is depressed. Enclosed within the wand is a stiff but malleable, retractable wire stylet. When the stiff wire stylet is retracted, the wand becomes pliable, permitting the ETT to advance easily into the trachea. This may well be the most important feature of this lightwand device, since it significantly improves its ease of use and intubation success rate.

The retractable wire stylet stiffens the wand sufficiently so that it can be shaped in the form of a field hockey stick (Figure 11-6). This configuration directs the bright light of the bulb against the anterior wall of the larynx and trachea. In addition, the hockey stick configuration enhances maneuverability during intubation and facilitates the placement of the ETT through the glottic opening. However, once through the glottis, the field hockey stick configuration can impede further advancement of the tube into the trachea. Retraction of the stiff wire stylet produces a pliable ETT-TL unit, permitting its advancement into the trachea until the transilluminated glow reaches the sternal notch, a point known to be midtrachea.

11.3.4   How do you prepare the Trachlight™ device?

One of the authors (ORH) had significant involvement in the development of the TL, as reflected in the following narrative describing intubation technique using the TL. Although the Trachlight™ device is no longer available, a newer version of the device is currently being developed. In addition, the technique described can be applied to other lightwand device that employs the concept of transillumination-guided tracheal intubation. As with any intubation technique, regular use of a TL improves the clinician's performance and intubation success rates, and reduces the risk of complications.

Lubrication of the internal wire stylet of the wand using silicone fluid (Endoscopic Instrument Fluid, ACMI, Southborough, MA) ensures its easy retraction during intubation. The wand should also be lubricated with the same silicone fluid to facilitate retraction of the wand following the ETT placement. The rail gear of the TL handle should always be inspected for missing fragments (prior to loading of the stylet, after retraction of the stylet).[38] Cutting the ETT to a length of 26 cm is recommended to facilitate maneuverability of the ETT-TL during oral tracheal intubation. The wand is then inserted into the ETT and the tube attached to the handle. The length of the wand is adjusted by sliding the wand along the handle to position the light bulb close to, but not protruding beyond, the tip of the ETT. With the TL in place, the ETT-TL unit is bent to a 90-degree angle just proximal to the cuff of the tube in the shape of a field hockey stick (Figure 11-6). Even though the degree of bend should be individualized to the patient, a 90-degree angle generally makes the intubation considerably easier and projects the maximum light intensity toward the surface of the skin as the device traverses the glottis and trachea, producing a well-defined exterior-circumscribed glow. If the TL is bent to 45 degrees, the maximum light intensity will be directed down the trachea. For obese patients or patients with short necks, a more acute bend (>90 degrees) provides better transillumination. Although it is the author's experience that the recommended length of the TL from bend to tip of 6.5 to 8.5 cm is suitable for most patients, some investigators have suggested that the length from bend to tip is best established by matching it to the patient's thyroid prominence-to-mandibular angle distance.[39]

11.3.5   How do you use the Trachlight™ to perform tracheal intubation?

Although the practitioner usually stands at the head of the table or bed during lightwand intubation, it is possible to employ this technique from the front or side of the patient, in the prehospital environment for instance. When the head is in the sniffing position, the epiglottis is in close contact with the posterior pharyngeal wall making it more difficult for the TL to advance behind the epiglottis. It is preferable that the patient's head and neck be positioned in a neutral or slightly extended position.

In most cases, patients can be intubated easily under ambient lighting conditions.[40] In very thin patients, the light intensity is so bright that it is possible to mistakenly interpret an esophageal intubation as an intratracheal placement. It is therefore recommended that intubations using the TL in otherwise normal individuals be carried out under ambient light. Dimming room lights may be advantageous in obese patients, patients with thick necks or dark skin, or when the technique is being learned. In settings where controlling the ambient lighting is not possible (eg, prehospital), it may be helpful to shade the neck with a towel or a hand.

Denitrogenation of the patient should precede all light-guided intubations. In an unconscious patient lying supine, the tongue falls posteriorly, pushing the epiglottis against the posterior pharyngeal wall (Figure 11-7). In order to have clear access to the glottic opening during intubation, it is necessary for the practitioner to grasp the jaw and lift it upward using the thumb and index finger of the nondominant hand. This lifts the tongue and

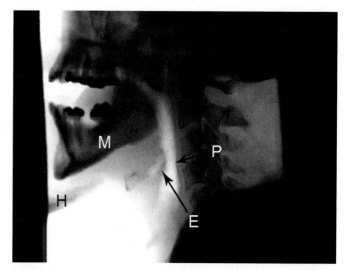

FIGURE 11-8. This radiological film of the upper airway shows that the jaw or mandibular (M) lift by the nondominant hand (H) can elevate the tongue and epiglottis (E) off the posterior pharyngeal wall (P), thus providing a clear passage for the endotracheal tube to enter the glottic opening.

epiglottis away from the posterior pharyngeal wall to facilitate placement of the tip of the ETT posterior to the epiglottis and into the glottic opening (Figure 11-8). The ETT-TL unit is then inserted into the midline of the oropharynx. The midline position of the ETT-TL is maintained while the device is advanced gently in a rocking motion along an imaginary anterior–posterior arc. When resistance to cephalad rocking of the handle is felt, the ETT-TL handle should be rocked forward (toward the feet) and the tip redirected toward the laryngeal prominence using the glow of the light as a guide. A faint glow seen above the laryngeal prominence indicates that the tip of the ETT-TL is located in the vallecula. When the tip of ETT-TL enters the glottic opening, a well-defined circumscribed glow can be seen in the anterior neck slightly below the laryngeal prominence (Figure 11-9). Retracting

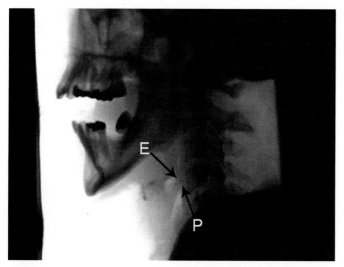

FIGURE 11-7. This radiological film of the upper airway shows that under anesthesia and with the patient lying supine, the tongue falls posteriorly, pushing the epiglottis (E) against the posterior pharyngeal wall (P).

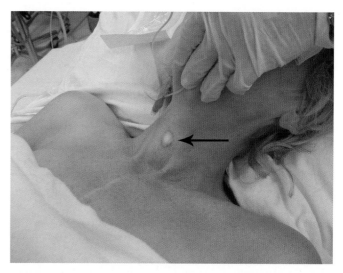

FIGURE 11-9. The ETT-TL is positioned in the midline and advanced gently in a rocking motion along an imaginary anterior–posterior arc. A bright, well-defined, circumscribed glow (arrow) is seen below the thyroid prominence when the ETT-TL enters the glottic opening.

the inner stiff wire stylet approximately 10 cm makes the ETT-TL tip more pliable, permitting advancement into the trachea with reduced risk of trauma. The ETT-TL is then advanced until the glow begins to disappear at the sternal notch, indicating that the tip of the ETT is approximately 5 cm above the carina in the average adult.[41] Following release of the locking clamp, the TL wand can be removed from the ETT.

Occasionally, the circumscribed glow cannot be readily seen in the anterior neck due to anatomical features such as morbid obesity or a short neck. Neck extension as described above may be helpful. Retraction of the breast or chest wall tissues together with spreading of the tissues around the trachea by an assistant enhances transillumination of the soft tissues in the anterior neck. Dimming the ambient light is seldom required.

Occasionally, following retraction of the wire stylet, the tip of the tube and lightwand can hang up on laryngeal structures, the cricoid ring, or a tracheal ring and cannot be advanced into the trachea readily. This is likely due to the fact that when an ETT is loaded along its natural curvature onto the Trachlight™, the tip of the ETT has a tendency to bend anteriorly upon retraction of the stiff internal stylet. While maintaining tube tip contact with the anterior airway, the clinician should rotate the ETT-TL 90 degrees or more to the right or the left side, permitting the tip of the ETT to alter the orientation of the tube tip perhaps enhancing the chance that the ETT will enter the trachea. Alternatively, immersing the ETT in warm saline solution prior to tracheal intubation will reduce its stiffness and the memory of its natural curvature. In addition, reverse loading of the ETT onto the Trachlight™ may minimize the tendency of the ETT tip to bend anteriorly while retracting the internal stiff stylet of the Trachlight™. The combination of softening and reverse loading of the ETT has been shown to overcome the problem of hang up during intubation with the Trachlight™.[42]

11.3.6 Can the Trachlight™ be used for nasotracheal intubation? How do you use the TL to perform a nasotracheal intubation?

In contrast to other commercially available lighted stylets, once the stiff internal wire stylet is removed, the wand of the TL becomes pliable and able to facilitate a light-guided nasotracheal intubation. When used with a nasal RAE (Ring, Aldair, and Elwyn) ETT, the inner wire stylet should be inserted halfway (about 15 cm) to allow unbending of the proximal curvature of the nasal RAE tube (Figure 11-10). Application of a vasoconstricting nasal spray to the nasal mucosa prior to intubation may help to minimize bleeding. The ETT-TL should be immersed in a bottle of warm sterile water or saline to soften the ETT and reduce the risk of mucosal damage during nasal intubation. Water-soluble lubricant is applied to the nostril to facilitate entry of the ETT-TL through the nose. As with oral intubation, a jaw lift during intubation will elevate the tongue and epiglottis away from the posterior wall of the pharynx, facilitating the placement of the tip of the ETT behind the epiglottis and into the glottic opening. The TL is switched on once the tip of the ETT-TL has advanced into the oropharynx, positioned in the midline, and advanced gently using the light glow as a guide.

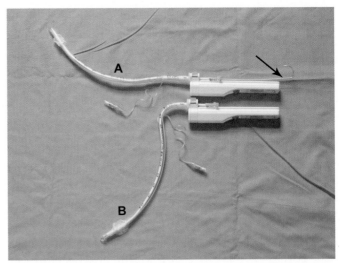

FIGURE 11-10. For light-guided nasal intubation using the Trachlight™, the internal wire stylet is generally removed so that the wand of the TL becomes pliable to facilitate nasotracheal intubation. However, if a nasal RAE tube is used, the proximal curvature of the nasal RAE tracheal tube will bend the pliable wand of the TL (B), making it difficult to control the tip of the tracheal tube during intubation. When the TL is used with a nasal RAE ETT, the wire stylet (arrow) should be retracted only halfway (about 15 cm) to allow unbending of the proximal curvature of the nasal RAE tube (A) to facilitate light-guided nasal intubation.

A faint glow seen above the laryngeal prominence indicates that the tip of the ETT-TL is located in the vallecula. A jaw lift and slight withdrawal of the ETT-TL will help to elevate the epiglottis and enhance the passage of the ETT-TL under it. When the ETT-TL enters the glottic opening, a well-defined circumscribed glow is seen in the anterior neck just below the thyroid prominence (Figure 11-11). Following the release of the locking clamp, the TL is withdrawn from the ETT. Correct tube placement should be confirmed using end-tidal CO_2 and auscultation.

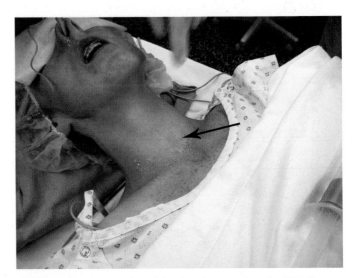

FIGURE 11-11. During nasotracheal intubation, when the ETT-TL enters the glottic opening, a well-defined circumscribed glow (arrow) is seen in the anterior neck just below the thyroid prominence.

11.3.7 What are the common problems with a blind or light-guided nasotracheal intubation? How do you overcome these problems?

Due to the natural curvature of the ETT, the tip of the tube often goes posteriorly into the esophagus during a blind or light-guided nasal intubation, despite external posterior pressure on the thyroid cartilage. To elevate the tip of the ETT anteriorly during intubation, it is sometimes necessary to flex the neck of the patient while advancing the ETT-TL slowly. In the event that flexing the neck of the patient is contraindicated, inflating the ETT cuff with 20 mL of air will help to elevate the ETT tip and align it with the glottis during intubation.[40,43,44] Alternatively, the use of a directional-tip tube, such as an Endotrol™ tube (Mallinckrodt Critical Care, Inc., St. Louis, MO), flexes the tube tip anteriorly and into the glottis.[45] In certain circumstances (eg, tube tip impingement in the posterior nasopharynx), nasotracheal intubation using the TL can be performed safely with the stiff, internal stylet in place.[46] This technique may be associated with fewer head-neck manipulations and deliver better control of the tip of the ETT.

11.3.8 What are the limitations of the Trachlight™ intubating technique?

The TL intubating technique requires transillumination of the soft tissues of the anterior neck without visualization of the laryngeal structures. Therefore, TL should not be used in patients with known abnormalities of the upper airway, such as tumors, polyps, infection (eg, epiglottitis, retropharyngeal abscess), and trauma to the upper airway, or if there is a foreign body in the upper airway. In these cases, alternative intubating techniques using direct or indirect vision should be considered. TL should also be used with caution in patients in whom transillumination of the anterior neck may not be adequate, such as patients who are grossly obese or with a limited neck extension. However, these contraindications and precautions must be weighed in the light of the urgency of achieving a patent airway in any patient whose ventilation may be compromised and urgent intubation is required. Clearly, this light-guided technique should not be attempted with an awake, uncooperative patient unless a bite block is used to prevent damage to the device or injury to the practitioner.

Since its introduction in 1995, the TL has been used extensively in many countries. While the potential risks of damage to the glottic opening during tracheal intubation using a nonvisual intubating technique is real, there have been no serious complications reported. Aoyama et al used a nasally placed bronchoscope to visualize the airway during TL intubation. They reported that the epiglottis may be pushed into the laryngeal inlet by the ETT-TL during a TL intubation.[47] Fortunately, the epiglottis usually spontaneously returned to its correct position. They also reported that structures around the glottic opening, including the epiglottis and the arytenoids, were transiently displaced during the placement of the ETT using the TL. The investigators concluded that there are potential risks of laryngeal damage in addition to the down folding of the epiglottis during the ETT placement using the TL, but such occurrences do not appear to cause permanent damage.

Other investigators have identified a reduced incidence of sore throat in patients intubated using the TL compared to laryngoscopic intubation.[40]

Intubation using a lightwand device has other potential risks. Stone et al reported disconnection of the light bulb from a lightwand requiring retrieval from a major bronchus.[48] However, the lightwand device employed in this instance (Flexilum™) was not designed or recommended for tracheal intubation. A later version of the same device solved the problem of bulb loss into the trachea by encasing stylet and bulb in a tough plastic sheath (Tubestat™). In contrast to the older lightwand devices, it is extremely unlikely that the light bulb will be detached from the TL, since the light bulb is firmly attached to the durable plastic sheath of TL. In fact, since its introduction in 1995, there have been no reported cases of detached light bulb from the TL. Although rare, subluxation of the cricoarytenoid cartilage has been reported in a study using an older version of a lightwand (Tubestat™).[49] However, with the retractable wire stylet, the risk of damaging the arytenoid cartilage during TL intubation should be low.

11.3.9 Is there any clinical evidence to suggest that the Trachlight™ is an effective and safe intubating device?

A large clinical study involving 950 elective surgical patients conducted to determine the effectiveness and safety of orotracheal intubation using either the TL or direct-vision intubation using a laryngoscope[36,40] showed a statistically significant difference in the total intubation time between the groups (15.7 ± 10.8 vs 19.6 ± 23.7 seconds for TL and laryngoscopy, respectively). However, such a small difference is probably of little clinical importance. There was a 1% failure rate with the TL and 92% success rate on the first attempt, compared with a 3% failure rate and an 89% success rate on the first attempt using the laryngoscope. There were significantly fewer traumatic events and sore throats in the TL group compared to laryngoscopy patients. Tsutsui et al reported similar findings in a study with 511 patients.[50] TL intubation was highly successful (99%) with the majority of the successful intubations (93%) being accomplished after one attempt. Unsuccessful intubation even at the third attempt occurred in only three patients (1%).

In 1995, Hung et al reported the effectiveness of TL intubation in 265 patients with a difficult airway (206 patients with a documented history of difficult intubation or anticipated difficult airways and 59 anesthetized patients with an unanticipated failed laryngoscopic intubation).[51] Tracheal intubation was successful in all patients except two in the anticipated difficult laryngoscopic intubation group. Apart from minor mucosal bleeding (mostly from nasal intubation), no serious complications were observed in any of the study patients. The results of this study indicate that TL is an effective technique for placement of ETTs (nasally and orally) for patients with both anticipated or unanticipated difficult airways. Other investigators have reported successful use of the TL in patients with a difficult airway. These include patients with a history of limited mouth opening,[52] cervical spine abnormality,[53] Pierre-Robin syndrome,[54] and cardiac patients with a difficult airway.[55]

11.3.10   What are some of the potential uses of the Trachlight™?

Tracheal intubation can fail with TL as well as with the laryngoscope. However, one study of 950 patients showed that all TL failures were resolved with direct laryngoscopy.[40] Similarly, all failures of direct laryngoscopy were resolved with TL. These results suggest that a tracheal intubation success rate approaching 100% can be achieved by combining the techniques. This combined approach may be particularly useful when an unanticipated Cormack/Lehane (C/L) Grade 3 laryngoscopic view is encountered.[7] Instead of using a styletted ETT with a 90-degree bend, one might employ an ETT-TL with the same bend. Under direct laryngoscopy, the tip of the ETT-TL can be hooked under the epiglottis. A well-defined circumscribed glow seen in the anterior neck slightly below the laryngeal prominence indicates that the tip of the ETT is placed at the glottic opening. In the event that such a glow is not seen, the ETT-TL can be repositioned until it can be. The effectiveness of this combined technique has been reported by Agro et al.[56] In this study, the investigators successfully performed tracheal intubation in all 350 surgical patients studied with a simulated difficult airway using a combined laryngoscope/TL approach.

The TL has been combined successfully with other intubating techniques including intubation through the LMA Classic™,[57,58] use in conjunction with the intubating LMA (Fastrach™),[59] with the Bullard laryngoscope,[60,61] and with a retrograde intubating technique.[62]

Recently, the TL has been shown to be useful in identifying the intratracheal position of the ETT tip during percutaneous dilational tracheotomy.[63] The TL wand without the stiff wire stylet is passed through the in situ ETT matching the length numbers on the ETT to position the TL tip at the ETT tip. This simple technique may help to prevent inadvertent punctures of the ETT and/or its cuff, ensuring that adequate ventilation and oxygenation can be reinstituted during the percutaneous procedure if required. This technique is inexpensive and minimizes the risk of damaging expensive equipment ordinarily used during procedures such as the flexible bronchoscope. Used properly, it is possible that this simple light-guided technique can also be used to accurately determine when the tip of the ETT is above the surgical tracheotomy site as the tube is pulled back during surgical tracheotomy.

11.4   DIGITAL INTUBATION

11.4.1   What is digital intubation? When was it introduced?

Airway management has been revolutionized by the abundance of extraglottic devices that not only facilitate effective ventilation but also aid tracheal intubation. Despite these advances, certain situations may make the blind insertion of an ETT into the trachea using the digits of the hand (digital intubation or tactile orotracheal intubation) as a suitable alternative method of securing an airway.

It is believed that this technique was first described by Herholt and Rafn in 1796 in drowning victims. It surfaced as a viable method of intubation in the emergency medicine literature in the mid 1980s.[64,65] Blind digital intubation has also been used

to establish an airway during neonatal resuscitation[66] and as an adjunct in blind nasotracheal intubation.[67]

11.4.2   What are the indications for digital intubation?

The skill levels of the practitioner, coupled with previous experience in using the technique of blind digital intubation are important prerequisites for success. The importance of practicing this technique in nonemergency situations cannot be overemphasized. The risk of infectious disease transmission must always be borne in mind. Awake patients with an intact gag reflex are not suitable for this technique. Muscle paralysis may be helpful in certain situations. The following list briefly describes the clinical situations where blind digital intubation may be used to establish a patent airway:

a. Inadequate access to a patient that prevents standard laryngoscopic techniques from being used.

b. Lack or failure of other airway management devices.

c. Inability to secure an airway with laryngoscopic techniques or extraglottic devices.

d. In the setting of cervical spine instability in an unconscious patient.

e. When blood, secretions, vomitus, or pus make adequate visualization of the glottis impossible.

11.4.3   How do you perform digital intubation?

The skilled practitioner ensures that an oxygen source, rescue airway devices, suction, and emergency drugs are immediately at hand. In-line immobilization should be performed in the setting of cervical spine instability. Cricoid pressure should be applied where clinically indicated. Although digital intubation can usually be performed without other adjuncts (Figure 11-12), the classic description of

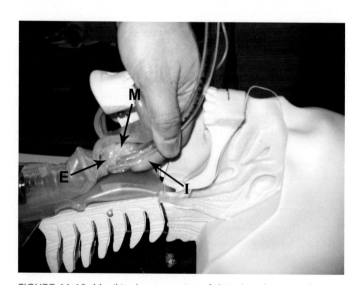

FIGURE 11-12. Manikin demonstration of digital intubation without using a stylet or intubating guide: the index and middle fingers of the nondominant hand are inserted into the mouth. Once the epiglottis (E) is palpated by the middle finger (M), it is lifted in an anterior direction. The index finger (I) of the nondominant hand is then flexed to guide the tracheal tube under the epiglottis and into the trachea.

blind digital intubation requires a malleable stylet to be inserted into the ETT.[68] The ETT is then bent into a shape such that it can elevate the epiglottis and enter the trachea. Alternatively, as the authors believe, an intubating guide (eg, the EI) together with an appropriately sized ETT is a simpler technique. The advantage of this latter technique is that it is easier to guide an EI through the glottic opening, and then railroad the ETT into the trachea than it is to place a stylet-ETT combination in the trachea. The intubating guide has a small external diameter and is easily manipulated with the fingers to enable passage through the vocal cords. In addition, the clicks felt as the intubating guide (eg, EI) advances over the tracheal rings combined with holdup will assist in confirmation that the EI has entered the trachea. The ETT with the malleable stylet is rigid and perhaps more likely to cause blunt trauma to the airway structures, especially if repeated manipulation is necessary for successful entry into the trachea.

To perform the procedure:

a. The patient's head should be placed in the sniffing position as for standard laryngoscopic intubation except in situations where cervical instability exists.

b. The practitioner stands or kneels adjacent to the patient (facing the patient's head) so that the nondominant side of the intubator is closest to the patient (Figure 11-13).

c. If available, an assistant can grasp and pull the tongue forward using gauze. This maneuver helps to lift the epiglottis anteriorly and makes palpation of the structures of the upper airway easier.

d. The practitioner then places the index and middle fingers of the nondominant hand into the patient's mouth. Once the epiglottis is palpated by the middle finger, it is lifted in an anterior direction.

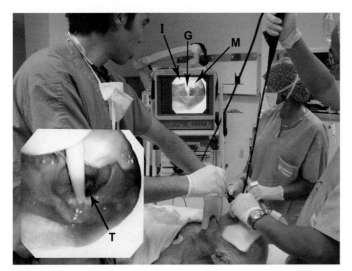

FIGURE 11-13. Digital intubation using an intubating guide: to visualize the technique of digital intubation, a flexible fiberoptic bronchoscope was placed through the right nostril into the nasopharynx of the patient. During the digital intubation, the index and middle fingers of the nondominant hand are inserted into the mouth. As shown in the monitor (and the enlarged insert), once the epiglottis is palpated by the middle finger (M), it is lifted in an anterior direction. The index finger (I) is then flexed to guide the intubating guide (G) under the epiglottis and into the trachea (T).

e. The intubating guide is then guided into the mouth along the palmar surface of the index finger of the nondominant hand.

f. The index finger of the nondominant hand is then flexed to steer the intubating guide under the epiglottis and into the trachea (Figure 11-13). Occasionally, the middle finger of the nondominant hand lifting the epiglottis has to be moved slightly laterally to allow successful passage of the intubating guide.

g. The clicks on the tracheal rings and holdup of the intubating guide on the lower bronchial tree serve as indicators of correct tracheal placement.

h. The ETT is then railroaded over the intubating guide into the trachea. Maintaining anterior displacement of the epiglottis facilitates ETT passage.

i. Confirmation of successful tracheal intubation should be determined by end-tidal CO_2 detection.

11.4.4 Can digital intubation be performed on a child?

Although the principles and techniques of digital intubation are similar, digital intubation can readily be performed without the use of a stylet or the EI in children. Hancock et al have employed this technique during neonatal resuscitation and accidental extubation scenarios.[66] Digital intubation of neonates and infants can be considered in situations where direct laryngoscopic techniques have failed, airway equipment failure has occurred, for meconium aspiration in the neonate, or during transport when inadequate access may preclude conventional techniques.

11.4.5 What are the limitations of digital intubation?

Although digital intubation is a simple and easy to learn technique, it is difficult to perform when the epiglottis cannot be identified or felt during intubation. This is particularly true for the patients who are excessively tall or with a full set of maxillary incisors and a small mouth opening. The procedure can also be difficult to perform if the practitioner has short or large fingers in relation to the patient's anatomy.

To minimize the risk of injury to the practitioner's fingers, digital intubation is generally contraindicated for patients who are awake and uncooperative. However, in emergency situations when limited equipment is available, a digital intubation may be an option with a bite block in place.

11.5 BLIND NASAL INTUBATION

11.5.1 What are the indications for blind nasal intubation?

The technique of blind nasal intubation was first popularized by Sir Ivan Magill and Stanley Rowbotham in the 1920s. This method of tracheal intubation has proved life saving in many difficult airway situations. Maintenance of spontaneous ventilation facilitates blind nasal intubation. The experience and skill of the practitioner are key determinants for success with this technique. The following is a list of indications for blind nasal intubation:

a. Elective oral, pharyngeal, and dental surgery

b. When the oral route is difficult or impossible (eg, limited mouth opening or severe masseter spasm)

c. Difficult airway—elective or unanticipated

11.5.2   What are the contraindications of blind nasal intubation?

The following may contraindicate blind nasal intubation, although all are relative:

a. Inadequate experience or skill of the practitioner

b. Base of the skull cranial fractures

c. Severe maxillofacial fractures with distorted nasal or midface anatomy

d. Known or suspected nasal obstruction secondary to pathology (eg, massive nasal polyps or tumors)

e. Bleeding diathesis secondary to hematological disease or anticoagulant medication

11.5.3   Which nostril should be used for blind nasal intubation?

As most practitioners are right handed, naturally, most would favor the use of the right hand to advance the ETT through the right nostril while using the left hand to feel the anterior neck to assess the position of the tip of the ETT during blind nasal intubation. In the absence of a septal abnormality (eg, a septal deviation), traditional teaching also suggests the right nostril over the left for nasal intubation.[69] It is generally felt that the left-facing bevel of the tracheal tube is the main cause of nasal trauma. The mucosa over the turbinates is highly vascular and can be easily traumatized. It is likely that the mucosa over the left turbinate is particularly at risk during left-sided intubation since the bevel tends to impact directly against it. So, to minimize trauma, most practitioners would insert the ETT with the bevel facing the flat nasal septum rather than facing the irregularly shaped turbinates along the lateral wall of the nasal cavity. However, others consider that the tip of the tracheal tube is more likely to cause nasal trauma than the bevel and therefore it is more reasonable to have the tip of the ETT to advance alongside the septal mucosa during intubation. Hence, some practitioners choose to advance the ETT through the left nostril during nasal intubation. Unfortunately, no scientific evidence currently exists to suggest that one nostril is safer than the other for nasal intubation in patients with a normal nasal anatomy.[70] Instead of debating which is the preferred nostril to minimize the risk of injury, it is perhaps more important to properly prepare the ETT (eg, selecting an appropriate size ETT and softening the ETT in warm saline or water) and the patient (eg, apply vasoconstrictor to the nostrils prior to performing the

nasal intubation), resist excessive force during intubation, and change to a different nostril or use a smaller ETT when it becomes necessary.

11.5.4   How do you perform a blind nasal tracheal intubation?

The answer to this question is largely determined by the indication for tracheal intubation. In elective situations, the nares are best prepared with a vasoconstrictor (though there is little evidence that this maneuver reduces bleeding or enhances success rates) and a local anesthetic of choice. In emergency situations with life-threatening hypoxemia, this may not be possible. The potential for severe epistaxis with airway hemorrhage must always be borne in mind. Rescue airway equipment including extraglottic devices and surgical airway kits should be available. Vital sign monitors are attached and the patient is fully denitrogenated if practical prior to the procedure being undertaken. Cervical spine precautions and cricoid pressure should be instituted as indicated. Maintenance of spontaneous ventilation is preferred to assist with successful tracheal intubation. Confirmation of tracheal tube placement is obtained by the usual clinical criteria as well as CO_2 detection methods. Some practitioners fully insert their little finger to gently dilate the nostril, minimize bleeding on tube insertion, and identify mid nares or posterior nares anatomical abnormalities that would preclude use of that nostril.

To perform the procedure:

a. Insert the appropriate size ETT into the naris.

b. Gently advance the ETT. If resistance is met, do not use excessive force. This may mean that the tip of the ETT has entered the depression in the nasopharynx where the eustachian tube enters (see Chapter 3). Consider switching to the alternative nostril.

c. Listen for breath sounds as you advance the ETT. The author has successfully used a stethoscope attached to the ETT adaptor to auscultate for breath sounds during the procedure. The BAAM whistle (*Beck Airway Airflow Monitor*, Great Plains Ballistics, Inc., Lubbock, TX) to provide an auditory cue in the form of a to and fro whistle to facilitate nasotracheal intubation coupled with an Endotrol™ ETT (Mallinckrodt Medical Inc. Argyle, NY) has been reported.[71] Careful inspection of the neck can also provide useful clues to the location of the tip of the ETT.

d. In the event that esophageal entry occurs repeatedly, the ETT can be withdrawn to the hypopharynx and the cuff of the ETT inflated to produce anterior displacement of the ETT tip toward the glottic opening.[44] Neck flexion is a commonly used maneuver to aid in passage of the ETT into the trachea if the ETT repeatedly impinges anterior to the epiglottis. Neck extension is employed if the ETT repeatedly passes posterior to the glottis into the esophagus. An Endotrol™ ETT as described above may also be used in this situation.[71] Clearly, this maneuver should not be performed in patients with known or suspected cervical pathology.

e. Confirm ETT placement once tracheal entry is suspected.

11.6   RETROGRADE INTUBATION

11.6.1   What is retrograde intubation and when was it introduced?

In 1960, two surgeons, Butler and Cirillo, reported the first retrograde intubation in surgical patients through an existing tracheotomy opening.[72] The technique was subsequently modified by Waters who performed a cricothyroid membrane puncture using a Touhy needle.[73] Waters inserted an epidural catheter through the Touhy needle and advanced it cephalad so that the catheter was brought out through the mouth. An ETT was then advanced over the epidural catheter into the trachea while pulling both ends of the catheter taut. After the ETT entered the trachea, the catheter was pulled out through the oral cavity.

11.6.2   How do you perform a retrograde intubation?

To improve success rates for this technique, many modifications have been suggested since its introduction. For instance, the use of a guide wire rather than an epidural catheter, even though the authors continue to prefer an epidural catheter because it is substantially cheaper, more pliable, and perhaps less traumatic.

11.6.2.1   Equipment

Although a preassembled kit is commercially available, the list of equipment necessary for the retrograde intubation is summarized in Table 11-1.

11.6.2.2   Patient Preparation

In contrast to the sniffing position advocated for laryngoscopic intubation, the patient's head and neck should be in a neutral or relatively extended position to favor an epiglottic position that is off the posterior pharyngeal wall. The epiglottis is almost in contact with the posterior pharyngeal wall when the head is in the sniffing position, making it difficult for the ETT to go underneath the epiglottis. In obese patients or patients with an extremely short neck, placing a pillow under the shoulders and neck may be useful.

11.6.2.3   The "Classic" Technique

This technique can be used in patients who are awake under topical anesthesia with sedation or under general anesthesia.[62,74] Although a cricothyroid membrane puncture can be performed using a blunt tip Touhy needle, the Angiocath is less traumatic and substantially easier to use. The cricothyroid membrane is punctured at an angle 90 degree to the skin using the 18-gauge Angiocath (or needle) in the midline position. Correct tracheal placement can be confirmed by aspirating a free stream of air bubbles in a fluid-filled syringe. Once the tracheal lumen is entered, the Angiocath needle is removed, leaving the catheter behind. The Angiocath catheter is then angled at 45 degree in a cephalad direction through which a 21-gauge epidural catheter (or a guide wire) can be inserted and advanced cephalad into the oropharynx. The epidural catheter can be readily retrieved from the mouth using the Magill forceps. After the removal of the Angiocath catheter from the anterior neck, and to avoid accidentally pulling the epidural catheter (or the guide wire) through, a hemostat is attached to the distal end of the epidural catheter or guide wire at the skin entry point. Similarly, a hemostat is attached to the epidural catheter or wire where it emerges from the mouth. The epidural catheter or guide wire is then inserted into the ETT. Lubrication of the tip of the ETT will facilitate its entry into the glottic opening. To elevate the tongue and epiglottis away from the posterior pharyngeal wall, the tongue of the patient is then gently pulled forward by an assistant if the procedure is performed under general anesthesia. While pulling the epidural catheter or the guide wire taut from both ends by an

◖ TABLE 11-1

Equipment Necessary to Facilitate Light-Guided Retrograde Intubation

EQUIPMENT	FUNCTION
Chlorhexidine or other antiseptic solutions	To minimize risk of infection
An appropriately sized tracheal tube	For tracheal intubation
An 18-gauge needle or intravenous Angiocath	Cricothyroid membrane puncture
A 5 mL fluid-filled syringe	Aspiration of free air
21-gauge epidural catheter (Portex) or a 110 cm long guide wire (0.038 in diameter)	To guide the ETT into the trachea
A tapered anterograde guide catheter is required for the guide wire technique 70 cm	To facilitate the ETT into the trachea
Magill forceps and a laryngoscope	To retrieve the epidural catheter from the oral cavity
Two hemostats	To hold the epidural catheter or guide wire
4 × 4 gauze	To hold the tongue forward during intubation
Water-soluble lubricant	To lubricate the tip of the ETT

assistant, the ETT is inserted into the oropharynx in the midline position. When the tip of the ETT enters the glottic opening, the tension of the epidural catheter at the distal end should be relaxed and the ETT can be advanced gently into the trachea. (For the guide wire technique, the guide wire should be removed before advancing the ETT into the trachea.) While leaving the epidural catheter in place, correct placement of ETT is confirmed using end-tidal CO_2. The epidural catheter is then removed through the mouth end of the ETT.

11.6.3 What other techniques can be used to improve the success rate of the retrograde intubation?

While retrograde intubation is simple technique, the success rate of tracheal intubation is unacceptably low. In a study involving 35 cadavers, Lenfant et al[75] reported a success rate of 69% using the conventional guide wire technique. The investigators suggested that failures were likely due to incorrect positioning of the endotracheal tube. In addition, because of the short distance between the cricothyroid membrane and the vocal cords, the depth of insertion of the ETT is not much (<10 mm in adults[74]), and accidental extubation can easily occur during the removal of the guide wire with this technique.

A number of technique modifications have been suggested to improve the success rate of the retrograde intubation. These include the insertion of the epidural catheter (or guide wire) through the Murphy eye of the endotracheal tube[76] from outside to inside to increase the length of ETT actually in the trachea, the use of a subcricoid puncture[77] for the same reason, pulling rather than guided technique,[78] and employing a multilumen catheter guide.[79] To increase the stiffness and allow easier negotiation of the ETT through the oropharynx into the trachea, a tapered tip anterograde guide catheter (eg, pediatric tube changer) placed over the guide wire has been suggested to improve the effectiveness of retrograde intubation.[74,80] Although these modifications are useful, they do not overcome the difficulty of determining the location of the tip of the ETT during intubation. Simultaneous visualization of the ETT passage can be achieved if a flexible endoscope is placed through the nose beforehand.

Retrograde intubation using a guide wire passed retrograde through the working channel of a flexible bronchoscope has also been shown to be effective as the tip of the ETT can be guided into the glottis under indirect vision.[81-83] However, the bronchoscope is expensive and the retrograde passage of the guide wire through the working channel of the bronchoscope can potentially damage the internal lining of the channel.[84] In addition, visualization of the laryngeal structures through a bronchoscope can also be difficult in the presence of blood and secretions.

The tip of the ETT can also be guided into the trachea using transillumination. The placement of the bulb of a lightwand at the tip of the ETT during retrograde intubation may assist ETT advancement. A bright circumscribed glow can be readily seen in the anterior neck when the tip of the ETT enters the glottic opening and advances to the cricothyroid membrane puncture site, potentially improving the success rate of the technique. The light-guided retrograde intubating technique using the flexible Trachlight™

(without the stiff internal stylet) has been shown to be effective and safe in patients with cervical spine instability.[62]

11.6.5 What is the clinical utility of the retrograde intubation?

While retrograde intubation is not often considered to be a technique of choice, it remains a useful and effective technique. The technique can be performed either under general anesthesia or awake with skin infiltration and topical anesthesia.[62,74] In both the original and revised American Society of Anesthesiologists Difficult Airway Algorithms,[85,86] retrograde intubation is recommended as an alternative method of intubation when encountering a difficult tracheal intubation if the patient's lungs can still be ventilated. In other words, retrograde intubation can play an important role in the management of a "cannot intubate, but can ventilate" failed airway. It can also be used in patients with a predicted difficult laryngoscopic intubation but no anticipated difficulties in BMV, such as patients with cervical spine instability.[62]

11.6.6 What are the complications of the retrograde intubation?

While the retrograde intubation is an effective intubating technique, it has some potential complications. Although rare, complications, such as sore throat, hoarseness, bleeding (puncture site and peritracheal hematomas), subcutaneous emphysema, upper airway obstruction (secondary to subcutaneous emphysema), pneumothorax, pneumomediastinum, pretracheal abscess, and trigeminal nerve trauma have been reported with retrograde intubation.[74] Fortunately, most of these complications are minor and self-limiting. It should be emphasized that, compared to the Touhy needle, the use of an 18-gauge Angiocath or needle has made the cricothyroid membrane puncture substantially easier to perform and less traumatic compared to the Touhy needle. In addition, to avoid wound contamination by the oral bacterial flora, the epidural catheter or guide wire should be removed from the cephalad end wherever possible following intubation.

11.7 SUMMARY

Although tracheal intubation under direct vision using a laryngoscope remains the conventional method of tracheal intubation, it is challenging in a small percentage of patients. Many alternative techniques have been developed over the last several decades to improve the success rate. However, these techniques often require expensive equipment, specialized skills, and are sometimes not particularly useful for patients in an emergency situation with limited resources.

Nonvisual intubating techniques occupy an important role in airway management. Over the last several decades, these nonvisual techniques have been shown to be effective and safe in securing an airway. However, as with all technical skills, one has to recognize that there is a learning curve and a skills maintenance requirement for all of these techniques to be of clinical utility.

REFERENCES

1. Bair AE, Filbin MR, Kulkarni RG, Walls RM. The failed intubation attempt in the emergency department: analysis of prevalence, rescue techniques, and personnel. *J Emerg Med*. 2002;23:131-140.

2. Konrad C, Schupfer G, Wietlisbach M, Gerber H. Learning manual skills in anesthesiology: is there a recommended number of cases for anesthetic procedures? *Anesth Analg*. 1998;86:635-639.

3. Mulcaster JT, Mills J, Hung OR, et al. Laryngoscopic intubation: learning and performance. *Anesthesiology*. 2003;98:23-27.

4. Macintosh RR. An aid to oral intubation (letter). *BMJ*. 1949;1:28.

5. Venn PH. The gum elastic bougie. *Anaesthesia*. 1993;48:274-275.

6. El-Orbany MI, Salem MR, Joseph NJ. The Eschmann tracheal tube introducer is not gum, elastic, or a bougie. *Anesthesiology*. 2004;101:1240.

7. Cormack RS, Lehane J. Difficult tracheal intubation in obstetrics. *Anaesthesia*. 1984;39:1105-1111.

8. Hagberg CA. Special devices and techniques. *Anesthesiol Clinic North America*. 2002;20:907-932.

9. Marciniak D, Smith CE. Emergent retrograde tracheal intubation with a gum-elastic bougie in a trauma patient. *Anesth Analg*. 2007;105:1720-1721, table of contents.

10. Braude D, Webb H, Stafford J, et al. The bougie-aided cricothyrotomy. *Air Med J*. 2009;28:191-194.

11. Reardon R, Joing S, Hill C. Bougie-guided cricothyrotomy technique. *Acad Emerg Med*. 2010;17:225.

12. Moscati R, Jehle D, Christiansen G, et al. Endotracheal tube introducer for failed intubations: a variant of the gum elastic bougie. *Ann Emerg Med*. 2000;36:52-56.

13. Hodzovic I, Latto IP, Wilkes AR, et al. Evaluation of Frova, single-use intubation introducer, in a manikin. Comparison with Eschmann multiple-use introducer and Portex single-use introducer. *Anaesthesia*. 2004;59: 811-816.

14. Levitan R, Ochroch EA. Airway management and direct laryngoscopy: a review and update. *Crit Care Clin*. 2000;16:373-388.

15. Weiss M. Management of difficult tracheal intubation with a video-optically modified Schroeder intubation stylet. *Anesth Analg*. 1997;85:1181-1182.

16. Dutta A, Kumra VP, Sood J, Swaroop A. Guided tactile probing: a modified blind orotracheal intubation technique for the problem-oriented difficult airway. *Acta Anaesthesiol Scand*. 2005;49:106-109.

17. Bokhari A, Benham SW, Popat MT. Management of unanticipated difficult intubation: a survey of current practice in the Oxford region. *Eur J Anaesthesiol*. 2004;21:123-127.

18. Combes X, Le Roux B, Suen P, et al. Unanticipated difficult airway in anesthetized patients: prospective validation of a management algorithm. *Anesthesiology*. 2004;100:1146-1150.

19. Nolan JP, Wilson ME. Evaluation of the gum elastic bougie. *Anaesthesia*. 1992;47:878-881.

20. Nolan JP, Wilson ME. Orotracheal intubation patients with potential cervical spine injury. *Anaesthesia*. 1993;48:630-633.

21. Annamaneni R, Hodzovic I, Wilkes AR, Latto IP. A comparison of simulated difficult intubation with multiple-use and single-use bougies in a manikin. *Anaesthesia*. 2003;58:45-49.

22. Jones I, Roberts K. Towards evidence based emergency medicine: best BETs from the Manchester Royal Infirmary. Difficult intubation, the bougie and the stylet. *Emerg Med J*. 2002;19:433-434.

23. Nocera A. A flexible solution for emergency intubation difficulties. *Ann Emerg Med*. 1996;27:665-667.

24. Phelan MP. Use of the endotracheal bougie introducer for difficult intubations. *Am J Emerg Med*. 2004;22:479-482.

25. Morton T, Brady S, Clancy M. Difficult airway management in English emergency departments. *Anaesthesia*. 2000;55:485-458.

26. Henderson JJ, Popat MT, Latto IP, Pearce AC. Difficult Airway Society guidelines for management of the unanticipated difficult intubation. *Anaesthesia*. 2004;59:675-694.

27. Kidd JF, Dyson A, Latto IP. Successful difficult intubation. Use of the gum elastic bougie. *Anaesthesia*. 1988;43(6):437-438.

28. Arndt GA, Cambray AJ, Tomasson J. Intubation bougie dissection of tracheal mucosa and intratracheal airway obstruction. *Anesth Analg*. 2008;107: 603-604.

29. Kadry M, Popat M. Pharangeal wall perforation—an unusual complication of blind intubation with a gum elastic bougie. *Anaesthesia*. 1999;54:393-408.

30. Smith BL. Haemopneumothorax following bougie-assisted tracheal intubation. *Anaesthesia*. 1994;48:91.

31. Gardner M, Janokwski S. Detachment of the tip of a gum-elastic bougie. *Anaesthesia*. 2002;57:88-89.

32. Tuzzo DM, Frova G. Application of the self-inflating bulb to a hollow intubating introducer. *Minerva Anestesiol*. 2001;67:127-132.

33. Yamamura H, Yamamoto T, Kamiyama M. Device for blind nasal intubation. *Anesthesiology*. 1959;20:221.

34. Ainsworth QP, Howells TH. Transilluminated tracheal intubation. *Br J Anaesth*. 1989;62:494-497.

35. Ellis DG, Stewart RD, Kaplan RM, et al. Success rates of blind orotracheal intubation using a transillumination technique with a lighted stylet. *Ann Emerg Med*. 1986;15:138-142.

36. Vollmer TP, Stewart RD, Paris PM, et al. Use of a lighted stylet for guided orotracheal intubation in the prehospital setting. *Ann Emerg Med*. 1985;14: 324-328.

37. Nishiyama T, Matsukawa T, Hanaoka K. Safety of a new lightwand device (Trachlight): temperature and histopathological study. *Anesth Analg*. 1998;87: 717-718.

38. Hosokawa K, Nakajima Y, Hashimoto S. Chipped rail gear of a lightwand device: a potential complication of tracheal intubation. *Anesthesiology*. 2008;109: 355; discussion 356.

39. Chen TH, Tsai SK, Lin CJ, et al. Does the suggested lightwand bent length fit every patient? The relation between bent length and patient's thyroid prominence-to-mandibular angle distance. *Anesthesiology*. 2003;98:1070-1076.

40. Hung OR, Pytka S, Morris I, et al. Clinical trial of a new lightwand (Trachlight™) to intubate the trachea. *Anesthesiology*. 1995;83:509-514.

41. Stewart RD, LaRosee A, Kaplan RM, Ilkhanipour K. Correct positioning of an endotracheal tube using a flexible lighted stylet. *Crit Care Med*. 1990;18: 97-99.

42. Hung OR, Tibbet JS, Cheng R, Law JA. Proper preparation of the Trachlight and endotracheal tube to facilitate intubation. *Can J Anaesth*. 2006;53:107-108.

43. Chung YT, Sun MS, Wu HS. Blind nasotracheal intubation is facilitated by neutral head position and endotracheal tube cuff inflation in spontaneously breathing patients. *Can J Anaesth*. 2003;50:511-513.

44. Gorback MS. Inflation of the endotracheal tube cuff as an aid to blind nasal endotracheal intubation [letter]. *Anesth Analg*. 1987;66:913.

45. Asai T. Endotrol tube for blind nasotracheal intubation (Letter). *Anaesthesia*. 1996;50:507.

46. Agro F, Brimacombe J, Marchionni L, Carassiti M, Cataldo R. Nasal intubation with the Trachlight. *Can J Anaesth*. 1999;46:907-908.

47. Aoyama K, Takenaka I, Nagaoka E, Kadoya T, Sata T, Shigematsu A. Potential damage to the larynx associated with light-guided intubation: a case and series of fiberoptic examinations. *Anesthesiology*. 2001;94:165-167.

48. Stone DJ, Stirt JA, Kaplan MJ, McLean WC. A complication of lightwand-guided nasotracheal intubation. *Anesthesiology*. 1984;61:780-781.

49. Debo RF, Colonna D, Dewerd G, Gonzalez C. Cricoarytenoid subluxation: complication of blind intubation with a lighted stylet. *Ear Nose Throat J*. 1989;68:517-520.

50. Tsutsui T, Setoyama K. A clinical evaluation of blind orotracheal intubation using Trachlight in 511 patients. *Masui*. 2001;50:854-858.

51. Hung OR, Pytka S, Morris I, et al. Lightwand intubation: II. Clinical trail of a new lightwand to intubate patients with difficult airways. *Can J Anaesth*. 1995;42:826-830.

52. Favaro R, Tordiglione P, Di Lascio F, et al. Effective nasotracheal intubation using a modified transillumination technique. *Can J Anaesth*. 2002;49:91-95.

53. Inoue Y, Koga K, Shigematsu A. A comparison of two tracheal intubation techniques with Trachlight and Fastrach in patients with cervical spine disorders. *Anesth Analg*. 2002;94:667-671, table of contents.

54. Iseki K, Watanabe K, Iwama H. Use of the Trachlight for intubation in the Pierre-Robin syndrome. *Anaesthesia*. 1997;52:801-802.

55. Gille A, Komar K, Schmidt E, Alexander T. Transillumination technique in difficult intubations in heart surgery [Article in German]. *Anasthesiol Intensivmed Notfallmed Schmerzther*. 2002;37:604-608.

56. Agro F, Benumof JL, Carassiti M, Cataldo R, Gherardi S, Barzoi G. Efficacy of a combined technique using the Trachlight together with direct laryngoscopy under simulated difficult airway conditions in 350 anesthetized patients. *Can J Anaesth*. 2002;49:525-526.

57. Asai T, Latto IP. Use of the lighted stylet for tracheal intubation via the laryngeal mask airway. *Br J Anaesth*. 1995;75:503-504.

58. Asai T, Oldham T, Latto IF. Unexpected difficulty in the lighted stylet-aided tracheal intubation via the laryngeal mask. *Br J Anaesth*. 1996;76:111-112.

59. Fan KH, Hung OR, Agro F. A comparative study of tracheal intubation using an intubating laryngeal mask (Fastrach) alone, or together with a lightwand (Trachlight). *J Clin Anesth*. 2000;12:581-585.

60. Gutstein HB. Use of the bullard laryngoscope and lightwand in pediatric patients. *Anesthesiol Clinic North America.* 1998;16:795-812.

61. McGuire G, Krestow M. Bullard assisted trachlight technique. *Can J Anaesth.* 1999;46:907.

62. Hung OR, Al-Qatari M. Light-guided retrograde intubation. *Can J Anaesth.* 1997;44:877-882.

63. Addas BM, Howes WJ, Hung OR. Light-guided tracheal puncture for percutaneous tracheostomy. *Can J Anaesth.* 2000;47:919-922.

64. Stewart RD. Tactile orotracheal intubation. *Ann Emerg Med.* 1984;13:175.

65. Stewart RD. Digital intubation. In: Dailey RH, Simon B, Stewart RD, et al, eds. *The Airway: Emergency Management.* St. Louis: Mosby; 1992.

66. Hancock PJ, Peterson G. Finger intubation of the trachea in newborns. *Pediatrics.* 1992;89:325-327.

67. Korber TE, Henneman PL. Digital nasotracheal intubation. *J Emerg Med.* 1989;7:275-277.

68. Murphy MF, Hung O. Blind digital intubation. In: Benumof JL, ed. *Airway Management: Principles and Practice.* 1st ed. Philadelphia, PA: Mosby-Year Book Inc; 1996, 277-281.

69. Aitkenhead AR, Smith G. *Textbook of Anaesthesia.* Edinburg: Churchhill Livingstone; 1998.

70. Smith JE, Reid AP. Identifying the more patent nostril before nasotracheal intubation. *Anaesthesia.* 2001;56:258-262.

71. Cook RT, Jr., Stene JK, Marcolina B, Jr. Use of a Beck Airway Airflow Monitor and controllable-tip endotracheal tube in two cases of nonlaryngoscopic oral intubation. *Am J Emerg Med.* 1995;13:180-183.

72. Butler FS, Cirillo AA. Retrograde tracheal intubation. *Anesth Analg.* 1960;39:333-338.

73. Waters DJ. Guided blind endotracheal intubation. *Anaesthesia.* 1963;18:159.

74. Dhara SS. Retrograde tracheal intubation. *Anaesthesia.* 2009;64:1094-1104.

75. Lenfant F, Benkhadra M, Trouilloud P, Freysz M. Comparison of two techniques for retrograde tracheal intubation in human fresh cadavers. *Anesthesiology.* 2006;104:48-51.

76. Bourke D. Modification of retrograde guide for endotracheal intubation. *Anesth Analg.* 1974;53:1013-1014.

77. Shantha TR. Retrograde intubation using the subcricoid region. *Br J Anaesth.* 1992;68:109-112.

78. Abdou-Madi MN, Trop D. Pulling versus guiding: a modification of retrograde guided intubation. *Can J Anaesth.* 1989;36:336-339.

79. Dhara SS. Retrograde intubation—a facilitated approach. *Br J Anaesth.* 1992;69:631-633.

80. Tobias R. Increased success with retrograde guide for endotracheal intubation. *Anesth Analg.* 1983;62:366-367.

81. Carlson CA, Perkins HM. Solving a difficult intubation. *Anesthesiology.* 1986;64:537.

82. Przybylo HJ, Stevenson GW, Vicari FA, et al. Retrograde fibreoptic intubation in a child with Nager's syndrome. *Can J Anaesth.* 1996;43:697-699.

83. Rosenblatt WH, Angood PB, Maranets I, et al. Retrograde fiberoptic intubation. *Anesth Analg.* 1997;84:1142-1144.

84. Ovassapian A, Mesnick PS. The art of fiberoptic intubation. *Anesthesiol Clinic North America.* 1995;13:391-409.

85. American Society of Anesthesiologists Task Force on Management of the Difficult Airway. Practice guidelines for the difficult airway. *Anesthesiology.* 1993;78:597-602.

86. American Society of Anesthesiologists Task Force on Management of the Difficult Airway. Practice guidelines for management of the difficult airway: an updated report by the American Society of Anesthesiologists Task Force on Management of the Difficult Airway. *Anesthesiology.* 2003;98:1269-1277.

SELF-EVALUATION QUESTIONS

11.1. Which of the following conditions does not affect the effectiveness of light-guided intubation using a lightwand?

A. morbid obesity

B. foreign body in the upper airway

C. retropharyngeal abscess

D. blood and secretion in the oropharynx

E. large goiter in the anterior neck

11.2. Which of the following modifications has not been shown to improve the success rate of the retrograde intubation?

A. the use of a subcricoid puncture

B. the use of a guide wire passing through the working channel of a flexible bronchoscope

C. the use of a flexible lightwand

D. the use of a guide wire instead of an epidural catheter

E. the insertion of the guide wire through the "Murphy" eye of the endotracheal tube during intubation

11.3. Which of the following is **not** a characteristic feature of the Eschmann Tracheal Tube Introducer (gum-elastic bougie)?

A. The Eschmann Introducer is 60 cm long.

B. The Eschmann Introducer has a J (coudé) tip (a 35-degree angle bend) at the distal end.

C. The Eschmann Introducer has a hollow lumen with two side ports.

D. The Eschmann Introducer is a reusable device.

E. The Eschmann Introducer consists of a core of tube woven from polyester threads covered with a resin layer.

CHAPTER (12)

Extraglottic Devices for Ventilation and Oxygenation

Chris Hinkewich, Orlando R. Hung, and Thomas J. Coonan

12.1 CASE PRESENTATION

A 57-year-old man was admitted for a laparoscopic appendectomy for acute appendicitis. He was otherwise healthy apart from essential hypertension, for which he took hydrochlorothiazide. He had fasted for more than 12 hours.

On examination, he was lying on a stretcher in a moderate amount of pain. He was hemodynamically stable. His height was 183 cm and his weight was 80 kg. His airway examination demonstrated a Mallampati score of II, mouth opening of 4.5 cm, thyromental distance of 6 cm, and good jaw protrusion. He had a full set of teeth, was not obese, and was estimated to be easy to ventilate with a bag and a mask. His cardiac and respiratory examinations were normal.

The patient was premedicated with intravenous midazolam 1 mg and, fentanyl 200 mcg, and this was followed by denitrogenation with 100% oxygen by facemask. As he did not have any indicators of a difficult airway, a decision was made to induce anesthesia with propofol 200 mg and rocuronium 50 mg. Bag-mask-ventilation (BMV) was established with an oral airway. Initial evaluation with direct laryngoscopy using a Macintosh laryngoscope showed a Cormack/Lehane Grade 3 view. The first attempt with direct laryngoscopy employing a tracheal introducer (bougie) resulted in an esophageal intubation. BMV was reestablished and a Glidescope was prepared. When the Glidescope was inserted, only the posterior arytenoids could be visualized, and several attempts with a styleted endotracheal tube and a tracheal introducer were unsuccessful (and were associated with a small amount of bleeding in the oropharynx).

At this point, the decision was made to attempt flexible bronchoscopy. Unfortunately, BMV became more difficult, the patient's oxygen saturation dropped into the low 80s, and it became necessary to insert nasal and oral pharyngeal airways and begin a two-hand and two-person BMV technique. A #4 Laryngeal Mask Airway Classic was rapidly prepared and inserted without complication, at which point it became possible to easily ventilate the patient. Sevoflurane was selected to maintain anesthesia, and to manage escalating tachycardia and hypertension. A 6.0 mm ID Microlaryngeal tracheal tube (MLT, [Covidien-Nellcor, Boulder, CO]) was loaded onto a flexible bronchoscope, which was then inserted through the LMA and into the glottic opening. The MLT was advanced into the trachea over the bronchoscope. After confirmation of correct placement by auscultation and capnograph recording, the decision was made to leave both the endotracheal tube and LMA in place for the duration of the procedure.

The surgery was uneventful and the patient emerged from anesthesia fully awake, warm, with adequate analgesia, and with no residual neuromuscular blockade. The difficult airway cart was brought to the room. However, the patient was extubated without complication, although he did complain of a sore throat in the post-anesthetic care unit, which gradually improved. He was later informed of the difficulty and provided with a notice to inform any subsequent practitioner of his difficult airway.

12.2 INTRODUCTION

12.2.1 What are extraglottic devices? Why do we need these devices?

Difficulties in airway management are associated with significant morbidity and mortality,[1] and it is crucial that practitioners responsible for airway management continue to refine existing skills, and acquire new knowledge and skills as they become available. Two decades ago, ventilation and oxygenation were achieved primarily via a facemask, or an endotracheal tube (ETT).

While BMV is seemingly simple to perform, it has limitations.[2] Tracheal intubation has been considered to be the gold standard for providing effective ventilation, while at the same time providing protection from the aspiration of gastric contents. However, tracheal intubation is a skill that is not easily mastered[3] and requires regular practice. Employing an extraglottic device (EGD) to successfully facilitate gas exchange may be a more easily acquired skill for the nonexpert airway practitioner.

In contrast to a mask placed on the face to provide bag-mask-ventilation (BMV), an EGD establishes a direct conduit for air to flow when placed in the periglottic area. The terminology has been somewhat confusing since some have referred to these devices as "supraglottic airway devices," although many have components that extend infraglottically (eg, the Combitube, the Laryngeal Tube [King LT in North America] and the EasyTube).[4] Hence, we agree with Brimacombe that the term extraglottic devices, or EGDs, is the more appropriate terminology.

EGDs vary in size, shape, and material. Most have balloons, or cuffs, that upon inflation can provide a reasonably tight seal in the upper airway. As illustrated in the case presentation, these EGDs (including the LMA Classic™) have been used successfully as rescue airway devices. There is clear evidence of their effectiveness and safety in providing ventilation and oxygenation. During the last two decades, these devices have changed the landscape of contemporary airway management, securing a place in the most recent iteration of the American Society of Anesthesiologists' (ASA) Difficult Airway Management Algorithm.[5]

12.2.2   Do manufacturing standards exist for EGDs to ensure patient safety?

The American Society for Testing and Materials Standards (ASTM) Committee F29 on Anesthetic and Respiratory Equipment has proposed the establishment of standards related to EGDs used in human subjects. A task group has proposed the standardization of terminology, design, production, manufacturing, testing, labeling, and promotion. Devices produced according to the proposed ASTM standards will:

- Facilitate unobstructed access of respiratory gases to the glottic inlet by displacing tissue

- Not require a (external) facial seal to maintain airway patency

- Terminate in a 15/22 mm connector to facilitate positive pressure ventilation via an anesthetic breathing system

- Be capable of maintaining airway patency when the (15/22 mm) airway connector is open to ambient atmosphere

- Minimize the escape of airway gases to the atmosphere

12.2.3   What EGDs are commercially available?

Many EGDs have been introduced.[4] The best known are the Laryngeal Mask Airway Classic™ (LMA-C), ProSeal™ Laryngeal Mask Airway (PLMA), Laryngeal Mask Airway Fastrach™ (LMA-FT), and Combitube™ (CBT). A number of more recently developed EGDs such as the Laryngeal Tube™ (LT), CobraPLA™ (CPLA),

Airway Management Device™ (AMD), LaryVent™ (LV), Cuffed Oropharyngeal Airway™ (COPA), PAxpress™ (PAX), Air-Q™ device, Ambu® AuraOnce Laryngeal Mask, Portex® Soft Seal Laryngeal Mask, and iGel™ are also gaining acceptance.

This is an evolving field with many new reusable and disposable EGDs introduced every year. This chapter will review the commonly used EGDs which also have sufficient information available in the literature, but it should not be considered an exhaustive review of all available devices. It should be emphasized that some devices (eg, the COPA and PAxpress™) are no longer being manufactured. The authors have elected to include them, as these devices have played a role in the evolution of EGDs; their limitations have informed the evolution of this class of devices.

12.3   LARYNGEAL MASK AIRWAY CLASSIC

12.3.1   What is the LMA? When was it introduced?

The LMA (LMA North America Inc., San Diego, CA [Figure 12-1]) was designed in 1981 by Dr Archie Brain, as he searched for a device that was easier to use and more effective than the face mask, and less invasive than an ETT. The LMA is designed to cover the periglottic area and provide continuity of airflow between the environment and the lungs. The device has a wide-bore tube connecting to an oval inflatable cuff that seals around the larynx. It is currently available in eight different sizes for use in patients ranging from neonates to large adults. Typically, a #3 LMA is used in teenagers and small adult females, while #4, #5, and #6 are used in average and large size adults.

During the last two decades, more than 2500 published articles and an estimate of more than 200 million patient uses have provided sufficient evidence to demonstrate the safety and efficacy of the device in airway management.[6,7] The LMA is now specified in the American Society of Anesthesiologists' Difficult Airway Management Algorithm.[5] Moreover, the LMA has a role in emergency airway management during CPR, the transport of the critically ill patient, and in the intensive care unit.[8,9] Although the LMA is a potentially useful device in situations in which tracheal intubation and mask ventilation are not possible (can't intubate, can't ventilate [CICV])[5], it should never be used as a substitute for a surgical airway (see Chapters 2 and 40). While

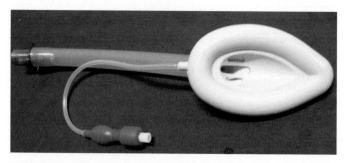

FIGURE 12-1. The LMA Classic™ has a wide-bore tube connected to an oval inflatable cuff that seals around the larynx.

this device can provide adequate ventilation and oxygenation, it does not protect the airway from aspiration, and it does not easily allow for the removal of pulmonary secretions. Therefore, when employed as a rescue device, the LMA can only be considered a temporizing measure, until a more definitive and protective airway is secured.

12.3.2   What is the proper way to insert the LMA?

While many techniques have been suggested for the insertion of the device, including the midline approach, the lateral approach, and the thumb technique,[10] the authors recommend the following steps:

1. To minimize the risk of down-folding the epiglottis, it is recommended that the cuff be completely deflated.

2. The LMA cuff should be well lubricated with a water-soluble lubricant.

3. Provided that there is no contraindication to moving the cervical spine, the patient's head and neck should be placed in a sniffing position. A head tilt will help to open the mouth.

4. In order to have clear access to the glottic opening and minimize down-folding of the epiglottis, it is recommended that the practitioner perform a jaw lift using the thumb and index finger of the nondominant hand. This lifts the tongue and epiglottis away from the posterior pharyngeal wall to facilitate placement of the LMA. The LMA should be inserted into the mouth with the index finger placed at the mask-tube junction, pressing the cuff against the hard palate, and advancing the LMA into the oropharynx following the natural curve of the posterior pharyngeal wall. The dimensions and design of the device allow the tip of the LMA to wedge into the hypopharynx. A definite resistance should be felt when the tip of the LMA enters the hypopharynx. Occasionally, resistance is encountered during insertion because of backward folding of the cuff also called 'tip roll'. Sweeping a finger behind the cuff to redirect it inferiorly into the laryngopharynx can usually overcome this problem.[11]

5. Following placement, the cuff should be inflated with the minimal volume of air necessary to achieve an adequate seal. However, this just-seal volume may not be adequate to seal the hypopharynx from the esophagus.[10] Therefore, most practitioners commonly inflate the cuff with more volume. In general, approximately 20 mL is required for #3, 30 mL for #4, and 40 mL for #5 LMA. Seal characteristics may be improved by ensuring that the LMA is secured in the midline of the mouth, and the head and neck placed in a neutral position.

6. The LMA should be fixed in position by taping it to the face, or by attaching it to the anesthesia breathing circuit.[12]

12.3.3   What is the proper way to remove the LMA?

In its normal position, the LMA is less stimulating than an ETT and is generally well tolerated by most patients on emergence. Many studies have compared removal under deep anesthesia versus while awake. Although airway obstruction appears to be less frequent if the device is removed with the patient awake, this technique is associated with more coughing, laryngospasm, biting, and hypersalivation.[13] While much controversy remains, it is the opinion of the authors that, in adults, the LMA should be removed awake. This is particularly true if mask ventilation is expected to be difficult. Many pediatric airway practitioners prefer removal under deep anesthesia, as children are more prone to laryngospasm.

It is unclear whether the LMA should be removed with the cuff deflated or inflated. Some recommend an inflated cuff because of its capacity to remove secretions that accumulate above the device from the oral cavity.[14] Others argue that the cuff should be deflated to minimize trauma and damage to the cuff itself. Brimacombe recommends the removal of the LMA with the cuff partially deflated.[13]

12.3.4   What are the advantages and disadvantages of using the LMA as opposed to an endotracheal tube?

Brimacombe conducted a meta-analysis of randomized prospective trials involving 2440 patients comparing the LMA with other forms of airway management, including tracheal intubation.[15] He reported many advantages of the LMA including rapidity and ease of placement, particularly for inexperienced operators; improved hemodynamic stability on induction and during emergence; minimal rise in intraocular pressure following insertion; reduced anesthetic requirements for airway tolerance; lower frequency of coughing during emergence; improved oxygen saturation during emergence; and a lower incidence of sore throat in adults.

An additional advantage of the LMA is its utility as a rescue device and during resuscitation.[16] Further, studies have shown that the LMA has less impact on mucociliary clearance than an ETT, and may reduce the risk of retention of secretions, atelectasis, and pulmonary infection.[17]

The major disadvantage of the LMA is its inability to seal the larynx and protect against aspiration, gastric insufflation, and air leak with positive pressure ventilation.[15] The mask is designed in such a way that the distal end of the device is intended to become wedged into the upper esophageal sphincter. However, in reality, the distal end may lie anywhere from the nasopharynx to the hypopharynx.

The magnitude of potential gastric insufflation probably depends on the airway pressure generated and the position of the LMA. However, very large series have shown that positive pressure ventilation with the LMA is both safe and effective, with no episodes of gastric dilatation in 11,910 LMA anesthetics under both spontaneous and positive pressure ventilation.[18]

According to a meta-analysis involving 547 LMA publications, the incidence of gastric aspiration associated with the use of the laryngeal mask airway is rare (0.02%),[19] and most of these cases had predisposing risk factors for pulmonary aspiration. However, fatal aspiration of gastric content has recently been reported,[20] and so proper assessment for aspiration risk prior to the use of the LMA is imperative. Most airway practitioners hesitate appropriately to use the LMA in patients with a history of hiatal hernia, gastroesophageal reflux, in obstetrical patients, or in patients with a bowel obstruction. Careful placement of the device, and vigilance at emergence of anesthesia, may attenuate the risk of gastric aspiration.

12.3.5   Is it safe to use the LMA for positive pressure ventilation?

Over the last two decades, the use of a face mask to facilitate the administration of anesthesia has largely been replaced by the LMA. Originally felt to be most appropriate for nonparalyzed patients with spontaneous ventilation, a survey done in the United Kingdom in the mid 1990s showed that 5236 of 11,910 patients (44%) underwent positive pressure ventilation (PPV) through the LMA.[18] While a few studies have reported the successful use of the LMA for PPV in a variety of patient populations and procedures,[21-23] they involved mostly small numbers of patients, with few large prospective randomized trials.[24] Recently, Bernardini et al compared the risk of pulmonary aspiration in a study involving 65,712 patients with positive pressure ventilation via an ETT (30,082 procedures) compared to an LMA (35,630 procedures).[25] Although three pulmonary aspirations occurred in the LMA group compared to seven with the ETT, there were no deaths related to these pulmonary aspirations. The investigators concluded that, while there was a selection bias related to contraindications and exclusions to the use of the LMA in their study group, the use of a laryngeal mask airway was not associated with an increased risk of pulmonary aspiration, compared with an ETT in this selected population.

Based on the current evidence, the LMA appears to be effective and probably safe for positive pressure ventilation in patients with normal airway resistance and compliance, and normal tidal volumes. However, gastroesophageal insufflation may occur when the LMA is used in conjunction with, and in the presence of, decreased pulmonary or chest wall compliance.[26,27]

Pressure-controlled ventilation (PCV) rather than volume-controlled ventilation (VCV) may provide effective mechanical ventilation in patients with high airway pressure, or reduced lung compliance, while at the same time minimizing the risk of gastric insufflation with the LMA.[28] It must be reemphasized that, although rare, cases of serious and even fatal gastric aspiration associated with the use of LMA have been reported.[20,29-31] Because of the potential for serious complications, more evidence with studies involving a large number of patients may be needed to confirm the safety of the use of the LMA for PPV.[24]

12.3.6   How are LMAs used appropriately in clinical practice?

Since its introduction in 1988, the LMA has been used in more than 200 million patients worldwide[7] and it has largely replaced the ETT and face mask for patients undergoing simple and uncomplicated surgical procedures. The extensive use of the LMA is a reflection of its overwhelming effectiveness and safety in a variety of age groups and surgical procedures. The LMA has also been shown to be effective and safe for elective caesarean section in nonobese parturients, though its use for this indication is controversial.[32]

A meta-analysis of currently available data shows that the LMA is safe and effective for pediatric airway management.[33] Furthermore, the LMA has been used successfully in the management of large numbers of difficult pediatric airways associated with a variety of congenital anomalies.

The LMA was approved for resuscitation by the European Resuscitation Council in 1996,[34] and the American Heart Association in 2000.[35] However, the possibility of gastric insufflation, related to high peak airway pressure, continues to be a concern in these patient populations, similar to those managed with BMV.

Brimacombe summarized the current evidence with respect to the use of the LMA in the management of the difficult and failed airway.[36] With the exception of airway pathology that may interfere with the LMA placement or seal, there is a considerable body of evidence to support the use of the LMA in both predicted and unpredicted difficult airways.[5]

The LMA also provides a conduit for tracheal intubation using either a blind technique, a transillumination technique (using the Trachlight™ without the stylet),[37,38] or a flexible bronchoscope (FB). Intubation success rates through the LMA have been found to be similar for patients with both normal and abnormal airways.[39]

The flexible laryngeal mask airway (FLMA) was specifically designed for use in ear, nose, and throat; head and neck; and dental surgery. It has been used for adenotonsillectomy,[40] laser pharyngoplasty,[41] and dental extraction.[42] The device consists of a Classic LMA bowl connected to a floppy, a wire-reinforced tube with a slightly narrower bore than the LMA Classic™. The long, flexible, narrow bore tube provides better surgical access to the oropharyngeal cavity than the standard laryngeal mask airway. The technique for placement of the FLMA is similar to that for the LMA.

The reusable LMA Classic™ is the *original* LMA. Variations on the original include:

- LMA Fastrach™, also known as the Intubating LMA (ILMA), and also available in a disposable form (Figure 12-2)

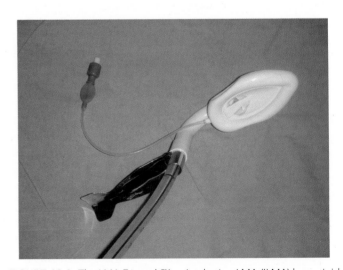

FIGURE 12-2. The LMA Fastrach™ or Intubating LMA (ILMA) has a rigid curved metal airway tube with a manipulating handle, an epiglottis-elevating bar, a deeper bowl, and a ramp that directs an endotracheal tube up and into the larynx, enhancing the success rate of blind intubation. In this figure, a dedicated wire-reinforced silicone-tipped tracheal tube (TT) is inserted into the metal lumen of the ILMA. When the horizontal black line on the TT meets the proximal end of the ILMA, the tip of the TT will emerge from beneath the epiglottis-elevating bar.

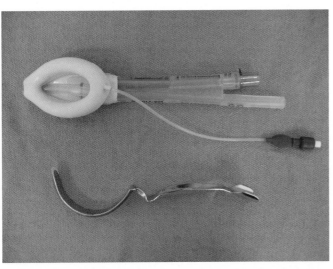

FIGURE 12-3. The LMA ProSeal™ incorporates a drainage tube placed lateral to the airway tube and a second dorsal cuff. The drainage tube travels from the proximal end of the device through the bowl opening into the upper esophagus. It permits the insertion of standard nasogastric tubes to facilitate the drainage of gastric contents. Also shown is the metal introducer employed to facilitate placement of the PLMA.

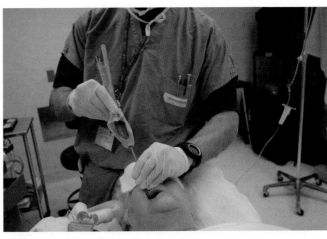

FIGURE 12-5. The tracheal introducer-guided insertion technique of the LMA ProSeal™ follows the placement of the tracheal introducer into the esophagus under direct vision with a laryngoscope and is guided into position by placing the tracheal introducer through the esophageal conduit.

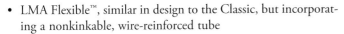

- LMA Flexible™, similar in design to the Classic, but incorporating a nonkinkable, wire-reinforced tube
- LMA ProSeal™, a device that has improved seal characteristics and incorporates a gastric drainage capability (Figures 12-3, 12-4, and 12-5)
- LMA Unique™, a single-use device virtually identical to the Classic (Figure 12-6)
- LMA Supreme™, a new disposable device that incorporates the insertion advantages of the Fastrach™, with the seal characteristics of the ProSeal™ (Figure 12-7)

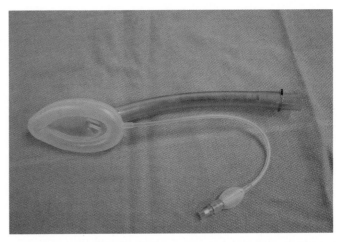

FIGURE 12-6. The LMA Unique™ is a single-use device virtually identical to the Classic with aperture bars.

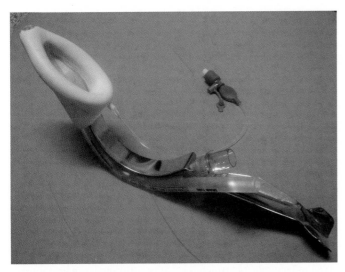

FIGURE 12-4. This figure shows the LMA ProSeal™ loaded onto the introducer. The distal end of the metal introducer is placed in an insertion strap on the PLMA and the airway tube is folded around the introducer and clipped into a proximal matching slot.

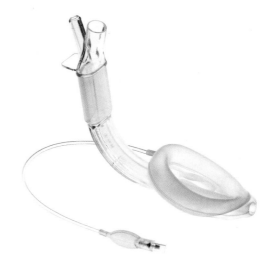

FIGURE 12-7. The LMA Supreme™ is a new disposable device that incorporates the insertion advantages of the Fastrach™ and the seal characteristics of the LMA ProSeal™.

12.4   FASTRACH™ INTUBATING LARYNGEAL MASK AIRWAY

12.4.1   What is the LMA Fastrach™, or Intubating LMA, and why was it developed?

While it is possible to intubate the trachea through an LMA, success rates are variable. Accordingly, an Intubating LMA (LMA Fastrach™, or Intubating LMA (ILMA), LMA North America Inc., San Diego, CA [Figure 12-2]) was designed by Dr Brain. The device has a rigid metal-curved airway tube with a guiding handle, an epiglottis-elevating bar, a deeper bowl, and ramp that directs an ETT up and into the larynx. The device is easy to use, is associated with high success rates of intubation, and has received widespread acceptance. The ILMA is a reusable device which can be cleaned and sterilized using an autoclave. A disposable device has also been recently introduced.

12.4.2   How is tracheal intubation performed using the ILMA?

Tracheal intubation through the ILMA can be achieved blindly. To facilitate the insertion of an ETT through the ILMA, the following steps are recommended:

1. Lubricate the posterior side of the ILMA and the ETT (including the connector of the tracheal tube) with a water-soluble lubricant. Ensure that the ETT slides easily through the ILMA.

2. With the patient in a sniffing position, open the airway by using a head tilt. It should be emphasized that the insertion of an ILMA may be difficult if the interincisor gap is less than 20 mm.

3. Grasp the metal handle of the ILMA and insert the device straight back over the tongue to the back of the oropharynx. Then advance the cuff into the hypopharynx following the palatopharyngeal curve by rotating the device using the metal handle and maintaining gentle pressure against the palate. Once in place, inflate the cuff to achieve a seal for manual ventilation. The metal handle may be used to manipulate the device to achieve a seal to ensure adequate ventilation and oxygenation. The device should be gently rotated in the sagittal plane (commonly known as the first Chandy maneuver) to establish optimally unobstructed ventilation.[43]

4. While a number of ETTs, including the Mallinckrodt Hi-Lo PVC tube, can be used for tracheal intubation, the dedicated wire-reinforced silicone-tipped tracheal tube (TT) supplied with the ILMA has been shown to give the highest success rates.[44] With the black vertical line on the tube facing the operator, insert the tube into the metal lumen of the ILMA until the horizontal black line on the tracheal tube meets the proximal end of the ILMA metal tube (Figure 12-2). At this point, the tip of the TT is just emerging from beneath the epiglottis-elevating bar. Resistance will be felt as the TT elevates this bar exiting the distal end of the ILMA, and entering the patient's glottis.

5. Tracheal placement is confirmed in the usual manner. Manipulation of the ILMA by lifting the device from the posterior pharyngeal wall using the metal handle (the second Chandy maneuver) may enhance successful passage in the event of failure. This manuever helps to prevent the TT from colliding with the arytenoids and minimizes the angle between the aperture of the ILMA and the glottis.[45]

Some evidence suggests that the ILMA in situ produces sufficient pressure on the posterior hypopharyngeal wall to potentially compromise mucosal blood flow.[46] For this reason, except perhaps in an airway rescue or resuscitation situation, it is recommended that the device be withdrawn over the TT. A stabilizing rod is provided with the ILMA to hold the TT in position while the ILMA is withdrawn.

Many investigators have studied the effectiveness of the blind intubating technique through the ILMA. The reported mean (range) first-time and overall success rate is 73% (53-100) and 90% (44-100), respectively.[46] Several factors that *decrease* success rates of blind intubation through the ILMA technique have been identified: the use of a #3 ILMA, instead of #4 or #5 ILMA, for adult male patients; the application of cricoid pressure; lifting the ILMA handle; the use of a collar; and an inexperienced practitioner.

12.4.3   What other techniques have been described to enhance success rates for tracheal intubation through the ILMA?

Several studies have been published evaluating the effectiveness of a laryngoscope to assist ILMA intubation. The overall success rate appears to be no better than the blind technique. Light-guided techniques employing a flexible lightwand (Trachlight™) have also been investigated, and have demonstrated improved success rates.[47,48] Lightwand-guided intubation through the ILMA has a first-time and overall success rate of 84% and 99%, respectively.[46] Recently, Wong et al[49] reported the successful use of the Trachlight-assisted Fastrach intubation in a patient with a difficult airway secondary to the Hallermann-Streiff syndrome. In out-of-hospital tracheal intubation by an emergency physician, Dimitriou et al has shown that a flexible lightwand-guided tracheal intubation through the ILMA had a high success rate, with no failures in 37 patients.[50]

Pandit et al[51] found that bronchoscopic-guided intubation had a higher success rate (95%) through the ILMA than through the LMA (80%), although the time to intubation was longer with the flexible bronchoscope (FB)-assisted technique, compared to the blind technique (74 seconds vs 49 seconds). Overall, in a range of studies, flexible bronchoscope-guided intubation through the ILMA has a first time and overall success rate of 87% and 96%, respectively. However, following a failed blind technique, flexible bronchoscope-guided intubation through the ILMA has a success rate of only 86%.[46]

Agro et al[52] reported the use of a shorter fiberoptic device, Shikani Seeing Eye Stylet™, (Clarus Medical, Minneapolis, MN, USA) to facilitate a Fastrach intubation. Although tracheal intubation was successful, the investigators commented that the major limitation of the Shikani device was its inability to control the direction of the tip of the device.

Using the Patil Intubation Guide (Anesthesia Associates Inc., San Marcos, CA, USA), a whistle diaphragm to detect breath sounds, Osborn successfully intubated the trachea through the ILMA under topical anesthesia in a patient with a recent cervical spine fusion.[53] In 2005, a case series was published describing the successful use of the airway whistle with the ILMA in four patients with known difficult airways.[54]

12.4.4   What are the indications for the ILMA?

The ILMA alone does not prevent the aspiration of gastric contents and may produce hypopharyngeal mucosal ischemia if it is left in place for a prolonged duration. Therefore, its role in routine airway management may be limited. However, when used as a temporizing measure, it is a highly effective device in the emergency environment, as an adjunct to failed or difficult BMV, and as a rescue device in the failed airway. Brain has suggested that the ILMA may not be indicated when the patient is anticipated to be an easy intubation (easy direct laryngoscopy), but may be of considerable benefit when the glottis is high and anterior (difficult direct laryngoscopy). Furthermore, recent studies have confirmed earlier findings that ventilation and intubation through the LMA Fastrach™ can be successfully achieved in obese patients with BMI greater than 30.[55,56]

With respect to emergency medical services (EMS) and prehospital care, the importance of early and effective airway control is universally acknowledged. Tracheal intubation under direct laryngoscopy is associated with a number of practical problems in prehospital trauma and there is evidence to suggest that the ILMA may play an important role in the prehospital setting, in securing the airway of trauma patients with a head injury.[57,58]

In a recent study by Gercek et al,[59] the degree of cervical spine movement of three common methods of tracheal intubation in patients with C-spine injuries (direct laryngoscopy [DL], ILMA, and FB) were compared using real-time, three-dimensional ultrasonography in healthy elective surgical patients with manual in-line immobilization. They showed that manual in-line immobilization reduced the cervical spine range of motion during different intubation procedures to a limited extent: the least diminution (ie, the greatest C-spine movement) occurred with DL (with an overall flexion/extension range of 17.57 degrees), versus significantly less C-spine movement with ILMA use (overall flexion/extension range of 4.60 degrees), and FB use (overall flexion/extension range of 3.61 degrees—oral, 5.88 degrees—nasal). Furthermore, the mean ($\pm$ SD) total time required for intubation was shortest for the ILMA (16.5 $\pm$ 9.76 seconds), followed by DL (27.25 $\pm$ 8.56 seconds), and the longest for both FB techniques (oral: 52.91 $\pm$ 56.27 seconds, nasal: 82.32 $\pm$ 54.06 seconds).

The prime role of the ILMA lies in managing the airway of patients with a difficult or a failed airway. From a retrospective study involving 254 patients with difficult airways, including patients with either Cormack/Lehane Grade 4 views, immobilized cervical spines, stereotactic frames, or airways distorted by surgery or radiation therapy, the clinical experience with the ILMA (both elective and emergency use) has been largely positive.[45,60]

The Difficult Airway Society (UK) guidelines for management of the unanticipated difficult tracheal intubation in the nonobstetric adult patient without upper airway obstruction now include the ILMA.[61]

The LMA C-trach™ was a modification of the ILMA (Fastrach™) fitted with a fiberoptic camera to allow continuous visualization of the airway. When compared to the ILMA, it was shown to have a higher first attempt success rate, but a longer insertion time.[62] This device is no longer available on the market, largely due to its cost.

12.5   PROSEAL™ LARYNGEAL MASK AIRWAY

12.5.1   What is the PLMA? How does it differ from the LMA?

The PLMA (Intavent Orthofix, Maidenhead, UK [Figure 12-3]) is a laryngeal mask variant that incorporates several modifications to the LMA:

- An esophageal conduit is incorporated to provide access to the esophagus and the gastrointestinal tract to minimize the risk of aspiration. This incorporated conduit renders a dual tube look to the device.

- A second cuff on the dorsal aspect of the PLMA is intended to enhance the seal characteristics of the device.

- The PLMA lacks mask aperture bars, and (like the ILMA) has a deeper bowl which makes the migration of the epiglottis into the distal lumen of the device less likely.

- The PLMA also has a flexible wire-reinforced airway tube to improve flexibility and minimize kinking, and a bite-block to reduce the danger of bite-induced airway obstruction, or tube damage.

The drainage conduit traverses the bowl of the cuff on its way to the upper esophagus, in an effort to reduce the risk of gastric insufflation when positive pressure is applied to the airway. Standard gastric tubes (≤ 18 French [Fr] gauge) can be accommodated by the conduit to facilitate gastric decompression. An accessory vent under the drainage tube is intended to prevent the pooling of secretions and can act as an accessory ventilation port.[63]

Employing moderate force to advance the laryngeal cuff forward into the periglottic tissues may improve the airway seal. The dual-tube arrangement seems to reduce the incidence of accidental device rotation during anesthesia. This feature enhances the ability to secure the device in position, giving greater confidence for use in longer procedures.

12.5.2   How is the PLMA placed?

The technique of insertion of the PLMA is similar to that of the LMA. While there is no randomized controlled study comparing the placement technique of the PLMA, with or without a muscle relaxant, it has recently been shown that successful placement of the PLMA requires deeper anesthesia when compared with the LMA.[64,65]

Three insertion techniques for the PLMA have been advocated:

1. The Introducer-Assisted Insertion Technique: Prior to its placement, the PLMA is loaded onto an introducer by placing the distal end of a metal introducer in an insertion strap on the PLMA (Figure 12-4). The airway tube is folded around the introducer and fitted into a proximal matching slot. The head and neck of the patient should be placed in a sniffing position. Following the placement of the PLMA, the introducer is removed as the PLMA is held in position.

2. The Digital Technique: Similar to the LMA, the digital technique involves the placement of the index finger under the insertion strap during the insertion of the PLMA. Rotating the PLMA 90 degrees in the mouth until resistance is felt at the hypopharynx was found to be more successful and associated with a decrease in blood staining on the device, and in the incidence of sore throat.[66]

3. The Tracheal Introducer-Guided Insertion Technique: This is probably the most reliable technique to optimally place the tip of the PLMA cuff in the hypopharynx.[67] A well-lubricated tracheal introducer (eg, an Eschmann tracheal introducer) is placed into the esophagus under direct vision with a laryngoscope. The PLMA is guided into position by placing the tracheal introducer through the esophageal conduit (Figure 12-5). While this technique enjoys a high success rate, it is time-consuming, and probably more stimulating and traumatic.

In a recent study, Eschertzhuber et al[68] compared these three insertion techniques in patients with simulated difficult laryngoscopy using a rigid neck collar. Insertion was more frequently successful with the Eschmann tracheal introducer technique (ETI) at the first attempt (ETI—100%, digital—64%, introducer-assisted technique—61%). The time taken for successful placement was similar among groups on the first attempt. However, it was shorter for the ETI technique after three attempts (ETI 31 ± 8 seconds, digital 49 ± 28 seconds, introducer-assisted technique 54 ± 37 seconds).

Proper placement of the PLMA can be confirmed by a number of techniques. Air leak through the drainage tube at low airway pressures suggests malposition of the PLMA. Although air leaks are ordinarily easily detected by auscultation, or by feeling air exiting the drainage tube, a small volume leak is probably best detected by the soap bubble test.[69] Three other tests have been suggested to check the patency of the drainage tube, including passing a gastric tube through the drainage tube; passing an FB through the drainage tube; and performing a suprasternal notch tap while observing a soap bubble, or lubricant, at the proximal end of the drainage tube.[70]

12.5.3   What are the advantages of the PLMA, compared to the LMA?

In principle, the PLMA would be expected to reduce the aspiration risk when compared to the LMA. Laboratory (and cadaver) evidence are supportive of the theoretical efficacy of the PLMA.[71] However, clinical evidence is lacking, largely because the incidence of aspiration of gastric contents with the LMA is so low (0.02%), and a randomized controlled clinical trial with a large patient population is needed. Aspiration of gastric contents has been reported with the PLMA,[72] and malposition of the PLMA has been identified as a cause of the aspiration.[73]

The design of the PLMA cuff significantly improves airway seal when compared to the LMA. The larger, softer, wedge-shaped PLMA cuff enables the anterior cuff to better adapt to the shape of the pharynx.[74] Most believe that pressure exerted on the pharyngeal mucosa by the cuffs of LMAs is the cause of sore throat seen with the device. Compared to the LMA, PLMA intracuff pressures are lower and airway seal pressure higher for any given intracuff volume.[75] Moreover, pressure exerted on the hypopharyngeal mucosa has been found to be below that considered critical for mucosal perfusion.

Perhaps the greatest limitation of the use of the LMA in small children is that the seal is often inadequate for positive pressure ventilation, even at high intracuff pressures. This does not appear to be as significant a limitation when the PLMA is used in these patients. In a series of studies comparing the PLMA to the LMA in children of various ages, Goldmann et al showed that the first-time insertion of the PLMA was more successful, was associated with a seal sufficient to permit maximal tidal volume with positive pressure ventilation, produced less gastric insufflation, and provided an improved bronchoscopic laryngeal view compared to the LMA.[76-79] Another comparison study between PLMA and LMA in neonates and infants showed similar success rates, but higher tidal volumes and leak pressures for the PLMA.[80] A larger study by Lopez-Gil of children aged 1 to 16 showed equivalence of ease of insertion, endoscopic confirmed position and mucosal trauma between the PLMA and LMA, but better sealing pressures and less gastric insufflations with the PLMA.[81] Finally, Goldmann et al demonstrated that positive end-expiratory pressure (PEEP) could safely be applied using the PLMA in children.[82]

12.5.4   What are the disadvantages of the PLMA?

It is generally felt that the PLMA is more difficult to place than the LMA. The success rate for first-time PLMA insertion is lower than the first-time insertion success rate for the LMA (average success rate of 85% with a range from 81% to 100% for the PLMA vs average success rate of 93% with a range of 89% to 100% for LMA).[74] It is possible that the insertion difficulty may in part be related to the larger, deeper, and softer cuff of the PLMA. Although the learning curve for the insertion of the PLMA has not been studied, it has been suggested that 20 to 30 insertions of the PLMA are required before competency is achieved.[74]

12.5.5   What are the potential clinical uses of the PLMA?

The improved airway seal characteristics and touted lower risk of gastric aspiration of the PLMA compared to the LMA has expanded its applicability to surgical procedures that would not have been considered safe had an LMA been employed. These procedures include laparoscopy,[83] open abdominal surgery, surgery in patients with obesity, and in patients with gastroesophageal reflux.[74] A recent study by Hohlreider et al demonstrated less postoperative nausea, vomiting, airway morbidity, and analgesic requirements for the PLMA than the tracheal tube in females undergoing breast and gynaecological surgery.[84]

The PLMA has been used to provide ventilation and oxygenation in patients with a history of difficult laryngoscopic intubation.[85,86] Recently, a number of investigators reported the successful use of the PLMA to rescue a failed airway in obstetrical patients after a failed intubation.[71,87-89]

A number of studies, involving volunteers under general anesthesia[90] and manikins have shown that the PLMA may play an important role in airway management in the trauma setting. Although supported by laboratory evidence,[91] there are no clinical case reports of the use of the PLMA in the trauma setting. As well, the role of the PLMA shows favorable promise for CPR, but needs further investigation.

12.5.6   What is the LMA Supreme™ and what is its clinical utility compared the PLMA?

The LMA Supreme™ (Intavent Orthofix, Maidenhead, UK) is a new, single-use, latex-free, LMA device with a drainage tube (Figure 12-7). It was designed to combine the desirable features of both the Intubating LMA (ease of insertion, because of the rigid anatomically shaped airway tube made of medical-grade polyvinyl chloride) and the PLMA™ (higher seal pressures and gastric access).[92] The cuff of the LMA Supreme (LMAS) is designed to provide higher seal pressures than the LMA Classic or Unique. In an early clinical study involving 70 patients, Ali et al[93] reported that the LMAS is superior to the LMA Classic because of its ease of insertion, with low cuff pressure and high oropharyngeal leakage pressure. However, several recent clinical studies comparing the LMAS and PLMA reported conflicting findings.[92,94,95] While studies conducted by Verghese[92] and Hosten[95] reported that both LMAS and PLMA had similar leak pressures, Lee et al[94] found that the oropharyngeal leak pressure and the maximum achievable tidal volume are lower with the LMAS than with the PLMA. However, there was no difference in the efficacy in ventilation and safety between the LMAS and PLMA in these studies.

Because of the ease and speed of successful insertion, higher glottic seal pressures, and ability to access gastric contents, Verghese et al[92] suggested that the LMAS may have a role in airway management in cardiopulmonary resuscitation (CPR), and in the cannot intubate, cannot ventilate scenario currently recommended for the LMA Classic.[5]

12.6   THE COMBITUBE™

12.6.1   What is CBT and how does it differ from the LMA?

The Combitube (CBT) (Tyco-Healthcare-Kendall-Sheridan, Mansfield, MA [Figure 12-8]) is an easily inserted and highly efficacious EGD. It is specified in the ASA Difficult Airway Algorithm as a primary rescue device in CICV situations.[5] It also has been used successfully during CPR and in trauma patients.

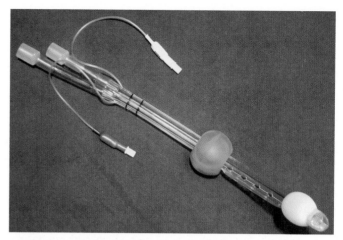

FIGURE 12-8. The Combitube™ is a double-lumen airway, with one lumen for ventilation and the other for access to the GI tract. The oropharyngeal balloon is designed to be positioned just behind the posterior part of the hard palate, sealing both the mouth and nose. A smaller cuff seals the esophagus. Two printed ring marks at the proximal end of the tube indicate appropriate depth of insertion when the upper teeth or alveolar ridges are situated between these two marks.

The CBT is a double-lumen airway, one of which is open at both ends, as with a normal ETT. The other consists of an open proximal lumen and a distal blocked lumen, which resembles an esophageal obturator airway.[96-100] The device has two balloons designed to trap the glottis between them. An oropharyngeal balloon is designed to be positioned just behind the posterior part of the hard palate. Once inflated, this balloon presses the base of the tongue in a ventro-caudal direction and the soft palate in a dorso-cranial direction, sealing the oral and nasal airways from behind. Another smaller cuff seals the esophagus once inflated. Perforations between the two balloons in the distally blocked lumen permit the egress of air or oxygen when positive pressure ventilation is applied to a proximal port. Two circumferential rings printed on the proximal end of the tube indicate that the device has been inserted to the proper depth when the upper teeth or alveolar ridges are situated between these two marks. The CBT is available in two sizes: the CBT 37F SA (small adult), to be used in patients 4 to 6 ft in height (approximately 120 to 180 cm); and the CBT 41F, for patients taller than 6 ft (approximately >180 cm).

12.6.2   How is the CBT inserted?

Insertion is facilitated by bending the CBT between the balloons for a few seconds before insertion to mimic the curvature of the pharynx. It is made more pliable if heated to body temperature, perhaps attenuating its blunt trauma potential. Placement of the CBT is most readily performed with the patient's head placed in a neutral position,[99] although some clinicians prefer slight extension or flexion. The classical sniffing position is usually not helpful. In the fully awake patient, sedation and topical anesthesia are necessary to ensure that the patient does not react to the insertion. To elevate the tongue and epiglottis, a jaw lift is performed by grasping the lower jaw with the thumb and forefinger. The CBT is inserted blindly along the surface of the tongue with initial gentle downward, curved, dorso-caudal movement, and then directed parallel to the patient's horizontal plane until the printed ring marks lie between the upper and lower teeth, or alveolar ridges in edentulous patients. After insertion, the oropharyngeal balloon of the CBT 37F is inflated with 85 mL of air through a blue pilot balloon. The corresponding filling volume for the CBT 41F is 100 mL. Then the distal balloon is inflated with approximately 10 mL of air.

With blind insertion, the CBT is successfully placed in the esophagus in more than 95% of cases. Ventilation is achieved via the longer blue connector (No. 1), leading to the blocked lumen which contains perforations at the level of the larynx, between the two balloons. The trachea is effectively ventilated because the nose, mouth, and esophagus are sealed by the two balloons. The second tracheoesophageal lumen of the CBT can be used for decompression of the esophagus and stomach, thereby minimizing the risk of aspiration.

Auscultation of breath sounds over the chest, the absence of gastric insufflation, end-tidal CO_2 detection, and esophageal detection devices can all assist in the confirmation of correct positioning.[101,102]

Should the CBT enter the trachea on blind insertion, it can function like a standard ETT and there will be no need for inflation of the pharyngeal cuff. Ventilation can be achieved through the shorter, unobstructed clear tube (No. 2), leading to the tracheal lumen.

Although it is rare, ventilation may be impossible through either the proximal or distal lumen. This usually signifies that the CBT has been placed too deeply, with the obturator lumen positioned in the esophagus and the oropharyngeal balloon obstructing the entrance to the larynx. After deflation of the balloons, the CBT should be withdrawn approximately 2.0 to 3.0 cm. While the CBT may be inserted blindly, the use of a laryngoscope is recommended whenever possible.

12.6.3   What are the advantages of the CBT, compared to the LMA?

The CBT was designed primarily for use in CPR,[97,103] even by nonmedical personnel. It has been demonstrated to permit effective ventilation during routine surgery, as well as in the ICU.[104] Most believe that the principal role of the CBT is in emergency airway control when tracheal intubation is not immediately possible.[105-108] The CBT may be kept in situ for up to 8 hours and allows controlled mechanical ventilation at inflating pressures as high as 50 cm H_2O (see aspiration potential below). The CBT can be replaced by deflation of the oropharyngeal balloon and insertion of an ETT either under direct laryngoscopy, or by indirect view using a flexible bronchoscope placed anterior, or lateral to the CBT.

Several case reports describe the successful use of the CBT in cases of unanticipated difficult airways.[109-111] Thus, it is not surprising that the American Society of Anesthesiologists (ASA) task force on difficult airway management lists the CBT, along with the laryngeal mask airway as CICV rescue methods.[5,112] Consequently, the CBT should be part of a portable kit for the management of difficult airways.

A major advantage of the CBT over conventional tracheal intubation is that the device can be inserted with the head and neck in a neutral position. Additionally, it requires only modest mouth opening for insertion, and its tubular profile permits insertion in situations that cannot be negotiated by more bulky devices. The CBT can be inserted from a variety of angles making it useful in awkward environments (eg, a patient who is trapped in a vehicle, see Chapter 16). The CBT may be of special benefit in patients with massive bleeding or regurgitation, when visualization of the vocal cords is impossible. While protection from aspiration is not absolute, the CBT may be more effective in this regard, due to much higher sealing pressures than the traditional LMA.[113]

12.6.4   What are the disadvantages of the CBT?

The CBT was not designed to replace other devices for routine surgery. While the esophageal cuff offers some protection against the reflux of gastric contents into the periglottic area, the level of protection against aspiration does not approach that of a cuffed ETT.

The suctioning of tracheal secretions is impossible when the CBT is in the esophageal position. To address the issue of secretions and suctioning, Krafft et al proposed a modification in the CBT in which the two anterior, proximal perforations of the CBT are replaced by a single, larger, ellipsoid-shaped hole that allows for fiberoptic access of the trachea, tracheal suctioning, and tube exchange over a guide wire.[114] It should be noted that recently developed flexible bronchoscopes (eg, Storz, Tuttlingen, Germany) with a small outer diameter (3.0 mm OD) allow passage through the unmodified pharyngeal perforations.

Contraindications to the use of the CBT include: an intact gag reflex, airway obstruction by foreign bodies, tumors, or swelling, the presence of known esophageal disease, and the prior ingestion of caustic substances.

Complications associated with the use of CBT have been reported.[115,116] In a retrospective study of 1139 patients requiring resuscitation using the CBT, four cases of subcutaneous emphysema, pneumomediastinum, and pneumoperitoneum associated with the CBT during prehospital management were reported.[116] The reason for these complications appeared to be hyperinflation of the distal balloon (20-40 mL), although external chest compression and continuous positive-pressure ventilation may also have been factors. Other rare complications include transient cranial nerve dysfunction,[117] esophageal rupture,[118] and tongue engorgement.[119]

12.6.5   What are the potential clinical uses of the CBT?

The CBT is an easy-to-use, rapidly inserted emergency airway device that has performed satisfactorily in many circumstances. It is accepted as a primary rescue device in CICV situations, as well as for CPR, and in trauma patients. The CBT has been recommended in Practice Guidelines for Management of the Difficult Airway of the ASA.[5] It has also been recommended in the Guidelines for Cardiopulmonary Resuscitation and Emergency Cardiac Care of the American Heart Association (AHA). In 2000, the CBT was upgraded by the AHA as a class IIa device. Furthermore, the CBT may provide an element of protection in patients at risk for aspiration, and it may be of benefit for patients in whom manipulation of the cervical spine is hazardous or impossible. Successfully placed, the device is capable of facilitating adequate ventilation and oxygenation, and in most instances is as effective as endotracheal intubation.[120]

12.7 LARYNGEAL TUBE (KING LT AIRWAY®)

12.7.1 What is a LT and how does it differ from LMA?

The laryngeal tube airway (VBM Medizintechnik, Sulz am Neckar, Germany [Figure 12-9]), also known as the King LT Airway® in North America, is an EGD that was introduced to the European market in 1999.[121] It is similar in appearance and function to the CBT, and is available in three configurations (see below). The fundamental configuration of the LT is a silicone airway tube with ventilation outlet perforations lying between two cuffs, pharyngeal and esophageal. As opposed to the CBT, the LT has a single pilot balloon connected to both cuffs and a single 15 mm standard male adapter. The airway tube is short and "J" shaped with an average diameter of 1.5 cm leading to a blind tip. The device requires a mouth opening of at least 23 mm for its insertion. After device placement, the proximal cuff should lie in the hypopharynx and the distal cuff in the upper esophagus. Both cuffs are high volume-low pressure in design to establish an adequate seal, while minimizing the risk for ischemic mucosal damage. Two ventilation outlets are located between the two cuffs, in the anterior aspect of the tube. The proximal outlet is protected by a V-shaped deflection in the pharyngeal cuff, such that when with the cuff is inflated, soft tissue is deflected from this opening, helping to maintain a patency. There are two side holes near the distal outlet.

Even though the two cuffs are supplied by a single inflation pilot balloon apparatus, the design of the inflation system allows the pharyngeal cuff to fill first, stabilizing the position of the tube.[121] Once the pharyngeal cuff has molded to the anatomy of the patient, the esophageal cuff inflates. The amount of air for cuff inflation is specific to tube size and is indicated on a syringe that is included in the package. Six sizes, suitable for neonates up to large adults, are available. Safe inflation of the dual cuffs may be enhanced with the aid of a cuff pressure gauge and ought to be limited to 60 cm H_2O.

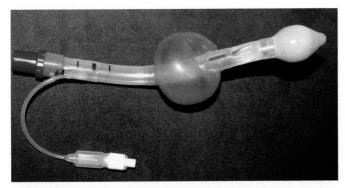

FIGURE 12-9. The laryngeal tube airway consists of a silicone airway tube with two ventilation outlet perforations lying between two cuffs, a single pilot balloon, and a 15 mm male adapter.

Since its introduction in 1999, the LT has undergone considerable changes in design. Presently, there are several versions of the laryngeal tube: standard reuseable laryngeal tube, single-use laryngeal tube (LT-D), laryngeal tube-Suction II, and single-use laryngeal tube-Suction II (LTS-D).[122] Similar to the PLMA, the laryngeal tube- Suction has two lumens: one for ventilation and the other serves as a conduit to the esophagus and stomach.

12.7.2 How is a LT inserted?

An appropriately sized LT should be selected based on the patient's weight and height. Prior to insertion, the cuffs should be completely deflated and well lubricated. The device should be inserted with the patient's head and neck in a sniffing position.[122] The head is extended on the neck with the nondominant hand, to open the mouth. The LT is then inserted blindly in the midline, with the tip pressed against the hard palate and then advanced along the palate into the hypopharynx until resistance is felt, at which point a proximal horizontal black line should be aligned with the front teeth. The device is usually easily inserted with insertion times comparable to those reported for the LMA.[123] While a number of studies reported easier and faster insertion of the LT compared to the CBT by the prehospital care personnel and trainees, these studies used only manikins and not patients.[124,125] Clinical studies are necessary to confirm these findings.

The device provides a patent airway in the majority of patients following the first insertion attempt and success does not require extensive training.[126,127] Indicators of correct placement include end-tidal carbon dioxide detection, auscultation of bilateral breath sounds, absence of gastric insufflation, and adequate chest movement. Capnographic waveform analysis may be of particular use in confirming proper position of the LT. A brief period of positive pressure ventilation (PPV) may also confirm proper alignment of the LT and the absence of obstruction.

Correct placement of the LT may also be verified using a light-wand (Trachlight™). The Trachlight™ (without the internal stiff wire stylet) is inserted into the LT and advanced until a faint glow can be seen above the thyroid prominence. This indicates that the tip of the lightwand is just above the laryngeal inlet. The lightwand is then advanced further until a well-defined circumscribed glow is seen in the anterior neck, slightly below the thyroid prominence, indicating entrance into the glottis and correct positioning of the LT. Incorrect positioning would demonstrate a lateral glow, or a glow with a halo, indicating malpositioning of the ventilation orifice. The LT should be removed with the patient either deeply anesthetized, or totally awake. In an awake patient, the LT should be removed only when airway protective reflexes have completely returned.

12.7.3 What are the advantages of the LT, compared to the LMA and the CBT?

Insertion of this device is relatively easy and successful in most patients on the first attempt. The soft tip minimizes mechanical trauma on insertion and high volume/low pressure cuffs provide a good seal and protection against mucosal ischemic damage.

A single pilot balloon confers an element of simplicity and speed in emergency situations. Other advantages of LT include:

1. The adequacy of ventilation with the LT is comparable to that obtained with other EGDs. The ease of insertion and high quality of the seal achieved may confer a preferred role for the LT in airway management during cardiopulmonary resuscitation.[126]

2. The LT can be used successfully in children as young as 2 years old, with superior seal pressures and equivalent ease of insertion.[128]

3. The esophageal cuff of the laryngeal tube may provide an element of protection against the reflux of gastric contents into the periglottic area and the tube-Suction options permit gastric decompression. Both of these features may reduce the risk of aspiration, relative to the LMA Classic.[129,130]

4. Due to the form and length of the device, an unintended tracheal intubation should not occur.

12.7.4   What are the disadvantages of the LT?

1. Protection from aspiration is less than that offered by a cuffed ETT, and in high aspiration risk situations tracheal intubation remains necessary. While the newer laryngeal tube-Suction II, and single-use laryngeal tube-Suction II (LTS-D) may have the potential to provide some protection from aspiration, presently there are no clinical data available.

2. The intracuff pressure may increase by as much as 15 cm H_2O within 30 minutes after its insertion if nitrous oxide is employed, due to the diffusion of this gas into the cuff. Manometric monitoring of the cuff pressure has been suggested.[131]

3. Position adjustments to ensure airflow continuity may be required more frequently in obese patients.[132]

Positive pressure ventilation through the LT may provide inadequate ventilation in patients who require high pulmonary inflation pressures.

1. The mouth opening required for LT insertion is at least 23 mm.

2. As with any EGD, the LT may not be effective in the presence of anatomic distortion of the upper airway, such as lesions of the epiglottis or laryngopharynx.

3. The LT is less effective than the LMA in children younger than 10 with respect to ease of ventilation and endoscopic view through the device.[133]

12.7.5   What are the potential clinical uses of the LT?

In anesthetic practice, the LT can be used in patients who are candidates for face mask or LMA-delivered anesthesia. It may also find a role in the failed airway, similar to that of the LMA and the CBT.

The dimension and position of the ventilation holes and the protection offered by the overhanging cuff block permits the insertion of a suction catheter, endotracheal tube exchange device, FB, or an Eschmann introducer, over which an ETT may be passed.[134]

12.8   LARYVENT™

12.8.1   What is the LV and how does it differ from the LMA?

The LV (B+P Beatmungs-Produkte GmbH, Seelscheid, Germany) consists of a single tube with a standard male connector, two cuffs with a single pilot balloon, and a ventilation outlet. The superior cuff lies in the hypopharynx and the ventral part of the cuff contains the orifice for ventilation. The inferior cuff is smaller and should lie at the level of the upper esophageal sphincter. As with other EGDs, the insertion of the LV is a blind technique and appears to have a rapid learning curve, similar to that of the LT.

12.8.2   How do you insert the LV?

Prior to the use of the LV, the cuffs should be tested by inflating 50 mL of air. During insertion, the tip of the LV should be introduced along the posterior wall of pharynx and advanced until resistance is felt. The cuffs should then be inflated with 50 mL of air. If there is resistance to filling, the LV has been introduced too deeply and should be retracted 2 to 3 cm before reattempting cuff inflation.

12.8.3   What are the advantages of the LV, compared to the LMA?

The advantages of the LV are similar to those of the LMA Unique, and LT, with comparable provision of ventilation and oxygenation, at least in early clinical experience.[126,135]

12.8.4   What are the disadvantages of the LV?

More complex handling, resulting in a significantly higher failure rate, and postoperative patient discomfort suggest that the LV may not be the first choice in routine anesthesia practice.[135]

12.8.5   What are the potential clinical uses of the LV?

The role and advantage of the LV are similar to those of the LT. The precise advantages have not yet been defined by clinical trials.

12.9   AIRWAY MANAGEMENT DEVICE™

12.9.1   What is the AMD and how does it differ from the LMA?

The AMD (Nagor Limited, Isle of Man; manufactured by Biosil Ltd, Cumbernauld, UK [Figure 12-10]) is a newly introduced EGD.[136] The AMD consists of a clear silicone dual lumen tube that is concave ventrally with inflatable oropharyngeal and hypopharyngeal cuffs. An oval ventilation port is located in the ventral

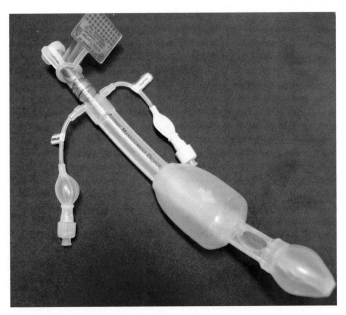

FIGURE 12-10. The Airway Management Device™ is a clear silicone tube with hypopharyngeal and oropharyngeal cuffs. An oval hole located between the two cuffs in the ventral part of the device allows ventilation.

part of the device opposite the laryngeal inlet. The connector at the proximal end of the tube is Y-shaped incorporating two ports: one for anesthetic gas delivery and providing access for suction catheters, an FB or an Eschmann introducer; and the second for a channel into the esophagus for suction. When fully inflated, the upper cuff fills, elevating the tongue and epiglottis. The cuffs have independent inflation controls, which are color coded. The shape of the cuffs ensures correct orientation in the airway and prevents both lateral movement and rotation of the tube. The AMD is available in several sizes: 3.0 to 3.5 for patients weighing 30 to 60 kg, and size 4.0 to 5.0 for patients more than 60 kg.

12.9.2 How is the AMD inserted?

The insertion technique is similar to other EGDs. Both cuffs of the AMD should be well lubricated, the pharyngeal cuff should be fully deflated, and the esophageal cuff should have 5.0 to 9.0 mL of air. This closes the esophageal cuff channel through a unique constriction mechanism and permits atraumatic insertion. The AMD, held in the dominant hand, is inserted in the midline of the mouth in a caudal direction until it seats properly in the hypopharynx. The pharyngeal cuff is then inflated with 50 to 80 mL of air. Like all EGDs, proper placement should be confirmed after insertion.

12.9.3 What are the advantages of the AMD compared to the LMA?

A key feature of this device lies in the access it provides to the esophagus when the esophageal cuff is partially deflated. A suction catheter can be introduced through the device without interrupting ventilation to aspirate the esophagus, and provides an element of protection against aspiration.

12.9.4 What are the disadvantages of the AMD?

Compared with other EGDs, the AMD device is somewhat difficult to insert and airway trauma is possible.[136-138] Cook et al reported a first-time success rate of 66% in establishing an airway, with an average of 0.56 manipulations per patient and a primary failure rate of 11%.[137] The AMD also had an increased incidence of loss of airway during anesthesia.[139] While the AMD may provide protection against aspiration, presently there are no data to support the claim.

12.9.5 What are the potential clinical uses of the AMD?

While the dynamic relationship between the hypopharyngeal cuff and the esophageal suction port is interesting, the precise advantage of the AMD is difficult to define at this time.

12.10 PERILARYNGEAL AIRWAY (COBRAPLA™)

12.10.1 What is the CPLA and how does it differ from the LMA?

The CobraPLA (CPLA) (Engineered Medical Systems, Inc., Indianapolis, IN [Figure 12-11]) consists of a breathing tube with a circumferential inflatable cuff proximal to a ventilation outlet, a 15 mm standard adapter, and a distal widened cobra-shaped head designed to separate soft tissues and to allow ventilation of the trachea. Once in place, the cobra head lies in front of the laryngeal inlet. Internal to the cobra head, a ramp directs ventilation into the trachea. A soft grill shields the inferior aperture of the device in an attempt to deflect the epiglottis anteriorly. The bars of the grill are sufficiently flexible to permit an ETT to pass easily. The cuff is shaped such that it resides in the hypopharynx at the base of the tongue and, when inflated, raises the base of the tongue exposing the laryngeal inlet and affects an airway seal. The unique shape of the distal part of the device allows it to slide easily along the hard palate during insertion, and to move soft tissues away from the laryngeal inlet once in place.

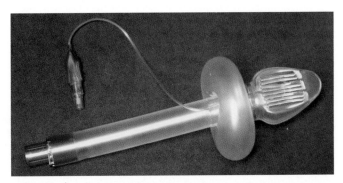

FIGURE 12-11. The CobraPLA™ consists of a breathing tube with a circumferential inflatable cuff proximal to the ventilation outlet portion, a 15 mm standard adapter, and a distal widened *Cobra head* designed to separate the soft tissues of the hypopharynx and permit ventilation.

The CPLA is available in eight sizes and it can be used in small children, including neonates.[140] Size selection is governed by the weight of the patient. Generally, #3 is used in most female patients, #4 for most men, and #5 for larger men. When one is unsure which size is best, or when learning placement technique, selecting the lower size is recommended. In general, larger sizes require considerably higher cuff pressures to produce an acceptable seal compared to the smaller sizes.[141]

Recently, several modifications of the original design of the CPLA have been introduced.[140] The second-generation CPLA has a distal curve in the breathing tube to avoid kinking, and softer material to facilitate insertion and minimize trauma. The Cobra PLUS has a temperature probe to measure core temperature and a gas sampling line for the three smallest pediatric sizes.

12.10.2   How do you insert the CPLA?

The CPLA is simple to insert, though some more difficulty is encountered in the obese.[142] Prior to insertion, the pharyngeal cuff is fully deflated and folded back against the breathing tube. The back of the cobra head and cuff are lubricated, taking care that the lubricant does not obstruct the grille. The patient's head is placed in the sniffing position. A jaw lift is performed and the distal end of the CPLA is directed straight back through the mouth between the tongue and hard palate. Modest neck extension (without a jaw lift maneuver) may aid the passage of the device as it turns toward the glottis at the back of the mouth. Once the CPLA traverses the back of the mouth, it usually turns caudally toward the larynx with minimal resistance, as the flexible distal tip guides the device downward. The CPLA is properly seated above the glottis when modest resistance to further distal passage is encountered. Once inserted, the flexible tip lies behind the arytenoids, the cuff lies in the hypopharynx at the base of the tongue, and the ramp lifts the epiglottis. Then the cuff is inflated until the leak with positive pressure ventilation disappears. Indicators of correct placement are absence of leak on auscultation of the neck, bilateral breath sounds, absence of gastric insufflation, easily produced chest movement, and positive carbon dioxide detection. Exceeding a peak airway pressure of 25 cm H_2O with positive pressure ventilation is not recommended, even when testing for ventilation and cuff seal, because of the risk of gastric insufflation.

If the CPLA is not inserted far enough, inflation of the cuff may cause the tongue to protrude from the mouth of the patient. In this situation, the cuff should be deflated and the device advanced further or a smaller sized CPLA selected. It is possible to advance the cobra head beyond the laryngeal inlet, in which case ventilation will not be possible. The CPLA should be removed awake with the airway protective reflexes intact.

12.10.3   What are the advantages of the CPLA, compared to the LMA?

The tube of the CPLA has a larger lumen than most EGDs and may be particularly useful in directing flexible endoscope-assisted tracheal intubation,[143,144] especially when larger ETTs are indicated. An ETT of 8.0 mm ID can be advanced through the sizes 4 to 6 CPLA.[140] In addition, it has been made short enough that its removal after insertion of an ETT is greatly facilitated.

As with similar EGDs, a Trachlight™ with the rigid internal stylet removed can be used in lieu of an FB to facilitate tracheal intubation. Although less reliable, blind tracheal intubation through the CPLA using a generic ETT introducer (eg, the Eschmann introducer) may be possible.

Like many other EGDs, the insertion technique is simple and has been accomplished by personnel with little or no experience. Several small clinical studies reported that the CPLA has better airway sealing characteristics compared to the LMA.[145,146] During gynecological laparoscopy, the CPLA provided similar insertion characteristics, but higher airway-sealing pressures than the LMA Classic.[147] However, Park et al[148] showed that gastric insufflation, or ventilatory difficulty, may occur following the change of the position of the head and neck when using the CobraPLA, as compared to PLMA. A number of reports have supported the use of the CPLA in the CICV situation, a factor related to the unique design of the device.[140,142,149]

Khan et al[150] reported successful use of the CPLA for ventilation following failed attempts in placing an LMA in patients with face and neck contractures, as well as limited mouth opening.

12.10.4   What are the disadvantages of the CPLA?

In comparison with trials for the LMA Classic and LMA Unique, the CPLA took slightly longer to insert and macroscopic blood occurred more frequently on the CPLA, seen on up to 40% of the devices after removal.[143,146,147] Although blood staining has been detected more frequently with the CPLA compared with other EGDs, there were no differences in airway morbidity.[151] Therefore, the clinical significance of these findings is uncertain.

The CPLA is not appropriate for patients with low lung compliance or increased airway resistance. The major disadvantage of the device is that it does not protect against aspiration and does not secure the airway as effectively as an ETT.[152] The mask aperture bars probably have no anatomical utility and predispose to herniation of the pharyngeal structures on insertion and while in situ.[151]

Although it is rare, aspiration associated with use of the CPLA has been reported.[152,153] In fact, Cook et al[152] terminated the CPLA evaluation study after two cases of serious pulmonary aspiration with the use of the CPLA, suggesting that the CPLA should be avoided in patients at risk of aspiration.

12.11   THE STREAMLINED PHARYNX AIRWAY LINER™

12.11.1   What is the SLIPA and how does it differ from the LMA?

The SLIPA (SLIPA Med, Cape Town, South Africa [Figure 12-12]) is a disposable EGD. It is designed for airway management during controlled ventilation.[154,155] The peculiar shape of the device provides a seal without the use of an inflatable cuff.

The body of the SLIPA is shaped like a hollow boot with *toe*, *bridge*, and *heel* prominences, designed to engage the mucosal

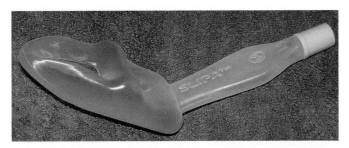

FIGURE 12-12. The SLIPA is shaped like a hollow boot with *toe*, *bridge*, and *heel* prominences, designed to engage the patient's pharynx. The hollow design feature permits the entrapment of liquids such as secretions, blood, and gastric fluids, thus preventing aspiration.

lining of the patient's pharynx. Its hollow configuration and shape permit the entrapment of secretions, blood, or gastric contents in the device, theoretically reducing the risk of aspiration. The device is formed from soft plastic material, flexible enough to allow easy insertion. The hollow chamber flattens to facilitate insertion. After placement, the *toe* should sit in the hypopharynx. The *bridge*, with its two lateral bulges, fits into the pyriform fossae, displacing tissue away from the posterior pharyngeal wall. The *heel* of the chamber anchors the SLIPA in position by sliding over the soft palate and into the nasopharyngeal opening. Toward the toe side of the bridge are smaller lateral bulges that coincide with the inferior cornus of the hyoid bone designed to relieve pressure on relevant nervous tissue, such as the superior laryngeal branch of the vagus.

12.11.2   How is the SLIPA inserted?

The SLIPA is inserted similarly to the LMA. The patient's head and neck should be placed in a sniffing position. Held in the dominant hand, the SLIPA is inserted in the midline of the mouth, pressed against hard palate, and advanced until resistance is felt. A jaw lift may facilitate placement. The crescent shape of the toe minimizes the risk of downward folding of the epiglottis, which may lead to airway obstruction. The toe of the device slips easily into the esophagus, where it creates a seal. After placement, the SLIPA returns to its preinsertion shape.

12.11.3   What are the advantages and disadvantages of the SLIPA, compared to the LMA?

Although there is a theoretical lower risk of gastric insufflation relative to the LMA, this has not been shown in studies. In one small study, Lange et al found that there was actually a higher rate of gastric insufflations with SLIPA compared to LMA (19% vs 3%).[156]

12.11.4   What are the potential clinical uses of the SLIPA device?

Based on the current available evidence, the SLIPA appears to have comparable efficacy and complications as the LMA, and may be used as a primary airway device for short surgical procedures.[140] While the SLIPA may have a potential lower risk of aspiration in the presence of PPV, there are few clinical trials in this regard.

12.12   CUFFED OROPHARYNGEAL AIRWAY

12.12.1   What was the COPA and how did it differ from the LMA?

The COPA (Mallinckrodt Medical, Athlone, Ireland [Figure 12-13]) was first described in 1992 by Greenberg,[157] and was intended for use during anesthesia in spontaneously breathing patients. The device is a modified Guedel airway, with an inflatable distal cuff, and a proximal 15 mm connector. The flange at the proximal end is fitted with two posts for securing a strap, used to stabilize the device in the mouth against the upper teeth or gums. The device is no longer manufactured and is presented for historical purposes only. The COPA was available in four sizes: 8, 9, 10, and 11 (the numbers refer to the length of the shaft of the device, ie, the distance in centimeters between the flange and the distal tip).

12.12.2   How was the COPA inserted?

The COPA was inserted in the same fashion as a Guedel airway, with a rotating movement.

12.12.3   What are the advantages of the COPA, compared to the LMA?

Agrò et al[158] demonstrated the ability of the COPA to guide an ETT into the trachea employing a light-guided technique with a lightwand. After confirming proper placement, the lightwand was removed and a tube exchange catheter (TE) was inserted through the COPA into the trachea. The patients were then paralyzed and ventilation through the TE reconfirmed. The COPA was removed leaving the TE in situ for the ETT to be guided into place. This combined technique was successful in 6 out of 10 patients.

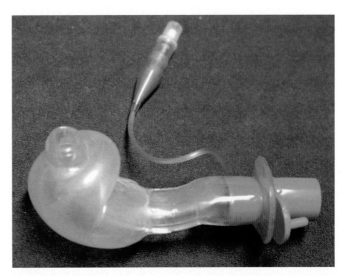

FIGURE 12-13. The cuffed oropharyngeal airway (COPA) was a modified Guedel airway with an inflatable distal cuff and a proximal 15 mm connector. The flange at the proximal end was fitted with two posts for a securing strap to stabilize the device in the mouth against the upper teeth or gums.

12.12.4 What were the disadvantages of the COPA?

The COPA was contraindicated in patients at risk for aspiration. Compared to the LMA, the COPA appeared to have a higher incidence of postoperative sore throat, as well as jaw and neck pain.[159] The COPA required more airway manipulations than the LMA in order to maintain patency.[160]

12.12.5 What were the potential clinical uses of the COPA?

The simplicity of the COPA was its most compelling feature, enhancing its utility in many environments. It is smaller than most other devices suggesting it might be particularly useful in patients with restricted mouth opening. The COPA could be used to assist with the placement of an ETT, although the success rates were low.

12.13 PHARYNGEAL AIRWAY EXPRESS™

12.13.1 What was the PAX and how does it differ from the LMA?

Like the COPA, this device is no longer manufactured. The PAX (Vital Signs, Totowa, NJ) was an EGD invented by Douglas Mongeon of Orange Park Acres, California. The PAX was made from polyvinyl chloride and was intended for single use. It consisted of a single curved tube with an inflatable cuff to be positioned in the proximal pharynx, and a noninflatable, gilled, conical tip at the distal end. The tip forms a no-pressure seal in the hypopharynx that was designed to minimize gastric insufflation and regurgitation. Between the cuff and tip on the inner curve was a rectangular vent that faced anteriorly toward the glottic inlet. The distal half of the vent had three vertical gills to prevent epiglottic intrusion and device obstruction. The internal diameter of the airway tube was about 12 mm. The maximum recommended cuff inflation volume was 60 mL. There was only one size for adults weighing greater than 41 kg.

12.13.2 How was the PAX inserted?

Prior to insertion, the cuff was deflated and lubricated. During insertion, the PAX was held in the dominant hand like a pen. The mouth was opened with the nondominant hand and the PAX advanced into the pharynx until resistance was felt. The cuff was then inflated with the pilot balloon until a seal sufficient to permit ventilation was achieved, or the maximum cuff inflation volume reached.

12.13.3 What were the advantages of the PAX, compared to the LMA?

The insertion success rate for the PAX was high and it was an effective ventilatory device, with a low risk of gastric insufflation.[161] Mondello et al[162] evaluated the PAX in 91 patients undergoing surgery and demonstrated that the device provided safe and effective airway control during mechanical ventilation in all but one case.

12.13.4 What were the disadvantages of the PAX?

This device was associated with a relatively high incidence of mucosal trauma. Further, mucosal pressures with the device in place may exceed pharyngeal perfusion pressure.

The PAX had a moderately high failure rate when lightwand-guided intubation was attempted and produced more marked changes in hemodynamic variables when compared with those produced by the LMA.[163]

12.14 IGEL

12.14.1 What is the iGel and how does it differ from the LMA?

The iGel (Intersurgical Ltd., Wokingham, UK) is a single-use extraglottic device that is made of a thermoplastic elastomer gel. It has a noninflatable cuff which can anatomically seal the pharyngeal, laryngeal, and perilaryngeal structures with a minimal risk of compression trauma. The device has an elliptical cross-sectional–shaped tube with a slight curve longitudinally to facilitate insertion and minimize axial rotation once it is placed (Figure 12-14). It also has an independent gastric drainage tube and an integral bite block. It is single use and available in sizes 3 to 5. A size 4 is recommended by the manufacturers for patients between 50 and 90 kg, making it the most common size for the normal adult population.

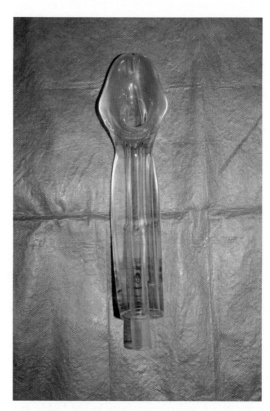

FIGURE 12-14. The iGel device has a noninflatable cuff and an elliptical cross-sectional–shaped tube with a slight curve longitudinally to facilitate insertion. In addition, it also has an independent gastric drainage tube and an integral bite block.

12.14.2   How is the iGel inserted?

With the patient's head and neck placed in a sniffing position, the well-lubricated iGel is placed in the mouth and passed along the posterior pharynx until resistance is felt.[164] Insertion does not require an introducer or placement of the finger into the mouth, as the device is simply pushed into place. A 45-degree twist can be employed to facilitate insertion. The cuff does not require the inflation of air following placement.

12.14.3   What are the advantages of the iGel, compared to the LMA?

The insertion process requires one fewer step, as there is no air required for cuff inflation. The elastomer gel may provide a more efficient seal around the larynx after warming to body temperature.[165] In addition, the gel-filled cuff may potentially cause less direct trauma or pressure damage to the oropharyngeal mucosa. Unfortunately, at present, there are no clinical data to confirm this potential advantage.

The iGel has a gastric drainage tube which may offer added protection against the aspiration of regurgitated stomach contents. Two separate case reports have confirmed that this drainage tube provided protection against aspiration.[165,166] However, in a case series of 280 patients reported by Gibbison et al,[167] three patients had regurgitation while using the iGel. Although the iGel completely protected the airway from aspiration of regurgitated stomach contents in two of these patients, it did not provide complete protection in the third patient. The investigators concluded that the efficacy of the drainage tube has not been confirmed, and further study is required to determine the safety profile of the device.

12.14.4   What are the disadvantages of the iGel?

In a clinical evaluation study with 100 patients, Gatward et al[168] found that the airway seal offered by the iGel is inferior to other EGDs, such as the PLMA. In a cadaver study, Schmidbauer et al[169] showed that both the LMA Proseal and LMA Classic provided a better seal of the esophagus than the iGel airway. If there is a leak around the iGel, it may have to be replaced with a different size, since there is no option of adding or withdrawing air from the cuff.

The drainage tube of the iGel is significantly smaller than the drainage tube of the PLMA. For instance, a 12 Fr gauge catheter can be inserted through the size 4 iGel compared to a 16 Fr catheter for a size 4 PLMA.[168] It is unknown if the smaller drainage tube is adequate to provide equivalent protection of aspiration, compared with other EGDs with a larger drainage tube.

12.14.5   What are the clinical uses of the iGel?

Compared with seven other extraglottic airway devices (Airway Management Device™, CobraPLA™, Combitube™, Laryngeal Tube, Laryngeal Tube Disposable (LTD), Laryngeal Tube Suction II (LTS II), and the SLIPA™), the iGel has been shown to perform the best for ease of insertion into the airway during training on manikins by 10 anesthesiologists.[170]

In a clinical evaluation study involving 100 patients, Gatward et al[168] reported that the iGel was successfully inserted in all patients and allowed effective controlled ventilation in 98%. The investigators also commented that, while the airway seal offered by the iGel may be inferior to other EGDs, such as the PLMA, it is still sufficient for controlled ventilation in the vast majority of patients. Rates of failure, manipulations required, and complications were also very low for the iGel in that study. In another prospective observational study with 71 patients, Richez et al[171] confirmed the efficacy and safety of the iGel airway device.

The iGel has been successfully used to provide ventilation in patients with a difficult airway in a number of case reports. Michalek et al[172] reported successful placement of the iGel under general anesthesia in two uncooperative patients with an anticipated difficult intubation (Hunter and Waardenburg syndromes). Oxygenation and ventilation were maintained using the iGel which was then used as a conduit for tracheal intubation using a pediatric flexible bronchoscope (FB).

Joshi et al[173] reported the use of the iGel as an airway rescue in a patient with scleroderma and predicted difficult intubation. Under general anesthesia, ventilation was difficult with a bag-mask, the LMA Classic, and the LMA Proseal but ventilation was achieved easily with a size 4 iGel. Others have also reported the use of the iGel as a rescue airway device.[174]

While these are encouraging results, more clinical studies with larger patient populations are needed to confirm these findings.

12.15   SUMMARY

During the last two decades, EGDs, such as the Laryngeal Mask Airway™ and the Combitube™, have been shown to be effective and safe devices for delivering effective oxygenation and ventilation. In addition, many studies have shown that these devices can be used successfully to rescue patients with a failed airway. These devices are now recommended by authorities such as the American Society of Anesthesiologists (ASA) (Difficult Airway Management Algorithm) and the Difficult Airway Society (UK) for this indication.

The major disadvantage of all EGDs is their inability to completely seal the larynx and protect against aspiration. In addition, poor seal by any of these devices can lead to air leak on positive pressure ventilation and gastric insufflation. Newer designs of EGD, such as the Intubating LMA (or LMA Fastrach™), LMA Proseal™, LMA Supreme™, and the King LTS-D have been developed to attempt to address these concerns.

As a result of the widespread acceptance and popularity of the original LMA, many newly designed, reusable, and disposable EGD devices have been introduced. Although many preliminary clinical studies have demonstrated the efficacy and safety of these devices, most of them involved only a small number of patients. More clinical studies with larger patient populations are needed to confirm these findings. Finally, these devices are not only effective airway management and airway rescue devices, but they can be used and learned easily, in contrast to bag-mask-ventilation and endotracheal intubation. It is entirely reasonable to expect that these devices will supplant BMV as a rescue airway maneuver.

REFERENCES

1. Caplan RA, Posner KL, Ward RJ, Cheney FW. Adverse respiratory events in anesthesia: a closed claims analysis. *Anesthesiology.* 1990;72:828-833.

2. Langeron O, Masso E, Huraux C, et al. Prediction of difficult mask ventilation. *Anesthesiology.* 2000;92:1229-1236.

3. Mulcaster JT, Mills J, Hung OR, et al. Laryngoscopic intubation: learning and performance. *Anesthesiology.* 2003;98:23-27.

4. Brimacombe J. A proposed classification system for extraglottic airway devices. *Anesthesiology.* 2004;101:559.

5. Practice guidelines for management of the difficult airway: an updated report by the American Society of Anesthesiologists Task Force on Management of the Difficult Airway. *Anesthesiology.* 2003;98:1269-1277.

6. Bogetz MS. Using the laryngeal mask airway to manage the difficult airway. *Anesthesiol Clin North America.* 2002;20:863-870, vii.

7. Cook TM. The classic laryngeal mask airway: a tried and tested airway. What now? *Br J Anaesth.* 2006;96:149-152.

8. Kokkinis K. The use of the laryngeal mask airway in CPR. *Resuscitation.* 1994;27:9-12.

9. Stone BJ, Leach AB, et al. The use of the laryngeal mask airway by nurses during cardiopulmonary resuscitation: results of a multicentre trial. *Anaesthesia.* 1994;49:3-7.

10. Brimacombe JR. Placement phase. In: Brimacombe JR, ed. *Laryngeal Mask Anesthesia.* Philadelphia, PA: W.B. Saunders, Elsevier Ltd.; 2005:191-240.

11. Garcia-Pedrajas F, Monedero P, Carrascosa F. Modification of Brain's technique for insertion of laryngeal mask airway. *Anesth Analg.* 1994;79:1024-1025.

12. Bignell S, Brimacombe J. LMA stability and fixation. *Anaesth Intensive Care.* 1994;22:746.

13. Brimacombe JR. *Emergence Phase in Laryngeal Mask Anesthesia.* Philadelphia, PA: Saunders, Elsevier Ltd; 2005:265-270.

14. Deakin CD, Diprose P, Majumdar R, Pulletz M. An investigation into the quantity of secretions removed by inflated and deflated laryngeal mask airways. *Anaesthesia.* 2000;55:478-480.

15. Brimacombe J. The advantages of the LMA over the tracheal tube or facemask: a meta-analysis. *Can J Anaesth.* 1995;42:1017-1023.

16. Benumof JL. Laryngeal mask airway and the ASA difficult airway algorithm. *Anesthesiology.* 1996;84:686-699.

17. Keller C, Brimacombe J. Bronchial mucus transport velocity in paralyzed anesthetized patients: a comparison of the laryngeal mask airway and cuffed tracheal tube. *Anesth Analg.* 1998;86:1280-1282.

18. Verghese C, Brimacombe JR. Survey of laryngeal mask airway usage in 11,910 patients: safety and efficacy for conventional and nonconventional usage. *Anesth Analg.* 1996;82:129-133.

19. Brimacombe JR, Berry A. The incidence of aspiration associated with the laryngeal mask airway: a meta-analysis of published literature. *J Clin Anesth.* 1995;7:297-305.

20. Keller C, Brimacombe J, Bittersohl J, Lirk P, von Goedecke A. Aspiration and the laryngeal mask airway: three cases and a review of the literature. *Br J Anaesth.* 2004;93:579-582.

21. Keller C, Sparr HJ, Brimacombe JR. Positive pressure ventilation with the laryngeal mask airway in non-paralysed patients: comparison of sevoflurane and propofol maintenance techniques. *Br J Anaesth.* 1998;80:332-336.

22. Keller C, Sparr HJ, Luger TJ, Brimacombe J. Patient outcomes with positive pressure versus spontaneous ventilation in non-paralysed adults with the laryngeal mask. *Can J Anaesth.* 1998;45:564-567.

23. Maltby JR, Beriault MT, Watson NC, Fick GH. Gastric distension and ventilation during laparoscopic cholecystectomy: LMA-Classic vs. tracheal intubation. *Can J Anaesth.* 2000;47:622-666.

24. Sidaras G, Hunter JM. Is it safe to artificially ventilate a paralysed patient through the laryngeal mask? The jury is still out. *Br J Anaesth.* 2001;86:749-753.

25. Bernardini A, Natalini G. Risk of pulmonary aspiration with laryngeal mask airway and tracheal tube: analysis on 65,712 procedures with positive pressure ventilation. *Anaesthesia.* 2009.

26. Devitt JH, Wenstone R, Noel AG, O'Donnell MP. The laryngeal mask airway and positive-pressure ventilation. *Anesthesiology.* 1994;80:550-555.

27. Johannigman JA, Branson RD, Davis K, Jr., Hurst JM. Techniques of emergency ventilation: a model to evaluate tidal volume, airway pressure, and gastric insufflation. *J Trauma.* 1991;31:93-98.

28. Natalini G, Facchetti P, Dicembrini MA, Lanza G, Rosano A, Bernardini A. Pressure controlled versus volume controlled ventilation with laryngeal mask airway. *J Clin Anesth.* 2001;13:436-439.

29. Griffin RM, Hatcher IS. Aspiration pneumonia and the laryngeal mask airway. *Anaesthesia.* 1990;45:1039-1040.

30. Ismail-Zade IA, Vanner RG. Regurgitation and aspiration of gastric contents in a child during general anaesthesia using the laryngeal mask airway. *Paediatr Anaesth.* 1996;6:325-328.

31. Nanji GM, Maltby JR. Vomiting and aspiration pneumonitis with the laryngeal mask airway. *Can J Anaesth.* 1992;39:69-70.

32. Han TH, Brimacombe J, Lee EJ, Yang HS. The laryngeal mask airway is effective (and probably safe) in selected healthy parturients for elective Cesarean section: a prospective study of 1067 cases. *Can J Anaesth.* 2001;48:1117-1121.

33. Brimacombe JR. Pediatrics. In: *Laryngeal Mask Anesthesia.* Philadelphia, PA: Saunders, Elsevier Ltd; 2005:357-389.

34. Guidelines for the basic management of the airway and ventilation during resuscitation. A statement by the Airway and Ventilation Management Working Group of the European Resuscitation Council. *Resuscitation.* 1996;31:187-200.

35. The American Heart Association. Guidelines 2000 for Cardiopulmonary Resuscitation and Emergency Cardiovascular Care. Part 11: neonatal resuscitation. *Circulation.* 2000;102:1343-1357.

36. Brimacombe JR. Difficult airway. In: Brimacombe JR, ed. *Laryngeal Mask Anesthesia.* Philadelphia, PA: Saunders, Elsevier Ltd.; 2005:305-355.

37. Agro F, Brimacombe J, Carassiti M, Marchionni L, Morelli A, Cataldo R. Use of a lighted stylet for intubation via the laryngeal mask airway. *Can J Anaesth.* 1998;45:556-560.

38. Hung OR. Light-guided tracheal intubation through the laryngeal mask airway. *Anesth Analg.* 1997;85:1415.

39. Langenstein H. The laryngeal mask airway in the difficult intubation. The results of a prospective study. *Anaesthesist.* 1995;44:712-718.

40. Williams PJ, Bailey PM. Comparison of the reinforced laryngeal mask airway and tracheal intubation for adenotonsillectomy. *Br J Anaesth.* 1993;70:30-33.

41. Sher M, Brimacombe J, Laing D. Anaesthesia for laser pharyngoplasty—a comparison of the tracheal tube with the reinforced laryngeal mask airway. *Anaesth Intensive Care.* 1995;23:149-153.

42. Quinn AC, Samaan A, McAteer EM, Moss E, Vucevic M. The reinforced laryngeal mask airway for dento-alveolar surgery. *Br J Anaesth.* 1996;77:185-188.

43. Brain AI, Verghese C, Addy EV, Kapila A. The intubating laryngeal mask. II: a preliminary clinical report of a new means of intubating the trachea. *Br J Anaesth.* 1997;79:704-709.

44. Wong JK, Tongier WK, Armbruster SC, White PF. Use of the intubating laryngeal mask airway to facilitate awake orotracheal intubation in patients with cervical spine disorders. *J Clin Anesth.* 1999;11:346-348.

45. Ferson DZ, Rosenblatt WH, Johansen MJ, et al. Use of the intubating LMA-Fastrach in 254 patients with difficult-to-manage airways. *Anesthesiology.* 2001;95:1175-1181.

46. Brimacombe JR. Intubating LMA for airway intubation. In: Brimacombe JR, ed. *Laryngeal Mask Anesthesia.* Philadelphia, PA: Saunders, Elsevier Ltd.; 2005:469-504.

47. Chan PL, Lee TW, Lam KK, Chan WS. Intubation through intubating laryngeal mask with and without a lightwand: a randomized comparison. *Anaesth Intensive Care.* 2001;29:255-259.

48. Fan KH, Hung OR, Agro F. A comparative study of tracheal intubation using an intubating laryngeal mask (Fastrach) alone or together with a lightwand (Trachlight). *J Clin Anesth.* 2000;12:581-585.

49. Wong DT, Woo JA, Arora G. Lighted stylet-guided intubation via the intubating laryngeal airway in a patient with Hallermann-Streiff syndrome. *Can J Anaesth.* 2009;56:147-150.

50. Dimitriou V, Voyagis GS, Grosomanidis V, Brimacombe J. Feasibility of flexible lightwand-guided tracheal intubation with the intubating laryngeal mask during out-of-hospital cardiopulmonary resuscitation by an emergency physician. *Eur J Anaesthesiol.* 2006;23:76-79.

51. Pandit JJ, MacLachlan K, Dravid RM, Popat MT. Comparison of times to achieve tracheal intubation with three techniques using the laryngeal or intubating laryngeal mask airway. *Anaesthesia.* 2002;57:128-132.

52. Agro FE, Antonelli S, Cataldo R. Use of Shikani flexible seeing stylet for intubation via the intubating laryngeal mask airway. *Can J Anaesth.* 2005;52:657-658.

53. Osborn IP. The intubating laryngeal mask airway (ILMA) is assisted by an old device. *Anesth Analg.* 2000;91:1561-1562.

54. Rich JM. Recognition and management of the difficult airway with special emphasis on the intubating LMA-Fastrach/whistle technique: a brief review with case reports. *Proc (Bayl Univ Med Cent).* 2005;18:220-227.

55. Frappier J, Guenoun T, Journois D, et al. Airway management using the intubating laryngeal mask airway for the morbidly obese patient. *Anesth Analg.* 2003;96:1510-1515, table of contents.

56. Roblot C, Ferrandiere M, Bierlaire D, et al. Impact of Cormack and Lehane's grade on intubating laryngeal mask airway Fastrach using: a study in gynaecological surgery. *Ann Fr Anesth Reanim.* 2005;24:487-491.

57. Asai T, Matsumoto H, Shingu K. Awake tracheal intubation through the intubating laryngeal mask. *Can J Anaesth.* 1999;46:182-184.

58. Mason AM. Use of the intubating laryngeal mask airway in pre-hospital care: a case report. *Resuscitation.* 2001;51:91-95.

59. Gercek E, Wahlen BM, Rommens PM. In vivo ultrasound real-time motion of the cervical spine during intubation under manual in-line stabilization: a comparison of intubation methods. *Eur J Anaesthesiol.* 2008;25:29-36.

60. Langeron O, Semjen F, Bourgain JL, Marsac A, Cros AM. Comparison of the intubating laryngeal mask airway with the fiberoptic intubation in anticipated difficult airway management. *Anesthesiology.* 2001;94:968-972.

61. Henderson JJ, Popat MT, Latto IP, Pearce AC. Difficult Airway Society guidelines for management of the unanticipated difficult intubation. *Anaesthesia.* 2004;59:675-694.

62. Liu EH, Goy RW, Lim Y, Chen FG. Success of tracheal intubation with intubating laryngeal mask airways: a randomized trial of the LMA Fastrach and LMA CTrach. *Anesthesiology.* 2008;108:621-626.

63. Keller C, Brimacombe J, Kleinsasser A, Loeckinger A. Does the ProSeal laryngeal mask airway prevent aspiration of regurgitated fluid? *Anesth Analg.* 2000;91:1017-1020.

64. Handa-Tsutsui F, Kodaka M. Propofol concentration requirement for laryngeal mask airway insertion was highest with the ProSeal, next highest with the Fastrach, and lowest with the Classic type, with target-controlled infusion. *J Clin Anesth.* 2005;17:344-347.

65. Kodaka M, Okamoto Y, Koyama K, Miyao H. Predicted values of propofol EC50 and sevoflurane concentration for insertion of laryngeal mask Classic and ProSeal. *Br J Anaesth.* 2004;92:242-245.

66. Hwang JW, Park HP, Lim YJ, Do SH, Lee SC, Jeon YT. Comparison of two insertion techniques of ProSeal laryngeal mask airway: standard versus 90-degree rotation. *Anesthesiology.* 2009;110:905-907.

67. Howath A, Brimacombe J, Keller C. Gum-elastic bougie-guided insertion of the ProSeal laryngeal mask airway: a new technique. *Anaesth Intensive Care.* 2002;30:624-627.

68. Eschertzhuber S, Brimacombe J, Hohlrieder M, et al. Gum elastic bougie-guided insertion of the ProSeal laryngeal mask airway is superior to the digital and introducer tool techniques in patients with simulated difficult laryngoscopy using a rigid neck collar. *Anesth Analg.* 2008;107:1253-1256.

69. O'Connor CJ, Jr., Stix MS. Place the bubble solution with your fingertip. *Anesth Analg.* 2002;94:763-764.

70. O'Connor CJ, Jr., Borromeo CJ, Stix MS. Assessing ProSeal laryngeal mask positioning: the suprasternal notch test. *Anesth Analg.* 2002;94:1374-1375; author reply 1375.

71. Cook TM, Nolan JP. Failed obstetric tracheal intubation and postoperative respiratory support with the proseal laryngeal mask airway. *Anesth Analg.* 2005;100:290; author reply 290-291.

72. Cook TM, Brooks TS, Van der Westhuizen J, Clarke M. The Proseal LMA is a useful rescue device during failed rapid sequence intubation: two additional cases. *Can J Anaesth.* 2005;52:630-633.

73. Brimacombe J, Keller C. Aspiration of gastric contents during use of a ProSeal laryngeal mask airway secondary to unidentified foldover malposition. *Anesth Analg.* 2003;97:1192-1194, table of contents.

74. Cook TM, Lee G, Nolan JP. The ProSeal laryngeal mask airway: a review of the literature. *Can J Anaesth.* 2005;52:739-760.

75. Keller C, Brimacombe J. Mucosal pressure and oropharyngeal leak pressure with the ProSeal versus laryngeal mask airway in anaesthetized paralysed patients. *Br J Anaesth.* 2000;85:262-266.

76. Goldmann K, Jakob C. Size 2 ProSeal laryngeal mask airway: a randomized, crossover investigation with the standard laryngeal mask airway in paediatric patients. *Br J Anaesth.* 2005;94:385-389.

77. Goldmann K, Jakob C. A randomized crossover comparison of the size 2½ laryngeal mask airway ProSeal versus laryngeal mask airway-Classic in pediatric patients. *Anesth Analg.* 2005;100:1605-1610.

78. Goldmann K, Roettger C, Wulf H. Use of the size 3 ProSeal laryngeal mask airway in children. Results of a randomized crossover investigation with the Classic laryngeal mask airway. *Anaesthesist.* 2006;55:148-153.

79. Goldmann K, Roettger C, Wulf H. The size 1(1/2) ProSeal laryngeal mask airway in infants: a randomized, crossover investigation with the Classic laryngeal mask airway. *Anesth Analg.* 2006;102:405-410.

80. Micaglio M, Bonato R, De Nardin M, et al. Prospective, randomized comparison of ProSeal and Classic laryngeal mask airways in anaesthetized neonates and infants. *Br J Anaesth.* 2009;103:263-267.

81. Lopez-Gil M, Brimacombe J, Garcia G. A randomized non-crossover study comparing the ProSeal and Classic laryngeal mask airway in anaesthetized children. *Br J Anaesth.* 2005;95:827-830.

82. Goldmann K, Roettger C, Wulf H. Use of the ProSeal laryngeal mask airway for pressure-controlled ventilation with and without positive end-expiratory pressure in paediatric patients: a randomized, controlled study. *Br J Anaesth.* 2005;95:831-834.

83. Maltby JR, Beriault MT, Watson NC, et al. The LMA-ProSeal is an effective alternative to tracheal intubation for laparoscopic cholecystectomy. *Can J Anaesth.* 2002;49:857-862.

84. Hohlrieder M, Brimacombe J, von Goedecke A, Keller C. Postoperative nausea, vomiting, airway morbidity, and analgesic requirements are lower for the ProSeal laryngeal mask airway than the tracheal tube in females undergoing breast and gynaecological surgery. *Br J Anaesth.* 2007;99:576-580.

85. Brimacombe J, Keller C. Awake fibreoptic-guided insertion of the ProSeal laryngeal mask airway. *Anaesthesia.* 2002;57:719.

86. Brown NI, Mack PF, Mitera DM, Dhar P. Use of the ProSeal laryngeal mask airway in a pregnant patient with a difficult airway during electroconvulsive therapy. *Br J Anaesth.* 2003;91:752-754.

87. Awan R, Nolan JP, Cook TM. Use of a ProSeal laryngeal mask airway for airway maintenance during emergency Caesarean section after failed tracheal intubation. *Br J Anaesth.* 2004;92:144-146.

88. Keller C, Brimacombe J, Lirk P, Puhringer F. Failed obstetric tracheal intubation and postoperative respiratory support with the ProSeal laryngeal mask airway. *Anesth Analg.* 2004;98:1467-1470, table of contents.

89. Vaida SJ, Gaitini LA. Another case of use of the ProSeal laryngeal mask airway in a difficult obstetric airway. *Br J Anaesth.* 2004;92:905; author reply 905.

90. Asai T, Murao K, Shingu K. Efficacy of the ProSeal laryngeal mask airway during manual in-line stabilisation of the neck. *Anaesthesia.* 2002;57:918-920.

91. Genzwuerker HV, Roth H, Schmeck J. Comparing laryngeal mask airway ProSeal and laryngeal tube. *Anesth Analg.* 2003;96:1535; author reply 1535-1536.

92. Verghese C, Ramaswamy B. LMA-Supreme—a new single-use LMA with gastric access: a report on its clinical efficacy. *Br J Anaesth.* 2008;101:405-410.

93. Ali A, Canturk S, Turkmen A, et al. Comparison of the laryngeal mask airway Supreme and laryngeal mask airway Classic in adults. *Eur J Anaesthesiol.* 2009;26:1010-1014.

94. Lee AK, Tey JB, Lim Y, Sia AT. Comparison of the single-use LMA supreme with the reusable ProSeal LMA for anaesthesia in gynaecological laparoscopic surgery. *Anaesth Intensive Care.* 2009;37:815-819.

95. Hosten T, Gurkan Y, Ozdamar D, et al. A new supraglottic airway device: LMA-supreme, comparison with LMA-Proseal. *Acta Anaesthesiol Scand.* 2009;53:852-857.

96. Agro F, Frass M, Benumof JL, Krafft P. Current status of the Combitube: a review of the literature. *J Clin Anesth.* 2002;14:307-314.

97. Frass M, Frenzer R, Zdrahal F, et al. The esophageal tracheal combitube: preliminary results with a new airway for CPR. *Ann Emerg Med.* 1987;16:768-772.

98. Urtubia R, Aguila C. Combitube: a new proposal for a confusing nomenclature. *Anesth Analg.* 1999;89:803.

99. Urtubia RM, Aguila CM, Cumsille MA. Combitube: a study for proper use. *Anesth Analg.* 2000;90:958-962.

100. Walz R, Davis S, Panning B. Is the Combitube a useful emergency airway device for anesthesiologists? *Anesth Analg.* 1999;88:233.

101. Butler BD, Little T, Drtil S. Combined use of the esophageal-tracheal Combitube with a colorimetric carbon dioxide detector for emergency intubation/ventilation. *J Clin Monit.* 1995;11:311-316.

102. Wafai Y, Salem MR, Baraka A, et al. Effectiveness of the self-inflating bulb for verification of proper placement of the Esophageal Tracheal Combitube. *Anesth Analg.* 1995;80:122-126.

103. Frass M, Frenzer R, Rauscha F, Schuster E, Glogar D. Ventilation with the esophageal tracheal combitube in cardiopulmonary resuscitation. Promptness and effectiveness. *Chest.* 1988;93:781-784.

104. Frass M, Frenzer R, Mayer G, et al. Mechanical ventilation with the esophageal tracheal combitube (ETC) in the intensive care unit. *Arch Emerg Med.* 1987;4:219-225.

105. Bishop MJ, Kharasch ED. Is the Combitube a useful emergency airway device for anesthesiologists? *Anesth Analg.* 1998;86:1141-1142.

106. Brimacombe J, Berry A. The oesophageal tracheal combitube for difficult intubation. *Can J Anaesth.* 1994;41:656-657.

107. Mercer M. The role of the Combitube in airway management. *Anaesthesia.* 2000;55:394-395.

108. Staudinger T, Tesinsky P, Klappacher G, et al. Emergency intubation with the Combitube in two cases of difficult airway management. *Eur J Anaesthesiol.* 1995;12:189-193.

109. Banyai M, Falger S, Roggla M, et al. Emergency intubation with the Combitube in a grossly obese patient with bull neck. *Resuscitation.* 1993;26:271-276.

110. Deroy R, Ghoris M. The Combitube elective anesthetic airway management in a patient with cervical spine fracture. *Anesth Analg.* 1998;87:1441-1442.

111. Klauser R, Roggla G, Pidlich J, Leithner C, Frass M. Massive upper airway bleeding after thrombolytic therapy: successful airway management with the Combitube. *Ann Emerg Med.* 1992;21:431-433.

112. American Society of Anesthesiologists Task Force on Management of the Difficult Airway. Practice guidelines for the difficult airway. *Anesthesiology.* 1993;78:597-602.

113. Bercker S, Schmidbauer W, Volk T, et al. A comparison of seal in seven supraglottic airway devices using a cadaver model of elevated esophageal pressure. *Anesth Analg.* 2008;106:445-448, table of contents.

114. Krafft P, Roggla M, Fridrich P, et al. Bronchoscopy via a redesigned Combitube in the esophageal position. A clinical evaluation. *Anesthesiology.* 1997;86:1041-1045.

115. Calkins TR, Miller K, Langdorf MI. Success and complication rates with prehospital placement of an esophageal-tracheal combitube as a rescue airway. *Prehosp Disaster Med.* 2006;21:97-100.

116. Vezina D, Lessard MR, Bussieres J, et al. Complications associated with the use of the Esophageal-Tracheal Combitube. *Can J Anaesth.* 1998;45:76-80.

117. Zamora JE, Saha TK. Combitube rescue for Cesarean delivery followed by ninth and twelfth cranial nerve dysfunction. *Can J Anaesth.* 2008;55:779-784.

118. Bagheri SC, Stockmaster N, Delgado G, et al. Esophageal rupture with the use of the Combitube: report of a case and review of the literature. *J Oral Maxillofac Surg.* 2008;66:1041-1044.

119. McGlinch BP, Martin DP, Volcheck GW, Carmichael SW. Tongue engorement with prolonged use of the esophageal-tracheal Combitube. *Ann Emerg Med.* 2004;44:320-322.

120. Frass M, Rodler S, Frenzer R, et al. Esophageal tracheal combitube, endotracheal airway, and mask: comparison of ventilatory pressure curves. *J Trauma.* 1989;29:1476-1479.

121. Agro F, Cataldo R, Alfano A, Galli B. A new prototype for airway management in an emergency: the Laryngeal Tube. *Resuscitation.* 1999;41:284-286.

122. Asai T, Shingu K. The laryngeal tube. *Br J Anaesth.* 2005;95:729-736.

123. Dorges V, Ocker H, Wenzel V, Schmucker P. The laryngeal tube: a new simple airway device. *Anesth Analg.* 2000;90:1220-1222.

124. Huter L, Schwarzkopf K, Rodiger J, et al. Students insert the laryngeal tube quicker and more often successful than the esophageal-tracheal combitube in a manikin. *Resuscitation.* 2009;80:930-934.

125. Tumpach EA, Lutes M, Ford D, Lerner EB. The King LT versus the Combitube: flight crew performance and preference. *Prehosp Emerg Care.* 2009;13:324-328.

126. Finteis T, Genzwuerker HV, Hinkelbein J, et al. LMA-Unique, SoftSeal, LTD and LaryVent: bench model comparison of 4 single-use supraglottic airway devices to facemask ventilation. *Respiration.* 2004;21:65(A-262).

127. Wiese CH, Bahr J, Graf BM. "Laryngeal Tube-D" (LT-D) and "Laryngeal Mask" (LMA)]. *Dtsch Med Wochenschr.* 2009;134:69-74.

128. Genzwuerker HV, Fritz A, Hinkelbein J, et al.Prospective, randomized comparison of laryngeal tube and laryngeal mask airway in pediatric patients. *Paediatr Anaesth.* 2006;16:1251-1256.

129. Asai T, Murao K, Shingu K. Efficacy of the laryngeal tube during intermittent positive-pressure ventilation. *Anaesthesia.* 2000;55:1099-1102.

130. Marquez X, Marquez A. A new laryngeal tube. *Anesth Analg.* 2003;96:1842.

131. Asai T, Kawachi S. Pressure exerted by the cuff of the laryngeal tube on the oropharynx. *Anaesthesia.* 2001;56:911-912.

132. Agro FE, Galli B, Cataldo R, et al. Relationship between body mass index and ventilation with the Laryngeal Tube(R) in 228 anesthetized paralyzed patients: a pilot study. *Can J Anaesth.* 2002;49:641-642.

133. Bortone L, Ingelmo PM, De Ninno G, et al. Randomized controlled trial comparing the laryngeal tube and the laryngeal mask in pediatric patients. *Paediatr Anaesth.* 2006;16:251-257.

134. Genzwuerker HV, Vollmer T, Ellinger K. Fibreoptic tracheal intubation after placement of the laryngeal tube. *Br J Anaesth.* 2002;89:733-738.

135. Dörges V, Francksen H, Bein B, et al. Disposable laryngeal tube vs. laryvent. *Anesthesiology.* 2004;101:A568.

136. Johnson R, Bailie R. Airway management device (AMD) for airway control in percutaneous dilatational tracheostomy. *Anaesthesia.* 2000;55:596-597.

137. Cook T, Nolan JP, Gupta KJ, Gabbott DA. The Airway Management Device (AMD) is not "reliable and safe". *Anaesthesia.* 2002;57:291.

138. Mandal NG. A new device has to be safe and reliable too. *Anaesthesia.* 2001;56:382-383.

139. Pay LL, Lim Y. Comparison of the modified Airway Management Device with the Proseal laryngeal mask airway in patients undergoing gynaecological procedures. *Eur J Anaesthesiol.* 2006;23:71-75.

140. Hooshangi H, Wong DT. Brief review: the Cobra Perilaryngeal Airway (CobraPLA) and the Streamlined Liner of Pharyngeal Airway (SLIPA) supraglottic airways. *Can J Anaesth.* 2008;55:177-1785.

141. Agro F, Barzoi G, Carassiti M, Galli B. Getting the tube in the oesophagus and oxygen in the trachea: preliminary results with the new supraglottic device (Cobra) in 28 anaesthetised patients. *Anaesthesia.* 2003;58:920-921.

142. Agro F, Carassiti M, Barzoi G, et al. A first report on the diagnosis and treatment of acute postoperative airway obstruction with the CobraPLA. *Can J Anaesth.* 2004;51:640-641.

143. Gaitini L, Yanovski B, Somri M, et al. A comparison between the PLA Cobra and the Laryngeal Mask Airway Unique during spontaneous ventilation: a randomized prospective study. *Anesth Analg.* 2006;102:631-636.

144. Kusaka Y, Uda R, Son H, Akatsuka M. Successful fiberoptic tracheal intubation via Cobra PLA in a patient with an epiglottic tumor. *Masui.* 2009;58:474-476.

145. Wronska-Sewruk A, Nestorowicz A, Kowalczyk M. Classic laryngeal mask airway vs COBRA-PLA device for airway maintenance during minor urological procedures. *Anestezjol Intens Ter.* 2009;41:73-77.

146. Andrews DT, Williams DL, Alexander KD, Lie Y. Randomised comparison of the Classic Laryngeal Mask Airway with the Cobra Perilaryngeal Airway during anaesthesia in spontaneously breathing adult patients. *Anaesth Intensive Care.* 2009;37:85-92.

147. Galvin EM, van Doorn M, Blazquez J, et al. A randomized prospective study comparing the Cobra Perilaryngeal Airway and Laryngeal Mask Airway-Classic during controlled ventilation for gynecological laparoscopy. *Anesth Analg.* 2007;104:102-105.

148. Park SH, Han SH, Do SH, et al. The influence of head and neck position on the oropharyngeal leak pressure and cuff position of three supraglottic airway devices. *Anesth Analg.* 2009;108:112-117.

149. Agro F, Barzoi G, Galli B. The CobraPLA in 110 anaesthetized and paralysed patients: what size to choose? *Br J Anaesth.* 2004;92:777-778.

150. Khan RM, Maroof M, Johri A, et al. Cobra PLA can overcome LMA failure in patients with face and neck contractures. *Can J Anaesth.* 2005;52:340.

151. van Zundert A, Brimacombe J, Kamphuis R, Haanschoten M. The anatomical position of three extraglottic airway devices in patients with clear airways. *Anaesthesia.* 2006;61:891-895.

152. Cook TM, Lowe JM. An evaluation of the Cobra Perilaryngeal Airway: study halted after two cases of pulmonary aspiration. *Anaesthesia.* 2005;60:791-796.

153. Farrow C, Cook T. Pulmonary aspiration through a Cobra PLA. *Anaesthesia.* 2004;59:1140-1141; discussion 1141-1142.

154. Miller DM, Lavelle M. A streamlined pharynx airway liner: a pilot study in 22 patients in controlled and spontaneous ventilation. *Anesth Analg.* 2002;94:759-761, table of contents.

155. Miller DM, Light D. Laboratory and clinical comparisons of the Streamlined Liner of the Pharynx Airway (SLIPA) with the laryngeal mask airway. *Anaesthesia.* 2003;58:136-142.

156. Lange M, Smul T, Zimmermann P, Kohlenberger R, Roewer N, Kehl F. The effectiveness and patient comfort of the novel streamlined pharynx airway

liner (SLIPA) compared with the conventional laryngeal mask airway in ophthalmic surgery. *Anesth Analg.* 2007;104:431-434.

157. Greenberg RS, Toung T. The cuffed oropharyngeal airway—a pilot study. *Anesthesiology.* 1992;77:A558.

158. Agro F, Cataldo R, Carassiti M, et al. COPA as an aid for tracheal intubation. *Resuscitation.* 2000;44:181-185.

159. Brimacombe JR, Brimacombe JC, Berry AM, et al. A comparison of the laryngeal mask airway and cuffed oropharyngeal airway in anesthetized adult patients. *Anesth Analg.* 1998;87:147-152.

160. Girgin NK, Kahveci SF, Yavascaoglu B, Kutlay O. A comparison of the laryngeal mask airway and cuffed oropharyngeal airway during percutaneous dilatational tracheostomy. *Saudi Med J.* 2007;28:1139-1141.

161. Dimitriou V, Voyagis GS, Iatrou C, Brimacombe J. The PAxpress is an effective ventilatory device but has an 18% failure rate for flexible lightwand-guided tracheal intubation in anesthetized paralyzed patients. *Can J Anaesth.* 2003;50:495-500.

162. Mondello E, Casati A. A prospective, observational evaluation of a new supraglottic airway: the PAXpress. *Minerva Anestesiol.* 2003;69:517-522, 522-525.

163. Casati A, Vinciguerra F, Spreafico E, et al. The new PA(Xpress) airway device during mechanical ventilation in anaesthetized patients: a prospective, randomized comparison with the laryngeal mask airway. *Eur J Anaesthesiol.* 2004;21:667-669.

164. Intersurgical: i-gel User Guide. 2009.

165. Gabbott DA, Beringer R. The iGEL supraglottic airway: a potential role for resuscitation? *Resuscitation.* 2007;73:161-162.

166. Liew G, John B, Ahmed S. Aspiration recognition with an i-gel airway. *Anaesthesia.* 2008;63:786.

167. Gibbison B, Cook TM, Seller C. Case series: protection from aspiration and failure of protection from aspiration with the i-gel airway. *Br J Anaesth.* 2008;100:415-417.

168. Gatward JJ, Cook TM, Seller C, et al. Evaluation of the size 4 i-gel airway in one hundred non-paralysed patients. *Anaesthesia.* 2008;63:1124-1130.

169. Schmidbauer W, Bercker S, Volk T, Bogusch G, Mager G, Kerner T. Oesophageal seal of the novel supralaryngeal airway device I-Gel in comparison with the laryngeal mask airways Classic and ProSeal using a cadaver model. *Br J Anaesth.* 2009;102:135-139.

170. Jackson KM, Cook TM. Evaluation of four airway training manikins as patient simulators for the insertion of eight types of supraglottic airway devices. *Anaesthesia.* 2007;62:388-393.

171. Richez B, Saltel L, Banchereau F, et al. A new single use supraglottic airway device with a noninflatable cuff and an esophageal vent: an observational study of the i-gel. *Anesth Analg.* 2008;106:1137-1139, table of contents.

172. Michalek P, Hodgkinson P, Donaldson W. Fiberoptic intubation through an I-gel supraglottic airway in two patients with predicted difficult airway and intellectual disability. *Anesth Analg.* 2008;106:1501-1504, table of contents.

173. Joshi NA, Baird M, Cook TM. Use of an i-gel for airway rescue. *Anaesthesia.* 2008;63:1020-1021.

174. Sharma S, Scott S, Rogers R, Popat M. The i-gel airway for ventilation and rescue intubation. *Anaesthesia.* 2007;62:419-420.

SELF-EVALUATION QUESTIONS

12.1. Which of the following is **NOT** true about the laryngeal tube (King LT)?

A. It cannot be used in patients with a history of latex allergy.

B. The laryngeal tube has two cuffs (pharyngeal and esophageal), but a single balloon for pressure control.

C. The laryngeal tube requires a mouth opening of at least 23 mm for its insertion.

D. The laryngeal tube cuffs should be inflated to a pressure up to 60 cm H_2O using a manometer if possible.

E. A well-lubricated endotracheal tube can be passed blindly through the airway lumen of the LT.

12.2. Which of the following is **NOT** true with the use of the laryngeal mask airway?

A. In general, approximately 20 mL is required to inflate the cuff for a #3, 30 mL for a #4, and 40 mL for a #5 LMA.

B. The LMA should be inserted into the mouth with the index finger placed between the mask-tube junction.

C. The LMA cuff should be pressed against the hard palate during the insertion into the oropharynx.

D. Prior to insertion, the cuff should be completely deflated.

E. To facilitate placement, the LMA should be lubricated using lidocaine gel.

12.3. In comparison with tracheal intubation, which of the following is **NOT** an advantage of the LMA?

A. improved hemodynamic stability on induction and during emergence

B. no risk of gastric aspiration

C. reduced anesthetic requirements for airway tolerance

D. lower frequency of coughing during emergence

E. a lower incidence of sore throat in adults

CHAPTER (13)

Surgical Airway

Gordon O. Launcelott and Liane B. Johnson

13.1 INTRODUCTION

In 1799, as George Washington lay dying of life threatening upper airway obstruction, one of his physicians, Elisha Cullen Dick, argued against further bloodletting and for tracheotomy. In retrospect this was the only lifesaving option available. It was not attempted and the President succumbed.[1]

Indications for surgical airway access vary from the elective through to impending airway compromise, and finally to the true emergency *cannot intubate, cannot oxygenate* scenario. This chapter will deal primarily with techniques of surgical airway access that the practitioner can use to deal with the difficult airway that presents either in the form of impending airway compromise or, the life-threatening emergency.

13.1.1 Why cricothyrotomy and not tracheotomy?

The higher complication rate of emergency tracheotomy, compared to cricothyrotomy,[2] results from the fact that the trachea is situated deeper in the neck, the posterior tracheal wall lacks the protection of a circumferential cricoid cartilage (increasing the risk of esophageal perforation), there is a greater abundance of adjacent vascular structures, and there is a proximity of the thyroid gland and lung. The palpable, often visible, surface landmarks of the thyroid and cricoid cartilages and the ability to accomplish the task faster, with a minimum of equipment, make emergency cricothyrotomy more attractive than tracheotomy, for the surgeon and nonsurgeon alike.[3]

As a consequence, all of the techniques to be discussed with the exception of percutaneous dilational tracheotomy (see Chapter 31) and possibly needle insufflation in children will involve access to the airway through the cricothyroid membrane (CTM).

13.1.2 What is the history of cricothyrotomy?

Surgical access to the airway has its origins in ancient times but it was the pandemic of *morbus strangulatorius* in Europe at the beginning of the 19th century that began its modern evolution. The French surgeon, Pierre Bretonneau, first attempted to relieve the laryngeal obstruction of this infectious laryngo-tracheal bronchitis by tracheotomy in 1818, finally meeting with success in 1825.[4] His paper, published in 1826, gave the disease entity the name diphtheria,[5] from the Greek *diphthera* meaning leather. This was in recognition of the thick, leathery, blue-white upper respiratory tract membranes characteristic of the disease.[6] In the 20 years that followed, Armand Trousseau, Joseph Récamier, and MP Guersant, honed the technical aspects of bronchotomy[7]—laryngotomy and tracheotomy—and by 1851 Trousseau published his experience in 222 cases, 127 of whom survived.[8]

In the United States, Chevalier Jackson published further refinements to the technique in 1909.[9] Ten years later (1921), he published a paper attributing the devastating complication of subglottic stenosis to high tracheotomy, concluding that the only acceptable point of access to the airway was below the first tracheal ring and that high tracheotomy should be abandoned.[10] Jackson was a figure of immense authority[11] and it is not surprising that high tracheotomy, or cricothyrotomy, was relegated to almost total obscurity for close to five decades.

Brantigan and Grow[3] renewed interest in the approach following publication of their 1976 paper. The impetus for the study came from anecdotal experience during the early days of cardiac surgery. Grow, a student of Chevalier Jackson, looked to cricothyrotomy as a way to avoid contamination of median sternotomy wounds by pathogens tracking down the shared mediastinal tissue planes from open tracheotomy sites. He began performing cricothyrotomy, initially in emergency situations, and later electively when it was evident to him that subglottic stenosis did not appear to be a problem.

Grow and Brantigan reported their experience in 655 cricothyrotomies performed over an 8-year period. Duration of intubation ranged from 1 to less than 40 days, with an average of 7 days. Their results showed minimal complications and no cases of subglottic stenosis. Subsequently, several authors,[12-14] including a recent prospective study,[15] reported similar findings in patients not previously subjected to prolonged endotracheal intubation, or suffering from any acute laryngeal pathology. Talving et al reviewed 30 years (between 1978 and 2008) of published literature to determine the rates of subglottic stenosis following emergency cricothyrotomy.[16] Twenty studies (17 retrospective reports and 3 prospective, observational series) with a total of 1124 patients, including 368 trauma patients, were reviewed. With follow-up periods ranging between 2 and 60 months, the rate of subglottic stenosis among survivors was 2.2 % and 1.1% among emergency trauma patients.[16] While acknowledging that a well-designed prospective investigation is needed, the authors concluded that no study to date has demonstrated any benefit of routine conversion to tracheotomy.

The discrepancy between the observations of Jackson in the 1920s and the modern authors results from several factors that reflect the two eras, separated by over half a century. Most of the surgical indications for a surgical airway in Jackson's era were inflammatory in nature; cricothyrotomy in the presence of inflammation is now well recognized to predispose to subglottic stenosis. In addition, high tracheotomy was a much more complex procedure than the modern cricothyrotomy, involving division of the cricoid or thyroid cartilages. The lack of antibiotics, and the primitive design of the tracheostomy tubes available in the 1920s, undoubtedly compounded the situation.[17]

As cricothyrotomy is more advantageous for its speed, safety, and simplicity,[18] access through the CTM is the technique of choice in emergency surgical airway management.

In spite of literature to the contrary, the devastating complication of subglottic stenosis associated with cricothyrotomy still compels most clinicians to convert to tracheotomy as soon as possible.

13.1.3 What anatomy do I have to know to perform these procedures?

Access to the airway through the CTM requires a practical knowledge of the anatomy of the larynx, particularly the surface landmarks, as well as the important adjacent structures in the neck.

In most adult males, the thyroid notch (Adam's apple) is a prominent feature, which identifies the superior aspect of the thyroid cartilage. With the neck extended, palpation inferiorly from this point will often allow the practitioner to identify the inferior margin of the thyroid cartilage and the ring-shaped cricoid

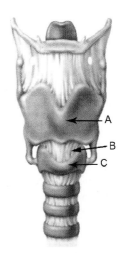

FIGURE 13-1. Anatomy of the larynx and trachea: (A) the thyroid cartilage; (B) the cricothyroid membrane; and (C) the cricoid cartilage.

cartilage below (Figure 13-1). Between the inferior margin of the thyroid and the cricoid cartilages is the CTM. The size of the membrane in adults is 22 to 33 mm wide and 9 to 10 mm high.[19] The vocal cords are attached to the internal anterior surface of the thyroid cartilage, approximately 1 cm above the upper border of the cricothyroid membrane.[20] Care should be exercised in placing instruments superior to the cricothyroid incision for this reason. The only important vascular structure in the vicinity of the CTM is the superior thyroid artery, which, in 54% of people, courses on its lateral border.[21] The left and right cricothyroid arteries, branches of their respective superior thyroid arteries, course medially and traverse the upper half of the CTM,[21] anastomosing in the midline. Injury to this vessel can be avoided by entering the CTM in its inferior half. Caution also dictates that the incision should not extend laterally greater than 1 cm.[17]

Other important anatomical structures include the hyoid bone and the thyroid gland and isthmus. The airway itself is suspended by the hyoid bone lying superior to the thyroid cartilage. Identifying the hyoid bone is important to avoid mistaking the thyrohyoid space for the cricothyroid membrane. In patients with poorly palpable surface anatomy, the location of the hyoid bone can be estimated by extending a line from the mentum posteriorly, half the distance between the mentum and the angle of the mandible.[22]

The thyroid gland has a pyramidal lobe, in 40% of patients[23] that may extend as high as the hyoid bone and could be at risk of injury during cricothyrotomy.

13.1.4 How can I predict whether access through the CTM will be difficult?

Although there is no formal evidence, it is intuitive that anything interfering with either physical access to the larynx, or the ability to appreciate the landmarks of the larynx, will make CTM puncture difficult. This includes factors such as previous surgery, fixed cervical spine flexion deformity, hematoma, obesity, radiation to the neck, laryngotracheal malignancy, or tumor. **SHORT** (Surgery/Spine, Hematoma, Obesity, Radiation, and Tumor) is a useful mnemonic to remind practitioners of the factors that may be associated with a difficult surgical airway (see Section 1.6.4).

13.1.5   So, what do I need to do to get ready?

The following are common to all techniques of surgical access by way of the CTM:

a. Antisepsis and local anesthetic infiltration: If time permits, every effort should be made to use aseptic technique and infiltrate the proposed surgical site with local anesthetic.

b. Positioning the patient: The patient is ideally placed in the supine sniffing position, with the head extended to best expose the surface landmarks of the larynx. In an emergency situation, particularly in the setting of severe upper airway obstruction, it may be necessary to position the patient semi-recumbent, or fully erect.

c. Immobilization of the larynx and identification of the CTM: Immobilization of the larynx and identification of the CTM is most effectively accomplished by the right-handed practitioner standing on the right side of the patient. The left (nondominant) hand is used to stabilize the larynx by grasping the body of the thyroid cartilage between the thumb and middle finger, leaving the index finger free to palpate the cartilaginous structures (Figure 13-2). If the laryngeal notch is palpable, the index finger is moved caudad along the thyroid cartilage, in the midline, until the fingertip dips off its inferior aspect. Should surface landmarks be difficult to appreciate, the level of the cricothyroid membrane can be estimated as follows: with the head in neutral position, the fifth finger is placed in the suprasternal notch; with all fingers in juxtaposition, the location of the index finger will approximate the level of the CTM.[24] In addition, skin creases in the anterior neck may represent a useful visual landmark for estimating the level of the CTM. Hung et al demonstrated that with the head in the neutral position, in patients with two neck creases inferior to the mentum, the second skin crease was a median distance of 2.0 mm above the cricoid cartilage (Figure 13-3).[25]

For transtracheal catheter and Seldinger techniques, some right-handed practitioners will choose to stand over the right shoulder or at the head of the patient, immobilizing the larynx and identifying

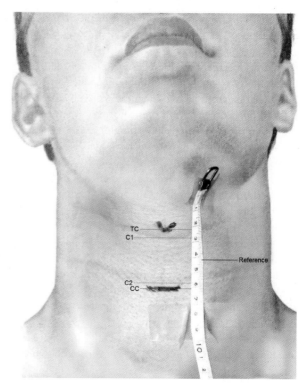

FIGURE 13-3. Surface landmarks of the anterior neck: thyroid cartilage (TC), first skin crease below mentum (C1), second skin crease below mentum (C2), and cricoid cartilage (CC).

the CTM, as described earlier. Others will choose to stand on the left side of the patient for these techniques, immobilizing the larynx and identifying the CTM with the left hand from below. This permits the practitioner to use the right hand to pass implements through the CTM in a caudad direction and in a more dextrous fashion. Primary immobilization of the larynx by the left hand, from below, also minimizes trauma to the thyroid cartilage by promoting retraction of the cricoid ring inferiorly, rather than superior retraction on the thyroid cartilage.

13.2   TECHNIQUES

Five methods of surgical access to the airway will be outlined:

1. Open cricothyrotomy
2. Seldinger cricothyrotomy
3. Transtracheal catheter ventilation
4. Percutaneous dilational tracheotomy

13.2.1   Can you walk me through each method...step by step?

13.2.1.1   Open Cricothyrotomy

Equipment: The instruments required are a scalpel with a #11 blade; a tracheal hook; Armand Trousseau dilator; and a 5.0 mm ID cuffed endotracheal tube, or a small, cuffed tracheotomy tube (Figure 13-4).

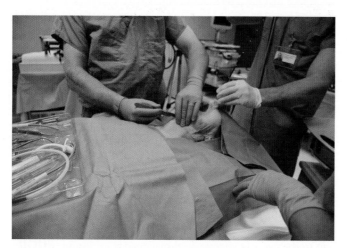

FIGURE 13-2. Open cricothyrotomy in a cadaver: The left (nondominant) hand is used to stabilize the larynx by grasping the body of the thyroid cartilage between the thumb and middle finger, leaving the index finger free to palpate the cartilaginous structures.

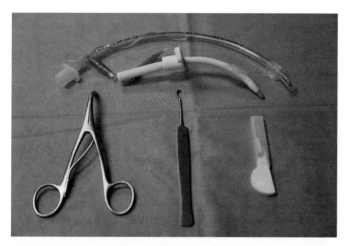

FIGURE 13-4. Equipment required for an open cricothyrotomy: a scalpel with a #11 blade; a tracheal hook; Armand Trousseau dilator; and a small, cuffed tracheal tube (or a cuffed tracheotomy tube).

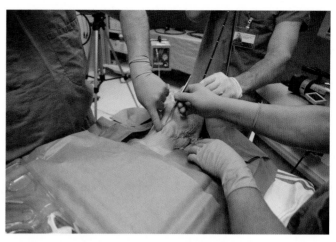

FIGURE 13-6. Open cricothyrotomy in a cadaver: retraction with a tracheal hook superiorly.

Technique: It should be clearly appreciated by the practitioner that the technique of emergency cricothyrotomy is primarily a tactile and *not* a visual technique. With the patient positioned and landmarks identified, the following are steps to a successful standard surgical cricothyrotomy technique:

1. A 4.0 cm vertical, midline skin incision (Figure 13-5)
2. A transverse incision of the CTM at the superior border of the cricoid cartilage
3. Retraction with a tracheal hook (Figure 13-6) either superiorly, with potential trauma to the vocal cords or thyroid cartilage, or inferiorly, with less risk and perhaps better exposure
4. Insertion of the Trousseau dilator (Figure 13-7)
5. Caudal placement of a 5.0 mm ID cuffed endotracheal tube, or a small, cuffed tracheotomy tube (Figure 13-8)
6. Inflation of the cuff, ensuring the proper position and removal of the hook and dilator

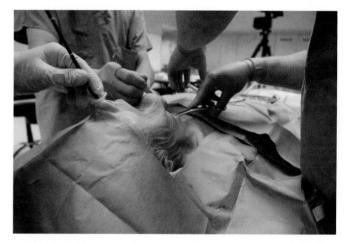

FIGURE 13-7. Open cricothyrotomy in a cadaver: insertion of the Trousseau dilator.

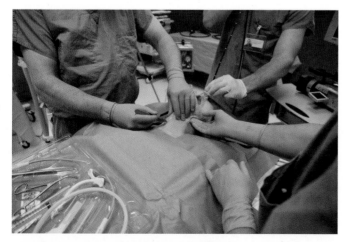

FIGURE 13-5. Open cricothyrotomy in a cadaver: A 4 cm vertical, midline skin incision is made followed by a transverse incision of the CTM at the superior border of the cricoid cartilage.

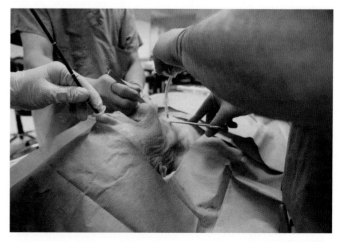

FIGURE 13-8. Open cricothyrotomy in a cadaver: The tracheotomy tube is inserted into the trachea through the Trousseau dilator.

Prior to securing the tube, it is important to confirm proper placement by ETCO$_2$ and/or by auscultation. A chest X-ray should be obtained, as soon as conveniently possible, to determine adequate tube position and to rule out any parenchymal lung injury, or pneumothorax. Current recommendations view a cricothyrotomy as a temporizing, lifesaving measure. The patient should undergo conversion to a traditional tracheotomy once stabilized.

13.2.1.2 Seldinger Cricothyrotomy Technique

The majority of practitioners are familiar with the Seldinger technique and most will be more comfortable with this approach.

> Equipment: There are several cricothyrotomy kits designed with this technique in mind and all with similar contents. They contain a scalpel blade, a syringe, an 18-gauge catheter over needle and/or a thin-walled introducer needle, a guidewire, a dilator, and a cuffed airway catheter (Figure 13-9).

> Technique: As access to the airway is achieved through the cricothyroid membrane, the anatomic considerations and patient positioning are the same as for open cricothyrotomy. The technique is summarized as follows:

1. Vertical midline stab incision through the skin overlying the CTM.

2. Caudal insertion of an 18-gauge needle attached to a syringe (Figure 13-10).

3. Confirmation of needle placement by aspirating air, followed by removal of the needle and syringe.

4. Insertion of the guidewire (Figure 13-11) and removal of the catheter, leaving the guidewire in the trachea.

5. After making a small cut of the CTM along the guidewire (Figure 13-12), the cuffed airway catheter loaded onto the dilator is advanced as a single unit, over the wire and into the airway (Figures 13-13 and 13-14).

6. Removal of the dilator and securement of the tube.

7. Confirmation of proper tube placement by ETCO$_2$ and/or by auscultation.

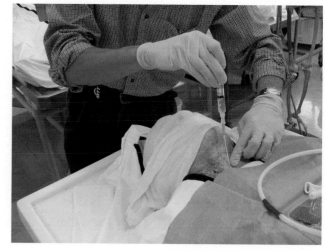

FIGURE 13-10. Seldinger cricothyrotomy in a cadaver: Following a vertical midline stab incision through the skin overlying the CTM, an 18-gauge needle attached to a syringe is inserted through the CTM.

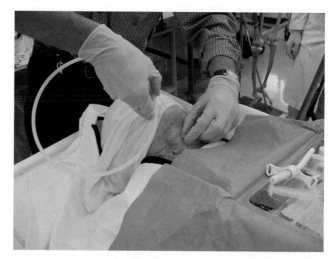

FIGURE 13-11. Seldinger cricothyrotomy in a cadaver: After confirming accurate needle placement by aspirating air, the needle and syringe are removed. A guidewire is inserted into the trachea through the catheter.

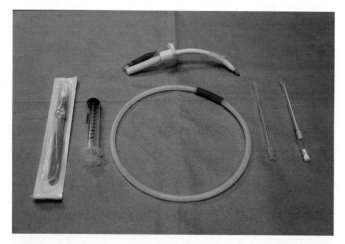

FIGURE 13-9. Equipment for Seldinger cricothyrotomy: a scalpel blade, a syringe, an 18-gauge catheter over needle and/or a thin-walled introducer needle, a guidewire, a dilator, and a cuffed airway catheter.

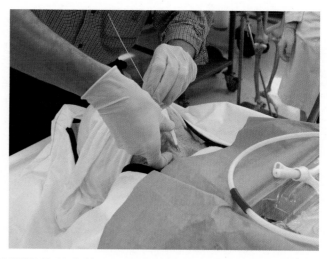

FIGURE 13-12. Seldinger cricothyrotomy in a cadaver: A small cut of the CTM is made along the guidewire.

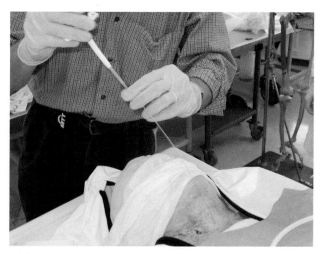

FIGURE 13-13. The airway catheter loaded onto the dilator is advanced as a single unit through the guidewire.

It should be noted that the Universal Cook Critical Care Melker Cricothyrotomy kit contains equipment to perform both open and Seldinger techniques. Once again, current teaching recommends securing a formal tracheotomy, once the patient is stabilized.

13.2.1.3   Transtracheal Catheter Ventilation

The passage of a 12 to 14 gauge catheter through the CTM for the purposes of establishing an emergency airway is a temporizing method at best. It provides short-term oxygenation until a definitive airway can be established. Many variations of this technique have been used in general relation to availability of equipment. One such technique is summarized as follows:

1. Caudal insertion of 14 g IV catheter, with syringe attached, through the CTM

2. Confirmation of position by aspiration air, and advancement of the catheter to its hub, while removing the needle and syringe

3. Oxygenation utilizing one of several options

4. Ensuring that there is sufficient time for egress of gas, in order to prevent hypercapnea/hypoxia and air trapping

Options that are available for delivery of O_2 include jet ventilation, the O_2 flush valve on the anesthetic machine, and the anesthesia circuit itself. As mentioned, it is essential that there is sufficient time and an available route for egress of gas. An assistant should be instructed to manage the upper airway with all necessary maneuvers, including LMA, or other airway, and appropriate airway maneuvers.

Gaufberg and Workman recommend that ventilation with this technique should not exceed 20 minutes in adults and 40 minutes in children.[26] It is also the only recommended emergency surgical airway, other than tracheotomy, in children under the age of 12 years.

13.2.1.3.1   Transtracheal Jet Ventilation

For the purposes of simplicity, only classic transtracheal jet ventilation (TTJV) and TTJV with the ENK modulator will be considered here.

Many operating rooms have access to a commercially available jet ventilator, consisting of a high-pressure connector, high-pressure hosing, an in-line regulator, a jet ventilation toggle switch, and a Luer-Lock connector. This device is powered by central wall oxygen at 50 psi (15 L·min⁻¹) and subject to an in-line regulator. Activation of the toggle switch, in a controlled fashion, allows oxygen to be safely jetted through the transtracheal catheter into the airway.

An O_2 tank regulator powers another form of TTJV system, with similar high-pressure hosing, jet injector, and Luer-Lock connector. A low flow tank regulator, as on the E cylinder O_2 transport tanks, can achieve a maximum pressure of 120 psi with the flow meter set at 15 L·min⁻¹. When the jet is activated briefly, very high flows are generated and can result in satisfactory tidal volumes through 14-gauge catheters over 0.5 second.[27]

For all systems, chest rise and fall, and the pulse oximeter response, are noted as a measure of ventilatory adequacy.

13.2.1.3.2   ENK Flow Modulator

The ENK flow modulator (Figure 13-15) permits transtracheal ventilation by tubing connected to the O_2 flush valve on an anesthesia machine, or on a wall-mounted flow meter. The device is

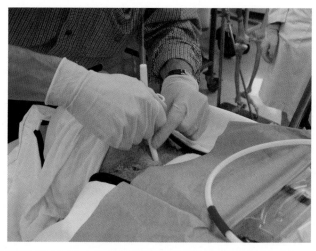

FIGURE 13-14. The airway catheter loaded onto the dilator is advanced through the guidewire into the trachea.

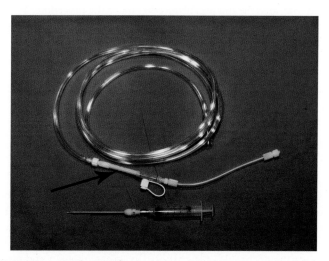

FIGURE 13-15. The ENK flow modulator: The device is equipped with a series of five holes (arrow) that can be occluded in a measured fashion to direct flow through the device to the patient.

equipped with a series of five holes that can be occluded in a measured fashion to direct flow through the device to the patient. As with TTJV, chest rise and fall is noted as a measure of ventilatory adequacy.

13.2.1.4   Percutaneous Dilational Tracheotomy

There is an increase in popularity of using percutaneous dilational tracheotomy (PDT) following Ciaglia's[28] 1985 publication. Limited to elective, bedside procedures, the current widespread use of this technique has revealed it to be safe, rapid, with minimal overall procedural morbidity.[15] In fact, the overall complication rate is low and comparable to traditional surgical tracheotomy.[29]

The procedure was initially performed as a blind technique relying on knowledge of surface landmarks. Adjuncts, such as the lightwand[30] (Trachlight™, Laerdal Medical Inc., Wappingers Falls, NY) and the flexible bronchoscope (FFB), can enhance the ease of performing the procedure while minimizing complications, such as paratracheal placement of the tracheotomy tube, pneumothorax, and loss of airway control upon withdrawal of the ETT.[31]

A summary of the Seldinger-based procedure with the Ciaglia Blue Rhino (Cook Inc., Bloomington, IN) is as follows:

1. Skin incision and palpation of cricoid and proximal tracheal rings
2. Flexible bronchoscopic (FB) visualization to retract the ETT and monitor insertion of a catheter over needle device between the second and third, or third and fourth, tracheal rings
3. Application of the Seldinger technique with J-guidewire and a single tapered dilator
4. Insertion of a size-appropriate tracheostomy tube
5. Confirmation of the intratracheal placement with the FB

PDT should be performed by a team of experienced practitioners familiar with the use of the FB and with the traditional surgical approach. Avoidance of the obese patient with poorly defined neck anatomy, acute laryngeal pathology, complete airway obstruction, previous neck surgery, or C-spine flexion deformity will increase the overall success rate of the procedure. For a complete review, and application of the technique, please refer to Chapter 31.

13.3   OTHER CONSIDERATIONS

13.3.1   Are there any contraindications to performing a surgical airway?

In the emergency situation when gas exchange cannot be established, a surgical airway is mandatory to prevent catastrophe. As such, there are no contraindications to a surgical airway. There are, however, certain issues that deserve consideration.

In acute or chronic inflammatory laryngeal pathology, and neoplastic disease, cricothyrotomy will likely be more difficult to perform and be subject to a greater incidence of subglottic stenosis.

Obesity, injuries, and deformities of the neck may either distort the anatomy and/or render surface landmarks difficult to palpate; and uncontrolled hemorrhage may complicate the situation in the anticoagulated patient. Cricotracheal separation is an absolute contraindication to any procedures that utilize the CTM.

13.3.2   What are the concerns in establishing a surgical airway in patients with a deep neck infection?

Deep space neck infections are most common in the extremes of age. Underlying medical problems often accompany the afflicted elderly patient. Deep space infections can either variably occlude, or shift the airway, rendering what should be an easily managed airway into an emergency. Caution dictates that airway management should be performed in a controlled environment, preferably the operating room. A CT scan, if feasible, would greatly facilitate understanding of the altered anatomy, but this may not be feasible in the severely compromised airway.

In the moderately affected airway, topical anesthesia and awake FB-assisted intubation is the method of choice. If the airway is severely compromised, with total airway obstruction a possibility, an awake surgical airway is the procedure of choice—to ensure a secure airway until the infection and its source can be treated.

13.3.3   Do you have any concerns in establishing a surgical airway in children?

In children, as the laryngeal prominence does not develop until adolescence, surface landmarks are more difficult to palpate. The vertical dimension of the cricothyroid membrane is considerably smaller in children than adults, with the result that an endotracheal tube may permanently damage the cartilaginous structures. There is an increased risk that the cricoid cartilage, the only completely circumferential supporting laryngeal structure, and the narrowest part of the airway in the child, may be damaged. In addition, the airway of the child is more malleable, making posterior perforation a greater risk and the laryngeal mucosa more vulnerable to injury and subglottic stenosis.[17] For all of these reasons, in an emergency situation, if transglottic tracheal tube placement cannot be accomplished, needle cricothyrotomy, or tracheotomy, is the method of choice in children 12 years of age or younger.[32]

13.3.4   What are the pros and cons of using noncuffed and cuffed tracheal tube for surgical airway?

The greatest risk of prolonged cricothyrotomy intubation is the development of subglottic stenosis (SGS). Underlying medical illness and/or an element of gastro-esophageal reflux, in conjunction with the mechanical disruption of intubation, may contribute to the development of SGS. Modern tracheostomy tubes are less likely to produce an inflammatory response in the mucosal airway, while low-pressure cuffs reduce mechanical trauma and its sequelae.

Cuffed tubes provide a seal in the airway to allow delivery of larger tidal volumes with lower airway pressures. However, cuffed tubes may be more difficult to insert in an emergency situation, due to their bulk and the risk of snagging the cuff on the edge of the surgical incision. This may tear the cuff and prevent an effective seal. It is critical that the simplest, safest, speediest, and most effective technique be used to reestablish an airway. Thus, a small, noncuffed tube would be adequate for the primary goal of salvage and provision of oxygenation.

As patients requiring a surgical airway may have decreased lung compliance, positive pressure ventilation through a noncuffed ETT can result in gas escaping from the proximal airway, resulting in inadequate ventilation. For this reason either the Cook cuffed airway catheter or #5 cuffed ETT are the tracheal tubes of choice when establishing an emergency surgical airway.

13.4   COMPLICATIONS

13.4.1   What immediate and delayed complications should I be aware of?

In most studies, complication rates are higher for emergency than elective cricothyrotomy. In a series of 38 emergency cricothyrotomies, McGill et al[22] reported an overall complication rate of 40%. The most-frequent complication identified by this group was misplacement of the endotracheal tube through the thyrohyoid membrane (ie, above the larynx), instead of through the CTM. Other complications included execution time greater than 3 minutes, unsuccessful tube placement, and significant hemorrhage. One patient suffered a longitudinal fracture of the thyroid cartilage, due to attempted placement of an 8.0 mm ID tube, resulting in significant long-term morbidity. In a similar series in 1989, Erlandson[33] reported a complication rate of 23%, related primarily to incorrect tube placement (10%) and hemorrhage (8%). Miklus et al[34] reported on 20 patients requiring emergency cricothyrotomy in the field. In this study, there were no complications of tube misplacement, significant hemorrhage, or long-term morbidity in survivors. Gillespie et al reviewed 35 patients requiring emergency surgical airway over a 6-year period and noted no differences in the overall complication rate between emergency tracheotomy and cricothyrotomy. Of particular note was that there were no long-term complications in the patients that received cricothyrotomy and were not subsequently converted to tracheotomy.[35]

Although rare, fatal hemorrhages have been reported as a result of laceration of the cricothyroid artery.[36] As this artery courses closer to the thyroid cartilage, there is a greater risk of hemorrhage if the incision is made in the upper half of the CTM.

Other complications include subglottic stenosis, dysphonia due to laryngeal damage, tracheal cartilage fracture, endobronchial intubation, pulmonary aspiration, recurrent laryngeal nerve injury, esophageal perforation, and tracheo-esophageal fistula.[17]

Tissue emphysema (including subcutaneous and mediastinal emphysema) and barotrauma (including tension pneumothorax) have been reported as complications of jet ventilation and establishment of a surgical airway.[37,38] Weymuller[39] cautions that only practitioners experienced with TTJV should attempt it in emergency airway management. He describes kinked or displaced transtracheal catheters, incoordination of respiratory effort, outlet obstruction, and distal airway secretions as the major problems encountered.

13.5   SUMMARY

When confronted with the difficult airway, it should be recognized that there are a multitude of techniques available to the practitioner. The wise practitioner is intimately familiar with the noninvasive techniques of difficult airway management and avoids the temptation to unnecessarily substitute surgical methods for the less invasive approaches.

Even within the parameters of the techniques of surgical airway access, it is evident that the practitioner needs to decide which is most appropriate for the clinical situation at hand. Dilational percutaneous tracheotomy is an elective technique, whereas cricothyrotomy is a technique designed to address the true airway emergency. Some catheter insufflation techniques have the advantage of simplicity but all are temporizing at best. This remains the procedure of choice in children under 12 years, where cricothyrotomy is considered a relative contraindication.

What is of vital importance for the practitioner is to recognize that *cannot intubate, cannot oxygenate* scenario can occur in a variety of clinical settings. As such, the practitioner needs to have in place the necessary knowledge, the necessary equipment, and the clinical confidence to act.

As it is unlikely that sophisticated gadgetry will be available in all circumstances, it is vital for the practitioner to be familiar with the technique that will most likely be successful with the minimum of equipment; this technique is undoubtedly cricothyrotomy. Commercial kits are now available that can be used for either open, or Seldinger techniques, packaged as one. These kits, or a suitable facsimile, should be available in all areas where the expert airway practitioner may be called upon to provide airway management, whether in the operating room, the emergency department, the Intensive Care Unit, or the hospital ward.

REFERENCES

1. Morens DM. Death of a president. *N Engl J Med.* 1999;341:1845-1849.
2. Ger R, Evans JT. Tracheostomy: an anatomico-clinical review. *Clin Anat.* 1993;6:337-341.
3. Brantigan CO, Grow JB, Sr. Cricothyroidotomy: elective use in respiratory problems requiring tracheotomy. *J Thorac Cardiovasc Surg.* 1976;71:72-81.
4. Salmon LF. Tracheostomy. *Proc R Soc Med.* 1975;68:347-356.
5. Brettoneau P. *Des Inflammations Speciales du Tissu Muquex.* Paris: Cr evot; 1826.
6. Merriam-Webster Online Dictionary. http://www.m-w.com/cgi-bin/dictionary?book=Dictionary&va=diphtheria&x=14&y=16.
7. Alberti PW. Tracheotomy versus intubation. A 19th century controversy. *Ann Otol Rhinol Laryngol.* 1984;93:333-337.
8. Trousseau A. Nouvelles recherches sur la tracheotomie. Paris: Halteste;1851.
9. Jackson C. Tracheotomy. *Laryngoscope.* 1909;19:285-290.
10. Jackson C. High tracheotomy and other errors: the chief cause of chronic laryngeal stenosis. *Gynaecol Obstet.* 1921;32:392.
11. Clerf LH. Chevalier Jackson. *Arch Otolaryngol.* 1966;83:292-296.
12. Boyd AD, Romita MC, Conlan AA, et al. A clinical evaluation of cricothyroidotomy. *Surg Gynecol Obstet.* 1979;149:365-368.

13. Greisz H, Qvarnstorm O, Willen R. Elective cricothyroidotomy: a clinical and histopathological study. *Crit Care Med.* 1982;10:387-389.

14. Holst M, Hedenstierna G, Kumlien JA, Schiratzki H. Elective coniotomy. A prospective study. *Acta Otolaryngol.* 1983;96:329-235.

15. Francois B, Clavel M, Desachy A, et al. Complications of tracheostomy performed in the ICU: subthyroid tracheostomy vs surgical cricothyroidotomy. *Chest.* 2003;123:151-158.

16. Talving P, DuBose J, Inaba K, Demetriades D. Conversion of emergent cricothyrotomy to tracheotomy in trauma patients. *Arch Surg.* 2010;145:87-91.

17. Boon JM, Abrahams PH, Meiring JH, Welch T. Cricothyroidotomy: a clinical anatomy review. *Clin Anat.* 2004;17:478-486.

18. Mace SE. Cricothyrotomy. *J Emerg Med.* 1988;6:309-319.

19. Kress TD, Balasubramaniam S. Cricothyroidotomy. *Ann Emerg Med.* 1982;11:197-201.

20. Bennett JD, Guha SC, Sankar AB. Cricothyrotomy: the anatomical basis. *J R Coll Surg Edinb.* 1996;41:57-60.

21. Dover K, Howdieshell TR, Colborn GL. The dimensions and vascular anatomy of the cricothyroid membrane: relevance to emergent surgical airway access. *Clin Anat.* 1996;9:291-295.

22. McGill J, Clinton JE, Ruiz E. Cricothyrotomy in the emergency department. *Ann Emerg Med.* 1982;11:361-364.

23. Blumberg NA. Observations on the pyramidal lobe of the thyroid gland. *S Afr Med J.* 1981;59:949-950.

24. Walls RM. Cricothyroidotomy. *Emerg Med Clin North Am.* 1988;6:725-736.

25. Hung OR, Kwofie K, Hung CR, Hung DR. The use of neck surface landmarks ("Launcelott creases"). 14th World Congress of Anesthesiologists. 2008.

26. Gaufberg SV, Workman TP. New needle cricothyroidotomy setup. *Am J Emerg Med.* 2004;22:37-39.

27. Gaughan SD, Ozaki GT, Benumof JL. A comparison in a lung model of low- and high-flow regulators for transtracheal jet ventilation. *Anesthesiology.* 1992;77:189-199.

28. Ciaglia P, Firsching R, Syniec C. Elective percutaneous dilatational tracheostomy. A new simple bedside procedure: preliminary report. *Chest.* 1985;87:715-719.

29. Feller-Kopman D. Acute complications of artificial airways. *Clin Chest Med.* 2003;24:445-455.

30. Addas BM, Howes WJ, Hung OR. Light-guided tracheal puncture for percutaneous tracheostomy. *Can J Anaesth.* 2000;47:919-922.

31. Freeman BD, Isabella K, Lin N, Buchman TG. A meta-analysis of prospective trials comparing percutaneous and surgical tracheostomy in critically ill patients. *Chest.* 2000;118:1412-1418.

32. Elliott WG. Airway management in the injured child. *Int Anesthesiol Clin.* 1994;32:27-46.

33. Erlandson MJ, Clinton JE, Ruiz E, Cohen J. Cricothyrotomy in the emergency department revisited. *J Emerg Med.* 1989;7:115-118.

34. Miklus RM, Elliott C, Snow N. Surgical cricothyrotomy in the field: experience of a helicopter transport team. *J Trauma.* 1989;29:506-508.

35. Gillespie MB, Eisele DW. Outcomes of emergency surgical airway procedures in a hospital-wide setting. *Laryngoscope.* 1999;109:1766-1769.

36. Schillaci CR, Iacovoni VF, Conte RS. Transtracheal aspiration complicated by fatal endotracheal hemorrhage. *N Engl J Med.* 1976;295:488-490.

37. Sanchez TF. Retrograde intubation. Anesthesiology. *Clin N Am.* 1995;13:439-476.

38. Smith RB, Schaer WB, Pfaeffle H. Percutaneous transtracheal ventilation for anaesthesia and resuscitation: a review and report of complications. *Can Anaesth Soc J.* 1975;22:607-612.

39. Weymuller EA, Jr, Pavlin EG, Paugh D, Cummings CW. Management of difficult airway problems with percutaneous transtracheal ventilation. *Ann Otol Rhinol Laryngol.* 1987;96:34-37.

SELF-EVALUATION QUESTIONS

13.1. All of the following are reported complications of a surgical airway **EXCEPT**

   A. hemorrhage

   B. fracture of the thyroid cartilage

   C. subglottic stenosis

   D. vocal cord damage

   E. mediastinal emphysema

13.2. Which of the following is **NOT** a useful predictor of a difficult cricothyrotomy?

   A. fixed cervical spine flexion deformity

   B. previous surgery of the neck

   C. previous radiation to the neck

   D. neck hematoma

   E. female gender

13.3. Which of the following is **NOT** true about establishing a surgical airway in children?

   A. A greater risk of posterior perforation while performing a surgical airway in children.

   B. A greater incidence of subglottic stenosis.

   C. The laryngeal prominence does not develop until adolescence.

   D. The height of the cricothyroid membrane is considerably larger in children than adults.

   E. Increase risk of cricoid cartilage damage.

SECTION ③ — Case Studies in Difficult and Failed Airway Management

CHAPTER 14

What Is Unique about Airway Management in the Prehospital Setting?

Mark Vu, David Petrie, John M. Tallon, and Michael F. Murphy

14.1 CASE PRESENTATION

On a stormy night in the countryside, a 72-year-old male driver falls asleep at the wheel and strays into oncoming traffic. A transport truck trying to avoid him strikes his small car. The car is crushed with the driver trapped inside. Emergency medical services (EMS) are activated. Basic life support (BLS) medics and firefighters arrive on scene within 10 minutes. The patient is conscious with a Glasgow Coma Score of 13, BP 80/40 mm Hg, HR 100 bpm, RR 26 breaths per minute, and O_2 saturations of 82% prior to oxygen therapy.

14.2 UNIQUE PREHOSPITAL ISSUES

14.2.1 What level of airway management can we expect from prehospital care providers?

"A" is the cornerstone in the ABCs, which form the foundation of BLS training for all prehospital care providers. The type of training and skill sets vary significantly from country to country and the provider mix varies from one jurisdiction to the next in any country. For clarity, we will define four discrete levels of airway management provided in an EMS system. Each level assumes proficiency in the skills of the previous one:

- First aid providers or "first responders"—trained to apply supplemental O_2 by face mask and perform artificial ventilation, typically bag-mask-ventilation (BMV), although in some jurisdictions extraglottic devices (EGDs) may be preferred at this level as first-line devices in place of BMV.

- BLS providers—more experienced with BMV, and these providers use EGDs, particularly Combitube™, King LT™, and Laryngeal Mask Airways (LMA) in some systems.

- Advanced life support (ALS) providers—typically perform laryngoscopy and endotracheal intubation with or without the use of facilitating drugs, such as sedative-hypnotics and neuromuscular blocking agents.

- Critical care providers (eg, typically air medical transport or critical care transport team members)—are permitted to perform rapid sequence intubation (RSI) using a laryngoscope and, usually, other advanced airway techniques such as cricothyrotomy. In some jurisdictions (most notably Europe and Australia), physicians are often members of these teams.

14.2.2 How are airway management protocols and equipment determined in prehospital care systems?

In most North American systems, prehospital care providers perform delegated medical acts based on standardized medical protocols. In many European systems, physicians may be the usual prehospital care providers and, therefore, are less likely to be dependent on protocols. While protocols ought to reflect best clinical evidence, from a practical perspective they are often limited by cost, training, competency maintenance, and space constraints.

Protocols approved by the medical director of the EMS system determine the equipment necessary in prehospital care practice.

The type and range of equipment available for managing the difficult airway in the prehospital setting are typically limited when compared to emergency department (ED) and operating room settings. Even the availability of basic equipment such as the endotracheal tube introducer (ETI; eg, the intubating stylet or the Eschmann tracheal introducer, also know as the gum-elastic bougie),[1] laryngoscope blades, and endotracheal tubes (ETT) in an array of types and sizes may be limited. Alternate intubating devices, such as the Intubating Laryngeal Mask Airway (ILMA or LMA Fastrach™) or lightwands (eg, Trachlight™), often are not available due to cost, resterilization, and issues of skills maintenance. Rescue devices, such as the esophageal–tracheal Combitube™, Laryngeal Mask Airway Classic (LMAC), and the LMA Unique™ (the disposable LMA), are becoming more popular because they are relatively inexpensive, disposable, and easy to use.[2,3] However, extra-tracheal ventilation devices may not be appropriate in some clinical situations, particularly if adequate ventilation calls for an increase in peak airway pressure beyond the seal capabilities of the device, if the patient is sufficiently responsive to reject the device, or if protection against aspiration is mandatory.[4] Surgical airway management devices[5] must be available in any system providing RSI. Critical care EMS systems often differ from many ground systems because they carry more advanced equipment, such as the Glidescope® video laryngoscope, or other devices.

14.2.3   What unique environmental considerations do prehospital care providers face when managing the airway?

The airway provider is often confronted with an array of circumstances unique to the field environment:

- A chaotic scene
- A dangerous scene (eg, flood, fire, radiation, electrical wires down, toxic environment, assailant on the loose, etc)
- Access to the patient and the airway which may be challenging due to a variety of factors:
  - An ongoing extrication
  - Position of the patient (eg, seated, upside down, etc). In nontrauma airway management, positioning may also present a problem (eg, intubation performed lying prone and leaning on the elbows). Even with the patient on a stretcher in an ambulance or helicopter, an ideal position for airway management may be difficult to achieve.
- Other uncontrollable environmental conditions:
  - Darkness inhibits full airway assessment and obscures subtle nonverbal communication cues among providers.
  - Bright sunlight may present similar problems, especially when tracheal intubation is performed using a laryngoscope or a lighted stylet.
  - Extremes of weather may present problems for both patient and care provider
  - An uncontrolled violent scene in which tactical EMS may be deployed with police required to limit access to patients.

- Spectators, family, or friends of patients may require skilled handling.
- Lack of other essential equipment for airway management, for example, suction.
- Uncontrolled human behavior in the prehospital setting may further interfere with airway management decisions and procedures:
  - Distraught relatives challenge the focus of prehospital care providers.
  - Knowledgeable and skilled assistants are seldom available.
  - Well-meaning first-aid providers or bystander physicians may hamper efforts with inappropriately timed comments or actions.

Finally, management of an airway in the prehospital environment may have to be carried out in the most adverse of surroundings and circumstances, for example, a crime scene, on a dance floor, in a stadium, and so on.

Back to our case: ALS responders arrive on the scene 15 minutes later. The patient's level of consciousness is falling and he remains hypotensive. BLS providers have skillfully assisted ventilations with the BMV while other skilled rescuers attempt to extricate the patient from the wreckage. The GCS is now 9, BP 80/40 mm Hg, HR 120 bpm, and O_2 saturation 88%.

14.3   AIRWAY CONSIDERATIONS

14.3.1   What are the patient factors that influence airway management decisions of a prehospital care provider?

There are three related elements governing airway management in the field environment: time, anatomy, and the clinical state of the patient.

14.3.1.1   Time Factors: When Is It Better to Wait?

All emergency airway management situations share this feature. In other words, they are context sensitive (see Chapter 6). Consider, for example, the following two cases:

- A 40-year-old man with sudden collapse, GCS 6, with no cough or swallowing reflex, O_2 saturations of 99%, and normal airway anatomy.
- The same 40-year-old man in a house fire who has stridor, O_2 saturations of 70%, and evidence of upper airway burns. Both patients have clear indications for securing the airway, though the approach in the prehospital setting would be quite different.

In the first patient above, the decision to intubate immediately will depend upon the anatomical assessment and time considerations. For example, if the transport time to a hospital is very short, it might be prudent to wait (ie, maximize O_2 with BMV, protect with suction) until arrival at the ED where a proper and controlled neuroprotective RSI can be done. Training must emphasize that airway management means gas exchange and it does not always require intubation. We must avoid the trap of the *technical imperative*—just because it can be done, it should be done. In fact, there is growing evidence that in certain situations prehospital intubation may not necessarily improve outcome.[6,7]

On the other hand, in the second patient, despite predicted difficulty with laryngoscopy, time is critical. A quick decision must be made and the provider must confidently follow the Emergency Difficult Airway Algorithm (Figure 2-5, Chapter 2).

14.3.1.2 Anatomic Factors: Predicting the Difficult Airway

The airway assessment is essentially an attempt to predict difficult laryngoscopy and intubation, difficult bag-mask-ventilation, difficult EGD, and difficult cricothyrotomy based on an examination of external anatomic features (see Sections 1.6.1, 1.6.2, 1.6.3, and 1.6.4). This evaluation is as crucial a component of prehospital airway management as it is in hospital. It permits the airway provider to make appropriate airway management plans (Plans A, B, and C) that are most likely to be successful.

The patient with acceptable oxygen saturations and a short transport time displaying predictors of difficult laryngoscopy and intubation might be better served by a rapid transport to the nearest ED with more resources. Should clinical or time considerations preclude this, the Emergency Difficult Airway Algorithm directs one to weigh carefully whether RSI, sedation, or awake intubation would be most appropriate. If any of these is unsuccessful, one should move promptly to the Failed Airway Algorithm (Chapter 2, Figure 2-6). Situations in which difficulty is predicted and airway management is urgently indicated are better handled by an early call through dispatch for scene backup.

Most prehospital ALS and critical care providers are familiar with the necessity for an airway evaluation prior to each intubation, particularly if medications are to be administered to facilitate the procedure. However, this may be limited to predictors of difficult laryngoscopy and intubation rather than difficulty in other airway techniques (see Chapter 1), such as difficult mask-ventilation and difficult surgical airway.

14.3.1.3 Clinical Factors: How Do the Clinical Condition and Presumed Diagnosis Affect Airway Management Decisions?

There are two clinical considerations in managing a difficult airway in the field setting: the indication for intubation and the underlying pathology.

Indications for endotracheal intubation in the prehospital environment are similar to those in any other emergency.[8]

1. Failure to maintain adequate oxygenation
2. Failure to maintain adequate ventilation (CO_2 removal)
3. Failure to protect the airway
4. The need for neuromuscular blockade
5. The anticipated clinical course

In practice, many patients may have more than one indication for intubation.

Underlying pathology: The indications for intubation among various EMS systems may differ. The most common indication (up to two-thirds of all intubations) in a typical ground EMS system is cardiac arrest.[9] The remainder tend to be split evenly among respiratory failure (asthma, chronic obstructive lung disease, congestive heart failure, pulmonary embolism, pneumonia, anaphylaxis), nontrauma CNS conditions (coma, intracranial bleed/stroke, seizure, overdose), trauma (head injury, chest injury, neck injury, blood loss causing shock), and shock states (sepsis, cardiogenic, hypovolemic).

Helicopter EMS (HEMS) (also called rotorcraft air medical transport [AMT]) rarely responds to primary cardiac arrest. These critical care teams are trained to manage cases that require more advanced airway procedures.

In certain circumstances, a patient may have an indication for intubation but circumstances, such as predicted difficult airway and a short transport time to the ED, may sanction BMV and suction until intubation is possible. The weighing of risk versus benefit is illustrated in the example above (40-year-old man with a collapse and a short transport time vs burn with long transport time). Even in the face of an accepted indication for intubation, the potential benefits of prehospital intubation must be weighed within the context of time, anatomic and clinical factors.

14.3.2 What alternatives do prehospital providers have in managing a difficult airway?

Effective BMV technique (including two-handed mask hold requiring two providers if available or necessary) is essential to the prehospital care provider, particularly when the airway could be difficult and the transport time is relatively brief.

Despite considerable controversy in the literature, the gold standard for definitive airway control remains the correct intratracheal placement of a cuffed ETT. According to the "Recommended Guidelines for Uniform Reporting of Data from Out-Of-Hospital Airway Management,"[10] there are four methods by which this can be achieved: direct oral laryngoscopy and intubation, nasotracheal intubation, oral rescue techniques (eg, LMA), and surgical rescue techniques (transtracheal jet ventilation and cricothyrotomy). These four methods may each be modified by five variables:

- Oral approach—no facilitating sedative drugs or paralytics
- Nasal approach—no facilitating sedative drugs or paralytics
- Sedation-facilitated intubation—without the use of paralytics
- RSI—with the use of paralytics and induction agents
- Other intubation techniques (eg, digital, lighted stylet, etc)

The actual number of options available to a given EMS system is limited by protocols, training, and equipment.

There is ample evidence that endotracheal intubation is not a benign intervention in the hands of inexperienced personnel.[11-13] Newer airway devices such as the LMA, King LT™, and the Combitube™ have been introduced and validated in the prehospital care setting.[4,14-20] These devices may be employed in two ways: as an alternative to endotracheal intubation in the cardiac arrest (or deeply comatose) patient by BLS providers[4,15,19,21] or as a rescue device in the setting of failed intubation by ALS or critical care providers.[14,16]

An emerging alternative to endotracheal intubation in the respiratory failure patient is prehospital noninvasive ventilation. Several case series have shown continuous positive airway pressure (CPAP) or bi-level ventilation to be feasible and potentially beneficial in the prehospital setting.[22-24] Further study is necessary to validate its effectiveness and safety.

14.3.3   What are the challenges in terminology associated with prehospital airway management?

Increasing attention is being paid to the many aspects of prehospital airway management. Research, discussion, education, and innovation in both devices and approaches have expanded. It is quite apparent that one approach does not fit all clinical situations in the ideal in-hospital environment, so it is folly to assume that it is less complex in the prehospital setting in which there are more variables to consider. The clinical choices involved in airway management in the field setting may well be limited by personnel training, the realities of maintaining competence, and the devices and drugs available to field personnel. Using patient outcome, rather than procedural outcome as the measure of success of airway management, one can begin to construct some useful definitions.

Inaccurate use of terms in three different risk/benefit clinical issues often make the selection of the best airway management method to proceed with in any clinical situation difficult. The three spectrums of risk/benefit are:

1. Pharmacology: which drug or combination of drugs should be administered?

2. Procedure/equipment: what procedure/equipment to use to facilitate the placement of a device?

3. Device: what device is most appropriate to oxygenate/ventilate the patient?

These confusions often lead to incorrect comparisons in research studies. If these three components are teased out from each other, it becomes apparent that interpretation of the results of a study comparing RSI versus EGDs is difficult in the case of Rapid Sequence Airway (RSA: a technique identical to RSI, only an EGD is employed as opposed to laryngoscopy and intubation).[25] The exact terminology eventually used is less important than the need to achieve consensus and consistency. However, separating these three decision points will be imperative, recognizing that the initial decision or plan may change with evolving clinical situations.

The most obvious use of vague terminology is in the area of the pharmacology of airway management. Many drugs and combinations of drugs can be used in facilitating prehospital airway procedures, particularly in what has been called rapid-sequence intubation,[26] rapid-sequence airway,[25] drug-facilitated intubation,[27] drug-assisted intubation,[28] deep sedation vs awake intubation,[29] and others. For simplicity, these variations can be grouped into three categories:

1. Rapid-sequence, in which paralysis is preceded by an induction agent appropriate to the clinical state of the patient and the situation

2. Sedation, in which the intent is to provide sedation, analgesia, or both

3. Awake, in which topical anesthesia of the upper airway allows for less sedative dose

It might be said that clinically the difference between 2 and 3 above is qualitative; but the intent, and therefore the use of drugs, is clearly different. A lack of understanding of these differences can be both educationally confusing and clinically catastrophic. The use of deep sedation in the patient with a difficult airway without backup plans and essential equipment can lead to apnea, aspiration, a failed airway, and poor patient outcome.

14.3.4   Should tracheal intubation even be performed in the field?

Both in and out of the hospital, inadequate ventilation and oxygenation have been identified as primary contributors to preventable mortality. It would seem reasonable, then, to assume that endotracheal intubation should be the gold standard in prehospital airway management. However, there has been considerable controversy as to whether patients requiring endotracheal intubation should have tracheal intubation performed in the field or deferred until arrival at hospital. There are several issues that arise from this controversy:

• Trauma victims—There continues to be skepticism as to whether the intubation of trauma victims in the field improves survival. During the 1980s, it was generally felt that invasive airway management was ineffective in improving survival in urban environments but might be effective in longer transport environments.[30] Studies published during the nineties gave conflicting results.[31-36] It might, at the very least, be anticipated that endotracheal intubation would be advantageous in patients with severe head injury. Early studies provided no clear direction[7,37-42] and a recent large trauma registry study found that prehospital intubation was associated with adverse outcomes after severe head trauma.[7] However, covariate adjustment in the same study suggests that management of the airway by an air medical team may improve outcomes. Unfortunately, as Zink and Maio pointed out in an accompanying editorial, this is a retrospective association rather than a causation study.[43]

• Cardiac arrest—In cardiac arrest patients, the issue of efficacy of ETT remains unresolved.[44-48] To further add to the controversy, a study involving out-of-hospital cardiac arrest victims showed that patients who received CPR with only chest compressions had comparable survival outcome compared to those who received chest compression and mouth-to-mouth ventilation.[49]

A large prospective study to determine the incremented benefit of introducing ALS (including intubation) to a previously optimized system did not show a mortality benefit in cardiac arrest patients.[50]

- Children—Early studies in children showed that tracheal intubation by paramedics was associated with higher failure and complication rates than that in adults.[51] Results of subsequent studies have confirmed these early findings.[6,32,52-55] The only prospective trial to investigate the effectiveness of ground paramedic in performing tracheal intubation in children showed that there was no increase in survival following endotracheal intubation (ETI) as compared to that in the group treated with BMV.[6] This same study revealed concerns about ETI displacement and inability to recognize this catastrophic complication.[6] Many authorities maintain that these latter studies reflect inadequate training of paramedical personnel in tracheal intubation of children. Furthermore, the literature does not resolve whether the field intubation of children with head injuries improves their outcome.[56,57] In the final analysis, the emergency intubation of children is an uncommon and anxiety-provoking event for most paramedics. Both of these factors are likely to increase performance stress and failure rates, compared to the intubation of adults.

Recent studies have presented data and formed conclusions that challenge the basic, time-honored dogma of EMS airway management and question the best approach to the compromised airway in the prehospital environment. Furthermore, the development of other airway adjuncts (eg, Combitube™, King LT™, LMA™, and CPAP) coupled with a reemphasis on standard BMV has changed the priority for prehospital endotracheal intubation and is a clear sign of maturity and success of the EMS.

It is becoming clear that airway management training and maintenance of competency programs are vital, as they will affect both the psychomotor skill development and decision making. Other issues such as equipment availability, the air versus ground environment, and the logistics associated with rural versus urban critical care transport/EMS suggest that a single, rigid approach to EMS airway management is inappropriate and cannot be supported.

Now to our case: ALS medics are unsuccessful in obtaining a definitive airway. Two IVs have been started and a normal saline (NS) bolus administered. The patient has just been extricated (30 minutes later), boarded, and collared. The HEMS critical care crew has just landed at the scene. The patient now has a GCS of 7, a clenched jaw, BP 90/60 mm Hg, HR 120 bpm, and an O_2 saturation of 90% with assisted BMV with oxygen supplement.

14.4 MANAGEMENT OF THE AIRWAY IN THIS CASE

14.4.1 Prehospital RSI—what does the evidence show?

The HEMS crew on the scene has the training and capability to perform an RSI on appropriate patients as part of their clinical mandate. This includes the use of an induction agent, followed in rapid sequence by a neuromuscular blocking agent in order to optimize intubating conditions to promote successful insertion of an ETT.[26]

Until recently, the evidence in the EMS literature has not supported the use of RSI. Several recent, well-designed studies of ground systems have consistently shown suboptimal outcomes, or no difference in outcome, in patients suffering acute severe head injury in whom RSI is used to facilitate endotracheal intubation.[6,7,12,37,58] Head injury was deliberately chosen in these studies because prior reports have suggested that optimal oxygenation and ventilation of these patients improve outcomes. Therefore, it was assumed that successful endotracheal intubation would demonstrate a benefit.[59] A case-control study of prehospital RSI of the severely head-injured patients in 2003 identified increased mortality and morbidity in the RSI group when compared to patients who had tracheal intubation performed in the ED following transport without RSI.[58]

There have been attempts to determine the reasons for the poor outcomes associated with RSI in ground EMS services.

These explanations have included:

- Increased on-scene time (average 15 minutes in one study)[60]
- Lack of adequate training of the paramedics[6,41,58]
- Inappropriate hyperventilation and unrecognized hypoxia during induction
- Paralysis and attempts at intubation[12]

Despite recent studies showing the lack of efficacy of RSI in the ground EMS systems, a distinct pattern of improved outcomes has emerged in the subpopulation of those patients in whom air medical transport (HEMS) had been utilized.[7,61-64] It would appear that the key to improved outcomes lies in the initial training and maintenance of competence (cognitive and psychomotor skills) for the prehospital providers.

14.4.2 How should a critical care transport team proceed with the management of the airway in this patient?

The HEMS crew elects to perform RSI using succinylcholine (1.5 mg·kg⁻¹) and etomidate (0.2 mg·kg⁻¹). A Grade 3 view of the laryngeal structures is obtained with no improvement of the view with the use of laryngeal manipulation. An Eschmann introducer is placed into the trachea and a 7.5-mm ID ETT is passed over it. A colorimetric end-tidal CO_2 ($ETCO_2$) detector confirms tracheal tube placement. Adequate oxygen saturation is maintained during the procedure, and postintubation systolic blood pressure is 90 mm Hg. To prevent hyperventilation, $ETCO_2$ monitoring is instituted postintubation and during transport.

Other options for the pharmacologic approach to RSI in this patient could include rocuronium as the paralytic (1.0 mg·kg⁻¹); ketamine (thought to be relatively contraindicated in head injury, although there is no evidence to support this) and propofol (relatively contraindicated in hypovolemia) as the induction agents; or a 50-50 mixture of these two induction agents.

Because of its slow onset and associated hypotensive side effects, midazolam is not recommended as an induction agent in EMS. Although the concept of nonparalytic RSI has been enshrined in some EMS systems, tracheal intubation after the administration of an induction agent alone (without paralytic agent) is not supported by the literature and is not generally recommended.[65] In fact, success rates in intubation are generally lower and complications are higher with deep sedation when compared with RSI.[66-68]

It should be emphasized that full C-spine immobilization ought to be maintained during the intubation procedure. In the event tracheal intubation failed, most EMS providers in this setting would use an EGD (eg, King LT™, LMA™, Combitube™). Cricothyrotomy (or an alternative percutaneous technique in young children) is a technique used by most advanced EMS providers. Continuous monitoring of oxygen saturation and ETCO$_2$ should be maintained during transport in order to prevent hypoxemia, inadvertent hyperventilation, or extubation.

14.4.3   How do prehospital providers confirm and maintain intratracheal placement of the ETT?

The consequences of an unrecognized, misplaced ETT may be devastating. Given the chaotic environment, the difficulty in employing the usual clinical verification signs, and the increased movement and transfer of the patient, it is more difficult to recognize an esophageal intubation in the prehospital setting than elsewhere. The exact number of unrecognized esophageal intubations is uncertain since many EMS systems do not gather these data. Inadvertent esophageal intubation rates in EMS have ranged from 1%[69] to 25%[70] based on verification of tube positioning by emergency physicians on arrival at the hospital. Very low rates are found in systems with specific tube verification protocols, ETCO$_2$ monitoring, and ongoing performance improvement to ensure compliance. Unacceptably high rates are found when such protocols are not in place or tube placement verification devices are not available.

Prehospital care providers can confirm correct placement of the ETT in three ways: clinically, with mechanical esophageal detector devices (EDD), or with an ETCO$_2$ detector. Clinical signs include visualization of the tube going through the vocal cords, mist condensation on the ETT, auscultation of lungs and stomach, and so on. Esophageal detection devices (EDDs) may take the form of a bulb or syringe aspiration device (Figures 14-1A and B). Carbon dioxide detectors may be colorimetric (Figure 14-2), digital capnometers, or continuous graphic display capnographs. End-tidal CO$_2$ verification of correct ETT placement is the standard of care in EMS.[71]

The limitations of each of these techniques must be recognized. Carbon dioxide detection techniques tend to be less accurate in identifying correct placement of the ETT in patients with circulatory arrest, with reported false-negative rates (carbon dioxide not detected, tube in the trachea) as high as 30% to 35%.[72] In patients with some circulation, carbon dioxide detection is reliable in confirming correct placement 99% to 100% of the time.[72-76]

Unlike carbon dioxide detection techniques, the EDD is not dependent on the presence of pulmonary blood flow. While some prehospital care systems use this device instead of carbon dioxide

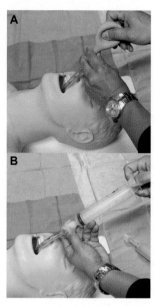

FIGURE 14-1. Esophageal detection devices (EDD): (A) the bulb type of EDD and (B) the syringe type of EDD.

detection, the failure to detect esophageal intubation can be as high as 20%, suggesting that it should not be the only verification method used.[77] Physical examination techniques to verify placement of an ETT in the trachea, while neither sensitive nor specific, remain important adjuncts to carbon dioxide detection and EDD, particularly in patients in cardiac arrest.

Finally, the migration of an ETT from the trachea to the esophagus during transport is an ever-present hazard. It has been demonstrated that the continuous monitoring of exhaled carbon dioxide during the prehospital phase of care minimizes the risk of unrecognized displacement.[78]

In summary, while carbon dioxide detection remains the most reliable method of verifying tracheal placement of the ETT in prehospital care, the use of several methods of confirmation is superior to just one method.

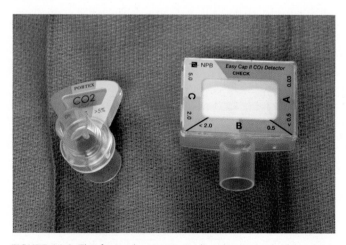

FIGURE 14-2. This figure depicts a typical qualitative end-tidal carbon dioxide detection device.

14.4.4 What is the postintubation care of this patient?

After successful endotracheal intubation, the ETT should be secured properly. It is also important to monitor oxygenation, ventilation, and hemodynamics continuously. Hyperventilation and the associated drop in $PaCO_2$ will adversely impact cerebral perfusion in patients with closed head injuries, and hypotension in head-injured patients has a significant negative impact on survival.[59] It is also critical to consider the additive impacts of positive-pressure ventilation and sedative/hypnotic medications on hemodynamic stability. Transition from negative-pressure, spontaneous ventilation to positive-pressure, assisted ventilation increases intrathoracic pressure and decreases venous return to the heart. In the context of prehospital patients with hypovolemia, this change in respiratory physiology can have a significant negative effect on blood pressure. Moreover, loss of sympathetic tone after induction of anesthesia with hypnotic agents commonly results in a drop in blood pressure. The anticipated change in hemodynamics following intubation should be carefully monitored in order to protect end-organ perfusion. Strategies to support hemodynamics include rapid volume administration (used by BLS and ALS providers) and the use of vasoactive agents, such as phenylephrine (used by CCT or physician providers).

14.5 SUMMARY

Airway management in the prehospital arena is difficult and fraught with realities that are unique to the environment. Individuals who provide prehospital airway management may vary widely in their training and experience. Although BMV is difficult to perform and may be replaced by extraglottic devices which are easier to perform and equally as effective, BMV will continue to play a crucial role in prehospital airway management.

Induction and neuromuscular blocking agents are widely used in prehospital care. It would appear that health-care providers (and systems), who have extensive training in airway management, intubate frequently, and participate in intensive skills maintenance and quality programs have improved intubation success rates and patient outcomes compared to those who do not. As with any airway practitioner employing these procedures, it is crucial that medications are used correctly in appropriate patients (ie, not in patients predicted to have a difficult airway) and the airway practitioner is capable of rescuing the airway (Plan B and Plan C) should Plan A fail (the Failed Airway).

Finally, initial and continuous confirmation of ETT placement by capnometry, the use of EDDs, and clinical methods represent the current standard of care in the prehospital arena.

REFERENCES

1. Phelan MP, Moscati R, D'Aprix T, Miller G. Paramedic use of the endotracheal tube introducer in a difficult airway model. *Prehosp Emerg Care.* 2003;7:244-246.
2. Davis DP, Valentine C, Ochs M, Vilke GM, Hoyt DB. The Combitube as a salvage airway device for paramedic rapid sequence intubation. *Ann Emerg Med.* 2003;42:697-704.
3. Swanson ER, Fosnocht DE, Matthews K, Barton ED. Comparison of the intubating laryngeal mask airway versus laryngoscopy in the Bell 206-L3 EMS helicopter. *Air Med J.* 2004;23:36-39.
4. Rumball CJ, MacDonald D. The PTL, Combitube, laryngeal mask, and oral airway: a randomized prehospital comparative study of ventilatory device effectiveness and cost-effectiveness in 470 cases of cardiorespiratory arrest. *Prehosp Emerg Care.* 1997;1:1-10.
5. Marcolini EG, Burton JH, Bradshaw JR, Baumann MR. A standing-order protocol for cricothyrotomy in prehospital emergency patients. *Prehosp Emerg Care.* 2004;8:23-28.
6. Gausche M, Lewis RJ, Stratton SJ, et al. Effect of out-of-hospital pediatric endotracheal intubation on survival and neurological outcome: a controlled clinical trial. *JAMA.* 2000;283:783-790.
7. Wang HE, Peitzman AB, Cassidy LD, Adelson PD, Yealy DM. Out-of-hospital endotracheal intubation and outcome after traumatic brain injury. *Ann Emerg Med.* 2004;44:439-450.
8. Walls RM. The decision to intubate. In: Walls RM, Murphy MF, eds. *Manual of Emergency Airway Management.* Philadelphia, PA: Lippincott Williams and Wilkins; 2008:1-7.
9. Wang HE, Kupas DF, Paris PM, Bates RR, Yealy DM. Preliminary experience with a prospective, multi-centered evaluation of out-of-hospital endotracheal intubation. *Resuscitation.* 2003;58:49-58.
10. Wang HE, Domeier RM, Kupas DF, Greenwood MJ, O'Connor RE, National Association of EMS Physicians. Recommended guidelines for uniform reporting of data from out-of-hospital airway management: position statement of the National Association of EMS Physicians. *Prehosp Emerg Care.* 2004;8:58-72.
11. Deakin CD. Prehospital management of the traumatized airway. *Eur J Emerg Med.* 1996;3:233-243.
12. Dunford JV, Davis DP, Ochs M, Doney M, Hoyt DB. Incidence of transient hypoxia and pulse rate reactivity during paramedic rapid sequence intubation. *Ann Emerg Med.* 2003;42:721-728.
13. Nolan JD. Prehospital and resuscitative airway care: should the gold standard be reassessed? *Curr Opin Crit Care.* 2001;7:413-421.
14. Blostein PA, Koestner AJ, Hoak S. Failed rapid sequence intubation in trauma patients: esophageal tracheal combitube is a useful adjunct. *J Trauma.* 1998;44:534-547.
15. Calkins MD, Robinson TD. Combat trauma airway management: endotracheal intubation versus laryngeal mask airway versus combitube use by Navy SEAL and Reconnaissance combat corpsmen. *J Trauma.* 1999;46:927-932.
16. Della Puppa A, Pittoni G, Frass M. Tracheal esophageal combitube: a useful airway for morbidly obese patients who cannot intubate or ventilate. *Acta Anaesthesiol Scand.* 2002;46:911-913.
17. Doerges V, Sauer C, Ocker H, Wenzel V, Schmucker P. Airway management during cardiopulmonary resuscitation—a comparative study of bag-valve-mask, laryngeal mask airway and combitube in a bench model. *Resuscitation.* 1999;41:63-69.
18. Dorges V, Ocker H, Wenzel V, et al. Emergency airway management by non-anaesthesia house officers—a comparison of three strategies. *Emerg Med J.* 2001;18:90-94.
19. Genzwuerker HV, Dhonau S, Ellinger K. Use of the laryngeal tube for out-of-hospital resuscitation. *Resuscitation.* 2002;52:221-224.
20. Tanigawa K, Shigematsu A. Choice of airway devices for 12,020 cases of non-traumatic cardiac arrest in Japan. *Prehosp Emerg Care.* 1998;2:96-100.
21. Tanigawa K, Takeda T, Goto E, Tanaka K. Accuracy and reliability of the self-inflating bulb to verify tracheal intubation in out-of-hospital cardiac arrest patients. *Anesthesiology.* 2000;93:1432-1436.
22. Craven RA, Singletary N, Bosken L, Sewell E, Payne M, Lipsey R. Use of bilevel positive airway pressure in out-of-hospital patients. *Acad Emerg Med.* 2000;7:1065-1068.
23. Kallio T, Kuisma M, Alaspaa A, Rosenberg PH. The use of prehospital continuous positive airway pressure treatment in presumed acute severe pulmonary edema. *Prehosp Emerg Care.* 2003;7:209-213.
24. Mosesso VN, Jr, Dunford J, Blackwell T, Griswell JK. Prehospital therapy for acute congestive heart failure: state of the art. *Prehosp Emerg Care.* 2003;7:13-23.
25. Braude D, Richards M. Rapid Sequence Airway (RSA)—a novel approach to prehospital airway management. *Prehosp Emerg Care.* 2007;11:250-252.
26. Walls RM. Rapid sequence intubation. In: Walls RM, Murphy MF, eds. *Manual of Emergency Airway Management.* Philadelphia, PA: Lippincott Williams and Wilkins; 2008:23-35.

27. Wang HE, Kupas DF, Paris PM, Yealy DM. Factors associated with the use of pharmacologic agents to facilitate out-of-hospital endotracheal intubation. *Prehosp Emerg Care*. 2004;8:1-9.

28. Frascone RJ, Pippert G, Heegaard W, Molinari P, Dries D. Successful training of HEMS personnel in laryngeal mask airway and intubating laryngeal mask airway placement. *Air Med J*. 2008;27:185-187.

29. Kovacs G, Law JA. How to do awake intubations—oral and nasal. In: Kovacs G, Law JA, eds. *Airway Management in Emergencies*. New York: McGraw-Hill; 2008:151-167.

30. Pepe PE, Stewart RD, Copass MK. Prehospital management of trauma: a tale of three cities. *Ann Emerg Med*. 1986;15:1484-1490.

31. Adnet F, Lapostolle F, Ricard-Hibon A, et al. Intubating trauma patients before reaching hospital—revisited. *Crit Care*. 2001;5:290-291.

32. Eckstein M, Chan L, Schneir A, Palmer R. Effect of prehospital advanced life support on outcomes of major trauma patients. *J Trauma*. 2000;48:643-648.

33. Frankel H, Rozycki G, Champion H, Harviel JD, Bass R. The use of TRISS methodology to validate prehospital intubation by urban EMS providers. *Am J Emerg Med*. 1997;15:630-632.

34. Karch SB, Lewis T, Young S, Hales D, Ho CH. Field intubation of trauma patients: complications, indications, and outcomes. *Am J Emerg Med*. 1996;14:617-619.

35. Liberman M, Mulder D, Sampalis J. Advanced or basic life support for trauma: meta-analysis and critical review of the literature. *J Trauma*. 2000;49:584-599.

36. Ruchholtz S, Waydhas C, Ose C, Lewan U, Nast-Kolb D; Working Group on Multiple Trauma of the German Trauma Society. Prehospital intubation in severe thoracic trauma without respiratory insufficiency: a matched-pair analysis based on the Trauma Registry of the German Trauma Society. *J Trauma*. 2002;52:879-886.

37. Bochicchio GV, Ilahi O, Joshi M, et al. Endotracheal intubation in the field does not improve outcome in trauma patients who present without an acutely lethal traumatic brain injury. *J Trauma*. 2003;54:307-311.

38. Garner A, Crooks J, Lee A, Bishop R. Efficacy of prehospital critical care teams for severe blunt head injury in the Australian setting. *Injury*. 2001;32:455-460.

39. Garner A, Rashford S, Lee A, Bartolacci R. Addition of physicians to paramedic helicopter services decreases blunt trauma mortality. *Aust N Z J Surg*. 1999;69:697-701.

40. Murray JA, Demetriades D, Berne TV, et al. Prehospital intubation in patients with severe head injury. *J Trauma*. 2000;49:1065-1070.

41. Ochs M, Davis DP, Hoyt DB. Lessons learned during the San Diego paramedic RSI Trial. *J Emerg Med*. 2003;24:343-344.

42. Winchell RJ, Hoyt DB. Endotracheal intubation in the field improves survival in patients with severe head injury. Trauma Research and Education Foundation of San Diego. *Arch Surg*. 1997;132:592-597.

43. Zink BJ, Maio RF. Out-of-hospital endotracheal intubation in traumatic brain injury: outcomes research provides us with an unexpected outcome. *Ann Emerg Med*. 2004;44:451-453.

44. Adnet F, Jouriles NJ, Le Toumelin P, et al. Survey of out-of-hospital emergency intubations in the French prehospital medical system: a multicenter study. *Ann Emerg Med*. 1998;32:454-460.

45. Bissell RA, Eslinger DG, Zimmerman L. The efficacy of advanced life support: a review of the literature. *Prehosp Disaster Med*. 1998;13:77-87.

46. Eisen JS, Dubinsky I. Advanced life support vs basic life support field care: an outcome study. *Acad Emerg Med*. 1998;5:592-598.

47. Mitchell RG, Guly UM, Rainer TH, Robertson CE. Can the full range of paramedic skills improve survival from out of hospital cardiac arrests? *J Accid Emerg Med*. 1997;14:274-277.

48. Rainer TH, Marshall R, Cusack S. Paramedics, technicians, and survival from out of hospital cardiac arrest. *J Accid Emerg Med*. 1997;14:278-282.

49. Hallstrom A, Cobb L, Johnson E, Copass M. Cardiopulmonary resuscitation by chest compression alone or with mouth-to-mouth ventilation. *N Engl J Med*. 2000;342:1546-1553.

50. Stiell IG, Wells GA, Field B, et al. Advanced cardiac life support in out-of-hospital cardiac arrest. *N Engl J Med*. 2004;351:647-656.

51. Aijian P, Tsai A, Knopp R, Kallsen GW. Endotracheal intubation of pediatric patients by paramedics. *Ann Emerg Med*. 1989;18:489-494.

52. Boswell WC, McElveen N, Sharp M, et al. Analysis of prehospital pediatric and adult intubation. *Air Med J*. 1995;14:125-127; discussion 127-128.

53. Brownstein D, Shugerman R, Cummings P, Rivara F, Copass M. Prehospital endotracheal intubation of children by paramedics. *Ann Emerg Med*. 1996;28:34-39.

54. Su E, Mann NC, McCall M, Hedges JR. Use of resuscitation skills by paramedics caring for critically injured children in Oregon. *Prehosp Emerg Care*. 1997;1:123-127.

55. Vilke GM, Steen PJ, Smith AM, Chan TC. Out-of-hospital pediatric intubation by paramedics: the San Diego experience. *J Emerg Med*. 2002;22:71-74.

56. Cooper A, DiScala C, Foltin G, Tunik M, Markenson D, Welborn C. Prehospital endotracheal intubation for severe head injury in children: a reappraisal. *Semin Pediatr Surg*. 2001;10:3-6.

57. Suominen P, Baillie C, Kivioja A, Ohman J, Olkkola KT. Intubation and survival in severe paediatric blunt head injury. *Eur J Emerg Med*. 2000;7:3-7.

58. Davis DP, Hoyt DB, Ochs M, et al. The effect of paramedic rapid sequence intubation on outcome in patients with severe traumatic brain injury. *J Trauma*. 2003;54:444-453.

59. Chesnut RM, Marshall LF, Klauber MR, et al. The role of secondary brain injury in determining outcome from severe head injury. *J Trauma*. 1993;34:216-222.

60. Ochs M, Davis D, Hoyt D, Bailey D, Marshall L, Rosen P. Paramedic-performed rapid sequence intubation of patients with severe head injuries. *Ann Emerg Med*. 2002;40:159-167.

61. Ma OJ, Atchley RB, Hatley T, Green M, Young J, Brady W. Intubation success rates improve for an air medical program after implementing the use of neuromuscular blocking agents. *Am J Emerg Med*. 1998;16:125-127.

62. Murphy-Macabobby M, Marshall WJ, Schneider C, Dries D. Neuromuscular blockade in aeromedical airway management. *Ann Emerg Med*. 1992;21:664-668.

63. Sing RF, Rotondo MF, Zonies DH, et al. Rapid sequence induction for intubation by an aeromedical transport team: a critical analysis. *Am J Emerg Med*. 1998;16:598-602.

64. Slater EA, Weiss SJ, Ernst AA, Haynes M. Preflight versus en route success and complications of rapid sequence intubation in an air medical service. *J Trauma*. 1998;45:588-592.

65. Werman HA, Schwegman D, Gerard JP. The effect of etomidate on airway management practices of an air medical transport service. *Prehosp Emerg Care*. 2004;8:185-190.

66. Lieutaud T, Billard V, Khalaf H, Debaene B. Muscle relaxation and increasing doses of propofol improve intubating conditions. *Can J Anaesth*. 2003;50:121-126.

67. McKeating K, Bali IM, Dundee JW. The effects of thiopentone and propofol on upper airway integrity. *Anaesthesia*. 1988;43:638-640.

68. McNeil IA, Culbert B, Russell I. Comparison of intubating conditions following propofol and succinylcholine with propofol and remifentanil 2 micrograms kg-1 or 4 micrograms kg-1. *Br J Anaesth*. 2000;85:623-625.

69. Bozeman WP, Hexter D, Liang HK, Kelen GD. Esophageal detector device versus detection of end-tidal carbon dioxide level in emergency intubation. *Ann Emerg Med*. 1996;27:595-599.

70. Katz SH, Falk JL. Misplaced endotracheal tubes by paramedics in an urban emergency medical services system. *Ann Emerg Med*. 2001;37:32-37.

71. O'Connor RE, Swor RA. Verification of endotracheal tube placement following intubation. National Association of EMS Physicians Standards and Clinical Practice Committee. *Prehosp Emerg Care*. 1999;3:248-250.

72. MacLeod BA, Heller MB, Gerard J, et al. Verification of endotracheal tube placement with colorimetric end-tidal CO_2 detection. *Ann Emerg Med*. 1991;20:267-270.

73. Grmec S. Comparison of three different methods to confirm tracheal tube placement in emergency intubation. *Intensive Care Med*. 2002;28:701-704.

74. Li J. Capnography alone is imperfect for endotracheal tube placement confirmation during emergency intubation. *J Emerg Med*. 2001;20:223-229.

75. Ornato JP, Shipley JB, Racht EM, et al. Multicenter study of a portable, hand-size, colorimetric end-tidal carbon dioxide detection device. *Ann Emerg Med*. 1992;21:518-523.

76. Takeda T, Tanigawa K, Tanaka H, et al. The assessment of three methods to verify tracheal tube placement in the emergency setting. *Resuscitation*. 2003;56:153-157.

77. Hendey GW, Shubert GS, Shalit M, Hogue B. The esophageal detector bulb in the aeromedical setting. *J Emerg Med*. 2002;23:51-55.

78. Silvestri S, Ralls GA, Krauss B, et al. The effectiveness of out-of-hospital use of continuous end-tidal carbon dioxide monitoring on the rate of unrecognized misplaced intubation within a regional emergency medical services system. *Ann Emerg Med*. 2005;45:497-503.

SELF-EVALUATION QUESTIONS

14.1. Rapid-sequence intubation by nonphysician prehospital care providers

  A. is regulated by federal statute

  B. is safe in adults but not children

  C. is well established for paramedics

  D. is supported by the available evidence for critical care prehospital providers

  E. will replace EGDs in the foreseeable future

14.2. All of the following statements about *nonparalytic RSI* are correct **EXCEPT**

  A. Some jurisdictions permit paramedics to employ this technique.

  B. It has been proven to be safer than paralytic RSI.

  C. It employs an induction agent at full dose but no neuromuscular blocking agent.

  D. It provides an inferior view of the glottis.

  E. It is felt to be more humane than intubating patients awake.

14.3. All of the following statements regarding qualitative, colorimetric end-tidal carbon dioxide determination in EMS are correct **EXCEPT**

  A. Continuous monitoring is indicated to identify inadvertent extubation during transport.

  B. These devices enable one to adhere to the standard of care for confirmation of endotracheal intubation.

  C. These devices are almost totally unreliable in patients having suffered a cardiac arrest.

  D. They are more effective than esophageal detector devices in confirming endotracheal placement.

  E. They are neither better nor worse than capnograpy in confirming correct endotracheal tube placement.

CHAPTER (15)

Airway Management of a Patient with Traumatic Brain Injury

J. Adam Law, Edward T. Crosby, and Andy Jagoda

15.1 CASE PRESENTATION

An advanced life support emergency services unit brought a 35-year-old man into the emergency department (ED) backboarded and collared. The patient was an unrestrained driver who was ejected from his car when it ran off the road and hit a tree. When a paramedic team arrived 10 minutes after the crash, the patient had a blood pressure (BP) of 90/50 mm Hg, heart rate (HR) 100 beats per minute (bpm), respiratory rate (RR) 20 breaths per minute, and oxygen saturation (SpO_2) 96% on room air. His Glasgow Coma Scale (GCS) score was 7 (opened eyes to pain 2, moaned 2, abnormal flexion 3). Pupils were equal and reactive, and his mouth was clenched closed. The patient was given oxygen via a nonrebreathing face mask. Although the patient exhibited periods of extreme agitation with combative behavior during transport, intravenous (IV) access was obtained and an infusion of Lactated Ringers was begun.

15.2 PREHOSPITAL CARE

After ensuring scene safety, the immediate management of the patient with traumatic brain injury (TBI) in a field setting should focus on stabilizing and maintaining oxygenation and blood pressure. All head-injured patients have potential cervical injury and should be immobilized. A fundamental premise in prehospital care is to anticipate and prepare for eventualities such as vomiting, seizures, and aberrations of blood pressure or oxygenation.

15.2.1 Should tracheal intubation be performed in the field for this patient?

In this patient, ensuring oxygenation via a patent airway is of paramount importance. Indications for a field intubation include inadequate ventilation or oxygenation despite supplemental oxygen administration or the inability of the patient to protect the airway. A relative indication for intubation is the risk of losing the airway during transport. Transport time and type of transport, that is, ground versus aeromedical, must be taken into consideration. Studies of the outcome of prehospital intubations have yielded conflicting results[1,2,3-5] and, as discussed in Chapter 14, prehospital airway management protocols are currently being further investigated. In the case presented, the patient was maintaining oxygenation and ventilation. His clinical course could not be certain, and it was reasonable for the field team to consider tracheal intubation. However, the patient had clenched teeth and was predicted to pose a difficult laryngoscopic intubation based on his short neck and cervical spine immobilization. A decision to intubate would involve the use of a rapid-sequence intubation (RSI) protocol; considering the short transport time, RSI was not indicated.

15.2.2 What additional considerations are imposed by field conditions?

Several other priorities in clinical care must be addressed by the field team after initial patient stabilization.

15.2.2.1 Circulation

Hypotension is a critical factor associated with an increased morbidity and mortality in patients with head injuries.[6,7] Blood pressure in the field should be monitored closely with the goal of avoiding hypotension (systolic BP <90 mm Hg in adults); if present, it should be corrected immediately. This patient presented with a field BP of 90/60 mm Hg. As hypotension is strongly associated with poor outcomes in TBI patients, fluid resuscitation becomes a priority. However, the field team must weigh the benefit of delaying transport from the field to secure an IV with the risk of delayed transport to a trauma center. Ideally, IV access should be attempted as the patient is expeditiously transported to the trauma center. It should be emphasized that isolated brain injury rarely accounts for hypotension in trauma patients with multisystem injury;[8] rather, if present, hemorrhage must always be suspected.

15.2.2.2 Neurologic Disability: ICP and C-spine

ICP: The GCS of seven, 10 minutes after the injury, is not predictive of the patient's clinical course or prognosis (other than the increased likelihood of C-spine injury). The patient did not have unequivocal evidence of increased intracranial pressure (ICP) since the pupils were equal and reactive and the motor response was decorticate, not decerebrate. As such there was no indication for paramedics to provide any intervention for managing elevated ICP with modalities such as intubation/hyperventilation, mannitol, or hypertonic saline.[9]

A potential pitfall in the management of the TBI patient is to assume that trauma is entirely responsible for altered mental status. Consideration must be given to the reversible causes of altered mental status, that is, hypoglycemia and drug toxicity, in addition to hypoxemia and hypotension.

C-spine immobilization: All patients with blunt trauma to the torso or neurological dysfunction should be suspected of having spinal cord injury until proven otherwise. Although neurologic impairment is fully manifest at the time of injury in most patients with vertebral injury,[10] the implications of an unidentified spine injury are such that routine use of immobilization devices is indicated. Secondary neurological injuries are reported to occur in 10% to 30% of patients with delayed diagnosis, who are not immobilized at time of entry into care[11,12] and in 2% to 10% of those who are immobilized.[13] Three recent studies suggest that the probability of associated C-spine injury is at least tripled with GCS scores of 8 or less.[14-16] Studies of techniques for optimal cervical immobilization have supported the use of a rigid cervical collar that incorporates the upper thorax, stabilization blocks on either side of the head, and a long spine board for transport.[17,18] Spinal immobilization is not without consequence in that patients are at risk of aspirating if they seize, vomit, or lose protective airway mechanisms. In addition, collars have been consistently demonstrated to increase ICP and may worsen intracranial pressure dynamics in patients with head injury,[19-23] probably by interference with cerebral venous drainage.[24] With the history of TBI and GCS of 7, the presented patient was at significant risk of cervical spine trauma and required full cervical spine immobilization.

15.2.2.3 Analgesia/Sedation

Patients with severe head injuries can experience episodes of agitation and combativeness, both of which tend to increase intracranial pressure, and can pose safety risks to both the patient and the field paramedic crew. Sedatives, such as benzodiazepines and opioid analgesics, are typically employed but, if given, the GCS score should first be determined, and the status of oxygenation and ventilation closely monitored after administration.

15.2.2.4 Transport Decisions

A priority in the early management of patients with moderate or severe brain injuries is transportation to the closest facility providing immediate access to neuroimaging and neurosurgical services. Patients with severe TBI transported to trauma centers without the availability of prompt neurosurgical care are at risk of a poor outcome.[7] Acute subdural hematomas in patients with severe TBI are associated with a 90% mortality if evacuated more than 4 hours after injury, but only 30% mortality if evacuated earlier.[25,26] Consequently, it is recommended that field emergency medical services (EMS) systems operate under strict ground and aeromedical trauma transport protocols. Commonly accepted criteria for transport of head-injured patients to a trauma center include severity of injury, a respiratory rate less than 10, systolic blood pressure less than 90 mm Hg, and a GCS score less than 12.

15.3 EMERGENCY DEPARTMENT MANAGEMENT

The ambulance arrived at the emergency department (ED) after a 15-minute transport. While the patient was being transferred onto the gurney in the trauma bay, it was noted that he was obese (5 ft 8 in [172 cm], 275 lb [125 kg], BMI 42.3 kg·m⁻²), he had blood coming out of his right ear, and his cervical collar was riding high up over his short neck. His BP was now 130/80 mm Hg, HR 110 bpm, RR 24 breaths per minute, SpO_2 was 90% on a nonrebreathing facemask, and he had snoring respirations. His blood sugar was 110 mg/dL (6.1 mmol·L⁻¹). His GCS score had decreased to 6 (2 for opened eyes to pain only, 2 for moans, and 2 for intermittent decerebrate posturing). At this point, it was noted that his right pupil was 8 mm and unreactive; his left pupil was 4 mm and reacted sluggishly. He moved all four extremities with no asymmetry. A quick airway evaluation revealed that his teeth were still clenched; he had a 6 cm thyromental span and 4 cm hypothyroid distance. There was no evidence of blunt trauma to the neck, and the cricothyroid membrane was identifiable and palpable in the midline. Two large-bore IVs were secured, blood was drawn, and sent for chemistries and type and cross match. Spun hematocrit was 45%. Portable chest and pelvis radiographs in the trauma bay were normal. Cross-table lateral x-rays of the C-spine showed good alignment and no prevertebral soft tissue swelling. A focused assessment with sonography in trauma (FAST) examination of the abdomen was performed, which showed no free fluid in the abdomen. A stat neurosurgery consult was ordered. Personnel from diagnostic imaging called, saying that they were ready to image the patient once he was stabilized. While the trauma team was deciding the best approach to securing the airway and managing the suspected increased intracranial pressure, the patient had a 30-second tonic-clonic seizure and desaturated to a SpO_2 of 80%.

15.3.1   What elements of airway management must be considered in this patient?

The immediate priority in this patient is reoxygenation, due to evidence suggesting that even a single episode of hypoxemia can worsen the prognosis in the patient with TBI.[6,7] The patient should receive assisted bag-mask-ventilation with 100% O_2. Once the SpO_2 is again well above 90%, attention can be turned to formulating a plan for tracheal intubation. Unless the seizure spontaneously terminates within 1 to 2 minutes, pharmacologic intervention with lorazepam would be indicated.

From the perspective of airway management, trauma patients secured on a backboard with cervical immobilization can appear very intimidating. In fact, however, formal airway assessment may point to little anticipated difficulty (see Sections 1.6.1, 1.6.2, 1.6.3, and 1.6.4). In this patient's case, his obesity predicts an increased likelihood of difficult bag-mask-ventilation (BMV).[27-29] Direct laryngoscopy may be difficult due to the patient's short neck and the cervical spine immobilization: manual in-line neck stabilization (MILNS) increases the likelihood of obtaining a poor (eg, Cormack/Lehane Grade 3) view at laryngoscopy.[30] Any trismus will likely resolve with muscle relaxant administration, if these are employed. Extraglottic device insertion may be difficult, but should succeed. Finally, while obesity can make trans-tracheal access difficult, in this patient, the cricothyroid membrane was easily palpable, suggesting easy access.

15.3.2   How are you going to proceed with tracheal intubation?

With a reasonable expectation of successful laryngoscopic intubation and the availability of a backup Plan B (eg, bag-mask-ventilation, extraglottic device use, or cricothyrotomy) should intubation fail, RSI should be used in this uncooperative patient. This plan confers the advantages of optimal intubating conditions with skeletal muscle relaxation while helping to reduce the risk of seizure activity or any laryngoscopy and intubation-induced increases in ICP, through the use of induction agents.

15.3.3   What are your goals during tracheal intubation of the TBI patient with C-spine precautions?

Our goals are to achieve tracheal intubation expeditiously while avoiding secondary neurologic injury by (1) maintaining oxygenation; (2) avoiding decreases in cerebral perfusion pressure; and (3) minimizing movement of the head and neck. Attention must also be directed toward prevention of gastric content aspiration.

15.3.4   How are cerebral perfusion pressure, intracranial pressure, cerebral blood flow, and autoregulation related; what changes TBI, and how can we modify these changes?

Elevated ICP is associated with worse outcomes in traumatic brain injury. While its early recognition and management have not been conclusively linked to improved outcome, it is prudent to avoid any further increases in ICP in the brain-injured patient.

Intracranial pressure reflects the state of the contents of the fixed housing of the intracranial vault. The three normal contents of the vault are brain tissue, cerebrospinal fluid (CSF), and blood. Intracranial blood volume is directly related to cerebral blood flow. This flow is normally kept relatively constant over a wide range of blood pressures by cerebral autoregulation; as blood pressure varies, cerebral vasoconstriction or vasodilatation occurs to maintain constant blood flow, and in turn volume. However, the brain's ability to autoregulate blood flow over a range of blood pressures is impaired or lost in TBI.

A second mediator of cerebral blood flow is blood carbon dioxide tension. As blood carbon dioxide tension rises, so will cerebral blood flow, leading to increased intracranial blood volume and thereby ICP. While aggressive hyperventilation in the patient with TBI is no longer recommended in the absence of signs of brain herniation,[7,31] attention should be paid throughout the airway management process to maintaining normocarbia.

Cerebral perfusion pressure (CPP) is the driving force for blood flow to the brain, and is measured by the difference between the mean arterial blood pressure (MAP) and the ICP, so that CPP = MAP − ICP. In the patient with disrupted autoregulation, decreases in MAP will decrease CPP while increases in MAP, if not accompanied by equivalent increases in ICP, may be beneficial because of the increase in driving pressure for oxygenation of brain tissue. It is generally recommended that the ICP be maintained below 20 mm Hg, MAP between 100 and 110 mm Hg,[31] and CPP at or above 70 mm Hg. Hypotension leading to a decrease in CPP, even for a very brief period, is especially harmful, and along with hypoxia, has been shown to be an independent predictor of increased mortality and morbidity in patients with a TBI.[6,7]

15.3.5   How does airway management affect intracranial pressure dynamics?

Laryngoscopy and intubation may cause an increase in ICP indirectly through an increase in blood pressure (with disrupted autoregulation) or through a direct effect on ICP. Both laryngoscopy and placement of an endotracheal tube result in afferent discharges that increase sympathetic activity and release of catecholamines, that is, the reflex sympathetic response to laryngoscopy (RSRL). A catecholamine surge may occur, especially with multiple attempts at laryngoscopy, potentially leading to increased heart rate and blood pressure. In the patient with TBI who has impaired autoregulation, such a blood pressure surge may contribute to an increase in ICP. This fact underscores the importance of using drugs to mitigate this RSRL.

15.3.6 What effects on ICP can be expected from medications commonly used during airway management in the emergency department?

Pharmacologic agents used to aid in airway management must be selected with consideration of their effects on CPP. Prior to intubation, a modest fluid bolus will help maintain blood pressure, while vasopressors such as ephedrine or phenylephrine should also be immediately available to treat postintubation hypotension. Pretreatment, induction, and paralytic agents used to attenuate a rise in ICP and/or facilitate intubation in the patient with TBI have been discussed in detail in Chapter 4. It should be noted that if a longer acting muscle relaxant is used to facilitate tracheal intubation or maintain postintubation paralysis, formal monitoring for ongoing seizure activity should be instituted in this patient.

15.4 CERVICAL SPINE CONSIDERATIONS

Victims of major trauma often require several interventions, including definitive airway control, before a full assessment of the cervical spine (C-spine) is possible. Without radiographic evidence of an intact C-spine, an unstable injury should be assumed and airway management undertaken accordingly.

15.4.1 What range of cervical spine movement is considered within physiologic limits?

In order to interpret the data on the effects of airway manipulations on movement of the cervical spine, the amount of motion that would indicate spinal instability should be defined. Panjabi and White have suggested that horizontal motion (anteroposterior [A-P] displacement) of one vertebral body on another exceeding 20% of vertebral body width (or 3.5-mm in an adult, corrected for x-ray magnification); greater than 11 degrees of relative angulation of adjacent cervical vertebrae; or greater than 1.4 mm of distraction on resting lateral radiography of the subaxial cervical spine is abnormal and would indicate instability.[32-34] Preexisting cervical abnormalities such as spinal stenosis could have neurologic consequences within these anatomic limits.[35]

15.4.2 What effect does direct laryngoscopy and intubation have on movement of the normal C-spine?

Radiographic studies on live and cadaveric subjects with intact C-spines demonstrate that direct laryngoscopy (DL) causes considerable extension between the occiput and C2. Most extension (about 12 degrees) occurs between the occiput and C1, with slightly over half as much (approximately 7 degrees) between C1 and C2.[36-47] A total of about 6 degrees of extension occurs from C2 to C5.[37-40,46,47] From C5 to the cervicothoracic junction, a small amount (about 8 degrees) of flexion occurs.[38-40] Actual tube passage causes slight

additional superior rotation between the occiput and C1, but little other movement.[36,46] There is some evidence that exposing only a minimum view during laryngoscopy (eg, seeking only a view of the posterior cartilages, but not of the cords) will reduce occiput-C2 extension.[36,46,48,49]

15.4.3 What effects do basic airway maneuvers have on movement of a normal C-spine?

Several radiographic studies have looked at the effects of basic airway-opening maneuvers and bag-mask-ventilation on C-spine movement. One cadaver study performed with no applied MILNS found that chin lift and jaw thrust caused as much extension at C1 to C2 as oral laryngoscopic intubation.[50] A second cadaver study, using backboard, cervical collar, and tape found that significantly more cervical spine displacement occurred with bag-mask-ventilation (BMV) than with either oral or nasal tracheal intubation.[51] However, a more recent study using elective surgical subjects with their heads taped in a neutral position found BMV to cause significantly less cervical spine movement than DL at each of the occiput-C1, C1-C2, C2-C5, and C5-T1 motion segments.[40] Although sometimes conflicting in their results, these studies can at least be taken as an indication that appropriate cervical spine precautions should be applied during all phases of airway management in those patients at risk of C-spine injury.

15.4.4 What are the effects of basic airway maneuvers in models of an injured C-spine?

Donaldson et al[50] studied the motion that occurred during various airway maneuvers in a series of six cadavers with a surgically created unstable C1-C2 segment. With the head stabilized, they found that preintubation maneuvers (chin lift and jaw thrust) caused more narrowing of the space available for the spinal cord (SAC) than DL or blind nasal intubation. In a subsequent cadaver series, this time with an unstable C5-C6, the same investigators demonstrated a trend toward chin lift/jaw thrust causing as much movement as DL.[52] Aprahamian also studied a cadaveric specimen with a posteriorly destabilized C5-C6 segment, and similarly reported that chin lift/jaw thrust caused as much or more movement at the site of injury as oral or nasal intubation.[53] Brimacombe et al determined cervical spine motion for six airway management techniques in cadavers with a posteriorly destabilized third cervical (C3) vertebra. Here again, both chin lift/jaw thrust and oral intubation with DL caused significant A-P displacement of the unstable segment,[54] although the movements were within the previously described physiologic limits.

While these studies on basic airway maneuvers provide reassuring evidence that DL is unlikely to cause more movement than preintubation maneuvers, they also reinforce that appropriate precautions against movement be instituted well before a tracheal intubation attempt.

15.4.5 How effective is manual in-line neck stabilization (MILNS) in preventing C-spine motion in normal patients and injury models?

Manual in-line neck stabilization (MILNS) appears to restrain overall spinal movements occurring during DL in patients and cadaveric specimens with normal spines to within physiological levels, and has less impact on airway interventions than do other forms of immobilization.[37,49,55] In injury models, Lennarson reported that MILNS did not completely eliminate movement at the injury level during intubation of a cadaver model with either posterior or complete ligamentous C4-C5 disruption; however, the movements recorded during interventions were within physiological limits.[46,56] Gerling evaluated the effect of MILNS as well as cervical collar immobilization on spinal movement during direct laryngoscopy in a cadaver model with a C5-C6 transection injury. Although there was less A-P displacement measured with application of MILNS compared with collar (7.5% of vertebral body width vs 13.7%), overall the magnitude of movement was small and within physiological range. There was no difference in axial distraction or angular rotation.[57] Turner studied 10 cadavers surgically destabilized at C4-C5. MILNS did not significantly change the median motion seen during DL in any of angulation, distraction, or A-P displacement at the unstable level.[35]

Two recent comprehensive reviews on the topic support the notion that while there may be some reduction in overall C-spine motion with MILNS, movement at individual motion segments, including sites of injury, may in fact not be significantly restrained by stabilization.[58,59] As Aprahamian[53] stated about collar immobilization in 1984, it may be that MILNS should simply be taken as a caution sign of a possible neck injury, and to then use gentle and precise airway maneuvers to minimize C-spine movement.[59]

15.4.6 How does applied MILNS impact ease of direct laryngoscopy?

Many trauma patients presenting to the emergency department arrive on a backboard immobilized with rigid cervical collar, sandbags, and tape. Unfortunately, any immobilization technique that restricts mouth opening will make laryngoscopy more difficult. In one study, 64% of patients immobilized with a collar, tape, and sandbags presented at Grade 3 or 4 view with DL, compared to only 22% of patients undergoing MILNS, with cervical collar removed.[30] Other studies concur that direct laryngoscopy in patients stabilized with cervical collars will result in a greater than 50% incidence of Grade 3 or 4 views.[57,60] Goutcher et al studied the effect of semirigid cervical collars on mouth opening in awake volunteers. Mean mouth opening of 40 mm without a collar decreased to 26 to 29 mm with cervical collar, and in a quarter of the subjects, mouth opening was reduced to 20 mm or less.[61] A common pattern of practice is therefore to loosen or open the rigid collar during laryngoscopy after the application of MILNS. In general, when MILNS is substituted for a rigid cervical collar, the direct laryngoscopic view should improve, with a quoted incidence of Grade 3 or 4 views between 20%[47,62-64] and 50%.[65-67] Thiboutot randomized elective surgical patients to standard sniffing position or MILNS for DL. In this series, the incidence of Grade 3 or 4 views in the MILNS group exceeded 50%, and 50% of patients could not be intubated within 30 seconds, compared to 5.7% without MILNS.[65] The consistent message from the literature is that MILNS application is associated with difficult direct laryngoscopy; strategies to improve laryngeal view and facilitate tracheal intubation during the application of MILNS have been reported and will be discussed subsequently.

15.4.7 Why is traction no longer used during MILNS?

Older publications make reference to using in-line traction when C-spine precautions were indicated. However, traction forces applied during MILNS may endanger the spinal cord if there is a serious ligamentous injury. Lennarson noted distraction at the site of a complete ligamentous injury when traction forces were applied for the purposes of spinal stabilization during direct laryngoscopy.[56] Similarly, Kaufmann demonstrated that in-line traction applied during radiographic evaluation resulted in spinal column lengthening and distraction at the site of injury in four recently deceased patients with ligamentous disruptions.[68] Bivins also studied the effect of in-line traction during orotracheal intubation in four victims of blunt traumatic arrest, who had unstable spinal injuries.[69] Traction applied to reduce subluxation at the site of injury resulted in both distraction and posterior displacement at the fracture site. Current recommendations promote the use of in-line stabilization and *not* traction during airway interventions requiring C-spine precautions.

15.4.8 Does the choice of direct laryngoscope blade impact the degree of C-spine movement during laryngoscopy?

A number of studies have reported cervical spine movement caused by different laryngoscope blades. Two studies in elective surgical patients found significantly less (by about 3 degrees) head extension with Miller, as compared with Macintosh blade laryngoscopy.[42,70] However, other studies have failed to demonstrate a difference in motion between the two blades.[51,55,71] Studies with the levering tip McCoy/CLM-type blades have also generated conflicting results: some have found significantly less C-spine movement with use of the activated blade when compared to a Macintosh[48,72] while others have not.[57,73]

In cadaver injury models, one study showed that Miller blade laryngoscopy resulted in significantly less axial distraction (1-2 mm) at the level of a surgically created C5-C6 transection than the Macintosh, but no difference in angular rotation or A-P displacement.[57] However, Aprahamian's study of a single cadaver, also with an unstable C5-C6 injury, reported no difference between Macintosh and Miller blades.[53] At present, there is no evidence that Miller blade use is preferred in the patient at risk from a C-spine injury.[74]

15.4.9 Is any direct laryngoscopy blade superior for exposing the glottis with applied MILNS?

To date, there is no convincing evidence that either curved or straight blades are superior to the other for exposing the laryngeal inlet during direct laryngoscopy with applied MILNS. However, a number of studies suggest that laryngoscopy using the levering tip McCoy/CLM blade with the tip activated may be helpful when a poor view is obtained in the setting of MILNS. Three studies report improvement of a Grade 3 view to 2 or better in 83% (with applied MILNS);[75] 86% (MILNS with cricoid pressure);[76] and 92% (rigid cervical collar) of cases respectively.[77]

15.4.10 How do alternatives to DL impact cervical spine movement during tracheal intubation?

Many of the alternatives to DL appear to cause less movement of the cervical spine during tracheal intubation. Laryngoscopy and intubation with the Bullard laryngoscope has been shown to result in significantly less C-spine movement than DL with Macintosh[37,71,78] or Miller blades.[71] Similarly, intubation with the Pentax airway scope (AWS) results in significantly less upper C-spine movement than DL with both attempted full[44,79] and minimal view[80] exposure of the cords. C-spine movement during AWS use is further reduced with prior passage of a bougie via the blade's delivery channel.[81] Compared with the Macintosh blade, Airtraq-facilitated intubation appears to cause significantly less movement at some, but not all C-spine motion segments.[39,41] The use of a Glidescope video laryngoscope (GVL) results in some reduction in midcervical spine movement compared with DL, but elsewhere movement is similar.[40,47] Studies with the Bonfils and Shikani optical stylets have concluded that less C-spine movement occurred with the optical stylets, compared to Macintosh blade DL,[38,78,82] as is the case with the Trachlight™-lighted stylet.[40,83] LMA Fastrach-facilitated enabled intubation results in less upper C-spine extension than direct laryngoscopy,[84,85] although mask insertion, cuff inflation, and intubation exerts significantly more pressure against C3 than other techniques, and may result in some posterior displacement of the upper cervical spine.[54,86] Tracheal intubation using a flexible bronchoscope laryngoscope results in less movement of the head and neck compared to direct laryngoscopy,[85] GVL,[87] and LMA Fastrach[54]-faciliated intubation in anesthetized patients, and a comparable amount to Trachlight intubation.[45] However, this information must be tempered with the appreciation that flexible bronchoscopes are expensive, can be more difficult to use, particularly in the presence of blood and secretions, and can be time-consuming in emergencies.[36] Flexible bronchoscopes are generally used if an awake intubation is elected, an option that permits the advantage of postintubation neurologic reassessment. Despite the evidence that there are lesser degrees of spinal movement when tracheal intubation is facilitated by some of the alternative devices, there is no evidence that neurological outcomes are altered by their use in the patient at risk with a C-spine injury.

15.4.11 How do adjuncts and alternatives to DL compare for successful intubation of the patient undergoing MILNS?

The tracheal tube introducer (TTI) is a valuable adjunct to DL in the patient undergoing MILNS. Nolan and colleagues randomized half of 157 patients undergoing MILNS in the operating room to attempted primary visual passage of the tube, or prior passage of a TTI.[63] Although the technique was quicker overall, 11 patients in the visual group required greater than 45 seconds for intubation, and there were five failures. All five failures were successfully intubated with adjunctive use of the TTI.

Other studies of the Bullard laryngoscope,[37] Glidescope videolaryngoscope,[64] Pentax AWS,[64,88,89] and Airtraq[90] or optical stylets[66,91] have documented one or more of a significantly improved laryngeal visualization,[63,64,88,89] better success rate,[66,89,91] or lower intubation difficulty score (IDS[92])[64,88-90] compared to Macintosh blade DL in the patient undergoing MILNS or wearing a cervical collar.

Several series evaluating LMA Fastrach use in patients with applied rigid collars have reported intubation success rates comparable to those obtained in unrestrained elective surgical patients[93-95]: the one study reporting a poor success rate under these conditions had included cricoid pressure in the study protocol.[96] Compared with the LMA Fastrach in a prospective study of elective surgical patients with applied MILNS, intubation with the Trachlight™ was quicker and resulted in a significantly higher success rate.[97]

In general, most of the alternatives to DL used in the patient undergoing MILNS cause less neck movement and sometimes enable easier visualization and/or tracheal intubation. For those with access to the devices and skill in their use, these may be a good option for such conditions, although compared to DL there are no data indicating an outcome benefit.

15.4.12 Is cricoid pressure contraindicated in patients with potential C-spine injury?

Radiographic studies have generally found that cervical spine movement with application of cricoid pressure is within physiologic limits. In a study of cadavers with intact cervical spines, with 40N of cricoid pressure and radiographs for assessment, Gabbott et al found a median A-P displacement of only 0.8 mm.[98] In a study of cadavers with an unstable C-spine at the C5-C6 level, Donaldson reported 0.64 mm of A-P displacement, 3.6 degrees of angulation and 1 mm of distraction with cricoid pressure application,[52] and no significant movement at the injury level in a second study using cadavers with instability at the C1-C2 segment.[50]

The decision to apply cricoid pressure in the patient with TBI must be considered in the context of both its risk of C-spine movement and other detrimental effects. Cricoid pressure may prevent successful BMV or interfere with efforts to place or ventilate through an LMA.[99] This likely results from obstruction of the airway by the applied pressure; the loss of airway patency may also shorten the time to desaturation even in the absence of ventilation.[100] A recent review has suggested that cricoid pressure may also increase difficulty experienced during airway management with

DL, the lightwand, and the flexible fiberoptic bronchoscope.[99] Thus, although cricoid pressure appears to result in radiographic movement that is within physiologic limits,[32] it may be prudent to reconsider its use in patients with known unstable lesions at or near the level of the cricoid cartilage, or in those in whom difficulty with bag-mask-ventilation or tracheal intubation has been encountered.

15.4.13 Does administration of an induction agent and/or a muscle relaxant by itself have any effect on the C-spine?

Historically, concern has been raised that administration of an induction agent and muscle relaxant to the patient with a C-spine injury could release any splinting of an unstable segment by adjacent muscle spasm. However, there is no readily available objective evidence for a clinically significant degree of cervical spinal movement due solely to induction agent and muscle relaxant administration.

15.4.14 How are extraglottic (rescue) ventilation devices impacted by C-spine precautions?

During insertion, the LMA Classic transiently exerts as much pressure on the upper cervical vertebrae as the LMA Fastrach.[86] In a cadaver model of a destabilized C3 segment, both the LMA Fastrach™ and LMA Classic™ caused significant posterior displacement of the unstable segment, yet significantly less than that caused by Combitube™ insertion.[54] Available data suggest that the Combitube™ can be difficult to insert with the neck held in-line[101] and is likely to cause spinal movement.[54] In comparison with the LMA Fastrach, the laryngeal tube was found to have a lower first-time insertion success rate in a series of patients with in-line stabilization and required more time to successfully establish ventilation.[102] However, it must be recognized that extraglottic devices are vital rescue oxygenation tools in difficult situations, and in spite of the potential for difficult insertion or C-spine movement, the benefits of their use in reoxygenating a hypoxemic patient will often outweigh the potential risk, particularly if care is taken to minimize such movement.

15.4.15 What effect does cricothyrotomy have on C-spine movement?

Surgical cricothyrotomy was originally advocated as a preferred airway intervention in patients at risk for cervical spine injury (CSI), rather than orotracheal intubation, and is now deemed to be an appropriate alternative if oral or nasal routes cannot be used or are unsuccessful. Although long considered safe in the presence of a CSI, the effect on C-spine movement of surgical cricothyrotomy has not been well studied. Gerling studied cervical spine movement during open surgical cricothyrotomy in a series of 13 cadavers with a complete C5-C6 transection.[103] A-P displacement was limited to 6.3% of C5 body width (1-2 mm), and axial distraction to less than 1 mm across the C5-C6 injury during the

procedure. Earlier, using a similar injury model in a single cadaver, Donaldson et al reported that A-P displacement was limited to 0.9 mm during tracheotomy.[52] As these movements are within physiological levels, values from both studies would likely be clinically irrelevant.

15.4.16 How safe is it to intubate the trachea of the patient with a potential C-spine injury?

There is no evidence that endotracheal intubation using direct laryngoscopy with in-line stabilization increases the risk of neurologic injury in patients with unstable cervical spine fractures.[104-106] Traditionally, oral intubation using direct laryngoscopy was deemed dangerous because it was thought to cause excessive spinal movement with the potential for secondary injury.[62] It was thought that such secondary injury could be avoided by the careful performance of nasotracheal intubation or cricothyrotomy. Although there were no data at that time to support this thesis and later data would seem largely to refute it, this hypothesis had achieved a sufficiently widespread acceptance as to be labeled a "therapeutic legend of emergency medicine" by Rosen.[107] McLeod and Calder reviewed the use of the direct laryngoscope in patients with spinal injury or pathology.[108] With the possible exception of one case,[109] they concluded after review and analysis of the case reports that it was unlikely that the use of the direct laryngoscope was the cause of the myelopathies reported. The potential for aggressive direct laryngoscopy with unrestricted spinal movement to cause neurological injury in spine-injured patients has been shown in two further case reports.[109,110] However, the message that these reports emphasize the need for spine stabilization in patients at risk of a C-spine injury until such injury is ruled out or definitive therapy for diagnosed CSI is implemented, and not that careful direct laryngoscopy is contraindicated.

15.4.17 Is direct laryngoscopy acceptable for intubation of the patient with a cervical spine injury?

There is clearly a difference of opinion in the literature regarding the optimal means of securing the airway by tracheal intubation in patients with cervical spine injury. Many authors have reported on the use of the direct laryngoscope in the management of patients with cervical spine injury for both elective and emergency intubations.[104-106,111-116] Most of these studies are limited both by their small sample size and their retrospective nature. However, they do reveal that neurological deterioration in spine-injured patients is uncommon after airway management when appropriate care is provided, even in high-risk patients undergoing urgent tracheal intubation. These studies are not sufficient to rule out the possibility that airway management provided in isolation or as part of a more complex clinical intervention, even provided with the utmost care, may rarely result in neurological injury.

The use of a direct laryngoscope following induction of anesthesia in the patient with a head injury is deemed an appropriate practice option by the American College of Surgeons as outlined in the manual of Advanced Trauma Life Support Program (ATLS, 2004) for doctors and by experts in trauma, anesthesia, and neurosurgery[105,106,108,117-126] and by the Eastern Association for the Surgery of Trauma.[125] Advantages of the direct laryngoscope in this setting include its effectiveness, the ability to visualize and remove upper airway foreign bodies during use and clinician familiarity; many anesthesia practitioners are not similarly skilled with other practice options.[127] Enthusiasm has been expressed by neuroanesthesia experts for the exclusive use of the flexible bronchoscope to facilitate tracheal intubation in patients with a CSI, citing this as the optimal practice option.[128] However, it is worth noting that over 40% of American anesthesiologists admit that they are not comfortable using a flexible bronchoscope for airway management.[127] Further, it should be recognized that significant difficulties may be experienced during the use of the bronchoscope, even by persons skilled in its use, during airway management in patients with a CSI.[129] Carefully performed direct laryngoscopy with appropriate MILNS in the trauma patient at risk for a C-spine injury can be considered a pattern of practice within the standard of care.

15.4.18 Is there anything else that might make airway management more difficult in the patient with a C-spine injury?

A small number of case reports and case series document the association of prevertebral retropharyngeal hematomas with some injuries of the upper C-spine, particularly with a hyperextension injury, as anterior elements of the spinal column are disrupted.[130-133] Such patients may present with symptoms of dysphagia and dyspnea, with the potential for difficult laryngoscopy due to anterior displacement of the laryngeal inlet.

15.5 POSTINTUBATION CONSIDERATIONS

15.5.1 What are the postintubation considerations in the head-injured patient?

Objective confirmation (eg, with an end-tidal CO_2 monitor) of tracheal placement of the ETT is essential. Recognizing the importance of maintaining CPP, blood pressure should be reassessed after airway interventions and any unacceptable drop corrected with fluid and/or vasopressors. Pupils should be reassessed. After checking for optimal position of the tip of the ETT, the tube should be firmly fixed to the patient, as a number of transfers will occur (eg, to the diagnostic imaging department and thereafter to the ICU or operating room). However, tight ties encircling the neck should be avoided. If the patient's blood pressure permits, a slight head-up position can be achieved by placing the stretcher in the reverse Trendelenberg position. This will promote venous drainage and may reduce elevated ICP.

Mechanical ventilation in the patient with elevated ICP is based on optimizing oxygenation and avoiding ventilation mechanics (eg, positive end-expiratory pressure [PEEP] or high peak inspiratory pressure [PIP]) that would increase ICP.

Controlled hyperventilation to a $Paco_2$ of approximately 30 mm Hg was formerly recommended for the early management of elevated ICP. It was believed that reduction in $Paco_2$ tensions in the brain led to vasoconstriction and decreased cerebral blood flow, thereby decreasing ICP. However, a growing body of research provides evidence that routine hyperventilation results in worse outcomes in TBI patients, possibly due to alterations in regional cerebral blood flow resulting in accumulations of neurotoxic agents, for example, lactate and glutamate.[134] The Brain Trauma Foundation Guidelines for the Management of Severe Traumatic Brain Injury now recommends that prophylactic hyperventilation be avoided, and that patients with severe TBI be ventilated in such a way as to target not less than the lower limits of normocapnia ($Paco_2$ of 35-40 mm Hg).[135] A similar approach seems prudent in patients with nontraumatic elevations of ICP (eg, cerebral hemorrhage). Hyperventilation to a $Paco_2$ of 30 mm Hg should be used only when osmotic agents and CSF drainage are not effective in managing an acute rise in ICP accompanied by patient deterioration, and utilized only until signs of herniation (eg, decerebrate posturing or a fixed dilated pupil) resolve.

Unless early and frequent neurological examinations are required (eg, by a neurosurgeon to decide whether there is sufficient persisting neurological functioning to warrant an attempt at surgical evacuation of a massive subdural hematoma), long-term sedation and paralysis will permit effective, controlled mechanical ventilation and other necessary interventions. Sedation and paralysis can also help mitigate the stimulating effects of the tube in the trachea and will eliminate any possibility of the patient coughing or bucking. A full paralyzing dose of a competitive neuromuscular blocking agent, such as rocuronium 1.0 mg·kg^{-1}, may be given, along with an initial dose of a sedative agent such as a benzodiazepine. Subsequent doses of approximately one-third of the initial dose of both agents should be given if the patient shows evidence of increased sympathetic activity or initiating motor movement. The pharmacologically paralyzed patient at risk of seizures should be monitored with EEG.

15.5.2 What happened to this patient?

As outlined earlier in Section 15.3, the patient's airway was fully assessed. The decision was taken to perform rapid-sequence intubation. Preparations included ensuring qualified help and requisite airway equipment were at hand, together with a briefing of the team about the Plan B approach should difficulty be encountered. An assistant was delegated to provide in-line immobilization of the C-spine, following which the front of the patient's rigid collar was removed. Denitrogenation was provided with a tightly fitting face mask, and induction medications were administered followed by application of cricoid pressure and administration of the skeletal muscle relaxant. For intubation, direct laryngoscopy was performed with a Macintosh #4 blade, with the practitioner attempting to expose only the posteriormost aspect of the laryngeal inlet. A tracheal tube introducer was then placed above the exposed arytenoid cartilages[63], followed by endotracheal tube (ETT) passage over the introducer with the laryngoscope blade still in situ. Tracheal placement of the ETT was confirmed with a disposable end-tidal CO_2 detector, whereupon cricoid pressure was released. The anterior aspect of the rigid cervical collar was reapplied, and MILNS was released. Vital signs were reassessed, with particular reference to the blood pressure. Decisions were then made about ongoing sedation and skeletal muscle relaxation and arrangements were made for patient transfer to the diagnostic imaging department.

15.6   SUMMARY

Airway management of the patient with a head injury must be undertaken with an appreciation of the importance of avoiding secondary injury to both brain and C-spine. Hypoxemia and hypotension must be avoided and formal C-spine precautions must be observed. However, apart from these directives, the practitioner should take comfort in the knowledge that as long as reasonable precautions are undertaken, familiar airway interventions are within the standard of care for the patient with potential C-spine injury, including rapid-sequence intubation, bag-mask-ventilation, and intubation using careful direct laryngoscopy. To the practitioner experienced in their use, alternative intubation techniques (eg, lightwand, rigid fiberoptic laryngoscope, and flexible bronchoscope) may permit tracheal intubation with less C-spine movement, although evidence is lacking of improved clinical outcome compared to use of direct laryngoscopy with MILNS. Awake intubation of the patient with a known C-spine injury confers the opportunity to reevaluate the patient's neurologic status postintubation. Irrespective of technique chosen, airway management in this setting should not proceed before a formal airway evaluation has been performed, needed personnel have been assembled and briefed, and airway equipment for the chosen and Plan B and C approaches has been readied.

REFERENCES

1. Winchell RJ, Hoyt DB. Endotracheal intubation in the field improves survival in patients with severe head injury. Trauma Research and Education Foundation of San Diego. *Arch Surg.* 1997;132:592-597.
2. Davis DP, Hoyt DB, Ochs M, et al. The effect of paramedic rapid sequence intubation on outcome in patients with severe traumatic brain injury. *J Trauma.* 2003;54:444-453.
3. Davis DP, Peay J, Serrano JA, et al. The impact of aeromedical response to patients with moderate to severe traumatic brain injury. *Ann Emerg Med.* 2005;46:115-122.
4. Rajani RR, Ball CG, Montgomery SP, Wyrzykowski AD, Feliciano DV. Airway management for victims of penetrating trauma: analysis of 50,000 cases. *Am J Surg.* 2009;198:863-867.
5. Cobas MA, De la Pena MA, Manning R, Candiotti K, Varon AJ. Prehospital intubations and mortality: a level 1 trauma center perspective. *Anesth Analg.* 2009;109:489-493.
6. Chesnut RM, Marshall LF, Klauber MR, et al. The role of secondary brain injury in determining outcome from severe head injury. *J Trauma.* 1993;34:216-222.
7. Badjatia N, Carney N, Crocco TJ, et al. Guidelines for prehospital management of traumatic brain injury 2nd edition. *Prehosp Emerg Care.* 2008;12(Suppl 1): S1-52.
8. Mahoney EJ, Biffl WL, Harrington DT, Cioffi WG. Isolated brain injury as a cause of hypotension in the blunt trauma patient. *J Trauma.* 2003;55:1065-1069.
9. *Guidelines for Prehospital Management of Traumatic Brain Injury.* New York: Brain Trauma Foundation Press; 1998.
10. Colterjohn NR, Bednar DA. Identifiable risk factors for secondary neurologic deterioration in the cervical spine-injured patient. *Spine.* 1995;20: 2293-2297.
11. Reid DC, Henderson R, Saboe L, Miller JD. Etiology and clinical course of missed spine fractures. *J Trauma.* 1987;27:980-986.
12. Davis JW, Phreaner DL, Hoyt DB, Mackersie RC. The etiology of missed cervical spine injuries. *J Trauma.* 1993;34:342-346.
13. Harrop JS, Sharan AD, Vaccaro AR, Przybylski GJ. The cause of neurologic deterioration after acute cervical spinal cord injury. *Spine.* 2001;26: 340-346.
14. Holly LT, Kelly DF, Counelis GJ, Blinman T, McArthur DL, Cryer HG. Cervical spine trauma associated with moderate and severe head injury: incidence, risk factors, and injury characteristics. *J Neurosurg.* 2002;96: 285-291.
15. Demetriades D, Charalambides K, Chahwan S, et al. Nonskeletal cervical spine injuries: epidemiology and diagnostic pitfalls. *J Trauma.* 2000;48: 724-727.
16. Tian HL, Guo Y, Hu J, et al. Clinical characterization of comatose patients with cervical spine injury and traumatic brain injury. *J Trauma.* 2009;67: 1305-1310.
17. Rosen PB, McSwain NE, Jr, Arata M, Stahl S, Mercer D. Comparison of two new immobilization collars. *Ann Emerg Med.* 1992;21:1189-1195.
18. Graziano AF, Scheidel EA, Cline JR, Baer LJ. A radiographic comparison of prehospital cervical immobilization methods. *Ann Emerg Med.* 1987;16:1127-1131.
19. Davies G, Deakin C, Wilson A. The effect of a rigid collar on intracranial pressure. *Injury.* 1996;27:647-679.
20. Kolb JC, Summers RL, Galli RL. Cervical collar-induced changes in intracranial pressure. *Am J Emerg Med.* 1999;17:135-137.
21. Ho AMH, Fung KY, Joynt GM, Karmakar MK, Peng Z. Rigid cervical collar and intracranial pressure of patients with severe head injury. *J Trauma.* 2002;53:1185-1188.
22. Mobbs RJ, Stoodley MA, Fuller J. Effect of cervical hard collar on intracranial pressure after head injury. *ANZ J Surg.* 2002;72:389-391.
23. Hunt K, Hallworth S, Smith M. The effects of rigid collar placement on intracranial and cerebral perfusion pressures. *Anaesthesia.* 2001;56: 511-513.
24. Stone MB, Tubridy CM, Curran R. The effect of rigid cervical collars on internal jugular vein dimensions. *Acad Emerg Med.* 2009 Dec 15. [Epub ahead of print].
25. Seelig JM, Becker DP, Miller JD, et al. Traumatic acute subdural hematoma: major mortality reduction in comatose patients treated within four hours. *N Engl J Med.* 1981;304:1511-1518.
26. Haselsberger K, Pucher R, Auer LM. Prognosis after acute subdural or epidural haemorrhage. *Acta Neurochir (Wien).* 1988;90:111-116.
27. Langeron O, Masso E, Huraux C, et al. Prediction of difficult mask ventilation. *Anesthesiology.* 2000; 92: 1229-1236.
28. Yildiz TS, Solak M, Toker K. The incidence and risk factors of difficult mask ventilation. *J Anesth.* 2005;19:7-11.
29. Kheterpal S, Han R, Tremper KK, et al. Incidence and predictors of difficult and impossible mask ventilation. *Anesthesiology.* 2006;105:885-891.
30. Heath KJ. The effect of laryngoscopy of different cervical spine immobilisation techniques. *Anaesthesia.* 1994;49:843-845.
31. Moppett IK. Traumatic brain injury: assessment, resuscitation and early management. *Br J Anaesth.* 2007;99:18-31.
32. White AI, Panjabi M. Clinical biomechanics of the spine. 2nd ed. Philadelphia, PA: JB Lippincott; 1990.
33. Panjabi MM, Chen NC, Shin EK, Wang JL. The cortical shell architecture of human cervical vertebral bodies. *Spine (Phila Pa 1976).* 2001;26: 2478-2484.
34. Panjabi MM, Thibodeau LL, Crisco JJ, 3rd, White AA, 3rd. What constitutes spinal instability? *Clin Neurosurg.* 1988;34:313-339.
35. Turner CR, Block J, Shanks A, Morris M, Lodhia KR, Gujar SK. Motion of a cadaver model of cervical injury during endotracheal intubation with a Bullard laryngoscope or a Macintosh blade with and without in-line stabilization. *J Trauma.* 2009;67:61-66.
36. Sawin PD, Todd MM, Traynelis VC, et al. Cervical spine motion with direct laryngoscopy and orotracheal intubation. An in vivo cinefluoroscopic study of subjects without cervical abnormality. *Anesthesiology.* 1996;85:26-36.

37. Watts AD, Gelb AW, Bach DB, Pelz DM. Comparison of the Bullard and Macintosh laryngoscopes for endotracheal intubation of patients with a potential cervical spine injury. *Anesthesiology.* 1997;87:1335-1342.

38. Turkstra TP, Pelz DM, Shaikh AA, Craen RA. Cervical spine motion: a fluoroscopic comparison of Shikani optical stylet vs Macintosh laryngoscope. *Can J Anaesth.* 2007;54:441-447.

39. Turkstra TP, Pelz DM, Jones PM. Cervical spine motion: a fluoroscopic comparison of the AirTraq laryngoscope versus the Macintosh laryngoscope. *Anesthesiology.* 2009;111:97-101.

40. Turkstra TP, Craen RA, Pelz DM, Gelb AW. Cervical spine motion: a fluoroscopic comparison during intubation with lighted stylet, GlideScope, and Macintosh laryngoscope. *Anesth Analg.* 2005;101:910-915, table of contents.

41. Hirabayashi Y, Fujita A, Seo N, Sugimoto H. A comparison of cervical spine movement during laryngoscopy using the Airtraq or Macintosh laryngoscopes. *Anaesthesia.* 2008;63:635-640.

42. LeGrand SA, Hindman BJ, Dexter F, Weeks JB, Todd MM. Craniocervical motion during direct laryngoscopy and orotracheal intubation with the Macintosh and Miller blades: an in vivo cinefluoroscopic study. *Anesthesiology.* 2007;107:884-891.

43. Mentzelopoulos SD, Tzoufi MJ, Papageorgiou EP. The disposition of the cervical spine and deformation of available cord space with conventional- and balloon laryngoscopy-guided laryngeal intubation: a comparative study. *Anesth Analg.* 2001;92:1331-1336.

44. Hirabayashi Y, Fujita A, Seo N, Sugimoto H. Cervical spine movement during laryngoscopy using the airway scope compared with the Macintosh laryngoscope. *Anaesthesia.* 2007;62:1050-1055.

45. Houde BJ, Williams SR, Cadrin-Chenevert A, et al. A comparison of cervical spine motion during orotracheal intubation with the trachlight(r) or the flexible fiberoptic bronchoscope. *Anesth Analg.* 2009;108:1638-1643.

46. Lennarson PJ, Smith D, Todd MM, et al. Segmental cervical spine motion during orotracheal intubation of the intact and injured spine with and without external stabilization. *J Neurosurg.* 2000;92:201-206.

47. Robitaille A, Williams SR, Tremblay MH, Guilbert F, Thériault M, Drolet P. Cervical spine motion during tracheal intubation with manual in-line stabilization: direct laryngoscopy versus GlideScope videolaryngoscopy. *Anesth Analg.* 2008;106:935-941, table of contents.

48. Sugiyama K, Yokoyama K. Head extension angle required for direct laryngoscopy with the McCoy laryngoscope blade. *Anesthesiology.* 2001;94:939.

49. Hastings RH, Wood PR. Head extension and laryngeal view during laryngoscopy with cervical spine stabilization maneuvers. *Anesthesiology.* 1994;80:825-831.

50. Donaldson WF, 3rd, Heil BV, Donaldson VP, Silvaggio VJ. The effect of airway maneuvers on the unstable C1-C2 segment. A cadaver study. *Spine.* 1997;22:1215-1218.

51. Hauswald M, Sklar DP, Tandberg D, Garcia JF. Cervical spine movement during airway management: cinefluoroscopic appraisal in human cadavers. *Am J Emerg Med.* 1991;9:535-538.

52. Donaldson WF, 3rd, Towers JD, Doctor A, et al. A methodology to evaluate motion of the unstable spine during intubation techniques. *Spine.* 1993;18:2020-2023.

53. Aprahamian C, Thompson BM, Finger WA, Darin JC. Experimental cervical spine injury model: evaluation of airway management and splinting techniques. *Ann Emerg Med.* 1984;13:584-587.

54. Brimacombe J, Keller C, Kunzel KH, Gaber O, Boehler M, Pühringer F. Cervical spine motion during airway management: a cinefluoroscopic study of the posteriorly destabilized third cervical vertebrae in human cadavers. *Anesth Analg.* 2000;91:1274-1278.

55. Majernick TG, Bieniek R, Houston JB, Hughes HG. Cervical spine movement during orotracheal intubation. *Ann Emerg Med.* 1986;15:417-420.

56. Lennarson PJ, Smith DW, Sawin PD, Todd MM, Sato Y, Traynelis VC. Cervical spinal motion during intubation: efficacy of stabilization maneuvers in the setting of complete segmental instability. *J Neurosurg.* 2001;94:265-270.

57. Gerling MC, Davis DP, Hamilton RS, et al. Effects of cervical spine immobilization technique and laryngoscope blade selection on an unstable cervical spine in a cadaver model of intubation. *Ann Emerg Med.* 2000;36:293-300.

58. Crosby ET. Airway management in adults after cervical spine trauma. *Anesthesiology.* 2006;104:1293-1318.

59. Manoach S, Paladino L. Manual in-line stabilization for acute airway management of suspected cervical spine injury: historical review and current questions. *Ann Emerg Med.* 2007;50:236-245.

60. MacQuarrie K, Hung OR, Law JA. Tracheal intubation using Bullard laryngoscope for patients with a simulated difficult airway. *Can J Anaesth.* 1999;46:760-765.

61. Goutcher CM, Lochhead V. Reduction in mouth opening with semi-rigid cervical collars. *Br J Anaesth.* 2005;95:344-348.

62. Walls RM. Orotracheal intubation and potential cervical spine injury. *Ann Emerg Med.* 1987;16:373-374.

63. Nolan JP, Wilson ME. Orotracheal intubation in patients with potential cervical spine injuries. An indication for the gum elastic bougie. *Anaesthesia.* 1993;48:630-633.

64. Malik MA, Maharaj CH, Harte BH, Laffey JG. Comparison of Macintosh, Truview EVO2, Glidescope, and Airwayscope laryngoscope use in patients with cervical spine immobilization. *Br J Anaesth.* 2008;101:723-730.

65. Thiboutot F, Nicole PC, Trepanier CA, et al. Effect of manual in-line stabilization of the cervical spine in adults on the rate of difficult orotracheal intubation by direct laryngoscopy: a randomized controlled trial. *Can J Anaesth.* 2009;56:412-418.

66. Byhahn C, Nemetz S, Breitkreutz R, Wissler B, Kaufmann M, Meininger D. Brief report: tracheal intubation using the Bonfils intubation fibrescope or direct laryngoscopy for patients with a simulated difficult airway. *Can J Anaesth.* 2008;55:232-237.

67. Santoni BG, Hindman BJ, Puttlitz CM, et al. Manual in-line stabilization increases pressures applied by the laryngoscope blade during direct laryngoscopy and orotracheal intubation. *Anesthesiology.* 2009;110:24-31.

68. Kaufman HH, Harris JH, Jr, Spencer JA, Kopanisky DR. Danger of traction during radiography for cervical trauma. *JAMA.* 1982;247:2369.

69. Bivins HG, Ford S, Bezmalinovic Z, Prince HM, Williams JL. The effect of axial traction during orotracheal intubation of the trauma victim with an unstable cervical spine. *Ann Emerg Med.* 1988;17:25-29.

70. Hastings RH, Hon ED, Nghiem C, Wahrenbrock EA. Force and torque vary between laryngoscopists and laryngoscope blades. *Anesth Analg.* 1996;82:462-468.

71. Hastings RH, Vigil AC, Hanna R, et al. Cervical spine movement during laryngoscopy with the Bullard, Macintosh, and Miller laryngoscopes. *Anesthesiology.* 1995;82:859-869.

72. Konishi A, Sakai T, Nishiyama T, et al. Cervical spine movement during orotracheal intubation using the McCoy laryngoscope compared with the Macintosh and the Miller laryngoscopes. *Masui.* 1997;46:124-127.

73. MacIntyre PA, McLeod AD, Hurley R, Peacock C. Cervical spine movements during laryngoscopy. Comparison of the Macintosh and McCoy laryngoscope blades. *Anaesthesia.* 1999;54:413-418.

74. Grossman D, Schriger DL. Immobilization technique and blade choice in the endotracheal intubation of trauma patients: Miller time or much ado about nothing? *Ann Emerg Med.* 2000;36:351-353.

75. Uchida T, Hikawa Y, Saito Y, Yasuda K. The McCoy levering laryngoscope in patients with limited neck extension. *Can J Anaesth.* 1997;44:674-676.

76. Laurent SC, de Melo AE, Alexander-Williams JM. The use of the McCoy laryngoscope in patients with simulated cervical spine injuries. *Anaesthesia.* 1996;51:74-75.

77. Gabbott DA. Laryngoscopy using the McCoy laryngoscope after application of a cervical collar. *Anaesthesia.* 1996;51:812-814.

78. Wahlen BM, Gercek E. Three-dimensional cervical spine movement during intubation using the Macintosh and Bullard laryngoscopes, the bonfils fibrescope and the intubating laryngeal mask airway. *Eur J Anaesthesiol.* 2004;21:907-913.

79. Maruyama K, Yamada T, Kawakami R, et al. Upper cervical spine movement during intubation: fluoroscopic comparison of the AirWay Scope, McCoy laryngoscope, and Macintosh laryngoscope. *Br J Anaesth.* 2008;100:120-124.

80. Maruyama K, Yamada T, Kawakami R, Hara K. Randomized cross-over comparison of cervical-spine motion with the AirWay Scope or Macintosh laryngoscope with in-line stabilization: a video-fluoroscopic study. *Br J Anaesth.* 2008;101:563-567.

81. Takenaka I, Aoyama K, Iwagaki T, et al. Approach combining the airway scope and the bougie for minimizing movement of the cervical spine during endotracheal intubation. *Anesthesiology.* 2009;110:1335-1340.

82. Rudolph C, Schneider JP, Wallenborn J, Schaffranietz L. Movement of the upper cervical spine during laryngoscopy: a comparison of the Bonfils intubation fibrescope and the Macintosh laryngoscope. *Anaesthesia.* 2005;60:668-672.

83. Konishi A, Kikuchi K, Sasui M. Cervical spine movement during light-guided orotracheal intubation with lightwand stylet (Trachlight). *Masui.* 1998;47:94-97.

84. Waltl B, Melischek M, Schuschnig C, et al. Tracheal intubation and cervical spine excursion: direct laryngoscopy vs. intubating laryngeal mask. *Anaesthesia.* 2001;56:221-226.

85. Sahin A, Salman MA, Erden IA, Aypar U. Upper cervical vertebrae movement during intubating laryngeal mask, fibreoptic and direct laryngoscopy: a video-fluoroscopic study. *Eur J Anaesthesiol.* 2004;21:819-823.

86. Keller C, Brimacombe J, Keller K. Pressures exerted against the cervical vertebrae by the standard and intubating laryngeal mask airways: a randomized, controlled, cross-over study in fresh cadavers. *Anesth Analg.* 1999;89:1296-1300.

87. Wong DM, Prabhu A, Chakraborty S, et al. Cervical spine motion during flexible bronchoscopy compared with the Lo-Pro GlideScope. *Br J Anaesth.* 2009;102:424-230.

88. Malik MA, Subramaniam R, Churasia S, et al. Tracheal intubation in patients with cervical spine immobilization: a comparison of the Airwayscope, LMA CTrach, and the Macintosh laryngoscopes. *Br J Anaesth.* 2009;102:654-661.

89. Enomoto Y, Asai T, Arai T, et al. Pentax-AWS, a new videolaryngoscope, is more effective than the Macintosh laryngoscope for tracheal intubation in patients with restricted neck movements: a randomized comparative study. *Br J Anaesth.* 2008;100:544-548.

90. Maharaj CH, Buckley E, Harte BH, Laffey JG. Endotracheal intubation in patients with cervical spine immobilization: a comparison of Macintosh and Airtraq laryngoscopes. *Anesthesiology.* 2007;107:53-59.

91. Kihara S, Yaguchi Y, Taguchi N, et al. The StyletScope is a better intubation tool than a conventional stylet during simulated cervical spine immobilization. *Can J Anaesth.* 2005;52:105-110.

92. Adnet F, Borron SW, Racine SX, et al. The intubation difficulty scale (IDS): proposal and evaluation of a new score characterizing the complexity of endotracheal intubation. *Anesthesiology.* 1997;87:1290-1297.

93. Komatsu R, Nagata O, Kamata K, Yamagata K, Sesler DI, Ozaki M. Intubating laryngeal mask airway allows tracheal intubation when the cervical spine is immobilized by a rigid collar. *Br J Anaesth.* 2004;93:655-659.

94. Moller F, Andres AH, Langenstein H. Intubating laryngeal mask airway (ILMA) seems to be an ideal device for blind intubation in case of immobile spine. *Br J Anaesth.* 2000;85:493-495.

95. Ferson DZ, Rosenblatt WH, Johansen MJ, et al. Use of the intubating LMA-Fastrach in 254 patients with difficult-to-manage airways. *Anesthesiology.* 2001;95:1175-1181.

96. Wakeling HG, Nightingale J. The intubating laryngeal mask airway does not facilitate tracheal intubation in the presence of a neck collar in simulated trauma. *Br J Anaesth.* 2000;84:254-256.

97. Inoue Y, Koga K, Shigematsu A. A comparison of two tracheal intubation techniques with Trachlight and Fastrach in patients with cervical spine disorders. *Anesth Analg.* 2002;94:667-671, table of contents.

98. Helliwell V, Gabbott DA. The effect of single-handed cricoid pressure on cervical spine movement after applying manual in-line stabilisation—a cadaver study. *Resuscitation.* 2001;49:53-57.

99. Neilipovitz DT, Crosby ET. No evidence for decreased incidence of aspiration after rapid sequence induction. *Can J Anaesth.* 2007;54:748-764.

100. Hardman JG, Wills JS, Aitkenhead AR. Factors determining the onset and course of hypoxemia during apnea: an investigation using physiological modelling. *Anesth Analg.* 2000;90:619-624.

101. Mercer MH, Gabbott DA. Insertion of the Combitube airway with the cervical spine immobilised in a rigid cervical collar. *Anaesthesia.* 1998;53:971-974.

102. Komatsu R, Nagata O, Kamata K, et al. Comparison of the intubating laryngeal mask airway and laryngeal tube placement during manual in-line stabilisation of the neck. *Anaesthesia.* 2005;60:113-117.

103. Gerling MC, Davis DP, Hamilton RS, et al. Effect of surgical cricothyrotomy on the unstable cervical spine in a cadaver model of intubation. *J Emerg Med.* 2001;20:1-5.

104. Talucci RC, Shaikh KA, Schwab CW. Rapid sequence induction with oral endotracheal intubation in the multiply injured patient. *Am Surg.* 1988;54:185-187.

105. Shatney CH, Brunner RD, Nguyen TQ. The safety of orotracheal intubation in patients with unstable cervical spine fracture or high spinal cord injury. *Am J Surg.* 1995;170:676-679; discussion 679-680.

106. Suderman VS, Crosby ET, Lui A. Elective oral tracheal intubation in cervical spine-injured adults. *Can J Anaesth.* 1991;38:785-789.

107. Rosen P, Wolfe RE. Therapeutic legends of emergency medicine. *J Emerg Med.* 1989;7:387-389.

108. McLeod AD, Calder I. Spinal cord injury and direct laryngoscopy—the legend lives on. *Br J Anaesth.* 2000;84:705-709.

109. Hastings RH, Kelley SD. Neurologic deterioration associated with airway management in a cervical spine-injured patient. *Anesthesiology.* 1993;78:580-583.

110. Liang BA, Cheng MA, Tempelhoff R. Efforts at intubation: cervical injury in an emergency circumstance? *J Clin Anesth.* 1999;11:349-352.

111. Meschino A, Devitt JH, Koch JP, Szalai JP, Schwartz ML. The safety of awake tracheal intubation in cervical spine injury. *Can J Anaesth.* 1992;39:114-117.

112. Holley J, Jorden R. Airway management in patients with unstable cervical spine fractures. *Ann Emerg Med.* 1989;18:1237-1239.

113. Rhee KJ, Green W, Holcroft JW, Mangili JA. Oral intubation in the multiply injured patient: the risk of exacerbating spinal cord damage. *Ann Emerg Med.* 1990;19:511-514.

114. Scannell G, Waxman K, Tominaga G, Barker S, Annas C. Orotracheal intubation in trauma patients with cervical fractures. *Arch Surg.* 1993;128:903-905; discussion 905-906.

115. Wright SW, Robinson GG, 2nd, Wright MB. Cervical spine injuries in blunt trauma patients requiring emergent endotracheal intubation. *Am J Emerg Med.* 1992;10:104-109.

116. Norwood S, Myers MB, Butler TJ. The safety of emergency neuromuscular blockade and orotracheal intubation in the acutely injured trauma patient. *J Am Coll Surg.* 1994;179:646-652.

117. Richards CF, Mayberry JC. Initial management of the trauma patient. *Crit Care Clin.* 2004;20:1-11.

118. Ball PA. Critical care of spinal cord injury. *Spine.* 2001;26:S27-S30.

119. Urdaneta F, Layon AJ. Respiratory complications in patients with traumatic cervical spine injuries: case report and review of the literature. *J Clin Anesth.* 2003;15:398-405.

120. Ivy ME, Cohn SM. Addressing the myths of cervical spine injury management. *Am J Emerg Med.* 1997;15:591-595.

121. Gajraj NM, Chason DP, Shearer VE. Cervical spine movement during orotracheal intubation: comparison of the Belscope and Macintosh blades. *Anaesthesia.* 1994;49:772-774.

122. Crosby ET. Tracheal intubation in the cervical spine-injured patient. *Can J Anaesth.* 1992;39:105-109.

123. Abrams K, Grande C. Airway management of the trauma patient with cervical spine injury. *Curr Opin Anaesth.* 1994;7:184-190.

124. Hastings RH, Marks JD. Airway management for trauma patients with potential cervical spine injuries. *Anesth Analg.* 1991;73:471-482.

125. Dunham CM, Barraco RD, Clark DE, et al. Guidelines for emergency tracheal intubation immediately after traumatic injury. *J Trauma.* 2003;55:162-179.

126. Gajraj N, Pennant J, Giesecke A. Cervical spine trauma and airway management. *Curr Opin Anaesthesiol.* 1993;6:369-374.

127. Ezri T, Szmuk P, Warters RD, Katz J, Hagberg CA. Difficult airway management practice patterns among anesthesiologists practicing in the United States: have we made any progress? *J Clin Anesth.* 2003;15:418-422.

128. Chesnut RM. Management of brain and spine injuries. *Crit Care Clin.* 2004;20:25-55.

129. McGuire G, el-Beheiry H. Complete upper airway obstruction during awake fibreoptic intubation in patients with unstable cervical spine fractures. *Can J Anaesth.* 1999;46:176-178.

130. Penning L. Prevertebral hematoma in cervical spine injury: incidence and etiologic significance. *AJR Am J Roentgenol.* 1981;136:553-561.

131. Biby L, Santora AH. Prevertebral hematoma secondary to whiplash injury necessitating emergency intubation. *Anesth Analg.* 1990;70:112-114.

132. Shiratori T, Hara K, Ando N. Acute airway obstruction secondary to retropharyngeal hematoma. *J Anesth.* 2003;17:46-48.

133. Myssiorek D, Shalmi C. Traumatic retropharyngeal hematoma. *Arch Otolaryngol Head Neck Surg.* 1989;115:1130-1132.

134. Marion DW, Puccio A, Wisniewski SR, et al. Effect of hyperventilation on extracellular concentrations of glutamate, lactate, pyruvate, and local cerebral blood flow in patients with severe traumatic brain injury. *Crit Care Med.* 2002;30:2619-2625.

135. Guidelines for prehospital management of traumatic brain injury, 2nd edition. *Prehosp Emerg Care.* 2007;12:S1-S52.

SELF-EVALUATION QUESTIONS

15.1. Which of the following is contraindicated during intubation of the trauma patient undergoing C-spine precautions with manual in-line neck stabilization (MILNS)?

A. removal of the front of the cervical collar

B. oral intubation using direct laryngoscopy

C. cricoid pressure

D. external laryngeal manipulation

E. none of the above

15.2. Which of the following airway interventions has been shown to improve neurologic outcome in the head-injured patient with a potential cervical spine injury?

A. performing an awake fiberoptic intubation

B. performing manual in-line neck stabilization during intubation attempts

C. use of an alternative to direct laryngoscopy such as a Glidescope

D. avoiding transient oxygen desaturation

E. all of the above

15.3. Which of the following statements concerning the head-injured patient is **TRUE**?

A. Improved neurological outcome is associated with the avoidance of direct laryngoscopy for intubation in this population.

B. The unconscious head-injured patient (GCS <8) has a threefold chance of cervical spine injury.

C. Avoidance of cervical spine movement during airway management is more important than avoiding transient hypoxemia and hypotension.

D. The safest way of performing tracheal intubation is proven to be the flexible bronchoscope.

E. The use of muscle relaxants for intubation of these patients is contraindicated because they will interfere with subsequent neurological evaluation.

CHAPTER (16)

Airway Management of an Unconscious Patient Who Remains Trapped inside the Vehicle Following a Motor Vehicle Collision

Tom C. Phu, Orlando R. Hung, and Ronald D. Stewart

16.1 CASE PRESENTATION

A 23-year-old driver is involved in a motor vehicle crash (MVC) in which her car has collided with an oncoming vehicle. On arrival at the scene, the emergency medical services (EMS) field team estimates a prolonged extrication time and difficult airway problem, and calls for EMS physician-on-call back-up. Upon arriving at the scene, you note that she appears to be unconscious inside the vehicle and is not making effective respiratory efforts. She is slumped back against her seat.

16.2 PATIENT CONSIDERATIONS

16.2.1 According to the advanced trauma life support (ATLS) guidelines, what are the immediate issues that need to be addressed?

The prehospital environment can be an unpredictable and unstable environment for the patient and the EMS practitioner. Thus, prior to the initiation of resuscitation protocols, scene safety must be assessed and assured. Assessment and management of the airway, breathing, and then circulation (ABCs) follows Advanced Trauma Life Support Guidelines (ATLS).[1] After scene safety, for the critically injured patient, airway management remains the

greatest priority and challenge. In this unconscious patient, rapid extrication from the vehicle is unlikely, so airway assessment and management must be performed immediately while the patient is still in the vehicle.

In this patient, the practitioner must assume that the patient has suffered a severe traumatic brain injury (TBI). Oxygenation and ventilation in the setting of severe TBI is of utmost importance in initiating treatment as prolonged hypoxia and hypercapnia are associated with increased morbidity and mortality. Associated injuries are likely in this patient: cervical spine injury; cardiothoracic injuries such as pneumothorax, hemothorax, flail chest, cardiopulmonary contusions, and cardiac tamponade; as well as intrabdominal injuries. Once the airway is adequately managed, the EMS team will need to assess the patient for these injuries, while recognizing that a complete assessment and definitive intervention will require expeditious transport to adequate in-hospital facilities.

16.2.2 How does this prehospital setting affect your management of this patient?

Field management of this patient's airway is second only to scene safety considerations. The scenario described is an example of a worst-case situation and the field environment will have a significant impact on the options and interventions available. The practitioner will not be able to make the same judgments or carry out the same assessments possible in a controlled hospital environment. In this context, the practitioner will have to choose the optimal method of airway management in this patient while considering other options, should the primary attempt fail. While prehospital intubation has traditionally been used as the definitive airway in the field environment, there is growing evidence that it may be associated with no patient benefit at best[2] and possibly an increased risk of adverse patient outcomes[3,4] at worst. If tracheal intubation is found to be difficult or impossible, or beyond the skill set of the responder, the use of alternative airway techniques, including the extraglottic devices (EGDs), should be considered.

16.2.3 What are the indications for airway management in this patient?

Life-threatening ventilatory insufficiency will lead to cardiorespiratory arrest if not corrected promptly—particularly in the context of a severe TBI and elevated ICP. Furthermore, airway management is indicated in this patient in order to protect from hypoxia and aspiration.

16.2.4 Are there any special considerations in this case?

There are several important considerations which should guide the prehospital practitioner in managing this patient's airway. These include: a critically injured patient and the need to immediately secure the airway, TBI, limited patient access, and limited resources. The fact that the patient is trapped and the confines of the vehicle restrictive will not allow for controlled intubation conditions. Direct laryngoscopy (DL) is likely contraindicated in such surroundings in the immediate management of this patient's airway. Furthermore, Mort et al, found a positive correlation between the number of laryngoscopic intubation attempts (≤2 vs >2) and complications, including hypoxemia, regurgitation of gastric contents, aspiration, bradycardia, and cardiac arrest.[5] These data suggest that EMS practitioner should limit the number of intubation attempts in this patient—and perhaps avoid attempting laryngoscopic intubation in this patient and alternative methods would be indicated. Airway interventions should be instituted quickly and would include other airway adjuncts if initial intubation attempts fail. Securing an airway must be undertaken in a planned and expeditious manner.

If the patient is obtunded but still has intact airway reflexes (eg, gag reflex), any attempt at airway manipulation may lead to biting, gagging, and the vomiting of gastric contents. Airway reflexes will also make more difficult attempt at airway intervention.

16.2.5 How would you alleviate the airway obstruction?

Several simple maneuvers can be used to alleviate an airway obstruction. These include a chin lift, jaw thrust, head tilt, and tongue pull. Some of these simple steps may involve significant movement of the C-spine (see Chapter 15). Although a jaw thrust, or pulling the tongue forward, is traditionally felt to be associated with the least cervical movement, cadaver studies have shown it is still associated with some C-spine movement and should be performed carefully.[6] However, in this emergency situation, in which

the failure to oxygenate and ventilate this patient may result in greater risk to hypoxic brain injury and perhaps death, the practitioner must weigh the risk of cervical spine movement against the risk of failure to provide oxygenation and ventilation.

Application of a face mask with oxygen supplementation should be performed at a minimum. In the absence of adequate respiratory effort, ventilation and oxygenation must be provided to the patient immediately by bag-mask-ventilation (either one person or two person), if possible, while planning for a more definitive airway. An oropharyngeal airway may help to alleviate airway obstruction.

16.2.6 How would you assess the patient's airway? Are traditional means of airway assessment valid in the unconscious patient?

Several airway measurements exist as tools to predict a difficult laryngoscopy (see Chapter 1). Unfortunately, these assessment tools are not useful in the prehospital environment in which on-scene factors (patient positioning, poor patient access, smoke, fumes, fire, and environmental hazards) as well as uncooperative or unconscious patients may prevent EMS practitioner from performing these assessments.

The overall appearance of this patient should first be assessed. Specifically, on-site practitioner should assess the patient for signs of inadequate ventilation, as manifested by signs of gasping, use of accessory muscles, indrawing, cyanosis, and so on. Airway evaluation in this patient should then proceed to a search for airway trauma and signs of injury to the head and neck.

The practitioner should assume airway management will be difficult and should be ready to use alternative airways techniques, should early intubation attempts fail.

16.3 AIRWAY MANAGEMENT

16.3.1 Is this patient likely to be difficult to oxygenate? Why?

Airway management must be initiated prior to extrication. BMV may be made more difficult if there is blood or teeth, or foreign bodies in the airway. If the patient is upright or there is limited access to the face, oxygenation will be a challenging task and the practitioner may find two-person BMV (see Chapter 7 for details) will facilitate ventilation/oxygenation in this patient. While the acronym "MOANS" (see Section 1.6.1) may be useful to predict difficulties with BMV in conscious cooperative patients, it is not useful for this patient. The effect of trauma to the head and neck on BMV can be unpredictable, but does not preclude an initial attempt at BMV to oxygenate the patient. It is also reasonable to use an extraglottic device (EGD), such as the laryngeal mask airway (LMA), if the BMV fails. Unfortunately, the effectiveness of ventilating a patient using the LMA may be equally unreliable following facial trauma.

Blind airway techniques should be avoided in patients with a facial trauma as it may be associated with injuries to the airway and a potentially distorted anatomy. However, in the presence of hypoxemia, coupled with limited resources, a blind or nonvisual airway technique may be considered to ensure ventilation and oxygenation, provided that it is performed cautiously by a skilled practitioner.

16.3.2   What are your airway options in this patient?

Managing the airway of this patient will be challenging due to the critical injuries sustained by this patient and the unpredictable environment. The options that should be considered by the initial EMS practitioners will depend on their skills and level of training. To avoid significant complications, advanced airway techniques, including alternative techniques, should be attempted only by skilled and experienced EMS practitioners. Practitioners with basic airway skills should use basic airway maneuvers, including jaw thrust and tongue pull. Jaw thrust maneuvers should be used with caution because of the risk of cervical spine injury. However, to minimize the risk of hypoxemia or hypoventilation, it would be reasonable to perform a gentle jaw thrust to improve ventilation/oxygenation when a chin-lift does not appear to clear the obstructed airway. Practitioners with appropriate airway training might, in addition to the above maneuvers, consider the use of EGDs, such as the various types of LMA devices (LMA Classic™, intubating LMA, LMA ProSeal™), Laryngeal Tubes, and Combitube™ among others. The availability of these devices in various EMS organizations may determine the specific EGD used.

Practitioners with advanced airway training may consider the use of endotracheal intubation, ranging from DL to the use of the intubating LMA, lightwand (eg, Trachlight™), and surgical cricothyrotomy. Endotracheal intubation may be fraught with risks and complications in this patient, particularly with practitioners who do not routinely perform the procedure. These complications including esophageal intubation, aspiration, hypoxemia add further trauma to the airway.

Regardless of the level of airway training, multiple intubation attempts should be avoided if initial attempts at intubation are unsuccessful, as repeated attempts will increase the risk of hypoxemia and mortality.

16.3.3   What is the role of the extraglottic devices in managing the airway of this patient?

There are several extraglottic devices (EGDs) which can be used as rescue airways. These include the LMA and its variants (such as the LMA Fastrach™ and the LMA ProSeal™), Combitube™, Laryngeal Tube (King LT™), and others.

Insertion and use of the LMA is described in Chapter 12. The LMA and its variants are advantageous in this patient because it can be inserted while facing the patient who may be upright and difficult to access and may provide an effective rescue airway to oxygenate the patient. While there are many other EGDs that can be used in this setting, most practitioners are familiar with the LMA and perhaps, it should be the device of choice. The LMA is also useful because it can provide a conduit for subsequent endotracheal intubation (LMA Classic™ and LMA Fastrach™).

Although intubation using the LMA to guide the endotracheal tube (ETT) into the trachea can be performed using either the LMA Classic™ or the LMA Fastrach™ (intubating LMA), it is much easier to advance the ETT through the LMA Fastrach™. (See Table 16-1 for appropriate ETT sizes.)

The LMA Fastrach™ is designed with a rigid handle to facilitate its insertion. When correctly positioned, the LMA Fastrach™ is designed to direct the ETT into the trachea. Reported intubation success rates using the LMA Fastrach™ range from 82% to 99.3%.[8] Although the LMA Fastrach™ comes with a specifically designed silicone-wire-reinforced tracheal tube, a recent report found no difference in the success rates in intubation through the LMA Fastrach™ when the silicone-wire ETT was compared to a warmed standard polyvinyl chloride ETT.[9] However, the necessity of warming an ETT, especially in the prehospital environment, makes it a less attractive option.

When used together with the LMA Fastrach™, the Trachlight™ (see Section 12.4.3) has been shown to facilitate confirmation of tracheal placement of the ETT and improve the success rate of tube placement.[10] There is a growing consensus that the LMA Fastrach™ may be a useful airway alternative in the prehospital environment due to its rapid learning curve,[11] high success rate of insertion, and its ability to ventilate and oxygenate the patient, as well as to facilitate intubation.

The Combitube™ (see Section 12.6) is a double-lumen EGD which can be easily inserted as a rescue device in this patient. Several reports suggested that it can play an important role in trauma airway management.[12-15] Its correct use depends on determining its position either in the esophagus (>90% of insertions) or the trachea and ventilating the patient via the correct lumen. Incorrect use can lead to significant complications, including insufflation of the stomach with aspiration, esophageal and pharyngeal trauma, and subsequent rupture.[15] Its use is contraindicated in the presence of esophageal or pharyngeal injuries.[11]

The Laryngeal Tube (see Section 12.7) is a single-lumen EGD device with a distal and proximal cuff. In between the two cuffs are ventilation ports which allow for oxygenation of the patient. The Laryngeal Tube (LT) has been shown to be easily inserted with minimal airway trauma. However, there are few peer-reviewed studies examining the role of the LT in the trauma patient. Some

▸ TABLE 16-1

Appropriate ETT Sizes for Intubation via LMA-Classic

LMA-CLASSIC SIZE (in mm)	ENDOTRACHEAL TUBE SIZE (in mm ID)
4	6.0
5	7.0
LMA Fastrach™ (3, 4, and 5)	Up to 8.0

studies have suggested inexperienced prehospital practitioners have a 78% to 100% success rate of insertion in anesthetized patients.[16] In prehospital cardiac arrest patients, the LT was successfully inserted in 83% of patients.[17] Like other EGDs, the LT is not designed to protect against aspiration, so similar precautions to other EGDs should be considered. However, the recent introduction of the single-use Laryngeal Tube with suction and drainage option (LTS-D) may provide protection against aspiration.[18] While it appears that LT is an effective EGD, its role in trauma airways remains to be determined.

16.4 OTHER CONSIDERATIONS

16.4.1 Discuss the role of EGDs in the trauma patient

EGDs are gaining popularity in managing the airway of the trauma patient when the trachea cannot be intubated.[19-22] Martin et al examined the use of the LMA in the prehospital environment; the authors reported a success rate of 94% in trauma patients.[21] All successful insertions were performed in 10 seconds or less. The authors investigated the effectiveness of the LMA in providing adequate oxygenation and ventilation in these patients and found that, during transport, patient oxygen saturations ranged from 97% to 100% while the end-tidal CO_2 ranged from 24 to 35 mm Hg.[21] These data support a role for the LMA, and other EGDs (although most studies have only examined the role of LMAs), as tools for oxygenation and ventilation in trauma patients when tracheal intubation in the field was unsuccessful.

To address the issue of aspiration with EGDs, multiple devices have been developed with alternate channels that would allow for drainage of regurgitated gastric contents.[23] The LMA ProSeal™ (see Section 12.5 for details) contains a drainage tube that extends into the upper esophagus at the distal end of the device.[23] Multiple case reports suggest that the LMA ProSeal™ is effective[24,25] at minimizing, although not eliminating, aspiration risk.[26,27]

The Combitube™ also has the potential to protect the airway from aspiration of gastric contents. Using dye within the oropharynx, Mercer recently showed that the Combitube™ could protect the airway in most anesthetized patients.[28] However, tracheal soiling was seen in 7% (2/27) of the studied patients.[28] Similarly, using a pH probe in the trachea, Hagberg et al[29] reported evidence of low pH in the trachea in 1 of 25 anesthetized patients (4%) using a Combitube™, suggesting possible microaspiration of acidic gastric contents.

Recently, dual-lumen laryngeal tubes with suction and drainage (LTS-D and LTS-II) have been introduced. While these devices may allow easy ventilation and aspiration protection,[18] large clinical studies are needed to assess their effectiveness in doing so.

In summary, while these EGDs are effective rescue devices to provide oxygenation and ventilation in trauma patients, and may play an important role in providing oxygenation and ventilation in patients with difficult or impossible intubation, they do not ensure protection against the risk of aspiration of gastric contents.

16.4.2 What are your concerns with transporting this patient with an EGD as an airway?

EGDs are effective devices for ventilation; however, there are a few considerations to keep in mind during transport.

First, these devices cannot ensure complete protection of the airway against the risks of aspiration, although many studies have not reported a significant incidence.[21,22,30] There have been case reports of the successful use of the LMA ProSeal™ and LMA Supreme™ as a rescue airway in trauma,[7] suggesting that it may play a role in the prehospital environment. At this time, the lack of well-designed studies of EGDs in the trauma setting would suggest supporting their use as rescue devices only if endotracheal intubation fails.

A second concern regarding the use of EGDs in the prehospital management of the trauma patient relates to the risk of malpositioning during transport. Any change in the positioning of the EGD may impair its ability to provide effective oxygenation and ventilation and the practitioner must continuously monitor the positioning and effectiveness of the EGD during transport. The application of cervical collars to maintain in-line cervical stabilization may also cause the EGDs to shift or cause airway obstruction during transport.[22]

16.4.3 What are your options for endotracheal intubation in this patient?

Laryngoscopic intubation may be difficult until the patient is extricated from the vehicle. Even then, the condition of the patient in the field environment may be adverse to the successful placement of an ETT under DL. In the clinical situation in which the patient cannot be removed from the vehicle, the options for endotracheal intubation include lightwand-guided intubation, digital intubation, and intubation through an LMA or the LMA Fastrach™. However, it should be noted that techniques not requiring direct visualization, such as the lightwand, increase the potential for airway trauma. Thus, intubation with either direct laryngoscopy (if possible) or using the LMA Fastrach™ is preferable to attempts at intubation with the lightwand.

16.4.4 Discuss the pros and cons of lightwand (Trachlight) intubation in this patient

Light-guided intubation using a lightwand has been shown to be an effective and safe technique for both oral and nasal-tracheal intubation.[31-33] The technique of intubation using the lightwand (Trachlight™) has been described in Chapter 11.[34,35]

Because of its limitations as a nonvisualizing technique, the lightwand should be reserved for situations in which alternative airway techniques are difficult or impossible. These include limited mouth opening and patient factors that would make surgical cricothyrotomy impossible (eg, lack of equipment, trauma to the anterior neck, making impossible to identify landmark, etc). In the absence of these factors, other airway management techniques would be more advantageous than the lightwand, including direct laryngoscopy and the use of EGDs (+/– intubation).[32,33,36]

The disadvantages of the lightwand in this patient include possibility of a traumatized airway, and ambient lighting may make the use of a lightwand difficult. Since we are unable to rule out a traumatic airway in this patient, the use of the lightwand may lead to delays in securing the airway and may further increase the risk of hypoxemia, morbidity, and mortality.

16.4.5   Digital intubation

Digital intubation (or tactile orotracheal intubation) involves the insertion of an ETT into the trachea using the fingers. It should be performed only by trained practitioners. Digital-guided intubation has been described previously (see Chapter 11). It is a safe and effective technique for airway management in the prehospital setting in an unconscious patient, requiring minimal equipment and patient access.[37,38]

While facing the patient, the clinician pulls the patient's tongue forward using the dominant hand. The nondominant hand is then inserted into the oropharynx where the epiglottis can be palpated and lifted superiorly using the long finger. An Eschmann Tracheal Introducer (ETI) (if available) can then be inserted into the airway with the dominant hand. The Eschmann Tracheal Introducer is then guided anteriorly into the trachea with the index finger of the nondominant hand. Confirmation of tracheal placement of the ETI can be done in the usual manner (eg, tracheal clicks and the hold up). The ETT can then be advanced over the ETI and into the trachea, employing the nondominant hand to guide the ETT over the tongue into the trachea. The ETI is then removed and positioning of the ETT in the trachea is confirmed using auscultation and end-tidal CO_2. If an ETI is not available, an ETT with stylet can be advanced into the airway and guided into the trachea (see Section 11.4). Digital intubation can also be performed using the lightwand in lieu of the ETI. This allows the practitioner to confirm placement using tactile and visual cues.

There are relatively few studies examining the role of digital intubation in the management of a patient's airway. Stewart reported that digital intubation is a simple and useful airway technique in the prehospital environment because it can be performed with minimal head and neck movement and with a cervical collar in place.[38] The presence of blood or secretions in the airway does not seem to influence its success. Similarly, Hardwick and Bluhm, in their series, report successful intubation in 58 out of 66 patients in the prehospital setting.[37]

Digital intubation is an effective airway technique that, while possible, should be reserved only for those skilled in this technique. It cannot be used in patients with intact airway reflexes.

16.4.7   Would nasotracheal intubation be suitable for this patient?

Blind nasal intubation would not be the first choice for airway management in this patient because of potential basal skull fracture and lack of respiratory efforts. However, in the event that the patient's condition is deteriorating rapidly, and multiple attempts at the airway have been made, it may be reasonable to consider the blind nasal technique while concurrently preparing for a surgical cricothyrotomy if the practitioner is skilled with these techniques.

16.4.8   Surgical cricothyrotomy

If the airway cannot be secured (either by endotracheal intubation or with the use of an EGD), and ventilation is unsuccessful or inadequate, securing the airway using a surgical technique is indicated. Delays in proceeding to a surgical airway following a series of failed attempts at airway control, is an important cause of morbidity and mortality. Surgical airways, such as surgical cricothyrotomy (SC), should be performed only by those familiar with the techniques. Studies in prehospital airway management have reported success rates of 82% to 100% when performed by trained paramedics, nurses, or physicians. Complication rates vary from 0% to 27%.[39] Details of performing SC are described in Chapter 13. The practitioner should be aware that obese patients, or those with abnormal anatomy (eg, hematoma, trauma to the neck, previous surgery, and radiation), might make identifying the cricothyroid membrane difficult. SC can be performed using either the open or Seldinger technique. To facilitate SC, there are a number of cricothyrotomy kits available (eg, Cook Critical Care, Bloomington, IN). If possible, a cuffed cricothyrotomy tube should be used to ensure effective ventilation following its placement.

While SC may not be performed often in the prehospital environment, there is evidence that it can be performed, with reasonable success, should prehospital responders be appropriately trained.[39-41] In their retrospective review of SC performed by paramedics, Fortune et al found that paramedics who were trained in SC were able to perform the technique with 64% of patients arriving in the emergency department with acceptable SC airways.[41] A further 16% required minor manipulation in the emergency department.

If cricothyrotomy kits are not available, SC can be performed with a scalpel, an Eschmann Tracheal Introducer (gum elastic bougie) and an endotracheal tube.[42,43] In these reports, the authors describe the insertion of an Eschmann Tracheal Introducer (ETI) following a skin and cricothyroid membrane incision. The ETT is then guided over the ETI and acts as its own dilator of the cricothyroid membrane. The advantage of this technique is that it does not require a cricothyrotomy kit, has only three steps, and can be done quickly in an emergency. Similar to all airway management techniques, this three-step cricothyrotomy technique needs to be taught prior to its use in the field.

16.4.9   What would your overall approach be in the management of this patient's airway?

The management of this patient's airway must take into consideration the safety of the scene, the skills of the practitioner, the equipment available, the critical nature of this patient's injuries, and the urgency of establishing an airway. Emergency medical systems (EMS) can vary significantly in both structure and quality of care. North American EMS organizations are paramedic-based systems while other EMS organizations incorporate physicians (often anesthesiologists) and other health professionals. The variability between skill levels of prehospital practitioners precludes a generic algorithm appropriate for all responders. Rather, it would be more appropriate to have protocols based on the skill level of the practitioner.[17]

Initial attempts at airway management, appropriate for responders of all skill levels, should involve simple maneuvers which may alleviate the obstructed airway or facilitate further airway interventions. This includes a jaw thrust, tongue pull, and/or insertion of an oropharyngeal airway (OPA). Chin lifts may be considered necessary, but one should proceed with caution and recognize the potential impact of cervical spine movement in a patient with a high risk of cervical spine injury.

If the patient initiates any respiratory effort with these maneuvers, attempts at supporting the patient's airway while extrication proceeds may be sufficient—particularly if the responder has training only in basic airway management. Insufficient ventilation in this situation may necessitate assistance with BMV. This may require two-person BMV to ensure adequate delivered volumes.

Responders possessing training beyond basic skills may continue with BMV or consider the use of other adjuncts. The LMA Laryngeal Tube™, or Combitube™ are the most commonly used prehospital airway alternatives. The skill levels required to ensure proper insertion and adequate ventilation are variable. The insertion success rates to allow adequate ventilation for the LMA Classic™ may vary between 64% and 100% when inserted by respiratory therapists and EMS providers.[17,44,45] The LMA Fastrach™ may be a useful alternative because of its ease of insertion, high success rate, and ability to ventilate as well as facilitate intubation.[17] In their observational study of prehospital intubations by paramedics using either the intubating LMA or direct laryngoscopy, McCall et al[46] found that the rate of successful intubation of unconscious patients was 88% with the intubating LMA and 63% with DL. Nakazawa et al[8] demonstrated successful intubations between 82% and 99.3% with the intubating LMA. Overall success rates, including those requiring more than one attempt, were not statistically different at 91% for DL and 92% with the intubating LMA.[46] In a simulation of a difficult airway, Reeves et al[47] examined the rates of successful insertion of the intubating LMA by ambulance officers, physicians with intubating experience, and physicians without intubation experience. Most importantly, they found that 100% of patients were successfully ventilated with the intubating LMA. The respective failure rates of intubation (not ventilation) in the groups were 7% (ambulance officers with intubating experience), 20% (physicians with intubating experience), and 16% (physicians without intubating experience).[47] While the study by Reeves et al involved only a small group of participants, the results are consistent with other studies which suggest that success insertion rates are high with the intubating LMA in individuals with varying levels of airway management skills.[17] In this situation, ventilation and oxygenation may be all that is needed until the patient can be extricated and transported to hospital. In the event that tracheal intubation is needed, the intubating LMA may facilitate the ETT placement.

The LMA ProSeal™ (see Section 12.5) is a variant of the LMA with the potential ability to passively drain gastric contents via its esophageal vent.[48] There have been case reports of the drainage tube allowing for drainage of gastric contents during active vomiting.[25,49]

Conversely, there have also been case reports of aspiration despite the use of the LMA ProSeal™.[48]

The use of the combitube™ (see Section 12.6) in prehospital care has been well described.[17] Its insertion does require training and, thus, its use should be reserved for the trained practitioner. Esophagus placement occurs 95% of the time with the remaining 5% resulting in translaryngeal placement. Successful insertion and ventilation ranges from 79% to 82.4%.[17]

The practitioner with advanced training in airway management may feel comfortable using additional airway techniques beyond those already described (maneuvers to relieve airway obstruction, EGDs). Additional options, reserved for practitioners with advanced skills in airway management, include digital intubation and surgical cricothyroidotomy as described earlier.

As with all airway management techniques, successful ventilation and oxygenation should be confirmed using colorimetry or capnography.

16.5 SUMMARY

Prehospital airway management of an unconscious, apneic patient trapped in a vehicle is one of the most challenging situations for airway practitioners. Options in airway management are generally limited. The selection of an airway technique must depend on the field conditions, patient's condition, available resources, and the skills of the practitioner.

The focus of the practitioner should be on maintaining oxygenation and ventilation until the patient can be extricated to facilitate further assessment and management. The approach should begin with basic airway techniques including jaw thrust, chin lift, and the provision of oxygen via BMV. Practitioners with more advanced training can employ alternative airways including the EGDs, or may attempt intubation. Multiple attempts should be avoided for fear of increasing the risk of hypoxemia, hypercarbia, airway trauma, and mortality. If intubation is deemed appropriate, alternative intubating techniques such as digital intubation, intubating LMAs may be considered, but only by practitioners with advanced airway skills. Others with less experience or training should focus on basic airways skills and getting further assistance. Surgical cricothyrotomy may be necessary if oxygenation and ventilation is inadequate despite other techniques. It can be performed with either commercially available cricothyrotomy kits or, in emergency situations; the three-step technique can be used.

REFERENCES

1. American College of Surgeons. Advanced Trauma Life Support program for doctors: ATLS. Chicago, IL: American College of Surgeons; 2009.
2. Cobas MA, De la Pena MA, Manning R, Candiotti K, Varon AJ. Prehospital intubations and mortality: a level 1 trauma center perspective. *Anesth Analg* 2009;109:489-493.
3. Bochicchio GV, Ilahi O, Joshi M, Bochicchio K, Scalea TM. Endotracheal intubation in the field does not improve outcome in trauma patients who present without an acutely lethal traumatic brain injury. *J Trauma*. 2003;54:307-311.
4. Davis DP, Peay J, Sise MJ, et al. The impact of prehospital endotracheal intubation on outcome in moderate to severe traumatic brain injury. *J Trauma*. 2005;58:933-939.

5. Mort TC. Emergency tracheal intubation: complications associated with repeated laryngoscopic attempts. *Anesth Analg*. 2004;99:607-613.

6. Donaldson WF, 3rd, Heil BV, Donaldson VP, Silvaggio VJ. The effect of airway maneuvers on the unstable C1-C2 segment. A cadaver study. *Spine*. 1997;22:1215-1218.

7. Grier G, Bredmose P, Davies G, Lockey D. Introduction and use of the ProSeal laryngeal mask airway as a rescue device in a pre-hospital trauma anaesthesia algorithm. *Resuscitation*. 2009;80:138-141.

8. Nakazawa K, Tanaka N, Ishikawa S, et al. Using the intubating laryngeal mask airway (LMA-Fastrach) for blind endotracheal intubation in patients undergoing cervical spine operation. *Anesth Analg*. 1999;89:1319-1321.

9. Kundra P, Sujata N, Ravishankar M. Conventional tracheal tubes for intubation through the intubating laryngeal mask airway. *Anesth Analg*. 2005;100:284-288.

10. Fan KH, Hung OR, Agro F. A comparative study of tracheal intubation using an intubating laryngeal mask (Fastrach) alone or together with a lightwand (Trachlight). *J Clin Anesth*. 2000;12:581-585.

11. Langeron O, Birenbaum A, Amour J. Airway management in trauma. *Minerva Anestesiol*. 2009;75:307-311.

12. Blostein PA, Koestner AJ, Hoak S. Failed rapid sequence intubation in trauma patients: esophageal tracheal combitube is a useful adjunct. *J Trauma*. 1998;44:534-537.

13. Mercer MH, Gabbott DA. Insertion of the Combitube airway with the cervical spine immobilised in a rigid cervical collar. *Anaesthesia*. 1998;53:971-974.

14. Mercer MH, Gabbott DA. The influence of neck position on ventilation using the Combitube airway. *Anaesthesia*. 1998;53:146-150.

15. Vezina MC, Trepanier CA, Nicole PC, Lessard MR. Complications associated with the Esophageal-Tracheal Combitube in the pre-hospital setting. *Can J Anaesth*. 2007;54:124-128.

16. Kurola JO, Turunen MJ, Laakso JP, et al. A comparison of the laryngeal tube and bag-valve mask ventilation by emergency medical technicians: a feasibility study in anesthetized patients. *Anesth Analg*. 2005;101:1477-1481.

17. Berlac P, Hyldmo PK, Kongstad P, Kurola J, Nakstad AR, Sandberg M. Pre-hospital airway management: guidelines from a task force from the Scandinavian Society for Anaesthesiology and Intensive Care Medicine. *Acta Anaesthesiol Scand*. 2008;52:897-907.

18. Wiese CH, Bartels U, Schultens A, et al. Using a Laryngeal Tube Suction-Device (LTS-D) Reduces the "No Flow Time" in a Single Rescuer Manikin Study. *J Emerg Med*. 2009.

19. Greene MK, Roden R, Hinchley G. The laryngeal mask airway. Two cases of prehospital trauma care. *Anaesthesia*. 1992;47:688-689.

20. Martin SE, Ochsner MG, Jarman RH, Agudelo WE. Laryngeal mask airway in air transport when intubation fails: case report. *J Trauma*. 1997;42:333-336.

21. Martin SE, Ochsner MG, Jarman RH, Agudelo WE, Davis FE. Use of the laryngeal mask airway in air transport when intubation fails. *J Trauma*. 1999;47:352-357.

22. Matioc AA, Wells JA. The LMA-unique in a prehospital trauma patient: interaction with a semirigid cervical collar: a case report. *J Trauma*. 2002;52:162-164.

23. Brain AI, Verghese C, Strube PJ. The LMA "ProSeal"—a laryngeal mask with an oesophageal vent. *Br J Anaesth*. 2000;84:650-654.

24. Evans NR, Llewellyn RL, Gardner SV, James MF. Aspiration prevented by the ProSeal laryngeal mask airway: a case report. *Can J Anaesth*. 2002;49:413-416.

25. Mark DA. Protection from aspiration with the LMA-ProSeal after vomiting: a case report. *Can J Anaesth*. 2003;50:78-80.

26. Brimacombe J, Keller C. Aspiration of gastric contents during use of a ProSeal laryngeal mask airway secondary to unidentified foldover malposition. *Anesth Analg*. 2003;97:1192-1194.

27. Koay CK. A case of aspiration using the proseal LMA. *Anaesth Intensive Care*. 2003;31:123.

28. Mercer MH. An assessment of protection of the airway from aspiration of oropharyngeal contents using the Combitube airway. *Resuscitation*. 2001;51:135-138.

29. Hagberg CA, Vartazarian TN, Chelly JE, Ovassapian A. The incidence of gastroesophageal reflux and tracheal aspiration detected with pH electrodes is similar with the Laryngeal Mask Airway and Esophageal Tracheal Combitube—a pilot study. *Can J Anaesth*. 2004;51:243-249.

30. Rosenblatt WH. Airway management. In: Barash PG, Cullen BF, Stoelting RK, eds. *Clinical Anesthesia*. 4th ed. Philadelphia, PA: Lippincott Williams & Wilkins; 2001:601,606-608.

31. Hung OR, Pytka S, Morris I, et al. Clinical trial of a new lightwand device (Trachlight) to intubate the trachea. *Anesthesiology*. 1995;83:509-514.

32. Hung OR, Pytka S, Morris I, Murphy M, Stewart RD. Lightwand intubation: II—clinical trial of a new lightwand for tracheal intubation in patients with difficult airways. *Can J Anaesth*. 1995;42:826-830.

33. Hung OR, Stewart RD. Lightwand intubation: I—a new lightwand device. *Can J Anaesth*. 1995;42:820-825.

34. Agro F, Hung OR, Cataldo R, Carassiti M, Gherardi S. Lightwand intubation using the Trachlight: a brief review of current knowledge. *Can J Anaesth*. 2001;48:592-599.

35. Davis L, Cook-Sather SD, Schreiner MS. Lighted stylet tracheal intubation: a review. *Anesth Analg*. 2000;90:745-756.

36. Vollmer TP, Stewart RD, Paris PM, Ellis D, Berkebile PE. Use of a lighted stylet for guided orotracheal intubation in the prehospital setting. *Ann Emerg Med*. 1985;14:324-328.

37. Hardwick WC, Bluhm D. Digital intubation. *J Emerg Med*. 1984;1:317-320.

38. Stewart RD. Tactile orotracheal intubation. *Ann Emerg Med*. 1984;13:175-178.

39. Gerich TG, Schmidt U, Hubrich V, Lobenhoffer HP, Tscherne H. Prehospital airway management in the acutely injured patient: the role of surgical cricothyrotomy revisited. *J Trauma*. 1998;45:312-314.

40. Bair AE, Panacek EA, Wisner DH, Bales R, Sakles JC. Cricothyrotomy: a 5-year experience at one institution. *J Emerg Med*. 2003;24:151-156.

41. Fortune JB, Judkins DG, Scanzaroli D, McLeod KB, Johnson SB. Efficacy of prehospital surgical cricothyrotomy in trauma patients. *J Trauma*. 1997;42:832-836.

42. MacIntyre A, Markarian MK, Carrison D, Coates J, Kuhls D, Fildes JJ. Three-step emergency cricothyroidotomy. *Mil Med*. 2007;172:1228-1230.

43. Smith MD, Katrinchak J. Use of a gum elastic bougie during surgical cricothyrotomy. *Am J Emerg Med*. 2008;26:738 .

44. Kokkinis K. The use of the laryngeal mask airway in CPR. *Resuscitation*. 1994;27:9-12.

45. Leach A, Alexander CA, Stone B. The laryngeal mask in cardiopulmonary resuscitation in a district general hospital: a preliminary communication. *Resuscitation*. 1993;25:245-248.

46. McCall MJ, Reeves M, Skinner M, Ginifer C, Myles P, Dalwood N. Paramedic tracheal intubation using the intubating laryngeal mask airway. *Prehosp Emerg Care*. 2008;12:30-34.

47. Reeves MD, Skinner MW, Ginifer CJ. Evaluation of the intubating laryngeal mask airway used by occasional intubators in simulated trauma. *Anaesth Intensive Care*. 2004;32:73-76.

48. Hung O, Murphy M. Unanticipated difficult intubation. *Curr Opin Anaesthesiol*. 2004;17:479-481.

SELF-EVALUATION QUESTIONS

16.1. A 23-year-old driver is involved in a motor vehicle crash (MVC). She is trapped inside the vehicle and appears to be unconscious and is not making effective respiratory efforts. She is slumped back against her seat. How would you immediately manage this patient?

A. Extricate him/her from the vehicle for definitive management.

B. Insert a nasal/oral airway and attempt positive pressure ventilation.

C. Obtain a definitive airway by intubating the patient.

D. Scene survey, followed by maneuvers to relieve airway obstruction and attempts at BMV.

E. This patient is impossible to intubate and surgical cricothyroidotomy is indicated.

16.2. Which of the following statements of the use of EGDs in managing the trauma airway is **INCORRECT**?

   A. Aspiration is a small risk and therefore EGDs are an effective first-line airway in trauma.

   B. EGDs are an effective rescue device should intubation be delayed or unsuccessful.

   C. EGDs can act as an alternative to intubation.

   D. EGDs are effective airways in the trauma patient during transport.

   E. All EGDs have been well studied in the trauma population and are proven to be effective.

16.3. The Lightwand/Trachlight™ can be used as an airway adjunct on its own or it can be combined with which one of the following techniques to facilitate intubation?

   A. direct laryngoscopy

   B. digital intubation

   C. intubation via an LMA

   D. nasotracheal intubation

   E. all of the above

CHAPTER 17

Airway Management of a Motorcyclist with a Full-Face Helmet Following a Crash

Mark P. Vu and Orlando R. Hung

17.1 CASE PRESENTATION

A 29-year-old male motorcyclist presents to the emergency department (ED) after being involved in a high-speed motor vehicle crash (MVC). The motorcyclist was traveling at approximately 65 km·h^{-1} (40 miles per hour) when he drove through an intersection and collided with a car. Although damage to the car was minimal, the motorcycle was severely damaged and the patient was found approximately 50 m (160 ft) from the point of impact. The patient's vital signs at the scene were: HR 110 beats per minute (bpm), BP 120/70 mm Hg, RR 24 breaths per minute, and SpO$_2$ 93% on room air. Paramedics placed the patient on a spine board and transferred him to the ED. In the ED, he complains of pain in his chest, difficulty breathing, and pain in his legs. He is wearing a nonmodular full-face helmet. His vital signs are found to be HR 120 bpm, BP 110/50 mm Hg, RR 32 breaths per minute, SpO$_2$ 89%, and he is becoming confused. There is clinical evidence of a compound fracture of his right femur.

17.2 PATIENT CONSIDERATIONS

17.2.1 What are the initial steps in the management of this patient?

The general principles of trauma care and resuscitation apply to this patient. An initial, rapid survey of the patient's vital functions including his airway, breathing, and circulation (the A-B-Cs) is undertaken.[1] Large-bore intravenous access, oxygen, and basic monitoring (pulse oximetry, ECG, and serial blood pressure readings) are

instituted quickly. If the helmet cannot be easily or safely removed for the primary survey, supplemental oxygen may be provided by placing an inverted simple face mask through the opening in the helmet. His airway assessment shows that he is wearing a full-face, nonmodular type motorcycle helmet, obscuring his mouth from view. His nose and nares are visible above the line of the face shield portion of the helmet, and his anterior neck is visible and displays normal anatomy. Rapid examination of his chest demonstrates equal air entry bilaterally and his pulses are equal. Although this patient is protecting his airway, is breathing, and has an adequate blood pressure, he may require intervention to control his airway and breathing urgently after completion of the primary survey.

17.2.2 Are there recommendations in the Advanced Trauma Life Support® guidelines for the removal of helmets prior to transport?

There is currently no consensus regarding whether prehospital personnel should routinely remove a patient's helmet prior to transport to hospital. Individual patient factors and coexisting injuries will guide the decision to remove the patient's helmet. If possible, the helmet should remain in place unless emergency airway or respiratory support is needed, in which case the helmet should be carefully removed in a manner that minimizes cervical spine motion. Most helmet removal techniques endorse a two-person approach: one person stabilizes the patient's head from below while another person carefully removes the helmet from above.[2] Prehospital personnel should be encouraged to consult with a hospital-based receiving physician if questions regarding patient care exist.

17.2.3 Are there recommendations in the ATLS® guidelines for the removal of helmets once the patient has arrived in hospital?

There is also no consensus on when or how a patient's helmet should be removed once the patient arrives in hospital. If the patient's condition permits, the helmet can remain in place during the trauma assessment to minimize the potential for cervical spine movement. After a careful neurological assessment, and if the patient is in stable condition, removal of the helmet under fluoroscopy may be considered. If the patient's condition necessitates emergency airway or breathing support, the risks of providing airway management with the helmet in place should be carefully weighed against the risks of emergency removal of the helmet. These issues will be discussed later in this chapter.

17.2.4 Following a high-speed motorcycle crash, what other injuries might you anticipate for this patient?

Anticipating and identifying coexisting medical conditions in patients is important for practitioners. Alcohol is often a factor in motorcycle crashes and should be suspected in all cases.[3] A recent prospective study of 150 patients admitted to the emergency surgical service following a motor vehicle crash showed that 37% were intoxicated with blood alcohol concentration (BAC) greater than or equal to 100 mg·dL^{-1} or 0.1%[4] (1% BAC by volume = 10 mg·mL^{-1}, and the BAC legal limit is between 0.08% and 0.1% depending on the Province or State). Other causes for the crash should also be considered, including cerebrovascular accident, cardiac event, seizure, or intoxication from substances other than alcohol. A focused survey of the patient as suggested by the Advanced Trauma Life Support (ATLS®) guidelines will help to identify injuries that will significantly affect airway management decisions. Airway practitioners should presume that this group of patients will have a full stomach and are at high risk for a cervical spine injury. Also, patients with open-face type helmets are at higher risk of sustaining facial injuries, but these injuries are still possible in patients wearing full-face helmets. A rigorous assessment of the oropharynx, nasal passages, and ears is often difficult in patients wearing helmets and the benefits of a nasotracheal approach to endotracheal intubation should be weighed against the risks of this procedure in this population of patients.

17.3 AIRWAY CONSIDERATIONS

17.3.1 What types of helmets worn by motorcyclists are potentially problematic for airway management?

Motorcycle helmets can be grouped into two categories in the context of airway management: open-face and full-face. Open-face helmets cover the cranium, sometimes cover the ears, but do

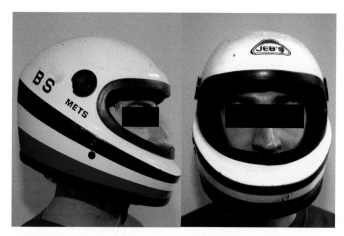

FIGURE 17-1. Full-face type helmets present a challenge to airway practitioners. The patient's mouth is completely obscured by the face shield portion of the helmet. In general, the nose and neck are readily accessible (right). However, in some types of full-face helmets, access to the nose may be limited.

not cover the neck, chin, mouth, or nose. These features make them less protective to the patient in the event of a crash. There is an increase in the likelihood of serious anterior neck and facial injuries affecting airway anatomy, but concurrently renders airway assessment and intervention more straightforward. Full-face helmets are more protective to patient's face in the event of a crash, but are a major hindrance to airway assessment and intervention since access to the mouth is practically impossible (Figure 17-1). Moreover, removal of full-face helmets can be difficult, resulting in potentially significant cervical spine motion.[5,6] A recent study was conducted to evaluate the cervical spinal movement during the removal of a full-face helmet in 10 fresh cadavers with an experimental unstable fractured odontoid. Under fluoroscopy, there was significant movement of C1-C2 during helmet removal and dislocation of C1-C2 in two cases.[7] Although the clinical significance of these findings in live patients is unknown, this study suggests that there is a potential risk of spinal cord injury in a patient during the removal of a full-face helmet.

An important variation on the full-face helmet is the modular full-face helmet (Figure 17-2). The design of this helmet allows the movement of the face shield portion of the helmet away from the face. This helmet design allows the effective conversion of a full-face helmet into an open-face configuration, making airway management with the helmet in place more feasible.

17.3.2 Should helmets always be removed in order to provide airway management?

Removal of helmets for airway management is case dependent. There is currently no consensus on whether helmets should be routinely removed prior to airway management in trauma patients. There are concerns that cervical spine movement during helmet removal may be significant. Although the evidence of cervical spine movement during helmet removal has been supported by radiographic studies in cadavers, its clinical

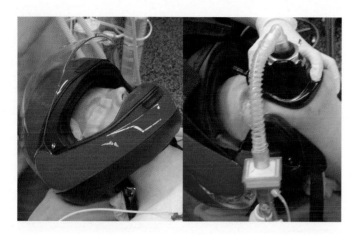

FIGURE 17-2. Modular type helmets allow more options for airway interventions (left). Displacement of the face shield cephalad (right) allows full access to the patient's nose, mouth, and neck as well as ventilation using a face mask.

importance remains unknown. In prehospital care, removal of helmets by paramedics is standard prior to airway management. However, in sports medicine it is currently recommended that emergency medical personnel have the tools to remove face shields in order to provide airway management with the helmet in place.[8] Hospital-based airway practitioners should expect situations in which prehospital personnel have deferred definitive airway management until arrival at the hospital and therefore should be prepared for any scenario.

17.3.3 Describe a systematic approach to manage the airway of a patient wearing a motorcycle helmet

When a patient is wearing a motorcycle helmet, assessment of their airway should be completed in the standard fashion aiming to assess the feasibility of providing oxygenation and ventilation by: (1) bag-mask, (2) extraglottic device (EGD), (3) tracheal intubation by direct laryngoscopy, or (4) via a surgical airway. The first part of the assessment of a patient wearing a motorcycle helmet is identifying whether the helmet is open- or full-face configuration.

In a patient wearing an open-face helmet, airway management can be performed with the helmet in place and the patient's head can be manually stabilized by an assistant to minimize movement of the head and neck. Bag-mask-ventilation, extraglottic device insertion, tracheal intubation, and surgical airway access are commonly straightforward in this scenario. If the open-face helmet has a visor, it can be removed to optimize line-of-sight during direct laryngoscopy.

In a patient wearing a full-face helmet, the practitioner must now determine whether the helmet is a modular type or not. If it is a modular type full-face helmet, the helmet may be left in place and the face shield portion can be carefully retracted superiorly to expose the face and neck. Once this is done, the airway can be managed with considerations similar to an open-face style helmet. It should be noted that a retracted face shield might obscure the line-of-sight during direct laryngoscopy. Alternative orotracheal intubating devices such as the Trachlight™ lighted-stylet, a

video laryngoscope, or a rigid/flexible fiberoptic intubation device are potentially useful.

In a patient wearing a full-face helmet that is not modular, several important issues must be carefully considered. Bag-mask-ventilation and extraglottic device insertion are practically impossible because access to the mouth and face is extremely limited by the face shield. Direct laryngoscopy is also impossible for the same reason. Access to the neck for a surgical airway is often possible and the anatomical landmarks for cricothyrotomy should be carefully assessed. At this juncture, the practitioner should decide: (1) Can the helmet be removed prior to airway management; and (2) Should the helmet be removed prior to airway management? In many cases it may be most appropriate to remove the helmet prior to airway interventions since this provides practitioners with the opportunity to properly assess the patient and optimally expose all relevant anatomy. Although there is no consensus on the proper technique for helmet removal, most authors advocate a two-person technique as described earlier. Some helmets have special mechanisms to facilitate emergency removal. Instructions can sometimes be found written on the sides of the helmet and may prove useful. Once the helmet is removed, oxygenation and ventilation can be provided in the standard fashion.

17.3.4 Should the endotracheal intubation be performed awake?

The patient wearing a motorcycle helmet, especially a full-face helmet, has significant predictors of difficult airway management. Bag-mask-ventilation is impossible in patients wearing full-face helmets and is suboptimal in patients wearing open-face helmets because of full-stomach considerations. Laryngoscopy is difficult or impossible with full-face helmets, as is EGD insertion. In light of this, an awake intubation approach should be considered and is a reasonable option in cooperative patients. When possible, an awake look direct laryngoscopy can be a useful adjunct to the airway assessment as well. Unfortunately, awake intubation in this group of patients is challenging because they are often uncooperative and have significant secretions in their airway, limiting the efficacy of topical anesthesia. Practitioners must consider the benefits of an awake technique and be prepared to proceed to an alternative plan.

17.4 DIFFICULT SITUATIONS—WHEN THE HELMET CANNOT BE REMOVED

17.4.1 Describe how you would provide oxygenation and ventilation in a situation where you cannot remove a nonmodular, full-face helmet?

Arguably the most challenging situation for a practitioner is when a patient wearing a full-face helmet needs oxygenation and ventilation but the helmet cannot be removed easily. Many circumstances can make helmet removal difficult or impossible.

Examples of such situations include patients with foreign objects penetrating the helmet and embedded in the skull and patients in whom removal of the helmet causes them extreme pain or distress, or individuals trapped in confined spaces where the helmet cannot be removed (eg, race car). A systematic assessment of the airway management options for this patient will show that bag-mask-ventilation is impossible because the helmet's face shield obscures the mouth and chin. Similarly, insertion of an EGD is practically impossible because access to the mouth is also limited. The two remaining options are (1) surgical airway using a cricothyrotomy or (2) nasotracheal intubation. Rapid assessment of the surgical landmarks relevant to cricothyrotomy, either percutaneous or open, is essential since this part of the patient's airway is usually unobstructed by the helmet or face shield. Securing the airway by a nasotracheal route is relatively simple and potentially useful and lifesaving. Airway practitioners familiar with nasotracheal intubation techniques should review the contraindications to this approach, such as evidence of basal skull fracture, prior to proceeding. Blind nasal intubation in a spontaneously breathing patient has a reasonable success rate by experienced practitioners. A recent report showed that blind nasal intubating technique has a 90% success rate for prehospital trauma patients requiring an endotracheal tube.[9,10] However, the success of blind nasotracheal intubation is limited by practitioner familiarity. A flexible lightwand, such as the Trachlight™, loaded on a nasotracheal tube can be effectively used to achieve endotracheal intubation in a patient wearing a full-face helmet.[11] In this technique, transtracheal illumination using the lightwand indirectly confirms proper placement of the nasotracheal tube.[12] If blood is present in the airway, the potential for a false passage in the airway makes a blind technique relatively contraindicated. Using a flexible bronchoscope can be a helpful guide, especially in situations where blind techniques are contraindicated, but its efficacy may be limited by the presence of blood or secretions in the airway. Flexible endoscopic intubation can be performed with the patient awake and the nasopharyngeal mucosa topically anesthetized or with the patient under general anesthesia and muscle relaxed. The risks of each approach should be considered in the context of the patient's comorbidities and the practitioner's familiarity with the techniques.

Airway practitioners are strongly advised to consider a "double set up" plan that includes both a primary intubation approach (eg, a light-guided nasotracheal intubation, flexible bronchoscope, etc) and a secondary back up surgical approach for the patient wearing a full-face helmet that cannot be removed. Since the patient's neck is almost always accessible regardless of the type of helmet worn, a double set up facilitates prompt airway control via a surgical access in case the primary plan is unsuccessful. Two separate equipment trays should be prepared: the first contains all the equipment needed for oral or nasotracheal access; the second tray contains all the instruments needed for a surgical airway. Having a second skilled practitioner available who is familiar with surgical airway access is ideal. Prior to initiating the airway intervention, the patient should be optimally positioned, the neck should be prepped, and the airway management team should agree on clear trigger points that identify when the primary approach has failed and the secondary approach is to be undertaken (ie, surgical airway).

17.4.2 How do you perform a light-guided nasotracheal intubation for this patient if it becomes necessary?

An appropriate size uncut endotracheal tube (ETT) should be used. While it is not possible to warm and soften the ETT in this emergency situation, generous lubrication of the ETT will facilitate nasal intubation and minimize injury. The Trachlight™ (or a flexible lightwand) is prepared as previously described (see Section 11.3.6) with the stiff internal wire stylet removed so that the ETT/Trachlight™ (ETT/TL) unit is pliable and suitable for nasal intubation. Ideally, a vasoconstrictor, for example, xylometazoline hydrochloride (Otrivin) nasal spray (if available and time permits), should be administered prior to the insertion of the ETT/TL through the nostril. Following the placement of the ETT-TL tip into the nasopharynx, it is advanced gently into the glottic opening using the transillumination of the soft tissues of the anterior neck. As it is not possible to perform a jaw lift with the full-face helmet in place, a gentle jaw thrust with minimal neck movement can be performed by an assistant to elevate the tongue and epiglottis. Using the light glow, the tip of the ETT-TL is then guided to the glottic opening. When the tip of the endotracheal tube enters the glottic opening, a bright circumscribed glow can be seen readily just below the thyroid prominence and the ETT-TL unit is then advanced into the trachea.

To demonstrate the effectiveness and safety of light-guided nasotracheal intubation using the Trachlight™ device in patients wearing full-face helmets, we successfully performed this light-guided nasotracheal technique in healthy consented patients undergoing elective oromaxillofacial surgery requiring nasotracheal intubation.[11] A BMW System IV motorcycle helmet was used to demonstrate feasibility. With the open-face helmet, ventilation could be achieved easily via a face mask under anesthesia (Figure 17-2). Prior to tracheal intubation, the helmet was in the full-face configuration. Trachlight™ nasotracheal intubation was performed using the technique described earlier. With a gentle jaw thrust, the ETT-TL was then inserted through the nostril and into the nasopharynx. When the tip entered the glottic opening, a bright circumscribed glow was seen in below the thyroid prominence (Figure 17-3). Tracheal intubation was successful in all six patients.

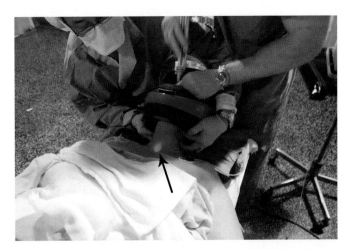

FIGURE 17-3. Light-guided nasotracheal intubation using a Trachlight™ through a full-face modular type helmet (BMW System IV helmet). With a gentle jaw thrust, the ETT-TL was inserted through the nostril and into the nasopharynx. When the tip entered the glottic opening, a bright circumscribed glow (arrow) was seen in below the thyroid prominence.

The mean time to intubation was 22.0 ± 12.1 seconds. Transient nasal mucosal bleeding was the only observed complication.

Occasionally, the tip of the ETT-TL will repeatedly go posteriorly into the esophagus. To overcome this problem, the tip of the ETT can be easily elevated anteriorly by flexing the neck. However, movement of the neck should be avoided for this patient with a potential cervical spine injury. It is also possible to elevate the tip of the ETT anteriorly and align it with the glottis by inflating the endotracheal tube cuff of the ETT in the hypopharynx with 20 mL of air.[13] The tip of the ETT-TL can then be guided by transillumination toward the glottic opening. When the tip enters the glottic opening, a bright circumscribed glow is seen in below the thyroid prominence. At this point, the endotracheal tube cuff should be deflated to allow the advancement of ETT-TL further into the trachea. Following the inflation of the cuff, endotracheal tube placement should be confirmed using auscultation and the presence of end-tidal CO_2.

17.4.3   Would your approach to airway management change for a patient who is wearing a football helmet or hockey helmet?

The approach to a patient who is wearing a different type of protective helmet is similar. Sports helmets can be open-face, full-face, and can have various styles of face shields. Many of these face shields can be easily removed with simple tools, such as a screwdriver. For example, the cage of a football helmet can be easily removed using a cage removal tool that can instantly convert a caged and unmanageable airway into an accessible airway. Current recommendations suggest that injured athletes requiring emergency medical care should have their face shields removed and their helmets left in place for airway management.[14,15] This highlights the fact that sports helmets have face shields or cages that are easily removed and takes heed of research suggesting that cervical spine motion is lessened when the helmet is left in place.

17.5   SUMMARY

Airway management in patients wearing a helmet can present a major challenge to practitioners. The principles of airway management remain the same regardless of whether or not the patient is wearing a helmet; however the type of helmet can significantly impact the options available to practitioners. It is worth remembering that almost all patients wearing a helmet are trauma patients, and so the usual considerations of full stomach, head injury, and cervical spine precautions are applicable. If a patient's airway can be managed with the helmet in place, this is often a safer option if an unstable cervical spine injury is suspected. Removing a helmet prior to airway management is often appropriate to optimize intubating conditions, but should be done carefully. Rarely, situations occur where a patient's helmet cannot be removed but oxygenation and ventilation must be provided, and practitioners must have a plan and the skills to deal with this challenging situation.

REFERENCES

1. American College of Surgeons. Committee on Trauma. Advanced Trauma Life Support program for doctors: ATLS. 8th ed Chicago, IL: American College of Surgeons; 2009.
2. Tintinalli, JE, ed. *Emergency Medicine: A Comprehensive Study Guide.* New York: McGraw Hill Professional Publishing; October 2003.
3. Hurt, HH, Ouellet, J, Thom, DR. Motorcycle Accident Cause Factors and Identification of Countermeasures. Vol 1. Technical Report, Traffic Safety Center. Los Angeles: University of Southern California; 1981.
4. Mancino M, Cunningham MR, Davidson P, Fulton RL. Identification of the motor vehicle accident victim who abuses alcohol: an opportunity to reduce trauma. *J Stud Alcohol.* 1996;6:652-658.
5. Kolman JM, Hung OR, Beauprie IG, et al. Evaluation of cervical spine movement during helmet removal. *Can J Anesth.* 2003;50:A18.
6. Brimacombe J, Keller C, Kunzel KH, Gaber O, Boehler M, Pühringer F. Cervical spine motion during airway management: a cinefluroscopic study of the posteriorly destabilized third cervical vertebrae in human cadavers. *Anesth Analg.* 2000;5:1274-1278.
7. Laun RA, Lignitz E, Haase N, Latta LL, Ekkernkamp A, Richter D. Mobility of unstable fractures of the odontoid during helmet removal. A biomechanical study. *Unfallchirург.* 2002;105(12):1092-1096.
8. Waninger KN. On-field management of potential cervical spine injury in helmeted football players: leave the helmet on! *Clin J Sport Med.* 1998;2:124-129.
9. Dauphinee K. Nasotracheal intubation. *Emerg Med Clin North Am.* 1988;6(4):715-723.
10. Weitzel N, Kendall J, Pons P. Blind nasotracheal intubation for patients with penetrating neck trauma. *J Trauma.* 2004;56(5):1097-1101.
11. Vu M, Guzzo A, Hung O, Morrison A. A novel method for endotracheal intubation in patients wearing full-face helmets. World Congress of Anesthesiologists. 2004:CD014.
12. Hung OR, Pytka S, Morris I, et al. Clinical trial of a new lightwand device (Trachlight) to intubate the trachea. *Anesthesiology.* 1995;83(3):509-514.
13. Gorback MS. Inflation of the endotracheal tube cuff as an aid to blind nasal endotracheal intubation [letter]. *Anesth Analg.* 1987;66:913.
14. Laprade RF, Schnetzler KA, Broxterman RJ, et al. Cervical spine alignment in the immobilized ice hockey played. A computed tomography analysis of the effect of helmet removal. *Am J Sports Med.* 2000;23(6):800-803.
15. Swenson TM, Lauerman WC, Blanc RO, Donaldson WF, Fu FH. Cervical spine alignment in the immobilized football player. Radiographic analysis before and after helmet removal. *Am J Sport Med.* 1997;25(2):226-230.

SELF-EVALUATION QUESTIONS

17.1. You are about to perform a tracheal intubation in an unconscious, 29-year-old male motorcycle driver who was involved in a high-speed MVC. His open-face helmet is in place, his airway examination is favorable, and he has no predictors of difficult bag-mask-ventilation, extraglottic device insertion, or laryngoscopy. Regarding his helmet, which of the following statements is true?

A. A skilled assistant should maintain in-line stabilization of the patient's head and neck during the airway intervention.

B. If the open-face style helmet is not obstructing the line-of-sight for laryngoscopy, it may remain in place during the airway intervention.

C. A rapid sequence induction (RSI) technique with a muscle relaxant is a reasonable choice to facilitate endotracheal intubation.

D. All of the above are true.

17.2. A 20-year-old motorcycle driver is involved in a high-speed MVC. He is brought to your hospital on a spine board still wearing his full-face style helmet. His vital signs are stable and he is cooperative. He complains of pain in his left leg and his neck. You should:

A. Remove his helmet immediately and provide supplemental oxygen.

B. Carefully remove the helmet by yourself and ask the patient to inform you of any discomfort.

C. Ask the patient to carefully remove the helmet himself while you assist him.

D. Complete your primary survey assessment, provide oxygen through his helmet if necessary, and complete lateral C-spine x-rays with the helmet in place prior to removing the helmet with the assistance of a skilled colleague.

17.3. You assess a 50-year-old male motorcyclist who was involved in a high-speed MVC. He is wearing a modular full-face helmet with the face shield retracted. He is unconscious, breathing spontaneously, and is receiving oxygenation and ventilation via a Combitube™ placed in the field by paramedics after multiple failed attempts at laryngoscopy. He is obese and has a full beard. His SpO_2 on FiO_2 1.00 is 87%, BP 110/70 mm Hg, HR 100 bpm, RR 24 breaths per minute, assisted. You quickly review this case with a colleague and decide that your safest plan to establish a definitive airway is:

A. Leave the Combitube™ in place indefinitely.

B. Replace the Combitube™ with an LMA.

C. Give succinylcholine, remove the Combitube™, and replace it with an orotracheal tube under direct laryngoscopy.

D. Perform a cricothyrotomy with the Combitube™ in place and the patient breathing spontaneously.

CHAPTER (18)

Airway Management of a Morbidly Obese Patient Suffering from a Cardiac Arrest

Saul Pytka and Idena Carroll

18.1 CASE PRESENTATION

A 67-year-old woman presents to the emergency department (ED) by ambulance with a 3-hour history of increasing dyspnea associated with chest pain. She has a history of coronary artery disease, hypertension, and hyperlipidemia, but no known allergies. Her medications include atenolol, low-dose aspirin, atorvastatin, acetaminophen with codeine, and nitroglycerin spray as needed. Prior to notifying the emergency medical services, the patient had used three sprays of nitroglycerin every 5 to 10 minutes with no relief.

She is placed on 10 L·min^{-1} oxygen by face mask and is transported to the hospital. Upon arrival at the ED, her vital signs are heart rate (HR) 113 beats per minute (bpm) and irregular, respiration rate (RR) 31 breaths per minute, blood pressure 85/45 mm Hg, and SaO$_2$ 86%. On examination, she appears to be in severe respiratory distress and is unable to speak more than three to four words in one breath. She is morbidly obese with an estimated weight of over 137 kg (300 lb) and is 151 cm (5 ft) tall with a body mass index (BMI) of 60 kg·m^{-2}. Chest auscultation reveals faint breath sounds with crackles over the entire lung fields, a significant decrease in air entry in both bases combined with mild wheezing. Other findings include 1+ bilateral ankle edema, S$_4$ heart sound, and a grade III/VI systolic murmur radiating to the axilla. Her jugular venous pressures (JVP) cannot be assessed because of her marked obesity and short neck. Her electrocardiogram reveals a pattern consistent with an acute antero-lateral myocardial infarction. The chest x-ray shows poor inflation and is also consistent with pulmonary edema.

Following the initial assessment, it is noticed that the SaO$_2$ decreases to 81% and her respirations increase to 35 to 40 breaths per minute. Pink froth appears from her mouth.

As you prepare for airway intervention, she loses consciousness. The monitor shows pulseless ventricular tachycardia. What do you do to secure the airway at this time?

18.2 INTRODUCTION

18.2.1 Define obesity

Obesity is the presence of an excess of body fat when compared to average values for age and gender. When the percentage of body fat exceeds 15% to 18% in men, or 20% to 25% in women, the individual is considered obese. Unfortunately, measuring body fat is not practical as it requires sophisticated techniques.

The ideal body weight (IBW) has been used frequently in clinical settings to define obesity:

$$\text{IBW (kg)} = \text{height (cm)} - x$$

where x is 100 for males and 105 for females.

Patients who weigh 20% above IBW are considered overweight, and they are considered morbidly obese if their weight is 200% above the calculated IBW.[1]

The World Health Organization (WHO) has utilized body mass index (BMI) as the international method of classifying obesity.[2] It has become the standard method for defining obesity.

$$\text{BMI}[3] = \text{body weight (kg)}/\text{height}^2 \text{ (m)}$$

Using the BMI, obesity is categorized as follows[4]:

• A person is considered overweight with a BMI of 25 to 29.9 kg·m^{-2}.

- Obese individuals have a BMI greater than 30 kg·m^{-2}.

- Morbidly obese individuals have a BMI greater than 35 kg·m^{-2}.

- Super-morbidly obese individuals have a BMI greater than 55 kg·m^{-2}.

It has been well established that obesity is associated with multiple medical issues including hypertension, heart disease, congestive heart failure, diabetes mellitus, stroke, obstructive sleep apnea, an increased incidence of perioperative wound infection, and respiratory complications.

Recently, a more important predictor of long-term outcome has been shown to be the type of fat distribution, rather than BMI. "Male" or "android pattern central obesity" (trunk and abdomen) has been shown to correlate more with negative outcomes and increased risk of cardiac disease and premature death than "female pattern", gynecoid obesity (peripheral).

"Metabolic syndrome" (Syndrome X) describes truncal obesity as being a waist to hip ratio of greater than 0.9 in men, or greater than 0.85 in women, or a waist circumference of greater than 40 in (approximately 100 cm) in men and 35 in (approximately 88 cm) in women. This syndrome is associated with glucose intolerance (type II diabetes), hypertension, dyslipidemia, microalbuminuria, prothrombotic states, and proinflammatory states (eg, elevated C-reactive protein) and represents a particularly high-risk group for the development of cardiovascular and cerebrovascular diseases.[5,6]

Reducing the degree of obesity has been shown to favorably impact the progression of these disorders.[7,8]

18.2.2   What are the anatomic and physiologic factors that might contribute to the difficulty of airway management in the morbidly obese patient?

Numerous factors have been implicated as contributing to difficult bag-mask-ventilation, extraglottic device (EGD) use, laryngoscopy and intubation, and the performance of a surgical airway in this population. These include large breasts (male and female), excess adipose tissue in the face and cheeks, short neck, large tongue, redundant palatal and pharyngeal tissue, superior and anterior larynx, limited mouth opening, limited access to the anterior neck, and limited cervical spine mobility.[4]

Experience and the literature, suggest that, based on weight alone, morbidly obese patients do not represent a difficult airway (see Chapter 1). Even when a morbidly obese patient has favorable airway assessment parameters (ie, Mallampati I, full range of motion of neck, adequate mouth opening, etc), other factors can make airway intervention more challenging.

There is a significant decrease in tolerable apnea time in obese, compared with that of nonobese subjects. This decrease occurs in a linear fashion as obesity increases and relates to both a decreased respiratory reserve and an increase in metabolic requirements.[9] This decreased respiratory reserve is the result of a decrease in functional residual capacity combined with a closing capacity that intrudes on tidal volume ventilation.[9,10] Furthermore, the high FiO_2 employed in all intubations induces absorption atelectasis, further reducing the

amount of lung tissue available for gas exchange. Because of these factors, precipitous oxygen desaturation occurs when the patient is rendered apneic during airway management.[10] Data from Jense suggest that, during rapid sequence induction (RSI) in the morbidly obese patient, apneic time before the development of hypoxemia permits only one intubation attempt before hypoxemia ensues.[9]

The morbidly obese patient also has a restrictive lung defect resulting in a decreased vital capacity, expiratory reserve volume, and inspiratory capacity.[9,11] Auler et al found that morbidly obese patients under general anesthesia show a higher resistance throughout the respiratory system.[12]

The presence of morbid obesity is considered by many to be a predictor for difficult mask ventilation.[4,9,13] Adequate bag-mask-ventilation (BMV) requires an open airway and a tight mask seal. The difficulty of creating a patent airway in the morbidly obese and maintaining a competent mask seal in the face of elevated airway pressures sufficient to overcome the restrictive defect imparted by obesity mitigate against effective BMV. Anterior translation of the mandible (jaw thrust) to affect airway opening has been shown to be more difficult and less effective in the obese.[14] In the cited study, nine nonobese and nine obese subjects were anesthetized and given neuromuscular blocking agents. Once apneic, and with steady airway pressure applied via a nasal device, the oropharynx and velopharynx (nasopharynx) were visualized with an endoscope. The cross-sectional areas were measured, both in the resting state and with a jaw thrust applied. In both groups of patients, the jaw thrust improved the cross-sectional area of the oropharynx. However, while an improvement with the jaw thrust maneuver occurred in the measurements of the velopharynx in the nonobese population, no improvement was noted to occur with this maneuver in the obese patients. The authors found that obstruction persisted in the lateral plane rather than the in the A-P dimension, and postulated that this was due to the redundant soft tissue around the tonsillar pillars closing in from the sides as the tonsillar pillars were stretched antero-posteriorly. This may explain why CPAP or PEEP augments ventilation in the obese patient, as both laterally splint the airway.[14,15] It may also explain why the LMA has been found to be an effective rescue device in the obese population (see later).

18.2.3   What are the special considerations in patients with obstructive sleep apnea?

About 5% of morbidly obese patients have obstructive sleep apnea (OSA).[4] In studying over 6000 subjects, Nieto[16] reported that the majority of patients with OSA are not obese. Consequently, questioning patients regarding OSA should not be reserved for only the obese. The presence of snoring may be the only indicator of OSA in the general population. Snoring and obesity are important predictors for difficult BMV.[13]

Although difficult to quantify, a direct correlation may exist between difficult tracheal intubation and OSA.[17] Some controversy exists, however, and opposing data are present in the literature. In their study, Neligan et al showed that OSA is not a risk factor for difficult intubation. They did show, however, that male gender as well as high Mallampati scores (≥III) did predict difficulty in establishing an airway.[18] Chung et al followed up with sleep studies on a number of patients who were found to be difficult or failed intubations at the time of surgery. Sixty-six percent of these were subsequently diagnosed with OSA.[19]

In patients with OSA, airway patency is disturbed by relaxation of pharyngeal dilator muscles during sleep. The upper airway is soft, pliable, and narrow in these patients, which makes it collapsible during sleep. Turbulent air flow through these structures produces vibrations (snoring) and collapse (apnea).[20] This obstruction continues until the level of sleep is interrupted and the individual regains pharyngeal muscle tone. This snoring-obstruction-apnea cycle can be exacerbated by drugs or alcohol. Consequently, sedatives, particularly the long-acting agents given in the perioperative period, can have a pronounced deleterious effect on the ability of this patient population to maintain airway patency when asleep.[4] There is little question that these factors lead to increased perioperative risk for morbidity and mortality. Numerous papers address the management issues surrounding the perioperative care of this patient population.[21] Unfortunately, most of it is expert opinion, rather than evidence based. A useful reference is the published guidelines by the American Society of Anesthesiologists. Again, these are positions based primarily on expert consensus.

The obesity hypoventilation syndrome (OHS), also known as Pickwickian syndrome, is characterized by chronic respiratory insufficiency, with both obstructive and restrictive features on pulmonary function testing. Chronic hypoxemia and hypercarbia, polycythemia, somnolence, pulmonary hypertension, and right ventricular dysfunction (cor pulmonale) characterize this condition. These patients all exhibit a marked reduction in hypoxic and hypercarbic drives, measuring one-sixth and one-third the response to that of controls.[22] Although some similarities exist between OSA and OHS, they are not the same disease. As pointed out earlier, not all patients with OSA are obese, and patients with OHS do not necessarily have OSA. Due to the significant underlying pulmonary and cardiac dysfunction with the OHS population, they are at significant perioperative risk.

18.2.4   Is tracheal intubation more difficult in morbidly obese patients?

There is some disagreement as to whether morbid obesity predicts difficult intubation. The incidence of difficult intubation in the morbidly obese population has been reported to be approximately 13% to 20 %.[23-25]

However, in a study of 100 morbidly obese patients with BMIs of greater than 40 kg·m^{-2}, Brodsky et al[26] concluded that obesity, per se, was not a predictive factor in determining difficulty of intubation. Of the many parameters measured in the study population, the only two that correlated with difficult laryngoscopy following rapid-sequence induction with cricoid pressure were large neck circumference and high Mallampati scores. A neck circumference (measured at the level of the thyroid cartilage) of 40 cm was associated with a 5% incidence of difficult intubation. In the same study, difficult intubations were encountered in 35% of patients with a neck circumference of 60 cm.[26] Of interest, larger neck circumference has also been associated with increasing severity of obstructive sleep apnea.[27]

In a separate study, Ezri also found that obesity, by itself, was not a predictor of difficult intubation.[28]

18.3   AIRWAY MANAGEMENT PREPARATION

18.3.1   Are obese patients at increased risk of aspiration?

Obesity has been frequently listed as a risk factor for aspiration. However, recently this belief has been challenged by a number of studies that have found no increase in gastric volumes or acidity in obese subjects.[29,30] Maltby et al[31] demonstrated that gastric emptying was no different in obese than in nonobese patients and suggested that the same guidelines for fasting can be applied to both patient populations. Aspiration risks and prophylaxis should be applied in the obese patients using the same criteria as in the nonobese. For a detailed discussion of aspiration and risks, see Chapter 5.

18.3.2   How should the morbidly obese patient be positioned for airway management?

Because of the decreased oxygen reserve in this patient population, it is crucial to position these patients carefully for tracheal intubation prior to induction of anesthesia. Appropriate positioning prior to the induction of anesthesia can significantly reduce the apnea time required for intubation as well as increase the oxygen reserve. While recent literature has questioned the advantage of the sniffing position over simple head extension,[32] these studies still advocate the sniffing position for obese patients. Proper sniffing position has been defined as head extension and a 35 degree flexion of the neck onto the chest.[33]

Achieving adequate sniffing position in a patient of ideal body weight may mean only placement of a pillow under the neck and extending the head. However, in a morbidly obese patient, optimal position often requires building a ramp of sheets or towels under the shoulders, neck, and head (Figures 18-1 and 18-2). This is referred to as "extreme sniffing" or "ramped" position. As an alternative to blankets, towels, and pillows, the Troop® Elevation Pillow can be used (see Figure 49-2). A comparison study of 60 morbidly obese patients by Collins et al,[34] demonstrated a significant improvement of laryngoscopic grade in patients in the "ramped" position. Determinants of proper "ramped" positioning have been described as follows: at least a 90 degree angle between the mandible and chest; the face higher than the chest; external auditory meatus at the same horizontal level as the sternal angle.[34]

A second and important positioning principle involves the use of the reverse Trendelenberg position. Bed placement of 30 degree head-up tilt increases functional residual capacity (FRC) and compliance (both lung and chest wall), thereby permitting greater degrees of pulmonary oxygen reserve.[35] Adding continuous positive airway pressure (CPAP) of 10 cm of H_2O pressure has been shown to be an effective maneuver in reducing the degree of atelectasis associated with induction. Patients receiving positive

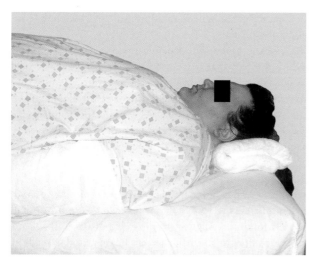

FIGURE 18-1. This picture shows a morbidly obese patient lying in a supine position with the neck and head resting on a regular pillow. It is difficult to access the mouth as well as perform direct laryngoscopy in this patient lying in this position.

end-expiratory pressure (PEEP)/CPAP prior to induction can be expected to have higher PaO_2 values than control groups that have not undergone the maneuver.[36,37]

18.3.3 How should medications be dosed in the morbidly obese patient?

When determining the dosage of a drug, the ideal body weight (IBW) or lean body weight (LBW) are generally used. The LBW is a measured value, but can be estimated by the formula:

$$LBW = (a) \text{ (weight)} - b \text{ (weight}^2/[100 \times \text{height}])^2$$

where a and b = 1.1 and 128, respectively, for men, and 1.07 and 148, respectively, for women, weight in kg, and height in m.[38]

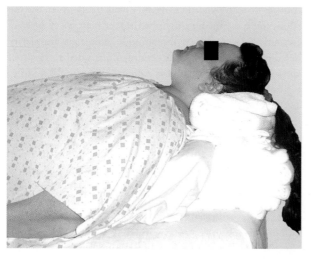

FIGURE 18-2. This picture shows a morbidly obese patient lying in a supine position with the shoulder, neck, and head resting on a stacked ramp of hospital linen. This is an optimal position for airway management and laryngoscopic intubation for obese patients as the external auditory meatus is at the same horizontal level as the sternal angle.[31]

The ideal body weight (as presented earlier), can be approximated by a simple formula.

$$IBW \text{ (kg)} = \text{height (cm)} - x$$

where x is 100 for males and 105 for females.[1]

The use of total body weight (TBW) to calculate the dose is particularly problematic for lipophylic drugs. For some lipophylic agents, the use of TBW leads to an over calculation of the required dosage, and hence toxicity.

Perhaps the best way to calculate the appropriate dose of these agents is to employ the adjusted body weight (ABW):

$$ABW^{39} = IBW + 0.4 \text{ (TBW} - IBW)$$

There are a number of reasons for not using the TBW in calculating drug dosing. In the obese person, not all of the excess weight is fat. Lean mass is increased in the obese person, and represents 20% to 40% of the increased weight and in addition, blood supply to adipose tissues is quite low, accounting for only 5% of cardiac output. For all practical purposes, protein binding (a major influence on volume of distribution) in obese patients is similar to that in those who are nonobese.[40]

18.4 AIRWAY MANAGEMENT

18.4.1 Discuss the appropriate methods for denitrogenation of the morbidly obese patient

While the term preinduction oxygenation or "preoxygenation" has been used by most to reflect denitrogenation of the lungs, it is more appropriate to use the term "denitrogenation," as it more accurately reflects the desired end result of nitrogen being washed out of the lungs. Two denitrogenation methods have been described and are equally effective for the obese patient.[9] They include: (1) four vital capacity breaths of 100% oxygen and (2) breathe 100% oxygen normally (tidal-volume breathing) through a snug-fitting facemask for 5 minutes. Denitrogenation employing CPAP with 100% oxygen showed no significant difference when compared with standard denitrogenation techniques in one study,[10] but proved beneficial in another.[36]

18.4.2 How effective is the laryngeal mask airway in the obese patient?

A number of studies and case reports have been published recently, illustrating the effectiveness of the various laryngeal mask devices in providing ventilation and oxygenation in obese patients. Doyle and colleagues reported the management of the airway in a patient weighing 445 kg (980 lb and BMI of 163 kg·m⁻²). After failing awake tracheal intubation using a flexible bronchoscope, they successfully placed a size 5 LMA ProSeal™ awake and anesthesia was induced using sevoflurane.[41] A surgical airway was then performed.

In a study involving 60 obese patients (BMI >30), Natalini et al have shown that both LMA Classic™ and LMA Proseal™ are effective in providing mechanical ventilation.[42] In another efficacy study of the LMA ProSeal™ (LMAP) in the morbidly obese, Keller[43] induced anesthesia in 60 morbidly obese (BMI >35 kg·m^{-2}) patients and inserted an LMAP. Insertion of the LMAP was successful in all patients, 90% on the first attempt, and the remaining 10% on the second attempt. Following adequate oxygenation, the LMAP was removed, and laryngoscopic intubation was successful in 54 patients (90%) on the first attempt and four patients (7%) on the second attempt. Failure to intubate the trachea occurred in the remaining two patients (3%). These patients had the LMAP reinserted and the surgery proceeded using the extraglottic airway. No significant hypoxemia was reported in any patient during the study.

Frappier et al[44] studied 118 morbidly obese surgical patients with BMIs of greater than 45 kg·m^{-2}. Following induction, all initially underwent laryngoscopy to determine the Cormack/Lehane grade. Subsequently, they all underwent attempted tracheal intubation using the intubating laryngeal mask airway (ILMA). Tracheal intubation was successful in 114 patients (96.3%). Laryngoscopic intubation was successful for the remaining four patients with failed ILMA attempts. No correlation between laryngoscopic grade and failure with the ILMA was evident.

18.4.3 What are the plans to secure the airway of this patient?

Pulseless ventricular tachycardia renders this patient a crash airway (Chapter 2). Airway management of this patient should take into account the principles discussed earlier. Management of the cardiac emergency should be guided by the most recent ACLS guidelines provided by the American Heart Association. This would include initiation of cardiac compressions and defibrillation as indicated.

As with any emergency intubation, every effort is made to ensure that the first attempt is the best attempt:

• Best person
• Best position
• Best paralysis
• Best BURP
• Best length and type of laryngoscope blade

If possible, placing the patient in a ramped position (Figure 18-2) with reverse Trendelenberg immediately has the potential to improve pulmonary mechanics, improve the success of BMV, and optimize the ability to provide preintubation oxygenation saturations. Help should be summoned and adjuncts and alternative airway devices, such as the rigid fiberoptic laryngoscopes or video laryngoscopes (Plan B and Plan C), should be immediately available. Direct laryngoscopy may not be difficult, unless there is a history of difficult intubation (OSA, previously failed intubation, etc) or predictors of difficulty, such as a thick neck or a high Mallampati score elicited before collapse.

Induction agents are not indicated in the crash airway. Neuromuscular-blocking agents (eg, succinylcholine) may be required in the event the first attempt at oral intubation fails and residual muscle tone is suspected to be a factor contributing to that failure (see Crash Intubation Algorithm, Chapter 2). However,

it is of questionable benefit to administer succinylcholine in the presence of a pulseless VT.

The risk of aspiration depends upon a number of factors, including the fact that it is an emergency, her stomach is likely to be full either from gastric juices or gas from attempts at bag-mask-ventilation, and a positive history of gastro-esophageal reflux disease (GERD), to name a few. As failed or difficult intubation increases the risk of aspiration, cricoid pressure is employed while managing the airway. However, if intubation or airway management proves difficult in the presence of cricoid pressure, the pressure can, and should be released. It is important to recognize that cricoid pressure has never been proven to be protective, and has been demonstrated to render airway management more difficult in some situations (see Chapter 5 for detailed discussion).

If the decision to intubate her trachea was to be made prior to her arrest, the choice to use neuromuscular-blocking agents to facilitate that intubation would depend on the level of confidence one has that the airway can be secured. Inherent in this is the anticipated ease of oxygenation with BMV or EGD in the event that intubation fails. If the decision is made to paralyze, the selection and dosing of induction agents should be based on the hemodynamic stability of the patient. Should effective gas exchange not be possible, an awake look may be employed to further evaluate the potential for a successful intubation (see Chapter 2).

18.4.4 What are the rescue options for the failed airway in the morbidly obese patient?

The first rescue from failed BMV is improved BMV. BMV is likely to be difficult in this patient due to soft tissue collapse of the upper airway, difficult or impossible mask seal, and noncompliant lungs due to her obesity and pulmonary edema. Having an experienced assistant to facilitate two-handed BMV technique may be crucial (see Chapter 7 for details).

Management decisions in the face of the failed airway depend on whether it is a 'can't intubate, can ventilate' failed airway or a 'can't intubate, can't ventilate' (CICV) failed airway. In the former situation, there is time and the practitioner may select an EGD or an alternative airway device or technique of greatest familiarity. As discussed earlier, the LMA has been demonstrated to be an effective device in the morbidly obese patient due to its ability to splint the airway. If found to be effective, ventilation and oxygenation can be facilitated. However, with the high pressures that may be required, adequate ventilation may prove to be challenging. In that scenario, switching to an intubating LMA (LMA Fastrach™) may allow subsequent intubation. Another option, particularly if one already has an LMA Classic™ in place, is to employ the Cook Aintree® Intubation Catheter (AIC). The AIC is a hollow catheter that slides over a flexible bronchoscope (FB).[45] This technique allows use of the FB to facilitate intubation even in the situation where the practitioner has only low or average skills with the flexible scope. The loaded scope can then be passed through the LMA Classic™ and advanced through the vocal cords and into the trachea. The LMA Classic™ and the bronchoscope are removed, leaving the AIC behind. An endotracheal tube (ETT) can then be advanced over the AIC and the catheter removed, leaving the ETT in place.

In the latter situation (CICV), there is no time and a cricothyrotomy must be performed. While preparing to perform the surgical airway, an EGD may be attempted concurrently.

In the CICV situation, it is appropriate to use alternative intubating techniques, such as the intubating LMA, the Bullard Laryngoscope, or the Glidescope® guided by the skill of the practitioner. These devices have been shown to be effective in tracheal intubation in morbidly obese patients.

Due to the short, thick neck, performing a surgical airway in this morbidly obese patient would undoubtedly prove to be difficult.

18.5   SUMMARY

The incidence of morbid obesity is increasing in our society, posing both long- and short-term risks to the patient requiring airway management. Associated medical conditions affecting vital organ system reserve influence our decision making when airway management is required. Obesity alone may not predict difficult laryngoscopy, therefore, highlighting the importance of thorough airway examination. However, a thick neck or high Mallampati scores do predict difficulty with laryngoscopic intubation in obese patients. Difficulty with mask-ventilation is common. Preparation for failure is important. The various airway devices highlighted in this chapter have been shown to be effective in the obese patient.

It should be expected that rapid desaturation and hypoxemia may occur following induction and paralysis. However, proper positioning to maximize FRC and recruit alveoli and proper denitrogenation practices will minimize desaturation.

Drug dosing adjustments due to obesity remains poorly understood for many agents. If time permits, careful *titration to effect* with intravenous induction agents may prove to be effective and safer than dosing according to body weight.

Finally, the recognition of failure is crucial, as is the recognition of what type of failure has occurred. Management pathways are guided by how much time there is, and the experience of the practitioner.

REFERENCES

1. Zeman F. *Clinical Nutrition and Dietetics.* 2nd ed. New York: MacMillan Publishing Company; 1991:470-516.
2. World Health Organization, ed. *Report of WHO Consultation on Obesity. Preventing and Managing the Global Epidemic.* Geneva: WHO; June 3-5, 1998.
3. Bray GA. Pathophysiology of obesity. *Am J Clin Nutr.* 1992;55:488S-494S.
4. Adams JP, Murphy PG. Obesity in anaesthesia and intensive care. *Br J Anaesth.* 2000;85:91-108.
5. Deen D. Metabolic syndrome: time for action. *Am Fam Physician.* 2004;69:2875-2882.
6. Mitka M. Metabolic syndrome recasts old cardiac, diabetes risk factors as a "new" entity. *JAMA.* 2004;291:2062-2063
7. Anderson JW, Konz EC. Obesity and disease management: effects of weight loss on comorbid conditions. *Obes Res.* 2001;9(Suppl 4):326S-334S.
8. Kenchaiah S, Evans JC, Levy D, et al. Obesity and the risk of heart failure. *N Engl J Med.* 2002;347:305-313.
9. Jense HG, Dubin SA, Silverstein PI, O'Leary-Escolas U. Effect of obesity on safe duration of apnea in anesthetized humans. *Anesth Analg.* 1991;72:89-93.
10. Cressey DM, Berthoud MC, Reilly CS. Effectiveness of continuous positive airway pressure to enhance pre-oxygenation in morbidly obese women. *Anaesthesia.* 2001;56:680-684.
11. Doyle DJ, Arellano R. Upper airway diseases and airway management: a synopsis. *Anesthesiol Clin North America.* 2002;20:767-787, vi.
12. Auler JO, Jr, Miyoshi E, Fernandes CR, Bensenor FE, Elias L, Bonassa J. The effects of abdominal opening on respiratory mechanics during general anesthesia in normal and morbidly obese patients: a comparative study. *Anesth Analg.* 2002;94:741-748.
13. Langeron O, Masso E, Huraux C, et al. Prediction of difficult mask ventilation. *Anesthesiology.* 2000;92:1229-1236.
14. Isono S, Tanaka A, Tagaito Y, Sho Y, Nishino T. Pharyngeal patency in response to advancement of the mandible in obese anesthetized persons. *Anesthesiology.* 1997;87:1055-1062.
15. Rothfleisch R, Davis LL, Kuebel DA, deBoisblanc BP. Facilitation of fiberoptic nasotracheal intubation in a morbidly obese patient by simultaneous use of nasal CPAP. *Chest.* 1994;106:287-288.
16. Nieto FJ, Young TB, Lind BK, et al. Association of sleep-disordered breathing, sleep apnea, and hypertension in a large community-based study. Sleep Heart Health Study. *JAMA.* 2000;283:1829-1836.
17. Hiremath AS, Hillman DR, James AL, Noffsinger WJ, Platt PR, Singer S. Relationship between difficult tracheal intubation and obstructive sleep apnea. *Br J Anaesth.* 1998;80:606-611.
18. Neligan PJ, Porter S, Max B, Malhotra G, Greenblatt EP, Ochroch EA. Obstructive sleep apnea is not a risk factor for difficult intubation in morbidly obese patients. *Anesth Analg.* 2009;109:1182-1186.
19. Chung F, Yegneswaran B, Herrera F, Shenderey A, Shapiro CM. Patients with difficult intubation may need referral to sleep clinics. *Anesth Analg.* 2008;107:915-920.
20. Loadsman JA, Hillman DR. Anaesthesia and sleep apnoea. *Br J Anaesth.* 2001;86:254-266.
21. Gross JB, Bachenberg KL, Benumof JL, et al. Practice guidelines for the perioperative management of patients with obstructive sleep apnea: a report by the American Society of Anesthesiologists Task Force on Perioperative Management of patients with obstructive sleep apnea. *Anesthesiology.* 2006;104:1081-1093.
22. Zwillich CW, Sutton FD, Pierson DJ, Greagh EM, Weil JV. Decreased hypoxic ventilatory drive in the obesity-hypoventilation syndrome. *Am J Med.* 1975;59:343-348.
23. Buckley FP, Robinson NB, Simonowitz DA, Dellinger EP. Anaesthesia in the morbidly obese. A comparison of anaesthetic and analgesic regimens for upper abdominal surgery. *Anaesthesia.* 1983;38:840-851.
24. Juvin P, Lavaut E, Dupont H, et al. Difficult tracheal intubation is more common in obese than in lean patients. *Anesth Analg.* 2003;97:595-600.
25. Voyagis GS, Kyriakis KP, Dimitriou V, Vrettou I. Value of oropharyngeal Mallampati classification in predicting difficult laryngoscopy among obese patients. *Eur J Anaesthesiol.* 1998;15:330-334.
26. Brodsky JB, Lemmens HJ, Brock-Utne JG, Vierra M, Saidman LJ. Morbid obesity and tracheal intubation. *Anesth Analg.* 2002;94:732-736.
27. Katz I, Stradling J, Slutsky AS, Zamel N, Hoffstein V. Do patients with obstructive sleep apnea have thick necks? *Am Rev Respir Dis.* 1990;141:1228-1231.
28. Ezri T, Medalion B, Weisenberg M, Szmuk P, Warters RD, Charuzi I. Increased body mass index per se is not a predictor of difficult laryngoscopy. *Can J Anaesth.* 2003;50:179-183.
29. Juvin P, Fevre G, Merouche M, Vallot T, Desmonts JM. Gastric residue is not more copious in obese patients. *Anesth Analg.* 2001;93:1621-1622.
30. Harter RL, Kelly WB, Kramer MG, Perez CE, Dzwonczyk RR. A comparison of the volume and pH of gastric contents of obese and lean surgical patients. *Anesth Analg.* 1998;86:147-152.
31. Maltby JR, Pytka S, Watson NC, Cowan RA, Fick GH. Drinking 300 mL of clear fluid two hours before surgery has no effect on gastric fluid volume and pH in fasting and non-fasting obese patients. *Can J Anaesth.* 2004;51:111-115.
32. Adnet F, Borron SW, Lapostolle F, Lapandry C. The three axis alignment theory and the "sniffing position": perpetuation of an anatomic myth? *Anesthesiology.* 1999;91:1964-1965.
33. Benumof JL. Comparison of intubating positions: the end point for position should be measured. *Anesthesiology.* 2002;97:750.
34. Collins JS, Lemmens HJ, Brodsky JB, Brock-Utne JG, Levitan RM. Laryngoscopy and morbid obesity: a comparison of the "sniff" and "ramped" positions. *Obes Surg.* 2004;14:1171-1175.
35. Dixon BJ, Dixon JB, Carden JR, et al. Preoxygenation is more effective in the 25 degrees head-up position than in the supine position in severely obese patients: a randomized controlled study. *Anesthesiology.* 2005;102:1110-1115.
36. Coussa M, Proietti S, Schnyder P, et al. Prevention of atelectasis formation during the induction of general anesthesia in morbidly obese patients. *Anesth Analg.* 2004;98:1491-1495.

37. Perilli V, Sollazzi L, Modesti C, et al. Comparison of positive end-expiratory pressure with reverse Trendelenburg position in morbidly obese patients undergoing bariatric surgery: effects on hemodynamics and pulmonary gas exchange. *Obes Surg*. 2003;13:605-609.

38. Bouillon T, Shafer SL. Does size matter? *Anesthesiology*. 1998;89:557-560.

39. Erstad BL. Dosing of medications in morbidly obese patients in the intensive care unit setting. *Intensive Care Med*. 2004;30:18-32.

40. Cheymol G. Effects of obesity on pharmacokinetics implications for drug therapy. *Clin Pharmacokinet*. 2000;39:215-231.

41. Doyle DJ, Zura A, Ramachandran M, et al. Airway management in a 980-lb patient: use of the Aintree intubation catheter. *J Clin Anesth*. 2007;19:367-369.

42. Natalini G, Franceschetti ME, Pantelidi MT, Rosano A, Lanza G, Bernardini A. Comparison of the standard laryngeal mask airway and the ProSeal laryngeal mask airway in obese patients. *Br J Anaesth*. 2003;90:323-326.

43. Keller C, Brimacombe J, Kleinsasser A, Brimacombe L. The Laryngeal Mask Airway ProSeal as a temporary ventilatory device in grossly and morbidly obese patients before laryngoscope-guided tracheal intubation. *Anesth Analg*. 2002;94:737-740.

44. Frappier J, Guenoun T, Journois D, et al. Airway management using the intubating laryngeal mask airway for the morbidly obese patient. *Anesth Analg*. 2003;96:1510-1515.

45. Higgs A, Clark E, Premraj K. Low-skill fibreoptic intubation: use of the Aintree Catheter with the classic LMA. *Anaesthesia*. 2005;60:915-920.

SELF-EVALUATION QUESTIONS

18.1. Which of the following is **NOT** true about airway management in obese patients?

A. The presence of morbid obesity is a predictor for difficult mask ventilation.

B. Jaw thrust has been shown to be less effective in the obese patients.

C. Airway obstruction under anesthesia in obese patients even with the application of a jaw thrust is due to a decrease in the anterior-posterior dimension of the velopharynx (nasopharynx).

D. Precipitous oxygenation desaturation usually occurs shortly following the induction and paralysis of obese patients.

E. Morbidly obese patients do not represent a risk of difficult intubation, based on weight alone.

18.2. Which of the following is **NOT** true of obstructive sleep apnea (OSA)?

A. The majority of patients with OSA are obese.

B. Larger neck circumference has been associated with increased severity of obstructive sleep apnea.

C. The presence of snoring may be the only indicator of OSA in the general population.

D. In patients with OSA, airway patency is disturbed by relaxation of pharyngeal dilator muscles during sleep.

E. The snoring-obstruction-apnea cycle of OSA can be exacerbated by sedative and opioid medications including alcohol.

18.3. Which of the following airway techniques is **NOT** known to be difficult in obese patients?

A. bag-mask-ventilation

B. surgical airway

C. light-guided intubation using a Trachlight™

D. laryngoscopic intubation is obese patients with thick necks

E. ventilation using an LMA

CHAPTER 19

Airway Management with Blunt Anterior Neck Trauma

David A. Caro and Steven A. Godwin

19.1 CASE PRESENTATION

A 25-year-old man drives into an unseen wire while he is snowmobiling. The wire strikes his anterior neck and throws him from his snowmobile. Paramedics failed to place an endotracheal tube (ETT) in the field and he arrives in the emergency department (ED) immobilized on a long spine board, with a cervical collar in place. He is unconscious, unresponsive to painful stimuli, and with stridor. Initial vital signs include a heart rate of 120 beats per minute (bpm), a blood pressure of 160/90 mm Hg, a respiratory rate of 24 breaths per minute, and an oxygen saturation of 93% on room air. A non-rebreather oxygen mask is applied, and his oxygen saturation increases to 97%.

Palpation demonstrates no obvious subcutaneous air, but there is a large abrasion across the anterior and lateral areas of the neck (Figure 19-1). Palpation of the larynx demonstrates crepitus and slight anatomic distortion. Plans begin immediately to protect and secure the airway.

19.2 INITIAL PATIENT ASSESSMENT AND MANAGEMENT

19.2.1 What are the important considerations in evaluating this patient?

Upon arrival at the ED, the team should follow a protocol that is consistent with the guidelines of the Subcommittee of Advanced Trauma Life Support® of the American College of Surgeons Committee on Trauma.[1] Aggressive initial management and a high index of suspicion for associated injuries are key steps in the successful management of patients with this type of injury.

A young patient with no significant medical history should have adequate cardiorespiratory reserve. His initial oxygen saturation is concerning, but it improves with supplemental oxygen. His depressed level of consciousness could be due to a number of factors, and anoxic injury to the brain or spinal cord must be a consideration. His normotension, elevated pulse rate, and use of accessory muscles of respiration would suggest that his cervical cord is essentially intact. Despite two small studies which suggest that laryngotracheal injury is compatible with a normal cervical spine,[2,3] the airway practitioner must assume that this patient has a cervical spine fracture until proven otherwise.[4]

Other associated injuries can occur with this type of clothesline injury. These include facial laceration, laceration of the esophagus, and injury to the recurrent laryngeal nerve.[5] It is imperative to thoroughly evaluate the patient after first ensuring airway, breathing, and circulation.

19.2.2 What are the airway priorities in this patient?

Considerations in this patient include laryngeal fracture, tracheal disruption, and a hematoma which could impinge on the airway; all of these may be difficult to detect.[6] Blunt anterior neck trauma can influence all four choices of initial airway management in this patient: bag-mask-ventilation, use of the extraglottic devices (EGDs), laryngoscopy and intubation, and cricothyrotomy.

Difficulty with bag-mask-ventilation could stem from either anatomical upper airway distortion due to the trauma itself, tracheal disruption, or to trauma related to prior intubation attempts.

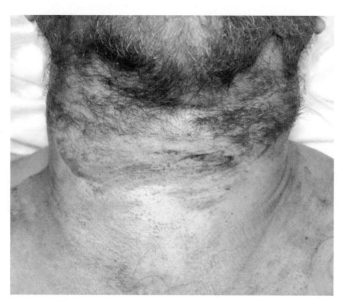

FIGURE 19-1. This picture shows that this clothesline injury patient has a large abrasion across the anterior and lateral areas of the neck.

Unfortunately, the use of EGDs may be contraindicated in the setting of supraglottic or glottic disruption, or distortion.[7,8]

Anticipate difficult laryngoscopy. Supraglottic or glottic distortion may hinder visualization of the vocal cords. In the event the practitioner elects to pursue direct laryngoscopy, a Miller blade may be the preferable blade, as it may provide better control of the epiglottis and a more direct line-of-sight vision.[9]

One must recognize that blunt anterior airway trauma may result in disruption of the trachea distal to the glottis. Tracheal transection may result in obstruction to tube passage or placement of the tube in a false passage through the tracheal disruption. Orotracheal laryngoscopy cannot detect this injury and may lead to a false sense of security relative to the ease of intubation.[10] One case series demonstrated six of seven tracheal disruptions to be at the cricothyroid/tracheal junction; four of these seven were successfully intubated while the others required emergency tracheotomy.[10]

Cricothyrotomy may be very difficult in laryngeal trauma, as normal anatomic landmarks may be distorted, making it difficult to identify the larynx, the cricothyroid membrane, and the cricoid ring. In addition, subcutaneous air may compromise the capacity to identify the trachea to perform percutaneous needle puncture and for this reason, an open surgical technique is the preferred surgical approach (see Chapter 13 for details).

19.3 AIRWAY MANAGEMENT

19.3.1 What should we consider in managing this patient's airway?

This airway is not a crash airway, but it is a difficult one. Difficulty is expected with bag-mask-ventilation and laryngoscopy; the airway is possibly disrupted and neck mobility is limited. Difficulty

can also be anticipated with EGD utilization and with cricothyrotomy (potential for hematoma and laryngeal/tracheal distortion).

Summoning help is the first step in the management of this patient. There is time to formulate a plan. The use of paralyzing agents or drugs that might lead to respiratory depression should be avoided in this patient. Conversely, coughing could worsen the injury, or could further compromise a traumatized spinal cord. Careful sedation and topical anesthesia is appropriate in this patient, and in-line stabilization of the cervical spine is an absolute requirement.

Typically, orotracheal intubation should be performed by the most experienced laryngoscopist immediately available. In addition, in-line stabilization of the cervical spine should be employed to guard against exacerbating an unstable cervical injury. Further, in a patient who has a potentially disrupted distal airway, the procedure of choice is intubation using a flexible bronchoscope (FB).[11,12] This technique permits visualization as one advances into the trachea and ensures that the endotracheal tube is not advanced into a blind passage. Orotracheal laryngoscopy, following the gentle placement of an Eschmann Introducer (EI) (gum-elastic bougie), may be a distant second choice.[1,13] The tactile response transmitted through the EI when it is slid against the tracheal rings may help to confirm that the EI is in the trachea and will guide the ETT into place.[14] Confirmation of correct placement with an FB is important, if feasible. A failed airway mandates a tracheotomy.

19.3.2 Step by step, what is the best way to intubate the trachea of this patient?

Equipment ought to be available to carry out bronchoscopic intubation, orotracheal intubation with an EI, and a tracheotomy. Tracheotomy equipment should be opened at the bedside and the patient's neck should be prepped and anesthetized. A bag-mask-ventilation device, Magill forceps, functioning suction, and airway adjuncts (such as oral and nasal airway devices) should be prepared.

Denitrogenation with a bag-mask-ventilation device is essential. A well-oxygenated patient gives the airway practitioner a cushion of time in the event it is needed. Steadily declining oxygen saturations may mandate assisted ventilation by a bag-mask. It is important to reiterate that EGDs are contraindicated in this patient as they may actually worsen the existing airway distortion. The inability to oxygenate with a bag-mask at any point mandates an immediate surgical airway. Pretreatment with intravenous medications is not indicated in this patient, unless other conditions exist that would mandate their use. Nebulized or atomized 4% lidocaine could be considered for use, provided that adequate denitrogenation can be carried out. Topical anesthesia will help to blunt the protective cough reflex that could aggravate cervical spine injury, or possibly disrupt the patency of a tenuous airway.

Numerous sedating agents may be considered, including ketamine, propofol, midazolam, or etomidate. Ketamine is a good choice for this patient as it carries the benefit of analgesia, along with sedation, with the rare complication of associated laryngospasm, or emergence reaction. Propofol and midazolam may have the advantage of practitioner's familiarity and ease of titration, although both drugs can potentially precipitate complete obstruction through a loss of muscle tone. The advantage of etomidate is its relative cardiovascular stability. However, the potential myoclonus associated with etomidate may place the potential unstable cervical spine and patency of a possible tenuous airway at risk.

Neuromuscular blocking agents ought to be avoided, as suggested earlier, although they may have a role in a crash airway. As mentioned earlier, the FB is the intubation technique of choice for this patient. The amount of time the practitioner has to perform bronchoscopy and intubation will depend on the ability to maintain oxygen saturation. Blood and secretions may make the procedure difficult. In the event a flexible bronchoscope is not readily available, and the patient requires urgent intubation, an oral direct laryngoscopy guided by an EI is a logical alternative. The EI may be gently inserted into the larynx, with the tip of the EI sliding across the tracheal rings to confirm intratracheal placement. However, because of the injury, the trachea may not be contiguous with the larynx. While an awake look may reveal that the glottis can be viewed, this does not guarantee that the trachea is contiguous with the larynx. An inability to visualize glottic structures on the awake look mandates a change of plan and precludes the use of neuromuscular blockade in all but the most extreme circumstances. Further, BURP (backwards, upwards, rightwards pressure) on the larynx may not be possible to do due to the trauma.

Unsuccessful oral intubation after three attempts, oxygen desaturation, or failure in ventilation indicates a failed airway. In this circumstance, tracheotomy is in order. Open tracheotomy is preferable to percutaneous techniques for the reasons stated earlier. This method allows the practitioner to identify the trachea and intubate under direct visualization. Blind attempts at finding the distal airway are rarely successful.[15,16]

19.4 OTHER CONSIDERATIONS

19.4.1 What are the concerns with ventilation and postintubation care?

Once intubated, confirmation of ventilatory exchange takes priority. The presence of end-tidal CO_2 indicates that the ETT is in the trachea and that the lower respiratory tree is being ventilated. Care must be taken to secure the ETT in place. Sedation is in order, as continued protection of the cervical spine until fracture, dislocation, and ligamentous disruption of the cervical spine have been ruled out. Paralysis may also be in order if this patient is endangering his spine by excessive movement.

19.4.2 What are potential postsurgical complications associated with clothesline injuries?

The outcome is generally very good if the patient survives the initial injury, and receives prompt aggressive resuscitation and airway management.[16] However, following the repair of the laryngotracheal and cervical spine injuries, several serious postoperative complications may occur. These include: mediastinal infection;

tracheoesophageal fistula; and subglottic stenosis.[5] In a retrospective review of clothesline injury in children and adolescents (on all-terrain vehicles), between 1998 and 2003, Graham et al reported that all patients (n = 7) had significant neck and/or facial lacerations, with long-lasting disfigurement.[17] One of the patients also had a functional impairment.

19.4.3 What other alternative should be considered if securing the airway is not possible for a patient with a clothesline injury?

Extracorporal circulation via a femoral-femoral cardiopulmonary bypass (CPB), placed with the use of local anesthesia and a portable unit, can be a lifesaving method of oxygenation and could have an important role in managing patients with a severely disrupted trachea. This can provide a safe solution for oxygenation when tracheal intubation or a surgical airway is either unsuccessful or too hazardous. However, a review of the literature did not reveal the use of CPB in airway compromise from clothesline injury. Furthermore, establishment of a femoral-femoral bypass requires at least 15 to 20 minutes, even in experienced hands,[18] making it impractical and difficult to apply in emergency situations.

19.5 SUMMARY

In summary, blunt anterior neck injury poses a unique challenge to airway management. Care must be taken to protect airway reflexes whenever an inability to intubate is anticipated. The airway practitioner must recognize many barriers to airway management which can prevent intubation, including an obstructing hematoma or a transected trachea. Intubation using a flexible bronchoscope is the ideal method of intubation in these patients, as the indirect visualization provides the reassurance that the trachea is contiguous.

REFERENCES

1. Butler AP, Wood BP, O'Rourke AK, Porubsky ES. Acute external laryngeal trauma: experience with 112 patients. *Ann Otol Rhinol Laryngol.* 2005;114(5): 361-368.
2. Aufderheide TP, Aprahamian C, Mateer JR, et al. Emergency airway management in hanging victims. *Ann Emerg Med.* 1994;24:879-884.
3. Penney DJ, Stewart AH, Parr MJ. Prognostic outcome indicators following hanging injuries. *Resuscitation.* 2002;54:27-29.
4. Nikolic S, Micic J, Atanasijevic T, Djokic V, Djonic D. Analysis of neck injuries in hanging. *Am J Forensic Med Pathol.* 2003;24:179-182.
5. LeJeune FE, Jr. Laryngotracheal separation. *Laryngoscope.* 1978;88:1956-1962.
6. Stassen NA, Hoth JJ, Scott MJ, et al. Laryngotracheal injuries: does injury mechanism matter? *Am Surg.* 2004;70:522-525.
7. Pollack CV, Jr. The laryngeal mask airway: a comprehensive review for the emergency physician. *J Emerg Med.* 2001;20:53-66.
8. Wakeling HG, Nightingale J. The intubating laryngeal mask airway does not facilitate tracheal intubation in the presence of a neck collar in simulated trauma. *Br J Anaesth.* 2000;84:254-256.
9. Arino JJ, Velasco JM, Gasco C, Lopez-Timoneda F. Straight blades improve visualization of the larynx while curved blades increase ease of intubation: a comparison of the Macintosh, Miller, McCoy, Belscope and Lee-Fiberview blades. *Can J Anaesth.* 2003;50:501-506.
10. Wu MH, Tsai YF, Lin MY, Hsu IL, Fong Y. Complete laryngotracheal disruption caused by blunt injury. *Ann Thorac Surg.* 2004;77:1211-1215.

11. O'Mara W, Hebert AF. External laryngeal trauma. *J La State Med Soc.* 2000;152: 218-222.
12. Heidegger T, Starzyk L, Villiger C, et al. Fiberoptic intubation and laryngeal morbidity: a randomized controlled trial. *Anesthesiology.* 2007;107:585-590.
13. Arndt GA, Cambray AJ, Tomasson J. Intubation bougie dissection of tracheal mucosa and intratracheal airway obstruction. *Anesth Analg.* 2008;107:603-604.
14. Steinfeldt J, Bey TA, Rich JM. Use of a gum elastic bougie (GEB) in a zone II penetrating neck trauma: a case report. *J Emerg Med.* 2003;24:267-270.
15. Shweikh AM, Nadkarni AB. Laryngotracheal separation with pneumopericardium after a blunt trauma to the neck. *Emerg Med J.* 2001;18:410-411.
16. Edwards WH, Jr, Morris JA, Jr, DeLozier JB, 3rd, Adkins RB, Jr. Airway injuries. The first priority in trauma. *Am Surg.* 1987;53:192-197.
17. Graham J, Dick R, Parnell D, Aitken ME. Clothesline injury mechanism associated with all-terrain vehicle use by children. *Pediatr Emerg Care.* 2006;22:45-47.
18. Belmont MJ, Wax MK, DeSouza FN. The difficult airway: cardiopulmonary bypass—the ultimate solution. *Head Neck.* 1998;20:266-269.

SELF-EVALUATION QUESTIONS

19.1. Following a blunt anterior neck injury, a patient presents with stridor and an oxygen saturation of 85%. What is the ventilation device of choice to attempt to enhance oxygenation after passive means have failed?

   A. laryngeal mask airway

   B. intubating laryngeal mask airway

   C. bag-valve-mask device

   D. King LT™ airway

   E. Combitube™

19.2. What percentage of live patients with blunt anterior neck trauma have an associated cervical spine injury?

   A. The literature is not clear.

   B. 5%.

   C. 10%.

   D. 15%.

   E. 20%.

19.3. What are the limitations of percutaneous cricothyrotomy in the setting of blunt anterior neck trauma with a concomitant laryngeal fracture?

   A. Subcutaneous air may mimic intratracheal air, providing false localization.

   B. Airway distortion may not allow readily identifiable, percutaneous airway structures.

   C. Distal tracheal disruption may not be identified.

   D. Advancement of the guidewire through the needle may be difficult.

   E. All of the above.

CHAPTER (20)

Airway Management in the Emergency Department

Michael F. Murphy and Ron M. Walls

20.1 CASE PRESENTATION

An unconscious 19-year-old morbidly obese man is brought into the emergency department (ED) by emergency health services (EHS) paramedics, having been found unresponsive at a fraternity initiation party. He had been drinking heavily, although the amount of alcohol consumed is unknown. The patient is unidentified and there is no available past medical history. Respirations are shallow, and paramedics have inserted a nasal trumpet and an oral airway and are assisting ventilation with a bag-mask. They had attempted oral and nasal intubation three times in the field but failed due to the patient being combative and obesity.

The vital signs are: blood pressure (BP) 114/70 mm Hg, heart rate (HR) 103 beats per minute (bpm), respiratory rate (RR) 8 to 10 breaths per minute and shallow, and oxygen saturation is 92% by assisted bag-mask-ventilation. The patient responds only to pain with purposeful movement. His blow by breath sample for ethanol reads at 220 mg/dL or 47.7 mmol·L^{-1} and his blood sugar is 90 mg/dL or 5 mmol·L^{-1}. There are no signs of trauma.

In summary, we have no information as to his identity, his history of present or past illnesses, history of allergies or medications, his past medical history, his family or social history, or what or how much might be in his stomach.

20.2 INTRODUCTION

20.2.1 What is it about managing the airway in the ED that makes it "different"?

Making crucial decisions in the face of incomplete information is fundamental to the practice of emergency medicine. Expert management of the emergency airway is a defining skill of emergency medicine. All necessary equipment and medications, including neuromuscular blocking agents, must be readily available to emergency practitioners who must be skilled in all aspects of airway management. Patients requiring immediate emergency airway management present, sometimes unexpectedly, to the ED. Many of the patients have characteristics associated with difficult laryngoscopy and intubation, but the urgency of the airway problem frequently prevents deferral or even consultation. Frequently, others have already tried and failed to manage the airway, resulting in trauma and other complications which compound the difficulty faced by the next practitioner. Such issues serve to highlight the importance of the verbal report given by field personnel as they deliver patients to an ED.

Accordingly, the emergency practitioner must be both capable and constantly prepared to undertake skilled and timely intervention in patients with compromised airways, and to plan an approach that takes into account all potential difficulties and incorporates within it backup plans (Plan B, Plan C, etc).

20.2.2   Who is primarily responsible for managing the airway in the ED?

Airway evaluation and management is the first priority of resuscitation, and establishing a patent airway and oxygenating the brain and vital organs takes precedence over all other activities. That is not to say that concurrent evaluation and management activities should not occur, it simply says "Do this first!" Identifying that the patient requires airway management does not necessarily mandate that the management be undertaken immediately; it simply establishes that early, deliberate airway management is indicated. In some cases, the patient will be apneic with an unprotected airway, and airway management will supersede virtually all other evaluation and management. In other cases, the examining practitioner will identify that early airway management is required, and plan to provide it early during the course of comprehensive and coordinated examination and intervention.

The emergency practitioner has final responsibility for ensuring definitive management of the airway for patients presenting to the ED, which might, at times, require the advice and help of consultants from anesthesia, or, more rarely, otolaryngology, or any of a number of other specialties.

20.2.3   What are the indications for tracheal intubation in the ED?

The indications for endotracheal intubation in the ED are straightforward:

- Inability of the patient to maintain the airway
- Failure to protect the airway
- Failure to effect adequate gas exchange
- A predictable deterioration in maintaining or possible loss of the airway, including the need for medications that might threaten airway maintenance or ventilation

Early establishment of a patent airway and provision of adequate oxygenation are critical to patient survival. Equally important is the ability to *predict* an impending loss of airway patency or gas exchange capability, particularly if the patient will be subjected to diagnostic studies in other specialty areas beyond the ED, or transported by land or air to another facility.

Subsequent decisions as to *how and when* the airway should be managed will depend on numerous factors, including the skills and experience of the practitioner, the equipment available, the condition of the patient, and the anatomy of the airway.

20.2.4   Is there a conceptual framework which the emergency practitioner or a consulting anesthesiologist employs in approaching the airway in the ED?

It is widely recognized that a conceptual framework focusing on rapid airway evaluation, critical action analysis and performance, and

facility with an array of airway management techniques minimizes the risk of failure and improves outcome.[1] To be precise, in an emergency, the airway practitioner must be capable of the following:

- Rapidly assessing the urgency of the situation and the patient's need for intervention
- Determining the best method of airway management for the particular circumstances at hand and having at least a backup plan in the event of failure
- Understanding the risks and benefits of each possible approach
- Deciding which pharmacological agents to use, in what order, and in what doses
- Managing the airway in the context of the patient's overall condition
- Using any of a number of airway devices to achieve a definitive airway while minimizing the likelihood, severity, and duration of hypoxemia or hypercarbia
- Recognizing when the planned airway intervention has failed and an alternative (rescue) technique is required
- Being able to rapidly identify when to call for assistance and what type of assistance might be required

20.3   HISTORY

20.3.1   How did airway management in the ED evolve to where it is today?

Emergency airway management for much of history consisted of various forms of back-pressure/arm-lift artificial respiration, or mouth-to-mouth, mouth-to-nose, and bag-mask-ventilation (BMV) by minimally trained providers until the 1960s when resuscitation research identified airway management failure as a crucial issue affecting outcome.[2-5] By the early 1970s, endotracheal intubation was recognized as an essential part of the skill set for physicians providing emergency care, but most physicians staffing emergency departments were trainees or practicing physicians with little or no formal training in emergency medicine. Intubation was generally accomplished without neuromuscular blocking agents, using either the oral or the nasal routes, sometimes requiring heavy sedation before airway management could be attempted. Intubation using a sedative, such as a benzodiazepine, often accompanied by an opioid, such as morphine, became a common practice despite its frequent failures and complications.

The advent of emergency medicine residency training programs in 1969 and the rapid growth of the specialty through the ensuing two decades established a large cadre of trained emergency medicine specialists and led to the rapid deployment of neuromuscular blockade to facilitate orotracheal intubation. By the late 1980s, the use of neuromuscular blockade for this purpose was well established in emergency medicine residency training programs, and had been dubbed "rapid sequence intubation" (RSI) in distinction to the anesthesia term "rapid sequence induction."[6] By the mid to late 1990s, neuromuscular blockade was widely used and it became evident that neuromuscular blockade not only made the technical task of intubation easier and faster, but also resulted in greater success with lower complication rates.[6]

However, a need clearly emerged for a consistent framework to identify patients at risk for difficult and possibly failed laryngoscopy and intubation, to develop a reliable approach to such patients, and to expand the rescue options beyond the single choice of cricothyrotomy.

The challenges facing emergency airway practitioners today include:

1. Restricting the use of neuromuscular blockade only to patients in whom there is a strong likelihood that tracheal intubation will be successful or that gas exchange can be maintained by some other technique in the event of failure

2. Selecting an alternative approach for those patients in whom a difficult or impossible intubation may be anticipated

3. Ensuring the success for alternative rescue devices or techniques in the event of intubation failure

20.4   UNIQUE FEATURES

20.4.1   How common is the difficult and failed airway in the ED?

Difficult airways are common in emergency practice, the incidence being as high as 20% of all emergency intubations. However, the incidence of intubation failure is quite uncommon, being in the 0.5% to 2.5% range. Moreover, the disaster of being unable to intubate or ventilate rarely occurs (0.1%-0.5%).[6]

It is crucial to realize that in the case of a difficult airway, the same standard applies as for a routine airway: the practitioner must secure the trachea with a cuffed endotracheal tube. In the case of a failed airway, the approach is focused on rescue and in keeping the patient alive and well oxygenated until the airway can be definitively secured.

Thus, the devices, techniques, and even the approach differ in these two situations. A difficult airway is managed in an anticipatory way; a failed airway is managed in a reactive way. In 2002, Walls coined the phrase "The Difficult Airway is something you anticipate; the Failed Airway is something you experience."[7]

20.4.2   What is unique about airway management in an ED?

Emergency airway management may be in an ED, or extend beyond the ED to those locations where emergency practitioners are called to manage airway, or to be directly responsible for their management by surrogate providers such as paramedics. These locations include the out-of-hospital setting, in-patient wards, intensive care units, diagnostic units such as x-ray or radiotherapy, and other sites.

Emergency airway management situations are characterized by several unique features:

• Clinical evaluation, rather than blood gases, is used to assess the adequacy of ventilation and judge the need for intubation in the acutely ill patient.

• The patient is usually at high risk for aspiration.

• The airway must be secured by a cuffed endotracheal tube. Canceling the case, awakening the patient, or significantly delaying airway management is not an option, nor in most cases, is any other form of airway management that does not protect the airway (beyond the temporary use of an extraglottic device).

• Crucial decisions must be made on the basis of less information than in almost any other setting. This, in fact, is the essence of emergency medicine and highlights the importance of expeditious and planned strategies for airway evaluation and management (see Chapters 1 and 2 for details).

• The need for intubation is ordinarily obvious, but in an emergency, the decision to intubate is often dependent on having knowledge of the natural course of the disorder or injury rather than on the patient's precise clinical status at the time of the evaluation. There are few other situations in medicine in which judgment and knowledge of the *anticipated clinical course* of a disorder are so crucial.

• Erring on the side of caution:
  ○ Intubate earlier rather than later. Be especially cautious of penetrating neck wounds with evidence of injury to the airway itself (subcutaneous air) or the vascular system (hematoma—it does not have to appear to be expanding). Both the presence of such injuries and their apparent time course are important. The patient who presents 12 hours after sustaining a penetrating neck injury has withstood the test of time. A similar-appearing injury 10 minutes after injury is an unknown, and must be assumed to present an imminent risk.
  ○ Do not paralyze a patient (ordinarily RSI) if you are not confident that you can oxygenate the patient successfully with a BMV unit or an EGD. If these fail, a surgical airway is required, and this procedure must be planned for. Anticipating this procedure requires assessing the difficulty for each approach to managing the airway prior to embarking on Plan A (see Chapter 2).
  ○ Do not sit on patients with upper airway obstruction or insist on taking the patient out of the ED (eg, to the CT scan or to the OR) unless it is absolutely clear that the patient's condition is stable enough and you are confident you can successfully secure the airway if needed. Observing the patient presents the risk that anatomy will worsen and obstruction will ensue, at which time the patient will be much more difficult to intubate and the need for doing so will be much greater.

20.4.3   How should one proceed in managing the airway in an emergency?

Once it has been decided that intubation is indicated, the focus must be on what kind of airway problem is present, and what the correct course of action is (see Chapter 2).

• Is this a "crash airway" situation in which the patient is unconscious, unresponsive, and near death?

• Is this a "difficult airway" in which one anticipates difficulty with bag-mask-ventilation, EGD use, laryngoscopy and intubation, or cricothyrotomy?

- If neither of these two situations exists, then an RSI is the method of choice.

- Has a failed airway supervened?

This systematic approach to airway management in the ED takes into account all possible presentations, and properly identifying the type of airway situation permits the practitioner to select an appropriate course of action. Algorithms that address these situations are expeditious management strategies often used in crisis and are described in Chapter 2.

20.5   SUMMARY

Rapid sequence intubation (RSI) by emergency practitioners is associated with a high rate of success and low incidence of complication. However, some patients should not be paralyzed and to successfully manage their airways will require alternative procedures, such as awake bronchoscopic intubation. The current challenge then is *how* to identify these patients in whom intubation or ventilation with bag-mask or extraglottic devices would not suffice.

In the case presented here, the emergency practitioner recognized multiple difficult airway indicators, including obesity, a large tongue, and a high larynx. Because the patient was adequately oxygenating via the bag-mask, and after assessment determined that there was not significant bleeding in the airway caused by the failed earlier intubation attempts, the patient received topical anesthesia with lidocaine (see Chapter 3) and underwent uneventful nasal intubation using a flexible bronchoscope. The patient did not require sedation, was ventilated for 2 hours, then weaned to a T-piece. He was extubated 12 hours after presentation and discharged home after evaluation by an alcohol-abuse counselor.

REFERENCES

1. Benumof J. The ASA difficult airway algorithm: new thoughts and considerations. 51st Annual Refresher Course Lectures and Clinical Update Program, #235. American Society of Anesthesiologists; 2000.
2. Daya M, Mariani R, Fernandes C. Basic life support. In: Dailey R, Simon B, Young G, Stewart R, eds. *The Airway: Emergency Management*. Philadelphia, PA: Mosby; 1992:39-61.
3. Safar P. Ventilatory efficacy of mouth-to-mouth artificial respiration: airway obstruction during manual and mouth-to-mouth artificial respiration. *J Am Med Assoc*. 1958;167:335-341.
4. Safar P, Mc MM. Mouth-to-airway emergency artificial respiration. *J Am Med Assoc*. 1958;166:1459-1460.
5. Safar P. History of cardiopulmonary resuscitation. *Acute Care*. 1986;12:61-62.
6. Walls R. Airway. In: Marx J, Hockberger R, Walls R, eds. *Rosen's Emergency Medicine: Concepts and Clinical Practice*. Philadelphia, PA: Mosby; 2009:2-20.
7. Murphy M, Walls RM. Identification of the difficult and failed airway. In: Walls RM, Murphy MF, eds. *Manual of Emergency Airway Management*. 3rd ed. Philadelphia, PA: Lippincott, Williams, Wilkins; 2008:81-93.

SELF-EVALUATION QUESTIONS

20.1. All of the following are indications for emergency tracheal intubation **EXCEPT**:

A. upper airway obstruction

B. failure to protect the airway

C. failure to maintain reasonable oxygen saturations

D. the need for hyperventilation

E. cardiac arrest

20.2. Responsibility for ensuring appropriate airway management in the ED:

A. rests with the most highly trained individual in the room

B. rests with the anesthesia practitioner, if present

C. is often unclear

D. rests primarily with the emergency practitioner of record

E. should be negotiated at the time

20.3. An unconscious 19-year-old morbidly obese man is brought in to the emergency department (ED) by emergency health services (EHS) paramedics, having been found unresponsive at a fraternity initiation party. He had been drinking heavily, although the amount of alcohol consumed is unknown. The patient is unidentified and there is no available past medical history. Respirations are shallow, and paramedics have inserted a nasal trumpet and an oral airway and are assisting ventilations with a bag-mask. They had attempted oral and nasal intubation three times in the field but failed due to the patient being combative and obesity. All of the following are acceptable strategies to employ in managing this airway **EXCEPT**:

A. moving the patient to the OR for airway management

B. intubating "earlier rather than later"

C. performing an awake look, then backing off to perform RSI

D. intubating awake even if you sense that you can paralyze the patient and be successful at intubation

E. delaying airway management at all costs until an anesthesia practitioner is present

CHAPTER (21)

Patient with Deadly Asthma Requires Intubation

Kerry B. Broderick and Richard D. Zane

21.1   CASE PRESENTATION

This 26-year-old man has a long history of severe asthma. His trachea has been intubated many times in the past for his asthma, most recently 2 months ago during which he spent a week in the intensive care unit (ICU). He arrives in the emergency department (ED) after an emergency medical service (EMS) transport of 15 minute during which he has been receiving continuous aerosolized salbutamol (albuterol, Ventolin) via a nebulizer. He arrives with marked respiratory distress. He is awake, diaphoretic, and is speaking in two-word sentences.

He is 5 ft 2 in (157 cm) tall and weighs 165 lb (75 kg). His vital signs are: respiratory rate (RR) 24 breaths per minute, heart rate (HR) 134 beats per minute (bpm), and blood pressure 110/60 mm Hg. His oxygen saturation is 89% on a non-rebreather and he is becoming fatigued. As he is receiving corticosteroid chronically for his asthma, he has a steroid body habitus with an edematous face and neck.

21.2   PATIENT EVALUATION

21.2.1   What are this patient's vital organ system reserves?

Cardiovascular reserve: This is a young patient who should have adequate cardiac reserve and there should be little concern with respect to systolic and diastolic cardiac function unless there is a significant carbon dioxide retention and respiratory acidosis which would resolve with adequate ventilation. However, depending on the length of time he has been acutely ill and how adequate his oral fluid intake has been, he is likely to be volume depleted. In combination with a decrease in venous return secondary air trapping and auto-PEEP (positive end-expiratory pressure) seen with acute asthma, the presence of hypovolemia can precipitate a significant hypotension, particularly if induction agents are used to facilitate intubation. The patient has been receiving a large amount of salbutamol, a medication with significant β_1-agonist properties. In combination with stress and hypercapnia, there is a significant arrhythmia potential from large amounts of salbutamol. Depending on how much β_1-agonist he has been taking, there is a high likelihood that he is also relatively hypokalemic due to the cellular shifting of potassium caused by the β_1-agonist. This may contribute to the potential for arrhythmia as well. When choosing induction agents for this patient, it is important to keep in mind that they all have negative inoptropic properties.

CNS reserve: There is nothing to indicate that this patient will respond abnormally to standard doses of induction agents, keeping in mind that he is obese and should be dosed accordingly. However, the practitioner ought to be watchful for agitation, confusion, or somnolence associated with carbon dioxide retention, in which case sensitivity to sedative hypnotic induction agents ought to be anticipated. Respiratory acidosis can potentiate myocardial depression associated with anesthesia induction agents.

Respiratory reserve: Patients with severe asthma have prolonged expiratory phases and air trapping.[1] Tidal volume is limited, with minimal or no respiratory reserve. Intubation may be indicated as these patients can become significantly fatigued and as such, are unable to maintain gas exchange on their own. Substantial ventilation-perfusion mismatch is present, which limits the ability to oxygenate and denitrogenate the lungs prior to induction. Preinduction hypoxemia will rapidly ensue following the administration of paralytics or induction agents.

21.3 AIRWAY EVALUATION AND MANAGEMENT OPTIONS

21.3.1 Employing the mnemonics suggested in Chapter 1, is this a difficult airway?

Yes! Facial and neck edema from chronic steroid dependence may make bag-mask-ventilation (BMV) difficult. In addition, this patient is obese and in status asthmaticus, both of which are associated with very high airway pressures that can be difficult or impossible to overcome with a positive-pressure BMV. Other than these factors, there appear to be no other predictors of a difficult BMV when applying the mnemonics MOANS (see Section 1.6.1).

Using the LEMON airway evaluation (see Section 1.6.2), the neck and face edema may make laryngoscopy difficult. As he has experienced many tracheal intubations in the past, in conjunction with corticosteroids and mechanical ventilation, subglottic stenosis is a possibility that must be considered. However, the geometry of his upper airway appears normal, and he has a Mallampati Class II airway. His neck appears to be freely mobile.

A recommended mnemonic to assist the assessment of the feasibility of using an extraglottic device (EGDs) is RODS (see Section 1.6.3). Restricted mouth opening is not an issue in this patient and upper airway obstruction is only a possibility. However, he has severe obstructive respiratory disease and his compromised pulmonary compliance, the "stiffness of the lungs," will seriously limit usefulness of an EGD just as BMV may be difficult.

While there are only a few indicators of a potentially difficult airway, he may not be an optimal candidate for a rapid-sequence intubation (RSI). A failed intubation in a hypoxemic person with very poor lung compliance would be a very dangerous situation. On the other hand, there is no reason to believe that a surgical airway would be difficult in this patient (SHORT, see Section 1.6.4). The decision to perform RSI should be in the context of the experience of the practitioner as well as the device(s) being used and availability of backup. For instance, the use of RSI may be very different if the practitioner is using a video laryngoscope instead of a standard laryngoscope.

21.3.2 Are there any other airway concerns in a patient with status asthmaticus?

This patient has no respiratory reserves, rapid oxygen desaturation, hypotension, and possible subglottic stenosis. The insertion of a tracheal tube in a person who is already in bronchospasm may exacerbate his condition.

21.3.3 Have we medically optimized his treatment prior to tracheal intubation?

For reasons already outlined, avoiding intubation would be the best option if at all possible. β_2-Agonists are the mainstay of treatment in asthma.[2] However, this patient has been on continuous bronchodilators for the 15-minute transport and had utilized his inhaler every 15 minutes at home prior to calling the paramedics. The addition of corticosteroid may be beneficial for this patient with an acute exacerbation of asthma,[3] although the delayed onset of action for corticosteroids will not be helpful in avoiding intubation in the immediate/emergent period.

21.3.4 What additional therapies are available to this patient?

Anticholinergics: Meta-analysis suggests that there is a modest benefit in adding this therapy to β_2-Agonists.[4] The benefits appear to outweigh the potential risks for the patient, so anticholinergics should be considered in this case.

Magnesium: Two meta-analysis have been performed analyzing the effect of IV magnesium on patients with asthma.[5,6] Seven trials were identified and the investigators conclude that magnesium has no confirmed role in the management of mild or moderate asthma. In severe asthma, there is evidence that magnesium improves pulmonary function and hospitalization rates, although there is no good evidence that in severe asthma magnesium decreases the need for intubation. Magnesium is unlikely to cause harm. However administration should not delay intubation or any other therapy.

Noninvasive ventilatory support (NIVS): One randomized trial and several small uncontrolled trials support the use of NIVS in acute asthma.[7] NIVS has been demonstrated to improve expiratory flow rates and reduce the need for hospitalization, although a recent meta-analysis by Ram et al concluded that routine use of NIVS in severe acute asthma could not be recommended.[8]

21.3.5 What are the possible options regarding airway management in this patient?

In this particular patient, and despite the reservations that have been mentioned, RSI by a skilled practitioner is probably the best choice. Planning ahead is crucial, as is deciding on a Plan B and C in the event Plan A should fail. While recognizing the limitations of denitrogenation prior to tracheal intubation (described earlier), the practitioner ought to administer as high an oxygen concentration as possible to the patient, employing a bag-mask unit if the patient can tolerate its use. As an added advantage, the practitioner can provide gentle assisted ventilation to the patient if he is able to tolerate it, taking care not to cause insufflation of the stomach, vomiting, or gagging. Rapid-sequence induction drugs chosen should be administered to the patient while he remains in a comfortable position, in this patient most commonly sitting upright. Once the patient loses consciousness, the patient can be placed in the supine position and laryngoscopy and intubation performed. A large, 8.0 mm ID or larger, endotracheal tube is preferred in order to reduce resistance and facilitate aggressive pulmonary toilet.

If time permits, patients with reactive airway disease or obstructive lung disease should be administered with 1.5 mg·kg⁻¹ of IV lidocaine 3 minutes before tracheal intubation in order to attenuate the reflex bronchospasm in response to airway manipulation, which is thought to be mediated via the vagus nerve.[9-11] The recommendation to use IV lidocaine in RSI protocols for the severe asthmatic is extrapolated from the results of studies employing healthy volunteers with a history of bronchospastic disease.[12-14] Unfortunately, there is also evidence that IV lidocaine does not protect against intubation-induced bronchoconstriction in asthma. In a prospective, randomized, double-blind, placebo-controlled trial of 60 patients, lidocaine and placebo groups were not different in their transpulmonary pressure and airflow immediately after intubation and at 5-minute intervals.[15] Until more data are available, it seems reasonable to minimize the risk of intubation-induced bronchoconstriction by using lidocaine premedication in the asthmatic if time and resources permit.

Ketamine is generally considered to be the induction agent of choice in the asthmatic patient because it increases circulating catecholamines and inhibits vagal outflow. In addition, it is a direct smooth muscle dilator and it does not cause histamine release.[16] While case reports of dramatic improvement in pulmonary function with ketamine have driven its popularity,[17,18] no randomized studies have been performed to demonstrate ketamine's superiority over other agents. In a case series, 19 of 22 asthmatic patients with active wheezing had a decrease in bronchospasm during ketamine-induced anesthesia.[19] In one prospective, placebo-controlled, double-blind trial of 14 mechanically ventilated patients with bronchospasm, the 7 patients treated with 1.0 $mg \cdot kg^{-1}$ ketamine had a significant improvement in oxygenation but no improvement in PCO_2 or lung compliance. In addition, the outcome (discharge from the ICU) was the same in both groups. The study population was heterogeneous, making conclusions of the benefit of ketamine difficult at best.[20] A randomized, double-blind, placebo-controlled trial of low-dose IV ketamine, 0.2 $mg \cdot kg^{-1}$ bolus followed by an infusion of 0.5 $mg \cdot kg^{-1} \cdot hour^{-1}$, in nonintubated patients with acute asthma failed to demonstrate a benefit in IV ketamine.[21]

Although evidence is limited, at the present time, based on its mechanism of action and safety profile, ketamine appears to be the best agent available for RSI in the asthmatic. Intravenous ketamine 1.5 $mg \cdot kg^{-1}$ should be given immediately before the administration of 1.5 $mg \cdot kg^{-1}$ of succinylcholine.

21.3.6   How would you intubate the trachea of this patient?

1. Preprocedure preparations:

The following difficult airway devices should be ready if available:

- An Eschmann Introducer (gum-elastic bougie)
- A fiberoptic or video laryngoscope if available
- A cricothyrotomy kit
- An intubating LMA™

The following drugs should be available:

- Lidocaine at 1.5 $mg \cdot kg^{-1}$ IV in syringes
- Ketamine at 1 to 2 $mg \cdot kg^{-1}$ in syringes
- Succinylcholine at 1.5 to 2 $mg \cdot kg^{-1}$ in prefilled syringes
- Sedation and paralytic agents for postintubation management

2. Cardiac monitors are applied along with pulse oximetry. Denitrogenation is achieved using high-flow oxygen with the patient sitting.

3. Lidocaine is administered IV at 1.5 $mg \cdot kg^{-1}$. This should be given about 3 to 5 minutes prior to the actual laryngoscopy if time and resources permit.

4. Ketamine is administered IV and the patient is observed until unconscious. This should take 1 to 2 minutes.

5. Succinylcholine is administered. The patient is placed supine with the head and neck placed in a sniffing position. Cricoid pressure is applied if not contraindicated. The patient is observed for fasiculations.

6. Laryngoscopy is performed. The cords are visualized easily and the endotracheal tube (ETT) is passed and secured.

7. Capnography is used to confirm correct tracheal placement.

8. Postintubation drugs are administered for sedation and paralysis.

21.4   ADDITIONAL CONSIDERATIONS

21.4.1   What are the appropriate ventilator settings for this patient following tracheal intubation?

All asthmatic patients have obstructed small airways and dynamic alveolar hyperinflation with varying amounts of end-expiratory residual intra-alveolar gas and pressure (auto-PEEP or intrinsic PEEP). Elevations in auto-PEEP increase the risk for baro/volutrauma. Reversal of airflow obstruction and decompression of end-expiratory filled alveoli are the primary goals of early mechanical ventilation in the asthmatic. The former requires continuous in-line nebulization with increasingly higher doses of β_2-agonists until reversal is objectively measured (decrease in peak and plateau airway pressures) or unacceptable side effects are produced. Safe, uncomplicated alveolar decompression requires a prolonged expiratory time (I:E of 1:4 to 1:5). This is achieved by using smaller tidal volumes than usual, with a high inspiratory flow (IF) rate to shorten the inspiratory cycle time, permitting a longer expiratory phase.[22]

The initial goal of ventilator therapy in the asthmatic patient is to improve arterial oxygen tension to adequate levels without inflicting barotraumas on the lungs or increasing auto-PEEP. Initial tidal volume should be reduced as necessary, to avoid barotrauma and air trapping. The speed at which a mechanical breath is delivered in liters per minute, typically 60 $L \cdot min^{-1}$, is called the IF rate. In asthma, the initial IF should be increased to 80 to 100 $L \cdot min^{-1}$ with a decelerating flow pattern. A pressure control paradigm is preferred over volume control. If volume control is chosen, the ideal waveform is one of deceleration rather than constant (square). The ventilation rate should be relatively low in order to allow sufficient time for alveolar decompression. It is acceptable to permit the maintenance or gradual development of hypercapnia through reduced minute ventilation, as this reduces the potential for barotrauma. High intrathoracic pressure caused by air trapping may compromise cardiac output and produce hypotension and therefore should be avoided.[23,24]

The highest measured pressure at peak inspiration is the peak inspiratory pressure (PIP). The compliance of the lungs, chest wall, ventilatory circuit, and ventilator; the resistance of the ETT; and the effect of mucous plugs all contribute to the PIP. This reading has an inconsistent predictive value for baro/volutrauma but ideally should be kept under 50 cm H_2O. A sudden rise in PIP should be interpreted as indicating tube blockage, mucus plugging, or pneumothorax until proven otherwise. A sudden, dramatic fall in PIP may indicate extubation.

The measured intra-alveolar pressure during a 2 to 4 second end inspiratory pause is referred to as the plateau pressure (P_{plat}). Values less than 30 cm H_2O are best and are not usually associated with baro/volutrauma. Measurement and trending of P_{plat} are excellent objective tools to confirm optimal ventilator settings and the patient's response as well as the reversal of airflow obstruction. If initial ventilator settings disclose a P_{plat} of more than 30 cm H_2O, consider lowering minute ventilation and increasing IF, both of which will prolong expiratory time and attenuate hyperinflation. If P_{plat} is unavailable, PIP may be used as a surrogate.

Most patients in status asthmaticus who require intubation are initially hypercapnic. The concept of controlled hypoventilation (permissive hypercapnia) promotes *gradual* development (over 3-4 hours) and maintenance of hypercapnia (PCO_2 up to 90 mm Hg) and acidemia (pH as low as 7.2). This is done primarily to decrease the risk of ventilator-related lung injury and prevent hemodynamic compromise as a result of increasing intrathoracic pressure from auto-PEEP or intrinsic PEEP ($PEEP_i$). Permissive hypercapnia is usually accomplished by reducing minute ventilation, increasing IF rate to 80 to 120 L·min^{-1}, and paralyzing and heavily sedating (usually paralyzing) patients who otherwise would not tolerate these settings. Permissive hypercapnia may be instrumental in promoting prolonged expiratory times and reducing auto-PEEP.[25,26]

21.4.2   What are the initial ventilator settings for this patient?

1. Determine the patient's ideal body weight.

2. Set a tidal volume of 6 to 8 mL·kg^{-1} with an FiO_2 of 1.0 (100% oxygen).

3. Set a respiratory rate of 8 to 10 breaths per minute.

4. Set an inspiratory to expiratory ratio of 1:4 to 1:5. Pressure control is preferred. If using the pressure control, the I:E ratio is adjusted directly by the I:E ratio parameter, or by adjusting the inspiratory time parameter. If using volume control, the I:E ratio can be adjusted by increasing the peak flow rate, and the "ramp" inspiratory waveform should be selected. Peak IF can be as high as 80 to 100 L·min^{-1}.

5. Measure and maintain the plateau pressure at less than 30 cm H_2O or try to keep PIP at less than 50 cm H_2O.

6. Focus on the oxygenation and pulmonary pressures initially. If necessary, allow maintenance or gradual development of hypercapnia to avoid high plateau pressures and increasing auto-PEEP.

7. Assure continuous sedation with a benzodiazepine and paralysis with a nondepolarizing muscle relaxant. The practitioner may consider a continuous ketamine infusion for sedation and potential smooth muscle relaxation.

8. Continue in-line β$_2$-agonist therapy and additional pharmacologic adjunctive treatment based on the severity of the patient's illness and objective response to treatment.

21.5   SUMMARY

The patient with severe asthma constitutes a difficult airway even without features that might predict difficult laryngoscopy and intubation due to the fact that BMV and EGD rescue is likely to be difficult or impossible. A cuffed endotracheal tube in the trachea is essential to permit adequate positive pressure ventilation, and this suggests that rescue techniques, such as employing noncuffed tracheal devices, transtracheal jet ventilation, noncuffed Seldinger cricothyrotomy devices, and so on are of little use.

If the use of medications to facilitate intubation is contemplating, the practitioner should consider lidocaine and ketamine. A continuous infusion of ketamine may be of use following intubation. Postintubation hypotension ought to be expected and managed aggressively with fluids and vasopressor if indicated, recognizing tension pneumothorax as a cause of precipitous hemodynamic change. Ventilation strategies ought to include low volumes and respiratory rates with long expiratory times and slow peak IF rates. Arterial carbon dioxide levels are not of immediate concern, provided the arterial pH can be maintained at a level consistent with reasonable cardiac, liver, and renal function.

REFERENCES

1. Hall J, Schmidt G, Wood L, eds. *Principles of Critical Care*. 2nd ed. New York: McGraw-Hill; 1998:1671.
2. National Heart, Lung, and Blood Institute. *National Asthma Education and Prevention Program (NAEPP) Expert Panel Report 2: Practical Guide for the Diagnosis and Management of Asthma*. National Institutes of Health Publication 97–4053. Bethesda, MD: US Department of Health and Human Services; 1997.
3. Levy BD, Kitch B, Fanta CH. Medical and ventilatory management of status asthmaticus. *Intensive Care Med*. 1998;24:105-117.
4. Stoodley R, Aaron S, Dales R. The role of ipratropium bromide in the emergency management of acute asthma exacerbation: a meta-analysis of randomized clinical trials. *Ann Emerg Med*. 1999; 34:8-18.
5. Alter H, Koopsell T, Hilty W. Intravenous magnesium as an adjuvant in acute bronchospasm: a meta-analysis. *Ann Emerg Med*. 2000;36:191-197.
6. Rowe B, Bretzlaff J, Bourdon C, Bota G, Camargo C. Intravenous magnesium sulfate treatment for acute asthma in the emergency department: a systemic review of the literature. *Ann Emerg Med*. 2000;36:181-190.
7. Garpestad E, Brennan J, Hill NS. Noninvasive ventilation for critical care. *Chest*. 01 Aug 2007;132(2):711-720.
8. Ram FS, Wellington S, Rowe B, Wedzicha JA. Non-invasive positive pressure ventilation for treatment of respiratory failure due to severe acute exacerbations of asthma. *Cochrane Database Syst Rev*. 2005;1:CD004360.
9. Walls R. Lidocaine and rapid sequence intubation. *Ann Emerg Med*. 1996;27:528-529.
10. Gal T. Bronchial hyperresponsiveness and anesthesia: physiologic and therapeutic perspectives. *Anesth Analg*. 1994;78:559-573.
11. Gold M. Anesthesia, bronchospasm, and death. *Semin Anesth*. 1989;8:291-306.
12. Groeben H, Foster W, Brown R. Intravenous lidocaine and oral mexiletine block reflex bronchoconstriction in asthmatic subjects. *Am J Respir Crit Care Med*. 1997;156:1703-1704.
13. Groeben H, Silvanus M, Beste M, Peters J. Both intravenous and inhaled lidocaine attenuate reflex bronchoconstriction but at different plasma concentrations. *Am J Respir Crit Care Med*. 1999;159:530-535.
14. Downes H, Gerber N, Hirshman C. IV lignocaine in reflex and allergic bronchoconstriction. *Br J Anaesth*. 1980;52:873-880.

15. Maslow A, Regan M, Israel E, et al. Inhaled albuterol, but not intravenous lidocaine, protects against intubation-induced bronchoconstriction in asthma. *Anesthesiology.* 2000;93:1198-1204.
16. Huber F, Reeves J, Gutierrez J, Corssen G. Ketamine: its effect on airway resistance in man. *South Med J.* 1972;65:1176-1180.
17. Hommedieu C, Arens J. The use of ketamine for the emergency intubation of patients with status asthmaticus. *Ann Emerg Med.* 1987;16:568-571.
18. Rock M, de la Roca S, Hommedieu C, Truemper E. Use of ketamine in asthmatic children to treat respiratory failure refractory to conventional therapy. *Crit Care Med.* 1986;14:514-516.
19. Corssen G, Gutierrez J, Reves JG, Huber FC. Ketamine in the anesthetic management of asthmatic patients. *Anesth Analg.* 1972;51:588-596.
21. Hemmingsen C, Nielsen P, Odorica J. Ketamine in the treatment of bronchospasm during mechanical ventilation. *Am J Emerg Med.* 1994;12:417-420.
22. Howton J, Rose J, Duffy S, et al. Randomized, double-blind, placebo controlled trial of intravenous ketamine in acute asthma. *Ann Emerg Med.* 1996; 27:170-175.
23. Corbridge TC, Hall JB. Techniques for ventilating patients with obstructive pulmonary disease. *J Crit Illness.* 1994;9:1027-1032.
24. Tuxen D. Permissive hypercapnic ventilation. *Am J Respir Crit Care Med.* 1994; 150:870-874.
25. Wiener C. Ventilatory management of respiratory failure in asthma. *JAMA.* 1993; 269:2128-2131.
26. Bidani A, Tzouanakis A, Cardenas V, Zwischenberger J. Permissive hypercapnia in acute respiratory failure. *JAMA.* 1994;272:957-962.

SELF-EVALUATION QUESTIONS

21.1. Hypotension following RSI facilitated tracheal intubation of the deadly asthmatic may be due to all of the following **EXCEPT**:

   A. increased mean intrathoracic pressure associated with positive pressure ventilation

   B. hypovolemia related to reduced oral intake pre-presentation

   C. acute respiratory acidosis

   D. reduced systemic vascular resistance due to succinylcholine

   E. an acute tension pneumothorax

21.2. All of the following are true with respect to the pharmacologic management of asthma in the peri-intubation period **EXCEPT**:

   A. IV magnesium has been shown to decrease the need for intubation.

   B. Antimuscarinics such as glycopyrrolate have been shown to increase the viscosity of bronchial secretions, increase the incidence of mucous plugging, and should not be used in acute severe asthma.

   C. The evidence clearly supports the use of lidocaine in acute severe asthma.

   D. Ketamine is the induction drug of choice in acute severe asthma.

   E. IV magnesium in high doses leads to skeletal muscle weakness.

21.3. Which of the following characterizes the best way to mechanically ventilate an intubated patient with acute severe asthma?

   A. large tidal volumes and low ventilation rates

   B. small tidal volumes and low peak flow rates

   C. large tidal volumes and low peak flow rates

   D. small tidal volumes and high peak flow rates

   E. large tidal volumes and high peak flow rates

CHAPTER (22)

Patient in Cardiogenic Shock

Kerry B. Broderick

22.1 CASE PRESENTATION

A 62-year-old man presents to the emergency department by car complaining of chest pain, air hunger, and extreme weakness. He has a history of hypertension and an anterior wall myocardial infarction (MI) 2 years ago. His electrocardiogram shows a large anterolateral MI, and his chest radiograph shows vascular redistribution and mild interstitial edema. He is on beta blockers. His last echocardiogram was done 2 months ago and showed an ejection fraction of 25%.

His respiratory rate (RR) is 40 breaths per minute, heart rate (HR) 100 beats per minute (bpm), blood pressure 68/40 mm Hg, and his oxygen saturation is at 86% with a non-rebreather mask. He is intensely diaphoretic and has two-word dyspnea. He has a beard and a normal stature.

22.2 PATIENT EVALUATION

22.2.1 What is this patient's physiological reserve?

Many medications employed in airway management possess properties that affect cardiac and respiratory function. For this reason, it is critical that the practitioner evaluates the ability of these systems (physiological reserve) to withstand the effects of administered medications and procedures.

22.2.1.1 Cardiac Reserve

This patient is in cardiogenic shock with limited to no cardiac reserve. He has severe systolic dysfunction and almost certainly

the same degree of diastolic dysfunction. It appears that his sympathetic nervous system is working at maximum ability just to sustain his present vital signs.

22.2.1.2 CNS Reserve

There is nothing to indicate that this patient will have any CNS problems with induction agents.

22.2.1.3 Respiratory Reserve

This patient is in pulmonary edema and will have limited respiratory reserve. Denitrogenation prior to intubation may help but is of questionable value. He is already maximizing his respiratory effort and induction may precipitate acute hypoxemia.

22.2.2 How would you evaluate the airway of this patient for difficulty?

1. On MOANS-guided evaluation for difficult BMV (see Sections 1.6.1), you are uncertain that the patient can be ventilated by bag and mask. He has a thick beard and is likely to have gastric air distention due to his increased respiratory effort and air swallowing. His lungs will be stiff (reduced compliance) secondary to his interstitial pulmonary edema. This is of particular concern on initiating positive pressure ventilation following intubation with respect to a reduction in venous return.

2. On LEMON evaluation to predict difficult laryngoscopy and intubation (see Sections 1.6.2), *looking externally* his face and neck appear normal, although he has a beard and that may hide a small mandible. He cooperates for a Mallampati evaluation and appears to have a Grade II. He is not *obese*; his *neck* is freely mobile.

3. The mnemonic RODS can be used to guide the evaluation for difficulty in the use of extraglottic devices (EGD) (see Sections 1.6.3). His mouth opening is not restricted, upper airway obstruction is not anticipated, and his airway does not appear distorted or disrupted. However, as with bag-mask-ventilation, his lungs are stiff meaning that ventilation employing an EGD may be unsuccessful.

4. On SHORT evaluation for difficult surgical airway (see Sections 1.6.4), there is no history of previous neck surgery or evidence of anterior neck hematoma. He is not obese and there is no history of neck radiation or tumor.

In summary, this gentleman has little cardiac and respiratory reserve. Difficulty with oxygenation and ventilation via a bag-mask due to reduced lung compliance and poor mask seal secondary to his beard is predicted. However an EGD, endotracheal tube, or a surgical airway are not predicted to be difficult. Therefore, he is a reasonable candidate for rapid sequence intubation should one wish to employ that technique.

22.2.3   Are there other airway management concerns in the patient with cardiogenic shock?

Most medications used for sedation or induction of anesthesia have the potential to produce hypotension, less so perhaps with etomidate and ketamine than others. This patient has limited to no cardiac reserve, and medications that reduce cardiovascular performance are contraindicated. Induction agents, in particular, must be chosen carefully and in reduced dosages. Some would say that amnesia in situations such as this, rather than induction of anesthesia, is the goal in an effort to preserve cardiac performance to the extent possible. The administration of an opioid in an individual exhibiting signs of maximal sympathetic stimulation may be contraindicated in the face of actual or incipient hypovolemia or hypotension. Finally, the onset times of medications administered intravenously may be delayed due to low cardiac output, a particular concern with the muscle relaxant in a situation where rapid-sequence intubation is desired. Under this circumstance, it is prudent to consider succinylcholine over nondepolarizing agents to achieve rapid muscle relaxation.

22.2.4   How should we medically optimize this patient prior to intubation?

22.2.4.1   Diuretics and Vasodilators

This patient is hypotensive, and the concern is that induction and intubation may acutely worsen his hypotension, as may therapies used to treat pulmonary edema such as diuretics and vasodilators. Small doses of nitroglycerine and furosemide may help to relieve some of the cardiac stress due to the pulmonary edema but may aggravate the hypotension. Consider delaying the administration of these drugs until the decision is made regarding airway control and stabilization.

22.2.4.2   Noninvasive Ventilatory Support

Numerous small studies have demonstrated a beneficial effect of using noninvasive ventilatory support (NIVS) in patients with cardiac pulmonary edema (CPE). However, it has been argued that larger prospective trials are needed before firm conclusions can be drawn. A randomized prospective study of 39 patients with pulmonary edema showed a significant decrease in need for intubation ($p = .005$) in patients receiving CPAP compared to patients receiving standard medical care. However, there were no significant differences in mortality and hospital length of stay between the study groups.[1] An open, nonrandomized study involving 29 patients with NIVS showed that oxygen saturation increased from $73.8 \pm 11\%$ to $93 \pm 5\%$, mean pH increased from 7.22 ± 0.1 to 7.31 ± 0.07 ($p <0.01$), and $PaCO_2$ decreased from 62 ± 18.5 to 48.4 ± 11.5 mm Hg.[2] A randomized, controlled, prospective clinical trial with 27 patients comparing nasal CPAP to nasal bi-level positive airway pressure (BL-PAP) against historical controls for intubation rates and MI found that BL-PAP improved ventilation and vital signs more rapidly than CPAP. However, intubation rates, hospital stay, and overall mortality between these two modes of NIVS showed no significant differences in this study. There was a higher rate of MI in patients treated with BL-PAP (71%) as compared to CPAP (31%) and that found in the historical controls (38%).[3] A randomized prospective study of 40 patients comparing BL-PAP to high-dose isosorbide (HDI) reported that 80% of patients in the BL-PAP group required intubation as compared to 20% in the HDI group. In addition, there were more deaths (2 vs 0) and a higher MI rate (55% vs 10%) in the BL-PAP group compared to the HDI group. Unfortunately, this study was prematurely terminated.[4] One subsequent study comparing BL-PAP with mask-ventilation in patients with CPE failed to demonstrate an increase in MI or mortality in the BiPAP-treated group.[5] A meta-analysis of NIVS studies in pulmonary edema from 1983 through 1997 found that only 3 of 497 studies were sufficiently rigorous to fulfill study criteria. These three randomized control trials showed that NIVS patients had a decreased need for intubation (–26%, 95% CI, –13% to –38%), but the decrease in hospital mortality was not significant (–6.6%, +3% to –16%) as compared to standard therapy alone.[6]

In this case, it is necessary to carefully weigh the potential benefits of NIVS against the potential to increase mean intrathoracic pressure, which reduces venous return and cardiac output. Furthermore, it is apparent that intubation is indicated and therefore NIVS is unlikely to be a serious consideration.

22.3   AIRWAY EVALUATION AND MANAGEMENT OPTIONS

22.3.1   Which pharmacologic agents would you select for this case?

Drug selection in individuals who are moribund is particularly important, especially medications that have significant cardiopulmonary side effects.

22.3.1.1   Neuromuscular Blocking Agent

Recalling that circulation times in cardiogenic shock are prolonged, the muscle relaxant of choice for intubation is the one with the most rapid onset, succinylcholine, unless there is a contraindication. In the face of metabolic acidosis, as is almost certainly the case in this patient, the potassium may be elevated, but this ought not deter the use of succinylcholine. Longer-acting neuromuscular blocking agents, such as pancuronium, vecuronium, and rocuronium, may be employed postintubation to maintain paralysis. The relative sympathomimetic side effects of pancuronium may be of some benefit in this patient, although the degree of sympathetic activation that is evident indicates that this would be of marginal value.

22.3.1.2   Sedative/Induction Agent

The selection of an induction agent is more difficult. However, in this patient, one is more interested in amnesia than induction of anesthesia. Recognizing this as the goal, small doses of ketamine (10-20 mg) and midazolam (1-2 mg) are clearly preferable to the other induction agents. Small doses of etomidate may be used, although the amnestic effects of etomidate may be less intense than with those already mentioned. Agents such as thiopental or propofol may cause further deterioration in this patient's hemodynamic status and should not be used.

22.3.1.3   Cardiovascular Pressure Support

This patient is hypotensive, and it is likely that intubation and positive pressure ventilation will acutely worsen his hypotension. Therefore, vasopressors should be prepared and immediately available, recognizing that balanced α/β adrenergic agonists (epinephrine, norepinephrine, vasopressin) are preferable to α-agonists alone, particularly in a catecholamine-depleted heart, as in this patient.

Inotropic support should theoretically improve outcomes in patients who present with CPE. However, they can also cause tachycardia, dysrhythmias, increase myocardial oxygen demand, and myocardial ischemia, all of which may increase mortality. These medications should be used judiciously. There are two common inotropic classes, catecholamines and phosphodiesterase inhibitors (PDEIs). The catecholamine class includes dopamine, dobutamine, and norepinephrine. Dopamine and norepinephrine may provide blood pressure support by increasing systemic vascular resistance, which can actually worsen cardiac output. Dobutamine, while inducing some mild preload and afterload reductions, may also further lower the blood pressure. Catecholamines work through the adenoreceptors, which are often saturated with endogenous catecholamines due to the patient's condition. Therefore, higher than normal dosages may be needed in the CPE patient, and unfortunately these dosages are associated with a higher rate of adverse effects. Regarding vasopressin, one experimental study comparing dobutamine (DOB) to dobutamine-norepinephrine combination to arginine vasopressin (AVP) demonstrated that AVP further worsened shock by decreasing the cardiac output and systemic vascular resistance compared with DOB alone.[7]

PDEIs work by increasing intracellular cyclic-AMP, which produces a positive inotropic effect on the heart, induces peripheral vasodilation, and reduces pulmonary vascular resistance. Together, these effects produce preload, afterload, and cardiac output improvement.[8] Studies comparing milrinone to dobutamine in patients with severe CPE did not show any improvement in hospital length of stay or mortality.[9,10]

"Calcium sensitizer" levosimendan has been suggested and studied recently as an alternative to dobutamine for CPE.[11,12] In one study comparing the two agents, levosimendan produced greater improvement in cardiac output and pulmonary vascular pressures and a reduced 180-day mortality rate (26% vs 38%).[13] However, in the SURVIVE trial there was no decrease in 180-day mortality. There was significant reduction in B-type natriuretic peptide in the levosimendan group.[14]

22.3.2   So, how exactly would you handle the entire process?

1. Pre-procedure preparations:
   • Get the difficult airway devices ready
     ◦ Tracheal introducer
     ◦ Glidescope® or other video laryngoscopes
     ◦ Intubating LMA™ (Fastrach-LMA)
   • Ketamine 10 to 20 mg in syringes or midazolam 1 to 2 mg
   • Succinylcholine at 1.5 to 2.0 mg·kg^{-1} in prefilled syringes
   • Sedation and paralytic agents for postintubation
   • Epinephrine 10 µg·mL^{-1} or vasopressin 0.4 U·mL^{-1} in 10 mL syringes

2. The patient is seated initially. The cardiac monitors are applied along with pulse oximetry. The patient is denitrogenated.

3. Ketamine or midazolam is administered IV followed immediately by succinylcholine. The patient is then placed supine with the head and neck in a sniffing position. The patient is observed for fasiculations.

4. Laryngoscopy is performed. The cords are visualized and the endotracheal tube is placed and secured.

5. Capnography and auscultation are performed to confirm tracheal intubation.

6. Postintubation drugs are administered for sedation and paralysis to permit mechanical ventilation.

7. Postintubation hypotension is managed by reevaluating ventilation parameters, volume infusion, repeated small doses of epinephrine (10 µg per dose), or vasopressin (0.4 U per dose). Postintubation hypertension may be managed with small doses of propofol (10 mg per dose) or a nitroglycerine infusion.

22.4   ADDITIONAL CONSIDERATIONS

22.4.1   How should the patient be managed following tracheal intubation?

The initial goal of ventilator management in this patient is to maximize oxygenation and relieve the work of breathing while at the same time being sensitive to the adverse effects of positive-pressure ventilation on venous return. It is important to realize that the air hunger exhibited by this patient is in large measure related to the metabolic acidosis associated with cardiogenic shock as he attempts to remove carbon dioxide. The ventilator should be set at tidal volumes of 8 mL·kg^{-1}. PEEP should be started at about 5 cm H_2O and then be increased depending on the cardiovascular effects and oxygenation status of the patient. Careful and immediate attention to the peak and plateau pressures should guide the ventilator settings thus maximizing oxygenation.

22.4.1.1 Cardiovascular Considerations

The blood pressure should be monitored immediately after intubation, expecting that the patient's hypotension may be acutely worsened. Agents that should be considered have been discussed earlier. If they have been started, they may need to be titrated depending on the patient's blood pressure in the early postintubation period.

22.5 SUMMARY

Patients in cardiogenic shock are critically ill. Endotracheal intubation is often temporally associated with circulatory and cardiac arrest. Attention to detail is crucial. The maintenance of oxygenation, medication selection, dosage adjustments, and caution with respect to positive-pressure ventilation are exceedingly important in these patients.

REFERENCES

1. Bersten AD, Holt AW, Vedig AE, Skowronski GA, Baggoley CJ. Treatment of severe cardiogenic pulmonary edema with continuous positive airway pressure delivered by face mask. *NEJM*. 1991;325:1825-1830.
2. Hoffman B, Welte T. The use of noninvasive pressure support ventilation for severe respiratory insufficiency due to pulmonary oedema. *Intensive Care Med*. 1999;25:15-20.
3. Mehta S, Jay GD, Woolard RH, et al. Randomized, prospective trial of bilevel versus continuous positive airway pressure in acute pulmonary edema. *Crit Care Med*. 1997;25:620-628.
4. Sharon A. High-dose intravenous Isorsorbide-Dinitrate is safer and better than Bi-Pap ventilation combined with conventional treatment for severe pulmonary edema. *JACC*. 2000;36:832-836.
5. Levitt MA. A prospective, randomized trial of BiPAP in severe acute congestive heart failure. *J Emerg Med*. 2001;21:363-369.
6. Pang D, Keenan SP, Cook DJ, Sibbald WJ. The effect of positive pressure airway support on mortality and the need for intubation in cardiogenic pulmonary edema: a systematic review. *Chest*. 1998;114:1185-1192.
7. How O, Rosner A, Kildal AB. Dobutamine-norepinephrine, but not vasopressin, restores the ventriculoarterial matching in experimental cardiogenic shock. *Translat Res*. 2010;156:273-281.
8. Shipley JB, Tolman D, Hastillo A, Hess M. Milrinone: basic and clinical pharmacology and acute and chronic management. *Am J Med Sci*. 1996;311:286-291.
9. Yamani MH, Haji SA, Starling RC, et al. Comparison of Dobutamine-based and Milrinone-based therapy for advanced decompensated congestive heart failure: hemodynamic efficacy, clinical outcome, and economic impact. *Am Heart J*. 2001;142:998-1002.
10. Cuffe MS, Califf RM, Adams KF, Jr, et al. Short term intravenous milrinone for acute exacerbation of chronic heart failure: a randomized controlled trial. *JAMA*. 2002;287:1541-1547.
11. Nieminen MS, Akkila J, Hasenfuss G, et al. Hemodynamic and neurohumoral effects of continuous infusion of levosimendan in patients with congestive heart failure. *J Am Coll Cardiol*. 2000;36:1903-1912.
12. Slawsky MT, Colucci WS, Gottlieb SS, et al. Acute hemodynamic and clinical effects of levosimendan in patients with severe heart failure. *Circulation*. 2000;102:2222-2227.
13. Follath F, Cleland JG, Just H, et al. Efficacy and safety of intravenous levosimendan compared to dobtamine in sever low-output heart failure (the LIDO study): a randomized double-blind trial. *Lancet*. 2002;360:196-202.
14. Mebazza A, Nuemann MS, Packer M, et al. Levosimendan vs. dobutamine for patients with acute decompensated heart failure. *JAMA*. 2007;297:1883-1891.

SELF-EVALUATION QUESTIONS

22.1. With respect to noninvasive pulmonary ventilation (NIPV)

   A. Patients on NIPV have a higher rate on intubation than controls.

   B. Large randomized controlled studies have been conclusive.

   C. Meta-analysis have showed no significant decrease in hospital mortality.

   D. CPAP improves ventilation and vital signs more rapidly than Bi-PAP.

22.2. Hypotension following intubation in patients with cardiogenic shock is likely due to

   A. the underlying disease

   B. positive pressure ventilation

   C. respiratory acidosis

   D. the use of an induction agent

   E. all of the above

22.3. With respect to the selection of induction agents for patients in cardiogenic shock

   A. Etomidate demonstrates remarkable cardiovascular stability.

   B. Opioids are preferable to other induction agents as they offer impressive cardiac stability.

   C. No induction agent should be used because these patients have unstable hemodynamics.

   D. Amnesia rather than induction of anesthesia is a better endpoint if one is going to use an induction agent.

   E. Ketamine is preferable to etomidate or propofol as it maintains muscle tone.

CHAPTER 23

Airway Management in the Patient with Burns to the Head, Neck, Upper Torso, and the Airway

Robert J. Vissers

23.1 CASE PRESENTATION

The emergency department receives a call from the emergency medical services (EMS) about a burn victim coming to your facility in about 5 minutes. In an attempt to take his own life, a 40-year-old man, while locked inside his vehicle, set himself on fire with gasoline. The patient's arrival at hospital was delayed due to a prolonged extrication and transport time of about 1 hour. He had significant burns to the anterior trunk, thighs, head, and neck. The EMS personnel advise that a difficult airway ought to be anticipated.

Attempts to examine his airway, establish intravenous (IV) access, and oxygenate are foiled by his severely agitated and uncooperative state.

23.2 INITIAL ASSESSMENT AND MANAGEMENT

23.2.1 How can airway assessment and management, resuscitation, patient comfort, and cooperation be achieved?

The evaluation of the airway in a burn victim is crucial to patient management. Difficulties with bag-mask-ventilation (BMV), the use of extraglottic devices, laryngoscopy, and surgical airways may all be present and should be anticipated.

Despite extensive burns, these patients are often awake, alert, and in severe pain. They are likely to require significant fluid resuscitation early in the course of their care. However, unless there are associated injuries, the immediate priorities for burn victims are early airway control, fluid resuscitation, and pain management. Accurate assessment of the airway and the patient's underlying physiological status may be impossible, until control of pain and agitation is achieved. Immediate IV access is desirable to facilitate this. But, access may also be restricted by the location of the burns.

In this case, the patient arrived very agitated, in severe pain, and without IV access. Haldol and morphine were given intramuscularly to achieve cooperation. Due to the location of his burns, access was restricted to his lower extremities and groin, areas which were spared due to his seated position. While nursing staff attempted peripheral IV access in his feet, a right femoral venous catheter was placed under ultrasound guidance.

Limited IV access requires that conditions be used to optimize success. It is recommended that the most experienced practitioners be assigned to provide vascular access using ultrasound guidance through unburned skin. Attention to sterile technique is particularly important in this population as delayed infections represent a serious risk. Intravenous access through an overlying burn is not contraindicated, but is more difficult to locate landmarks, can be challenging to secure, and may become dislodged with subsequent tissue edema. An intraosseous line is an alternative access option in an emergency situation when intravenous access cannot be achieved.

23.2.2 Are there difficulties with bag-mask-ventilation that might be anticipated in this patient?

Anatomical features predictive of difficult BMV may be present as well in burn victims, although other barriers to effective ventilation with a bag-mask must be considered. This patient is not obese, not elderly, and there is no facial hair or edentulous state to

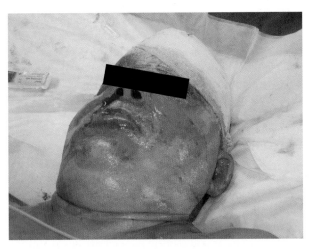

FIGURE 23-1. This photograph was taken shortly after the patient with burns to the head and neck presented to the emergency department.

suggest a poor seal. However, edema associated with the burn may have created anatomic changes affecting airway patency, airway resistance, and compliance. These may affect the ability to deliver adequate ventilation by either BMV or extraglottic devices.

Inspection of the face and neck revealed deep burns in this patient (Figure 23-1). The loss of skin elasticity was severe, restricting the mouth opening to several centimeters and preventing full movement of his jaw and extension of his neck. Further inspection revealed nasal hair singeing, pharyngeal erythema, and soot present in his posterior oropharynx. But, no swelling or stridor was appreciated.

While the indirect sign above strongly suggest the presence of thermal injury, the absence of facial burns, singed hairs, or carbonaceous sputum cannot reliably exclude the presence of supraglottic and laryngeal edema. When managing a significant burn injury which occurred in an enclosed space, even if the external examination is normal, one should assume airway swelling and inhalation injury are present and direct visualization is indicated (or warranted). The obstruction caused by thermal injury is related to progressive swelling and may also be complicated by skin sloughing. Early in the course of this evolving upper airway obstruction, BMV with positive-pressure manual ventilation may be able to overcome it. Bronchospasm and mucosal edema of the lower airways may accompany inhalation injury, further complicating attempts at bag-mask-ventilation. Fourth-degree burns (extend through the skin into underlying tissues) and deep third-degree burns to the chest may cause a significant reduction in chest wall compliance, particularly if the burn is circumferential. Eschar of the neck may prevent appropriate positioning of the patient for airway management. Emergency escharotomies of the chest or neck may be required (see later).

23.2.3 Are there issues with laryngoscopy and intubation that need to be considered in this patient?

The fundamental principle of airway management in the acute burn victim is early tracheal intubation and airway control, before conditions deteriorate. The intrinsic difficulties related to laryngoscopy uncovered with the LEMON assessment (see Section 1.6.2) remain relevant and need to be assessed. Reduced mouth opening, airway obstruction, and restricted neck mobility are the most common difficulties encountered. Edema caused by thermal injury to the perioral area, oropharynx, and glottis represents the primary difficulty in airway management. Associated swelling may obscure the upper airway and prevent visualization of the vocal cords. Mouth opening may be further reduced by loss of skin elasticity. Neck immobilization may be required if there is associated trauma to the cervical spine, or may be produced by neck eschar. Vocal cord edema is an independent predictor of need for intubation and has been associated with the presence of oral soot, facial burns, and the degree of body burns.[1]

This patient has a reduced ability to open the mouth. Despite the neck burn, mobility appears reasonable and there are no signs of a cervical fracture. The mechanism of an enclosed space burn, associated with facial burns and carbonaceous sputum, all strongly suggest the presence of thermal injury to the glottis. There is no stridor present. However, this is considered a late finding in an adult. Only 50% of patients with thermal injury to the airway present with hoarseness or respiratory distress, and only 20% will present with stridor.[1,2]

Despite the potential for difficult laryngoscopy in this patient, airway management should not be delayed and definitive airway control must be achieved urgently. The natural evolution of upper airway burn injury is progressive swelling, airway narrowing for 12 to 24 hours, and resolution in 3 to 5 days. Although significant airway edema may be present in the first 2 hours, visualization sufficient to permit intubation is usually possible at this time, and will only deteriorate with delay. Immediate airway evaluation and consideration of early intubation is strongly recommended. In a study of patients requiring transportation to a burn center, the most common findings were loss of or inability to secure intravenous access and inability to secure an airway.[3]

23.2.4 Are there physiologic issues which need be considered while managing the airway of this patient?

Other issues to consider in the burn patient are fluid resuscitation, the presence of trauma, and the presence of inhalation injury. Fluid resuscitation requirements in burn patients can be significant. There are a number of suggested formulas to guide volume replacement. But there is no demonstrated superiority in outcome among them and in general, most suggest approximately 4 mL·kg^{-1}·%BSA burn replacement in the first 24 hours. Despite much debate, studies have also failed to demonstrate a significant difference in patient outcome with the use of specific fluid regimens. The most important thing to remember regarding fluid management is the need for early replacement of the volume deficit to support tissue perfusion and to correct the metabolic acidosis.[4] The end points for resuscitation are debatable, but hourly urine output is a useful parameter for guiding fluid management. A urine output of 0.5 mL·kg^{-1}·h^{-1} or approximately 30 to 50 mL·h^{-1} in most adults and older children is desirable. In small children, the end point should be higher, approximately 1 mL·kg^{-1}·h^{-1}. Conversely, fluid overload is a potential concern in the initial resuscitation as overly aggressive fluid resuscitation can lead to unnecessary edema and pulmonary dysfunction. Too aggressive fluid resuscitation can also increase the need for escharotomies and extend the time required for ventilator support.

In this case, there is no history to suggest associated trauma, however, when the burn is associated with a blast injury, concurrent assessment of traumatic injuries will be necessary. The presence of associated injuries may enhance the need for early intubation, to facilitate therapy or operative intervention. Associated hemorrhagic shock will increase the need for aggressive volume resuscitation and the early consideration of blood replacement.

Inhalation injury may take up to 24 hours to become evident.[5,6] Due to the impressive heat exchange capacity of the upper airway, thermal injury is usually most significant above the vocal cords. However, heat-induced injuries may be present in the lower airway. Smoke inhalation can cause significant, progressive toxicity and hypoxemia by three mechanisms: the inhalation of gases causing hypoxia; airway inflammation from direct pulmonary toxins; and tissue hypoxia from systemic toxins such as cyanide and carbon monoxide. Any burn which takes place in an enclosed space, such as in the case of the patient described above, should raise the suspicion for inhalation and smoke injury. Chest radiography at presentation is a poor predictor of inhalation injury, since it is often normal initially. The presence of pulmonary infiltrates on initial evaluation suggests severe injury and a poor prognosis.[7]

23.2.5   How can carbon monoxide poisoning be identified?

Most pulse oximeters cannot reliably differentiate between oxygenated hemoglobin (HbO_2) and carboxyhemoglobin (COHb) and will give a spuriously high measurement of oxygen saturation. Reliance on pulse oximetry or a calculated SpO_2 (as may occur with arterial blood gas measurement) rather than hemoglobin oxygen saturation measured by co-oximeter (spectrophtometry) will fail to diagnose carbon monoxide poisoning, and will provide false reassurance that there is adequate issue oxygenation. An arterial blood gas specifying measured rather than calculated oxygen saturation should be obtained early in the course of management, and a COHb determination performed. High-flow oxygen through a non-rebreather mask should be applied immediately, regardless of the pulse oximetry reading. Depending on the level of COHb and patient presentation, other therapies, such as hyperbaric oxygen may be considered. The presence of significant carbon monoxide poisoning is another indication for early intubation to facilitate ventilation with 100% oxygen.[8]

23.3   AIRWAY MANAGEMENT CONSIDERATIONS

23.3.1   What would be the best way to manage this airway?

This patient represents potential difficulties to laryngoscopy and intubation, as well as ventilation with a bag-mask. Cricothyrotomy

is possible despite the burn but the open technique is preferred. Despite the difficulties discussed earlier, the extent of the burns, the involvement of the face and neck, and the potential for associated inhalation injury mandate definitive airway management. As stated previously, the fundamental principle is early airway intervention. Any existing difficulties will only become worse with delay.

Anticipating these difficulties, there are a few options possible in this patient. Regardless of the strategy employed, there needs to be a bedside rescue device and surgical airway available before proceeding with any airway management technique. With limited mouth opening and restricted neck movement in the patient described earlier, it is advisable to have a device at the bedside that may be inserted blindly. When mouth opening and neck extension is restricted by loss of skin elasticity, or oral swelling is anticipated, video laryngoscopy may be a preferred alternative to traditional laryngoscopy.

Rescue devices such as the lightwand (Trachlight™), the intubating LMA, the Combitube™, or a rigid fiberoptic laryngoscope, such as the Shikani scope or the Bullard laryngoscope, may be used in this setting. One case report describes the successful use of a Combitube™ in a patient with facial burns, reduced oral opening, and known tracheal stenosis.[9] Due to the potential for severe delayed facial edema, the placement of an oral tube is preferred over a nasal approach. However, severe oral swelling from local chemical burns (ingestions, Freon "huffing", etc) may prevent an oral approach, and blind nasotracheal or flexible bronchoscope-assisted nasal intubation may be the only nonsurgical option. Regardless of the intubating technique chosen, an open surgical cricothyrotomy kit should be available at the bedside.

Three approaches may be considered in this patient:

1. Inspection with the patient awake following topicalization and sedation using a laryngoscope or video laryngoscope. This technique has been well described in other chapters. If assessment suggests that the cords are likely to be visualized, the practitioner may undertake a rapid-sequence induction (RSI) technique. The urgency of the situation may preclude the use of an antisialagogue as it takes 15 to 20 minutes to be effective in enhancing a topical application of local anesthetic agent. A combination of IV midazolam and ketamine would be reasonable choices in this patient. The analgesic properties of ketamine are desirable and the potential for inhalation-induced bronchospasm favor this agent. Pain associated with this injury and respiratory distress may make it difficult to achieve an adequate level of cooperation unless high doses are used. Inability to gain cooperation without compromising ventilation may require the practitioner to move directly to RSI as outlined in option three, later.

2. Assessment of the airway with a flexible bronchoscope. The technique is similar to that described earlier, including topical anesthesia of the nares. This also requires a level of cooperation that cannot be achieved without sedation and analgesia. Utilizing the flexible bronchoscope, the practitioner may consider intubation over the scope, or proceeding to RSI if assessment suggests this is likely to be successful.

3. Another option is going directly to RSI. This may be considered if:
   A. Difficulty with laryngoscopy and intubation is not anticipated.
   B. The urgency or uncooperative state of the patient prevents the two options described earlier.
   C. Success was felt to be likely after an awake look.

The RSI procedure should not begin until Plan B and C are prepared and available at the bedside. Plan B should incorporate one of the rescue devices discussed earlier. Plan C should include rapid surgical cricothyrotomy. If difficulties are anticipated but urgency requires RSI, a double setup with the neck prepped and the surgical kit open is recommended. Attendance by another practitioner skilled in cricothyrotomy is desirable. An intubating stylet should be part of the initial laryngoscopic attempt, particularly since the glottic opening may be narrowed or difficult to visualize. Failure of laryngoscopy should be recognized early, allowing no more than three attempts. Persistent laryngoscopic attempts are unlikely to be successful and are associated with adverse outcomes. Instead, be prepared to move rapidly to Plan B or C.

23.3.2 If the airway appears normal on presentation, should the trachea be intubated prophylactically?

As described earlier, not all airway injuries manifest immediately. Edema and associated obstruction will continue for at least 24 hours. Significant generalized edema may progress over several days because of the increased microvascular permeability of all tissues and the significant fluid requirements of burn patients. Tracheal intubation and paralysis may be required to facilitate care such as escharotomies, wound management, associated traumatic injuries, and pain control. If patient transport is required, the initial presentation at the scene or hospital may offer the best conditions for airway management and tracheal intubation, and is strongly encouraged before transportation takes place.[3] Even if the upper airway is normal, progression of inhalation injury, particularly in the face of an increased work of breathing, may require tracheal intubation and positive-pressure ventilation. In the care of a burn patient, as a general rule, it is always better to intubate the trachea early than late.

23.3.3 Is cricothyrotomy contraindicated in a patient with burns involving the anterior neck?

No. In fact there are no absolute contraindications to a surgical airway when the patient cannot be oxygenated and the trachea cannot be intubated, since the alternative is death. Many of these patients have a tracheotomy in their course of treatment (see discussion later), even when burns involve the neck. However, endotracheal intubation is the preferred method of primary airway control. In patients with burns to the anterior neck, elective tracheotomy is generally delayed until 5 to 7 days after skin grafting.[10]

A cricothyrotomy remains the rescue airway of choice should attempts to secure the airway fail and the trachea cannot be ventilated. In this patient, the significant anterior neck burns have created a noncompliant skin and eschar, obscuring landmarks and causing difficulty with neck extension. An open cricothyrotomy technique using an adequate midline vertical incision, as opposed to a percutaneous Seldinger technique, is therefore recommended in this patient. This will serve as an escharotomy to release the contracted tissue and enhance the ability to identify the cricothyroid space by palpation through the wound.

23.4 POSTINTUBATION AND VENTILATION MANAGEMENT

23.4.1 How does the presence of an inhalation injury affect ventilation?

The clinical effects of inhalation injury include upper airway edema from thermal injury, capillary leak of fluids into the airways, bronchospasm from toxins, and small airway occlusion from sloughed mucosal debris and impaired ciliary clearance. This can lead to increased dead space, intrapulmonary shunting, and decreased lung and chest wall compliance. These problems are compounded if pulmonary infection supervenes.[5]

Bronchospasm may well respond to inhaled β_2-agonists. Air trapping can occur and adequate expiratory times should therefore be permitted. Vigorous pulmonary toilet will be required in the days following injury due to endobronchial debris, alveolar fluid, and infection. Positive end-expiratory pressure is often required to maintain small airway patency. Avoidance of excessive inflating pressures may be needed to avoid secondary lung injury. The concept of permissive hypercapnia has been associated with improved pulmonary outcomes in these patients.[11] Prophylactic steroids in the burn patient have not been associated with improved outcome and may increase mortality.

23.4.2 Are there other concerns specific to postintubation management in the burn victim?

Endotracheal tube stabilization in patients with facial burns can be challenging, particularly during debridement and grafting of facial burns. Methods of securing the tube to a nasogastric tube looped around the hard palate or nasal septum have been described.[12]

The role of tracheotomy in the management of inhalation injury and burns remains controversial.[13] Advantages include ease of pulmonary toilet and the avoidance of dislodged orotracheal tubes. A tracheotomy is more likely to be needed in patients with greater than 60% total body surface area burns and has been associated with an increased incidence of pulmonary infections.[14] The potential long-term sequelae, such as tracheal stenosis and fistula formation, will be major considerations in the decisions of the health-care team. The two emergency indications for a surgical airway are the failure to achieve tracheal intubation upon initial airway management, and if the endotracheal tube is inadvertently dislodged, the subsequent edema makes replacement impossible. Recognizing that significant airway edema will likely occur, cutting the endotracheal tube short is not advised. Great care should be taken to ensure tube security and prevent accidental extubation. Replacement of a defective endotracheal tube should be attempted only by employing a tube exchanger with rescue devices immediately available.

23.5   ADDITIONAL CONSIDERATIONS

23.5.1   When should escharotomy be considered in the burn patient?

Severe third-degree and fourth-degree burns cause the collagen in skin to lose its elasticity, shorten, and become rigid. When this occurs in the chest wall, particularly in circumferential burns, significant restrictive pulmonary mechanics can occur with a reduction in pulmonary compliance. Incisional escharotomy may be needed to improve compliance of the lungs and maintain ventilation. The same can be said of circumferential burns of the extremities in which circulation may be compromised.[15] Chest wall escharotomies are typically performed by a plastic surgeon, although they are easily performed by any physician if required as a lifesaving intervention. Vertical incisions are made bilaterally in the anterior axillary lines, from below the level of the clavicles to the lower rib margin. The top and bottom of the incisions are then joined to form a square across the chest. A tight neck eschar may draw the neck into flexion and impair ventilation. This may require a vertical incision from the sternal notch to the chin to release the constricting eschar.

Escharotomies do not take precedence over airway management, but in the case of significant circumferential chest burns with persistent ventilatory compromise, immediate escharotomies may be indicated, particularly if transport is contemplated.

23.5.2   Is succinylcholine contraindicated in acute burns?

The risk of lethal hyperkalemia following succinylcholine administration is well documented in patients with greater than 5% of body surface area (BSA) burned. The greatest risk would appear to be between 18 and 66 days postburn.[16,17] However, it should be noted that one author found that the risk of hyperkalemia was present just 9 days postburn.[18] It seems reasonable to consider succinylcholine safe if used 4 to 5 days after the burn is sustained and then not used until the burn is fully healed (see also Section 4.4.2.4). Rocuronium is an appropriate alternative. Burn injury has been associated with some resistance to the effects of nondepolarizing muscle relaxants over time, therefore higher doses of rocuronium (1.5 mg·kg^{-1}) have been described as effective in this setting.[19]

23.6   SUMMARY

Unless there is associated trauma, the immediate priorities for burn victims are early airway control, fluid resuscitation, and pain management. The acutely burned patient should always be evaluated for thermal airway injury and inhalation injury, particularly if the burn occurred in a confined space, more so if superheated steam is involved. Signs of upper airway obstruction ought to motivate further evaluation of the upper airway to determine if endotracheal intubation is indicated. Ventilatory failure is potentially multifactorial in these patients, being related to heat-induced upper airway obstruction, inhalation injury, and the acute reduction of compliance caused by chest wall eschar. Finally, as in all patients presenting to the ED, one must be vigilant for other associated injuries, such as blunt or penetrating trauma, as well as underlying medical conditions.

REFERENCES

1. Madnani DD, Steele NP, DeVries E. Factors that predict the need for intubation in patients with smoke inhalation injury. *Ear Nose Throat J*. April 2006;85(4): 278-280.
2. Darling GE, Keresteci MA, Ibanez D, Pugash RA, Peters WJ, Neligan PC. Pulmonary complications in inhalation injuries associated with cutaneous burn. *J Trauma*. 1996;40:83-89.
3. Klein MB, Nathans MB, Emerson D, Heimbach DM, Gibran NS. An analysis of the long-distance transport of burn patients to a regional burn center. *J Burn Care Res*. 2007;28:49-55.
4. Miller K, Chang A. Acute inhalation injury. *Emerg Med Clin NA*. 2003;21: 533-557.
5. Hettiaratchy S, Papini R. Initial management of a major burn: II—assessment and resuscitation. *BMJ*. Jul 10 2004;329(7457):101-103.
6. Tricklebank S. Modern trends in fluid therapy for burns. *Burns*. 2009;35: 757-767.
7. Masanes MJ, Legendre C, Lioret N, Saizy R, Lebeau B. Using bronchoscopy and biopsy to diagnose early inhalation injury. *Chest*. 1995;107:1365.
8. Ernst A, Zibrak JD. Carbon monoxide poisoning. *N Engl J Med*. 1998;339: 1603-1608.
9. Hagberg CA, Johnson S, Pillai D. Effective use of the esophageal tracheal Combitube following severe burn injury. *J Clin Anesth*. 2003;15:463-466.
10. Langford RM, Armstrong RF. Algorithm for managing injury from smoke inhalation. *BMJ*. 1989;299:902.
11. Sheridan RL, Kacmerek RM, McEttrick MM, et al. Permissive hypercapnia as a ventilatory strategy in burned children: effect on barotrauma, pneumonia and mortality. *J Trauma*. 1995;39:854-859.
12. Gray RM, Rode H. Intra-operative endotracheal tube stabilization for facial burns. *Burns*. 2010;36:572-575.
13. Jones WG, Madden M, Finkelstein J, Yurt RW, Goodwin CW. Tracheostomies in burn patients. *Ann Surg*. 1989;209:471-474.
14. Aggarwal S, Smailes S, Dziewulski P. Tracheostomy in burns patients revisited. *Burns*. 2009;35:962-966.
15. Sheridan RL. Scientific reviews: burns. *Crit Care Med*. 2002;30(11 Suppl): S500-514.
16. Gronert GA, Dotin LN, Ritchey CR, Mason AD, Jr. Succinylcholine-induced hyperkalemia in burned patients. II. *Anesth Analg*. 1969;48:958-962.
17. Schaner PJ, Brown RL, Kirksey TD, Gunther RC, Ritchie CR, Gronert GA. Succinylcholine-induced hyperkalemia in burned patients. 1. *Anesth Analg*. 1969; 48:764-770.
18. Viby-Mogensen J, Hanel HK, Hansen E, Graae J. Serum cholinesterase activity in burned patients. II: anaesthesia, suxamethonium and hyperkalaemia. *Acta Anaesthesiol Scand*. 1975;19:169-179
19. Han TH, Martyn JA. Onset and effectiveness of rocuronium for rapid onset of paralysis in patients with major burns: priming or large bolus. *Br J Anaesth*. 2009;102:55-60.

SELF-EVALUATION QUESTIONS

23.1. Airway burns

   A. are asymptomatic 50% of the time

   B. are associated with stridor 20% of the time

   C. are more common if the patient is trapped in an enclosed space at the time of the burn

   D. may progress to upper airway obstruction over 6 to 12 hours

   E. all of the above

23.2. The time course of upper airway swelling leading to total upper airway obstruction is

A. 1 to 3 hours

B. 5 to 8 hours

C. 12 to 24 hours

D. unpredictable

E. seconds to minutes

23.3. The risk of succinylcholine-induced hyperkalemia

A. is limited to patients with >20% third-degree burns

B. is causally related to burn-induced myoglobinuric renal failure

C. may be seen as early as 24 hours postburn

D. can be eliminated by pretreating with a nondepolarizing muscle relaxant

E. is a risk until the burn injury is fully healed

CHAPTER 24

Airway Management in a Patient with Angioedema

Michael F. Murphy, Genevieve MacKinnon, and David Petrie

24.1 CASE PRESENTATION

This 25-year-old black woman presents to the emergency department (ED) 2 hours after the onset of lip swelling that has progressed to difficulty in breathing. With the exception of newly diagnosed hypertension, she is otherwise well. Last week, her primary care physician began a course of a new antihypertensive medication, lisinopril. She has had no history of swelling and there is no family history of disorders characterized by swelling. Her vital signs are temperature 37°C, heart rate (HR) 100 beats per minute (bpm), respiratory rate (RR) 22 breaths per minute, blood pressure (bp) 165/90 mm Hg, and SpO_2 is 99% on 2 L·min^{-1} of O_2 by nasal prongs.

The patient is seated (Figure 24-1) with markedly edematous lips. She has a muffled voice (hot potato voice) and is unable to swallow her own secretions due to the swelling. There is no stridor. The remainder of the physical examination is unremarkable.

24.2 DIAGNOSIS AND INVESTIGATIONS

24.2.1 What is the pathophysiology of angioedema?

Angioedema is defined as the abrupt onset of non-pitting swelling of the skin, mucous membranes, and deep subcutaneous tissues, including the linings of the upper respiratory and intestinal tracts.[1] Angioedema develops because of a local increase in permeability of the submucosal or subcutaneous capillary vessels, causing local plasma extravasation. This is exacerbated by the release of vasoactive substances such as histamines, prostaglandins, bradykinins,

and cytokines.[2] Angioedema can be divided into hereditary angioedema (HAE) and acquired angioedema.

Hereditary angioedema is extremely rare, affecting 1 in 50,000 people.[2] It develops due to a C1 esterase inhibitor deficiency, which is inherited in an autosomal dominant pattern. This deficiency results in an abnormal increase in the activation of C1 and subsequently excessive formation of the enzyme kallikrein. The excess kallikrein transforms kininogen into kinins, including bradykinin. Bradykinin is highly vasoactive and produces the characteristic tissue swelling.[2] HAE is commonly precipitated by trauma and stress, and can recur. If the patient has known HAE, then treatment with fresh frozen plasma (FFP) is beneficial, as it contains C1 esterase inhibitor. In some centers, vapor-heated C1 inhibitor concentrate is available and is proving beneficial in recurrent attacks of HAE.[2]

Acquired angioedema is due to faulty activation of the complement and kallikrein–kinin systems. It comprises several types, including the traditional IgE-mediated allergic response, precipitated by exposure to an allergen (such as peanuts, antibiotics, and shellfish). Anaphylaxis is characterized by an acute onset and not only causes angioedema of the upper airways but also has a more systemic effect causing wheeze secondary to bronchoconstriction and hypotension secondary to vasodilation and third spacing.[3] Anaphylaxis (or anaphylactoid) reactions can cause angioedema through other mechanisms such as direct mast cell degranulation (opiates, radio-contrast media) or by altering arachidonic acid metabolism (benzoates, angiotensin-converting enzyme inhibitors [ACEIs], and nonsteroidal anti-inflammatory agents [NSAIDs]).[4,5]

The development of angioedema secondary to ACEIs is of particular interest.[4,5] In addition to inhibiting the conversion of angiotensin I to angiotensin II, the suppression of ACE results in

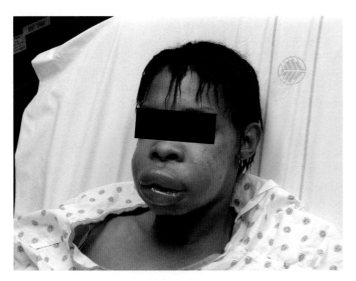

FIGURE 24-1. Patient with angioedema.

a decrease in the breakdown of bradykinin and substance P. As outlined earlier, this can result in severe tissue swelling.[1] ACEI-induced angioedema has a predilection for the head and neck,[2] rendering it a particular challenge in airway management. It appears that this drug effect is associated specifically with the class of drugs known as ACEIs,[2] although recently, angioedema has been demonstrated to occur with the angiotensin II receptor blockers (ARBs) as well.[6,7] Treatment with IV steroids, antihistamines, and subcutaneous epinephrine (0.3 mg) may be beneficial in allergy-induced angioedema, but has been shown to be ineffective in HAE and of limited use in ACEI and ARB-induced angioedema.[7,8] There is no role for FFP in ACEI or ARB-induced angioedema.

ACEI-induced angioedema affects more women than men in the United States and is most common among 40- to 50-year-olds. Close to half of those affected with angioedema are African American.[9] According to the literature, the incidence of ACEI-induced angioedema ranges from 0.1% to 0.2% of all patients taking this class of drugs.[1,2,10] However, ACEI-induced angioedema is the most common cause of angioedema seen in US EDs, accounting for 17% to 38% of all angioedema cases.[11] In the omapatrilat (a new ACEI) versus enalapril (OCTAVE) trial, the investigators found that there was an increased incidence of the disorder in African American patients, those older than 65, and those with a history of drug rash or seasonal allergies.[10] Approximately 50% of all ACEI-induced angioedema cases occur within 1 week of starting the medication, with the remainder occurring anywhere from weeks to years after starting the drug.[2]

24.2.2   What is the general clinical course of the disorder?

Patients with HAE usually report trauma, often minor (eg, dental visit), followed by tissue swelling. They can present with swelling in such widespread anatomic areas as the face, hands, arms, legs, GI tract, and genitalia, but often respond to treatment. In one large series, 10% of the patients with HAE required definitive airway intervention because of upper airway edema. The onset

of IgE-mediated anaphylaxis is rapid and often life threatening if not treated appropriately.[2] The clinical course of ACEI-induced angioedema is often subacute but always extremely unpredictable, and life-threatening presentations requiring airway interventions do occur and are reported in up to 20% of these patients.[2] According to the literature, between 0 and 22.2% of patients with angioedema will require intubation.[9] It is extremely difficult to predict which patients who present with a stable airway will progress to a requirement for airway intervention. Researchers from Boston[9] retrospectively analyzed cases of ACEI-related angioedema and determined that increasing age and oral cavity/oropharyngeal involvement predicted the need for airway intervention. These predictors had a sensitivity of 65.2% and specificity of 83.7%.

Since the clinical course of angioedema, especially ACEI-induced, is very unpredictable, it is recommended that these patients be admitted to an environment where they can be closely monitored for at least 24 hours.

24.2.3   What investigations might one employ to aid in the diagnosis and evaluate the severity of the disorder?

The severity of airway compromise on presentation will determine the extent of initial investigations of these patients, and thus the workup for HAE is typically undertaken after the acute episode has resolved. The unpredictable clinical course of this disorder demands that each of these patients be triaged as emergencies to a resuscitation area of the ED and attended to immediately by nursing and physician staff. Evaluation and management are carried out concurrently, as is appropriate in patients with life-threatening conditions. As a result, early airway intervention is strongly advised. It is often obvious that the airway is in immediate jeopardy and this should trigger calling for assistance and implementing a strategy to secure the airway, from either above or below (surgically). The decision for airway intervention will be based largely on the clinical signs of respiratory distress: air hunger, agitation, hypoxia, and especially muffled voice, difficulty swallowing saliva, and stridor.

If one has the luxury of time and possess the skill, severity may be assessed by flexible nasopharyngoscopy.[12] It is prudent to prepare for this procedure as though one were intending to perform an awake endoscopic-guided nasal intubation. This assumes that one has anesthetized the nasopharyngeal passage and inserted a nasotracheal tube through which the endoscope is passed in case the findings mandate intubation. It is preferable that the scope used for this procedure be of sufficient length and stiffness to guide an endotracheal tube into the trachea.[12] Repeated nasopharyngoscopic evaluation at regular intervals may be indicated in the event immediate endotracheal intubation is not necessary. Additionally, as with all upper airway emergencies, it is prudent to be prepared to undertake an immediate surgical airway in the event that diagnostic maneuvers trigger complete upper airway obstruction. This is often referred to as a *double set-up* in the context of airway management.

A portable cross-table soft tissue x-ray of the airway is seldom useful and it should be emphasized that this investigation *must not* delay care if the airway is compromised and *must not* mean that the patient has to leave the resuscitation area. These patients are always reluctant to lay flat for studies, such as CT scanning and MRI evaluations to be performed. This hesitancy ought to alert the practitioner that the degree of airway obstruction is significant, rendering such studies contraindicated. Arterial blood gases and other laboratory investigations are generally not helpful in the management of these patients.

24.3   AIRWAY MANAGEMENT

24.3.1   How does one decide that intubation is indicated?

This decision is most often made on clinical grounds and is based on the degree of upper airway obstruction present, and the pace at which it changes. Diagnostic studies, with the possible exception of flexible endoscopic evaluation of the airway, are not usually helpful in deciding when to intubate. As mentioned earlier, early airway intervention is the safest course of action,[13] particularly as the clinical course may be erratic and unpredictable. Although securing the airway should be the priority, some practitioners may consider a course of steroids and nebulized epinephrine in the hope of halting or reversing the progression of airway compromise.

Any evidence of upper airway obstruction, including a muffled voice, difficulty managing secretions, or stridor, ought to trigger urgent airway intervention. Other clinical signs motivating immediate intervention include: air hunger (dyspnea), confusion, agitation, or falling oxygen saturations.[14]

24.3.2   How should the airway be evaluated for difficulty?

These airways should always be considered difficult and managed according to the Difficult Airway Algorithm (see Chapter 2). Specifically, they fail the MOANS analysis (see Section 1.6.1) for difficult bag-mask-ventilation in that mask seal may be inadequate. But more importantly, adequate gas exchange may be prevented by edematous upper airway tissue, occluding the airway even in the face of high pressures generated by bag-mask devices. Gas exchange at the alveolar level may also be compromised by bronchoconstriction and increased fluid and secretions.

Based on the airway evaluation using the mnemonic RODS (see Section 1.6.3), the use of extraglottic devices (EGDs) will be difficult. Insertion of the device may not be possible and the larynx itself may be edematous to the point of obstruction. Furthermore, the EGD may not provide an effective seal in an edematous hypopharynx.

The failure of MOANS and RODS alone prohibits the use of paralytic agents, even if one felt that the LEMON analysis (see Section 1.6.2) might permit successful direct laryngoscopy and intubation. In other words, rapid-sequence intubation (RSI) is imprudent. An assessment for cricothyrotomy is appropriate in these patients, as this procedure may emerge as the preferred and primary intervention for airway management and may be performed awake under local anesthesia. In other words, if laryngoscopy is unsuccessful or impossible in a patient who is very difficult to ventilate using a bag-mask, and alternative intubating techniques, and extraglottic rescue devices are unlikely to work, the surgical option has to be considered early in the planning and execution of airway management.

24.3.3   How should this patient's airway be managed?

Some patients with angioedema have had prior episodes and may be able to provide some reassurance that this episode will resolve under close observation. However, such patients are few and the course of this disease is unpredictable. It is much more likely that the clinical course will be unpredictable and a more aggressive approach to airway management is therefore justified.

Management is driven by the Difficult Airway Algorithm (see Chapter 2). In the event that oxygen saturations are poor and cannot be improved, one is directed to the Failed Airway Algorithm and immediate cricothyrotomy. RSI is rarely an option in these patients. If there is time, the next step will depend on the practitioner's access to, and ability to use, a flexible bronchoscope (FB). If an experienced practitioner is available, then intubation using FB ought to be performed with immediate cricothyrotomy as backup. The nasal route for the FB-guided intubation mentioned earlier is ordinarily much easier for those who infrequently perform intubations. In the event one does not have, or cannot use, a flexible bronchoscope then an awake look employing a conventional laryngoscope may help create a more informed decision to intubate awake or to move to cricothyrotomy.

It is a difficult decision to use sedative hypnotic agents to facilitate airway evaluation and management in patients with upper airway obstruction in general and angioedema in particular. Patients with upper airway obstruction maintain their airways by using every airway muscle at their disposal, and even small doses of these sedative agents may precipitate a complete upper airway obstruction. In small titrated doses, ketamine may be preferable in that it maintains muscle tone and respiratory drive. The disadvantages of laryngeal sensitization, salivation, and confusion must be weighed against the positive aspects of using this drug.

The use of topical local anesthetic agents in patients with upper airway obstruction is also not without risk. Several cases have been reported in the last decade of topicalization converting partial upper airway obstruction to complete obstruction (see Section 3.3.2.1). However, a practitioner may have no choice but to employ topicalization in an attempt to secure the airway. Blind (nonvisual) techniques such as blind nasal intubation and light-guided techniques are relatively contraindicated due to the potential for airway distortion and the risk of producing further trauma and bleeding.

24.4   SUMMARY

The incidence of angioedema has increased dramatically over the past two decades with the introduction of angiotensin-converting enzyme (ACE) inhibitors and angiotensin receptor blockers (ARB) for the treatment of hypertension. The clinical course of an episode is unpredictable. For this reason, securing the airway early is generally a safer course than watching and waiting. Available therapies, including intravenous steroids and nebulized alpha agonists (eg, epinephrine), are of marginal value and ought not delay airway intervention. Intubation over a flexible bronchoscope may be the preferred technique, the nasal route being recommended for those who perform flexible bronchoscopic intubation infrequently. Alternatively, employing sedation and topical anesthesia may enable one to intubate using direct laryngoscopy. However, the Plan B option of cricothyrotomy performed under local anesthesia with the patient awake must be considered as a backup, or in some cases, even a primary method of securing the airway.

As with all cases of upper airway obstruction, one must appreciate that while the patient may have stable vital signs, the airway is exceedingly unstable!

REFERENCES

1. Muelleman RL, Tran TP. Allergy, hypersensitivity and anaphylaxis. In: Marx JA, Hockberger R, Walls R, eds. *Rosen's Emergency Medicine: Concept and Clinical Practice*. 5th ed. St. Louis: Mosby; 2002:1619-1634.
2. Kaplan AP, Greaves MW. Angioedema. *J Am Acad Dermatol*. 2005;53: 373-392.
3. Sampson HA, Munoz-Furlong A, Campbell RA, et al. Second symposium on the definition and management of anaphylaxis: summary report. *J Allergy Clin Immunol*. 117;391:1996.
4. Chiu AG, Krowiak EJ, Deeb ZE. Angioedema associated with angiotensin II receptor antagonists: challenging our knowledge of angioedema and its etiology. *Laryngoscope*. 2001;111:1729-1731.
5. Gannon TH, Eby TL. Angioedema from angiotensin converting enzyme inhibitors: a cause of upper airway obstruction. *Laryngoscope*. 1990;100: 1156-1160.
6. Haymore BR, Yoon J, Mikita CP, Klote MM, DeZee KJ. Risk of angioedema with angiotensin receptor blockers in patients with prior angioedema associated with angiotensin-converting enzyme inhibitors: a meta-analysis. *Ann Allergy Asthma Immunol*. 2008;101:495-499.
7. Simons FE, Gu X, Simons KJ. Epinephrine absorption in adults: intramuscular versus subcutaneous injection. *J Allergy Clin Immunol*. 2001;108:871-873.
8. Reid M, Euerle B. Angioedema. http://emedicine.medscape.com/article/135604-overview. Accessed June 20, 2011.
9. Zirkle M, Bhattacharyya N. Predictors of airway intervention in angioedema of the head and neck. *Otolaryngol Head Neck Surg*. 2000;123:240-245.
10. Kostis JB, Kim HJ, Rusnak J, et al. Incidence and characteristics of angioedema associated with enalapril. *Arch Intern Med*. 2005;165:1637-1642.
11. Roberts JR, Wuerz RC. Clinical characteristics of angiotensin-converting enzyme inhibitor-induced angioedema. *Ann Emerg Med*. 1991;20:555-558.
12. Bentsianov BL, Parhiscar A, Azer M, Har-El G. The role of fiberoptic nasopharyngoscopy in the management of the acute airway in angioneurotic edema. *Laryngoscope*. 2000;110:2016-2019.
13. Thompson T, Frable MA. Drug-induced, life-threatening angioedema revisited. *Laryngoscope*. 1993;103:10-12.
14. Bernstein S, Buckley PJ, Pollack CV, Walls R. Intubation strategies in patients with angioedema or intraoral obstruction: a multicenter study. *Acad Emerg Med*. 1999;6:518.

SELF-EVALUATION QUESTIONS

24.1. ACE-inhibitor-induced angioedema patients

A. usually respond to subcutaneous and aerosolized epinephrine

B. have a notoriously unpredictable clinical course with respect to the airway

C. can usually be safely observed as long as they do not have stridor

D. usually respond to high-dose intravenous steroids

E. can be managed with fresh frozen plasma

24.2. All of the strategies for definitive airway management are acceptable in patients with angioedema **EXCEPT**

A. awake intubation using a flexible bronchoscope

B. awake intubation under direct laryngoscopy

C. rapid-sequence intubation

D. cricothyrotomy

E. tracheotomy

24.3. Which of the following symptoms would suggest an obstructed airway with a diameter of 4.5 mm or less and necessitate definitive airway management?

A. stridor

B. muffled voice

C. oxygen desaturation

D. difficulty managing secretions

E. use of accessory muscles

CHAPTER (25)

Airway Management for Blunt Facial Trauma

David A. Caro and Aaron E. Bair

25.1 CASE PRESENTATION

A 40-year-old officer was thrown from his police boat causing him to strike his face on a concrete bridge abutment. He was found lying face down and unconscious by other officers on the scene. Upon paramedic arrival, his initial Glasgow Coma Scale (GSC) score was 9, with facial bleeding, and a tenuous airway. He was positioned so as to optimize airway patency and expeditiously transported to the nearest emergency department (ED).

The patient presented to the ED with sonorous respirations and an oxygen saturation of 95%, despite an inspired oxygen concentration (FiO$_2$) of 0.7. Vital signs included a pulse of 65 beats per minute (bpm), a blood pressure (bp) of 155/90 mm Hg, a respiratory rate of 12 breaths per minute, and a temperature of 37°C. Upon initial examination (Figure 25-1), he had ongoing oral and nasal hemorrhage; periorbital, nasal, and lip ecchymoses; mobility of his maxilla; and multiple broken teeth. The patient appeared somnolent and his GCS score was 9. In light of his injuries, and their mechanisms, cervical spine precautions were initiated in anticipation of tracheal intubation (for airway protection).

25.2 PATIENT ASSESSMENT

25.2.1 What are the airway evaluation considerations in this patient?

This patient presents with clinical issues that may influence his airway management. In addition to airway protection and maintenance, strategic management of his ventilation will likely be required.

As this is not a crash intubation situation, an evaluation of the airway for anticipated difficulty is possible.

The presence of mid-face instability and orofacial disruption will likely hinder the success of bag-mask-ventilation (BMV) due to a poor mask seal. Similarly, in the presence of soft tissue edema and foreign bodies (teeth, clots, etc.), use of an extraglottic device (EGD) may be difficult. Laryngoscopy will likely be complicated by the presence of blood, tissue edema, and possible airway disruption. In addition, the use of cervical spine precautions limits the ability to position the head and neck optimally during laryngoscopic intubation. His airway is classified as difficult, requiring the difficult airway algorithm to be employed.

25.2.2 What is the LeFort classification system?

Significant mid-face injuries that involve the maxilla and pterygoid plates can be categorized by the LeFort system (Figure 25-2). While fractures can be of mixed type, they are generally classified as follows: the fracture lines of a LeFort I fracture follow the course of the overlying nasolabial folds (ie, involve the maxilla inferior to the nose only); LeFort II fractures involve a larger portion of the maxillae, triangulating from the premolar region on both sides to the nasal bones; and LeFort III fractures include the zygomatic arches, thereby allowing for total mobility of the facial structures (craniofacial disjunction).

By definition, LeFort fractures require that the maxilla be fractured in two separate places, leaving an essentially free-floating segment of bone. This alters the structural integrity of the face and potentially complicates airway visualization. LeFort II and III fractures can significantly impair the airway practitioner's ability

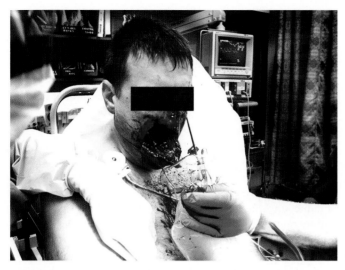

FIGURE 25-1. A photograph of the patient shortly after presentation to the ED.

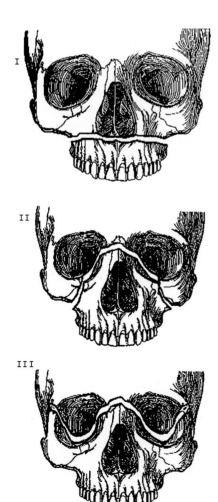

FIGURE 25-2. Diagram of the LeFort classification of facial fractures.

to ventilate the patient using a bag-mask, due to poor mask fit and associated obstruction of the nares.[1-3]

25.2.3 How is a basilar skull fracture different from a LeFort fracture?

Blunt facial and head trauma are often associated with other injuries, including basilar skull and cervical spine fractures. Basilar skull fractures most commonly involve the petrous portion of the temporal bone. However, the sphenoid and ethmoid bones can also be involved. The possibility of ethmoid fracture may be of particular concern, as a free passage may ensue between the nasal and intracranial cavities. Inadvertent intracranial placement of nasally introduced tubes and catheters has been reported, making the blind insertion of nasal airway devices contraindicated.[4,5]

25.2.4 How often is a major facial fracture associated with cervical spine injury?

The incidence of associated cervical spine fracture with severe blunt facial trauma ranges from 1% to 2.6% of patients.[6-9] This potential for associated cervical spine injury requires that, in the absence of the C-spine that has been fully cleared, the airway practitioner makes every effort to maintain the cervical spine in a neutral position. An assistant will be needed to maintain in-line cervical immobilization during attempts at laryngoscopy.

25.2.5 What other concerns do you have for this patient?

There are other issues for this patient. The patient has sustained a head injury that is moderately symptomatic. An increase in intracranial pressure (ICP), or even an intracranial hematoma, is possible. The principles of management for the brain-injured patient include the avoidance of hypotension and hypoxemia, as both are independently associated with aggravating secondary brain injury and higher patient mortality. In addition, gratuitous intracranial engorgement due to patient coughing should be controlled. Modulation of the patient's cerebral metabolic oxygen demand is desirable to mitigate increases in cerebral blood flow to areas of normal brain with the potential to cause an increase in ICP. Pretreatment with intravenous lidocaine and fentanyl should be considered prior to induction and paralysis in an effort to blunt further ICP rise with laryngoscopy. For induction, a cerebroprotective sedative (eg, propofol, benzodiazepines, or barbiturates) is warranted, but care must be taken not to induce hypotension that could exacerbate the patient's brain injury. Etomidate may be attractive because of its associated hemodynamic stability, and is neutral in its effects on ICP.[10-14] The choice of agents is of particular importance when caring for patients with a diminished cardiac reserve, such as those with severe cardiac disease, those who are critically ill, or patients who are elderly. These patients are more prone to a hypotensive response than are healthier patients with similar injuries. As this is not a crash intubation situation, an evaluation of the airway for anticipated difficulty is possible.

25.2.6 What investigations are warranted for this patient before proceeding to airway management?

The priority in managing patients with trauma is adequate gas exchange and oxygenation. Clearly, airway intervention takes precedence over any further investigations. Some may argue that a cross-table lateral cervical spine x-ray ought to precede airway intervention. However, since such an investigation would not alter the manner in which the airway is managed (in-line stabilization during laryngoscopy), it ought not delay airway management. Concurrent resuscitation and evaluation is the hallmark of trauma management, meaning that relevant investigations are underway at the same time intubation is undertaken and do not delay management.

25.3 AIRWAY MANAGEMENT

25.3.1 What are the airway management considerations one needs to be aware of?

The initial plan should anticipate both difficult laryngoscopy and difficult BMV. This is at least in part related to the potential for an unstable cervical spine prohibiting proper positioning of the airway by neck flexion or extension with the potential for spinal cord injury. The practitioner should also consider how the patient ought to be positioned for laryngoscopy, as the volume of bleeding and the mechanical stability of the airway might preclude lying the patient flat. An induction with full paralysis might be desirable, although it must be recognized that failure of both intubation and BMV is a significant possibility in this patient. In such a circumstance, the efficacy of many of the common alternative devices would also be compromised. Transillumination with the lightwand (eg, Trachlight™) could be problematic. The intubating laryngeal mask airway might be difficult to place. Vision with the Bullard™ laryngoscope, GlideScope®, or bronchoscope would be clouded in the presence of blood. Basic backups, such as the Combitube™, or surgical airway, would have to be available.

25.3.2 What procedure should be used to intubate the trachea of this patient?

Timing of positioning in anticipation of airway management is an important consideration. Upon arrival, the patient is able to maintain his airway as he is sitting up. This positioning allows blood and bone fragments to be somewhat displaced away from the airway. However, immediately placing the patient in a supine position strictly for concern of his cervical spine places his tenuous airway at undue risk. Given his mental status and host of injuries, one would anticipate that he would begin to obstruct his airway upon supine positioning. As such, consider denitrogenation in his original position of comfort. Manual in-line cervical immobilization can be quickly initiated in the sitting position. Once all preparations for the difficult airway have been made, the patient should be placed supine immediately preceding laryngoscopy.

With a deteriorating neurological status and a possible increase in ICP, Plan A is a standard approach to rapid-sequence intubation (RSI) with in-line cervical spine stabilization. Alternatively, if the airway is determined to be too difficult to proceed with RSI, an awake look may be employed as Plan A, realizing that the topical anesthesia will most likely fail due to the amount of blood in the airway. Paralysis and intubation would be indicated upon viewing glottic structures. Plan B would be an EGD and Plan C a surgical airway—in other words a "triple setup." Preparation begins by assembling standard intubating equipment, alternative airway devices, and a surgical airway kit. Denitrogenation with a non-rebreather oxygen mask should be initiated well in advance of induction. Uncontrolled epistaxis may impede this process, can lead to aspiration, and may require immediate packing, or cauterization. Adequate suctioning is essential.

Pretreatment with lidocaine, and an opioid should be given 3 minutes prior to intubation, time permitting. RSI will ordinarily include propofol or etomidate, followed by succinylcholine. Anti-aspiration maneuvers, such as Sellick maneuver, ought to be employed, although cautiously to avoid internal jugular vein compression and impeded venous return from the cranial vault. Dosages of the opioids and the induction agents should be moderated to avoid hypotension, particularly in the face of substantial sympathetic nervous system activation.

A sequence of predetermined steps should be employed if failure with laryngoscopy or oxygenation occurs. The alternative airway device of choice should be the one with which the practitioner has the most experience. An intubating LMA has particular advantage, as it may circumvent the problem of a traditional mask seal on top of a mobile maxilla. It can also be manipulated by the guiding handle to best fit the hypopharynx. As an additional backup, the patient's neck should be prepped, and cricothyrotomy equipment should be opened and ready for use, in the event that the preceding steps fail to secure the airway.

25.4 POSTINTUBATION MANAGEMENT

25.4.1 What other issues should be considered following tracheal intubation?

Stable hemodynamics, as well as intracranial dynamics with adequate cerebral perfusion, together with adequate oxygenation and ventilation, are mandatory for this patient. Serial arterial blood gas measurements to monitor for hypo- or hyperventilation are recommended. Continuous capnography, if available, can be useful in this setting. Importantly, during the time of initial evaluation in the ED, the patient should be adequately sedated and paralyzed to limit the possibility of accidental extubation.

25.5 SUMMARY

A maxillofacial injury can significantly impair both the ability to bag-mask-ventilate a patient and perform laryngoscopy. Careful consideration must be given to approach this difficult airway, which is complicated further by the significant risk of cervical spine injury, as well as brain injury. The lesson from this patient is to have multiple backup devices ready to use, along with a predetermined plan on how to employ them, in the event that the trachea cannot be intubated orally.

REFERENCES

1. Manson PN. Some thoughts on the classification and treatment of LeFort fractures. *Ann Plast Surg*. 1986;17:356-363.
2. Ghysen D, Ozsarlak O, van den Hauwe L, Van Goethem J, De Schepper AM, Parizel PM. Maxillo-facial trauma. *JBRBTR*. 2000;83:181-192.
3. McRae M, Frodel J. Midface fractures. *Facial Plast Surg*. 2000;16:107-113.
4. Martin JE, Mehta R, Aarabi B, Ecklund JE, Martin AH, Ling GS. Intracranial insertion of a nasopharyngeal airway in a patient with craniofacial trauma. *Mil Med*. 2004;169:496-497.
5. Schade K, Borzotta A, Michaels A. Intracranial malposition of nasopharyngeal airway. *J Trauma*. 2000;49:967-968.
6. Ardekian L, Gaspar R, Peled M, Manor R, Laufer D. Incidence and type of cervical spine injuries associated with mandibular fractures. *J Craniomaxillofac Trauma*. 1997;3:18-21.
7. Bayles SW, Abramson PJ, McMahon SJ, Reichman OS. Mandibular fracture and associated cervical spine fracture, a rare and predictable injury. Protocol for cervical spine evaluation and review of 1382 cases. *Arch Otolaryngol Head Neck Surg*. 1997;123:1304-1307.
8. Beirne JC, Butler PE, Brady FA. Cervical spine injuries in patients with facial fractures: a 1-year prospective study. *Int J Oral Maxillofac Surg*. 1995;24:26-29.
9. Haug RH, Wible RT, Likavec MJ, Conforti PJ. Cervical spine fractures and maxillofacial trauma. *J Oral Maxillofac Surg*. 1991;49:725-729.
10. Guldner G, Schultz J, Sexton P, Fortner C, Richmond M. Etomidate for rapid-sequence intubation in young children: hemodynamic effects and adverse events. *Acad Emerg Med*. 2003;10:134-139.
11. Gauss A, Heinrich H, Wilder-Smith HG. Echocardiographic assessment of the haemodynamic effects of propofol: a comparison with etomidate and thiopentone. *Anaesthesia*. 1991;46:99-105.
12. Jellish WS, Riche H, Salord F, Ravussin P, Tempelhoff R. Etomidate and thiopental-based anesthetic induction: comparisons between different titrated levels of electrophysiologic cortical depression and response to laryngoscopy. *J Clin Anesth*. 1997;9:36-41.
13. Bramwell KJ, Haizlip J, Pribble C, VanDerHeyden TC, Witte M. The effect of etomidate on intracranial pressure and systemic blood pressure in pediatric patients with severe traumatic brain injury. *Pediatr Emerg Care*. 2006;22(2):90-93.
14. Modica PA, Tempelhoff R. Intracranial pressure during induction of anaesthesia and tracheal intubation with etomidate-induced EEG burst suppression. *Can J Anaesth*. 1992;39(3):236-241.

SELF-EVALUATION QUESTIONS

25.1. After denitrogenation, attempts at RSI fail. The oxygen saturation decreases into the high 80% range. What is the next step in your management?

A. attempt to intubate by using Eschmann Introducer

B. change laryngoscope blade types

C. place an LMA

D. improve attempts at BMV with improved technique

E. cricothyrotomy

25.2. After multiple attempts at intubation and recognized inability to ventilate with either bag-mask or LMA, what is your next step in management?

A. Place an invasive airway (eg, open cricothyrotomy or percutaneous cricothyrotomy).

B. Call for assistance.

C. Attempt bronchoscopic-assisted intubation.

D. Support with bag-mask until awakening and resumption of spontaneous respirations.

E. Blind nasal intubation.

25.3. The incidence of associated cervical spine fracture with severe blunt facial trauma

A. is negligible

B. is not a concern provided a cervical collar that provides rigid immobilization is used

C. ranges from 1% to 2.6% of patients

D. in some studies approaches 20%

E. is unknown

CHAPTER (26)

Airway Management in a Patient with Ludwig's Angina

Kirk J. MacQuarrie and David Kirkpatrick

26.1 CASE PRESENTATION

A 32-year-old man (Figure 26-1) presented to the emergency department with dysphagia, dysphonia, and dyspnea. Further inquiry revealed a 1-week history of right-sided jaw pain. This was initially treated with oral antibiotics and analgesics by his family doctor while awaiting an appointment with his dentist. He saw his dentist the previous day and had an abscessed molar tooth extracted from his right mandible. Unfortunately, his pain continued and he developed swelling and fever, prompting him to present to the emergency department. His past medical history was unremarkable, and aside from his remaining prescription of the penicillin and hydromorphone, he was on no medications. He had no known allergies.

26.2 INTRODUCTION

26.2.1 Discuss the incidence and etiology of deep-neck infections in adults

The management of the patient whose airway is compromised due to a deep-neck infection is a challenge for even the most experienced practitioner. Fortunately for all, these are relatively rare. A typical ENT referral center may see one to three adult cases per year requiring airway management. As in this case, the deep-neck infection is often odontogenic. Intravenous drug abuse is another important cause. However, many cases of deep-neck infections do not have an identifiable etiology.[1] Diabetes mellitus may also be a risk factor and its presence tends to be associated with more aggressive infection.[2,3]

26.2.2 Do all deep-neck infections require airway intervention?

Most patients with deep-neck infections can be managed conservatively without surgical intervention and do not require intervention to maintain the patient's airway.[4,5] This conservative approach is similar to the management of adenotonsillar hypertrophy secondary to infectious mononucleosis, which will typically respond to steroids with or without antibiotics. Even epiglottitis in the adult population only rarely will require airway manipulation in the form of intubation or tracheotomy. Early deep-neck infections present usually as a cellulitis that can be successfully treated with antibiotics alone. Small, localized abscesses, such as peritonsillar abscesses, can often be treated with needle aspiration followed by antibiotics.

26.2.3 What is Ludwig's angina and how does it differ from retropharyngeal abscess?

This life-threatening infection of the floor of the mouth was first described in 1836 by Wilhelm Frederick von Ludwig. The condition has also been called "morbus strangulatorius", "angina maligna", and "garotillo" (Spanish for "hangman's loop"). These older terms reflect the high mortality, typically by total airway obstruction, in the days before antibiotics.

Ludwig's angina is defined as severe bilateral cellulitis and edema of the submandibular and sublingual spaces. *Woody* swelling of the submandibular area in a febrile patient with a history of jaw pain is the classic presentation. The infection may cause swelling of the tongue and epiglottis that will then impair the ability to swallow and clear secretions. Total airway obstruction may result from progressive swelling or from laryngospasm secondary

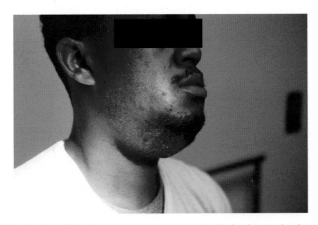

FIGURE 26-1. This 32-year-old man presented with dysphagia, dysphonia, and dyspnea. There was marked swelling of the right side of the neck. Due to marked discomfort, he was unable to protrude his tongue for proper pharyngeal evaluation.

to aspiration of pus secretions, or both.[6] Surgical intervention is usually required if abscess formation and airway compromise occur. Whereas most cases of deep-neck infections can be managed conservatively with antibiotics alone, true cases of Ludwig's angina typically require more aggressive intervention in terms of surgical drainage and definitive airway management. Treatment of Ludwig's angina is three-pronged and involves airway management, antibiotic therapy, and surgical drainage.

26.3 ASSESSMENT OF THE PATIENT

26.3.1 Why might airway management be difficult in patients with Ludwig's angina?

Patients with Ludwig's angina or a retropharyngeal abscess frequently have features that create difficulty with all aspects of airway management: bag-mask-ventilation (BMV), ventilation using extraglottic devices (LMA), laryngoscopy and tracheal intubation, and even performing a surgical airway.

Bag-mask-ventilation may be challenging in these patients for a number of reasons. Patients with stridor will have significantly decreased airway caliber, necessitating high airway pressures to produce adequate gas flow. It may not be possible to generate these pressures with BMV. Because of pain and anxiety, both the awake or obtunded patients may not tolerate application of the facemask and airway opening maneuvers due to pain and anxiety. It may prove difficult or impossible to open the airway of the sedated or unconscious patient due to loss of muscle tone and the resultant further narrowing of the airway. Copious secretions may increase the risk of laryngospasm, and tongue swelling may preclude use of an oral airway. A nasal airway is an option but bleeding could possibly trigger laryngospasm.

Upward displacement of the tongue by the infection can make insertion of any of the extraglottic rescue devices difficult or impossible. Although Brimacombe et al reported the successful use of a small Laryngeal Mask Airway (#2) as a rescue device for a hypoxic adult patient with quinsy,[7] extraglottic rescue devices for

failed BMV, even if they can be inserted, may be ineffective due to glottic edema.

Secretions and edema, particularly tongue swelling, will make direct laryngoscopy more difficult regardless of the type of blade chosen. Nuchal rigidity, trismus, or both may be improved with sedation or muscle relaxants but there is no guarantee that these agents will be effective. Blind intubation techniques, such as the intubating Laryngeal Mask Airway (LMA-Fastrach™, LMA North America Inc., San Diego, California) and light-guided intubation (Trachlight™, Laerdal Medical Corp., Wappingers Falls, New York) would not generally be considered for first-line use in these patients as these techniques run the risk of disrupting infected tissue and potentially soiling the airway. Furthermore, these nonvisual intubating techniques could result in laryngospasm during the intubation attempt. Typically these patients have heavy secretions and occasionally some bleeding, limiting the use of indirect visual techniques such as the flexible and rigid fiberscopes and video laryngoscopes. In true cases of Ludwig's angina, oral intubation with any instrument is frequently not an option due to limited oral access. Most experts would advocate either a nasal intubation or a surgical airway.

Unfortunately, performing a surgical airway in this patient population is difficult. The anatomy is often distorted due to swelling, and hyperemic tissues may increase the likelihood of bleeding. In some patients, the abscess may involve the area surrounding the trachea. Supine positioning of the patient to perform a surgical airway may worsen dyspnea and reduce the patient's cooperation.

To add to the difficulty of airway management in these patients, all possible options of ventilation and oxygenation involve some danger. The ultimate decision will be made based on the urgency of the clinical circumstance, the available resources, the careful setting of priorities, and the skill and experience of the airway team (anesthesia practitioner and surgeon).

26.3.2 Discuss the role of CT scan in assessing these patients

The advent of the CT scan has revolutionized the ability to accurately assess the swollen, inflamed neck. In addition to determining the severity of the infection involving different tissue planes and neck spaces, the resolution of the CT scan can help to differentiate between a cellulitis and an abscess. The CT scan can also determine the presence or absence of jugular vein thrombosis. Unfortunately, in the presence of a rapidly deteriorating airway, it is necessary to proceed with emergency airway management before a CT examination of the neck becomes available. Even in patients with stable airways, a CT scan may not be possible prior to definitive airway management because the patient may be unable to lie flat. In these cases, the CT scan is done to better determine the extent of the infection only after securing an airway.

26.3.3 Discuss the technique of nasopharyngoscopy and its role in the management of patients with deep-neck infections

Nasopharyngoscopy is a safe and simple technique which should become familiar to anesthesia practitioners, otolaryngologists, and emergency specialists. Following the application of topical vaso-constrictor and topical anesthetic (10% Xylocaine), the flexible nasopharyngoscope is passed into the nasopharynx. The glottis should not be anesthetized as this could trigger laryngospasm. With the flexible nasopharyngoscope, the glottis can be viewed from above without the risk of provoking laryngospasm. The technique is usually first done in the emergency department as part of the initial evaluation, and repeated at the bedside or in the operating room as required to provide an ongoing evaluation of the airway.

26.3.4   How was this patient assessed?

On examination, he appeared anxious and in severe discomfort. He was febrile with a temperature of 38.7°C (101.66°F). His respiratory rate was 26 breaths per minute. His heart rate was 104 beats per minute (bpm) and his blood pressure was 132/76 mm Hg. His oxygen saturation was 91% on 40% oxygen delivered through the facemask. He had a marked decrease in the range of motion of his neck. Significant swelling and erythema was observed extending from the right submandibular region, crossing the midline and down the neck to include his left upper chest.

In a lateral x-ray of the neck, marked submandibular and retropharyngeal swelling was seen, as well as a diminished airway caliber (Figure 26-2). Although potentially helpful, a CT scan was not done as it was felt that the patient could not tolerate lying flat, even for a short period of time.

Nasopharyngoscopy was performed in the emergency department (ED) by the ENT resident and revealed right lateral pharyngeal swelling and posterior displacement of the epiglottis obscuring the vocal cords.

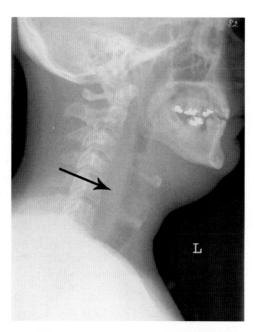

FIGURE 26-2. Although this lateral x-ray view of the head and neck did not show any obvious sign of airway obstruction, it showed an increase prevertebral soft tissue (swelling of the posterior pharyngeal wall) (arrow), an important diagnostic sign of retropharyngeal abscess.[18] There was also a loss of normal lordotic curvature of the spine.

26.3.5   How do you assess the severity of airway obstruction?

Airway obstruction is assessed clinically by history and physical examination, noting symptoms and looking specifically at signs, such as oxygen saturation, respiratory rate, stridor, tracheal tug, intercostal indrawing, and accessory muscle use. Lateral x-ray (Figure 26-2) and CT scan of the head and neck can quantify the degree of obstruction. It is also possible to examine the dynamic aspect of the obstruction through nasopharyngoscopy.

26.4   AIRWAY MANAGEMENT

26.4.1   What are the indications for establishing a definitive airway in patients with deep-neck infections?

Indications for definitive airway management in these patients are impending airway obstruction or sepsis. The decision to secure the airway is generally made by the ENT surgeon based on impending airway obstruction. There is some evidence that it may be prudent to intervene at an earlier stage in the diabetic patient.[3] In some instances, the ED physician may be forced into airway intervention if the patient is acutely decompensating (see Chapter 2, Crash Algorithm). Once the decision to intervene is made, anesthesia and ENT consultants, if not already involved, should be immediately consulted. These patients are ideally managed in the operating room, provided that the transfer is quick and complete airway obstruction is not imminent.

26.4.2   What was the plan in this case?

Given the severity of the obstruction and the patient's worsening symptoms, the decision was made to establish a definitive airway. Anesthesia was immediately consulted and the plan was made to proceed to the operating room for either endotracheal intubation or tracheotomy, followed by surgical drainage of the abscess.

26.4.3   Do these patients require a primary surgical airway or can an attempt be made to intubate from above?

Once the need to secure the airway has been established, the next decision is whether to attempt intubation from above (either oral or nasal) or to go directly to a surgical airway. In the stable patient, this generally refers to an awake tracheotomy done by an experienced surgeon. Local anesthesia with minimal sedation (eg, remifentanil 0.05-0.1 ug·kg^{-1}·min^{-1}) is usually all that is needed to ensure patient acceptance when the procedure is performed by a competent surgeon. In rare circumstances, an awake cricothyrotomy may be indicated if surgical expertise or time is not available. The choice of airway should be a joint decision of the anesthesia practitioner and surgeon based on the predicted difficulties of each of the following: bag-mask-ventilation, EGD ventilation, direct laryngoscopy, alternative intubation, and surgical access. The skill and experience of the airway team will also affect this decision. Potter et al[8] reviewed the literature in 2002 and found that the background of the involved surgeon had a significant influence on preferred management. They found primary surgical airways appeared to be favored by otolaryngologists, while oral and maxillofacial surgeons favored oral or nasal intubation.

26.4.4   Discuss the double set up and Plan C

In many cases, it will be reasonable to make a nonsurgical attempt to secure the airway. The specific route (awake, asleep, oral, and nasal) will be discussed later but it is critical to have a well-developed Plan B (and sometimes Plan C). The double set up is the recommended approach for most of these cases, meaning that the surgical team is ready to go should attempts fail to secure the airway from above. This may involve having the surgical team gowned and gloved, and the neck prepped. Many times a formal tracheotomy can be performed. But in the event of serious airway compromise, a cricothyrotomy may be a better choice.

The surgical airway typically represents Plan B and this may solve the airway problem. Surgical access could, however, prove difficult for any of the reasons discussed earlier. Loss of the airway during tracheotomy has been reported[9] and such an eventuality must be prepared for with Plan C. This will typically involve sedation (IV or inhalation) to facilitate patient cooperation, but in rare circumstances could require muscle relaxation and an attempt at direct laryngoscopy while attempts at obtaining surgical access continue.

26.4.5   Discuss the pros and cons of securing the airway in the awake or anesthetized patient

One must decide whether to perform tracheal intubation awake or asleep. As discussed earlier, these patients invariably have features that pose problems in airway management. The safest initial approach with these patients is to manage the airway while they are awake. Sedation may indeed be necessary in some cases, but it is preferred to keep the patient cooperative and spontaneously breathing. Reassurance and relieving the patient's fear and anxiety is crucial; repeated reassurance and a confident demeanor on the part of the practitioner are essential. As well, the patient will often need to be maintained in a sitting or semi-sitting position in order to help preserve the airway and increase comfort, thereby ensuring the patient's cooperation.

26.4.6   Discuss reasons why an awake intubation may be unsuccessful

While awake intubation remains the safest initial approach to airway management, it is important to realize that sudden deterioration may occur even in a fully awake or minimally sedated patient.[10,11,12] Reports of complete airway obstruction and some of failed bronchoscopic intubation emphasize the importance of managing these patients under double set up.[13] Inadequate airway anesthesia, practitioner's inexperience, over-sedation, copious secretions, bleeding are all reasons for failure of an attempt at awake intubation.

26.4.7   What is the plan if awake intubation fails or is not an option?

If an awake intubation fails or is not possible, then a complete, but rapid, reassessment of the situation is in order. The next safest approach may be an awake surgical airway, provided that the patient still has a patent airway and is at least minimally cooperative. In the rapidly deteriorating or actively uncooperative patient, a primary surgical airway may not be a practical alternative. It may then become necessary to induce general anesthesia in a patient with multiple predictors of difficulty with all aspects of airway management.

26.4.8   Discuss options if general anesthesia becomes necessary to secure the airway

Should it be necessary to induce general anesthesia, the ideal approach is a matter of opinion. There are pros and cons to all of the available choices. Induction of general anesthesia in this setting should always be done under double set up as discussed earlier.

Perhaps the classic approach is an inhalation induction in an attempt to induce general anesthesia while preserving spontaneous ventilation. Inhalation induction followed by direct laryngoscopy and intubation is a common practice in children with airway obstruction since awake intubation is rarely a practical option in children.

Inhalation induction of adults with airway obstruction may be more difficult in that the relatively longer excitement phase predisposes to aspiration, laryngospasm, or both. As anesthetic depth increases, complete airway obstruction can also occur due to the loss of muscle tone. Inhalation induction typically requires at least some degree of patient cooperation, but can be accomplished without.[14] As with awake intubation, it is critical to have a well-rehearsed backup plan (Plan B and C).

Preservation of spontaneous ventilation under anesthesia may also be accomplished utilizing IV agents. Compared to inhalation agents, it may be more difficult to preserve adequate spontaneous ventilation and achieve adequate depth of anesthesia using IV agents. Recent evidence suggests that remifentanil may be a more attractive IV sedation option. Machata et al have demonstrated excellent intubating conditions when remifentanil was used for conscious sedation.[15] A bolus of 0.75 ug·kg^{-1} followed by an infusion of 0.075 ug·kg^{-1}·min^{-1} provided good intubating conditions.

Rapid-sequence intubation (RSI) is unlikely to represent a first-line management option in these patients. However, in the event that the airway is completely lost, consideration should be given to use of muscle relaxants to facilitate intubation while attempts continue to achieve surgical airway access. RSI may also be considered for the actively uncooperative patient provided there is a double set up.

26.4.9   Discuss the pros and cons of "nasal or oral" intubation

Following the decision to attempt intubation from above, the next decision is whether to use the nasal or oral route. Each has its advantages and drawbacks.

The nasal route bypasses the tongue (which may be swollen) and often provides a convenient passage to the glottic opening. At one time, blind nasal intubation was a common choice in these patients, but with the general availability of flexible bronchoscopes, this technique is now seldom indicated. Furthermore, blindly advancing the endotracheal tube (ETT) into the glottic opening may rupture the abscess with resultant soiling of the trachea. The risk of epistaxis is a major concern with the nasal approach, as bleeding may hamper visualization and could trigger laryngospasm.

The oral approach avoids the risk of nasal bleeding and tube size is limited only by size of the glottic opening. Unfortunately, the massive tongue swelling combined with trismus, often seen in patients with Ludwig's, can make an oral intubation impossible.

26.4.10   How can one minimize the risk of bleeding associated with nasal intubation?

The risk of bleeding during nasal intubation can be minimized with the liberal use of topical vasoconstrictors (eg, xylometazoline) and by using a small ETT (7.0 mm inner diameter [ID] or smaller). Reinforced ETTs are more flexible and may cause less trauma and are therefore preferable in these patients. Regular ETTs (including nasal RAE ETTs) may be made less damaging to tissues by softening the tubes in warm saline prior to use.

The practice of dilating up the nasal passage using different sizes of nasal trumpets may also decrease bleeding and allow for passage of a larger tube. Following application of local anesthesia and vasoconstrictors, a small soft nasal airway lubricated with 2% lidocaine jelly can be inserted into the right nasal passage (larger in most people). If resistance is encountered, the left nares can be tried. The process can then be repeated with the next larger size airway. The goal is to get easy passage of at least a size 8 nasal airway. An ETT a half size smaller can then be used for the intubation. A larger tube (7.0 mm ID or greater) is advantageous in that it allows for insertion of the adult flexible bronchoscope with its superior optics and suction capabilities.

26.4.11   What is the best tool to facilitate intubation?

For the most part, the tool that one chooses to facilitate intubation in these patients is less important than the approach discussed earlier. The technique chosen should reflect the practitioner's skill, experience, and comfort with the technique, as well as the safety and practicality of the chosen technique. Nonvisual techniques are discouraged due to risks of soiling the airway and of possible laryngospasm. For reasons discussed earlier, techniques that allow visualization of the airway are preferred, usually either a direct-vision laryngoscopy or the flexible bronchoscope (FB). Other methods may be acceptable provided the practitioner is skilled in their use.

26.4.12   Discuss the advantages and disadvantages of flexible bronchoscopic intubation

Flexible bronchoscopic intubation (FBI) offers the advantage of being able to see *around the obstruction* and is usually well tolerated in the awake patient. Unfortunately, heavy secretions, bleeding, or both, may limit the usefulness of the FBI. In addition, as the ETT is advanced blindly over the bronchoscope during intubation, careful attention is required to avoid rupturing the abscess and soiling of the infective materials into the trachea. Use of the adult FBI can lessen the effect of secretions compared to the pediatric FBI but necessitates the use of at least a size 7.0 mm ID ETT. FBI may be more difficult in the unconscious patient with decreased muscle tone.

26.4.13   Discuss the advantages and disadvantages of direct laryngoscopy

Direct laryngoscopy will often be advantageous in the presence of heavy secretions. It can be performed quickly and is generally the technique of choice in the unconscious patient. Direct laryngoscopy is highly stimulating and may not be tolerated in the awake patient, particularly if much force is needed to expose the glottis.

26.4.14   Describe the plan to secure the airway in this case

In the operating room, the airway was reevaluated and, in consultation with the ENT surgeon, the decision was made to perform an awake nasal tracheal intubation under double set up.

The patient was positioned semi-sitting and standard monitors were applied. Supplemental oxygen was delivered with nasal prongs during preparation and airway anesthesia. A judicious dose of midazolam (0.5 mg bolus) was administered intravenously to reduce the patient's anxiety and improve cooperation. The neck was prepped and the surgical team was gowned and gloved, and ready to perform an emergency surgical airway (Plan B).

26.4.15   Discuss airway anesthesia for patients with Ludwig's angina

There are multiple techniques to anesthetize the airway and these are discussed in Chapter 3. The chosen technique depends largely on the preference of the practitioner. However, care must be taken to avoid early stimulation of the airway which can result in fatal laryngospasm.[7]

Inflammation and infection can, in theory, decrease the efficacy of local anesthetics due to changes in local pH. However, this is generally not of any clinical significance. Heavy secretions, bleeding, or both, can decrease the amount of local anesthetic that actually reaches the mucosa and this should be taken into account, but there are many reports of successful airway anesthesia in the presence of infection.[16]

26.4.16 How was airway anesthesia achieved in this case?

Airway anesthesia was achieved with a combination of lidocaine ointment and inhaled lidocaine. Xylometazoline (Otrivin nasal spray) was applied to both nasal passages in hopes of decreasing bleeding potential. Approximately 2.0 cm of 5% lidocaine ointment was applied to the back of the tongue with a tongue depressor. The DeVilbiss atomizer was then used to deliver 15 mL of 4% lidocaine as an aerosol via a nasal route. No attempts were made to specifically block the superior laryngeal nerve due to the possibility of disrupting the abscess and potentially soiling the airway.

26.4.17 How was this patient's airway secured?

The patient was asked to take a deep breath while occluding each nares. The right appeared more patent and was dilated up as described earlier (Section 26.4.10) so that a #8.0 nasal airway was easily accepted. A #7.0 reinforced ETT was then gently advanced into the nasopharynx. An adult 5.2 mm flexible bronchoscope was then passed through the ETT. After identifying the glottic opening, which was significantly deviated to the left, the bronchoscope was directed into the trachea and the ETT was then gently advanced off into the airway. Following CO_2 confirmation of successful tube placement, general anesthesia was induced with fentanyl and propofol.

Surgical drainage of the abscess was then accomplished without incident. Following 36 hours of ventilation in the ICU, the patient was uneventfully extubated and made a full recovery.

26.5 SUMMARY

It is clear that there is more than one approach to the management of the airway in these patients. The choice will be based on the particular patient presentation and the skills and experience of the airway team.

In 2002, Jenkins et al surveyed the management choices for the difficult airway by Canadian anesthesia practitioners.[17] Regarding the management of a patient unable to swallow due to a retropharyngeal abscess, 70% chose an awake approach, 23% chose inhalation induction, and only 7% chose an IV induction of anesthesia. While 37% chose direct laryngoscopy and 8% chose primary surgical airway, FBI was the initial technique chosen by 50% of the responders. A 2004 study by Bross-Soriano et al reported on 107 patients with Ludwig's angina over 18 years.[2] Surgical airway was required in 28%, when nasal intubation failed or was not possible.

Deep-neck infections with abscess formation resulting in airway compromise provide challenges for both the airway practitioner and the surgeon who are dependent upon each other for a successful outcome. The likelihood of a satisfactory result is enhanced by early involvement of the team planning an approach to such challenges.

REFERENCES

1. Parhiscar A, Har-El G. Deep neck abscess: a retrospective review of 210 cases. *Ann Otol Rhinol Laryngol.* 2001;110:1051-1054.
2. Bross-Soriano D, Arrieta-Gomez J, Prado-Calleros H. Management of Ludwig's angina with small neck incisions: 18 years of experience. *Otolaryngol Head Neck Surg.* 2004;130(6):712-717.
3. Boscolo-Rizzo P, Da Mosto MC. Submandibular space infection: a potentially lethal infection. *Int J Infect Dis.* 2009;13:326-333.
4. Mayor GP, Millan JM, Vidal AM. Is conservative treatment of deep neck space infections appropriate? *Head & Neck.* 2001;23(2):126-133.
5. Sichel JY, Dano I, Hoewald E, Biron A, Elishar R. Nonsurgical management of parapharyngeal space infections: a prospective study. *Laryngoscope.* 2002;112:906-910.
6. Neff SP, Merry AF, Anderson B. Airway management in Ludwig's angina. *Anaesth Intensive Care.* 1999;26:659-661.
7. Brimacombe J, Perry A, Van Duren P. Use of a size 2 LMA to relieve life-threatening hypoxia in an adult with quinsy. *Anaesth Intensive Care.* 1993;21:475-476.
8. Potter JK, Herford AS, Ellis E. Tracheotomy versus endotracheal intubation for airway management in deep neck space infections. *J Oral Maxillofac Surg.* 2002;60:349-354.
9. McGuire G, El-Beheiry H, Brown D. Loss of the airway during tracheostomy: rescue oxygenation and re-establishment of the airway. *Can J Ansth.* 2001;48(7):697-700.
10. Ho AMH, Chung DC, To EWH, et al. Total airway obstruction during local anesthesia in a non-sedated patient with a compromised airway. *Can J Anesth.* 2004;51(8):838-841.
11. Shaw IC, Welchew EA, Harrison BJ, Michael S. Complete airway obstruction during awake fiberoptic intubation. *Anaesthesia.* 1997;52:576-585.
12. McGuire G, El-Beheiry H. Complete upper airway obstruction during awake fiberoptic intubation in patients with unstable cervical spine fractures. *Can J Anesth.* 1999;46(2):176-178.
13. Pahl C, Yarrow S, Steventon N, Saeed NR, Dyar O. Angina bullosa haemorrhagica presenting as acute upper airway obstruction. *Br J Anaesth.* 2004;92:283-286.
14. Smith CE, Fallon WF. Sevoflurane mask anesthesia for urgent tracheostomy in an uncooperative trauma patient with a difficult airway. *Can J Anesth.* 2000;47(3):242-245.
15. Machata AM, Gonano C, Holzer A, et al. Awake nasotracheal fiberoptic intubation: patient comfort, intubating conditions, and hemodynamic stability during conscious sedation with remifentanil. *Anesth Analg.* 2003;97(3):904-908.
16. Ovassapian A, Tuncbilek M, Weitzel EK, Joshi CW. Airway management in adult patients with deep neck infections: a case series and review of the literature. *Anesth Analg.* 2005;100(2):585-589.
17. Jenkins K, Wong DT, Correa R. Management choices for the difficult airway by anesthesiologists in Canada. *Can J Anesth.* 2002;49(8):850-856.
18. Wholey MH, Bruwer AJ, Baker HL Jr. The lateral roentgenogram of the neck: with comments on the atlantoodontoid-basion relationship. *Radiology.* 1958;71:350-356.

SELF-EVALUATION QUESTIONS

26.1. What is Ludwig's angina?

   A. epiglottitis

   B. unstable angina

   C. deep-neck infection and edema involving the entire floor of the mouth

   D. lingual tonsillitis

   E. mediastinitis

26.2. Which of the following airway management strategies may be difficult in patients with a Ludwig's angina?

A. face-mask-ventilation

B. ventilation using extraglottic devices

C. direct laryngoscopy

D. surgical airway

E. all of the above

26.3. Which of the following is **NOT** an acceptable intubating technique in managing patients with Ludwig's angina?

A. surgical airway

B. flexible bronchoscopic intubation

C. intubation using an intubating LMA

D. laryngoscopic intubation

E. intubation using a GlideScope®

CHAPTER (27)

Airway Management in the Intensive Care Unit

Stephen Beed

27.1 CASE PRESENTATION

A grossly intoxicated and obese 52-year-old woman slips while leaving a restaurant, striking her head on a concrete step. She loses consciousness and while lying on her back vomits and aspirates. She is transported by ambulance to the emergency department (ED). By the time she reaches the ED, she is awake and complaining of difficulty in breathing. She is 5 ft (152 cm) tall and weighs 220 lb (100 kg). She has a heart rate (HR) of 122 beats per minute (bpm) (sinus rhythm on the cardiac monitor), respiratory rate (RR) of 28 breaths per minute (and labored), oxygen saturation (SpO_2) 90% (on a non-rebreather), and a blood pressure 154/88 mm Hg. Computed tomography (CT) of her head is negative and she has no other injuries. The patient is admitted to the intensive care unit (ICU) for management of her aspiration pneumonitis. Following admission to the ICU, she becomes more distressed and her oxygen saturation falls into the low 80s despite optimal medical management and attempts at noninvasive ventilation. The decision is made to intubate the trachea of the patient. Airway evaluation reveals a thyromental distance of 4 cm; she has both upper and lower dentures. The initial attempt to intubate her trachea awake is unsuccessful and is complicated by further vomiting and aspiration. A second attempt employing a rapid-sequence intubation (RSI) technique, including Sellick maneuver is successful. During the intubation, particulate matter in the pharynx is noted. The laryngeal view with external laryngeal manipulation is a Cormack/Lehane Grade 2. Tracheal placement is confirmed with end-tidal carbon dioxide ($ETCO_2$) detection. Bronchial lavage with a flexible bronchoscope (FB) is performed immediately after intubation.

The patient subsequently develops severe adult respiratory distress syndrome (ARDS) requiring deep sedation, with FiO_2 1.0 and pressure-controlled ventilation, adjusted by using ARDSNet

parameters[1-4] to the following: pressure level (PC) 20 cm H_2O, positive end-expiratory pressure (PEEP) 16 cm H_2O, FiO_2 1.0, tidal volume (TV) 500 to 550 mL, and RR 24 breaths per minute. She receives aggressive supportive care. On ICU day 5, corticosteroids are started and the patient subsequently improves. Her sedation is decreased and by day 7 she is switched to a PC of 18 cm H_2O, RR 24 to 30 breaths per minute, and TV 385 to 760 mL.

On day 11, the patient develops a new fever, an increased WBC, hypotension requiring inotropic support, and falling oxygen saturation requiring an increase in FiO_2 to 0.50. Bronchoscopy and CT scanning confirms a ventilator-associated pneumonia. On return from CT scan she self-extubates and within 30 minutes requires reintubation. This is accomplished by direct laryngoscopy following the application of topical airway anesthesia, and administration of 1 mg of midazolam, 50 μg of fentanyl. To facilitate tracheal intubation, a styletted orotracheal tube (OTT) and BURP (backwards, upwards, and right-side-orientated pressure on the larynx) are used. Broad-spectrum antibiotics are started. She undergoes a bedside percutaneous tracheotomy on day 13 and is weaned from ventilator support by day 20. She is transferred to the intermediate medical care unit on day 22.

27.2 UNIQUE AIRWAY ISSUES IN THE ICU

27.2.1 What is unique about the ICU patient?

Patients admitted to the ICU generally have limited physiologic reserve. They need minute-to-minute monitoring and treatment and usually require respiratory and/or hemodynamic support. Physicians choosing to practice in the ICU environment must possess excellent airway management skills for a variety of reasons. Some patients initially not intubated will decompensate while in ICU and require tracheal intubation. Others are admitted to the ICU having been intubated elsewhere and will be extubated (planned or unplanned) during their ICU stay. Still others, having been extubated, will fail and require reintubation. As with any intervention, an understanding of the dynamic and often subtle interplay between commonly utilized medications and the physiologic reserve of the compromised patient must be understood.

In addition to limited cardiopulmonary reserve, other important concerns, such as hepatic and renal dysfunction, a full stomach, and altered neurological function are also common in this patient population. Intensive care patients are as complex as the environment in which they are cared for. The practitioner tasked with airway management in this setting must be aware of these factors and make sound decisions, often very quickly, to improve patient outcome.

27.2.2   How common is airway management in ICU patients?

Airway management outside the controlled operating room environment carries higher risk to the patient for a variety of reasons including the acuity of the situation, the patient's limited physiologic reserve, and less access to advanced airway equipment. In addition, the delivery of this care is often by nonexperts or practitioners with limited experience.[5]

It is known that cardiac arrest outside of the operating room occurs frequently.[6] Furthermore, the incidence of cardiac arrest in the ICU setting is as high as 2%, much higher than the 0.068% rate in the operating room.[7] Chacko et al reported on critical incidents in a closed 18-bed, multidisciplinary unit over a 33-month period.[8] Airway-related incidents accounted for 32.8% of all reported incidents, with the most common being accidental extubation. In this study, there were 32 incidents (11.4% of those reported) that led to adverse outcomes, including 4 deaths, all of which were due to airway-related events.

Needham et al reported on factors which contributed to airway events that had been collected as part of the Intensive Care Unit Safety and Reporting System, a voluntary anonymous reporting system developed in conjunction with the Society of Critical Care Medicine and used in 18 ICUs across the United States over a 12-month period. There were 841 incidents reported with 78 airway events. More than half of the airway events were considered preventable and about 20% of the patients with airway reports sustained a physical injury and had an actual or anticipated prolonged hospital length of stay associated with the event. There was one death related to an airway event. Additionally, family dissatisfaction when these events occurred was common. Factors noted to limit airway events included adequate ICU staffing and the use of skilled assistants.[9]

27.2.3   Does the ICU environment influence how the patient's airway is managed in the ICU?

The American College of Critical Care Medicine describes three levels of intensive care: a Level One center provides comprehensive care across all disciplines and is typically located in a large urban hospital environment affiliated with an academic medical center; a Level Two center provides comprehensive care, but not in all disciplines; and a Level Three center can provide some intensive care support and stabilization of the critically ill patient.[10] Common to all such facilities is the need to manage the airway of the critically ill patient from time to time.

Perhaps more than in other environments, physical barriers may complicate the management of an airway crisis in the ICU. The presence of equipment (mechanical ventilators, monitors, infusion pumps, dialysis machines, etc) and vascular lines can make it difficult to even get to the head of the bed. Specialized apparatus for patient care (air beds, cervical spine collars, orthopedic frames, etc) in an already overcrowded environment also contribute to difficulty in accessing the airway or positioning the patient for optimal airway management, particularly in an emergency. Space limitations may make it difficult for other members of the resuscitation care team to access the patient. Finding room for the equipment needed for airway management such as the difficult airway cart and the bronchoscopy cart can also be a challenge (see Chapter 60).

27.2.4   Does the airway management skill set of ICU medical personnel have an impact on patient outcome?

Presently, physician staffing in the ICU varies widely from low-intensity models (no intensivists or elective consultation) to high-intensity models (eg, trained intensivists, mandatory intensivist consultations, or closed units).[11] The involvement of intensive care–trained physicians in the care of patients in the ICU can result in as much as a 30% decrease in mortality and decreased length of stay.[12,13]

Many intensive care practitioners have significant expertise in airway management. It seems intuitive that increased airway skills would lead to improved patient outcomes. Schmidt et al reported on 322 consecutive emergency tracheal intubations performed by anesthesiology residents during an ICU rotation, who were either supervised or not supervised by an attending anesthesiologist. Supervision was associated with a significant decrease in complications (6.15 vs 21.7%, $p = .001$).[14]

In a multicentered study done by Jaber et al, a review of 253 intubations in 220 patients was undertaken.[15] Their data confirm that emergency intubation is a high-risk intervention with at least one complication occurring in 71 cases (28%). There was severe hemodynamic collapse in 65 patients, severe hypoxemia in 66, and cardiac arrest occurred in 4 patients. There were two deaths within 30 minutes of intubation with two other patients dying within several days of requiring intubation. Additionally, greater then three attempts were required in 12% of patients. The only protective factor noted was an intubation performed by a junior resident who was also supervised by a senior (ie, two operators were present).[15] A recently published study reviewed the incidence of life-threatening complications occurring within 60 minutes of intubation in 203 consecutive intensive care unit patients.[16] The investigators found that with the implementation of an "ICU intubation bundle management protocol" (Table 27-1), there were significant decreases in life-threatening complications and

TABLE 27-1

Intubation Care Bundle Management

Preintubation
1. Presence of two operators
2. Fluid loading (isotonic saline 500 mL or starch 250 mL) in absence of cardiogenic pulmonary edema
3. Preparation of long-term sedation
4. Preoxygenation for 3 minutes with NIPPV in case of acute respiratory failure (FiO_2 100%, pressure support ventilation level between 5 and 15 cm H_2O to obtain an expiratory tidal volume between 6 and 8 mL·kg^{-1} and PEEP of 5 cm H_2O)

During intubation
5. Rapid-sequence induction: etomidate 0.2-0.3 mg·kg^{-1} or ketamine 1.5-3 mg·kg^{-1} combined with succinylcholine 1 to 1.5 mg·kg^{-1} in absence of allergy, hyperkalemia, severe acidosis, acute or chronic neuromuscular disease, burn patient for more than 48 hours and medullary trauma
6. Sellick maneuver

Postintubation
7. Immediate confirmation of tube placement by capnography
8. Norepinephrine if diastolic blood pressure remains = 35 mm Hg
9. Initiate long-term sedation
10. Initial protective ventilation: tidal volume 6-8 mL·kg^{-1} of ideal body weight, PEEP = 5 cm H_2O and respiratory rate between 10 and 20 cycles/min, FiO_2 100% for a plateau pressure = 30 cm H_2O.

NIPPV, noninvasive positive-pressure ventilation; PEEP, positive end-expiratory pressure; FiO₂, inspired oxygen fraction.

other complications, compared to the control phase during which the bundle protocol was not in use.

27.2.5 How should an ICU be equipped to manage the airway of critically ill patients?

The need to maintain a standard and difficult airway kit in the ICU deserves emphasis. A survey of ICUs revealed that most ICUs maintain an airway cart but only about 50% maintain a difficult airway cart, and less than 5% conform to the suggested list of equipment offered by ASA guidelines. Devices used to confirm tracheal intubation and detect esophageal intubation are present in 93% of ICUs but only routinely used in 68% of cases. Only 4% of ICUs had both a bulb syringe and $ETCO_2$ detectors as suggested by the American Heart Association.[17]

An FB is the most popular device selected for use in a difficult airway situation, even though it is immediately available less than one-third of the time. When surveyed, 51% of respondents thought the FB was the primary backup when conventional intubation fails. In a "cannot intubate, cannot ventilate" situation, 20% thought the FB was the method of choice, a laryngeal mask airway (present in only 50% of the airway kits) was chosen 36% of the time, and a cricothyrotomy was the first choice for only 32% of the respondents. The authors commented on the underutilization of the laryngeal mask airway (LMA) and the need for "continued efforts to educate medical personnel on airway management in the ICU setting."[17]

Respondents to this survey who were aware of an adverse airway-related outcome occurring in the previous year (43% were aware of morbidity and 20%, mortality) acknowledged much more frequently that they needed to restructure their airway management strategies than those who were unaware of such events.[17]

In addition to the equipment required to successfully intubate the trachea, there is clearly a place for extraglottic devices in the airway cart of an ICU. Any EGD is suitable for short-term rescue use in an ICU setting, although those designed for higher seal pressure, such as the LMA ProSeal and Supreme, King LT, and Combitube may be preferable. These EGDs have been discussed in more detail in Chapter 12.

27.3 PHARMACOLOGY OF DRUGS USED FOR AIRWAY MANAGEMENT IN THE ICU

27.3.1 What induction agents are commonly used in the ICU?

Attention to the hemodynamic effects of commonly used induction drugs is crucial in the critically ill patient and mandates careful selection of agents and doses. Published recommended induction doses generally apply to the healthy ambulatory population undergoing elective surgical procedures. These doses are excessive and dangerous in most ICU patients, especially those with limited cardiopulmonary reserve and/or hypovolemia. Coexistent hepatic or renal dysfunction may prolong the duration of pharmacological effects, depending on the metabolic and elimination pathways of the drug. Therefore, it is crucial to select the appropriate drug(s) and dosages, and have immediate availability of agents to support the circulation following induction.

The most commonly utilized induction drug is propofol. Significant hypotension (a 10%-40% decrease in systolic blood pressure) does occur related to direct myocardial depression and altered sympathetic output with decreased arterial tone. Blood pressure is better preserved with ketamine (0%-40% increase) or etomidate (0%-17% increase), so that these drugs may be better choices for induction.[18]

Etomidate's favorable cardiovascular profile makes it the induction agent of choice for the patient with minimal cardiovascular reserve. However, adrenocortical suppression, even after a single dose, has been well described.[19] Therefore, this drug has been abandoned as a long-term sedative in the ICU. The clinical significance of this adrenal suppression is unknown, but is a factor to be considered before choosing this drug as an induction agent in the critically ill patient.[20]

Ketamine is a direct myocardial depressant, although its indirect sympathomimetic effects result in a stable hemodynamic profile when used as an induction agent in patients with resilient cardiovascular and sympathetic nervous systems.[18] The option of administering this drug intramuscularly extends its utility, particularly in patients with no vascular access. The tachycardia and hypertension sometimes seen with ketamine's use may increase myocardial oxygen demand, a factor to be considered in the population at risk.[12] Ketamine can increase secretions which could theoretically precipitate laryngospasm or be problematic during awake upper airway examination in the difficult airway patient or during procedural sedation. Ketamine produces sedation, analgesia, and amnesia in low doses. Higher doses produce the dissociative state. Emergence dysphoria is not uncommon, although its incidence and intensity may be attenuated by combining ketamine with a small dose of benzodiazepine.[21] The relevance of this phenomenon following a single dose of ketamine for induction and airway management in ICU patients is unclear.

In a comparison of etomidate versus ketamine for rapid-sequence intubation in 655 acutely ill patients, there was no significant difference between the drugs in resulting intubating conditions, hemodynamic changes, or 28-day outcomes. In a subgroup of 232 patients, 116 in each group, adrenal insufficiency was assessed by measuring basal cortisol levels and response to adrenal corticotrophin hormone stimulation test. Adrenal insufficiency was significantly higher in the etomidate group than the ketamine group but there was no outcome difference.[20] Another group looked specifically at etomidate use in septic patients who were known to have a higher incidence of baseline adrenal insufficiency. They showed no statistically significant increase in hospital length of stay or mortality when etomidate was used for rapid-sequence intubation.[22] One further study reported on rapid-sequence intubation in emergency departments in 525 high-risk patients who were induced with etomidate, thiopental, or propofol. When outcome was controlled for preexisting risk, there was no difference in this cohort of patients attributable to the drug chosen for induction, although hypotension and the need for a vasopressor were greatest if propofol was used.[23]

27.3.2 Should opioids be used to facilitate tracheal intubation in the ICU?

Opioids can be helpful in attenuating the reflex sympathetic response to laryngoscopy (RSRL), and thus the hemodynamic responses to laryngoscopy.[24]

Due to the array of opioids available, choices can be made with respect to potency, speed of onset of drug effect, route of metabolism/excretion, and pharmacologic half-life. Although the blunting of adverse responses related to airway management may be of clinical value, this potential benefit must be balanced against the risks of attenuating existing sympathetic support of hemodynamics, respiratory depression, and the potential for chest wall rigidity.

Most opioids undergo oxidative metabolism in the liver, the capacity for which may be reduced in patients with end-stage liver disease. However, a single dose of opioids when employed in the pretreatment phase of an intubation does not require adjustment in patients with liver dysfunction. In contrast, prolonged infusions are associated with the risk of accumulation. The pharmacokinetics of some opioids are unaffected in liver disease and thus are reasonable choices for intubation if an opioid is needed.[25] This is particularly true for remifentanil, which has an alternative elimination pathway.

27.3.3 Do benzodiazepines have a role in airway management for the critically ill patient in the ICU?

Anxiety frequently accompanies dyspnea and respiratory distress. The anxiolytic properties of benzodiazepines, in addition to their antegrade amnesic effects and their ability to raise seizure threshold enhance their utility for airway management in the critically ill. However, as with all sedative hypnotic agents, benzodiazepines are respiratory depressants, depressing the slope of the CO_2 response curve and shifting it to the right.[26] Opioids and benzodiazepines potentiate each other's respiratory depressant activities when administered simultaneously.[27]

27.4 AIRWAY MANAGEMENT OPTIONS

27.4.1 What is the general approach to airway management in the critically ill patient?

Several options exist to manage most situations. Algorithms have been published to aid the practitioner in making these decisions. One such algorithm[28] emphasizes the importance of involving senior practitioners' help for the management of airways in the intensive care unit and highlights the need to differentiate between invasive versus noninvasive airway management approaches, includes the ASA difficult airway pathway (see Figures 2-1 and 2-2), and incorporates the use of advanced airway techniques for the management of these complex patients. Ultimately the route chosen is dictated by the needs of the patient and the beliefs and skills of the care team, with the caveat that practitioners responsible for these decisions possess the appropriate skills and experience. If time permits, this may entail a request for more experienced help.

The timeline of respiratory deterioration will strongly influence the approach. Acute decompensation may mandate immediate intervention (see Crash Airway Algorithm, Chapter 2). Drugs to facilitate intubation are not usually indicated in these cases but ancillary equipment may be required, particularly if intubation is anticipated to be difficult. On the other hand, clinical deterioration may be gradual, providing time to summon help as required and an opportunity to plan for a more methodical approach. This approach may include pharmacologic adjuncts, although while affording better intubating conditions, they may blunt or stop spontaneous ventilation.[27]

With a higher expected inability to effectively oxygenate and ventilate these critically ill patients, the importance of decision making is augmented with respect to the use of medications, particularly sedative hypnotics and muscle relaxants. For those reasons, most advise that these drugs should only be employed by those skilled in an array of airway rescue techniques.[29] As always, the decisions are the result of a risk-benefit analysis.

It has been shown repeatedly that in the hands of a skilled airway practitioner, the safest and most successful method is a rapid-sequence intubation (RSI) technique. However, this assumes that the practitioner has taken the necessary steps to evaluate the airway for difficulty beforehand (see Chapter 1), perhaps deferring the identified difficult airway to more skilled practitioners. Likewise, in the event that intubation, ventilation, or both fail, the practitioner must be capable of rescuing the airway (see Chapter 2). The ASA Difficult Airway algorithm is specifically designed to be used in the operation room (OR) environment and is of limited use in the ICU setting, though Mort recognizes that it may be of some use in this setting.[6,30]

In the event that RSI is contraindicated, the judicious use of medication may facilitate an awake intubation by providing better conditions for the practitioner while providing for patient comfort. As a general principle, the minimal amount of drug required to optimize intubating conditions and provide patient comfort during intubation should be used. The skills and experience of the practitioner and acuity of the situation will guide these decisions. The management decisions are best dictated by practitioner experience, rather than dogma.

27.4.2 How do you perform an awake tracheal intubation in the ICU?

Many patients requiring tracheal intubation in the ICU are managed with a combination of topical airway anesthesia and judicious doses of sedative agents. Lidocaine is the most commonly employed local anesthetic. Systemic absorption through oral and pharyngeal mucosa is rapid and thus toxicity is a consideration (see Chapter 3).[31]

A variety of approaches to the application of topical airway anesthesia have been successfully employed, with various delivery methods (see Chapter 3). Anxiety frequently accompanies the dyspnea seen in the hypoxemic patient and the prospect of an "awake" intubation is daunting, even for the patient in extremis. A small dose of benzodiazepine can be helpful, as can be small doses of opioids. Remifentanil has emerged as a popular adjunct to the traditional opioids in facilitating awake intubation (see Section 3.5). The availability of antagonists to opioids (naloxone) and

benzodiazepines (flumazenil) provides a small margin of safety if respiratory depression ensues, although this must not prevent the practitioner from exercising good clinical judgment. The ability to recognize and immediately deal with complications must be part of the armamentarium of the practitioner responsible for airway management.

27.4.3 Is RSI appropriate for tracheal intubation of the critically ill patient?

This question raises several issues related to the RSI technique that are more or less unique to the ICU environment:

- The patient is critically ill and may not tolerate predetermined bolus doses of induction agents.
- The critically ill patient typically has limited functional residual capacity (FRC), increased oxygen consumption, and tolerates apnea poorly.
- As discussed earlier, these patients are often difficult to position optimally for intubation.
- Plan B and Plan C alternatives may be also difficult (eg, intubating laryngeal mask ventilation may not be possible in patients with adult respiratory distress syndrome (ARDS) and severely reduced pulmonary compliance: the "S" of RODS (see Section 1.6.3).
- Access to the neck to perform a cricothyrotomy may be difficult or impossible.

The rapid administration of an induction agent and a fast-acting muscle relaxant provides optimal intubating conditions and is appropriate in patients who do not have an anticipated difficult tracheal intubation. This approach has been advocated in emergency medicine where it has been associated with high success rates, low complication rates, and a low failure rate provided meticulous attention is paid to the identification of the difficult airway.[29] Similar results can be expected with RSI use in the ICU as long as the practitioner is appropriately skilled in airway management.

Bag-mask-ventilation (BMV) is fundamental to airway management, particularly in the event RSI has failed. It is often said that the best rescue from failed BMV is improved BMV. A variety of factors in the critically ill patient affect the ability to provide effective BMV: physical factors, such as obesity; a crowded environment; illness-related conditions (eg, head and neck trauma, impaired GI motility, or gastric ileus); and pulmonary factors such as restrictive lung disease and reduced pulmonary compliance: both common in the ICU patient.

EGDs may be lifesaving in situations such as these provided that they are available and one has experience in using them. A number of authors have published the successful use of LMAs for difficult airway situations in the intensive care unit.[32] In particular, the Proseal LMA has found a place in the intensive care unit to facilitate weaning from controlled ventilation in patients with severe bronchospasm as well as to attenuate the hemodynamic response to extubation in intensive care unit patients.[33,34]

Most ICU patients receive infusions of multiple medications concurrently. The resultant confusion of infusion pumps and lines presents an array of risks related to the bolus administration of induction agents and muscle relaxants:

- Medication compatibility
- Unintended bolus of the baseline infusion medication
- Interruption of essential infusions

The use of dedicated injection port in a dedicated, free-flowing intravenous line is preferable for administration of drugs during airway management.

27.5   PREPARATION AND TRACHEAL INTUBATION FOR THIS PATIENT

27.5.1   Airway evaluation

During the initial assessment, this patient was in extremis. Difficulty with BMV ought to be anticipated due to her toothlessness, obesity, and reduced pulmonary compliance (see Section 1.6.1).

Laryngoscopy and intubation were not predicted to be especially difficult. However, on evaluation of the airway, she looked somewhat difficult due to her obesity; her thyromental distance was somewhat decreased, her decreased level of consciousness made assessment of her Mallampati score impossible, and there was concern that vomitus might have partially obstructed her airway. There was no evidence of limited neck mobility (see Section 1.6.2).

If required, an EGD was an option. However, this was somewhat problematic because of the presence of particulate matter after vomiting. In addition, poor pulmonary compliance related to body habitus and lung volume loss, or collapse, after aspiration can make ventilation difficult with an EGD (see RODS in Section 1.6.3). A surgical airway might be difficult due to the access issues presented by her obesity (see SHORT in Section 1.6.4).

27.5.2   Are there any medical considerations that may impact airway management of this patient?

The urgency of the situation when this patient was first encountered was related to marked hypoxemia refractory to high inspired concentrations of oxygen and a trial of noninvasive ventilation. An initial attempt at awake orotracheal intubation was unsuccessful. Due to the risk of further vomiting and aspiration in a patient with a decrease in level of consciousness and limited ability to cooperate, further attempts at an awake intubation were deemed unreasonable and an RSI was performed.

Increasingly, after successful tracheal intubation of the critically ill patient, protocols that call for minimal sedation are being employed. The need to alleviate patient stressors including pain, sleep deprivation, the irritation that accompanies the presence of invasive tubes and monitors, and therapeutic interventions mandate the use of sedatives, although their excessive use comes at a cost. The incorporation of sedation holidays has resulted in earlier extubation, decreased length of stay in ICUs, decreased

hospital length of stay, decreased complications such as infections, decreased incidence of delirium, and improved long-term neurocognitive function.[35,36]

The self-extubation in the ICU on day 11 presents a different array of considerations:

- There was more time to review the available options, including calling for airway management help if needed.
- Hemodynamic instability related to sepsis and hypotension provided relative contraindications to RSI.
- The patient was cooperative and as she was stable for 30 minutes following the accidental extubation, the care team had a fairly accurate assessment of her physiologic reserve.
- Knowledge of her previously successful tracheal intubation was available.

There were also some considerable physiologic challenges:

- She was borderline hypoxemic due to increased dead space ventilation, reduced FRC, and increased shunt fraction related to her pneumonia.
- Her fever, together with the increase in work of breathing associated with the resolving ARDS probably led to increased O_2 consumption.
- Her trachea had been intubated for 11 days presenting the possibility of upper airway edema.
- She likely had a gastric ileus and full stomach related to her immobility and the fact that she had been receiving sedatives and opioids.

27.5.3   How should you have performed tracheal intubation for this patient?

Before proceeding, the patient should be optimally positioned. If the practitioner has the appropriate knowledge to properly assess the airway, and skills to rescue the airway should intubation fail, then RSI becomes an option. A well-performed awake intubation can also be done, but with poor topical airway anesthesia or clumsy intubation attempts this can precipitate vomiting, as happened in this patient. In retrospect, a primary RSI technique controlling for the risk of regurgitation and aspiration may have served this patient better.

Had the intubation attempt failed during RSI and gas exchange could be maintained with BMV, a second attempt could be made, with options including a blade change, the use of an Eschmann introducer, or an alternative technique to direct laryngoscopy. If at any point gas exchange is not possible, the situation becomes a failed airway, and cricothyrotomy becomes the default response. An EGD should be placed while preparations are concurrently made for cricothyrotomy.

Later in her ICU stay, when the patient extubated herself, it was reasonable to permit a brief trial of spontaneous respiration. Reintubation could be performed under controlled circumstances if it failed. At the time of reintubation, the patient was slightly confused but cooperative. Her hemodynamic instability made her particularly susceptible to bolus dosing of induction medications. Judicious titration of a benzodiazepine to produce anxiolysis and amnesia coupled with topical anesthesia of the airway were employed. An opioid was used to attenuate the RSRL. A difficult airway cart with airway adjuncts, EGDs, and a flexible bronchoscope were immediately available at the bedside. Experienced help (ICU nurse, RT, and a senior resident) was present.

As recovery was expected to take some time, and as the patient had previously been on a ventilator for a significant period, an elective tracheotomy was done after the intubation. Doing this at the bedside averted the need to transfer the patient to an OR and consume valuable OR time (see Chapter 31 for details).

27.5.4 What are postintubation management issues in the ICU patient?

Intubation of the trachea is confirmed by watching the ETT pass through the glottis, but confirmation of tracheal placement should routinely be done using qualitative assessment of $ETCO_2$. The chest is auscultated and the ETT secured in place by ties. If the patient is considered to be at high risk of dislodging the ETT (copious secretions, craniofacial injury or deformity, bandages, full beard, morbid obesity), a commercially available oral tube holder (eg, the Endotracheal Tube Attachment Device [ETAD™], COS Medical, Inc. Atlanta, GA) should be used to secure the tube. A chest x-ray is routinely performed to identify where the tip of the ETT is positioned within the trachea (*not* to rule out esophageal intubation). Vital signs are continuously monitored throughout the procedure. A postintubation arterial blood gas is only done if the practitioner feels that is clinically indicated.

The postintubation *minimal sedation approach*, can include a combination of a continuous infusion of an opioid and a benzodiazepine, to allow for patient comfort as well as to optimize the efficiency of mechanical ventilation. More readily titratable drugs, such as propofol, can also be used so that depth of sedation can be lightened quickly and reliably. The use of muscle relaxants to facilitate intubation must be viewed separately from their use to facilitate mechanical ventilation. For mechanical ventilation, paralytics should be viewed as a last resort and they are unnecessary in most cases. The use of muscle relaxants may contribute to the development of "polyneuropathy of critical illness," a devastating complication with unfavorable patient outcomes. Nonetheless, in isolated cases, these drugs may be necessary.

27.6 EXTUBATION CONSIDERATIONS

27.6.1 Planned extubation for ICU patients

Clinical assessment by intensivists for extubation readiness by clinical criteria alone has been shown to be inadequate, so a myriad of parameters (eg, negative inspiratory force, forced vital capacity maneuver, tidal volume [TV], rapid shallow breathing index [f/TV], T piece trial, arterial blood gases—66 parameters in total) have been proposed to help predict the likelihood of successful extubation.[37] Such extubation planning, a routine part of intensive care, is generally considered to be effective, and results in reasonable reintubation rates.[38] Nonetheless, with a failure rate of 2% to 19%

for patients undergoing planned extubation, reintubation is occasionally necessary.[39] The majority of reports dealing with patients requiring reintubation describe an increase in patient morbidity.[40] Chapter 2 describes an Extubation Algorithm (see Figure 2-7) employing an endotracheal tube exchange catheter. Such devices may prove invaluable in the event that reintubation is required, particularly in patients with a difficult airway.

27.6.2 When should a tracheotomy be considered for an ICU patient?

The timing of tracheotomies for patients expected to require prolonged ventilatory support has been influenced by the technology available. The more rigid endotracheal tubes in the 1960s, with their increased risk of laryngeal injury, supported early tracheotomy. With the more pliable modern polyvinyl chloride (PVC) ETTs, more prolonged translaryngeal intubation is well tolerated and elective placement of a tracheotomy is sometimes delayed until after 2 or 3 weeks of intubation.[31,41] According to recent French and American studies, practices vary widely, showing great variability in indications, timing, and approach.[26,42,43]

At present, the timing of tracheotomy "remains one of professional judgment,"[31] although there is some evidence that early percutaneous tracheotomy (within 48 hours) is associated with lower mortality, morbidity, decreased length of mechanical ventilation, and length of ICU stay, relative to tracheotomy at 14 to 16 days postintubation.[40]

The challenge is to predict early in the ICU course those patients who might require prolonged ventilatory support (and who might then definitely benefit from needed surgical airway) versus those who will be successfully extubated with 10 to 14 days.

27.7 SUMMARY

The ICU is a highly specialized environment mandated to provide intense, continuous, active monitoring and treatment for the critically ill patient. Highly trained personnel focus their skills and resources to meet the needs of these patients. A particular challenge is in the area of expert airway management.

Increasing the proportion of units staffed with practitioners with airway skills (intensivists), lobbying for compliance with the ASA recommendations regarding airway management, providing necessary equipment for the difficult airway, identifying patients at risk of self-extubation, and encouraging the application of experience and skill in the approach to the airway needs of the critically ill will improve outcomes.

REFERENCES

1. Bernard GR, Artigas A, Brigham KL, et al. Report of the American-European consensus conference on ARDS: definitions, mechanisms, relevant outcomes and clinical trial coordinator. The Consensus Committee. *Intensive Care Med*. 1994;20:225-232.
2. American Thoracic Society, European Society of Intensive Care Medicine, Societe de Reanimation Langue Francaise International Consensus Conference in Intensive Care Medicine. Ventilator-associated lung injury in ARDS. *Intensive Care Med*. 1999;25:1444-1452.

3. Kallet RH, Jasmer RM, Pitter JF, et al. Clinical implementation of the ARDS network protocol is associated with reduced hospital mortality compared with historical controls. *Crit Care Med*. 2005;33:925-929.

4. Artigas A, Bernard GR, Carlet J, et al. The American-European Consensus Conference on ARDS, Part 2: Ventilatory, pharmacologic, supportive therapy, study design strategies, and issues related to recovery and remodeling. Acute respiratory distress syndrome. *Am J Resp Crit Care Med*. 1998;157: 1332-1347.

5. Boylan J, Cavanagh B. Emergency airway management competence vs. expertise. *Anesthesiology*. 2008;109:945-947.

6. Mort TC. The incidence and risk factors for cardiac arrest during emergency tracheal intubation: a justification for incorporating the ASA guidelines in the remote location. *J Clin Anesth*. 2004;16:508-516.

7. Olssen GI, Hallen B. Cardiac arrest during anesthesia: computer aided study of 250,542 anesthetics. *Acta Anesthesthesiol Scand*. 1988;32:653-654.

8. Chacko J, Raju H, Singh MK, Mishra RC. Critical incidents in a multidisciplinary intensive care unit. *Anaesth Intensive Care*. 2007;35:382-386.

9. Needham DM, Thompson DA, Holzmuller CG, et al. A system factors analysis of airway events from the Intensive Care Unit Safety Reporting System (ICUSRS). *Crit Care Med*. 2004;32:2227-2233.

10. Haupt MT, Bekes CE, Brilli RJ, et al. Task Force of the American College of Critical Care Medicine, Society of Critical Care Medicine. Guidelines on critical care services and personnel: recommendations based on a system of categorization of three levels of care. *Crit Care Med*. 2003;31: 2677-2683.

11. Pronovost PJ, Angus DC, Dorman T, et al. Physician staffing patterns and clinical outcomes in critically ill patient: a systematic review. *JAMA*. 2002;288: 2151-2162.

12. Birmeyer JD, Dimick JD. The Leapfrog group's patient safety practices 2003: the potential benefits of universal adoption. http://www.leapfroggroup.org/media/file/Leapfrog-Birkmeyer.pdf. Accessed June 20, 2011.

13. Dorman T, Angood PB, Angus DC, et al. American College of Critical Care Medicine. Guidelines for critical care medicine training and continuing medical education. *Crit Care Med*. 2004;32:263-272.

14. Schmidt UH, Kumwilaisak K, Bittner E, George E, Hess D. Effects of supervision by attending anesthesiologists on complications of emergency tracheal intubation. *Anesthesiology*. 2008;109:973-977.

15. Jaber S, Amraoui J, Lefrant JY, et al. Clinical practice and risk factors for immediate complications of endotracheal intubation in the intensive care unit: a prospective, multiple-center study. *Crit Care Med*. 2006;34:2355-2361.

16. Jabar S, Jung B, Corne P, et al. An intervention to decrease complications related to endotracheal intubation in the intensive care unit: a perspective multi-center study. *Intensive Care Med*. 2010;36:248-255.

17. Oliwas N, Mort T. National ICU difficult airway survey: preliminary results. *Anesthesiology*. 2003;99:A403.

18. Reves JG, Glass PSA, Lubarsky DA, McEvoy MD. Intravenous non-opiod anesthetics. In: Miller R, ed. *Miller's Anesthesia*. 6th ed. New York: Elsevier; 2005:323.

19. Lundy JB, Slane ML, Frizzi JD. Acute adrenaline insufficiency after a single dose of etomidate. *J Intensive Care Med*. 2007;22:111-117.

20. Jabre P, Combes X, Lapostolle F, et al. KETASED Collaborative Study Group. Etomidate versus ketamine for rapid sequence intubation in acutely ill patients: a multicentre randomised controlled trial. *Lancet*. 2009;374:293-300.

21. Chudnofsky C, Weber JE, Stoyanoff PJ, et al. A combination of midazolam and ketamine for procedural sedation and analgesia in adult emergency department patients. *Acad Emerg Med*. 2000;7:228-235.

22. Tekwani KL, Watts HF, Rzechula KH, Sweis RT, Kulstad EB. A perspective observational study of the effect of Etomidate on septic patient mortality and length of stay. *Acad Emerg Med*. 2009;16:11-14.

23. Baird CR, Hay AW, McKeown DW, Ray DC. Rapid sequence induction in the emergency department: induction drug and outcome of patients admitted to the intensive care unit. *Emerg Med J*. 2009;26:576-579.

24. Jeng CS, Lin CJ, Huang CH, et al. The optimal injection time of alfentanil for blunting circulatory response to tracheal intubation. *Acta Anaesthesiol Taiwan*. 2005;431:3-9.

25. Tegeder I, Lotsch J, Geisslinger G. Pharmacokinetics of opioids in liver disease. *Clin Pharmacokinet*. 1999;37:17-40.

26. Sunzel M, Paalzoq L, Breggren L, Eriksson I. Respiratory and cardiovascular effects in relation to plasma levels of midazolam and diazepam. *Br J Pharmacol*. 1988;25:561-569.

27. Bailey PL, Pace NL, Ashburn MA, et al. Frequent hypoxemia and apnea after sedation with midazolam and fentanyl. *Anesthesiology*. 1990;73:826-830.

28. Walz JM, Zayaruzny M, Heard SO. Airway management in critical illness. *Chest* 2007;131:608-620.

29. Blanda M. Emergency airway management. *Emerg Clin North Am*. 2003; 21:1-26.

30. American Society of Anesthesiologists. Practice guidelines for management of the difficult airway. An updated report by the American Society of Anesthesiologists Task Force on Management of the Difficult Airway. *Anesthesiology*. 2003;98:1269-1277.

31. Heffner JE. Tracheostomy application and timing. *Clin Chest Med*. 2003;24: 389-398.

32. Nixon T, Brimacombe J, Goldrick P, McManus S. Airway rescue with the Proseal laryngeal mask airway in the intensive care unit. *Anaesth Intensive Care*. 2003;31:475-476.

33. Russo SG, Goetz EB, Troche S, et al. LMA Proseal for elective postoperative care on the Intensive Care Unit prospective randomized trial. *Anesthesiology*. 2009;111:116-121.

34. Laver S, McKinstry C, Craft TM, Cook TM. Use of the Proseal LMA in the ICU to facilitate weaning from controlled ventilation in patients with severe episodic bronchospasm. *Eur J Anaesthesiol*. 2006;23:977-978.

35. King MS, Render ML, Ely WE, Watson PL. Liberation and animation strategies to minimize brain dysfunction in critically ill patients. *Semin Respirol Crit Care Med*. 2010;31(1):87-96.

36. Girard TD, Pandharipande PP, Ely W. Delirium in the intensive care unit. *Crit Care*. 2008;12:S3.

37. Meade M, Guyat G, Cook D, et al. Predicting success in weaning from mechanical ventilation. *Chest*. 2001;120:400S-424S.

38. Chevron V, Manard JF, Richard JC, et al. Unexplained extubation: risk factors of development and redictive criteria for reintubation. *Crit Care Med*. 1998;26:1049-1053.

39. MacIntyre N. Evidence based guidelines for weaning and discontinuing ventilatory support. A collective task force facilitated by the American College of Chest Physicians, American Association for Respiratory Care and the American College of Critical Care Medicine. *Chest*. 2001;120:375S-395S.

40. Mort T. Unplanned extubation outside the operating room: a quality improvement audit of hemodynamic and tracheal airway complications associated with emergency tracheal reintubation. *Anesth Analg*. 1998;86:1171-1176.

41. Rumbak MJ, Newton M, Truncale T, et al. A prospective randomized study comparing early percutaneous dilational tracheostomy to prolonged translaryngeal intubation (delayed tracheostomy) in critically ill medical patients. *Crit Care Med*. 2004;32:1689-1694.

42. Blot F. Indications timing and techniques of tracheostomy in 152 French ICUs. *Chest*. 2005;127:1347-1353.

43. Freeman BD, Borecki IB, Coopersmith CM, Buchman TG. Relationship between tracheostomy timing and duration of mechanical ventilation in critically ill patients. *Crit Care Med*. 2005;33:2513-2520.

SELF-EVALUATION QUESTIONS

27.1. Polyneuropathy is a possible side effect of prolonged use of which of the following agents:

A. propofol

B. ketamine

C. midazolam

D. vecuronium

E. etomidate

27.2. Cardiorespiratory depression is a predictable side effect of which of the following:

A. propofol

B. etomidate

C. ketamine

D. fentanyl

E. midazolam

27.3. Which of the following respiratory care statements is **NOT** true in the adult ICU patient population?

A. Tracheotomy within 14 days of prolonged intubation is desirable.

B. There is no evidence of an advantage of tracheotomy within 2 to 3 days.

C. Tracheotomy is likely unwarranted for intubation that is less than 2 weeks duration.

D. Distinct advantages have been shown with percutaneous tracheotomy at the bedside.

E. With the more pliable modern PVC ETTs, more prolonged translaryngeal intubation is well tolerated.

CHAPTER (28)

Management of Extubation of a Patient Following a Prolonged Period of Mechanical Ventilation

Richard M. Cooper

28.1 CASE PRESENTATION

A 60-year-old man with chronic obstructive lung disease, limited exercise tolerance, and new-onset pneumonia required tracheal intubation because of hypoxemic respiratory failure. Optimal positioning for direct laryngoscopy (DL) performed by an experienced practitioner using a Macintosh 3 blade yielded a Cormack/Lehane (C/L) 3 view, requiring the use of an Eschmann tracheal tube introducer (ETTI). After 6 days of assisted ventilation, he had now been weaned to an FiO_2 of 0.4, positive end-expiratory pressure of 5 cm H_2O, and pressure support of 5 cm H_2O. The pulmonary infiltrates were much improved. His respiratory rate was 24 breaths per minute. A cuff-leak test was performed.

28.2 EXTUBATION STRATEGIES

28.2.1 What is a high-risk extubation?

In anesthesia, and most likely in critical and emergency care, adverse respiratory events are more frequently associated with extubation than intubation.[1,2] Nonetheless, much less attention has been paid to the management of extubation. A stratification of risk associated with extubation has been proposed,[3] and although unsupported by controlled, randomized clinical trials, the need for an extubation strategy has been advocated by expert panels.[4,5] The extubation of patients, who were easily intubated and in whom no intervening event has occurred to jeopardize their airways, can be regarded as "low-risk extubations." Those who were easily intubated but who are at greater risk of requiring reintubation (due to hypoxemia, hypercapnia, inadequate clearance of secretions, inability to protect

their airway, or airway obstruction) are "intermediate-risk extubations." Those in whom airway management is likely to be challenging or complex if reintubation is required represent "high-risk extubations." The last group includes:

1. Patients with a difficult tracheal intubation (failure to visualize their glottis —C/L ≥ 3—requiring multiple attempts or alternative techniques).

2. Those with interval complications (airway edema, extrinsic compression, glottic injuries).

3. Those with clinical conditions associated with difficult ventilation and/or intubation. This latter group would include, for example, patients with paradoxical vocal cord motion, morbid obesity, obstructive sleep apnea, airway surgery, maxillofacial surgery (particularly when it involves inter-maxillary fixation), deep-neck infections, cervical surgery, angioedema, or prolonged intubation.[3]

For most patients, the risk of requiring reintubation is low. The results of three studies involving nearly 50,000 patients presenting for a wide variety of surgical procedures indicated that only 0.09% to 0.19% required reintubation.[6-8] Certain surgical procedures such as panendoscopy and a variety of head and neck operations are associated with a risk of required reintubation approximately 10 times higher (1%-3%).[9-13] Patients in critical care units often have limited physiologic reserve, altered secretions, or an impaired capacity to protect their airways. In this group of patients, required reintubation is substantially higher still.[14-16]

When patients require emergency reintubation, the airway practitioner may have limited clinical information, equipment, supportive personnel, or preparation time. Furthermore, the patient may be hemodynamically unstable with associated airway obstruction, hypoxemia, or acidosis. There may be a reluctance to administer paralytics when there is uncertainty about the probability of securing the airway. Topical anesthesia may be ineffective due to time constraints or the presence of secretions or edema. Thus a struggle could ensue between the practitioner and an agitated and possibly hypoxemic patient. Generally, any *urgent reintubation is likely to be more challenging than the original intubation procedure. If the original intubation had been difficult, the reintubation could be life threatening.*

28.2.2 What strategies can be used for the high-risk extubation?

For high-risk extubations, it is especially important that every effort be taken to ensure that conditions are optimal. Optimal conditions include oxygenation, ventilation, the ability to clear secretions, and protect and maintain patency of the airway. Even when such conditions are optimal, reintubation may be required. Assessment of the airway prior to removing the endotracheal tube (ETT) might include:

- Laryngoscopy with the ETT in situ, although this is of limited value and is unlikely to reveal the extent of periglottic edema or vocal cord movement. Direct visualization of the tube in situ does not ensure that reintubation by this technique will be successful.[17]

- Laryngeal examination adjacent to the ETT using a flexible bronchoscope (FB) has some of the same limitations as laryngoscopy.[18,19] Alternatively, an FB can be positioned within the ETT, and as the latter is withdrawn, an effort can be made to inspect the airway below and above the vocal folds. Unfortunately, this technique often fails. As the ETT is withdrawn, the patient may cough, swallow, or secretions may obscure the view. Even if a laryngeal view is achieved, it is likely to be too hurried to be of value. This technique is further limited by the need to withdraw the FB shortly after the examination.

- If an extraglottic airway device (EGD, eg, LMA) is inserted and the ETT is withdrawn, an FB can be passed through the EGD. This technique is compatible with either controlled or spontaneous ventilation, and it keeps extraglottic secretions from obscuring the view. It allows regulation of the FiO_2 and can facilitate reintubation should it be required. This technique does require a properly seated EGD and is hazardous if the airway is significantly compromised.

- An ETTI (Portex Limited, Hythe, UK) or METTRO Mizus obturator (Cook Critical Care, Bloomington, IN) can be introduced into the ETT. When the latter is withdrawn, the introducer can serve as a guide over which the ETT can be reintroduced if necessary. As in the case of intubating over an FB, ETT passage over the FB is not without challenges. Because these devices are solid, they cannot be used to insufflate oxygen or provide ventilation.

- A hollow tube exchanger can be introduced permitting airway access, a means of oxygen administration, and serving as an airway "stylet" should this prove necessary.

- If DL has or is likely to fail, reintubation using an alternative indirect technique such as video laryngoscopy may be extremely

helpful. This can be done in conjunction with a tube exchanger.[20] Mort found that 47/51 (92%) of recently extubated patients with a difficult airway were successfully reintubated over a tube exchanger, 87% on the first attempt; this contrasts with a first pass success rate using DL of 14% in patients requiring reintubation in whom the exchange catheter had already been removed. Oxygen saturations below 90% and 80%, the incidence of HR less than 40 accompanied by hypotension, multiple attempts, and esophageal intubation were also significantly higher in the group without exchange catheters.[14]

28.3 DEVICES TO ASSIST EXTUBATION

28.3.1 What types of hollow tube exchangers are available?

There are several commercial tube exchangers including the Cook Airway Exchange Catheter (C-AEC, Cook Critical Care), the Endotracheal Ventilation Catheter (ETVC, Cardiomed International),* and the Sheridan Tracheal Tube Exchanger (Hudson Respiratory Care). In addition to aiding tube passage, these hollow devices can be used to insufflate or ventilate should it become necessary. Devices with a secure proximal connection and multiple distal end holes are preferred (C-AEC and ETVC). In contrast, the ETTI and the METTRO Mizus airway obturator (Cook Critical Care) are solid and cannot serve as an oxygen conduit. All of these devices are introduced through the existing ETT, and the distance markings on the tube exchanger are aligned with those on the ETT to ensure the distal tip of the tube exchanger is located above the carina. The tube exchanger remains in the airway after the ETT is withdrawn.

28.3.2 How long should a tube exchanger remain in the airway?

Most patients tolerate the tube exchanger surprisingly well. It is generally possible for patients to speak, swallow, and cough with the device in situ.[21] Although most often used orally, tube exchangers are more easily secured (and better tolerated) when inserted nasally. A patient with an ETT tube in place for a short time usually tolerates the tube exchanger less well than one who has had an ETT in place for a longer duration. If the patient has been intubated for several hours, coughing may indicate that the catheter is near or beyond the carina. The distance marking should be checked and a chest x-ray performed to confirm correct placement. If the patient remains intolerant of the exchanger despite proper placement, it may be appropriate to remove the device, although the need for reintubation may not declare itself for several hours.[14] As patients with known or suspected difficult airways are more likely to be successfully reintubated with fewer complications if performed over a tube exchanger,[14] a more cautious approach

---

*The author was a consultant to Cook in the development of the C-AEC and the inventor of the ETVC (Cardiomed International). He receives no royalties or consultancy fees from either of these companies.

would be to encourage tolerance with the instillation of topical anesthesia through the tube exchanger. A specific or arbitrary time period to leave a tube exchanger in situ is not rational. It is this author's practice to leave the device in place until the concern for the airway is resolved. Any patient requiring a tube exchanger would require the vigilance and expertise of a post-anesthetic care unit (PACU), intensive care unit (ICU), or emergency department (ED). Furthermore, inexperienced personnel may confuse the tube exchanger with a gastric tube with disastrous consequences.

28.3.3 How is a tube exchanger used to support oxygenation or ventilation?

A tube exchanger can serve as a conduit for oxygen by insufflation; however, if used for more than a few hours, the oxygen should be humidified. Insufflation should be at low flows of 2 to 4 L·min^{-1} and may be used in lieu of a facemask or nasal cannulae. Insufflation should always be attempted before considering jet ventilation.

If insufflation fails to correct hypoxemia, reintubation may be necessary and insufflation may continue even while intubation is being attempted. If reintubation is delayed or prolonged and hypoxemia is persistent or worsening in spite of oxygen insufflation, jet ventilation should be considered. To avoid the morbidity associated with jet ventilation, the following points should be addressed:

- Confirm that the distal tip of the tube exchanger is appropriately positioned above the carina, since jet ventilation into the bronchus or oropharynx can produce barotrauma.

- Delegate an assistant to hold the catheter close to the lips or nose to ensure that the device does not get ejected during ventilation.

- Administration of a muscle relaxant with appropriate sedation (if tolerated) will facilitate both endotracheal intubation and jet ventilation and will lessen the risks of barotrauma.

- Attach the tube exchanger to the jet ventilator by means of a Luer-Lok adapter (the C-AEC, ETVC, and Sheridan JETTX have these).

- Using a pressure-reducing valve, select the lowest driving pressure that results in chest expansion. Wall pressure of 50 psi is equivalent to 3500 cm H_2O and can produce dramatic, life-threatening barotrauma very quickly.[22]

- Correct hypoxemia—this should be the primary objective. One breath causing adequate chest expansion may correct hypoxemia even though it may take a short while for this to become apparent.

- To avoid breath stacking, the chest must be carefully observed. Subsequent breaths should not be delivered until it is clear that the chest has recoiled to a resting volume.

- Facilitate exhalation by minimizing airway obstruction (vocal cord relaxation, optimal positioning, tongue displacement, suctioning, etc).[22]

- Jet ventilation may prove lifesaving, but it requires fastidious attention to detail to ensure that life-threatening complications do not develop.[23]

28.4 AIRWAY EDEMA

28.4.1 What factors lead to airway edema?

Airway edema is not restricted to the vocal folds. In children subglottic swelling is the greatest concern, whereas in adults glottic and supraglottic edema is the focus of concern. Patients may have airway swelling due to prone or Trendelenburg positioning, allergic or hereditary angioedema, and thermal injuries or generalized swelling as in anaphylaxis, anasarca, and massive volume overload. They may have sustained injury to their tongue, uvula, or epiglottis during tracheal intubation or as a result of subsequent trauma, such as suctioning or seizures.

Insertion of a round tube through a triangular glottis results in contact and pressure at the posteromedial aspect of the larynx.[19] Injury can occur very early but this is usually of little consequence. Excessive or prolonged pressure can result in perichondritis or chondritis, which heals poorly. Healing may result in fibrosis, producing subacute or chronic laryngeal or tracheal stenosis or an exuberant growth of granulation tissue. Early postextubation obstruction is likely to be a consequence of edema, bleeding, and occasionally granulation tissue or arytenoid dislocation.

Much has been written about the duration of intubation and resultant airway injuries. However, the association between duration and incidence of airway injuries remains controversial. Most would maintain that the longer the duration of intubation, the greater the likelihood of airway edema. Significant airway injury may, however, occur early as a result of inadequate ETT immobilization, persistent attempts to phonate or cough, gastroesophageal reflux, traumatic laryngoscopy or intubation, and vocal fold granulomas. Some authorities recommend laryngoscopy at approximately day 7 under general anesthesia, using telescopes and image magnification to assess the severity of injury. Only then can a judgment be made regarding the feasibility of extubation, prolonging translaryngeal intubation, or the need for a tracheotomy.[24]

28.4.2 What techniques are useful to assess airway edema?

We have discussed the limited value of DL with the ETT in situ in contrast to extubation under general anesthesia with DL and image magnification. An alternative approach consists of controlled visualization using a flexible bronchoscope through an EGD. DL with image magnification provides the best anatomical evaluation; the EGD/FB examination with spontaneous ventilation provides a good assessment of both form and function.

If tissue swelling is sufficiently severe, it may encroach on the ETT at any point along the length of the ETT. Prior to extubation, a cuff-leak test can be used to assess this. The oropharynx is suctioned and the cuff is slowly deflated. The patient is asked to inhale and exhale slowly as the ETT is occluded.[25] An audible leak indicates the flow of air around the ETT. This has been found to be a useful predictor of successful extubation in pediatric trauma and burn victims as well as children with croup[26] and is sensitive but not specific in predicting postextubation stridor and the need for reintubation in adults.[27] The cuff-leak test can be enhanced by quantifying the leak during controlled ventilation. Lower cuff-leak volumes are predictive of postextubation stridor, a need for reintubation, or both.[28,29] Engoren did not find this to be predictive in postoperative cardiothoracic surgical patients[30] although others have suggested that the cuff leak, expressed as a proportion of the delivered tidal volume, may have greater utility.[31-33]

28.4.3   Are there methods of reducing airway edema?

Studies involving the prophylactic benefit of *corticosteroids* to reduce postextubation stridor have yielded contradictory findings. The benefits may be restricted to high-risk patients and may require multiple doses.[34] *Elevation of the head of the bed* may be helpful. If the patient manifests signs or symptoms suggestive of airway obstruction, laryngospasm and upper airway obstruction should be considered. If these are excluded, *epinephrine* (5 mL of 1:1000 solution) by inhalation often results in rapid improvement of airway edema by means of transient local vasoconstriction. Epinephrine can be administered as tolerated, although caution must be observed in patients with hypertension, tachycardia, or conditions in which these are poorly tolerated. Rebound vasodilation can also occur. Additional management measures might include fluid restriction or diuretic therapy.

Being less dense than nitrogen, helium can be used as an alternative to nitrogen as a transport medium for oxygen when turbulent airflow is present. This mixture consists of a blend of oxygen and helium, typically 30:70, although the oxygen concentration can be enriched if required. The benefits are proportional to the concentration of helium and the extent to which turbulent flow is present. Helium–oxygen (heliox) can be used concurrently with head elevation, corticosteroids, and epinephrine. The benefits from heliox and epinephrine should be apparent within minutes. Deteriorating conditions should prompt reintubation.

28.5   TECHNIQUE OF REINTUBATION

28.5.1   How should reintubation over a tube exchanger proceed?

If conservative measures are ineffective and reintubation over a tube exchanger is required, the exchanger can serve as a jet stylet.[35] Oxygen supplementation begins with insufflation and, if necessary, progresses to jet ventilation. Depending upon the design of the device, the proximal connector can be removed to permit the loading of a replacement ETT. If the fit is tight, a water-soluble lubricant can be applied to the tube exchanger, although care must be taken to ensure that this does not interfere with secure handling. The tube exchanger must be long enough to ensure that the part protruding from the patient's mouth or nose is at least as long as the replacement ETT. If necessary, the ETT can be shortened. In general, the smaller the size difference between the outer diameter of the tube exchanger and the inner diameter of the replacement ETT, the easier reintubation is likely to be. The tube exchanger is held securely at the mouth or nose. The ETT is then passed over

the exchanger. Throughout the procedure, the clinical condition of the patient should be monitored and any additional medications to provide sedation, hemodynamic control, topical anesthesia, or neuromuscular blockade should be administered. The team should review the primary and contingency plans in advance. It may be prudent to request additional help or equipment. If oxygenation can be sufficiently maintained, there is no urgency.

A laryngoscope can be used to elevate the tongue and epiglottis to facilitate advancement of the ETT over the tube exchanger. Even more effective—particularly in the patient in whom DL is likely or known to be difficult—is the use of an indirect or video laryngoscope to facilitate the tube exchange.[20] This may permit laryngeal evaluation and visualized replacement of the ETT.

If glottic visualization cannot be achieved, the ETT is advanced over the tube exchanger as it might be over an FB, with tongue retraction or a jaw thrust. If resistance is encountered at the presumed depth of the glottic inlet, the ETT should be rotated counterclockwise, but force should never be applied. If the patient is still breathing spontaneously, the airway practitioner should wait for an inspiratory effort and advance the ETT as the vocal folds abduct. Frequently, the tube exchanger is inadvertently advanced while the ETT is being introduced. If the ETT has passed easily, the tube exchanger can be removed (or a capnograph can be attached to the tube exchanger prior to its removal), whereupon intratracheal placement of the ETT should be verified by capnography and auscultation.

28.5.2   What if reintubation over the tube exchanger fails?

If reintubation over the tube exchanger fails, several options exist. The adequacy of oxygenation by bag-mask or jet ventilation with the tube exchanger in situ should be assessed:

* *Oxygenation is adequate*: Time and expertise may permit the use of an alternative device, such as a flexible bronchoscope, a rigid fiberoptic scope, or a video laryngoscope. (These devices might also be considered prior to the removal of the ETT, along with the tube exchanger.) It is preferable to leave the tube exchanger in place, if possible, during the reintubation attempt. Alternatively, an Aintree catheter can be advanced over the pediatric AEC. The use of the Aintree catheter and a small (eg, 7.5 mm ID) ETT will minimize the discrepancy of the gap between the Aintree catheter and ETT and will facilitate tracheal reintubation.

* *Oxygenation or ventilation is inadequate:* If possible, confirm using a capnograph (or video laryngoscope) that the tube exchanger is still in the trachea.†

* If jet ventilation is available, it can be used as described above, but an assessment that the device has not become displaced should be made during the first breath. An assistant should

---

†Capnography does not guarantee intratracheal placement of a tube exchanger. Distal pharyngeal placement can also return a CO_2 waveform.

listen over the epigastrium to ensure the absence of air entry during ventilation. If this is successful, the next breath should ensure that the left lung is also ventilated, reducing the risk of barotrauma from endobronchial jet ventilation. If ventilation restores oxygenation, alternative plans can be put in place in a calm and efficient manner.

• If intubation over the tube exchanger was not successful, prior to its removal, reconsider the following:

A. Was a laryngoscope used to provide adequate tongue retraction?
B. Might the use of a smaller size ETT be possible?
C. Was a video or fiberoptic laryngoscope used in conjunction with the tube exchanger?
D. Was an Aintree catheter used together with the tube exchanger?

• If tongue retraction, a smaller size ETT, and a fiberoptic or video laryngoscope fail to facilitate reintubation and jet ventilation is not immediately available, assess the feasibility of bag-mask-ventilation (BMV) with the tube exchanger in situ. If this cannot be accomplished, the tube exchanger may be removed and further attempts made to achieve BMV.

• If BMV still cannot be achieved, the practitioner should refer to the Failed Airway (cannot intubate/cannot ventilate) Algorithm (see Section 2.5.5). Time is critical and if adequate ventilation cannot be achieved quickly, a surgical airway is mandatory. An extraglottic airway may be used if immediately available while preparing for a surgical airway.

28.5.3   How should ETT exchange of an intubated patient with a difficult airway proceed without a tube exchanger?

If a patient with a difficult airway requires replacement of an existing ETT and a tube exchanger is not available, an FB loaded with an ETT can be introduced alongside the existing ETT. The pharynx should be carefully suctioned. If the existing ETT still has an intact cuff, it can be deflated to allow FB passage alongside. Once tracheal access by the FB has been confirmed by visualizing tracheal rings and carina, the original tube can be withdrawn and the new ETT advanced over the FB.

For the patient requiring reintubation in whom DL had previously been difficult, video or fiberoptic laryngoscopy is particularly useful.[20]

28.6   TRACHEAL EXTUBATION

The trachea of the patient described at the beginning of this chapter was intubated using DL with an ETTI. The ETTI was placed blindly and successful placement cannot be guaranteed. In a recent study involving 11,257 adults, intubation by DL alone could not be accomplished in 100 patients. Nonvisualized intubation with an ETTI was successful in 80/89 cases; out of the successful intubations 50% required more than one attempt.[36] Though the authors regarded this as a validation of the ETTI strategy, the fact remains that it failed 10% of the time and required multiple attempts (after multiple attempts) in half of the patients.

Laryngoscopy that fails to reveal the larynx is a failed laryngoscopy, whether intubation succeeds or fails. Successful, blind intubation is a near miss. An extubation strategy should anticipate that reintubation might be required; reintubation may very well be more challenging than the initial intubation—the strategy should be to increase the likelihood of success and permit simultaneous intubation as well as oxygenation even if the glottis cannot be visualized. Extubation over a tube exchanger may best meet these objectives.

The patient demonstrated criteria that are associated with a successful wean from mechanical ventilation. However, such criteria are not synonymous with successful extubation. Demonstration of a large cuff leak reduces the likelihood of postextubation stridor or a need for reintubation. Examination of the vocal cords following extubation, either using an FB through an extraglottic airway device or by DL with image magnification, may provide additional certainty.

The oropharynx was suctioned, a cuff leak was demonstrated, a tube exchanger was inserted, the ETT was withdrawn, and the tube exchanger was secured to the patient's cheek and forehead. The exchanger was well tolerated and left in place for 3 hours during which time the patient continued to improve. He was able to talk and clear his secretions. The tube exchanger was then removed.

Had a cuff leak not been present, the options are less clear. A significant number of these patients would not require a tracheotomy. The patient can be taken to the operating room to have the glottis examined using DL and image magnification under general anesthesia with paralytics.[18] An alternative approach would be to use intravenous anesthesia and a short-acting muscle relaxant, followed by the insertion of an extraglottic device (EGD, eg, LMA) and extubation. The EGD would then be inflated as required; its position would be optimized using an FB. The relaxant would be allowed to wear off or be reversed, and spontaneous ventilation could resume. After extubation, flexible endoscopy through the lumen of the EGD would be used to assess the glottic appearance and function, while the adequacy of spontaneous ventilation would also be assessed.

Three outcomes might result:

• The assessment is unfavorable. Reintubation can be achieved over the FB using, for example, an Aintree catheter (Cook Critical Care) or a tube exchanger.[37,38] If reintubation is then contemplated, in this patient, a tracheotomy is probably indicated. This can be done at the bedside using one of several techniques, including percutaneous dilatational tracheotomy.[39]

• The examination is favorable. The sedation is discontinued and the EGD is removed when appropriate. There remains the possibility that reintubation will subsequently be required; however, the anatomy and glottic function have been assessed, and the patient has undergone a trial of extubation.

• The examination is indeterminate. A tube exchanger can be introduced and left in situ until the clinical status of the glottis is clarified.[38]

28.7 SUMMARY

The risk associated with tracheal extubation (or tube exchange) may be stratified into low, intermediate, and high risk depending upon the probability of complications, including the need for reintubation. A high-risk extubation exists when reintubation is likely to be difficult or very difficult to achieve; examples include conditions when a patient's airway access is limited by maxillomandibular or cervical fixation. It should be assumed that any emergency reintubation will be more challenging due to patient instability or limited resources. Strategies have been described to increase the probability of successful reintubation, including the substitution of an extraglottic airway and the use of a tube exchanger. Some tube exchangers have been designed to allow the administration of supplemental oxygen and ventilation. Jet ventilation through a small caliber catheter must be performed with care to avoid complications.

REFERENCES

1. Peterson GN, Domino KB, Caplan RA, Posner KL, Lee LA, Cheney FW. Management of the difficult airway: a closed claims analysis. *Anesthesiology.* 2005;103:33-39.
2. Asai T, Koga K, Vaughan RS. Respiratory complications associated with tracheal intubation and extubation. *British J Anaesth.* 1998;80:767-775.
3. Cooper RM, Hagberg CA. *Extubation and Changing Endotracheal Tubes, Benumof's Airway Management.* Philadelphia, PA: Mosby Elsevier; 2007: 1146-1180.
4. Crosby ET, Cooper RM, Douglas MJ, et al. The unanticipated difficult airway with recommendations for management. *Can J Anaesth.* 1998;45:757-776.
5. American Society of Anesthesiologists. Practice Guidelines for Management of the Difficult Airway: An Updated Report by the American Society of Anesthesiologists Task Force on Management of the Difficult Airway. *Anesthesiology.* 2003;98:1269-1277.
6. Hill RS, Koltai PJ, Parnes SM. Airway complications from laryngoscopy and panendoscopy. *Ann Otol Rhinol Laryngol.* 1987;96:691-694.
7. Rose DK, Cohen MM, Wigglesworth DF, DeBoer DP. Critical respiratory events in the postanesthesia care unit. Patient, surgical, and anesthetic factors. *Anesthesiology.* 1994;81:410-418.
8. Mathew JP, Rosenbaum SH, O'Connor T, Barash PG. Emergency tracheal intubation in the postanesthesia care unit: physician error or patient disease? *Anesth.Analg.* 1990;71:691-697.
9. Emery SE, Smith MD, Bohlman HH. Upper-airway obstruction after multilevel cervical corpectomy for myelopathy. *J Bone Joint Surg Am.* 1991;73: 544-551.
10. Tyers MR, Cronin K. Airway obstruction following second operation for carotid endarterectomy. *Anaesth Intensive Care.* 1986;14:314-316.
11. Levelle JP, Martinez OA. Airway obstruction after bilateral carotid endarterectomy. *Anesthesiology.* 1985;63:220-222.
12. Venna RP, Rowbottom JR. A nine year retrospective review of post operative airway related problems in patients following multilevel anterior cervical corpectomy. *Anesthesiology.* 2002;95:A1171.
13. Lacoste L, Gineste D, Karayan J, et al. Airway complications in thyroid surgery. *Ann Otol Rhinol Laryngol.* 1993;102:441-446.
14. Mort TC. Continuous airway access for the difficult extubation: the efficacy of the airway exchange catheter. *Anesth Anal.* 2007;105:1357-1362.
15. Gandia F, Blanco J. Evaluation of indexes predicting the outcome of ventilator weaning and value of adding supplemental inspiratory load. *Intensive Care Med.* 1992;18:327-333.
16. Demling RH, Read T, Lind LJ, Flanagan HL. Incidence and morbidity of extubation failure in surgical intensive care patients. *Crit Care Med.* 1988;16:573-577.
17. Ford RW. Confirming tracheal intubation—a simple manoeuvre. *Can Anaesth Soc J.* 1983;30:191-193.

18. Benjamin B, Cummings CW, Fredrickson JM, et al. *Laryngeal Trauma from Intubation: Endoscopic Evaluation and Classification, Otolaryngology: Head and Neck Surgery.* St. Louis, MO: Mosby-Year Book, Inc.; 1998: 2018-2033.
19. Benjamin BF, Holinger LM. Laryngeal complications of endotracheal intubation. *Ann Otol Rhinol Laryngol.* 2008;117:2.
20. Mort TC. Tracheal tube exchange: feasibility of continuous glottic viewing with advanced laryngoscopy assistance. *Anesth Anal.* 2009;108:1228-1231.
21. Cooper RM. The use of an endotracheal ventilation catheter in the management of difficult extubations. *Can J Anaesth.* 1996;43:90-93.
22. Cooper RM, Cohen DR. The use of an endotracheal ventilation catheter for jet ventilation during a difficult intubation. *Can J Anaesth.* 1994;41: 1196-1199.
23. Benumof JL. Airway exchange catheters: simple concept, potentially great danger. *Anesthesiology.* 1999;91:342-344.
24. Benjamin B. Prolonged intubation injuries of the larynx: endoscopic diagnosis, classification, and treatment. *Ann Otol Rhinol Laryngol Suppl.* 1993;160: 1-15.
25. Adderley RJ, Mullins GC. When to extubate the croup patient: the "leak" test. *Can J Anaesth.* 1987;34:304-306.
26. Kemper KJ, Izenberg S, Marvin JA, Heimbach DM. Treatment of postextubation stridor in a pediatric patient with burns: the role of heliox. *J Burn Care Rehabil.* 1990;11:337-339.
27. Fisher MM, Raper RF. The "cuff-leak" test for extubation. *Anaesthesia.* 1992;47: 10-12.
28. Miller RL, Cole RP. Association between reduced cuff leak volume and postextubation stridor. *Chest.* 1996;110:1035-1040.
29. Efferen LS, Elsakr A. Post-extubation stridor: risk factors and outcome. *J Assoc Acad Minor Phys.* 1998;9:65-68.
30. Engoren M. Evaluation of the cuff-leak test in a cardiac surgery population. *Chest* 1999;116:1029-1031.
31. Jaber S, Chanques G, Matecki S, et al. Post-extubation stridor in intensive care unit patients. Risk factors evaluation and importance of the cuff-leak test. *Intens Care Med.* 2003;29:69-74.
32. De Bast Y, De Backer D, Moraine JJ, Lemaire M, Vandenborght C, Vincent JL. The cuff leak test to predict failure of tracheal extubation for laryngeal edema. *Intensive Care Med.* 2002;28:1267-1272.
33. Sandhu RS, Pasquale MD, Miller K, Wasser TE. Measurement of endotracheal tube cuff leak to predict postextubation stridor and need for reintubation. *J Am Coll Surg.* 2000;190:682-687.
34. Shemie S. Steroids for anything that swells: dexamethasone and postextubation airway obstruction. *Crit Care Med.* 1996;24:1613-1614.
35. Bedger RC, Jr., Chang JL. A jet-stylet endotracheal catheter for difficult airway management. *Anesthesiology.* 1987;66:221-223.
36. Combes X, Le Roux B, Suen P, et al. Unanticipated difficult airway in anesthetized patients: prospective validation of a management algorithm. *Anesthesiology.* 2004;100:1146-1150.
37. Bogdanov A, Kapila A. Aintree intubating bougie. *Anesth Analg.* 2004;98: 1502.
38. Hsin ST, Chen CH, Juan CH, et al. A modified method for intubation of a patient with ankylosing spondylitis using intubating laryngeal mask airway (LMA-Fastrach)—a case report. *Acta Anaesthesiol Sin.* 2001;39: 179-182.
39. Gromann TW, Birkelbach O, Hetzer R. Balloon dilatational tracheostomy: initial experience with the Ciaglia Blue Dolphin method. *Anesth Analg.* 2009;108: 1862-1866.

SELF-EVALUATION QUESTIONS

28.1. Which of the following is a reliable method in assessing airway edema?

A. direct laryngoscopy

B. airway assessment using a flexible bronchoscope

C. performing a cuff-leak test

D. presence of facial edema

E. none of the above

28.2. Which of the following is **NOT** a useful step to minimize the morbidity associated with jet ventilation through a hollow tube exchanger?

A. ensure that the tip of tube exchanger is not positioned in the bronchus

B. avoid breath stacking

C. use the lowest driving pressure that results in chest expansion

D. avoid the administration of a muscle relaxant

E. facilitate exhalation by minimizing airway obstruction

28.3. Which of the following may be helpful to reduce airway edema?

A. elevation of the head of the bed

B. the use of nebulized epinephrine

C. fluid restriction

D. the use of diuretic therapy

E. all of the above

CHAPTER (29)

Airway Management of a Patient in a Halo Jacket Who Has Developed a Tracheal Tube Cuff Leak

Dietrich Henzler

29.1. CASE PRESENTATION

A 52-year-old worker of normal body habitus was injured in a fall from approximately 15 ft (5 m) of height. He sustained fractures to the vertebral bodies of C3 and C4, as well as a C5 transverse process fracture. He was retrieved by an ambulance team and admitted to the hospital in a hemodynamically stable condition. His breathing on admission was noted to be normal, albeit with decreased air entry to the right side. An infiltrate on chest x-ray was consistent with aspiration. Neurologically, the patient was awake and alert. He had evidence of a Brown-Sequard syndrome with an almost complete paralysis of his left limbs and a sensory deficit on his right.

The patient's neck had been placed in a rigid cervical collar at the scene and he was given oxygen via a face mask. Tracheal intubation was performed uneventfully by elective bronchoscopic intubation in the operating room (OR) for dorsal fixation of his C-spine. Completion of internal fixation by ventral stabilization was planned at a later date and in the interim the patient was placed in a halo frame for external fixation (Figure 29-1). He was then transferred to the intensive care unit (ICU) intubated and ventilated, as his oxygen requirements had increased to 60%. An aspiration pneumonia was suspected and he was sedated and ventilated according to a lung protective ventilation strategy.

Past medical history included hypertension, GERD, and a question of significant alcohol consumption.

By day 3 of his ICU admission, the pulmonary situation had improved marginally. He still required a FiO_2 of 0.45 and was breathing spontaneously with a pressure support of 12 cm H_2O and positive end-expiratory pressure (PEEP) of 10 cm H_2O. Attempts to wean the pressure support had failed at that point, resulting in tachypnea and oxygen desaturation. Thick purulent sputum was being suctioned from his endotracheal tube (ETT) twice per shift, and he was receiving empiric antibiotics to treat his presumed pneumonia.

Agitation had become a major issue, thought to be delirium tremens secondary to alcohol withdrawal. A cranial CT had ruled out posttraumatic intracerebral hemorrhage as the underlying cause. The patient was difficult to manage, often requiring more than one nurse at the bedside, and he had tried to remove lines and ETT with his functioning hand. For this reason he required passive restraints and sedation.

On day 4, the bedside nurse called urgently to report that the patient in his agitation had bitten off the pilot line to the ETT cuff. The cuff was leaking and the patient was being inadequately oxygenated, with a drop of SpO_2 to 87%.

29.2. PATIENT CONSIDERATIONS

29.2.1. Medical considerations

29.2.1.1. Is the Patient at Acute Risk of Suffering Harm?

Hemodynamics and gas exchange must be included in the assessment of the acute need for emergency treatment. While an SpO_2 of 87% is certainly abnormally low, it might not impose an acute danger to the patient on the short term. Two factors are important: whether the patient has organs at risk of hypoperfusion (and thus cellular hypoxia) and if sufficient oxygen carrying capacity exists to compensate for lower oxygen saturation.

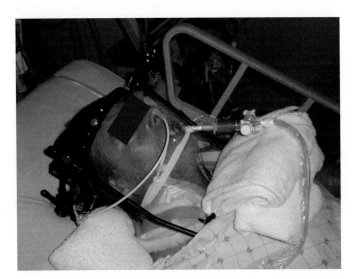

FIGURE 29-1. Patient with Halo frame for stabilization of cervical spine fractures (produced with permission).

Oxygen-carrying capacity (or oxygen delivery) depends on cardiac output, hemoglobin concentration, and hemoglobin oxygen saturation. The patient was slightly anemic (Hgb 110 g/dL), although with an increase in heart rate from 81 to 105 beats per minute following development of the cuff leak, some compensation had occurred by increasing cardiac output to maintain oxygen delivery.

The patient was not known to have coronary artery or cerebrovascular disease; he had no specific risk factors and was thus unlikely to have hypoperfusion of vital organs. As such, a borderline SpO_2 could be tolerated for a short period of time.

It was concluded that this patient needed urgent troubleshooting, but not necessarily an emergency ETT exchange, allowing a carefully planned procedure to prevent further harm.

29.2.1.2. Which Are the Management Options for Treatment?

In a prospective multicenter study involving 426 patients, Boulain[1] reported that self-extubation occurred in 46 patients (11%), and 18 of these patients did not require reintubation. Therefore, it is necessary to assess the patient's ability to breathe unassisted and determine the need for further ventilatory assistance. While it is possible that a subgroup of self-extubated patients not yet capable of completely breathing on their own may be amenable to noninvasive ventilaton (NIV), this patient's halo frame precluded NIV due to technical constraints.

Indicators for the ability to ventilate include respiratory rate, the patient's work of breathing, and gas exchange. In this patient, an increase in heart and respiratory rate and the decrease in SpO_2, combined with clearly visible usage of accessory muscles of respiration indicate the need for further ventilatory support. His respiratory failure was likely multifactorial, including the aspiration pneumonia as well as compromised intercostal and diaphragmatic muscular function due to his high spinal cord injury. As the patient needed further ventilatory assistance, an ETT exchange was indicated.

29.2.2. Airway considerations

29.2.2.1. What Should Be the Initial Management?

First, the patient should be placed on FiO_2 of 1.0 to improve oxygenation. This increased the SpO_2 to 91%, which helped to buy some time to adequately prepare for the procedure. Also, even though the leak prevailed, some degree of minute ventilation remained, as not all of the delivered tidal volume escaped and the patient continued spontaneous breathing efforts.

An attempt can be made to reestablish ventilation by fixing the pilot line. However, in this case, the line had multiple tears and could not be fixed.

Alternative approaches in the case of life-threatening hypoxemia should aim to temporarily restore oxygenation until a definitive airway can be placed. The existing tube, if ineffective, can be removed and the patient's respiratory efforts assisted with bag-mask-ventilation. Ventilation can be improved by use of an oropharyngeal airway. However, in most cases, even with a leaky cuff, some ventilation can be maintained by hyperventilating with high flows and respiratory rate (>30 breaths per minute), mimicking high-frequency ventilation.

The high-frequency oscillation (HFO) mode of ventilation can provide sufficient oxygenation even with a cuff leak. Indeed, during routine use of HFO, a cuff leak is sometimes purposefully used to improve ventilation. It is an ideal rescue maneuver in a situation where a patient desaturates and cannot be ventilated by other means. This option could be considered before a leaky tube was removed. HFO would be the preferred technique in this situation if a patient had profound gas exchange impairment, such as ARDS, to be used until arrangements for safe ETT exchange were made.

There should always be alternatives at hand in case the first attempt to reintubate the patient fails following removal of the faulty ETT. These can follow the ASA algorithm for the difficult airway and might include, but are not confined to, smaller ETTs, alternatives to DL, an appropriately sized EGD, and cricothyrotomy equipment. More help should be obtained as a difficult situation such as this can always be better managed with additional medical and nursing staff. Calling for additional expertise is not a sign of incompetence, but of professionalism!

29.2.2.2. How Might the Presence of a Halo Jacket Impact Airway Management?

The presence of a halo jacket can impact all facets of airway management. In this case, the trachea of the patient was first intubated by awake bronchoscopic intubation, and a direct laryngoscopic view had not been assessed thereafter. The halo jacket fixes the head in a neutral position, and prevents any flexion or extension of the neck (Figure 29-1). With direct laryngoscopy (DL), it is likely that at best a Cormack/Lehane (C/L) Grade 3 view will be achieved. Tracheal intubation is more likely to succeed with alternatives to DL, such as flexible or rigid fiber- or video-optic devices (see Chapters 9 and 10). Should intubation fail and the patient require oxygenation by positive pressure ventilation between attempts, BMV could also prove challenging due to decreased head extension, and for the same reason, EGD insertion may be difficult. Finally, cricothyrotomy is usually performed with the head extended, so this can also be expected to be somewhat more difficult in the patient with a halo jacket.

In this agitated and uncooperative patient, it is unlikely that an awake look DL assessment under topical airway anesthesia and light sedation will be an option. Alternative approaches must be considered.

29.2.2.3. What Other Risks Are Inherent in This Situation?

Enteral nutrition imposes an additional risk for aspiration while the airway is unprotected. Enteral feeds should be stopped immediately and the feeding tube suctioned to clear as much gastric content as possible.

An already agitated patient may well get more delirious if ventilatory support suddenly stops and hypoxemia develops. Sedation will also be needed to allow the patient tolerate the tube exchange procedure. On the other hand, should reintubation fail during tube exchange, preservation of spontaneous ventilation will add a margin of safety. When practical, nonpharmacological ways of calming the patient (talk-down and reassurance with the help of additional staff) cannot be overestimated. If needed, short-acting drugs such as propofol are preferred.

The reasons for the patient's continuing need for mechanical ventilation are weakness and pneumonia. Weakness alone as a cause of respiratory failure could be treated by noninvasive ventilation (NIV). However, in this case, severe agitation is a contraindication to NIV and as previously suggested the halo jacket will cause difficulty with its application. Pneumonia on the other hand causes edema, atelectasis, and ventilation-perfusion mismatch, resulting in hypoxemic respiratory failure. To aggravate the situation, the loss of PEEP due to the cuff leak will lead to even more atelectasis formation in unstable regions. Furthermore, functional residual capacity (FRC) will be reduced, increasing the patient's susceptibility to hypoxemia. As the combination of these factors increases the risk of hypoxemia within minutes, tube exchange should not be deferred for long.

Although a leak is clearly audible, other significant alterations of the airway should be anticipated. Mucosal swelling from inflammation and general edema, as well as displacement of tissue from the previous trauma may cause physical impediment to the placement of a new ETT or total obscuring of laryngeal inlet anatomy after the defective tube is removed.

29.3. MANAGEMENT PLAN

29.3.1. Which is the best strategy to secure the airway and avoid complications?

In evaluating the different options one has to consider the following key points:

- How much time is there to act?
- What equipment is available?

- Which technical skills are available?
- For the tube change, should spontaneous ventilation be maintained or ablated?

The first question has already been answered, as the patient is temporarily stable and should tolerate at least several minutes in the present situation. This will enable the necessary equipment to be obtained, as well as additional expertise. It may also allow the option of transferring the patient to the OR for the tube change, if great difficulty is anticipated.

In an ICU airway emergency, the needed equipment is rarely immediately available at the bedside. Contents and location of the airway equipment cart within the ICU should be well known. If the patient is stable and a difficult airway is anticipated, there may be time to obtain additional equipment from the OR.

Which procedure to choose will depend partially on the skills and experience of the attending practitioner. While there is much to be said for using familiar techniques and equipment, if time permits, additional expertise can be obtained to perform a less familiar technique (eg, tracheotomy), if indicated.

Preservation of spontaneous respiration during the tube change will provide the advantage of maintaining oxygenation for a short period of time should placement of the new ETT prove problematic after removal of the defective one. However, this patient is agitated, and will likely have to be deeply sedated for the procedure, putting him at risk of apnea. The downside of having an apneic patient would then occur without the upside of conditions optimized by a skeletal muscle relaxant. On the other hand, choosing to deliberately ablate spontaneous respirations with an induction dose of sedative/hypnotic and use of a skeletal muscle relaxant will provide for optimal conditions for the tube change but should occur only with an appreciation of (and preparations for) the difficulty that may be encountered during the procedure.

29.3.2. What options exist for exchanging the ETT?

As pointed out earlier, obstruction of the upper airway imposes a significant risk for the placement of a new endotracheal tube. Whenever tracheal extubation is required prior to reintubation with a new ETT, there is a chance that the new tube might not pass into the trachea. This could be caused by displaced, collapsed, or edematous tissue, which was previously held open by the ETT.

For the tube exchange, a number of options exist. With appropriate preparation, the defective tube can either simply be removed and a new one placed, or the procedure can occur over an airway exchange catheter. For the former option, as discussed earlier in Section 29.2.2.2, it must be appreciated that intubation by DL will most likely not succeed. Other options such as the lightwand, intubating laryngeal mask airway, or video laryngoscope, such as the Glidescope, are more likely to succeed, but (a) the equipment must be available and (b) the practitioner must be experienced in its use. Use of an airway exchange catheter would be judged preferable by many practitioners in this context, as following removal of the defective tube, a fairly rigid conduit remains in the trachea to guide the new tube to the appropriate location. In contrast to the Eschmann tracheal introducer (gum elastic bougie), the exchanger catheter has a hollow lumen with a connector, so that oxygenation can be provided should passage of the new tube fail. This might happen if the tip of the endotracheal tube impinges on soft tissue of the laryngeal inlet during blind advancement. Other complications are esophageal displacement[2] or pneumothorax, if used for jet ventilation.[3] Use of airway exchange catheters has been discussed in detail in Chapter 28.

If an experienced surgeon is immediately available, a surgical airway (cricothyrotomy or tracheotomy) will result in an almost 100% success rate, although it is the most invasive option. The complication rate, including risk of significant bleeding, false cannula passage, pneumothorax, and infection, has been quoted to be as high as 12.5% in elective tracheotomy[4] and even higher in emergencies. However, surgical airway in this setting would help avoid the risks inherent in a difficult tube change, and might be considered if time permits and there is a high probability that the patient will go on to tracheotomy anyway in the coming days or weeks. Otherwise, it will be a fallback option should other procedures fail for technical or time-critical reasons.

29.3.3. What medications can be used to facilitate the procedure?

The use of sedation in the ICU has decreased to much lower levels in recent years. Very few patients will tolerate a tube exchange without increasing their sedation, unless awake, cooperative, and topically well anesthetized. Compared to elective intubation in the operating room, the emergency intubation of critically ill patients carries a much higher risk of complications, for example, postintubation hemodynamic instability, which is associated with a significant mortality.[5] Vasomotor insufficiency, impaired organ perfusion and microcirculation, an increased sympathetic tone, and lower oxygen delivery (a combination of anemia, hypoxemia, and low cardiac output) place these patients at high risk for profound hypotension, arrhythmia, and myocardial hypoperfusion, to name just the most vital consequences of short-term instability. Careful planning and the choice of drugs have a great impact on preventing hemodynamic instability. Although difficult to predict whether a patient will develop hemodynamic instability, it is important to have a plan in place to treat this early, before it becomes life threatening. Generally, it is not the particular combination of drugs, but the way they are administered that has the greatest effect on preserving hemodynamic stability.

The choice of drugs should reflect the level of sedation desired, anticipated effects on hemodynamics, and their interactions with patient physiology. The ideal drug has a short duration of drug effect, is metabolized independently from liver and kidney function, has minimal cardiodepressant or vasodilating effects, and can be easily titrated to the desired degree of sedation. Often, no single drug has all these attributes, so a combination of drugs may be necessary.

Propofol is a readily titratable agent, increasingly used for long-term sedation in the ICU. It has dose-dependent cardiodepressant and vasodilating effects.

Benzodiazepines have classically been used for sedation in the ICU but tend to have a very long half-life, a dependency on liver metabolism, and the risk of creating delirium. Short-acting benzodiazepines, such as midazolam, are preferred for procedural sedation.

Etomidate is an ultra short-acting sedative with little effect on hemodynamics. Unfortunately, even a single dose can induce adreno-cortical depression, although the clinical significance of this remains uncertain.

Ketamine has sedative and analgesic properties, while respiratory function and hemodynamic stability are preserved. In contrast to other hypnotic drugs, it causes a dissociative state in which patients tolerate uncomfortable or painful stimuli. Ketamine can cause hallucinations, which has led to substantially decreased use for many years. However, due to the increasingly recognized importance of hemodynamic stability, ketamine has experienced a revival in recent years.

Opioids are standard analgesics often used as adjuncts for procedures such as tracheal intubation. While cardioprotective (by preventing tachycardia), in the context of a critically ill patient they can cause hypotension by suppressing sympathetic drive.

Muscle relaxants may be used in conjunction with a sedative/hypnotic agent to optimize intubating conditions provided an airway assessment has been performed that suggests tracheal intubation will succeed, or fallback options such as ventilation using a bag-mask or EGD will be possible should intubation fail. With a hemiparesis of 72 hours' duration, succinylcholine should be avoided in this patient.

29.4. PROCEDURE

29.4.1. What preparations were made for the tube exchange?

Tube exchange using an airway exchange catheter was the chosen technique, as the procedure is the least invasive combined with a good success rate. To help prevent soft tissue impingement during advancement of the new tube, a decision was made to do the exchange under indirect visualization of the glottis by videolaryngoscopy.[6] A Glidescope® was obtained from the operating room for the purpose. The plan was determined as follows:

1. A second person skilled in airway management (ie, respiratory therapist, physician) was called to the bedside.

2. At least one more nurse was called to assist with calming the patient, administering drugs, charting, or calling for additional help if needed.

3. Tube feeds were confirmed off, and the stomach suctioned through the nasogastric tube. A rigid suction catheter connected to the wall suction was placed close to the patient's head.

4. The bed was moved away from the wall to increase working space. The patient was placed in 30 degrees of head elevation.

5. A call was made to the OR to ensure that a surgeon would be immediately available if needed.

6. The following airway management supplies were gathered at the bedside: An adult-sized, 19 Fr Cook Airway Exchange Catheter with Rapi-Fit ventilation adapter; a complete conventional intubation kit with laryngoscopes and Macintosh 3 and 4 blades (lights checked); a Glidescope®; ETTs sizes 7 to 9 mm ID; oropharyngeal and nasopharyngeal airways; Ambu® bag with oxygen reservoir and face masks of appropriate size; a # 4 and # 5 LMA-Classic and LMA-Fastrach (intubating LMA); Xylocaine spray and gel; an emergency cricothyrotomy kit. An 8.5 mm ID ETT was opened and the outside lubricated with Xylocaine gel.

7. The following drugs were prepared: propofol infusion, fentanyl, midazolam, and rocuronium. An additional vasopressor was not deemed necessary as a norepinephrine infusion of $0.05\ \mu g\cdot kg^{-1}\cdot min^{-1}$ was running to maintain an adequate mean arterial pressure.

8. It was confirmed that the patient's FiO_2 had already been increased to 1.0. The patient was informed about the upcoming procedure.

29.4.2. Describe the airway exchange procedure

After all equipment and additional staff were present at the bedside, the propofol infusion was increased to 2.5 $mg\cdot kg^{-1}\cdot h^{-1}$ and a bolus of 100 µg of fentanyl was given IV. The patient went to sleep, dropping his MAP by 12 mm Hg, but continued to breathe. The norepinephrine infusion was increased to 0.07 $\mu g\cdot kg^{-1}\cdot min^{-1}$.

After hemodynamic stabilization, the tube change procedure began. The patient's 8.5 mm ID ETT was loosened from the fixation and held in position by the respiratory therapist. The oropharynx was then suctioned to remove secretions. The patient was disconnected from the ventilator and manually ventilated with a manual resuscitator.

Standing behind the patient's head, the second practitioner introduced the Glidescope® into the oropharynx without resistance and the glottis was easily visualized on the screen. Importantly, no direct force or jaw thrust had to be applied, which enabled the patient to tolerate the procedure without the need to further deepen sedation. The glottis was sprayed with two sprays of 10% Xylocaine. Then, without interrupting ventilation, the airway exchange catheter was introduced into the trachea via a suction port adapter. The centimeter markings on the ETT and airway exchange catheter were lined up, then the exchange catheter was advanced a further 5 cm (Figure 29-2). Too deep an insertion should be avoided to prevent bronchial injury. The defective ETT was then withdrawn while holding the airway exchange catheter in place. The new 8.5 mm ID ETT was then advanced over the exchange catheter under videoscopic vision. With minor manipulations of the ETT, tube passage through the glottis without impingement on soft tissue was accomplished, thus minimizing patient's discomfort and coughing. One practitioner held the Glidescope® in place, while the other advanced the ETT over the

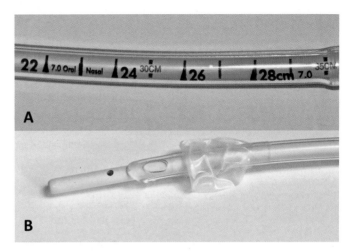

FIGURE 29-2. Markings on the endotracheal tube and the exchange catheter (A) indicating that the tip of the catheter exceeds the tube by 5 cm (B).

exchange catheter. The ETT cuff was inflated, and the exchange catheter and Glidescope® removed. The manual resuscitator was connected and ventilation resumed. Correct ETT placement was confirmed by $ETCO_2$ and auscultation. The procedural time without ventilation was less than 20 seconds, and the patient's SpO_2 dropped from 91% to 88%. The patient was then reconnected to the ventilator, which caused the SpO_2 to increase to 98%. Chest x-ray confirmed correct placement of the ETT tip 4 cm above the carina, and excluded pneumothorax or atelectasis.

29.5. SUMMARY

An ETT cuff leak is not necessarily an indication for immediate tube exchange, since sufficient ventilation to prevent acute hypoxemia can be maintained in most situations. A careful plan is important to safely restore mechanical ventilation without causing additional harm to the patient.

In a difficult airway situation, such as fixation of the neck in a halo frame, an exit strategy, for example, emergency surgical airway, should be in place. Additional staff and all equipment needed should be at the bedside before starting the procedure.

The procedure can be completed with or without sedative/hypnotic and paralysis. If sedation alone is selected, it should be titrated to achieve just the level needed to tolerate the procedure. Oversedation is associated with the risk of hemodynamic instability and complications. Topical anesthesia of the vocal cords helps to prevent coughing and decreases the need for sedation.

Use of an airway exchange catheter is a safe procedure with low risk of complications. Its success rate can be increased by additional use of videolaryngoscopy. The ETT is exchanged over the exchange catheter under indirect vision, helping avoid impingement of the tube's tip on laryngeal structures. After the exchange, correct tube placement should be confirmed and intrathoracic complications excluded by chest x-ray.

REFERENCES

1. Boulain T. Unplanned extubations in the adult intensive care unit: a prospective multicenter study. Association des Reanimateurs du Centre-Ouest. *Am J Respir Crit Care Med*. 1998;157:1131-1137.

2. Heininger A, Krueger WA, Dieterich HJ, et al. Complications using a hollow fiber airway exchange catheter for tracheal tube exchange in critically ill patients. *Acta Anaesthesiol Scand*. 2008;52:1031.

3. Nunn C, Uffman J, Bhananker SM. Bilateral tension pneumothoraces following jet ventilation via an airway exchange catheter. *J Anesth*. 2007;21:76-79.

4. Polderman KH, Spijkstra JJ, de Bree R, et al. Percutaneous dilatational tracheostomy in the ICU: optimal organization, low complication rates, and description of a new complication. *Chest*. 2003;123:1595-1602.

5. Mort TC. Complications of emergency tracheal intubation: hemodynamic alterations—part I. *J Intensive Care Med*. 2007;22:157-165.

6. Mort TC. Tracheal tube exchange: feasibility of continuous glottic viewing with advanced laryngoscopy assistance. *Anesth Analg*. 2009;108:1228-1231.

SELF-EVALUATION QUESTIONS

29.1. Which of the following methods is **NOT** suitable for the exchange of an endotracheal tube in a patient with anticipated difficult airway, such as in a halo jacket?

A. videolaryngoscopy

B. flexible bronchoscopic intubation

C. laryngoscopy with a Macintosh #3 blade

D. airway exchange catheter

E. tracheotomy

29.2. A possible complication during an airway exchange is

A. massive bleeding

B. increased abdominal pressure

C. acute respiratory failure

D. ventilator-associated pneumonia (VAP)

E. acute airway obstruction

29.3. All of the following can be tried if the tracheal tube cannot be advanced over the tube exchanger through the glottis **EXCEPT**:

A. counter-clockwise rotation of the tube

B. gentle pressure to force the tube through the glottis

C. lubrication of the tip of the tube

D. jaw thrust

E. assist with videolaryngoscopy

CHAPTER 30

Management of a Patient Admitted to the ICU with Impending Respiratory Failure due to a Suspected Infectious Etiology

David T. Wong

30.1 CASE PRESENTATION

A 47-year-old previously healthy male physician presented to hospital with the acute onset of fever, nonproductive cough, dyspnea, and malaise. As an intensive care unit (ICU) physician, he had intubated the trachea of a known Severe Acute Respiratory syndrome (SARS) patient in the emergency department 2 weeks earlier. He began to have respiratory symptoms 1 week later. He was admitted and placed in an isolation room. Both sputum and blood cultures were negative. In spite of empiric treatment with broad-spectrum antibiotics, his respiratory status progressively worsened over the next 24 hours, necessitating ICU admission. His vitals on admission to the ICU were respiratory rate (RR) 24 breaths per minute, heart rate (HR) 100 beats per minute (bpm), BP 130/90 mm Hg, and temperature 38.6°C. Oxygen saturation was 95% on an FiO_2 of 60%, and arterial blood gases (ABGs) revealed the following: pH 7.45, PCO_2 30, PO_2 60. With the PO_2 to FiO_2 ratio (PF ratio) determined to be 100, respiratory failure was diagnosed. The chest x-ray (CXR) showed progressive bilateral basal infiltrates. A complete blood count, electrolytes, creatinine, and liver function tests were all normal, but LDH was elevated. Neurological and cardiovascular systems were intact on examination.

Anesthesia was consulted regarding possible tracheal intubation for respiratory failure with an ARDS picture. The patient was agreeable to intubation. On airway examination he was noted to be of average body habitus (5 ft 10 in [176 cm] and 154 lb [70 kg]) with no obvious dysmorphic facial features. He had no beard and no history of obstructive sleep apnea. Although he was dyspneic, there was no evidence of stridor. With full dentition, the patient was able to open his mouth 5 cm, had a 4 cm thyromental

distance, and had a Mallampati Class III pharyngeal view. He exhibited good jaw protrusion, and head and neck mobility was unrestricted. The cricothyroid membrane was easily palpable in the midline.

30.2 MEDICAL CONSIDERATIONS

30.2.1 What airborne pathogens may pose serious danger to health care workers? What is the likely pathogen that caused the illness of the presented patient?

Health care workers (HCW) are at risk of coming in contact with respiratory secretions from patients with febrile respiratory illness of unknown etiology. There are a number of airborne viruses or bacteria that can pose a risk to HCW. For instance, active pulmonary tuberculosis carries a high risk of transmission to HCW. Similarly, active anthrax pulmonary infection may also pose a significant risk to HCW.

In general, most airborne viruses which can potentially infect HCW are not associated with high morbidity or mortality. In 2009, a new influenza A H1N1 virus (also known as swine flu) caused a worldwide pandemic affecting millions of patients. At the time of writing this chapter, there were over 375,000 confirmed cases with over 4500 deaths.[1] Fortunately, most infected patients ran a benign course. Rarely, patients presented to the hospital with a rapidly progressive severe pneumonia/ARDS picture.

The clinical picture presented in this patient is compatible with the diagnosis of Severe Acute Respiratory syndrome or SARS which is not transmitted through airborne pathogens.

30.2.2 What is the epidemiology of SARS? How did SARS come out of nowhere to affect thousands of people worldwide?

In November 2002, a cluster of atypical pneumonia cases of unknown etiology was discovered in Guangdong Province, China. In late February 2003, a symptomatic Chinese physician traveled to Hong Kong and transmitted the illness to others staying in the same hotel, initiating a worldwide epidemic. On March 12, 2003, the World Health Organization (WHO) issued a global alert warning of a wave of severe atypical pneumonia of unknown etiology.[2-4] On April 13, 2003, the causative agent for SARS was identified as a new coronavirus (SARS-CoV). By the end of July 2003, there were over 8000 cases of SARS worldwide with over 700 deaths.[5] Countries and regions with the highest case loads were China, Hong Kong, Taiwan, and Canada.

30.2.3 How is the SARS virus transmitted?

SARS is thought to be transmitted by respiratory droplets or by direct/indirect contact.[3] It is a moderately transmissible virus with a secondary infection rate of approximately 2.7 per case. The majority of SARS patients do not infect others while a small number of *super-spreaders* may be highly infectious.[6,7] There is no evidence of airborne transmission.

30.2.4 What are the risk factors for SARS viral transmission?

SARS patients develop nonspecific viral symptoms in the first week of their illness and respiratory symptoms in the second week, during which they are most infectious. Fowler et al assessed the risk factors for SARS transmission among 122 health care workers in a critical care setting.[8] They found that performing endotracheal intubation and caring for patients receiving noninvasive positive pressure ventilation were associated with 13 and 2.3 times the risk of acquiring infection compared to those who did not. Loeb et al studied risk factors for SARS transmission among 43 critical care nurses.[9] They found that assisting with intubation, suctioning prior to intubation, and manipulation of the oxygen mask were high-risk activities. In a third report, bag-mask-ventilation (BMV), endotracheal intubation, airway suctioning, noninvasive ventilation, and high-frequency oscillation were identified as high-risk procedures for SARS transmission in the ICU.[10]

30.2.5 What is the definition of SARS?

The WHO definition[11] of a *suspect SARS* patient is a person presenting after November 1, 2002 with a history of:

A. Fever >38°C

B. Cough and respiratory difficulty

C. Known exposure to a SARS patient or traveling in endemic area within 10 days of presenting illness

> ### TABLE 30-1

Symptoms of SARS Reported at Admission to Hospital

Fever	99.3%
Nonproductive cough	69.4%
Myalgia	49.3%
Dyspnea	41.7%
Headache	35.4%
Malaise	31.2%
Chills	27.8%
Diarrhea	23.6%
Nausea or vomiting	19.4%
Sore throat	12.5%
Arthralgia	10.4%
Chest pain	10.4%
Productive cough	4.9%
Dizziness	4.2%
Abdominal pain	3.5%
Rhinorrhea	2.1%

Source: Data from Booth CM, Matukas LM, Tomlinson GA, et al. Clinical features and short-term outcomes of 144 patients with SARS in the greater Toronto area. JAMA. 2003;289:2801-2809.

The WHO definition of a *probable SARS* patient is a suspect person with

A. Radiologic evidence of infiltrates consistent with pneumonia or respiratory distress syndrome *or*

B. One or more assays positive for SARS coronavirus *or*

C. Autopsy findings consistent with the pathology of respiratory distress syndrome without an identifiable cause

30.2.6 What is the typical clinical course of a SARS patient?

The incubation period is 2 to 5 days but can be up to 10 days.[12] The most common symptoms at admission to hospital are fever, nonproductive cough, myalgia, dyspnea, headache, malaise, chills, and diarrhea (Table 30-1). The majority of patients have unilateral or bilateral infiltrates on the chest radiograph. The overall death rate is 10% to 13%, but is as high as 50% in the 23% to 26% of patients requiring intensive care admission.[12-14] Risk factors for death include age, comorbidities, and APACHE II scores.[14]

30.3 PATIENT CONSIDERATIONS

30.3.1 What are the major considerations in this patient?

This patient fulfills the WHO definition of probable SARS and clinical criteria for ARDS (bilateral lung infiltrate with PF ratio ≤200 mm Hg). The patient has increased pulmonary shunting due to fluid-filled alveoli and atelectasis, leading to a high A-a gradient and a low PF ratio. He has little pulmonary reserve and is prone to the development of hypoxemia during intubation. He is also at risk of barotrauma (eg, pneumothorax) with positive pressure ventilation.

The patient is likely to have a depleted extracellular fluid volume due to his fasting status and large amounts of fluid loss from his respiratory system. This volume depletion, coupled with institution of positive pressure ventilation and removal of sympathetic drive puts him at risk of hypotension during and immediately following intubation.

30.3.2 What is the differential diagnosis of a patient with bilateral pulmonary infiltrates of unknown etiology?

The patient may be suffering from bacterial, viral, fungal, or parasitic pneumonia. Tuberculosis, *Pneumocystis carinii*, and atypical pneumonia such as mycoplasma and legionella are possibilities. In addition, bilateral lung infiltrates may be due to leaky pulmonary capillaries caused by diverse causes such as sepsis or pancreatitis. Of these causes, tuberculosis and SARS pose the highest risk of transmission to the health care workers and appropriate personal protection precautions should be exercised (see later).

30.4 AIRWAY CONSIDERATIONS

30.4.1 Is this patient predicted to have a difficult airway?

Airway examination should focus on the ability to provide ventilation and oxygenation through a bag-mask, an endotracheal tube, an extraglottic device, and a surgical airway. The mnemonics MOANS, RODS, LEMON, and SHORT described in Chapter 1 provide a useful framework to assess these aspects of the patient's airway. It should be emphasized that while the ASA task force on management of the difficult airway outlined 11 criteria for preoperative airway assessment for laryngoscopy and intubation,[15] no single airway test has perfect sensitivity or specificity in predicting difficult laryngoscopic intubation. In general, all single airway predictors share a common set of characteristics: low sensitivity, high specificity, and low positive predictive value. The combination of several airway predictors tends to improve the positive predictive value for difficult laryngoscopic intubation.

With reference to the airway examination presented in Section 30.1 earlier, it is apparent that this patient has several predictors of a difficult laryngoscopic intubation: borderline mouth opening, a reduced thyromental distance, and a Mallampati III classification. In combination, these characteristics place this patient at a *moderately* high risk for difficult laryngoscopy. However, alternative intubation devices, such as the intubating LMA (ILMA) or lighted stylet should be successful, and with adequate control of secretions, so should flexible or rigid fiberoptic devices or videolaryngoscopes. Bag-mask-ventilation if needed should be possible, although not optimal. Should extraglottic device placement and

use be required, decreased pulmonary compliance due to ARDS may present a problem with pop-off leak developing at higher airway pressures: availability of an LMA Pro-Seal or LMA Supreme might be advisable. Cricothyrotomy should be possible. Note that although some of these techniques are not desirable in the patient with SARS, their predicted success must still be assessed, particularly in the patient with predictors of difficulty.

30.4.2 What do you do differently when establishing an airway in a SARS patient?

A SARS patient poses a unique risk to health care workers due to its highly infectious nature and a high mortality rate for those infected. In developed countries such as Canada and Singapore, approximately 50% of SARS cases were health care workers involved in caring for SARS patients. The processes of tracheal intubation, bag-mask-ventilation, and suctioning were associated with the highest risk of acquiring SARS.[8-10] A cluster of nine health care workers who cared for a single SARS patient around the time of intubation in the ICU themselves developed SARS.[16]

In order to minimize the risk of SARS cross-transmission to health care workers, guidelines have been developed to reduce the risk of aerosolization of SARS droplets during the process of intubation.[3,17,18] It is critical that the health care worker apply and remove personal protection equipment (see Section 30.5.5) prior to and after intubation. In addition, bag-mask-ventilation, nebulization, and application of topical airway anesthesia are to be avoided. The patient should thus be sedated and paralyzed unless contraindicated. However, if a high potential for difficult laryngoscopy exists, there may be a conflict of priorities.

30.4.3 How are you going to approach this patient's airway?

This patient's situation presents us with a real dilemma. On the one hand, an awake intubation following application of topical airway anesthesia is generally considered to be the safest method of securing the airway in the patient presenting with potential difficult laryngoscopic intubation. On the other hand, to minimize the risk to health care personnel of SARS transmission, avoiding BMV is preferred, and paralysis of the patient will help avoid the potential for coughing. Protecting the patient and the health care worker are both important priorities.

Ultimately the method chosen for intubation is determined by how likely one is to encounter a failed airway situation (see Chapter 2). The possibility for such a situation will become evident as the patient is assessed for predictors of difficulty in all aspects of airway management. If the patient presents with evidence that airway control will be difficult using various techniques of endotracheal tube placement, bag-mask-ventilation, an extraglottic device, or cricothyrotomy, the practitioner should accept the risk of disease transmission and perform an awake intubation. However, in this case, as outlined in Section 30.4.1 earlier, the patient presents predictors of only moderate difficulty with laryngoscopy and no predictors of difficulty with alternative intubation (eg, ILMA, lighted stylet, flexible bronchoscope) equipment use.

Bag-mask and extraglottic device ventilation, if needed, will most likely be successful in spite of reduced pulmonary compliance. Cricothyrotomy should pose few problems.

Thus, a reasonable Plan A approach in this patient is to attempt tracheal intubation by direct laryngoscopy after induction using short-acting anesthetic and paralytic agents. The intubation should be undertaken by an experienced airway practitioner, wearing full protection, and with a full complement of alternative intubating devices. In addition, an extraglottic rescue device and cricothyrotomy equipment should be readily available in the room.

If direct laryngoscopy fails after one or two attempts, and oxygenation remains acceptable, Plan B calls for an alternative device to be used, in this case a video laryngoscope (eg, Glidescope) or a flexible bronchoscope. If intubation is not successful after three attempts, the patient should be awakened with the intention of proceeding with an awake intubation. If at any time between attempts oxygenation cannot be maintained with bag-mask-ventilation, Plan C calls for the immediate use of an EGD, such as an LMA ProSeal or LMA Fastrach™, while concurrently preparing to perform a cricothyrotomy in this *cannot intubate cannot oxygenate* situation.

30.5 PREPARATION AND PLANNING FOR ESTABLISHMENT OF AN AIRWAY IN THE SARS PATIENT

30.5.1 Where in the ICU should the patient be placed?

In order to minimize the spread of SARS virus, the patient should be placed in an isolation room, equipped with negative pressure ventilation.[3,17,18] The room should have a preentry room (anteroom) to allow application and removal of personal protection equipment.

30.5.2 Who should perform and who should assist with tracheal intubation?

Only those persons required to carry out the intubation should be permitted in the immediate vicinity of the patient. This team may consist of an experienced airway practitioner, respiratory therapist, and an ICU nurse. Students should be excluded. Additional personnel should stand by outside the room in the event that help or equipment is required during the airway management procedure. In this situation, this may include another individual with airway management expertise.

It is critically important that all team members are aware of Plan A, Plan B, and Plan C and have had the chance to rehearse the sequence of events prior to securing the airway.

30.5.3 What airway equipment should be available in the patient's room?

- *General equipment*: The room should contain a ventilator with hydrophobic filters (eg, PALL®) on the inspiratory and expiratory limbs, suction, capnography, oximetry, ventilation bag with expiratory filter, and oropharyngeal airway.[3]
- *Plan A equipment*: A laryngoscope handle, an appropriately sized curved and straight blade, a tracheal tube introducer (eg, Eschmann introducer), several sizes of endotracheal tubes, and endotracheal tube stylets.
- *Alternative (Plan B) rescue airway equipment*: The LMA, and at least two alternative intubation devices such as a flexible bronchoscope, lighted stylet, intubating laryngeal mask, or video laryngoscope, such as the Glidescope®.
- *Plan C equipment*: The equipment necessary to perform a surgical airway, as Plan C stipulates, ought to be immediately available and open.

30.5.4 What other equipment is considered essential?

Two functioning intravenous lines should be placed. Induction and emergency drugs should be prepared. Induction drugs consist of midazolam, fentanyl, propofol, succinylcholine, and a nondepolarizing muscle relaxant. Emergency drugs consist of atropine, ephedrine, phenylephrine, and epinephrine.[3]

30.5.5 How should health care workers dress in order to minimize SARS transmission?

All health care workers in direct contact with SARS patients should be wearing basic personal protection equipment (PPE). Enhanced PPE should be worn by all health care workers involved in high-risk procedures such as intubation[3,18] (Table 30-2).

Basic personal protection strategy consists of airborne precautions, contact precautions, and eye protection.

30.5.5.1 Basic PPE: Airborne Precautions

An N-95 mask or equivalent is used for airborne precaution. N-95 masks offer 8 hours of protection while PCM-2000 masks provide 4 hours. Touching the mask or lifting the mask to wipe the face with gloved fingers immediately contaminates the mask and it must be replaced. It is crucial that all staff who may be involved in the care of such patients be tested and trained for proper mask fitting well before they are needed. An improper mask fit may not provide airborne protection. A properly fitted N-95 mask can be a very uncomfortable experience for users who may need to wear them for a prolonged period of time.

30.5.5.2 Basic PPE: Contact and Eye Precautions

Contact precautions include double gloves, double gown, disposable hats, and shoe covers.[3] Following contact with each patient and removing gloves, an alcohol-based skin disinfectant should be used to wash hands. Eyes should be protected against contamination using disposable goggles or face shields.

TABLE 30-2

Infection Control for an ICU Patient Requiring Endotracheal Intubation[2]

Dress Precautions

Basic personal protection equipment
- N-95 or equivalent face mask
- Contact: gloves, gown, hat, shoe covers
- Eye protection: goggles or face shields
- Pens, pagers, or personal items should not be brought into or out of the room

Enhanced personal protection equipment for high-risk procedures
- Air-Mate® powered air purification respirator (PAPR) system
- Stryker T4 PAPR system

Environment/Equipment Precautions
- Isolation rooms
- Negative-pressure rooms preferable
- ICU rooms should be stocked with a full supply of airway and intubation equipment, induction and emergency drugs
- Equipment and stationary (eg, computer keyboard, pens, stethoscope) should be cleaned frequently with antiviral disinfectants
- Frequent hand washing with alcohol-based disinfectant
- No sharing of equipment

Airway and Ventilator Management
- Allow plenty of time to prepare for intubation
- The whole team to discuss and rehearse Plan A and Plan B for intubation
- Avoid topicalization of the airway
- Avoid nebulization therapy
- Avoid suctioning of an unprotected airway
- Avoid noninvasive positive pressure ventilation
- The most-experienced physician to perform intubation
- Minimize the number of personnel in the room during intubation
- Have a second parallel team on standby outside the room
- Sedate and paralyze patient prior to intubation unless contraindicated
- Use filters for Ambu bag and ventilator
- Ensure functioning scavenging system
- Usage of closed suctioning system

30.5.5.3 Enhanced PPE

Enhanced PPE consists of basic PPE plus powered air purification respirator (PAPR) systems.[18] They should be worn by all health care workers involved in high-risk procedures for these patients. One example of a commonly used PAPR system is the Air-Mate® (3M, St. Paul, MN). The Air-Mate® PAPR system consists of a belt-mounted powered air purifier (Figure 30-1, right) with a HEPA filter, connected via a tube to a light-weight head-piece (Figure 30-1, left). The HEPA filter removes particles of 0.3 to 15 μm with an efficiency of 98% to 100%.[5] Experience of several years' duration using the PAPR system in the bronchoscopy suite has revealed no documented disease transmission to health care workers. Chee et al reported their experience in Singapore among health care workers

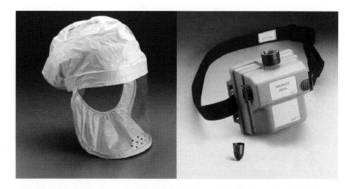

FIGURE 30-1. The Air-Mate® powered air purification respirator (PAPR) system consists of a belt-mounted powered air purifier (right) with a HEPA filter, connected via a tube to a light-weight head piece (left).

caring for SARS patients undergoing 41 surgical procedures.[19] With rigid adherence to basic and enhanced PPE, none of 124 health care workers directly exposed to SARS patients was infected.

It takes time to properly set up the room and apply PPE.[18] Therefore, it is crucial to be advised well in advance of patients requiring tracheal intubation. Furthermore, staff involved in the intubation must be trained and familiar with the personal protection equipment so that it can be applied properly and expeditiously, and removed properly to avoid contamination.

30.5.6 What conditions must be satisfied before proceeding with intubation?

Just before performing intubation, a checklist should be completed and Plans A, B, and C rehearsed so that all parties involved are absolutely clear as to each person's responsibilities and course of action until the airway is secured (Table 30-2).

The ventilator, monitors, airway equipment, suction, intravenous access, induction, and emergency drugs should be in the room. All equipment for Plans A, B, and C should be ready. The primary intubation team members apply basic and enhanced PPE including PAPR system and enter the patient's room. A second, parallel team is dressed and ready to enter the room if needed. A practitioner experienced in securing a surgical airway should be part of the second team on standby.

30.6 ACTUAL CONDUCT OF TRACHEAL INTUBATION

30.6.1 Describe the actual steps of tracheal intubation in this patient

The patient was denitrogenated while spontaneously breathing with FiO_2 of 1.0 for 5 minutes. At no time was positive pressure ventilation applied prior to intubation. Topicalization of the airway and nebulization of drugs were likewise avoided. The ventilator was set on volume control mode.

Once the patient was adequately denitrogenated, fentanyl 50 μg and midazolam 1 mg were given intravenously. A sleep dose of propofol was given followed by succinylcholine 1.5 mg·kg^{-1}.

After the patient was anesthetized and paralyzed, laryngoscopy was attempted with a MAC 3 blade. A Grade 3 laryngeal view was observed despite external laryngeal pressure and a head lift. The decision was made not to attempt blind intubation with direct laryngoscopy. Flexible bronchoscope-guided intubation was elected as the next option.

A propofol infusion was administered using a syringe pump at 100 μg·kg^{-1}·min^{-1}. Additional succinylcholine of 40 mg was given. The patient's vital signs were stable with a SpO_2 of 100%. Gentle tongue traction was performed by an ICU nurse. A 5.1 mm OD fiberscope was introduced orally and guided successfully through the larynx into the trachea under indirect visualization. A 7.5 mm ID endotracheal tube was advanced easily over the bronchoscope into the trachea. The endotracheal tube was positioned 3 cm above the carina and taped 22 cm at the teeth. The endotracheal

tube pilot balloon was inflated and a ventilation bag was used to ventilate the patient. A colorimetric CO_2 indicator further confirmed endotracheal placement of endotracheal tube.

30.7 OTHER CONSIDERATIONS

30.7.1 Outline your postintubation management

The patient's endotracheal tube was connected to the ventilator, and mechanical ventilation in a volume-control mode was begun.[20] As the patient's blood pressure and heart rate remained stable, the infusion of propofol was continued for patient sedation.

The airway management team proceeded to remove their PPE. Utmost care was taken to remove the gloves, gown, PAPR head gear, goggles, cap, and shoe covers in the proper sequence so that the health care workers' bodies were not contaminated.[3] Disposable equipment was discarded while reusable equipment such as the PAPR head gear was carefully wiped down using a disinfectant agent (eg, Virox®).

Any health care workers who participated in the care of the SARS patient were advised to be on high alert for the subsequent development of any symptoms or signs of SARS.[21]

30.7.2 Would precautions for other airborne pathogens differ in any way from SARS patients?

In general, HCW at risk of coming in contact with respiratory secretions from patients with febrile respiratory illness of unknown etiology should wear personal protection equipment including gloves, goggle, gown, and N-95 face mask.

As indicated earlier, the influenza A H1N1 virus (also known as swine flu) caused a worldwide pandemic with over 375,000 confirmed cases and over 4500 deaths in 2009.[21] The case-fatality ratio is significantly lower than SARS. Because it is a new virus, people have no immunity and can be infected upon exposure. The spectrum of clinical manifestation includes fever, cough, sore throat, malaise, myalgia, headache, and, occasionally, gastrointestinal symptoms. Fortunately, most patients diagnosed with H1N1 run a benign course, and rarely present with a severe pneumonia/ARDS picture.

The WHO recommends the following infection control measures[1]:

1. Before any contact with a patient with suspected H1N1 infection, basic PPE including surgical face mask gloves, goggle, and gown should be used.

2. For high-risk aerosol-generating procedures such as intubation or bronchoscopy, in addition to basic PPE, a N-95 face mask should be used.

Two antiviral drugs for influenza, oseltamivir and zanamivir, are available for treatment of pandemic influenza. Their efficacy in H1N1 infections is unknown as there are insufficient clinical data. An H1N1 vaccine has recently become available.

30.8 SUMMARY

In summary, the SARS epidemic and the recent H1N1 pandemic illustrate the rapidity and severity with which a new virus can strike worldwide. A global surveillance system for new infections and a national coordinated response must be in place should future viral infection alerts occur. There is a need in our health care system for emphasis on and compliance with ordinary infection-control measures such as hand washing, and the use of gloves, masks, and eye protection. Health care workers should be familiar, and hospitals must be equipped, with enhanced personal protection equipment should the need arise to care for suspected SARS patients. In order to minimize the risk of contamination and SARS transmission, they should be aware of the modifications of techniques for intubation. Much of what we have learned from the SARS epidemic can be used to improve our management of patients affected by viral or infectious outbreaks in the future.

REFERENCES

1. Pandemic (H1N1) 2009—update 72 http://www.who.int/csr/don/2009_10_30/en/index.html. Accessed October 31, 2009.
2. Chow KY, Lee CE, Ling ML, Heng DM, Yap SG: Outbreak of severe acute respiratory syndrome in a tertiary hospital in Singapore, linked to an index patient with atypical presentation: epidemiological study. *BMJ*. 2004;328:195.
3. Peng PW, Wong DT, Bevan D, Gardam M: Infection control and anesthesia: lessons learned from the Toronto SARS outbreak. *Can J Anaesth*. 2003;50:989-997.
4. Varia M, Wilson S, Sarwal S, et al: Investigation of a nosocomial outbreak of severe acute respiratory syndrome (SARS) in Toronto, Canada. *CMAJ*. 2003;169:285-292.
5. WHO: Summary of probable SARS cases with onset of illness from 1 November 2002 to 31 July 2003. http://www.who.int/csr/sars/country/table2004_04_21/en/. Accessed April 11, 2009.
6. Poutanen SM, Low DE, Henry B, et al: Identification of severe acute respiratory syndrome in Canada. *N Engl J Med*. 2003;348:1995-2005.
7. Shen Z, Ning F, Zhou W, et al: Superspreading SARS events, Beijing, 2003. *Emerg Infect Dis*. 2004;10:256-260.
8. Fowler RA, Guest CB, Lapinsky SE, et al: Transmission of severe acute respiratory syndrome during intubation and mechanical ventilation. *Am J Respir Crit Care Med*. 2004;169:1198-1202.
9. Loeb M, McGeer A, Henry B, et al: SARS among critical care nurses, Toronto. *Emerg Infect Dis*. 2004;10:251-255.
10. Scales DC, Green K, Chan AK, et al: Illness in intensive care staff after brief exposure to severe acute respiratory syndrome. *Emerg Infect Dis*. 2003;9:1205-1210.
11. WHO: Case definition for surveillance of Severe Acute Respiratory Syndrome (SARS). http://www.who.int/csr/sars/casedefinition/en/. Accessed April 11, 2009.
12. Booth CM, Matukas LM, Tomlinson GA, et al: Clinical features and short-term outcomes of 144 patients with SARS in the greater Toronto area. *JAMA*. 2003;289:2801-2809.
13. Choi KW, Chau TN, Tsang O, et al: Outcomes and prognostic factors in 267 patients with severe acute respiratory syndrome in Hong Kong. *Ann Intern Med*. 2003;139:715-723.
14. Lew TW, Kwek TK, Tai D, et al: Acute respiratory distress syndrome in critically ill patients with severe acute respiratory syndrome. *JAMA*. 2003;290:374-380.
15. Caplan RA, Benumof JL, Berry FA, et al: Practice Guidelines for management of the difficult airway. An updated report by the American Society of Anesthesiologists task force on management of the difficult airway. *Anesthesiology*. 2003;98:1269-1277.
16. Ofner M, Lem M, Sarwal S, Vearncombe M, Simor A: Cluster of severe acute respiratory syndrome cases among protected health care workers-Toronto, April 2003. *Can Commun Dis Rep*. 2003;29:93-97.
17. Kamming D, Gardam M, Chung F: Anaesthesia and SARS. *Br J Anaesth*. 2003;90:715-718.
18. Wong DT: Protection protocol in intubation of suspected SARS patients. *Can J Anaesth*. 2003;50:747-748.
19. Chee VW, Khoo ML, Lee SF, Lai YC, Chin NM: Infection control measures for operative procedures in severe acute respiratory syndrome-related patients. *Anesthesiology*. 2004;100:1394-1398.
20. Yam LY, Chen RC, Zhong NS: SARS: ventilatory and intensive care. *Respirology*. 2003;8 Suppl:S31-35.
21. Clinical management of human infection with new influenza A (H1N1) virus: Initial guidance. http://www.who.int/csr/resources/publications/swineflu/clinical_management/en/index.html. Accessed October 31, 2009.

SELF-EVALUATION QUESTIONS

30.1. Which of the following is considered the basic personal protection equipment in managing a patient with SARS?

A. N-95 or equivalent face mask

B. contact: gloves, gown, hat, shoe covers

C. eye protection: goggles or face shields

D. pens, pagers, or personal items should not be brought into or out of the room

E. all of the above

30.2. All of the following principles in managing the airway of a patient with SARS are true **EXCEPT**:

A. Awake bronchoscopic intubation is the preferred airway technique for all SARS patients with a potential difficult laryngoscopic intubation.

B. Intubation should be undertaken by an experienced airway practitioner, wearing full protection.

C. It is necessary to reduce the risk of aerosolization of SARS droplets during the process of intubation.

D. It is critical that the health care workers apply and remove personal protection equipment prior to and after intubating the patient.

E. Bag-mask-ventilation, nebulization, and application of topical airway anesthesia are to be avoided.

30.3. All of the following should be in the airway management team for patients with SARS **EXCEPT**:

A. an experienced airway practitioner

B. an experienced surgeon for a surgical airway

C. an experienced paramedic

D. an ICU nurse

E. a respiratory therapist

CHAPTER (31)

Performing an Elective Percutaneous Dilational Tracheotomy in a Patient on Mechanical Ventilation

Angelina Guzzo, Liane B Johnson, and Orlando R. Hung

31.1 CASE PRESENTATION

A 28-year-old, previously healthy woman was thrown off an all terrain vehicle (ATV) and sustained blunt trauma to her chest. Her injuries included a flail chest with fractures of the right first and second ribs, a pulmonary contusion, as well as a right femur fracture and ruptured spleen. Following a splenectomy on the first night, she stabilized hemodynamically and subsequently underwent an open reduction internal fixation of the femur. On the 10th day, she failed an extubation attempt due to hypoxemia. Currently she is being ventilated with a pressure support of 12 cm H_2O, positive end-expiratory pressure (PEEP) of 5 cm H_2O, and FiO_2 0.50. Her ABG shows pH 7.47, PCO_2 37, PO_2 60, and HCO_3 26 torr. Her respiratory rate is 20 breaths per minute (bpm). All other vital signs are stable. You have been consulted to help perform a tracheotomy.

31.2 INTRODUCTION

31.2.1 Why would you perform a tracheotomy on this patient?

Local changes occur in airway mucosal surfaces following as little as 2 hours of endotracheal intubation. These pathophysiologic changes include a well-documented progression of mucosal ulceration, pressure necrosis, granulation tissue with subsequent healing, fibrosis, and occasionally stenosis.[1,2] There exists no consensus on the ideal timing of performing a tracheotomy in the hope of minimizing long-term airway complications,[3] but standard practice dictates a range of 7 to 10 days following the initial intubation. Griffiths et al did a meta-analysis of five studies on early (0-7 days) versus late (= 8 days) tracheotomy.[4] No difference was shown in mortality and risk of pneumonia. Early tracheotomy decreased length of stay in the intensive care unit (ICU) and length of artificial ventilation. Dunham and Ransom showed no difference in mortality, pneumonia, or ventilator/ICU stay between early versus late tracheotomy except in patients with severe brain injury.[5] Thus, if prolonged intubation is predicted based on patient circumstances, such as a high spinal cord injury, then earlier conversion to tracheotomy may be considered.

31.2.2 What are the advantages of a tracheotomy over a prolonged translaryngeal intubation?

The potential advantages of a tracheotomy over a prolonged translaryngeal intubation include less direct endolaryngeal injury, a potentially decreased risk of nosocomial pneumonia in certain patient subgroups,[3,6] more effective pulmonary toilet, and possibly decreased airway resistance for promoting weaning from mechanical ventilation. Additional benefits include improved patient comfort, communication and mobility, increased airway security, decreased requirements for sedation, better nutrition, and earlier discharge from ICU.[7]

31.3 AIRWAY CONSIDERATIONS

31.3.1 If a tracheotomy is going to be performed anyway, why is it important to know whether this patient has a difficult airway or anatomical features associated with difficult laryngoscopic intubation?

In fact, it is *extremely* important to assess the airway prior to performing a tracheotomy. When performing either a surgical tracheotomy (ST) or a percutaneous dilational tracheotomy (PDT), during the procedure the indwelling endotracheal tube (ETT) must be carefully withdrawn above the tracheotomy site to accommodate insertion of the tracheostomy tube. During this maneuver there is a potential risk of premature extubation and need for controlled ventilation and reintubation. Ultimately, preparing for a successful procedure requires a thorough chart review, patient airway assessment, proper equipment preparation (including the difficult airway cart if the patient has a history of difficult laryngoscopic intubation), and proper patient positioning. Attention to these factors and having qualified, briefed assistants will help minimize the need for emergency airway access should unanticipated difficulty arise.

While the importance of assessment and preparation is well accepted in airway management, the dynamic nature of the upper airway anatomy is often overlooked. Surgical procedures or radiotherapy that alters skeletal or soft tissues of the head and neck can change the upper airway anatomy, making laryngoscopic intubation difficult. A high index of suspicion should be applied to patients who have undergone recent surgery of the temporomandibular joints and mandible, reconstructive orthognathic or cosmetic surgery, fusion of the cervical spine, or patients with severe burns to the head and neck.[8,9] For example, Coonan et al[10] reported a patient with an unanticipated difficult laryngoscopy secondary to contracture of the temporalis muscle causing ankylosis of the jaw several weeks following a temporal craniotomy. Many patients presenting for tracheotomy will have undergone recent surgery; in evaluating these patients, the potential for such dynamic changes to what may previously have been an easily managed airway should always be considered.

31.3.2 How would you assess this patient's airway?

The patient's chart should be reviewed to determine if there is a history of difficult laryngoscopic intubation or difficult bag-mask-ventilation. Chapter 1 has reviewed anatomic and physiologic factors which may predict difficulty with each. The neck should also be assessed for C-spine stability and other factors that could create difficult surgical conditions such as cervical flexion deformity, obesity, previous neck surgery or radiation therapy, active neck infection, or tumor.

31.4 PREPARATION AND TECHNIQUES

31.4.1 Describe the anatomy of the airway with respect to performing a percutaneous dilational tracheotomy

Surgical access to the airway through the trachea requires knowledge and recognition of surface anatomy landmarks of the larynx as well as the important adjacent structures in the neck. Most importantly, dexterity and familiarity with flexible bronchoscopy is essential as a guide to safely complete a PDT.

Easily palpable landmarks in the anterior neck include the following: the hyoid is situated high in the neck, just below the submental space, and provides a primary suspensory role for the airway; the thyroid notch, most prominent in adult males, identifies the superior aspect of the thyroid cartilage; the cricoid cartilage is the only complete ring and is bridged by the cricothyroid membrane to the inferior portion of the thyroid cartilage (Figure 31-1). With the neck extended, palpation inferiorly from the cricoid cartilage may reveal proximal tracheal rings and the thyroid gland. The vocal cords are protected by the body of the thyroid cartilage anteriorly and attach to the arytenoid cartilages which articulate from the posterosuperior margin of the cricoid ring.

An experienced practitioner must perform flexible bronchoscopy to identify the level of important internal laryngeal structures

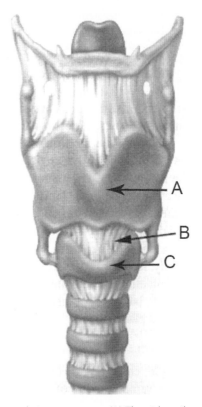

FIGURE 31-1. Surgical airway anatomy. (A) Thyroid cartilage. (B) Cricothyroid membrane. (C) Cricoid cartilage. Provided with permission from Walts et al (ref. 14).

(supraglottis, glottis, and subglottis) and to transilluminate the area between the second to fourth tracheal rings. In patients with poorly palpable surface anatomy, transillumination and visual confirmation of the guide needle will ensure proper positioning of the tracheostomy tube.

31.4.2 Compare and contrast the different sites at which surgical airway access can be performed

Surgical access to the airway can be gained at the cricothyroid space, subcricoid space, or between any of the tracheal rings. To secure an emergency airway rapidly, a cricothyrotomy is preferable because the cricothyroid membrane is superficial, easily identifiable, and thus easiest to access (see Chapter 13).[3] Controversy has existed about the long-term use of cricothyrotomy due to early reports of subglottic stenosis, limiting its use to emergency airway access.[11] However, reexploration of this notion in a recent prospective study involving 118 patients has shown the incidence and severity of complications to be similar between traditional tracheotomy and cricothyrotomy techniques.[11]

The first modern-day surgical tracheotomy (ST) performed by Chevalier Jackson in the early 1900s involved entering the trachea at the second or third tracheal ring.[12] He advocated avoiding the first and second tracheal rings due to a high incidence of subsequent subglottic stenosis.[13] Current consensus dictates that in ideal circumstances a tracheotomy is performed between tracheal rings two to four. Injury to the first ring or cricoid cartilage may increase the risk of subglottic stenosis, whereas placement too low may predispose to erosion of the anterior tracheal wall and possible creation of a tracheoinnominate fistula.[14]

The first percutaneous tracheotomy not requiring neck dissection was described in 1955 by Shelden,[15] during which a slotted needle was introduced blindly into the tracheal lumen. Several deaths occurred secondary to laceration of vital structures in proximity to the airway.[16] Toye and Weinstein[17] performed the first tracheotomy using a Seldinger technique where a single, tapered dilator was introduced with a recessed cutting blade. In 1985, Ciaglia[18] introduced a dilational Seldinger technique which has since been refined and has now become one of the most popular techniques for PDT.[19] Initially, PDT was performed in the immediate subcricoid space,[18] but in a follow-up publication the space between the first and second tracheal rings was advocated.[20] But, the more distal approach (beyond the second ring) was not recommended due to the risk of bleeding from the thyroid isthmus[20] or from puncture of an aberrant, high-riding innominate artery.

31.4.3 Describe the different techniques used to perform an elective surgical airway (for techniques to manage an emergency surgical airway, refer to Chapter 13)

31.4.3.1 Surgical Tracheotomy

ST is usually performed under general anesthesia in the operating room. The neck is extended to elevate the trachea into the neck (Figure 31-1). Depending on the length of the patient's neck, a horizontal incision is generally made crossing the midline approximately 2 cm above the sternal notch. The subcutaneous tissue and platysma muscle are divided transversely. The remainder of the dissection is performed longitudinally through the superficial cervical fascia and the linea alba dividing the strap muscles. Lateral retraction of the strap muscles often reveals the thyroid isthmus, which is commonly divided to provide better surgical access and to minimize the risk of bleeding by its manipulation.[14] Various types of tracheal incisions have been used. Quite frequently a superiorly based Bjork flap or window is made by unroofing the second or third tracheal ring.

To avoid damaging the indwelling ETT cuff during tracheotomy, it is a common practice to deflate the cuff and purposely advance the ETT distally into the right mainstem bronchus prior to making an incision in the trachea. Following tracheal access, the ETT is withdrawn under direct vision to just above the tracheotomy site by the airway practitioner. Superior retraction on the cephalad tracheal ring with a tracheal hook and spreading of the tracheal incision facilitates subsequent insertion of the tracheostomy tube.

Endotracheal positioning is confirmed by connecting the tracheostomy tube to the ventilatory circuit and monitoring for the presence of end-tidal CO_2. These final measures, in addition to assessing lung compliance and airway pressures, are ascertained prior to the complete removal of the ETT. The tracheostomy tube is then secured with sutures, and a tie passed around the neck.[14]

31.4.3.2 Percutaneous Dilational Tracheotomy

The PDT technique is easily performed at the bedside with two operators: one performing the tracheotomy while the second provides ventilation and oxygenation. It is essential to continuously monitor vital signs including pulse oximetry, blood pressure, heart rate, and rhythm. The patient should be ventilated with 100% oxygen throughout the procedure. The patient's current sedative regime can be supplemented with an opioid and an intravenous sedative/hypnotic such as a benzodiazepine or propofol.[21] It is important to maintain immobility during insertion of the needle to prevent inadvertent puncture of the posterior tracheal wall or coughing during the insertion of the tracheotomy tube, for example, through the use of a nondepolarizing muscle relaxant, such as rocuronium. For continued mechanical ventilation during the procedure, the cuff of the ETT is deflated and adjustments to tidal volume, respiratory rate, and PEEP are made to compensate for the air leak. At our institution, the patient is manually ventilated with a bag-mask device and 100% oxygen throughout.

Flexible bronchoscopy through the ETT to facilitate PDT insertion was introduced in 1989.[22] Bronchoscopy allows visualization of the needle entering the trachea, helping to confirm its location in the midline at the correct tracheal interspace, as well as ensuring that the ETT is not punctured or impaled and minimizing the risk of damaging the posterior tracheal wall.[19] In the case of accidental premature extubation, the bronchoscope can also be used to guide ETT reinsertion. There may also be a role for videoscopic bronchoscopy during teaching as there is a learning curve to performing PDT.[16] The disadvantages of flexible bronchoscopy include difficulties with ventilation and oxygenation leading to hypercarbia and hypoxia[19] and the potential for damage to the bronchoscope by the needle or guidewire.

Adjuncts, such as ultrasound and capnography, are increasingly being used to aid successful PDT. Ultrasound can help to determine the site of tracheal puncture prior to PDT, identifying structures at risk of hemorrhage such as variant arterial anatomy, primarily an aberrant innominate artery.[23] Kollig et al used ultrasound to determine the site of puncture followed by bronchoscopy; ultrasound findings changed the tracheal puncture site in 24% of the procedures.[24] Portable monitors are now available to quantify CO_2 at the bedside. Capnography and bronchoscopy have been shown to be equally effective to confirm tracheal needle placement.[25]

Prior to tracheal puncture, the ETT must be withdrawn to avoid cuff laceration or ETT impalement. Besides bronchoscopy, alternative methods have been advocated to confirm adequate ETT withdrawal before tracheal puncture. These include use of direct laryngoscopy with a tube exchanger, ETT cuff palpation, and premeasured blind withdrawal.[19] In 2000, our group described a technique using the Trachlight™ (Laerdal Medical Inc., Wappingers Fall, NY), a common and inexpensive intubation device, as an alternative to bronchoscopy to facilitate the PDT.

With the internal stiff wire removed from the Trachlight™, the pliable lightwand device is advanced into the ETT. In order to place the lightbulb of the Trachlight™ at the tip of the ETT, the number markings on the Trachlight™ wand shaft must be lined up with those on the ETT. Anterior neck transillumination[26] can then be used to confirm adequate withdrawal of the ETT prior to the needle puncture.

Since the original report of PDT by Ciaglia, the procedure has undergone three modifications. These include the movement of the tracheal cannulation site to one or two interspaces caudal to the cricoid cartilage; the use of bronchoscopy and the use of a single, bevelled dilator instead of multiple dilators.[19] While currently several kits are available for the Ciaglia single dilator technique, only the Ciaglia Blue Rhino™ kit (Cook Critical Care, Bloomington, IN) will be presented.

Under optimal conditions, the neck is extended and the surgical field is aseptically prepared (Figure 31-2A). The tracheostomy tube cuff must be checked for leaks and then well lubricated. The first or second tracheal interspace is located and local anesthetic injected (Figure 31-2B). A vertical skin incision is made in the

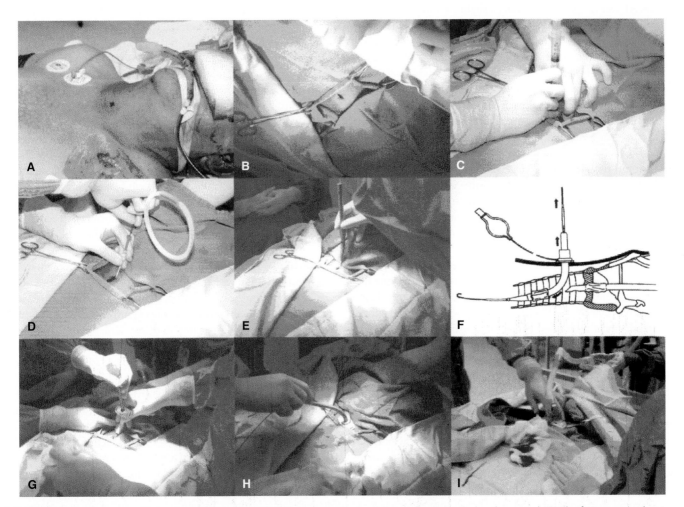

FIGURE 31-2. Percutaneous dilational tracheotomy. (A) Monitors are applied and the neck is extended and prepped. (B) The first or second tracheal interspace is identified. (C) An introducer needle is inserted with a syringe and aspirated until a free flow of air is obtained. (D) A J-tipped guide wire is guided into the trachea through the needle. (E) A dilator is advanced over the guide wire. (F and G) The tracheostomy tube is then inserted over the dilator and guide wire, and the tracheostomy tube and dilator are advanced as a unit into the trachea. (H) The dilator is then removed leaving the tracheostomy tube in situ. (I) The cuff of the tracheostomy tube is inflated and connected to the ventilator.
Fig 31-2F provided with permission from Cook Critical Care, Bloomington, IN.

midline from the level of the cricoid cartilage downward 1 to 1.5 cm. The wound is dissected bluntly to the subcutaneous fascia using a hemostat. The ETT should be withdrawn to 1 cm above the anticipated needle insertion site under bronchoscopic guidance. A 17-gauge sheathed introducer needle is advanced in a midline, posterior, and caudad direction. The tracheal air column is identified when air is aspirated into a fluid-filled syringe (eg, 2-3 mL of lidocaine) (Figure 31-2C). At this time the ETT is advanced and withdrawn 1 cm to verify that the needle does not concomitantly move, to rule out inadvertent impalement of the ETT. The outer sheath is then advanced into the trachea while the introducer needle is removed. The fluid-filled syringe is then reattached to the sheath and its position in the trachea is reconfirmed by free flow of air. To minimize the responses to the subsequent insertion of the dilator, the lidocaine in the syringe is instilled into the trachea. The syringe is removed and a 1.32 mm diameter J-tipped guide wire is advanced through the sheath into the trachea (Figure 31-2D). The sheath is then removed. Although not specified by the manufacturer, in our experience, it is beneficial to make a second cut around the guide wire with the scalpel to provide room for the dilator. A short 14 French introducing mini-dilator is advanced over the guide wire using a slight twisting motion and then removed. The Ciaglia Blue Rhino™ dilator, after soaking in water, is then advanced over the guide wire while maintaining the wire position (Figure 31-2E). The dilator and guide wire are advanced together into the trachea up to the black skin level mark. The dilator is withdrawn and advanced several times to help create the stoma, whereupon it is removed. The lubricated tracheostomy tube with its internal dilator is then inserted over the guide wire and advanced as a unit until it reaches the flange (Figure 31-2F and G). The guide wire and dilator are then removed, leaving the tracheostomy tube in situ (Figure 31-2H). The cuff is inflated and the tracheostomy tube's proximal connector is attached to the ventilator (Figure 31-2I). Once insertion into the trachea has been confirmed by end-tidal CO_2 detection, the translaryngeal ETT is removed.

Other PDT techniques have been developed.[7,19] The Rapitrach kit (Surgitech Medical, Sydney, Australia) used a dilating tracheotome with blades designed to slide over the guidewire into the trachea. To create a stoma, it was necessary to squeeze the blades open.[27] Unfortunately, the Rapitrach method resulted in a high rate of posterior tracheal wall and balloon cuff tears and was removed from the US market.[19] The Griggs technique uses a Howard-Kelly forceps that is introduced into the tracheal lumen with the guidewire.[28] A stoma is created when the forceps are opened, similar to the Rapitrach method, but without a cutting blade. This technique is popular in South America and Europe.[19] A third method is a translaryngeal approach developed by Fantoni and Ripamonti.[29] With this technique, a guide wire is inserted retrograde into the tracheal space and pulled out through the mouth. A trocar and tracheostomy tube with a pointed tip is then advanced over the wire and with traction applied to the guidewire, the trochar-tracheotosmy tube assembly is advanced through the mouth into the trachea. A pretracheal incision is then made over the skin so that the trocar end of the tracheostomy tube can be pulled through the anterior neck.

The trocar is then cut away leaving the tracheostomy tube in place. This technique avoids the downward direction of dilation and thus may minimize damage to the posterior tracheal wall.[19] A fourth method uses a single dilator from the Percutwist™ Tracheostomy Dilator Set (Rüsch, Kernen, Germany). This procedure uses a Seldinger technique in which a hydrophilically coated Percutwist™ dilator is moistened and advanced over a guide wire with a twisting motion to enlarge an opening in the anterior tracheal wall. A 9.0 mm ID tracheostomy tube is fitted with the insertion dilator and subsequently advanced over the guidewire into the trachea.[30] The Percutwist™ has had a higher rate of posterior wall puncture than the Ciaglia Blue Rhine technique.[31]

31.4.4 Describe and compare different tracheostomy tubes. Which tube would you choose for this patient?

In selecting a tracheostomy tube, patient anatomy and ventilatory needs must be considered. These needs will influence choice of tube internal diameter, length, cuff design, use of an inner cannula, and presence or absence of fenestrations. Sizing usually refers to the inner diameter (ID). The smallest outer diameter that satisfies the requirement for ventilation should be chosen.[14] Optimal sizing should aim for a tracheostomy tube approximately three-quarters of the diameter of the tracheal lumen.

In our case presentation, the indication for tracheotomy is prolonged intubation and ventilation, so a cuffed tube which seals the airway and prevents loss of tidal volume would be a good selection. One example of such a cannula is the No. 6 (6.0 mm ID) Shiley (Mallinckrodt, St. Louis, MO) with a large-volume, low-pressure, air-filled cuff[14] (Figure 31-3B). It is important to maintain an inflated cuff pressure of less than 30 cm H_2O to prevent tracheal mucosal ischemia and minimize the risk of erosion. Once the patient is weaned from the ventilator, conversion to a fenestrated tube (Figure 31-3C) might be appropriate because it reduces resistance to flow of air through the lumen of the tube, enabling vocalization.[14] Another option is to downsize the nonfenestrated tracheostomy tube which would also permit the patient to vocalize, while minimizing the risk of granulation tissue formation at the site of the fenestration. Excessive granulation tissue can cause tracheostomy tube obstruction and may also produce impressive bleeding from the airway. But, in general, the choice of a tracheostomy tube is often based on the practitioner's individual experience and preference.

Special consideration must be given to the obese patient. Standard tracheostomy tubes are unlikely to conform to the anatomy and thus a better choice is a flexible tube which is extra long and adjustable,[14] such as Bivona (Bivona Medical Technologies, Gary, IN) or Tracoe (TRACOE Medical GmbH, Frankfurt, Germany) tracheostomy tubes. The disadvantage of these tubes is that they have a single lumen without an inner cannula. They do have an advantage of minimizing risks of an inappropriately fitted tube, such as tube obstruction if too short, or necrosis of the anterior tracheal wall if too long.

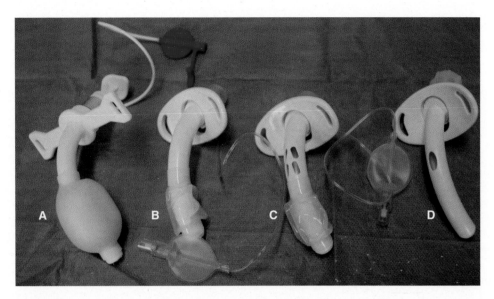

FIGURE 31-3. Tracheostomy tubes. (A) Bivona Foam-Cuf silicone tube (Bivona Medical Technologies, Gary, IN). (B) Shiley-cuffed nonfenestrated tube. (C) Shiley-cuffed fenestrated tube. (D) Shiley-uncuffed fenestrated tube (Shiley Mallinckrodt, St. Louis, MO).

31.4.5 What are the advantages of performing percutaneous dilational tracheotomy over surgical tracheotomy?

In general, the complications of PDT are few and are comparable to ST.[32] Theoretical advantages of PDT include a smaller skin incision, less dissection, and tissue trauma which may lead to less hemorrhage, fewer infections, fewer tracheal problems, and fewer cosmetic deformities. In addition, the procedure can be performed at the bedside in the ICU, by nonsurgical personnel, decreasing the risk of patient transport to the operating room with less overall cost and less use of human resources.[13,20,33] The disadvantages of performing PDT in the ICU relate mainly to lack of proper facilities and equipment. Poor lighting conditions and a crowded environment can also be hazardous. These risks can be minimized by proper preparation of a surgical set that includes drapes, tracheostomy tubes of various sizes, portable electrocautery, and a surgical lamp. A difficult airway cart should also be immediately available with appropriate anesthetic drugs, including muscle relaxants.

31.5 COMPLICATIONS

31.5.1 What are the contraindications to performing a percutaneous dilational tracheotomy?

Physiologic contraindications to PDT include a patient who is hemodynamically unstable, requires an FiO_2 greater than 0.60,

PEEP greater than 10 cm H_2O^6, or has an uncontrolled coagulopathy.[3] Anatomic contraindications include a previously documented difficult tracheal intubation, morbid obesity, obscure cervical anatomy, goiter, short thick neck, previous tracheotomy or neck surgery, cervical infection, facial and cervical trauma and fractures, halo traction, or known presence of subglottic stenosis.[3,6] However, PDT has been successfully performed in the morbidly obese and in those who had a previous tracheotomy.[34]

31.5.2 What are the complications of percutaneous dilational versus surgical tracheotomy?

Complications common to both percutaneous dilational tracheotomy (PDT) and surgical tracheotomy (ST) are listed in Table 31-1 and are summarized in a recent review by Engels et al.[35]

Three recent meta-analyses have been published comparing PDT to ST. Delaney et al identified 17 randomized trials with 1212 patients and concluded that PDT resulted in significantly fewer infections compared to ST.[36] In a pooled data analysis with 973 patients from 15 randomized control trials, Higgins and Punthakee also found that PDT had fewer wound infections, as well as less scarring and lower costs than ST. This difference was lost when only bedside procedures were considered. PDT did result in more decannulation and obstruction problems than ST.[37] Oliver et al analyzed 14 prospective and randomized controlled studies with 1273 patients and showed more early, minor complications with PDT than with bedside ST, but no difference in late complications.[38]

TABLE 31-1

Complications of Tracheotomy

INTRAOPERATIVE	POSTOPERATIVE (<24 HOURS)	UP TO 2 WEEKS	WEEKS TO MONTHS
Damage to great vessels	Tube dislodgement with loss of airway	Peristomal cellulitis	Suprastomal or tracheal granulation tissue with airway obstruction
Injury to posterior tracheal wall	Tube occlusion by dried secretions	Stomal granulation tissue	Poor stomal healing
Injury to cupula of lung with pneumothorax	Stomal hemorrhage	Stomal hemorrhage	Subglottic or tracheal stenosis
Tracheal ring rupture	Cuff leak		Tracheomalacia
Recurrent laryngeal nerve injury			Tracheoesophageal fistula
Paratracheal insertion			Tracheoinnominate fistula
Fire in the airway			

Source: References 3, 6, 14.

31.6   POSTTRACHEOTOMY MANAGEMENT

31.6.1   What should be done immediately after the placement of a PDT?

Following insertion of the tracheostomy tube, one must ensure that the tube is properly positioned and well secured until the tract has healed, in approximately 7 days. Because PDT is a dilational technique, creation of a false passage may easily occur. Should accidental decannulation occur within the first 7 days of PDT, and if a tracheal tube is needed, an oral ETT should be immediately placed instead of attempting reinsertion of a tracheostomy tube through the stoma.[39] Chest x-ray following the procedure is somewhat controversial; studies have shown that the incidence of pneumothorax following endoscopically guided PDT is less than 3%, although when nonguided, it may range up to 12%.[40] However, because no strong prospective data exist at this time, recommendations to exclude a routine chest x-ray cannot be made.

31.6.2   Discuss the special care of a tracheostomy tube

Surgical cannulation of the trachea will cause an increase in secretion production requiring frequent suctioning.[39] The suction catheter should be measured such that suctioning beyond the tip of the tracheostomy tube is not performed. If this simple measure is followed, then subsequent risks of deep suctioning will be eliminated. The potential trauma from deep suctioning includes tracheal excoriation, bleeding, ulceration and tracheitis, production of granulation tissue, and scarring of the bronchi and carina.

Creation of a tracheotomy bypasses the nose, so supplemental humidity and filtering of the air must be provided.[39] Humidity, in conjunction with tracheal irrigation, will help prevent encrusting of tracheal secretions and minimize mucus plugging of the tracheostomy tube. A filter may be placed on the tracheostomy tube to remove particulate matter in the air and from the ventilator.

The first tracheostomy tube change should be done once the tract is sufficiently mature to minimize the risk of creating a false passage. Although the timing varies with each center, it is generally done 5 to 7 days after an ST.[41] However, in our institution, the first tracheostomy tube change is done as early as 3 days. The first change after a PDT is usually at 7 days as the initial stoma is smaller and only created by a puncture.

31.7   SPECIAL CONSIDERATIONS

31.7.1   Should percutaneous dilational tracheotomy be performed in the pediatric population?

Traditionally PDT is not recommended for individuals younger than 16 years of age, the main drawbacks being the small airway diameter and the pronounced pliability of the cartilaginous framework. Fantoni and Ripamonti[42] have tried three different techniques in the pediatric population, one of which consisted of PDT guided by rigid bronchoscopy. This eliminated the main cartilaginous compliance issue seen in the pediatric population and elevated the trachea to a more superficial position, enabling cannulation. Ultimately, any technique used in the pediatric population should be performed in the operating room with specialized surgical staff and anesthesia support. Although the percutaneous dilational technique is still considered experimental in the pediatric patient population, in experienced hands and with the use of a rigid bronchoscope, an overall reduction in complications has been noted. These include smaller operative incisions in the skin and trachea, less blood loss, and virtual elimination of pleural dome injury and posterior wall trauma.[42]

31.7.2 Can you perform a PDT in a patient with subglottic stenosis?

Subglottic stenosis (SGS) is a known late complication of prolonged intubation or any type of tracheotomy. However, little has been published on the use of PDT in a patient with SGS. SGS is a graded problem, ranging from mild asymptomatic stenosis to complete obstruction. If the stenosis exceeds 50% to 75% of the lumen diameter, then the patient may be quite symptomatic, possibly requiring acute airway intervention. In known cases of SGS, optimal airway control may be achieved with an extra long, small, noncuffed pediatric ETT, or more likely a controlled tracheotomy performed on an awake patient or over a rigid bronchoscope.

It would be most imprudent to undertake PDT in the face of SGS as the vertical length, or thickness, of the stenosis may not be known even if the diameter is not significantly narrowed. To maximize patient safety and minimize otherwise preventable complications from PDT, this technique should not be used in a patient with known SGS.

31.7.3 What is the role of an extraglottic device in providing oxygenation and ventilation while performing the PDT?

To avoid the potential problem of an inadvertent puncture of the ETT cuff by the needle, tube transfixion, or accidental extubation, some reports suggest replacing the in situ ETT with an extraglottic device (EGD) shortly prior to the placement of the PDT. The laryngeal mask airway (LMA), intubating LMA™, LMA-ProSeal™, CobraPLA™, Airway Management device (AMD™), and the Combitube™ have all been used successfully during PDT placement during the last decade.[43-49]

While EGDs may have a theoretical advantage over the ETT in ventilating critically ill patients during PDT, they also have limitations, including difficult placement. In a prospective comparative study of PDT performed on patients with either an ETT or an LMA in situ, Ambesh et al showed that 33% of patients with LMAs during the PDT suffered potentially catastrophic complications.[50] These included loss of the airway, inadequate ventilation with hypoxemia, gastric distension, and regurgitation. In contrast, there were substantially fewer complications in the ETT group.

Until more clinical efficacy and safety data are available on the use of EGDs during PDT, in our opinion, the in situ ETT remains the best option during the procedure. In these critically ill patients who may have low lung compliance, airway edema, cervical spine instability, or a difficult airway, the ETT will provide a more secure airway during PDT. However, in the event that the airway is lost or accidental extubation occurs, EGDs may play an important role in oxygenating the patient while completing the PDT.

31.8 SUMMARY

To minimize airway complications, tracheotomy is often necessary for long-term mechanically ventilated patients in the intensive care setting. During the last two decades, elective percutaneous dilational tracheotomy (PDT) has been shown to be an effective and safe alternative to traditional surgical tracheotomy. Theoretical advantages of PDT over surgical tracheotomy include a smaller skin incision, less dissection, less tissue trauma, less hemorrhage, fewer infections, fewer tracheal problems, and less cosmetic deformity. In addition, the procedure can be performed at the bedside by nonsurgical personnel, decreasing the inherent risks of transporting patients to the operating room. However, practitioners should also be aware of the limitations and disadvantages of performing PDT in the intensive care unit. These include a lack of proper facilities and equipment, poor lighting conditions, and a crowded environment.

REFERENCES

1. Sue RD, Susanto I. Long-term complications of artificial airways. *Clin Chest Med.* 2003;24:457-471.
2. Liu H, Chen JC, Holinger LD, Gonzalez-Crussi F. Histopathologic fundamentals of acquired laryngeal stenosis. *Pediatr Pathol Lab Med.* 1995;15: 655-677.
3. Heffner JE. Tracheotomy application and timing. *Clin Chest Med.* 2003;24: 389-398.
4. Griffiths J, Barber VS, Morgan L, Young JD. Systematic review and meta-analysis of studies of the timing of tracheostomy in adult patients undergoing artificial ventilation. *BMJ.* 2005;330:1243.
5. Dunham CM, Ransom KJ. Assessment of early tracheostomy in trauma patients: a systematic review and meta-analysis. *Am Surg.* 2006;72:276-281.
6. Angel LF, Simpson CB. Comparison of surgical and percutaneous dilational tracheostomy. *Clin Chest Med.* 2003;24:423-429.
7. De Leyn P, Bedert L, Delcroix M, et al. Tracheotomy: clinical review and guidelines. *Eur J Cardiothorac Surg.* 2007;32:412-421.
8. Block C, Brechner VL. Unusual problems in airway management. II. The influence of the temporomandibular joint, the mandible, and associated structures on endotracheal intubation. *Anesth Analg.* 1971;50:114-123.
9. Boorin MR. Unanticipated difficult endotracheal intubation related to pre-existing chin implant and mandibular condylar resorption. *Anesth Analg.* 1997;84:686-689.
10. Coonan TJ, Hope CE, Howes WJ, Holness RO, MacInnis EL. Ankylosis of the temporo-mandibular joint after temporal craniotomy: a cause of difficult intubation. *Can Anaesth Soc J.* 1985;32:158-160.
11. Francois B, Clavel M, Desachy A, Puyraud S, Roustan J, Vignon P. Complications of tracheostomy performed in the ICU: subthyroid tracheostomy vs surgical cricothyroidotomy. *Chest.* 2003;123:151-158.
12. Bowen CP, Whitney LR, Truwit JD, Durbin CG, Moore MM. Comparison of safety and cost of percutaneous versus surgical tracheostomy. *Am Surg.* 2001;67:54-60.
13. Dulguerov P, Gysin C, Perneger TV, Chevrolet JC. Percutaneous or surgical tracheostomy: a meta-analysis. *Crit Care Med.* 1999;27:1617-1625.
14. Walts PA, Murthy SC, DeCamp MM. Techniques of surgical tracheostomy. *Clin Chest Med.* 2003;24:413-422.
15. Shelden CH, Pudenz RH, Freshwater DB, Crue BL. A new method for tracheotomy. *J Neurosurg.* 1955;12:428-431.
16. Powell DM, Price PD, Forrest LA. Review of percutaneous tracheostomy. *Laryngoscope.* 1998;108:170-177.
17. Toye FJ, Weinstein JD. Clinical experience with percutaneous tracheostomy and cricothyroidotomy in 100 patients. *J Trauma.* 1986;26:1034-1040.
18. Ciaglia P, Firsching R, Syniec C. Elective percutaneous dilatational tracheostomy. A new simple bedside procedure: preliminary report. *Chest.* 1985;87: 715-719.
19. deBoisblanc BP. Percutaneous dilational tracheostomy techniques. *Clin Chest Med.* 2003;24:399-407.
20. Ciaglia P, Graniero KD. Percutaneous dilatational tracheostomy. Results and long-term follow-up. *Chest.* 1992;101:464-467.
21. Schwann NM. Percutaneous dilational tracheostomy: anesthetic considerations for a growing trend. *Anesth Analg.* 1997;84:907-911.
22. Paul A, Marelli D, Chiu RC-J, Vestweber KH, Mulder DS. Percutaneous endoscopic tracheostomy. *Ann Thorac Surg.* 1989;47:314-315.
23. Al-Ansari MA, Hijazi MH. Clinical review: percutaneous dilatational tracheostomy. *Crit Care.* 2006;10:202.

24. Kollig E, Heydenreich U, Roetman B, Hopf F, Muhr G. Ultrasound and bronchoscopic controlled percutaneous tracheostomy on trauma ICU. *Injury.* 2000;31:663-668.

25. Mallick A, Venkatanath D, Elliot SC, Hollins T, Nanda Kumar CG. A prospective randomised controlled trial of capnography vs. bronchoscopy for Blue Rhino percutaneous tracheostomy. *Anaesthesia.* 2003;58:864-868.

26. Addas BM, Howes WJ, Hung OR. Light-guided tracheal puncture for percutaneous tracheostomy. *Can J Anaesth.* 2000;47:919-922.

27. Schachner A, Ovil J, Sidi J, Avram A, Levy MJ. Rapid percutaneous tracheostomy. *Chest.* 1990;98:1266-1270.

28. Griggs WM, Worthley LI, Gilligan JE, Thomas PD, Myburg JA. A simple percutaneous tracheostomy technique. *Surg Gynecol Obstet.* 1990;170:543-545.

29. Fantoni A, Ripamonti D. A non-derivative, non-surgical tracheostomy: the translaryngeal method. *Intensive Care Med.* 1997;23:386-392.

30. Frova G, Quintel M. A new simple method for percutaneous tracheostomy: controlled rotating dilation. A preliminary report. *Intensive Care Med.* 2002; 28:299-303.

31. Byhahn C, Westphal K, Meininger D, Gurke B, Kessler P, Lischke V. Single-dilator percutaneous tracheostomy: a comparison of PercuTwist and Ciaglia Blue Rhino techniques. *Intensive Care Med.* 2002;28:1262-1266.

32. Feller-Kopman D. Acute complications of artificial airways. *Clin Chest Med.* 2003;24:445-455.

33. Freeman BD, Isabella K, Lin N, Buchman TG. A meta-analysis of prospective trials comparing percutaneous and surgical tracheostomy in critically ill patients. *Chest.* 2000;118:1412-1418.

34. Ernst A, Critchlow J. Percutaneous tracheostomy—special considerations. *Clin Chest Med.* 2003;24:409-412.

35. Engels PT, Bagshaw SM, Meier M, Brindley PG. Tracheostomy: from insertion to decannulation. *Can J Surg.* 2009;52:427-433.

36. Delaney A, Bagshaw SM, Nalos M. Percutaneous dilatational tracheostomy versus surgical tracheostomy in critically ill patients: a systematic review and meta-analysis. *Crit Care.* 2006;10:R55.

37. Higgins KM, Punthakee X. Meta-analysis comparison of open versus percutaneous tracheostomy. *Laryngoscope.* 2007;117:447-454.

38. Oliver ER, Gist A, Gillespie MB. Percutaneous versus surgical tracheotomy: an updated meta-analysis. *Laryngoscope.* 2007;117:1570-1575.

39. Wright SE, VanDahm K. Long-term care of the tracheostomy patient. *Clin Chest Med.* 2003;24:473-487.

40. Gonzalez I, Bonner S. Routine chest radiographs after endoscopically guided percutaneous dilatational tracheostomy. *Chest.* 2004;125:1173-1174.

41. Tabaee A, Lando T, Rickert S, Stewart MG, Kuhel WI. Practice patterns, safety, and rationale for tracheostomy tube changes: a survey of otolaryngology training programs. *Laryngoscope.* 2007;117: 573-576.

42. Fantoni A, Ripamonti D. Tracheostomy in pediatrics patients. *Minerva Anestesiol.* 2002;68:433-442.

43. Dexter TJ. The laryngeal mask airway: a method to improve visualisation of the trachea and larynx during fibreoptic assisted percutaneous tracheostomy. *Anaesth Intensive Care.* 1994;22:35-39.

44. Lyons BJ, Flynn CG. The laryngeal mask simplifies airway management during percutaneous dilatational tracheostomy. *Acta Anaesthesiol Scand.* 1995;39: 414-415.

45. Verghese C, Rangasami J, Kapila A, Parke T. Airway control during percutaneous dilatational tracheostomy: pilot study with the intubating laryngeal mask airway. *Br J Anaesth.* 1998;81:608-609.

46. Craven RM, Laver SR, Cook TM, Nolan JP. Use of the Pro-Seal LMA facilitates percutaneous dilatational tracheostomy. *Can J Anaesth.* 2003;50:718-720.

47. Agro F, Carassiti M, Magnani C. Percutaneous dilatational cricothyroidotomy: airway control via CobraPLA. *Anesth Analg.* 2004;99:628.

48. Johnson R, Bailie R. Airway management device (AMD) for airway control in percutaneous dilatational tracheostomy. *Anaesthesia.* 2000;55:596-597.

49. Mallick A, Quinn AC, Bodenham AR, Vucevic M. Use of the Combitube for airway maintenance during percutaneous dilatational tracheostomy. *Anaesthesia.* 1998;53:249-255.

50. Ambesh SP, Sinha PK, Tripathi M, Matreja P. Laryngeal mask airway vs endotracheal tube to facilitate bedside percutaneous tracheostomy in critically ill patients: a prospective comparative study. *J Postgrad Med.* 2002;48:11-15.

SELF-EVALUATION QUESTIONS

31.1. You are an airway practitioner and have been asked to participate in a percutaneous dilational tracheotomy on the 28-year-old woman in the ICU. The surgeon has just inserted the tracheostomy tube and you are ventilating the patient using an Ambu bag through the ETT that you have pulled back to 1 cm above the tracheotomy insertion site. Once the tracheostomy tube is in place, you connect the Ambu bag to the tracheostomy tube and start to ventilate the patient. However, you notice that there is a lot of resistance to ventilation, the oxygen saturation is slowly declining, and there is some subcutaneous emphysema in the neck area. What is your immediate response?

A. Remove the tracheostomy tube and the ETT and begin BMV.

B. Tell the surgeon to reinsert the tracheostomy tube.

C. Tell the surgeon to prepare for a surgical cricothyroidotomy.

D. Remove the tracheostomy tube and push the indwelling ETT into the trachea 2 to 4 cm distally and ventilate through the ETT.

E. Assess the location of the tracheostomy tube using a fiberoptic bronchoscope.

31.2. You have secured the airway and placed the patient back on the ventilator. About 5 minutes later while you are catching up on your charting, the ventilator starts to alarm high airway pressures and the blood pressure has declined. Auscultation reveals decreased breath sounds on the right. What do you do next?

A. Administer 500 mL of Ringers lactate intravenously and vasopressor to raise the propofol-induced hypotension.

B. Call for a chest x-ray.

C. Use fiberoptic bronchoscopy to remove mucus plugs.

D. Do a needle decompression in the midclavicular line at the right second intercostal space of the chest.

31.3. Three days after the PDT was performed, as an anesthesiologist you are called urgently to the ICU because the tracheostomy tube was decannulated and despite attempts at BMV, the patient's oxygen saturation is 80%. Which of the following should you avoid?

A. Attempt BMV with two operators.

B. Insert an LMA.

C. Insert a Combitube.

D. Insert an ETT orally.

E. Reinsert the tracheostomy tube.

CHAPTER 32

Airway Management in an Uncooperative Down Syndrome Patient with an Upper GI Bleed

Michael F. Murphy

32.1 CASE PRESENTATION

This 33-year-old white female patient with Down syndrome (Figure 32-1) presented to the gastrointestinal (GI) service with a history of vomiting blood. You first encounter her when she is brought to the operating room at 22:00 hours with gross hematemesis and the general surgeon is going to attempt GI endoscopy to determine the site of bleeding and its cause, and attempts to stop it. Failing that, an open laparotomy is planned.

As she is being transferred to the operating room (OR) table, her only IV is inadvertently pulled out. In the past, she has had repeated episodes of aspiration pneumonia felt to be related to grossly carious teeth and is scheduled for a full mouth dental extraction in 2 weeks.

On examination, she is 5 ft 2 in (157.5 cm) tall and weighs 210 lb (96 kg) with a moderate developmental delay. Vital signs are: heart rate (HR) 122 beats per minute (bpm), blood pressure (BP) 100/80 mm Hg, and her oxygen saturation on *blow by oxygen* is 92% (she is combative and will not permit an oxygen mask to be applied). You suspect that she has aspirated some blood.

She is not cooperative and will not permit an IV to be restarted. She does not answer questions. She lies on her side with her head flexed forward and will not extend her neck when requested nor will she permit you to do so. She will not open her mouth as per your request and it seems that blood is everywhere.

According to the surgeon, her sister has cared for her for the past 20 years (parents are deceased). As far as her sister knows, she is perfectly healthy and has never had an anesthetic before. She is on no medication and has no allergies. Her past cardiac history is unremarkable according to the surgeon. She does not smoke.

Blood work done earlier in the day shows hemoglobin of 10.2 g/dL (102 mmol/L) and is otherwise normal.

She will require a general anesthetic with an endotracheal intubation. In addition, she is grossly uncooperative, is exhibiting some evidence of hypovolemia, has features indicative of a difficult airway, and has probably aspirated some blood.

32.2 PATIENT EVALUATION

32.2.1 What kind of vital organ system reserve does this patient have?

Cardiovascular reserve: The elevated pulse rate and the narrowed pulse pressure suggest an element of hypovolemia. You are hoping that the surgeon is correct and that she has no congenital heart disease (eg, an endocardial cushion defect).

CNS reserve: She is moderately developmentally delayed and anticipated to be combative on emergence. Her response to sedative hypnotic agents and ketamine for sedation is unpredictable.

Respiratory system reserve: She is moderately obese and is expected to have some restrictive lung disease with predictable consequences. In addition, she has probably aspirated blood and has a past history of repeated aspiration pneumonias. Her saturation on blow by oxygen is 92%. It is likely that she has limited oxygen reserves and will rapidly desaturate if she obstructs, or if she is paralyzed. Postoperative mechanical ventilation is a possibility. She is in extreme regurgitation and aspiration risk.

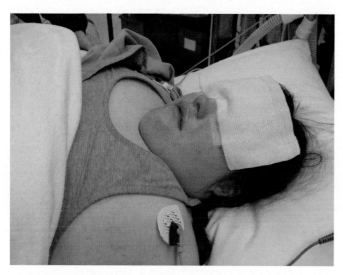

FIGURE 32-1. Patient with Down syndrome admitted to GI service department with a history of vomiting blood.

32.3   AIRWAY EVALUATION AND MANAGEMENT OPTIONS

32.3.1   Employing the mnemonics suggested in Chapter 1, does this patient have a difficult airway?

On MOANS-guided airway evaluation (see Section 1.6.1), you gain no confidence that you will be able to ventilate this patient using bag-mask-ventilation (BMV) when it becomes necessary. If her neck cannot be extended, a mask seal will be difficult. She is obese and the decrease in compliance may hinder BMV.

Employing LEMON (see Section 1.6.2) to assess the difficulty associated with laryngoscopy and intubation reveals that the *look* of this patient suggests difficulty. When you attempt to evaluate the geometry of her upper airway, you are unable to assess the volume of her mandibular space. This is particularly problematic in a person with Down syndrome (DS) in which the initial impression is that the tongue is relatively large for the volume of the mouth. You also have no idea where her larynx is relative to the base of her tongue. You are unable to evaluate a Mallampatti and get some idea as to airway access. Additionally, she is obese and you are unable to evaluate the degree of neck mobility.

The mnemonic for difficulties in using extraglottic devices (EGDs) is RODS (see Section 1.6.3). Whether there is restricted mouth opening or not is unknown. There does not appear to be any upper airway obstruction and the airway is neither distorted nor disrupted. As mentioned earlier, she is obese and the decreased compliance (stiff) may militate against successful ventilation with an EGD.

Finally, the patient should be assessed for a potentially difficult cricothyrotomy using the mnemonic SHORT (see Section 1.6.4). There is no history of prior anterior neck surgery, hematoma, or other overlying process that masks the anatomy. However, she is

obese, and in addition, one is unable to ascertain whether access to the anterior neck is possible. There is no history or evidence of radiation or tumor.

In summary, she has a potentially difficult airway and is not a candidate for a rapid-sequence induction, even though with a stomach potentially full of blood that would ordinarily be the preferred technique.

32.3.2   What other airway concerns do you have in patients with DS?

An increased incidence of subglottic stenosis in DS patients is well known.[1-4] This has been attributed, at least in part, to the increased incidence of regurgitation and aspiration in these patients during infancy and early childhood.[1] Therefore, these patients may require an endotracheal tube that is one to two sizes smaller than the standard size appropriate for the patient's age. In addition, the DS patient is predisposed to obstructive sleep apnea due to a relatively narrow nasopharynx and large tongue.[5,6]

C-spine subluxation is also seen in these patients and may be of concern in airway management.[7] Presently there is no consensus of opinion with respect to the need for preoperative radiological evaluation of the cervical spine for subluxation for patients with DS.

32.3.3   What are the airway management options?

This patient gives every indication that the management of her airway will be difficult. However, the more pressing problem is deciding how to pharmacologically manage her behavior without compromising her ability to maintain ventilation and oxygenation, to permit either an IV start and/or to gain control of the airway in a controlled fashion that minimizes the risk of aspiration.

Ideally, one would like to identify a preferable airway technique (Plan A), and two alternative methods (Plans B and C). However, with the limited airway evaluation, the most appropriate method chosen must have the *least* chance of producing apnea, aspiration, or a requirement for rapid action. In addition, the presence of copious amounts of blood in the airway is likely to render indirect visualization techniques (endoscopes, video laryngoscopes, optical stylets) to be of limited use. This really leaves one primary option for consideration: sedation and awake intubation employing a laryngoscope.

Plans B and C will likely include an EGD and the surgeon should be prepared to perform an immediate surgical airway if asked (a double set-up). One would be wise to consider the immediate availability of a lightwand (eg, Trachlight™) if the airway practitioner is sufficiently skilled in its use (see Chapter 11).

32.4   MANAGING THE AIRWAY

32.4.1   What are the pros and cons of the awake/sedated method?

Clearly the sedation and awake intubation approach is not without hazards. The use of sedative hypnotic agents in large oral or intramuscular dosages may provoke paradoxical excitement, or worse, lead to hypoventilation or apnea.

Ketamine is an attractive option. Seven mg·kg^{-1} (ideal body weight)[8-11] can be given orally with the expectation that the patient will be dissociated within 20 minutes, at least to the point that an IV can be placed. If the degree of cooperation is not sufficient after this dose, half the original dose can be repeated at 20 minutes.

Clearly this is not an option in this case. Four mg·kg^{-1} of ideal body weight IM produces reliable sedation and dissociation in approximately 5 minutes.[11-15]

The margin of safety with ketamine is greater than other sedative hypnotics, such as midazolam, as it preserves ventilatory function, muscle tone, and airway protective reflexes. The disadvantages of ketamine include the risk of laryngospasm, increase in secretions, emergence reactions, and postprocedure nausea and vomiting

32.4.2 How exactly would you manage the airway of this patient?

To prepare for airway management the neck of the patient is prepared in as sterile a fashion as the circumstances will allow and the surgeon and OR team are prepared to perform a surgical airway (double set-up). Ketamine 4 mg·kg^{-1} is then drawn up and ready to administer IM. Propofol 200 mg and succinylcholine 140 mg are also drawn up. Additionally, an assistant is prepared to place an IV on command if possible. A central line access kit is immediately available.

The following airway devices are immediately available for use:

- Styletted endotracheal tubes (ETTs) of various sizes (5, 6, and 7 mm ID)
- Two suctions with rigid suction handles
- LMA-Fastrach™ (Intubating LMA)
- Trachlight loaded onto a 7 mm ID ETT cut at 26 cm
- Video laryngoscope at the ready
- Flexible bronchoscope at the ready
- Topical local anesthetic spray (eg, 4% lidocaine in a syringe attached to a Mucosal Atomization Device [MAD])

The patient is then placed in the left lateral position on the OR table. An antisialogogue is not administered because it must be administered intramuscularly (see later). A pulse oximeter is applied when the patient permits, as is supplemental oxygen.

When all is ready, the ketamine is administered IM. Sufficient sedation/dissociation is typically achieved within 5 minutes. To permit an IV placement, gradual initiation of Sellick maneuver and an awake look is initiated. If the awake look indicates that orotracheal intubation is likely to be successful, then rapid-sequence intubation (RSI) may be performed, or if the patient is intubated immediately following the awake look, propofol can be administered rapidly after the airway is secured and confirmed. The dose of propofol administered must take into consideration the likelihood of hypovolemia.

Failure to visualize the airway adequately to intubate, or assure that intubation is possible if RSI is employed, in the face of ongoing acceptable oxygen saturations may lead one to resort to Plan B.

In the event adequate oxygen saturation cannot be maintained, a surgical airway is immediately performed.

32.4.3 How exactly was the airway of this patient managed?

After adequate sedation was achieved with IM ketamine, an awake look was performed in the left lateral decubitus position using a #3 Macintosh laryngoscope. About 50% of the glottis was visualized and tracheal intubation was achieved using a #7.0 ETT. After confirmation of the proper tracheal tube placement using end-tidal CO_2, the patient underwent volume resuscitation and sedation was carefully titrated using IV propofol. GI endoscopy revealed a bleeding duodenal ulcer. Hemostasis was achieved. The patient was transferred to the ICU intubated and ventilated for further evaluation of her presumed aspiration and ventilatory management.

32.5 ADDITIONAL CONSIDERATIONS

32.5.1 Should an antisialogogue be given when ketamine is employed?

As a general comment, antisialogogues are typically used whenever topical anesthesia of the oro- and hypopharynx is to be attempted because it minimizes the dilution of local anesthetic agent by saliva and improves the degree of topical anesthesia achieved. In this particular case, it was omitted because it would have required an IM injection.

Ketamine does stimulate tracheobronchial and salivary secretions, and this effect of the drug can potentially cause laryngospasm.[12] An antisialogogue, such as glycopyrrolate or atropine, is often given IM 15 to 20 minutes prior to the administration of ketamine to reduce these secretions. Glycopyrrolate is preferred because it produces less intense tachycardia. Unlike other tertiary-substituted antimuscarinics (scopolamine and atropine), glycopyrrolate is a polar quaternary-substituted ammonium compound, which does not cross the blood–brain barrier and therefore avoids the risk of producing confusion and sedation.

32.5.2 How common is laryngospasm with ketamine?

Laryngospasm is associated with all of the sedative hypnotics to some extent, including ketamine. The incidence of laryngospasm with ketamine is about 1% (ranging between 0.017% and 1.4% in various studies, including studies with data from over 11,000 patients).[13-16] It manifests as transient stridor. It is likely related to ketamine-induced sensitization of laryngeal reflexes, and in some cases is thought to be related to excessive upper respiratory secretions.[12] Thus, the recommendation has been made that an antisialogogue be coadministered with ketamine. Risk factors for laryngospasm include respiratory infection (fivefold increase) and age (three times greater risk in infants aged 1-3 months than the average).[17] One study of nearly 1200 pediatric patients with laryngospasm reported the incidence of complications as hypoxia 3.2%, aspiration 1.1%, and cardiac arrest 0.5%.[15]

32.5.3 How common are emergence reactions with ketamine?

Emergence delirium is the most common side effect of ketamine.[18] This response is thought to be caused by the drug's depression of CNS visual/auditory relay nuclei causing altered perception and interpretation of visual and auditory stimuli.[19] The occurrence of emergence reactions is associated with age (adults > children), gender (females > males), anxiety level, and psychological state prior to the procedure.[18,20,21] The incidence varies but may be as high as 10% to 30% in adults with a much lower occurrence in children. Severe agitation occurs in 1.6% and mild agitation in 17.6% of pediatric patients.[19] Emergence reactions are less common in older children (12.1% in those more than 5 years vs 22.5% in children under 5 years of age).[20]

Small doses of midazolam have been used to treat severe emergence reactions. However, the prophylactic coadministration of benzodiazepines is not recommended since they have no proven benefit, delay ketamine metabolism thereby prolonging recovery, may actually increase the incidence of recovery agitation in specific patient populations, and increase the risk of respiratory depression.[17,22-29]

32.5.4 Should these patients be recovered in a dark and quiet environment to prevent emergence reactions?

Whether or not a quiet, secluded environment which limits stimuli during the post-recovery period decreases the incidence of emergence reactions is debatable.[12] Some suggest that pre-procedure discussions with the patient (adult or child) have a greater impact on reducing the incidence of recovery agitation.[12,23] However, the prevailing impression is that less stimulation is advantageous.

32.5.5 How often do patients given ketamine vomit post-procedure?

Vomiting occurs in 6.7% of patients, which often persists into the recovery phase, and is also age related, being more common in younger children (12.5% incidence in children under 5 years vs 3.5% in those more than 5 years of age).[20] There have been no documented reports of clinically significant aspiration with ketamine when used in patients without contraindications.[26]

32.6 SUMMARY

This case study serves as a prototype for the uncooperative, difficult airway with a full stomach, has incipient hemodynamic instability, and is an emergency. Time to plan an approach is limited and hindered by the fact that the patient has no venous access. In an emergency, one does not have the luxury of time, and rigid adherence to the difficult and failed algorithms is advised.

Patient control is achieved with IM ketamine thereby allowing successful IV access. The difficult airway algorithm (Chapter 2) was employed to guide actions directed to managing the airway in this patient. At each step, the imperative is to ensure that adequate gas exchange occurs and one does not burn bridges.

REFERENCES

1. Boseley ME, Link DT, Shott SR, et al. Laryngotracheoplasty for subglottic stenosis in Down syndrome children: the Cincinnati experience. *Int J Pediatr Otorhinolaryngol.* 2001;57:11-15.
2. Mitchell RB, Call E, Kelly J. Diagnosis and therapy for airway obstruction in children with Down syndrome. *Arch Otolaryngol Head Neck Surg.* 2003;129:642-645.
3. Jacobs IN, Gray RF, Todd NW. Upper airway obstruction in children with Down syndrome. *Arch Otolaryngol Head Neck Surg.* 1996;122:945-950.
4. Miller R, Gray SD, Cotton RT, Myer CM, III, Netterville J. Subglottic stenosis and Down syndrome. *Am J Otolaryngol.* 1990;11:274-277.
5. Resta O, Barbaro MP, Giliberti T, et al. Sleep related breathing disorders in adults with Down syndrome. *Downs Syndr Res Pract.* 2003;8:115-119.
6. Dahlqvist A, Rask E, Rosenqvist CJ, Sahlin C, Franklin KA. Sleep apnea and Down's syndrome. *Acta Otolaryngol.* 2003;123:1094-1097.
7. Kanamori G, Witter M, Brown J, Williams-Smith L. Otolaryngologic manifestations of Down syndrome. *Otolaryngol Clin North Am.* 2000;33:1285-1292.
8. Rosenberg M. Oral ketamine for deep sedation of difficult-to-manage children who are mentally handicapped: case report. *Pediatr Dent.* 1991;13:221-223.
9. Younge PA, Kendall JM. Sedation for children requiring wound repair: a randomised controlled double blind comparison of oral midazolam and oral ketamine. *Emerg Med J.* 2001;18:30-33.
10. Turhanoglu S, Kararmaz A, Ozyilmaz MA, Kaya S, Tok D. Effects of different doses of oral ketamine for premedication of children. *Eur J Anaesthesiol.* 2003;20:56-60.
11. Zane R. The morbidly obese patient. In: Walls R, Murphy M, Luten R, Schneider R, eds. *Manual of Emergency Airway Management.* 2nd ed. Philadelphia, PA: Lippincott Williams and Wilkins; 2004:302-306.
12. Green S. Dissociative agents. In: Kraus B, Bructowicz R, eds. *Pediatric Procedural Sedation and Analgesia.* Philadelphia, PA: Lippincott, Williams and Wilkins; 1999:47-54.
13. Green SM, Johnson NE. Ketamine sedation for pediatric procedures: part 2, review and implications. *Ann Emerg Med.* 1990;19:1033-1046.
14. Green SM, Nakamura R, Johnson NE. Ketamine sedation for pediatric procedures: part 1, a prospective series. *Ann Emerg Med.* 1990;19:1024-1032.
15. Green SM, Rothrock SG, Lynch EL, et al. Intramuscular ketamine for pediatric sedation in the emergency department: safety profile in 1022 cases. *Ann Emerg Med.* 1998;31:688-697.
16. Green SM, Rothrock SG, Harris T, et al. Intravenous ketamine for pediatric sedation in the emergency department: safety profile with 156 cases. *Acad Emerg Med.* 1998;5:971-976.
17. Sachetti A, Gerardi M. Emergency department procedural sedation and analgesia. In: Strange G, Ahrens W, Lelyveld S, et al, eds. *Pediatric Emergency Medicine.* New York, NY: McGraw Hill; 2002:185-196.
18. Muse D. Conscious and deep sedation. In: Harwood-Nuss A, Wolfson A, Linden C, et al, eds. *The Clinical Practice of Emergency Medicine.* Philadelphia, PA: Lippincott, Williams and Wilkins; 2001:1758-1762.
19. Reeves J, Glass P, Lubarsky D. Nonbarbiturate intravenous anesthetics. In: Miller R, Cuehiara R, Miller E, et al, eds. *Anesthesia.* Philadelphia, PA: Churchill Livingstone; 2000:249-256.
20. Green SM, Kuppermann N, Rothrock SG, Hummel CB, Ho M. Predictors of adverse events with intramuscular ketamine sedation in children. *Ann Emerg Med.* 2000;35:35-42.
21. Hostetler MA, Davis CO. Prospective age-based comparison of behavioral reactions occurring after ketamine sedation in the ED. *Am J Emerg Med.* 2002;20:463-468.
22. Reich DL, Silvay G. Ketamine: an update on the first twenty-five years of clinical experience. *Can J Anaesth.* 1989;36:186-197.
23. White PF, Way WL, Trevor AJ. Ketamine—its pharmacology and therapeutic uses. *Anesthesiology.* 1982;56:119-136.

24. Wathen JE, Roback MG, Mackenzie T, Bothner JP. Does midazolam alter the clinical effects of intravenous ketamine sedation in children? A double-blind, randomized, controlled, emergency department trial. *Ann Emerg Med.* 2000;36:579-588.

25. Dachs RJ, Innes GM. Intravenous ketamine sedation of pediatric patients in the emergency department. *Ann Emerg Med.* 1997;29:146-150.

26. Green SM, Krauss B. Procedural sedation and analgesia. In: Roberts J, Hedges J, eds. *Clinical Procedures in Emergency Medicine.* Philadelphia, PA: Saunders; 2004:596-620.

27. Mace SE, Barata IA, Cravero JP, et al. Clinical policy: evidence-based approach to pharmacologic agents used in pediatric sedation and analgesia in the emergency department. *Ann Emerg Med.* 2004;44:342-377.

28. Strayer RJ, Nelson LS. Adverse events associated with ketamine for procedural sedation in adults. *Am J Emerg Med.* 2008;26:985-1028.

29. Melendez E, Bachur R. Serious adverse events during procedural sedation with ketamine. *Pediatr Emerg Care.* 2009;25:325-328.

SELF-EVALUATION QUESTIONS

32.1. Down syndrome patients are known to have the following attributes that may lead to failed intubation:

A. obstructive sleep apnea

B. large tongue

C. tendency to have subglottic stenosis

D. C-spine subluxation

E. all of the above

32.2. Ketamine used in the uncooperative patient:

A. aggravates the degree of cooperation because it is a dissociative agent.

B. produces such salivation that laryngospasm is a common problem.

C. is contraindicated because of the high incidence of emergency delirium.

D. can be administered po or IM.

E. midazolam has been proven to reduce the incidence of ketamine-induced emergency delirium in adults and children.

32.3. Oral or IM ketamine is useful in the management of the uncooperative patient. Which of the following is **TRUE**?

A. The dose of oral ketamine is 7.0 mg·kg^{-1}.

B. Midazolam prevents emergence reactions.

C. Glycopyrrolate should be coadministered with ketamine to prevent laryngospasm.

D. Ketamine is contraindicated in developmentally delayed individuals.

E. All of the above.

CHAPTER (33)

Airway Management in the Operating Room of a Patient with a History of Oral and Cervical Radiation Therapy

Ian R. Morris

33.1 CASE PRESENTATION

A 68-year-old man was found on CT to have a right lung nodule and paratracheal lymphadenopathy. He was then scheduled for diagnostic bronchoscopy and mediastinoscopy.

Twenty years ago, he was diagnosed with carcinoma of the right submandibular gland, and underwent excision of the gland, right radical neck dissection, and a course of radiotherapy. He quit smoking several years ago and has had hypertension for about 5 years. He has had a nonproductive cough for several months. His only medication is metoprolol.

On examination, he is in no distress at rest. His vital signs are: blood pressure (BP) 140/90 mm Hg, heart rate (HR) 70 beats per minute (bpm), and respiratory rate (RR) 18 breaths per minute. Oxygen saturation on room air is 96%. His weight is 94 kg and he is 170 cm tall. Auscultation of the chest reveals decreased breath sounds bilaterally but no rales or rhonchi, and normal heart sounds. No carotid bruits are evident.

Airway examination reveals a Mallampati IV classification. Mouth opening is 2.5 cm and mandibular protrusion is less than 1 cm. Full upper dentition is present but the mandible is edentulous. The thyromental distance is normal. Cervical spine extension is decreased. Palpation of the submandibular tissues (mandibular space) reveals a woody, indurated consistency. On inspection, telangiectasia and pallor of the submandibular skin are noted. The right neck has the typical appearance of a previous neck dissection. The mucosa of the tongue appears dry.

Laboratory data reveal normal electrolytes and a hemoglobin of 140 g·L⁻¹. ECG reveals nonspecific ST and T changes.

33.2 IS THIS PATIENT FIT FOR ANESTHESIA?

The patient has hypertension which is adequately controlled for his surgical procedure. Carcinoma of the lung is suspected on diagnostic imaging. He does not appear to require further medical optimization.

33.3 WHAT ANESTHETIC TECHNIQUE IS REQUIRED?

General anesthesia with endotracheal intubation is required for a brief but stimulating surgical procedure.

33.4 WHAT ANATOMIC AND PATHOPHYSIOLOGIC CHANGES OCCUR FOLLOWING RADIOTHERAPY TO THE STRUCTURES OF THE ORAL CAVITY AND NECK?

Radiotherapy inflicts a radiochemical injury to both normal and malignant cells.[1] The damage is related to the total radiation dose and the method of radiotherapy delivery. In order to achieve adequate tumor control, damage to normal tissues is inevitable.[1,2] *Acute* tissue toxicities from radiotherapy are considered to occur within 90 days of the commencement of treatment, and *late* effects beyond 90 days of treatment.[3] The late effects may not be manifested until years following the radiotherapy.[4] In general, tissues with rapidly dividing cell populations such as mucous membranes and skin demonstrate acute effects of radiation (mucositis, desquamation), whereas those with slowly proliferating cells such as connective tissue demonstrate late effects.[5] The severity of the late effects of radiation therapy in general cannot be predicted by the severity of the acute effects.[5] The mechanism of late tissue toxicity may be parenchymal or stromal cell death, or irradiation injury to the microvasculature.[5] Increased vascular permeability leads to deposition of fibrin in the perivascular interstitium and subsequent replacement by collagen.[6] An increase in collagen content can be seen as early as 1 week following irradiation.[6]

Following radiation therapy to the oral cavity, pharynx, or larynx, the mucous membranes can become erythematous within 1 week, and develop areas with white pseudomembranes (mucositis) at about 2 weeks.[5] The patches of mucositis may coalesce by the third week.[5] This acute mucosal reaction usually heals within 2 to 4 weeks following completion of radiotherapy, although ulceration and necrosis can occur.[4] Late effects of radiation on the mucosa are characterized by thinning or atrophy of the epithelium, telangiectasia, dryness, a loss of mucosal mobility, submucosal induration, and occasionally chronic ulceration and necrosis.[6] The mucosa is fragile and more susceptible than normal to mechanical injury.[5] Edema is seen in the subcutaneous or submucosal soft tissue in the early phase following radiotherapy, can persist for 6 to 12 months,[7] and can become chronic.[3,8] Fibrosis, one of the most common delayed radiation-associated manifestations, usually appears in subcutaneous tissues within 6 to 12 months of treatment,[5] although it can occur as early as 4 to 12 weeks.[6] The fibrosis tends to be slowly progressive,[5] nonhomogeneous, and variable in extent and severity from site to site.[9] The severity of the fibrosis increases when high total doses of radiation and large fraction sizes are used.[4] The risk of developing moderate to severe fibrosis has been reported to be about 40%.[3] The affected soft tissue loses elasticity and subcutaneous fat[6] and is indurated to palpation.[1,6] In the presence of moderate to severe fibrosis, contracture of the tissues also occurs.[1] In severe cases, the soft tissues develop a woody consistency and may form a hard mass fixed to skin and underlying muscle or bone (Figure 33-1).[5] Obstructive lymphedema may also be associated with fibrosis.[5] Radiation therapy to the neck can produce a limitation of neck extension (Figure 33-2).[6,10] High-dose irradiation of metastatic cervical lymphadenopathy results in more subcutaneous fibrosis in the neck than does a comparable dose in the absence of palpable lymphadenopathy.[5]

Hypothyroidism occurs in 5% to 10% of patients who undergo irradiation of the lower neck,[4] and fibrosis of the apical segments of the lungs can also occur.[5]

Voluntary muscle exposed to high-dose irradiation can also develop fibrosis, and when the muscles of mastication (the temporalis, masseter, and pterygoid muscles) are involved, trismus can be produced (Figure 33-3).[5] Trismus can be seen following radiotherapy for carcinoma of the nasopharynx or oropharynx. The temporomandibular joint itself is however relatively resistant to ankylosis secondary to radiation injury.[5] Fibrosis of the pharyngeal musculature can produce swallowing dysfunction[11] and a predisposition to aspiration.[2] Stenosis of the pharynx or supraglottic larynx can occur and lead to airway compromise (Figures 33-4 to 33-10).[5]

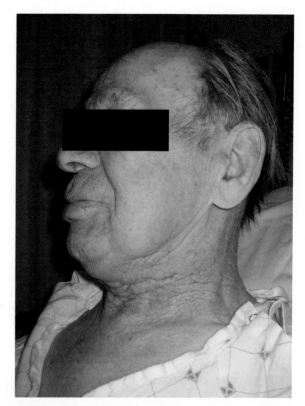

FIGURE 33-1. Appearance of the external neck following radiotherapy. The anterior neck demonstrates telangiectasia and a thickened appearance.

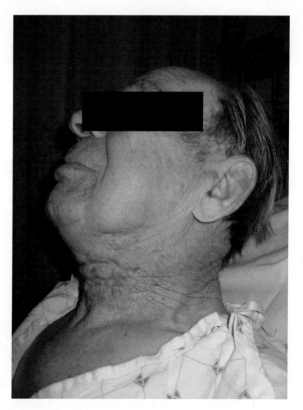

FIGURE 33-2. Limited cervical spine extension following radiotherapy.

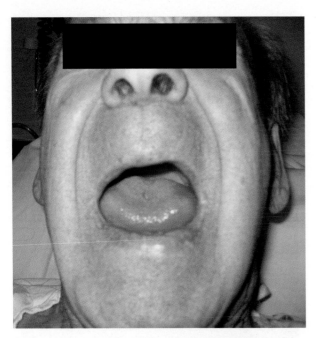

FIGURE 33-3. Limited mouth opening following radiotherapy.

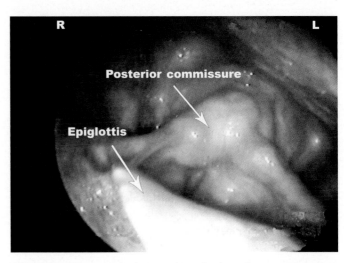

FIGURE 33-6. Laryngeal inlet view through a bronchoscope shows a normal epiglottis. Note the sharp leaf-like edge along the right lateral aspect.

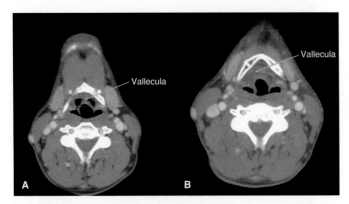

FIGURE 33-4. CT scans of the head and neck. (A) This CT scan shows normal soft tissues of the upper airway with normal vallecula. Note the bilateral air-filled depressions at this level. (B) This CT scan shows the post radiotherapy soft tissue swelling in the vallecula.

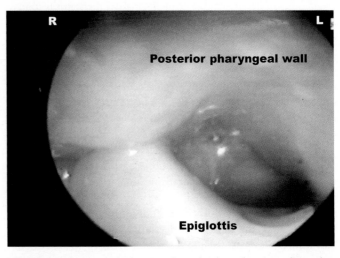

FIGURE 33-7. Laryngeal inlet view through a bronchoscope shows the appearance of the edematous epiglottis following radiotherapy.

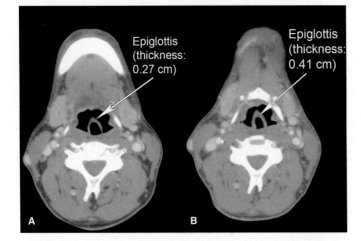

FIGURE 33-5. CT scans of the head and neck. (A) This CT scan shows normal soft tissues of the upper airway with normal vallecula. Note the bilateral air-filled depressions at this level. (B) This CT scan shows the post radiotherapy soft tissue swelling in the vallecula.

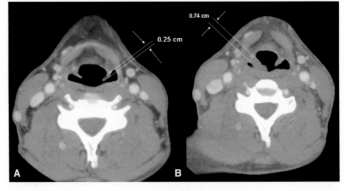

FIGURE 33-8. CT scans of the head and neck: (A) normal soft tissues of the upper airway with normal aryepiglottic folds (0.25 cm) and (B) thickening of the right aryepiglottic fold following radiotherapy (0.74 cm).

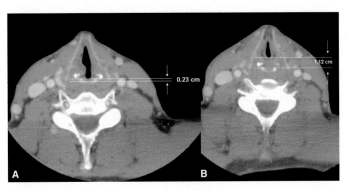

FIGURE 33-9. CT scans of the head and neck: (A) normal soft tissue thickness at the posterior commissure (0.23 cm) and (B) edema at the level of arytenoids cartilages and the posterior commissure (1.12 cm) following radiotherapy.

Laryngeal cartilage covered by normal mucous membrane usually tolerates conventional fractionated high-dose radiation therapy.[4,5] However, arytenoid edema, chrondritis, vocal cord palsy,[2] and rarely, chondronecrosis can occur (Figures 33-4[B], 33-5[B], 33-7, 33-8[B], 33-9[B], and 33-10).[1] Laryngeal edema can occur at any time following the completion of radiation therapy[12] and can produce airway compromise.[8] Laryngeal chondronecrosis has been reported to occur up to 22 years following radiotherapy.[8]

Radiation therapy also can produce vascular injury which includes intimal thickening, fragmentation of the internal elastic membrane, atheroma formation, and fibrosis of the media and adventitia.[5] A reduction in the microvascular network can ultimately lead to ischemia, and narrowing or obstruction of larger arteries can occur, as can occlusive thrombosis.[9] The changes in the vessel walls are similar to those associated with artherosclerosis due to aging.[6] Symptomatic carotid atherosclerosis can be a result of cervical irradiation and may require surgical intervention.[12]

Radiation injury to the salivary glands produces a decrease in saliva production and a change in the composition of saliva.[5] Typically, about 60% to 65% of the total salivary volume is produced by the parotid glands, 20% to 30% by the submandibular glands, and 2% to 5% by the sublingual glands.[5] The remainder of the salivary volume is produced by anonymous minor salivary glands distributed throughout the oral cavity and pharynx and which are variable from patient to patient.[5] The degree of salivary gland dysfunction depends on the volume of the salivary glands included in the radiation field and the total dose administered.[5] It is usually not possible to irradiate the pharynx or the upper jugular nodes without irradiating the submandibular glands; however, the parotid and submandibular glands can be partially shielded during treatment.[4] A significant reduction in salivary flow occurs within 1 week of fractionated radiotherapy to the head and neck.[5] Salivary flow may become barely measurable by the end of a 6- to 8-week course of treatment and the xerostomia may be permanent.[6] Xerostomia causes discomfort, alters taste acuity, and contributes to a deterioration in dental hygiene because the tissues become tender.[5] The diminished salivary flow has an altered electrolyte content and reduced pH, and promotes dental decay as the normal oral microflora is altered to a highly cariogenic microbial population.[5] In the absence of stringent measures to protect the teeth, caries can develop within 3 to 6 months and lead to complete destruction of the dentition within 3 to 5 years.[5] Dental extractions from an irradiated mandible can precipitate osteoradionecrosis.[4]

The patient presented here had palpable fibrosis of the submandibular tissues, decreased cervical extension, trismus, complete loss of mandibular dentition, and a dry mouth.

33.5   WHAT AIRWAY MANAGEMENT DIFFICULTIES CAN BE ANTICIPATED FOLLOWING RADIOTHERAPY TO THE ORAL CAVITY, PHARYNX, LARYNX, OR NECK?

Radiotherapy to the oral cavity, pharynx, larynx, or neck can produce limited mouth opening, limited cervical spine extension, and noncompliant immobile fibrotic soft tissue in the floor of the mouth and pharynx, as well as alteration of laryngeal anatomy. Airway management can be difficult in the presence of these anatomic changes. The degree of difficulty is dependent on the site and extent of the altered anatomy.

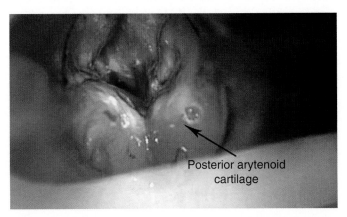

Posterior arytenoid cartilage

FIGURE 33-10. Laryngeal inlet view through a bronchoscope shows the appearance of the arytenoid cartilages and adjacent supraglottic area following radiotherapy. Note the extensive thickening and tissue distortion.

33.6   CAN VENTILATION BY FACE MASK OR EXTRAGLOTTIC DEVICE BE ANTICIPATED TO BE MORE DIFFICULT AFTER RADIOTHERAPY TO THE STRUCTURES OF THE UPPER AIRWAY?

In a review of 53,041 general anesthetics in which mask ventilation had been attempted, Kheterpal et al identified 77 cases of impossible mask ventilation (0.15%).[13] Of the subgroup of 310 patients with neck radiation, 3 could not be ventilated. Both univariate and multivariate analyses demonstrated neck radiation to be the most significant clinical predictor of impossible mask ventilation in this patient dataset. Of the 77 patients who were impossible to mask ventilate, 19 (25%) also demonstrated difficult intubation. However, the incidence of difficult intubation in the subgroup of patients with neck radiation was not provided.[13]

Giraud et al reported face mask ventilation to be easy after induction of general anesthesia in nine patients after oral or cervical radiation.[10] LMA placement was often difficult but was successful in all five patients who had received *oral* radiotherapy, and ventilation was satisfactory.[10] Two patients required lateral introduction of the LMA due to limitation of mouth opening.[10] LMA placement was easy in the four patients who had received *cervical* radiation, but positive-pressure ventilation was difficult.[10] On fiberoptic examination through the LMA, the vocal cords could not be visualized in any of these four patients due to vestibular-fold collapse. A large epiglottis was also seen in two of these patients. Muscle relaxation did not improve the laryngeal view. Ventilation was impossible in two of the four patients; however orotracheal intubation was successful. Fiberoptic intubation via the LMA was not attempted as the glottis could not be visualized. The authors theorized that the presence of the LMA in a narrowed, nondistensible hypopharynx may have compressed the larynx and thereby produced glottic collapse.[10]

Ferson et al reported the use of the Intubating LMA-Fastrach (ILMA) in 254 patients with difficult-to-manage airways of whom 40 had airway changes related to previous surgery, radiation therapy, or both.[14] In this subset of patients, the authors reported that correct positioning of the ILMA was more difficult, and 10 patients required the use of a smaller ILMA than that indicated by the patient's height and weight. There were no failures to insert the ILMA and ventilation was possible in all cases. Fiberoptically guided intubation through the ILMA was also successful in all 40 patients. The authors felt that a loss of elasticity due to fibrosis in the neck tissues caused positioning of the ILMA to be more difficult and suggested that fiberoptic guidance be used when attempting intubation through the ILMA in this group of patients.[14]

Langeron et al compared the efficacy of blind intubation through the ILMA with fiberoptic intubation in a group of 100 patients with anticipated difficult intubation undergoing scheduled surgery.[15] In this prospective randomized crossover study, following the induction of general anesthesia, intubation was initially attempted by blind intubation through the ILMA or fiberoptic intubation through an Ovassapian airway. In the event of failure of the first technique, the alternative technique was utilized. The first randomly assigned technique failed in seven patients, four in the fiberoptic group and three in the ILMA group. All were successfully intubated by the alternative technique. In the ILMA group, all three failures occurred in patients who had undergone previous cervical radiotherapy scheduled for ENT cancer surgery. In these patients, ventilation through the ILMA was not optimal for performing blind intubation, alignment of the ILMA was difficult, and increased leaks occurred during ventilation although oxygen desaturation did not occur. The authors concluded that the use of the ILMA could not be recommended in patients with previous cervical radiotherapy.[15]

Following cervical radiotherapy then, mask ventilation may be impossible[13] and the use of an LMA for airway management may not be successful due to obstruction at the level of the larynx.[10] Positioning of the ILMA[14,15] and ventilation through the ILMA may also be more difficult.[15] Laryngeal obstruction would also preclude ventilation using other extraglottic devices such as the Combitube™.

33.7 CAN ENDOTRACHEAL INTUBATION BE MORE DIFFICULT FOLLOWING ORAL OR CERVICAL RADIOTHERAPY?

Reduced mouth opening due to fibrosis of the muscles of mastication, reduced cervical spine extension, and fibrosis of the structures of the floor of the mouth can make visualization of the glottis by direct laryngoscopy difficult or impossible. Fibrotic subcutaneous and submucosal soft tissues lack compliance and may constitute a poorly mobile woody mass that cannot be elevated easily, if at all, on direct laryngoscopy. Post-irradiation atrophic mucosa is also easily traumatized and bleeding can readily occur. A thickened edematous epiglottis can obscure glottic visualization, and decreased vocal cord mobility may interfere with glottic cannulation (Figures 33-5[B], 33-7, and 33-9[B]). In the literature search performed for this chapter, no data on the incidence of difficult direct laryngoscopy associated with cervical radiation was found.

Tomioka et al reported ventilation by face mask under general anesthesia to be easy in a patient who had undergone radiotherapy for a pharyngeal tumor.[16] However, intubation with a #7.0 endotracheal tube was not possible due to tracheal stenosis, which Tomioka et al postulated, may have been produced by the radiation therapy.[16]

Yancey reported a Cormack/Lehane Grade III view with a #3 MacIntosh blade following induction of general anesthesia in a patient who had undergone left radical neck dissection and postoperative radiation 10 years previously.[17] A frozen larynx that was fibrotic and swollen was described. Intubation with a #3 Miller blade and a #6.5 endotracheal tube was difficult but successful.[17]

Alternative intubation techniques can also be more difficult following radiation-induced changes to the upper airway. The light-guided technique using a lightwand is best avoided in the presence of anatomic distortion of the airway.[18] Retrograde intubation may be feasible although laryngotracheal abnormality has been cited as a relative contraindication to this technique as well.[19] Limited mouth opening may preclude rigid fiberoptic techniques, and flexible fiberoptic intubation under general anesthesia may be more difficult in the presence of distorted anatomy and decreased mobility of the airway structures. Langeron et al reported failed blind intubation through the ILMA in patients who had cervical radiation.[15] However, Ferson et al reported successful fiberoptic intubation through the ILMA in patients who had airway changes secondary to radiotherapy.[14] No information on the efficacy of rigid fiberoptic intubation was found in the literature search performed for this chapter.

33.8 CAN A SURGICAL AIRWAY BE MORE DIFFICULT IN THIS GROUP OF PATIENTS?

Subcutaneous fibrosis in the neck can obscure surface anatomical landmarks, obliterate tissue planes, and make a surgical approach to the airway technically challenging (Figure 33-2). Percutaneous cricothyrotomy may fail in this setting, and tracheotomy may require more time to complete and be associated with more bleeding.[20]

33.9   WHAT SHOULD BE THE APPROACH TO AIRWAY MANAGEMENT IN THESE PATIENTS?

Neck radiation produces a wide spectrum of pathophysiology [13] and airway management of the patient following cervical or oral radiotherapy requires a careful airway assessment. The assessment should focus on the four dimensions of airway management as outlined by Murphy et al, and be used to predict potential difficulty with (1) face mask ventilation, (2) ventilation using an extraglottic device, (3) tracheal intubation, and (4) surgical access to the airway.[21]

If mask-ventilation and intubation are both predicted to be difficult after radiotherapy, then the airway should be secured with the patient awake. Should general anesthesia be induced in this setting and mask-ventilation be inadequate, rescue ventilation by means of an LMA may also fail.[10] The use of an LMA after *cervical* radiotherapy may in fact be contraindicated.[10] Furthermore, rescue by means of a surgical airway may also be difficult.[13,20] Topical anesthesia of the upper airway has been reported to produce transient glottic obstruction resulting in a profound reduction in maximum inspiratory and expiratory flows in some normal subjects,[22] and in the presence of preexisting airway compromise an increase in resistance to gas flow may be poorly tolerated.[23] Complete obstruction has been reported during topicalization and instrumentation of the airway.[20,24,25] However, awake fiberoptic intubation, in general, maintains a wide margin of safety and has been said to be the recommended method in the patient with predicted difficult intubation post radiotherapy. Nonetheless, extreme caution must be exercised in the presence of severe airway obstruction if complete obstruction is to be avoided.[10,26] Following radiotherapy to the floor of the mouth and/or pharynx, severe trismus may preclude oral intubation techniques, and in this setting awake nasal fiberoptic intubation may be the most reasonable alternative.

If mask-ventilation is predicted to be easy but intubation difficult, then fiberoptic intubation under general anesthesia may be considered, although anatomic distortion and decreased tissue mobility can make fiberoptic visualization more difficult. Fiberoptic intubation via an ILMA has been successful in the presence of radiotherapy-induced changes to the airway.[14] However, failure of blind intubation through the ILMA in this setting has been reported.[15]

In the presence of anatomic distortion but when intubation is predicted to be possible, inhalation induction of general anesthesia may be a reasonable option.[23,27,28] When an adequate depth of general anesthesia has been achieved, intubation can be performed during spontaneous ventilation utilizing a curved- or straight-blade laryngoscope, an operating laryngoscope such as the tubular Lindholm scope, or a rigid bronchoscope.[23,27] If intubation is not possible, tracheotomy can be performed under general anesthesia. Inhalation induction in the presence of airway compromise can

however be difficult.[23,28] Complete airway obstruction can occur and an emergency surgical airway may be required.[23,28] Meticulous attention to detail is necessary, in particular the maintenance of spontaneous ventilation and the avoidance of airway instrumentation until an adequate depth of general anesthesia is achieved.[23] The use of a nasal airway to alleviate obstruction at the level of the soft palate during inhalation induction may be helpful.[23]

Patients who have an extremely compromised airway, severe stridor, gross anatomic distortion, or a larynx that cannot be visualized on endoscopy should undergo awake tracheotomy performed under local anesthesia.[23,27,28]

33.10   HOW SHOULD THIS PATIENT'S AIRWAY BE MANAGED?

An anesthetic record from 2 years prior to this admission was available for review. Face mask ventilation had been recorded as *moderately* easy and intubation had been achieved using a lightwand *on the third attempt.*

Difficult direct laryngoscopy was predicted based on the examination of the airway (Mallampati IV, reduced mouth opening, limited mandibular protrusion, decreased cervical extension, woody induration involving the mandibular space). The predicted ease of face mask ventilation was also uncertain due to the presence of the submandibular induration and limited cervical extension. The recorded experience with face mask ventilation at the previous surgery is not reassuring. Ventilation by means of an LMA or other extraglottic device may be difficult as well in the presence of the existing anatomic distortion. Surgical access to the airway was not predicted to be difficult. An awake fiberoptic intubation was planned.

Routine monitors were attached and IV access established. No sedation was administered. The patient gargled and then expectorated 30 mL of 4% lidocaine. The Devilbiss atomizer was then used to administer 12 mL of 3% lidocaine aerosolized into the right nostril and the mouth. Five percent lidocaine paste was applied to the posterior one-third of the tongue, and an internal approach superior laryngeal nerve block was performed using Jackson forceps and cotton pledgets soaked in 4% lidocaine. The adult bronchoscope was then easily passed through the mouth into the trachea with the patient in the sitting position and using gentle tongue traction. A #8.5 endotracheal tube was then passed easily over the bronchoscope during maximum inspiration to widely abduct the vocal cords. The patient tolerated the intubation well. General anesthesia was then induced and bronchoscopy and mediastinoscopy performed uneventfully.

33.11   HOW SHOULD THIS PATIENT BE EXTUBATED?

Severe postextubation laryngeal obstruction due to laryngeal edema has been reported following hepatic resection in a patient who had previously undergone bilateral modified radical neck dissection and radiation therapy.[29] However, laryngeal edema was judged to be unlikely following this relatively brief surgical procedure in which the volume of IV fluid administered was small. Furthermore, no evidence of airway obstruction existed preoperatively.

The patient was therefore extubated fully awake in the semi-sitting position in the operating room immediately following surgery. The postoperative course was uneventful.

33.12   SUMMARY

Radiotherapy to the head and neck can produce limited mouth opening, limited cervical spine extension, noncompliant fibrotic soft tissue in the floor of the mouth and pharynx, and alteration of laryngeal anatomy. Airway management of the patient following cervical or oral radiotherapy therefore requires a careful airway assessment focused on the prediction of difficult mask ventilation, difficult extraglottic device utilization, difficult intubation, and difficult surgical airway. While complete obstruction has been reported during topicalization and instrumentation of the airway, awake fiberoptic intubation, in general, maintains a wide margin of safety and is the preferred method in the patient with predicted difficult mask ventilation and difficult laryngoscopic intubation post radiotherapy. Patients who have an extremely compromised airway, severe stridor, gross anatomic distortion, or a larynx that cannot be visualized on endoscopy should undergo awake tracheotomy performed under local anesthesia.

REFERENCES

1. Larson DL. Management of complications of radiotherapy of the head and neck. *Surg Clin North Am.* 1986;66:169-182.
2. Wu CH, Hsiao TY, Ko JY, Hsu MM. Dysphagia after radiotherapy: endoscopic examination of swallowing in patients with nasopharyngeal carcinoma. *Ann Otol Rhinol Laryngol.* 2000;109:320-325.
3. Trotti A. Toxicity in head and neck cancer: a review of trends and issues. *Int J Radiat Oncol Biol Phys.* 2000;47:1-12.
4. Vikram B. Complications of radiation therapy. In: Krespi YP, Ossoff RH, eds. *Complications in Head and Neck Surgery.* Philadelphia, PA: WB Saunders; 1993: 311-319.
5. Parsons J, Mendenhall WM, Million RR. Complications of radiotherapy for head and neck neoplasms. In: *Complications of Head and Neck Surgery.* New York: Thieme Medical Publishers, Inc.; 1995:194-229.
6. Cooper JS, Fu K, Marks J, Silverman S. Late effects of radiation therapy in the head and neck region. *Int J Radiat Oncol Biol Phys.* 1995;31: 1141-1164.
7. Gaitini LA, Fradis M, Vaida SJ, et al. Pneumomediastinum due to Venturi jet ventilation used during microlaryngeal surgery in a previously neck-irradiated patient. *Ann Otol Rhinol Laryngol.* 2000;109:519-521.
8. Weissler MC. Management of complications resulting from laryngeal cancer treatment. *Otolaryngol Clin North Am.* 1997;30:269-278.
9. Fajardo LF. Morphology of radiation effects normal times. In: Perez CA, Brady LW, eds. *Principles and Practice of Radiation Oncology.* Philadelphia, PA: J.B. Lippincott Company; 1992:114-123.
10. Giraud O, Bourgain JL, Marandas P, Billard V. Limits of laryngeal mask airway in patients after cervical or oral radiotherapy. *Can J Anaesth.* 1997;44: 1237-1241.
11. Mittal BB, Pauloski BR, Haraf DJ, et al. Swallowing dysfunction—preventative and rehabilitation strategies in patients with head-and-neck cancers treated with surgery, radiotherapy, and chemotherapy: a critical review. *Int J Radiat Oncol Biol Phys.* 2003;57:1219-1230.
12. Francfort JW, Smullens SN, Gallagher JF, Fairman RM. Airway compromise after carotid surgery in patients with cervical irradiation. *J Cardiovasc Surg (Torino).* 1989;30:877-881.
13. Kheterpal S, Martin L, Shanks AM, Tremper KK. Prediction and outcomes of impossible mask ventilation: a review of 50,000 anesthetics. *Anesthesiology.* 2009;110:891-897.
14. Ferson DZ, Rosenblatt WH, Johansen MJ, et al. Use of the intubating LMA-Fastrach in 254 patients with difficult-to-manage airways. *Anesthesiology.* 2001; 95:1175-1181.
15. Langeron O, Semjen F, Bourgain JL, et al. Comparison of the intubating laryngeal mask airway with the fiberoptic intubation in anticipated difficult airway management. *Anesthesiology.* 2001;94:968-972.
16. Tomioka T, Ogawa M, Sawamura S, et al. A case of post-radiation therapy patient with difficulty in intubation unexpected preoperatively. *Masui.* 2003; 52:406-408.
17. Yaney LL. Double-lumen endotracheal tube for one-lung ventilation through a fresh tracheostomy stoma: a case report. *AANA J.* 2007;75:411-415.
18. Hung OR, Stewart RD: Illuminating stylette (Lightwand). In: Benumof JL, ed. *Airway Management Principles and Practice.* St. Louis: Mosby, Inc.; 1996: 342-352.
19. Sanchez AF, Morrison DE. Retrograde intubation. In: Hagberg CA. *Handbook of Difficult Airway Management.* Philadelphia, PA: Churchill Livingstone; 2000: 115-148.
20. Ho AM, Chung DC, To EW, Karmakar MK. Total airway obstruction during local anesthesia in a non-sedated patient with a compromised airway. *Can J Anaesth.* 2004;51:838-841.
21. Murphy M, Hung O, Launcelott G, et al. Predicting the difficult laryngoscopic intubation: are we on the right track? *Can J Anaesth.* 2005;52:231-235.
22. Liistro G, Stanescu DC, Veriter C, et al. Upper airway anesthesia induces airflow limitation in awake humans. *Am Rev Respir Dis.* 1992;146:581-585.
23. Mason RA, Fielder CP. The obstructed airway in head and neck surgery. *Anaesthesia.* 1999;54:625-628.
24. McGuire G, el-Beheiry H. Complete upper airway obstruction during awake fibreoptic intubation in patients with unstable cervical spine fractures. *Can J Anaesth.* 1999;46:176-178.
25. Shaw IC, Welchew EA, Harrison BJ, Michael S. Complete airway obstruction during awake fibreoptic intubation. *Anaesthesia.* 1997;52:582-585.
26. Ovassapian A, Wheeler M. Flexible fiberoptic tracheal intubation. In: Hagberg CA, ed. *Handbook of Difficult Airway Management.* Philadelphia, PA: Churchill Livingstone; 2000:83-114.
27. Deam R, McCutcheon C. Management choices for the difficult airway. *Can J Anaesth.* 2003;50:623-624; author reply 624.
28. Wong DT, McGuire GP. Management choices for the difficult airway (Reply). *Can J Anaesth.* 2003:624.
29. Burkle CM, Walsh MT, Pryor SG, Kasperbauer JL. Severe postextubation laryngeal obstruction: the role of prior neck dissection and radiation. *Anesth Analg.* 2006;102:322-325.

SELF-EVALUATION QUESTIONS

33.1. Which of the following is **NOT** true with the airway management of a patient with a history of radiotherapy to the head and neck?

A. Surgical airway should be uncomplicated.

B. Limited mouth opening may preclude rigid fiberoptic intubating techniques.

C. Fibrosis of the structures of the floor of the mouth can make direct laryngoscopy difficult.

D. A decrease in vocal cord mobility may interfere with glottic cannulation.

E. In the presence of anatomic distortion of the airway, the light-guided technique using a lightwand is best avoided.

33.2. Which of the following is true with regard to the oxygenation and ventilation of a patient with a history of radiotherapy to the head and neck?

A. Face mask ventilation can be difficult.

B. The LMA may not ensure a patent airway following cervical radiotherapy.

C. Combitube™ placement can be difficult.

D. Glottic visualization by direct laryngoscopy may be impossible.

E. All of the above.

33.3. A patient with a history of radiotherapy to the head and neck is presented to the operating room for an excision of a small mass lesion in the oral cavity. During examination, he shows signs of an extremely compromised airway with severe stridor. Which of the following is the most appropriate technique to secure the airway?

A. fiberoptic intubation under general anesthesia

B. awake retrograde intubation under local anesthesia

C. awake intubation through an intubating LMA under local anesthesia

D. awake tracheotomy performed under local anesthesia

E. awake fiberoptic intubation under local anesthesia

CHAPTER (34)

Airway Management in Penetrating Neck Injury

Ian R. Morris

34.1 CASE PRESENTATION

A previously healthy 30-year-old man was shot at close range with a low-caliber handgun. A 911 call was placed immediately and paramedics were on the scene within 10 minutes. The victim was fully awake and cooperative. There was a single gunshot entrance wound in the midline at the level of the thyroid cartilage (Figure 34-1). The wound was about 5 mm in diameter and air was noted to be escaping from it. There was minimal bleeding. The patient complained of pain in the area of the anterior neck and the left scapula. He also complained of dyspnea and coughed up scant bloody sputum. He had no allergies, was on no medications, and was previously healthy.

Vital signs at the scene were: blood pressure (BP) 140/60 mm Hg, heart rate (HR) 90 beats per minute (bpm), respiratory rate (RR) 22 breaths per minute, oxygen saturation (SaO_2) was 97%. Glasgow Coma Scale was 15. One IV was placed in each upper extremity and oxygen was administered by non-rebreathing facemask (NRFM). The patient was immobilized on a spine board and transported to the emergency department (ED). Transport time was 20 minutes.

On arrival in the ED the patient was awake and responded appropriately. Vital signs were: BP 140/90 mm Hg, HR 96 bpm, RR 20 breaths per minute, SaO_2 was 98% on NRFM. He was hoarse, had scant hemoptysis, and complained of pain in the anterior neck and left scapular area. Air could again be appreciated escaping from the neck wound. There was minimal bleeding. Subcutaneous emphysema was palpable in the anterior neck but no hematoma was detected. No exit wound was identified. Air entry was decreased on auscultation of the left chest. The Glasgow Coma Scale was 15 and there were no neurologic deficits. The remainder of the examination was unremarkable.

34.2 INTRODUCTION

34.2.1 How common is penetrating neck injury?

Penetrating neck injury (PNI) has been reported to occur in 1% to 10% of all trauma patients[1,2] and in 0.4% to 5% of major penetrating trauma victims.[3] Not all PNIs involve vital structures. In a review of 26 reported series with a total of 4193 patients with PNI, there were 1285 vascular injuries (31%), 331 laryngotracheal injuries (8%), and 354 digestive (pharyngeal and esophageal) injuries (8.4%).[4] Others have reported vascular injury in 13.3% to 37%[2,5-7] of PNIs, aerodigestive tract injury in 6.3% to 18.5%,[6-9] and esophageal injury in 0.9% to 8%.[7,8,10,11] Pharyngoesophageal injury was reported by Thoma et al in 8.9% of PNIs.[6]

34.2.2 What is the mortality associated with PNI?

The mortality associated with PNI has been reported in multiple series and reviews to be between 0% and 11%.[1,4,5,7,12-22] A 2008 review reported that mortality rates from civilian PNIs was between 2% and 11%.[23]

Two series of patients with PNI have reported the mortality associated with vascular injury to be 0%[6] and 2.2%.[5] However, a mortality of 10% to 30% and approaching 50% has also been quoted for similar vascular injury.[2,23] In a review of 11 series with a total of 1584 cases, Arsensio et al[4] reported an average calculated mortality from penetrating carotid injury of 17%.

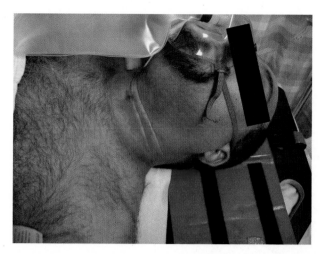

FIGURE 34-1. The 30-year-old man with gunshot wound of the neck.

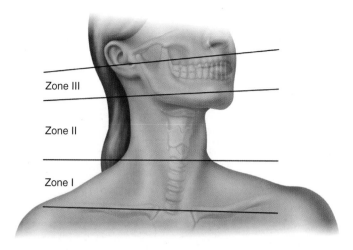

FIGURE 34-2. The three anatomic zones of the neck.

The mortality associated with penetrating laryngotracheal trauma has been reported to be 13.5%,[24] 3.5%,[25] 0%,[6] and 11.5%.[26] However, a mortality of 20%[27] to 40%[24] has also been quoted for penetrating laryngotracheal trauma.

The average calculated mortality for cervical esophageal wounds, most of which were penetrating, has been reported to be 10%.[4] An increase in mortality has been observed with delayed diagnosis.[2] A mortality associated with aerodigestive tract injury of 13% has also been reported.[28]

The mortality associated with PNI also varies with the mechanism of injury.[21] The mortality associated with high-velocity bullet wounds is greater than that associated with low-velocity bullet wounds which is greater than that associated with stab wounds.[21]

34.2.3 Why is knowledge of the anatomy of the neck important in PNI?

Penetrating injury to the aerodigestive tract, major vascular structures, or spinal cord in the neck can be life threatening.[7] No other region of the body contains so many vital structures in such a confined space.[7] Optimal evaluation and management of penetrating neck injury requires knowledge of the anatomy of the neck.[29]

The neck can be defined as that area located between the lower margin of the mandible and the superior nuchal line of the occipital

bone superiorly, and the suprasternal notch and the upper border of the clavicles inferiorly.[29] For the purpose of classification of penetrating neck injury, the neck has been divided into three anatomic zones[7,29] (Figure 34-2). Although Monson and others[30-33] have described the sternal notch as the boundary line between zones I and II, multiple other authors consider zone I to extend from the level of the clavicles and sternal notch to the cricoid cartilage[1-3,5-7,22,27,29,34,35] and zone II to extend from the level of the cricoid cartilage to the angle of the mandible. Zone III extends from the angle of the mandible to the base of the skull. Although the three zones of the neck have been said to refer to the area anterior to the sternocleidomastoid muscles,[7] posterior neck structures have also been included in this classification.[7,29]

The structures in zone I include the aortic arch, proximal carotid arteries, vertebral arteries, subclavian vessels, innominate vessels, apices of the lung, esophagus, trachea, brachial plexus, thoracic duct, and spinal cord (Figure 34-3). Important structures in zone II include the common, internal, and external carotids, the jugular veins, the larynx, the hypopharynx, and the proximal esophagus, as well as the spinal cord[2,7,29] (Figure 34-4). Important structures in zone III include the distal cervical, petrous, and cavernous portions of the internal carotid arteries, the vertebral arteries, the external carotid arteries and their major branches, the jugular veins, the *prevertebral* venous plexus, the pharynx, the spinal cord, and the facial nerves[2,7,29] (Figure 34-5).

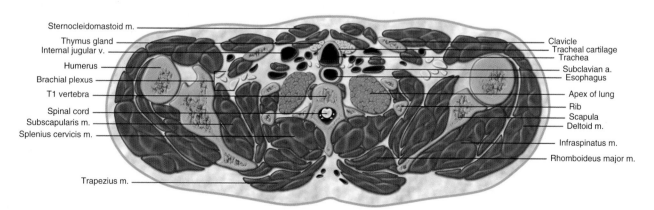

FIGURE 34-3. Anatomic structures in zone I of the neck as seen in transverse section.

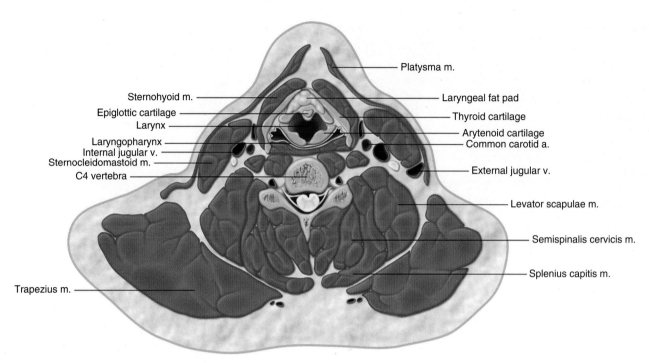

FIGURE 34-4. Anatomic structures in zone II of the neck as seen in transverse section.

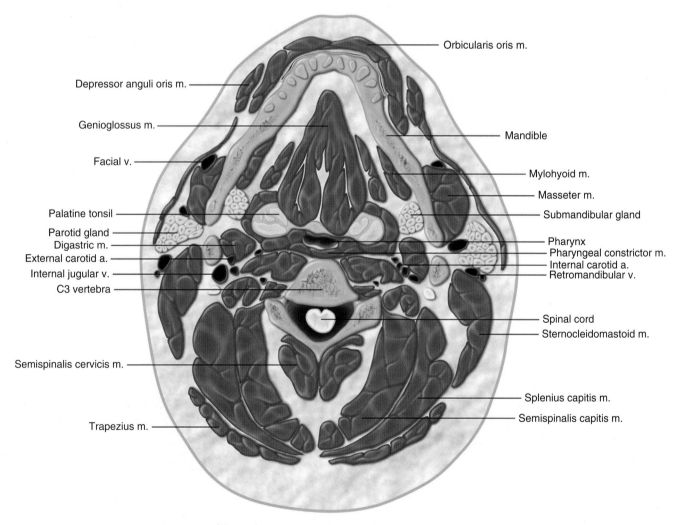

FIGURE 34-5. Anatomic structures in zone III of the neck as seen in transverse section.

The platysma, a thin superficial muscular sheet enclosed by the superficial fascia of the neck has often been cited as an important surgical landmark in the determination of whether a penetrating neck wound is superficial or deep.[2,29] Penetration of the platysma raises the potential of injury to a vital structure, and has been used as an indication for neck exploration. Deep to platysma is the deep cervical fascia, which is subdivided into the investing, pretracheal, and prevertebral layers.[2] The fascial compartments of the neck can limit external hemorrhage but when bleeding occurs within these closed compartments, airway compromise can be precipitated (Figure 34-6).

34.2.4 What are selective and mandatory neck explorations?

Management of penetrating injury to zone I is complicated by difficult surgical exposure and difficult proximal control of bleeding vessels.[2] Penetrating injury to zone III is similarly complicated by difficult surgical exposure and distal control of bleeding vessels.[2] Operative intervention for injury in zones I and III has traditionally been selective, based on physical examination and radiologic findings.[29]

The surgical management of penetrating injury to zone II has been controversial. Some authors have advocated mandatory exploration for wounds that penetrate the platysma, whereas others recommend a more selective approach to surgical neck exploration due to high negative finding rates using the mandatory approach.[5,7,11-16,18-21,29,36-42]

Penetrating neck trauma most commonly occurs in zone II[22] and requires emergency airway intervention in about one-third of cases.[22] In a series of 223 patients with PNI, Demetriades et al reported zone II injury in 47%, zone I injury in 18%, and zone III injury in 19%. More than one zone was involved in 16%.[5] Bell et al in a series of 120 patients reported 64% of PNI in zone II, 16% in zone I, and 20% in zone III.[7]

34.2.5 What are the mechanisms of PNI?

Forty-five percent of PNIs that penetrate the platysma have been reported to be caused by gunshot wounds (GSWs), 40% by stab wounds (SWs), and 4% by shotgun wounds (SGWs).[1,5] In a series of 203 patients with PNI, Thoma et al reported GSWs in 20.7% and SWs in 78.3%,[6] whereas Bell et al reported 25.8% GSWs and 52.5% SWs in a series of 120 patients.[7]

GSWs produce tissue destruction that is dependent on the kinetic energy of the projectile which is a function of the square of its velocity.[29] The projectile produces a crush effect on tissue that it contacts and a stretch effect on tissue surrounding the missile path.[43] High-velocity projectiles produce a greater blast effect and cause more extensive tissue destruction than low-velocity projectiles.[44] However, the amount of damage produced depends on the interaction of the projectile and the specific tissue affected, in addition to its velocity.[43] The site of the entry wound should be identified as well as the exit wound (if present), and consideration should be given to the path of the projectile.[2] GSWs are more likely to cause vascular, aerodigestive, and neurologic injuries than are stab wounds (73% vs 31%).[2,5] Transcervical GSWs (those that cross the midline) are also more likely to injure vital structures than GSWs that do not cross the midline.[2,17] For this reason mandatory exploration of transcervical wounds has been recommended,[45] although other authors have recommended a selective approach.[17]

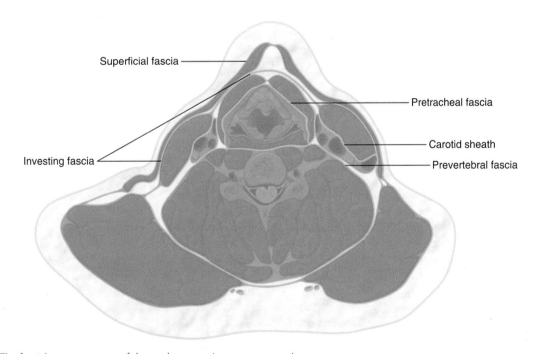

FIGURE 34-6. The fascial compartments of the neck as seen in transverse section.

34.3   CLINICAL ASSESSMENT

34.3.1   What are the essential elements of the clinical evaluation of PNI?

The initial evaluation of a PNI should follow the standard ABCs of resuscitation, followed by a systematic, rapid, and thorough secondary survey.[2] The presence of an expanding or pulsatile hematoma, active bleeding, hemorrhagic shock unresponsive to IV fluids, airway compromise, extensive subcutaneous (SC) emphysema, absent upper extremity pulse, or air bubbling through the wound mandates urgent operative intervention[2,7,22,29,46] and airway control.

In the hemodynamically stable patient without airway compromise, further diagnostic evaluation can be undertaken. The basis of this evaluation is the physical examination directed toward the identification of injury to the aerodigestive tract, the vasculature, and the nervous system.[2]

Physical signs indicative of vascular injury in addition to active bleeding, hemorrhagic shock, hematoma, or an absent upper extremity pulse noted earlier, include a carotid bruit or thrill, absent or decreased temporal or facial artery pulse, diminished ipsilateral radial pulse,[2,7] or signs of air embolism.[2] Abrupt onset of a stroke-type syndrome may herald vascular interruption, injury-induced thrombosis, or traumatic carotid or vertebral arterial dissection. Venous injury appears to be more common than arterial injury.[4] Physical examination alone has been reported to be a reliable indicator of clinically significant vascular injury.[7,46-49] In a retrospective review, Jarvik et al found no statistically significant difference between the sensitivities of clinical examination and angiography.[49] In a review of 145 cases of PNI, Sekharan et al found that of the 114 patients without hard signs of vascular injury, only one required operative repair.[50] Azuaje et al reported that physical examination alone had 93% sensitivity and 97% negative predictive value for vascular injury in a series of 216 patients.[51] Similarly, Demetriades et al reported that none of 160 patients without clinical signs of vascular injury had serious vascular injury that required treatment.[5] Thoma et al concluded that the absence of clinical signs and symptoms reasonably excluded vascular injury in their series of 203 patients.[6]

However, in a prospective study of 59 patients with a gunshot wound to the neck, Mohammed et al found physical examination alone to have a sensitivity of 57%, a specificity of 53%, a positive predictive value of 43%, and a negative predictive value of 67%.[52] Ten patients without clinical signs of vascular injury in fact had vascular injury.[52]

Hematoma is the most common sign, followed by shock and external bleeding.[7] Bleeding within the compartmentalized spaces of the neck can produce insidious displacement and distortion of the airway without external evidence. Airway obstruction can occur precipitously following a period of apparent quiescence, and airway control can be difficult.[22] Any evidence of direct vascular injury to the neck has been said to be justification for intubation.[22]

The signs and symptoms of aerodigestive injury include hoarseness or dysphonia, stridor, subcutaneous emphysema or crepitance, dyspnea, dysphagia, hemoptysis, tenderness on palpation of the larynx, and air bubbling from the wound.[2,7] Decreased breath sounds may be due to a hemothorax or pneumothorax.[2] The only hard clinical sign of laryngotracheal injury is air escaping from the neck wound.[8] Hoarseness is an indication of significant airway injury until proven otherwise.[27] Subcutaneous emphysema is a suspicious finding that requires further investigation[9] and violation of the aerodigestive tract must be assumed.[53] Demetriades et al reported that subcutaneous emphysema (clinical or radiological) was almost always present in penetrating aerodigestive tract injuries[8] and subcutaneous crepitus was the most common finding reported by Grewal et al in a series of 57 patients with penetrating laryngotracheal trauma.[25] An absence of signs or symptoms suggestive of aerodigestive trauma has been found to reliably exclude injuries requiring surgical repair in a series of 152 patients.[5] Emergency airway management has been required in 46% to 56% of patients with penetrating laryngotracheal injury.[24,25,27]

Esophageal injury due to penetrating neck trauma can be occult and difficult to diagnose on physical examination. Signs of esophageal trauma include dysphagia, odynophagia, hematemesis, SC crepitus, and retropharyngeal air on lateral neck radiograph.[2]

A thorough neurologic evaluation is necessary to detect or rule out penetrating injury to the central nervous system, cranial nerves, or peripheral nerves.[2] Complete spinal cord transection above C5 can lead to respiratory arrest, and injury below C5 can cause respiratory distress.[2] Injury to cranial nerve (CN) VII is manifested by facial weakness, CN XI by an inability to shrug the shoulders, and injury to CN XII by deviation of the tongue.[2] Injury to cervical nerve roots C5-C7 will manifest as sensory and motor deficit to the ipsilateral extremity.[2] Interruption of blood flow in the carotid or vertebral arteries can cause ischemic stroke.[2] The identification of spinal cord injury associated with PNI is important as immobilization has implications for airway management as well as physical examination.

It has been recommended that all patients with PNI be immobilized in a rigid cervical collar.[54] However, there are no reports of unstable cervical spine injury in PNI due to stab wounds, and a GSW to the neck would need to fracture the cervical vertebrae in two columns to create an unstable fracture.[55] The projectile would have to traverse the spinal cord to produce this injury and neurologic findings would be evident on physical examination[55] in the conscious examinable patient.

In a study reported by Klein et al, 33 of 183 patients with GSWs to the neck had cervical spine injuries.[56] However, only 1 of the 33 had a proven significant spinal injury with no neurologic findings on admission.[56] The authors concluded that immobilization is essential for patients with GSWs to the neck until radiologic evaluation is complete.[56] In a retrospective study by Medzon et al, 19 of 81 patients who had sustained a GSW to the head or neck had documented cervical spine fractures.[57] However, of the 65 patients who were alert and without neurologic deficits, only 3 had a fracture, none of which were unstable.[57] Sixteen of the 19 patients with fractures required acute airway management. The authors were reluctant to recommend removal of collar immobilization based on their data. However, they note that the likelihood of an unstable fracture in an alert and examinable patient without neurologic deficit is low.[57] They went on to suggest that the decision to remove the collar or discontinue spinal precautions should be individualized, and when emergency airway control is required, it would be reasonable to remove obstructive devices to permit more expeditious treatment.[57] In a retrospective review of 27 patients with PNI by Connell et al, 12 patients sustained a spinal cord injury, 1 due to a GSW and 11 from sharp weapons. Ten patients had obvious clinical evidence of spinal cord injury and two were in traumatic cardiac arrest. The authors concluded that fully conscious patients with isolated penetrating trauma and no neurologic deficit do not require spinal immobilization.[58]

Based on the available evidence, it appears unlikely that isolated PNI would produce an unstable cervical spine injury in the alert, examinable patient without a detectable neurologic deficit. Immobilization in this setting can interfere with airway management and can obscure findings on physical examination of the neck. In the presence of coincidental blunt trauma, an altered level of consciousness, or neurologic deficit, immobilization is indicated.

The patient presented here underwent cervical spine immobilization. He had the only hard clinical sign of laryngeal injury on clinical examination, air escaping from the entry wound in the anterior neck. There were no signs of vascular or neurologic injury.

34.4 AIRWAY MANAGEMENT

34.4.1 What airway management techniques are appropriate in PNI?

Airway management of the patient with penetrating neck trauma is intimidating and can be challenging even for the most skilled practitioners due to the coexistence of a potentially difficult airway and the need for rapid action.[1,22,55] In addition, the rarity of PNI means that the experience of any one practitioner in the management of this injury can be limited.[59] The need for airway control must be determined and the time available to achieve that control must be estimated. There must be a willingness to act quickly despite incomplete information as a delay in intervention can be hazardous,[22] and there must be an ability to improvise and change plans under rapidly changing circumstances.[27] Airway management decisions must be based on the patient's specific injuries, existing signs of airway compromise, the anticipated clinical course and risk of deterioration, the need for transport, and the patient's overall condition and level of cooperation, as well as planned diagnostic and therapeutic interventions.[3,22] On examination, evidence of injury to an air-containing structure in the neck (SC emphysema, stridor, dysphagia, odynophagia, respiratory distress), vascular injury (hematoma, active bleeding, shock, palpable thrill, carotid bruit, absent or diminished pulses), and spinal cord injury (motor and sensory deficit) must be evaluated. The likelihood of difficult direct laryngoscopy must also be assessed. Emergency airway management may be necessary to secure a patent airway, in preparation for operative intervention, or as a part of airway evaluation in selective management of PNI.[3] Emergency airway control is indicated in the presence of airway obstruction, respiratory failure, inability to protect the airway from aspiration, hemodynamic instability,[3] and hard signs of vascular injury that mandate emergency surgical intervention.[7,29] Edema, SC emphysema, or hematoma can produce sudden airway obstruction following a

period of relative quiescence, and anatomic distortion can make intubation or a surgical airway more difficult to perform.[22] The decision to observe a patient for impending airway compromise or to secure the airway to avoid a difficult intubation in the presence of anatomic distortion is a matter of clinical judgement.[22,55] This decision must be based on the evidence on clinical examination of significant vascular, aerodigestive tract, and neurologic injury, and it must be recognized that if one choses to observe, airway obstruction may be sudden, complete, and irreversible. If there is evidence of injury to an air-containing structure in the neck (larynx, trachea, pharynx, esophagus), positive-pressure bag-mask-ventilation may be hazardous and can produce increased anatomic distortion and airway obstruction.[2] Orotracheal intubation in the presence of laryngotracheal injury risks cannulation of a false passage, further disruption of damaged mucosa, and increased airway compromise.[8,44,60] If there is evidence of significant vascular injury, airway management is indicated.[22] A hematoma can expand in the deep tissue planes of the neck[22] and airway compromise may proceed insidiously only to be followed by rapid and catastrophic deterioration.[22]

The timing, place, and method of airway control depend on the type of neck injury, the cardio-respiratory condition of the patient, the available resources, and the experience and skills of the resuscitation team.[2,5]

Several investigators have reported experience with airway management in PNI. Shearer et al reviewed the records of 107 patients who required an artificial airway from a series of 282 patients admitted with PNI.[35] A surgical airway was the primary choice in 6%, RSI in 83%, awake bronchoscopic intubation in 7%, and blind nasal intubation in 4%. The success rates for these various techniques were: primary surgical, 100%; RSI, 98%; awake bronchoscopic, 100%; and blind nasal, 75%. Eight of the 107 patients had laryngotracheal injuries (8%) and 38 patients had vascular injuries (35.5%). RSI failed in two patients (2%) and a surgical airway was required. One blind nasal attempt failed (25%) and was followed by loss of the airway and death during attempted cricothyrotomy. Tracheotomy was performed as the primary airway in three of the eight patients with laryngotracheal injury. Of the nine patients who were hemodynamically unstable, five underwent a tracheotomy or cricothyrotomy in the ED. The authors concluded that airway control can be achieved in most patients with a penetrating neck injury by RSI or a surgical airway, and that a surgical airway should be strongly considered in patients who have wounds in proximity to the larynx who have stridor, dyspnea, hemoptysis, and SC emphysema.[35]

Mandavia et al conducted a retrospective study of ED intubations in patients presenting with PNI at a level I trauma unit over a 3-year period.[61] During the study period, 748 patients with PNI were evaluated in the ED, of whom 82 (11%) required immediate airway management. Twenty-four of these 82 patients were excluded due to pre-hospital cardiac arrest or intubation. In the remaining 58 patients (45 GSWs, 12 SWs, 1 MVA), 39 underwent RSI with a 100% success rate. Thirty-three patients required one attempt, four patients required two attempts, and two required three attempts. Oxygen desaturation (<90%) occurred in two patients. Five unconscious patients were intubated orally without paralysis, and two underwent emergency tracheotomy. Flexible bronchoscopic intubation was attempted in 12 patients and was successful in 9. The three remaining patients were successfully intubated by RSI, although one patient required two attempts and experienced oxygen desaturation to 79%. Both patients who underwent emergency tracheotomy had GSWs and were unable to phonate properly. One of these patients had a laryngeal injury confirmed by endoscopic laryngoscopy prior to tracheotomy. Oral endotracheal intubation was the definitive technique in 47 of the 58 patients and was successful 100% of the time it was employed. The authors concluded that RSI was safe and effective in all of the cases in which it was attempted, and that practitioners with airway expertise should consider using RSI in the setting of PNI.[61]

Eggen and Jorden reviewed the charts of 114 patients with penetrating injury that breeched the platysma.[30] The mechanism of injury was GSW in 59, SW in 39, shotgun wound (SGW) in 7, and miscellaneous in 9 patients. Sixty-nine patients required intubation, of whom 26 were intubated urgently. Urgent airway control was considered necessary in the presence of acute airway distress, airway compromise from blood or secretions, extensive SC emphysema, tracheal shift, or severe alteration of mental status. Eight of the 26 urgent intubations were initially unsuccessful, and six of these required an alternative technique. Four of these were failed oral intubation, three of whom were subsequently managed via the open wound, and one via a tracheotomy. Two of the six were failed nasotracheal intubations both of whom required emergency tracheotomy. Of the 26 patients who required urgent airway control, 9 required a tracheotomy and 5 of these patients had diffuse SC emphysema. Of the 98 patients with zone II injury, 22% required urgent airway control whereas all 3 patients with zone I injury and 5 of 13 (38%) with zone III injury required urgent airway control. The authors noted that a variety of approaches to airway management have been documented to be successful, and that no approach should be dismissed unless specific circumstances contraindicate it or make it technically impossible.[30] It should be noted that these cases occurred and that this study was published at a time when RSI was not widely practiced by emergency physicians.

Bell et al performed a retrospective analysis of 134 patients with PNI, of whom sixty-five sustained wounds that violated the platysma.[7] There were 31 patients with GSWs, 63 SWs, 13 flying glass injuries, and 15 who were impaled. Eight patients did not require airway management, except for the purpose of general anesthesia. Of the 59 patients who required emergency airway management, 48 were successfully intubated orally in the field. There were two failed intubations that required emergency tracheotomy on arrival, and seven additional tracheotomies were performed for airway compromise.[7]

Tallon et al performed a retrospective review of the airway management of PNI in a Canadian tertiary care center.[62] Nineteen patients were identified over the 11-year period of the study. Three patients were not intubated. Of the remaining 16, 5 were intubated in the pre-hospital setting, 6 in the ED, and 5 in the OR. Eight patients were intubated awake and eight others underwent RSI. No adverse airway-related outcomes were identified in either group.[62]

Thoma et al performed a prospective observational study of 203 patients with PNI who presented to Groote Schuur Hospital in Cape Town between July 2004 and July 2005.[6] Of these, 159 patients presented with stab wounds and 42 with low-velocity

gunshot wounds. A vascular injury was identified in 27 patients, pharyngoesophageal injury in 18, and an upper airway injury in 8. Four patients had a laryngeal injury and four had tracheal injuries. Twenty-five patients required surgical intervention, and eight additional patients had endovascular procedures. Six patients underwent tracheotomy, four of whom had airway compromise associated with oropharyngeal injury. One of the patients with laryngeal injury required tracheotomy and one patient with a complete C4 spinal cord injury required long-term ventilation. Patients with airway compromise and hemodynamic stability were intubated either by oral endotracheal intubation or if that failed, emergency cricothyrotomy. However, there were no failed intubations requiring a surgical airway. The details of the technique of intubation were not provided.[6]

Grewal et al retrospectively analyzed the records of all patients admitted to a level I trauma center who required operative management for penetrating laryngotracheal injury over a 15-year period.[25] Of the 57 patients with penetrating laryngotracheal injury, 32 had sustained GSWs and 25 had sustained SWs. Five patients were hemodynamically unstable on arrival. Emergency airway management was required in 32 of the 57 patients. Oral endotracheal intubation was performed in 14, cricothyrotomy in 3, and tracheotomy in 15. Eight of the emergency tracheotomies were performed in the ED. Forty-four patients underwent tracheotomy in the course of their resuscitation and management. The authors concluded that endotracheal intubation can be safely accomplished in selected patients with penetrating laryngotracheal injuries.[25] They suggested that patients with minor to moderate laryngotracheal injury can be safely intubated whereas patients with major laryngeal injuries required individualized management. If the expertise required to perform tracheotomy in the emergency department is limited, then cricothyrotomy was felt to be the safest alternative.[25]

In a retrospective review of laryngotracheal trauma at two major hospitals between 1996 and 2004, Bhojani et al identified 52 patients who had sustained penetrating laryngotracheal injury.[24] There were 26 GSWs and 24 SWs; 24 of the 52 patients required an emergency airway. Endotracheal intubation was performed in 20, tracheotomy in 3, and cricothyrotomy in 1. One patient, who was previously intubated, subsequently required emergency cricothyrotomy in the OR. Twelve of the patients who were intubated or who underwent cricothyrotomy required revision to tracheotomy. An additional seven patients required operative tracheotomy. The authors concluded that either routine intubation or a tracheotomy can be used to secure the airway.[24]

In a retrospective study of aerodigestive injuries of the neck, Vassiliu et al reviewed 1562 patients with neck trauma and identified 998 patients who had sustained penetrating injury.[9] There were 432 GSWs and 524 SWs during the 5-year study period. Blunt trauma produced aerodigestive injury in 7 patients, GSWs in 44, and SWs in 25. Forty-two patients with other penetrating mechanisms did not sustain aerodigestive injury. Forty of the seventy-six patients with aerodigestive injury required an emergency airway in the ED, one of whom had sustained blunt trauma. Orotracheal intubation was successful in 28 patients. In nine patients orotracheal intubation failed, and a cricothyrotomy was performed. Flexible endoscopic intubation was performed in three patients. Of the 38 patients with laryngotracheal trauma, 20 required an emergency airway in the ED. Flexible endoscopic nasotracheal intubation was performed in one patient. Of the remaining patients, RSI failed in five and a cricothyrotomy was performed. The failure rate for RSI was 23% in the GSW group and 20% in the SW group. Twenty-five of 49 patients with isolated pharyngoesophageal injuries required an emergency airway, 16 due to airway compromise secondary to pharyngeal hematoma, and 9 due to shock. RSI was successful in 17 of these 25 patients. A flexible endoscopic intubation was performed in three patients and a cricothyrotomy in five. The authors concluded that RSI is the easiest technique in most cases of aerodigestive injury. However, in the presence of large hematomas, RSI can be difficult and potentially dangerous.[9] If an RSI is undertaken, an experienced practitioner should be ready to perform a surgical airway, should the orotracheal intubation fail. In 22.5% of attempted RSI in this study, the airway was lost and a cricothyrotomy was necessary, highlighting the importance of the concept of a double set-up. The authors suggest that flexible endoscopic nasotracheal intubation is the safest approach provided that the patient has adequate cardiovascular stability.[9]

Bumpous et al performed a retrospective review of 16 patients with penetrating injury to the visceral compartment of the neck who were treated in a level I trauma center over an 8-year period.[28] There were nine handgun injuries, one shotgun injury, five stab wounds, one razor slash, and two victims of penetrating trauma associated with a motor vehicle accident. Three patients sustained zone I injury, eleven zone II injury, and two patients, zone III injury. Eleven patients sustained tracheal injury, six esophageal injury, and five laryngeal injury. Multiple sites of aerodigestive tract injury occurred in 13 patients. Tracheotomy was required in 12 of the 16 patients.

Gussack et al reported a series of 117 patients with PNI of whom 8 had penetrating laryngotracheal injury.[63] Of these eight patients with penetrating laryngotracheal injury, six underwent orotracheal intubation and two were intubated through the wound.[63] Four of those who underwent orotracheal intubation subsequently required tracheotomy. Both patients intubated through the wound required tracheotomy. No untoward effect occurred related to the orotracheal intubation.[63] The authors also reviewed an additional 392 cases of laryngotracheal trauma from 12 published series which included 123 cases of penetrating trauma. Seventy-three percent of the 392 cases required a tracheotomy. Gussack et al also reported a series of 12 patients with penetrating trauma to the laryngotracheal complex.[59] The mechanism of injury was GSW in five patients and SW in seven. Nine of the patients with penetrating laryngotracheal injury required active airway control and were orally intubated. Three required an emergency tracheotomy, two with SWs and one patient with a GSW. No intubation failures were reported. The authors felt that intubation is the primary method of airway control, and is generally more expeditious than tracheotomy in the majority of patients. However, they went on to state that the operator should move quickly to tracheotomy if intubation is difficult.[59] Cricothyrotomy was said to be relatively contraindicated if laryngeal trauma is suspected[59] although it is not clear that this is an evidence based position.

There is no uniform agreement on the airway management method of choice in penetrating neck injury.[3] Controversy persists and management varies from institution to institution.[2] The method chosen must depend on the practitioner's expertise with the various approaches[2] and, in general, the technique with which the practitioner is most comfortable is utilized.[55] However, familiarly with multiple approaches to secure the airway is required as success with any single technique is not guaranteed,[55] and back up plans must be in place should the primary technique fail.[22] In most cases, an orotracheal intubation is the easiest and most appropriate technique.[1,2] The use of rapid-sequence intubation in PNI was reported by Shearer et al with a success rate of 98%[35] and by Mandavia et al with a success rate of 100%.[61] Bell et al reported 2 failed and 48 successful oral intubations in PNI.[7] However, Eggen and Jorden reported 8 out of 26 initially unsuccessful intubations in PNI, 4 of which were failed oral intubation.[30] Gussack et al reported successful orotracheal intubation in penetrating laryngotracheal injury.[59,63] However, Vassiliu et al reported a failure rate of 22.5% with RSI in penetrating aerodigestive injury.[9] Rapid-sequence intubation can be difficult and potentially dangerous in the presence of PNI and should only be undertaken if judged likely to be successful and the personnel and equipment necessary to establish a surgical airway must be immediately available should the intubation fail (ie, a double set-up).

Awake flexible endoscopic intubation has been advocated as the safest method for most patients with PNI and should be considered in all cooperative patients with suspected airway injury.[3] However, this technique may only be feasible in stable patients who are not in severe respiratory distress, and is usually not possible in combative patients or when immediate airway control is required.[3,8] The nasal route may require less patient cooperation. The flexible endoscopic technique has the advantage that airway injuries may be identified and the endotracheal tube can be passed distal to the injury. The flexible bronchoscope can also be used to perform the intubation as part of a rapid-sequence intubation technique.[8] This variation of technique may be useful in combative patients who otherwise do not have predictors of difficult intubation.[8] In the moribund or apneic patient, or in the presence of massive upper airway bleeding, awake orotracheal intubation may be the most expeditious approach.[8]

If an airway must be immediately established and endotracheal intubation fails, then cricothyrotomy is indicated.[9,22,44,60] Conversion to tracheotomy can be performed as soon as the clinical situation permits.[44] Cricothyrotomy has also been considered to be contraindicated if the exact location of the airway injury is unknown[3] and tracheotomy had been advocated in this setting.[3] In the presence of laryngotracheal injury, if uncertainty exists about the difficulty or safety of intubation, an awake tracheotomy under local anesthesia can be performed under controlled conditions if the patient's condition permits.[2,44,60] However, an awake tracheotomy requires patient cooperation and the difficulties associated with the performance of a surgical airway in the presence of anatomic distortion in a restless hypoxic patient cannot be overemphasized.[8] In extreme circumstances in which a surgical airway is immediately required, most practitioners would consider a cricothyrotomy to be the procedure of choice.[30,39] and emergency tracheotomy is not considered an appropriate method to establish an emergency definitive airway.[27] Blind nasal intubation has been reported in the management of PNI with a success rate of 90%.[64] However, most authors agree that blind intubation techniques should not be used in PNI because of the risk of producing further injury and complete airway obstruction.[3]

34.4.2   How was the patient's airway managed?

The patient developed increasing respiratory distress following arrival in the ED. A surgeon, an anesthesiologist, and an emergency physician were at the bedside. Options for airway management were discussed. No bronchoscope was immediately available. The degree of respiratory distress rapidly increased and awake tracheotomy was not considered to be feasible. A rapid-sequence intubation (RSI) was initiated. The necessary equipment was opened and the surgeon was ready to perform a surgical airway should intubation fail.

On direct laryngoscopy a Grade 3 (epiglottis only) view was obtained with a #4 MacIntosh blade. The Eschmann tracheal introducer (bougie) was successfully passed on the first attempt and an 8.0-mm ID endotracheal tube (ETT) easily passed into the trachea over the bougie. Edema of the pharynx and larynx was noted. Endotracheal tube position was confirmed by colorimetric carbon dioxide analysis.

34.5   OTHER CONSIDERATIONS

34.5.1   What investigations are appropriate in the stable patient with PNI?

Patients who do not have airway compromise and who are hemodynamically stable should undergo further diagnostic evaluation based on the findings on physical examination.[7] The evaluation and management of PNI must also be tailored to the diagnostic capabilities in the individual institution and the experience and availability of personnel.[2] Stable patients who have suspected aerodigestive injury on examination require further investigation. Cervical spine and chest x-rays can be done as part of the initial trauma resuscitation. Flexible endoscopy is the investigation of choice for suspected laryngotracheal trauma.[8] Direct laryngoscopy may also be used in the evaluation of laryngeal trauma.[53,60] The diagnostic imaging procedure of choice in the evaluation of suspected laryngeal injury is high-resolution CT scanning, which provides the most complete radiologic assessment of the larynx.[60,65] However, CT scanning cannot be recommended as a replacement for triple endoscopy (pharyngolaryngoscopy, esophagoscopy, and bronchoscopy) in PNI[65] and controversy exists with regard to the utility of CT scanning in the evaluation of laryngeal injury.[44] The pharynx and cervical esophagus can be evaluated by endoscopy or contrast swallow studies or both modalities.[8] Rigid esophagoscopy may be more reliable than flexible esophagoscopy or esophagraphy for the diagnosis of cervical esophageal injury.[8] Catheter angiography continues to be the gold standard for the evaluation of suspected vascular injury and has well-documented efficacy.[7,66-69]

However, Rivers et al in a retrospective study concluded that the angiogram result did not alter management in zone II penetrating neck injuries.[70] Furthermore angiography is invasive and has an associated complication rate of 0.16% to 2.0%.[70] In a study of 223 patients with PNI, 176 underwent angiography.[5] Abnormalities were detected in 34 patients, of whom 14 required treatment of the vascular lesion.[5]

Helical and multislice CT angiography (CTA) has emerged as a fast and minimally invasive study for the evaluation of PNI.[7] This technology permits accurate evaluation of vascular and extravascular soft tissue and bone in less than 2 to 3 minutes and is readily available in most trauma centers.[7] Signs of vascular, aerodigestive, neurologic, and bony injury are well demonstrated by CTA.[7] Mazolewski et al, in a prospective study of zone II PNI, determined the sensitivity, specificity, positive predictive value (PPV), and negative predictive value (NPV) of CT angiography for significant injury to be 100%, 91%, 75%, and 100%, respectively.[71] Inaba et al in a prospective study of PNI reported that multidetector CT angiography (MCTA) achieved 100% sensitivity and 93.5% specificity in detecting all vascular and aerodigestive injuries.[72] Helical CTA (HCTA) has been compared to conventional angiography for the diagnosis of arterial injuries of the neck in several studies, and a sensitivity and specificity for HCTA as high as 90% to 100% has been reported.[7,71,73-75] In 2002, Munera et al reported a sensitivity of 100% and specificity of 98.6% in the evaluation of arterial injury in PNI.[76]

Color flow Doppler imaging and duplex ultrasonography have also been used in the evaluation of penetrating neck injury.[2,8,55]

X-rays of the cervical spine and chest revealed surgical emphysema in the neck, a left upper lung field opacity compatible with contusion or hemothorax, and a bullet fragment over the left scapula.

Following intubation the patient was taken to the CT scanner sedated and paralyzed. An enhanced CT scan revealed no vascular injury in the neck. Extensive surgical emphysema was present but no airway injury was identified.

34.5.2   What is the appropriate disposition of the patient with PNI?

Unstable patients are taken urgently to the OR. Stable patients without airway compromise undergo evaluation as directed by the physical examination. If a significant injury is identified, surgical management is undertaken as indicated. If no signs or symptoms of significant injury are present, and no injury is identified on further investigation, then observation is appropriate.

The patient was taken to the OR for neck exploration. In the OR, a rigid pharyngolaryngoscopy, flexible bronchoscopy, and flexible esophagoscopy were performed. No penetrating injury was identified although the cephaled trachea could not be examined due to presence of the ETT. Edema of the pharynx and larynx was again noted. On neck exploration penetrating injury to the trachea at the third and fourth tracheal rings was identified and repaired, and a tracheotomy was performed. The projectile tract was followed to the level of the cervical spine. Soft tissue disruption was noted in the tracheoesophageal groove and raised the likelihood of recurrent laryngeal nerve injury.

Nasopharyngoscopy was performed on postoperative day 2 and confirmed vocal cord palsy. The patient was decannulated on postoperative day 3.

On follow-up examination 1 month postoperatively, the patient had no shortness of breath but was still hoarse. Endoscopy revealed a persistently paralyzed vocal cord and minimal narrowing at the site of the tracheal injury.

34.6   SUMMARY

Optimal management of PNI requires knowledge of the anatomy of the neck, an understanding of the mechanism of injury, careful clinical examination, and investigation as directed by the physical examination. Management of the traumatized airway can prove to be the ultimate test of a practitioner's technical skills[27] and clinical judgment.

REFERENCES

1. Brywczynski JJ, Barrett TW, Lyon JA, Cotton BA. Management of penetrating neck injury in the emergency department: a structured literature review. *Emerg Med J.* 2008;25:711-715.
2. Kendall JL, Anglin D, Demetriades D. Penetrating neck trauma. *Emerg Med Clin North Am.* 1998;16:85-105.
3. Desjardins G, Varon AJ. Airway management for penetrating neck injuries: the Miami experience. *Resuscitation.* 2001;48:71-75.
4. Asensio JA, Valenziano CP, Falcone RE, Grosh JD. Management of penetrating neck injuries. The controversy surrounding zone II injuries. *Surg Clin North Am.* 1991;71:267-296.
5. Demetriades D, Theodorou D, Cornwell E, et al. Evaluation of penetrating injuries of the neck: prospective study of 223 patients. *World J Surg.* 1997;21:41-47; discussion 47-48.
6. Thoma M, Navsaria PH, Edu S, Nicol AJ. Analysis of 203 patients with penetrating neck injuries. *World J Surg.* 2008;32:2716-2723.
7. Bell RB, Osborn T, Dierks EJ, Potter BE, Long WB. Management of penetrating neck injuries: a new paradigm for civilian trauma. *J Oral Maxillofac Surg.* 2007;65:691-705.
8. Demetriades D, Velmahos GG, Asensio JA. Cervical pharyngoesophageal and laryngotracheal injuries. *World J Surg.* 2001;25:1044-1048.
9. Vassiliu P, Baker J, Henderson S, et al. Aerodigestive injuries of the neck. *Am Surg.* 2001;67:75-79.
10. McConnell DB, Trunkey DD. Management of penetrating trauma to the neck. *Adv Surg.* 1994;27:97-127.
11. Fogelman MJ, Stewart RD. Penetrating wounds of the neck. *Am J Surg.* 1956;91:581-593; discussion 593-596.
12. Ayuyao AM, Kaledzi YL, Parsa MH, Freeman HP. Penetrating neck wounds. Mandatory versus selective exploration. *Ann Surg.* 1985;202:563-567.
13. Belinkie SA, Russell JC, DaSilva J, Becker DR. Management of penetrating neck injuries. *J Trauma.* 1983;23:235-237.
14. Cabasares HV. Selective surgical management of penetrating neck trauma. 15-year experience in a community hospital. *Am Surg.* 1982;48:355-358.
15. Campbell FC, Robbs JV. Penetrating injuries of the neck: a prospective study of 108 patients. *Br J Surg.* 1980;67:582-586.
16. Cohen ES, Breaux CW, Johnson PN, Leitner CA. Penetrating neck injuries: experience with selective exploration. *South Med J.* 1987;80:26-28.
17. Demetriades D, Theodorou D, Cornwell E, et al. Transcervical gunshot injuries: mandatory operation is not necessary. *J Trauma.* 1996;40:758-760.
18. Golueke PJ, Goldstein AS, Sclafani SJ, Mitchell WG, Shaftan GW. Routine versus selective exploration of penetrating neck injuries: a randomized prospective study. *J Trauma.* 1984;24:1010-1014.
19. Meyer JP, Barrett JA, Schuler JJ, Flanigan DP. Mandatory vs selective exploration for penetrating neck trauma. A prospective assessment. *Arch Surg.* 1987;122:592-597.
20. Ngakane H, Muckart DJ, Luvuno FM. Penetrating visceral injuries of the neck: results of a conservative management policy. *Br J Surg.* 1990;77:908-910.
21. Ordog GJ. Penetrating neck trauma. *J Trauma.* 1987;27:543-554.
22. Walls RM, Vissers RJ. The traumatized airway. In: Benumof J, Hagberg CA, eds. *Benumof's Airway Management: Principles and Practice.* 2nd ed. Philadelphia, PA: Mosby Elsevier; 2007:939-960.
23. Bagheri SC, Khan HA, Bell RB. Penetrating neck injuries. *Oral Maxillofac Surg Clin North Am.* 2008;20:393-414.
24. Bhojani RA, Rosenbaum DH, Dikmen E, et al. Contemporary assessment of laryngotracheal trauma. *J Thorac Cardiovasc Surg.* 2005;130:426-432.
25. Grewal H, Rao PM, Mukerji S, Ivatury RR. Management of penetrating laryngotracheal injuries. *Head Neck.* 1995;17:494-502.
26. Minard G, Kudsk KA, Croce MA, et al. Laryngotracheal trauma. *Am Surg.* 1992;58:181-187.
27. Pierre EJ, McNeer RR, Shamir MY. Early management of the traumatized airway. *Anesthesiol Clin.* 2007;25:1-11,vii.
28. Bumpous JM, Whitt PD, Ganzel TM, McClane SD. Penetrating injuries of the visceral compartment of the neck. *Am J Otolaryngol.* 2000;21:190-194.
29. Britt LD, Weireter LJ, Cole FC. Management of acute neck injuries. In: Feliciano DV, Mattox KL, Moore EE, eds. *Trauma.* 6th ed. New York: McGraw-Hill; 2008.
30. Eggen JT, Jorden RC. Airway management, penetrating neck trauma. *J Emerg Med.* 1993;11:381-385.
31. Monson DO, Saletta JD, Freeark RJ. Carotid vertebral trauma. *J Trauma.* 1969;9:987-999.
32. Saletta JD, Lowe RJ, Lim LT, et al. Penetrating trauma of the neck. *J Trauma.* 1976;16:579-587.
33. Lee WT, Eliashar R, Eliachar I. Acute external laryngotracheal trauma: diagnosis and management. *Ear Nose Throat J.* 2006;85:179-184.
34. Roon AJ, Christensen N. Evaluation and treatment of penetrating cervical injuries. *J Trauma.* 1979;19:391-397.
35. Shearer VE, Giesecke AH. Airway management for patients with penetrating neck trauma: a retrospective study. *Anesth Analg.* 1993;77:1135-1138.
36. Apffelstaedt JP, Muller R. Results of mandatory exploration for penetrating neck trauma. *World J Surg.* 1994;18:917-919; discussion 920.
37. Bishara RA, Pasch AR, Douglas DD, et al. The necessity of mandatory exploration of penetrating zone II neck injuries. *Surgery.* 1986;100:655-660.
38. Carducci B, Lowe RA, Dalsey W. Penetrating neck trauma: consensus and controversies. *Ann Emerg Med.* 1986;15:208-215.
39. De la Cruz A, Chandler JR. Management of penetrating wounds of the neck. *Surg Gynecol Obstet.* 1973;137:458-460.
40. Dunbar LL, Adkins RB, Waterhouse G. Penetrating injuries to the neck. Selective management. *Am Surg.* 1984;50:198-204.
41. Lee C, May M, Sapote P, et al. Penetrating wounds of the neck: selective exploration. A study of 100 cases. *Trans Am Acad Ophthalmol Otolaryngol.* 1971;75:496-509.
42. Ashworth C, Williams LF, Byrne JJ. Penetrating wounds of the neck. Re-emphasis of the need for prompt exploration. *Am J Surg.* 1971;121:387-391.
43. Fackler ML. Wound ballistics. A review of common misconceptions. *JAMA.* 1988;259:2730-2736.
44. Butler AP, Wood BP, O'Rourke AK, Porubsky ES. Acute external laryngeal trauma: experience with 112 patients. *Ann Otol Rhinol Laryngol.* 2005;114:361-368.
45. Hirshberg A, Wall MJ, Johnston RH, Jr., Burch JM, Mattox KL. Transcervical gunshot injuries. *Am J Surg.* 1994;167:309-312.
46. Sriussadaporn S, Pak-Art R, Tharavej C, Sirichindakul B, Chiamananthapong S. Selective management of penetrating neck injuries based on clinical presentations is safe and practical. *Int Surg.* 2002;86:90-93.
47. Atteberry LR, Dennis JW, Menawat SS, Frykberg ER. Physical examination alone is safe and accurate for evaluation of vascular injuries in penetrating Zone II neck trauma. *J Am Coll Surg.* 1994;179:657-662.
48. Demetriades D, Charalambides D, Lakhoo M. Physical examination and selective conservative management in patients with penetrating injuries of the neck. *Br J Surg.* 1993;80:1534-1536.
49. Jarvik JG, Philips GR, 3rd, Schwab CW, Schwartz JS, Grossman RI. Penetrating neck trauma: sensitivity of clinical examination and cost-effectiveness of angiography. *AJNR Am J Neuroradiol.* 1995;16:647-654.
50. Sekharan J, Dennis JW, Veldenz HC, Miranda F, Frykberg ER. Continued experience with physical examination alone for evaluation and management of penetrating zone 2 neck injuries: results of 145 cases. *J Vasc Surg.* 2000;32:483-489.
51. Azuaje RE, Jacobson LE, Glover J, et al. Reliability of physical examination as a predictor of vascular injury after penetrating neck trauma. *Am Surg.* 2003;69:804-807.

52. Mohammed GS, Pillay WR, Barker P, Robbs JV. The role of clinical examination in excluding vascular injury in haemodynamically stable patients with gunshot wounds to the neck. A prospective study of 59 patients. *Eur J Vasc Endovasc Surg.* 2004;28:425-430.

53. Goudy SL, Miller FB, Bumpous JM. Neck crepitance: evaluation and management of suspected upper aerodigestive tract injury. *Laryngoscope.* 2002;112:791-795.

54. Pepe PE, Wyatt CH, Bickell WH, Bailey ML, Mattox KL. The relationship between total prehospital time and outcome in hypotensive victims of penetrating injuries. *Ann Emerg Med.* 1987;16:293-297.

55. Rathlev NK, Medzon R, Bracken ME. Evaluation and management of neck trauma. *Emerg Med Clin North Am.* 2007;25:679-694, viii.

56. Klein Y, Cohn SM, Soffer D, et al. Spine injuries are common among asymptomatic patients after gunshot wounds. *J Trauma.* 2005;58:833-836.

57. Medzon R, Rothenhaus T, Bono CM, Grindlinger G, Rathlev NK. Stability of cervical spine fractures after gunshot wounds to the head and neck. *Spine (Phila Pa 1976).* 2005;30:2274-2279.

58. Connell RA, Graham CA, Munro PT. Is spinal immobilisation necessary for all patients sustaining isolated penetrating trauma? *Injury.* 2003;34:912-914.

59. Gussack GS, Jurkovich GJ. Treatment dilemmas in laryngotracheal trauma. *J Trauma.* 1988;28:1439-1444.

60. O'Mara W, Hebert AF. External laryngeal trauma. *J La State Med Soc.* 2000;152:218-222.

61. Mandavia DP, Qualls S, Rokos I. Emergency airway management in penetrating neck injury. *Ann Emerg Med.* 2000;35:221-225.

62. Tallon JM, Ahmed JM, Sealy B. Airway management in penetrating neck trauma at a Canadian tertiary trauma centre. *CJEM.* 2007;9:101-104.

63. Gussack GS, Jurkovich GJ, Luterman A. Laryngotracheal trauma: a protocol approach to a rare injury. *Laryngoscope.* 1986;96:660-665.

64. Weitzel N, Kendall J, Pons P. Blind nasotracheal intubation for patients with penetrating neck trauma. *J Trauma.* 2004;56:1097-1101.

65. Atkins BZ, Abbate S, Fisher SR, Vaslef SN. Current management of laryngotracheal trauma: case report and literature review. *J Trauma.* 2004;56:185-190.

66. Hiatt JR, Busuttil RW, Wilson SE. Impact of routine arteriography on management of penetrating neck injuries. *J Vasc Surg.* 1984;1:860-866.

67. McCormick TM, Burch BH. Routine angiographic evaluation of neck and extremity injuries. *J Trauma.* 1979;19:384-387.

68. Reid JD, Weigelt JA, Thal ER, Francis H, 3rd. Assessment of proximity of a wound to major vascular structures as an indication for arteriography. *Arch Surg.* 1988;123:942-946.

69. Snyder WH, 3rd, Thal ER, Bridges RA, et al. The validity of normal arteriography in penetrating trauma. *Arch Surg.* 1978;113:424-426.

70. Rivers SP, Patel Y, Delany HM, Veith FJ. Limited role of arteriography in penetrating neck trauma. *J Vasc Surg.* 1988;8:112-116.

71. Mazolewski PJ, Curry JD, Browder T, Fildes J. Computed tomographic scan can be used for surgical decision making in zone II penetrating neck injuries. *J Trauma.* 2001;51:315-319.

72. Inaba K, Munera F, McKenney M, et al. Prospective evaluation of screening multislice helical computed tomographic angiography in the initial evaluation of penetrating neck injuries. *J Trauma.* 2006;61:144-149.

73. Gracias VH, Reilly PM, Philpott J, et al. Computed tomography in the evaluation of penetrating neck trauma: a preliminary study. *Arch Surg.* 2001;136:1231-1235.

74. LeBlang SD, Nunez DB, Rivas LA, Falcone S, Pogson SE. Helical computed tomographic angiography in penetrating neck trauma. *Emerg Radiol.* 1997:200-206.

75. Munera F, Soto JA, Palacio D, Velez SM, Medina E. Diagnosis of arterial injuries caused by penetrating trauma to the neck: comparison of helical CT angiography and conventional angiography. *Radiology.* 2000;216:356-362.

76. Munera F, Soto JA, Palacio DM, et al. Penetrating neck injuries: helical CT angiography for initial evaluation. *Radiology.* 2002;224:366-372.

SELF-EVALUATION QUESTIONS

34.1. Penetrating neck injury classification has divided the neck into three anatomic zones. Zone III extends from:

   A. the level of the clavicles and the sternal notch to the cricoid cartilage

   B. the level of the clavicles and the sternal notch to the thyroid cartilage

   C. the cricoid cartilage to the angle of the mandible

   D. the thyroid cartilage to the angle of the mandible

   E. the angle of the mandible to the base of the skull

34.2. The only hard clinical sign of laryngotracheal injury in penetrating trauma is:

   A. subcutaneous emphysema

   B. air escaping from the neck wound

   C. hoarseness

   D. hemoptysis

   E. stridor

34.3. In penetrating neck injury, the investigation of choice for suspected laryngotracheal trauma is:

   A. high-resolution CT scan

   B. direct laryngoscopy

   C. flexible fiberoptic endoscopy

   D. duplex ultrasonography

   E. catheter angiography

CHAPTER (35)

Intra-operative Accidental Dislodgement of the Endotracheal Tube in a Patient in Prone Position

Dennis Drapeau and Orlando R. Hung

35.1 CASE PRESENTATION

A 50-year-old obese man (120 kg, 173 cm, BMI 40 kg·m⁻²) was scheduled for lumbar spine instrumentation. Preoperative airway examination revealed no obvious indicators of difficult laryngoscopic intubation apart from the fact that he had a beard. Following induction of anesthesia with fentanyl, propofol, and rocuronium, a Cormack/Lehane Grade 2 laryngoscopic view was obtained with a #3 Macintosh blade. Laryngoscopic intubation was achieved easily while using backward, upward, and rightward pressure (BURP) externally on the larynx. After securing the endotracheal tube (ETT), the patient was then turned into the prone position for the surgical procedure. Two hours after the start of surgery, and after 1500 mL of blood loss and the administration of 4000 mL of crystalloid, a leak in the ventilation system was identified.

35.2 INTRODUCTION

35.2.1 What are your concerns when a patient is placed in the prone position for a surgical procedure?

Proper patient positioning for any medical procedure is an important consideration for a safe and successful outcome. The proper position provides for appropriate surgical access and guards against injury due to pressure points and strain on neurological and musculoskeletal structures. The prone position is most commonly required for surgical procedures on the spine, and for select procedures in neurosurgery, urology, and general surgery. This position

is complicated by an increased risk of stretch and pressure injury of nerves, cardiovascular instability, difficulty with ventilation, and problems with providing cardiopulmonary resuscitation as compared with a supine surgical position. Airway considerations for patients placed in the prone position may include difficult access to the airway, migration of the ETT (tip of the ETT moving cephalad or caudad with head extension and flexion, respectively), limited ability to reposition the head and neck for bag-mask-ventilation (BMV), and the potential development of airway edema.

This case represents one of the most challenging situations for airway practitioners: regaining control of the airway promptly with the patient in the prone position. Limited information is currently available in the literature to assist the airway practitioner with critical decision making should they encounter this situation.

35.3 INITIAL PATIENT MANAGEMENT

35.3.1 What is the differential diagnosis of the ventilation system leak?

A ventilation system leak is a fairly common occurrence during surgery and is usually easy to manage. However, it is more complex when it occurs in the prone patient due to the unique challenges it presents the airway practitioner and the dangerous or life-threatening situation that may develop for the patient.

In diagnosing and managing this situation, the source of the leak must be promptly determined. This is usually accomplished by inspecting all portions of the anesthesia circuit in an organized and sequential manner. With the prone patient, it is usually easier to start at the anesthesia machine and work your way to the patient. This would include checking flow rates, ventilator/bag volumes, valves, circuit tubing, and connections.

Leaks within the anesthesia machine or circuit may involve circuit disconnects, leaks around circuit connections or valves, and undetected holes in circuit components. Management of such leaks may include increasing the fresh gas flow, or replacing part or all of the anesthesia circuit or machine.

Potential leaks associated with an airway device include: (1) partial or complete dislodgement of the device; (2) inadequate volume in the ETT cuff; (3) disruption of the ETT cuff; and (4) a leak from the pilot cuff apparatus (pilot valve or tubing leak). Leaks from these causes may require reinsertion of the device, or removal of a defective airway device, and reinsertion of an appropriate replacement device.

35.3.2   If the ETT was found to be dislodged from the trachea, what is your initial management?

The goals of management are to regain control of the airway and to resume ventilation and oxygenation as soon as possible. If feasible, this should be achieved by turning the patient into the supine position. Operating room personnel must be informed of the emergency situation and additional help should be summoned. The difficult airway cart, the patient's stretcher or bed, and the resuscitation cart should be brought into the operating theater immediately. The surgical team should close the surgical wound as soon as possible to allow transfer of the patient to a stretcher in the supine position.

35.4   AIRWAY CONSIDERATIONS

35.4.1   If a stretcher is not immediately available, how do you provide ventilation to a patient in the prone position?

Options to regain control of the airway in a prone patient are similar to those in the supine patient. Bag-mask-ventilation (BMV) should be provided as soon as possible. However, BMV in the prone patient can be difficult due to limited access to the airway, difficult mask seal due to no occipital support to apply counter pressure to the head,[1] and lack of clinical experience performing BMV in a prone patient. It may be necessary to use a two-person BMV technique, with one person achieving a mask seal using both hands, while the second person provides manual ventilation. Provided that a good seal can be maintained between the mask and the patient's face, BMV should be reasonably easy in a patient lying prone as gravity tends to move the tongue away from the posterior pharyngeal wall. Obtaining a good seal for BMV may prove difficult in this case scenario as the patient has a beard. The authors therefore would recommend starting with two-person BMV technique (see Chapter 7) and quickly proceeding to alternative methods of ventilation should there be any difficulty obtaining an adequate seal for BMV.

If BMV is not possible, an extraglottic device (EGD), such as the laryngeal mask airway (LMA), can be used to provide emergency ventilation and oxygenation for a patient in the prone position. A number of investigators have reported successful use of EGDs (LMA and LMA-ProSeal™) to regain control of the airway and provide positive-pressure ventilation following endotracheal tube dislodgement in the prone position.[2,3] Insertion of the LMA in the prone patient should be attempted using the classic insertion technique recommended for patients in the supine position.[4] Successful insertion of the LMA may actually be easier in the prone position because gravity helps to move the tongue and epiglottis[5] away from the posterior pharyngeal wall and minimizes the risk of down folding of the epiglottis.

Other extraglottic devices (including the Combitube™ and LMA Supreme™[6] may be used while the patient is prone, depending on the skill and experience of the practitioner, as well as the available resources. However, there are currently no reports in the literature of the successful use of non-LMA-derived extraglottic devices for patients in the prone position.

35.4.2   Would you proceed with the surgical procedure, if adequate ventilation and oxygenation can be achieved following the successful placement of a LMA?

As mentioned, successful insertion of the LMA in patients in the prone position has been reported. Ng et al reported successful LMA insertion following induction of general anesthesia for brief surgical procedures in 73 prone adult patients.[5] However, difficulties were encountered with malposition of the LMA in four patients (5.5%), hypoventilation in two patients (2.7%), and bleeding in two patients (2.7%). Although these were considered to be minor problems, the authors clearly stated that successful insertion of the LMA in the prone position requires not only skill that comes from practice, but also the assurance that at any time the patient can be turned into the supine position should emergency airway management be necessary. Stevens reported successful use of the LMA in the prone position in 103 adult patients.[7] One patient regurgitated green emesis (without sequelae) and another patient had inadequate ventilation, requiring reinsertion of the LMA in the supine position. Brimacombe et al described using the ProSeal LMA successfully in 245 adult patients in the prone position, although 8 patients required a second attempt at insertion of the ProSeal LMA aided by a laryngoscope and bougie.[8] Herrick et al and Kee et al report incidences of airway obstruction of 3.5% and 3%, respectively, when the LMA was used in pediatric patients placed prone for radiotherapy.[9,10] It is probably reasonable to use the LMA for short surgical procedures in the prone position as long as there is still the option of repositioning the patient supine in the event that airway management becomes problematic. However, it would be unwise to use the LMA for obese patients or for long surgical procedures with the potential of massive bleeding and fluid shifts, such as in this case scenario. It is common to observe an increase in the airway pressure during the course of the surgery in the prone position, particularly when there is massive blood loss and fluid shifts. In this patient, the LMA should only be considered as a temporizing measure until a more definitive airway can be secured.

Therefore, the authors believe that it is necessary to replace the ETT prior to resuming the surgical procedure in this patient.

35.4.3 How do you manage a patient with a difficult airway who requires prone positioning?

Airway management of the patient with a difficult airway who requires surgery in the prone position poses unique challenges for the anesthesia practitioner. These issues can be categorized according to the etiology of the difficult airway: (1) anatomical characteristics making ventilation and/or tracheal intubation difficult; and (2) cervical spine instability. If difficult laryngoscopic intubation secondary to anatomical characteristics is predicted (LEMON, see Section 1.6.2), the technique utilized to manage the airway is dependent on whether or not ventilation can be readily provided by BMV, EGD, or a surgical airway, aspiration risk, the available resources, as well as the expertise of the practitioner. Once tracheal intubation has been achieved, the ETT must be carefully secured. The situation becomes more challenging when possible cervical spine instability or spinal cord damage exists. It is generally believed that awake bronchoscopic intubation and prone positioning of the patient prior to induction of anesthesia is ideal, because it allows verification of neurological integrity prior to surgery. However, there is no clinical evidence to support this practice. In a retrospective review of 150 patients with cervical spine injury, Suderman and Crosby found no difference in neurological outcomes following tracheal intubation awake or under general anesthesia, with or without in-line cervical spine immobilization[11] (see Chapter 15.4).

35.5 PREPARATION AND PLANS FOR TRACHEAL INTUBATION

35.5.1 Can intubation be performed in the lateral position?

While transfer of the patient to the supine position would be ideal, it could be difficult to achieve in a timely manner and is not without considerable risk to the patient depending on the situation. Therefore, it is desirable to have several alternative approaches for reestablishing tracheal intubation in this particularly difficult situation.

If it is feasible to place the patient in a lateral position, the left lateral decubitus is preferred by some practitioners for laryngoscopy and intubation, as gravity will help to displace the tongue to the left and facilitate visualization of the glottis.[1] However, others prefer the right lateral decubitus position as in this position, the operator's left arm has more room to maneuver during the procedure. The tongue can still be easily displaced by the laryngoscope in the right lateral decubitus position. Nathanson et al found tracheal intubation of a manikin in the lateral position to be more difficult than in the supine position.[12] The ease of intubation

increased with each subsequent attempt, indicating that operator experience was a confounding factor.[12] An assistant may be necessary to stabilize the head, neck, and body while performing an intubation in a patient in the lateral decubitus position.

Blind endotracheal intubation techniques using the intubating LMA (Fastrach™, LMA North America, San Diego) and the lighted stylet have also been described with a patient in the lateral position.[13-15] Experience with these intubation techniques will improve the operator's chance of success. Blind techniques should only be attempted after direct visualization techniques have failed, as anatomic distortion may be present.

35.5.2 What are the options for tracheal intubation in the prone position?

Reintubation while the patient is still in the prone position would eliminate the inherent risks associated with turning the patient. In addition to direct laryngoscopic intubation, alternative intubating techniques can be considered. These include the use of a flexible bronchoscope (FB), an intubating LMA (LMA Fastrach™, LMA North America Inc, San Diego, CA), light-guided intubation using the Trachlight™ (Laerdal Medical Corp., Wappingers Falls, New York), and digital intubation. However, there is limited clinical information with regard to the effectiveness and safety of these techniques in patients in the prone position.

Baer performed endotracheal intubation under direct laryngoscopy in the prone position in 200 patients undergoing lumbar surgery.[16] Two failed intubations occurred and these patients were then intubated in the lateral or supine positions, with difficulty.[16] This experience emphasizes the importance of airway assessment and management in the supine position when difficulty is predicted. We believe that tracheal intubation of patients in the prone position should be reserved for rescue situations and that elective intubation of patients requiring prone positioning should be performed in the supine position as this is most familiar to the airway practitioner.

Intubation in the prone position may be necessary if:

1. Ventilation and oxygenation are ineffective using BMV, the LMA, or the Combitube™.
2. Ventilation using BMV, the LMA, or the Combitube™ is adequate but a definitive airway is desired (eg, prolonged case, risk of aspiration).
3. Transfer of the patient to the supine position is impossible, or associated with extreme risk.

35.5.3 How can endotracheal intubation be performed in the prone position in the patient presented here?

Airway control in this case scenario can be reestablished by one of several techniques.

An intact ETT can be reinserted into the trachea by simple advancement, as long as the tip of the ETT is still in the glottis. This can be facilitated if a throat pack had been placed following the initial intubation. The ability to ventilate the patient through the ETT confirmed by the presence of an appropriate end-tidal CO_2 waveform indicates that simple advancement of the tube may be all that is required. If ventilation through the ETT is difficult, it may still be possible to advance the ETT into the trachea with the aid of a lighted stylet, FB, or a tube exchanger. When using a tube exchanger (airway exchange catheter), the intratracheal location of the tube exchanger should be verified by flexible bronchoscopy or by detecting an appropriate end-tidal CO_2 waveform when ventilating through the tube exchanger.

The tracheal tube should be replaced if there is evidence of tube damage and a significant leak exists. Small air leaks may be overcome by increasing inspired gas flow, if the remaining surgical time is short. The benefits of continuing the case without further airway manipulation must be weighed against potential further airway compromise and operating room contamination with anesthetic gases. Therefore, the anesthetic technique should be changed to TIVA, if required, should the anesthesia practitioner decide to proceed with the case in the presence of a small ETT leak. Larger leaks can be attenuated by the insertion of a throat pack, if not already present. If a throat pack was in place around the original ETT, it may be possible to pass a new ETT with a deflated cuff into the trachea through the cast (or track) made by the throat pack or it may be possible to change the tube over an airway exchange catheter. If these measures fail and airway control is lost, the throat pack should be removed if present and ventilation of the patient must be reestablished as soon as possible.

Tracheal intubation by direct laryngoscopy can be performed in the prone patient by the airway practitioner who is positioned at the head of the patient facing caudad and who uses the right hand to insert the laryngoscope into the pharynx and exposes the glottis (Figure 35-1). Operating the laryngoscope with the right hand while the practitioner faces the prone patient allows the laryngoscope blade to displace the tongue in the usual manner—away from the right side of the patient's mouth. The practitioner then uses the left hand to insert the ETT into the trachea. Alternately,

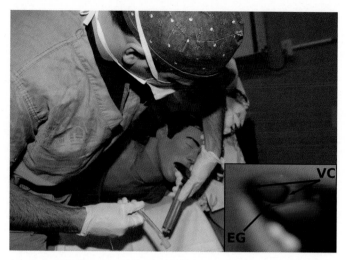

FIGURE 35-2. Laryngoscopic intubation of a manikin placed in the prone position: Laryngoscopic intubation can also be performed from the side (right) of the manikin. The inset shows the laryngoscopic view of this technique. The vocal cords (VC) and the epiglottis (EG) can be visualized easily.

direct laryngoscopy and intubation can be performed in a more conventional manner from either side of the patient (Figure 35-2). An assistant can turn the patient's head to the right and elevate the right shoulder slightly to facilitate access to the mouth. The head and neck can also be placed in the familiar sniffing position. This technique of laryngoscopic intubation in prone patients has been shown to be effective (99% success rate) and safe.[16]

Agrawal et al[17] described the successful use of the ILMA for tracheal intubation in a patient in the prone position who presented with injuries precluding supine positioning. The ILMA can also provide a conduit through which an ETT can be advanced into the trachea blindly, or with the aid of a lightwand, or the flexible bronchoscope (see Chapter 12). However, insertion of an intubating LMA (as compared to the LMA Classic™) can be difficult in the prone position. Alternatively, a 7.0 mm ETT could be passed through a classic LMA with FB guidance if the "aperture bars" are removed to allow easier passage of the ETT through the opening in the LMA.

35.5.4 Upon turning the patient into the supine position, bag-mask-ventilation is easy, but direct laryngoscopy reveals a Grade 3 view. What is the appropriate airway management?

A previously easy intubation may be difficult upon returning the patient to the supine position. Anatomic distortion of the airway can occur due to factors inherent to the surgical procedure, to the prone position, to trauma during the initial intubation, or to dislodgement of the ETT. Cervical vertebral fixation and surgical manipulation of oropharyngeal and neck tissues can alter airway anatomy. Bleeding into the airway and hematoma formation can be associated with neck surgery. Prolonged surgical procedures with significant blood loss may be associated with generalized edema due to fluid resuscitation. Direct pressure on facial and

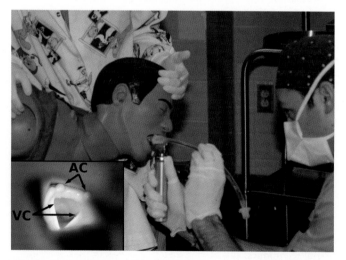

FIGURE 35-1. Laryngoscopic intubation of a manikin placed in the prone position: Laryngoscopic intubation can be performed from the front of the manikin with the right hand holding the laryngoscope. The inset shows the laryngoscopic view of this technique. The vocal cords (VC) and the arytenoid cartilages (AC) can be visualized easily.

neck structures and a dependent position compromise venous drainage and contribute to edema formation. Airway edema can alter the appearance of laryngeal structures and can make visualization of the larynx difficult.[18-20] Edematous tissues may also be more easily traumatized.

In this case scenario, the patient was placed in the supine position and direct laryngoscopy revealed a Grade 3 laryngoscopic view. The application of BURP[21] may improve the Cormack/ Lehane view.[22] If BURP does not improve the view of the glottis, alternative intubating techniques can be used, as long as effective ventilation and oxygenation can be provided by BMV. These techniques include the use of an Eschmann Introducer, lightwand (Trachlight™), intubating LMA, Glidescope™ (Keomed, Minnetonka, MN), Bullard laryngoscope, or FB. As each intubation attempt will likely decrease the chance of success on subsequent attempts, it is critical that the practitioner employs the technique with which he/she is most experienced. In general, in the presence of an abnormal upper airway (edema), tracheal intubation should be performed under direct or indirect vision, if at all possible. Use of the Eschmann Introducer can be considered to be a logical extension of direct laryngoscopy and has a high success rate in the presence of a Grade 3 view.[23] It is also helpful to use a smaller ETT and lubricate the inside and outside of the ETT to minimize the resistance to passage through the larynx and assist in passing the ETT over the introducer.

If a visual technique is unsuccessful but BMV is adequate, nonvisual intubation techniques may be used with great caution, while preparing the patient for a surgical airway.

The lightwand is an invaluable tool for airway management, but its utility in obese patients is limited. Furthermore, in this case scenario, the failed laryngoscopic intubation is probably secondary to airway edema and/or trauma. The use of a nonvisual intubating technique, such as the lightwand, would therefore likely be unsuccessful in this setting.

For the patient in this case scenario, BURP did not improve the glottic view (Cormack/Lehane Grade 3 view) and passage of an Eschmann Introducer was unsuccessful. Subsequent use of the Glidescope™ (Keomed, Minnetonka, MN) with a styletted endotracheal tube resulted in successful intubation and rest of the case proceeded uneventfully.

35.6 POSTINTUBATION AND VENTILATION MANAGEMENT

35.6.1 How can the tracheal tube be secured following intubation in a patient with a beard?

To minimize the risk of ETT dislodgement, it is imperative to secure the ETT properly, particularly for patients in a prone position. The most common method of securing the endotracheal tube is to tape it to the face. Unfortunately, the presence of facial hair, oils on the skin, perspiration, oropharyngeal secretions, and surgical skin preparation solutions can impair the adhesiveness of the tape. Generous use of waterproof tape and the use of multiple

attachment points can reinforce the bond to the patient's face. The application of tincture of benzoin to the skin may improve tape adhesion. Although adequate taping is required for the prone patient, complete sealing off of the mouth should be avoided, as oropharyngeal secretions should be allowed to drain out. This will minimize pooling of saliva and secretions, which may loosen the tape. In addition, the use of an antisialogogue (eg, glycopyrrolate) may be helpful as a preventive measure to minimize secretions. Placement of a throat pack in the oropharynx or a gauze bite block may also limit the amount of secretions available to disrupt the bond between the tape and the skin. However, the airway practitioner must always be aware of the potential for local pressure injury (eg, lingual nerve injury) associated with the use of these throat packs and bite blocks.[24,25]

Patients with facial hair often pose additional problems with securing the airway. For these patients, it may be best to tie the ETT around the neck with an umbilical tape. It is important not to tie the ETT too tightly and thereby obstruct venous return from the head. If the ETT cannot be tied around the neck (eg, cervical laminectomy or post-fossa craniotomy) other possible options to secure the ETT include: (1) suturing the ETT to the lips; (2) tying/suturing the ETT to the upper incisors (if present) or nares; and (3) shaving the patient's beard prior to induction of anesthesia.

35.7 OTHER CONSIDERATIONS FOR PATIENTS IN PRONE POSITION

35.7.1 How can airway edema be minimized in a patient in the prone position?

Tissue edema, particularly in dependent areas, can occur in surgical procedures involving significant blood loss and/or fluid shifts. Intra-operative dislodgement of the ETT in the prone patient with significant airway edema can be a disaster. Therefore, all attempts should be made to minimize the development of edema during procedures performed in the prone position. In lieu of large amounts of crystalloid solutions, it is perhaps prudent to administer colloid solutions, such as hydroxyethyl starch preparations. Although the efficacy of this approach has not been scientifically validated, it is our practice to use colloid solutions judiciously in order to limit crystalloid use to between 2 and 3 L in total.

Venous drainage of the head and neck can be optimized by keeping the head elevated if possible and avoiding compression or kinking of jugular veins. If the head must be turned to one side for airway or surgical access, the degree of rotation should be minimized.

35.4.4 How can airway edema be assessed and managed?

The development of edema in the hypopharynx and larynx while in the prone position can produce airway obstruction following extubation. Clinical signs, such as facial, orbital, or conjunctival edema, distended neck veins, and venous congestion of the head may indicate the presence of upper airway edema. The use of a flexible nasopharyngoscope to assess the extent of airway edema prior to tracheal extubation may be helpful,[26] although there have been no studies to confirm its utility.

There are no scientifically validated methods to assess the degree of postoperative airway edema or to predict post-extubation airway obstruction (see Section 28.4). However, the performance of a leak test prior to extubation in patients with suspected airway edema has been suggested.[27] The leak test measures the decrease in exhaled volume returned to the ventilator following deflation of the endotracheal tube cuff. A positive leak test (> 110 mL or > 10% of the tidal volume) has been shown to indicate that airway patency is sufficient to tolerate extubation without post-extubation stridor (PES) (99% specificity, 98% PPV), although a **negative** leak test is not predictive of the development of PES.[28] The leak test can also be performed by deflating the endotracheal tube cuff in a spontaneously breathing patient without ventilator support and then occluding the end of the ETT. The patient is observed for signs of an audible leak or coughing around the endotracheal tube. The absence of a leak and/or coughing are positive predictors for PES.[29] Multiple studies have found the leak test to be either helpful for predicting adverse events[30-32] or not,[33-35] but they all suffer from study design flaws. Therefore, airway practitioners should recognize the potential limitations of the cuff leak test as they apply it in clinical practice.

Laryngeal ultrasound may be an emerging method for assessing laryngeal anatomy. Lakhal et al showed a strong correlation between laryngeal ultrasound and MRI for measuring tracheal diameter at the cricoid ring in 27 young adults.[36] Ding et al reported a pilot study using a laryngeal ultrasound to predict post-extubation stridor in 41 patients.[37] The investigators used real-time ultrasonography to evaluate the air leak and to determine the relationship between the air column width during cuff deflation and the development of PES. The results of this study suggest that laryngeal ultrasonography could be a reliable, noninvasive method in the evaluation of laryngeal morphology and airflow through the upper airway. Other predictors of PES include length of intubation, female gender, body mass index, and ratio of ETT size to laryngeal diameter.[28,38] Kwon et al reported total operative time, and the volume of crystalloid and transfused blood given to be risk factors for delayed extubation.[39]

If the patient passes the leak test but still displays clinical evidence of facial and possible airway edema, it would be prudent to perform extubation over an endotracheal tube exchange catheter (Cook Critical Care, Bloomington, IN) to provide a means for ventilation should post-extubation airway obstruction occur. For patients failing the leak test, the authors recommend they should continue to be managed with an ETT in place until the airway edema resolves and a subsequent leak test is satisfactory. Although failing the leak test may not predict post-extubation problems with high specificity, using this approach provides for the greatest margin of safety for the patient. Appropriate treatment of airway edema includes elevation of the head and the use of steroids and diuretics. The efficacy of these measures has not yet been formally validated. Two recent meta-analyses[40,41] provided a comprehensive review of the effect of steroids on PES and showed that there is evidence to support multiple doses of steroids given 12 to 24 hours prior to extubation in adults for preventing PES in high-risk patients (as determined by the cuff leak test). The evidence for prophylactic steroids in neonates or children is heterogenous but shows a trend toward benefit and should be considered for high-risk patients.[41] Steroids may reduce the amount of airway edema and decrease the risk of post-extubation airway obstruction, however, evidence supporting a decreased rate of reintubation only exists in the pediatric population.[42-46]

35.7 SUMMARY

Of all the potential complications associated with prone positioning for a surgical procedure, managing a failed airway is probably the most challenging. The inability to ventilate and oxygenate the patient is life threatening for the patient and demands immediate action from the airway practitioner. Airway management for the prone patient starts by ensuring the tracheal tube is well secured initially to prevent later dislodgement. Every effort must be made to minimize airway edema while the patient is in the prone position. This is particularly important for long surgical procedures involving significant blood loss and fluid shifts.

In the event that the ETT is dislodged from the trachea, oxygenation should be promptly provided by bag-mask-ventilation, or through an extraglottic device such as the LMA, until endotracheal intubation is reestablished. Provided that oxygenation can be maintained, the choice of intubating technique is dependent on the available resources, the patient position, and the skills of the airway practitioner. All airway practitioners must have a strategy to manage a failed airway in a patient in the prone position. Special attention must be paid to the assessment of airway edema prior to tracheal extubation.

REFERENCES

1. Cupitt JM. Induction of anaesthesia in morbidly obese patients. *Br J Anaesth.* 1999;83:964-965.
2. Raphael J, Rosenthal-Ganon T, Gozal Y. Emergency airway management with a laryngeal mask airway in a patient placed in the prone position. *J Clin Anesth.* 2004;16:560-561.
3. Dingeman RS, Goumnerova LC, Goobie SM. The use of a laryngeal mask airway for emergent airway management in a prone child. *Anesth Analg.* 2005;100:670-671.
4. Brain A. Proper technique for insertion of the laryngeal mask. *Anesthesiology.* 1990;73:1053-1054.
5. Ng A, Raitt DG, Smith G. Induction of anesthesia and insertion of a laryngeal mask airway in the prone position for minor surgery. *Anesth Analg.* 2002;94:1194-1198.
6. Lopez AM, Valero R, Brimacombe J. Insertion and use of the LMA Supreme in the prone position. *Anaesthesia.* 2010;65:154-157.
7. Stevens WC, Mehta PD. Use of the Laryngeal Mask Airway in patients positioned prone for short surgical cases in an ambulatory surgery unit in the United States. *J Clin Anesth.* 2008;20:487-488.
8. Brimacombe JR, Wenzel V, Keller C. The ProSeal laryngeal mask airway in prone patients: a retrospective audit of 245 patients. *Anaesth Intensive Care.* 2007;35:222-225.
9. Herrick MJ, Kennedy DJ. Airway obstruction and the laryngeal mask airway in paediatric radiotherapy. *Anaesthesia.* 1992;47:910.
10. Kee WD. Laryngeal mask airway for radiotherapy in the prone position. *Anaesthesia.* 1992;47:446-447.
11. Suderman VS, Crosby ET, Lui A. Elective oral tracheal intubation in cervical spine-injured adults. *Can J Anaesth.* 1991;38:785-789.

12. Nathanson MH, Gajraj NM, Newson CD. Tracheal intubation in a manikin: comparison of supine and left lateral positions. *Br J Anaesth.* 1994;73:690-691.

13. Komatsu R, Nagata O, Sessler DI, Ozaki M. The intubating laryngeal mask airway facilitates tracheal intubation in the lateral position. *Anesth Analg.* 2004;98:858-861.

14. Cheng KI, Chu KS, Chau SW, et al. Lightwand-assisted intubation of patients in the lateral decubitus position. *Anesth Analg.* 2004;99:279-283.

15. Dimitriou V, Voyagis GS, Iatrou C, Brimacombe J. Flexible lightwand-guided intubation using the intubating laryngeal mask airway in the supine, right, and left lateral positions in healthy patients by experienced users. *Anesth Analg.* 2003; 96:896-898.

16. Baer K. [Is it much more difficult to intubate in prone position?]. [Article in Swedish]. *Lakartidningen.* 1992;89:3657-3660.

17. Agrawal S, Sharma JP, Jindal P, Sharma UC, Rajan M. Airway management in prone position with an intubating Laryngeal Mask Airway. *J Clin Anesth.* 2007; 19:293-295.

18. Farcon EL, Kim MH, Marx GF. Changing Mallampati score during labour. *Can J Anaesth.* 1994;41:50-51.

19. Samsoon GL, Young JR. Difficult tracheal intubation: a retrospective study. *Anaesthesia.* 1987;42:487-490.

20. Mallampati SR. Clinical sign to predict difficult tracheal intubation (hypothesis). *Can Anaesth Soc J.* 1983;30:316-317.

21. Knill RL. Difficult laryngoscopy made easy with a "BURP." *Can J Anaesth.* 1993;40:279-282.

22. Cormack RS, Lehane J. Difficult tracheal intubation in obstetrics. *Anaesthesia.* 1984;39:1105-1111.

23. Kidd JF, Dyson A, Latto IP. Successful difficult intubation. Use of the gum elastic bougie. *Anaesthesia.* 1988;43:437-438.

24. Evers KA, Eindhoven GB, Wierda JM. Transient nerve damage following intubation for trans-sphenoidal hypophysectomy. *Can J Anaesth.* 1999;46: 1143-1145.

25. Wang KC, Chan WS, Tsai CT, Wu GJ, Chang Y, Tseng HC. Lingual nerve injury following the use of an oropharyngeal airway under endotracheal general anesthesia. *Acta Anaesthesiol Taiwan.* 2006;44:119-122.

26. Bentsianov BL, Parhiscar A, Azer M, Har-El G. The role of fiberoptic nasopharyngoscopy in the management of the acute airway in angioneurotic edema. *Laryngoscope.* 2000;110:2016-2019.

27. Miller RL, Cole RP. Association between reduced cuff leak volume and postextubation stridor. *Chest.* 1996;110:1035-1040.

28. Kriner EJ, Shafazand S, Colice GL. The endotracheal tube cuff-leak test as a predictor for postextubation stridor. *Respir Care.* 2005;50:1632-1638.

29. Maury E, Guglielminotti J, Alzieu M, Qureshi T, Guidet B, Offenstadt G. How to identify patients with no risk for postextubation stridor? *J Crit Care.* 2004;19:23-28.

30. Chung YH, Chao TY, Chiu CT, Lin MC. The cuff-leak test is a simple tool to verify severe laryngeal edema in patients undergoing long-term mechanical ventilation. *Crit Care Med.* 2006;34:409-414.

31. Suominen P, Taivainen T, Tuominen N, et al. Optimally fitted tracheal tubes decrease the probability of postextubation adverse events in children undergoing general anesthesia. *Paediatr Anaesth.* 2006;16:641-647.

32. Wang CL, Tsai YH, Huang CC, et al. The role of the cuff leak test in predicting the effects of corticosteroid treatment on postextubation stridor. *Chang Gung Med J.* 2007;30:53-61.

33. Shin SH, Heath K, Reed S, Collins J, Weireter LJ, Britt LD. The cuff leak test is not predictive of successful extubation. *Am Surg.* 2008;74:1182-1185.

34. Suominen PK, Tuominen NA, Salminen JT, et al. The air-leak test is not a good predictor of postextubation adverse events in children undergoing cardiac surgery. *J Cardiothorac Vasc Anesth.* 2007;21:197-202.

35. Wratney AT, Benjamin DK, Jr., Slonim AD, He J, Hamel DS, Cheifetz IM. The endotracheal tube air leak test does not predict extubation outcome in critically ill pediatric patients. *Pediatr Crit Care Med.* 2008;9:490-496.

36. Lakhal K, Delplace X, Cottier JP, et al. The feasibility of ultrasound to assess subglottic diameter. *Anesth Analg.* 2007;104:611-614.

37. Ding LW, Wang HC, Wu HD, Chang CJ, Yang PC. Laryngeal ultrasound: a useful method in predicting post-extubation stridor. A pilot study. *Eur Respir J.* 2006;27:384-349.

38. Erginel S, Ucgun I, Yildirim H, Metintas M, Parspour S. High body mass index and long duration of intubation increase post-extubation stridor in patients with mechanical ventilation. *Tohoku J Exp Med.* 2005;207:125-132.

39. Kwon B, Yoo JU, Furey CG, Rowbottom J, Emery SE. Risk factors for delayed extubation after single-stage, multi-level anterior cervical decompression and posterior fusion. *J Spinal Disord Tech.* 2006;19:389-393.

40. Jaber S, Jung B, Chanques G, Bonnet F, Marret E. Effects of steroids on reintubation and post-extubation stridor in adults: meta-analysis of randomised controlled trials. *Crit Care.* 2009;13:R49.

41. Khemani RG, Randolph A, Markovitz B. Corticosteroids for the prevention and treatment of post-extubation stridor in neonates, children and adults. *Cochrane Database Syst Rev.* 2009:CD001000.

42. Markovitz BP, Randolph AG. Corticosteroids for the prevention of reintubation and postextubation stridor in pediatric patients: a meta-analysis. *Pediatr Crit Care Med.* 2002;3:223-226.

43. Meade MO, Guyatt GH, Cook DJ, Sinuff T, Butler R. Trials of corticosteroids to prevent postextubation airway complications. *Chest.* 2001;120: 464S-468S.

44. Anene O, Meert KL, Uy H, Simpson P, Sarnaik AP. Dexamethasone for the prevention of postextubation airway obstruction: a prospective, randomized, double-blind, placebo-controlled trial. *Crit Care Med.* 1996;24:1666-1669.

45. Darmon JY, Rauss A, Dreyfuss D, et al. Evaluation of risk factors for laryngeal edema after tracheal extubation in adults and its prevention by dexamethasone. A placebo-controlled, double-blind, multicenter study. *Anesthesiology.* 1992;77:245-251.

46. Lukkassen IM, Hassing MB, Markhorst DG. Dexamethasone reduces reintubation rate due to postextubation stridor in a high-risk paediatric population. *Acta Paediatr.* 2006;95:74-76.

SELF-EVALUATION QUESTIONS

35.1. Which of the following is **NOT** acceptable initial method to provide oxygenation and ventilation to the patient following dislodgement of the endotracheal tube (ETT) in the prone position?

A. advancing the ETT over a flexible bronchoscope into the trachea

B. establishing a surgical airway

C. insertion of a Laryngeal Mask Airway

D. bag-mask-ventilation

E. reintubation of the trachea using a laryngoscope

35.2. Following orotracheal intubation, which of the following is **NOT** an acceptable method of securing the endotracheal tube (ETT) in a patient with facial hair?

A. Tie the ETT around the neck with an umbilical tape.

B. Tie the ETT to the upper incisors.

C. Secure the ETT with a waterproof tape after the application of tincture of benzoin to the face.

D. Shave the patient's beard prior to induction of anesthesia.

E. None of the above.

35.3. Which of the following is most reliable in assessing postoperative airway edema in a patient who was placed prone for the procedure?

A. the amount of intra-operative fluid administered to the patient

B. the presence of facial edema

C. the leak test

D. flexible nasopharyngoscopy

E. none of the above

CHAPTER (36)

Lung Separation in the Patient with a Difficult Airway

Ian R. Morris

36.1 CASE PRESENTATION

A 50-year-old man presents with a 6-month history of progressive paraparesis. He had sustained a fall at work about 12 months ago and has complained of back pain since that time. He also complains of difficulty with urination and constipation over the past several weeks. Magnetic resonance imaging (MRI) reveals disc herniation at T10-T11 and spinal cord compression. He has been scheduled for T11 vertebrectomy, spinal cord decompression, and spinal instrumentation via a left thoracotomy. He is otherwise healthy. His medications include acetaminophen, and dexamethasone which has recently been added.

On examination, he is 173 cm (5 ft 8 in) tall and weighs 77 kg (170 lb). His vital signs are: blood pressure (BP) 140/80 mm Hg, heart rate (HR) 69 beats per minute (bpm) and regular, respiratory rate (RR) 16 breaths per minute, temperature 36.9°C, and oxygen saturation is 99% on room air. Examination of the lower extremities reveals 3/5 motor power in the left leg and 5/5 in the right leg. Sensation is altered below T11. The chest is clear to auscultation and the heart sounds are normal.

Airway examination reveals a Mallampati II classification, thyromental distance of 5 cm, mouth opening of 5 cm, mandibular mobility of 2 cm, normal cervical spine extension, and full dentition.

36.2 ANESTHESIA CONSIDERATIONS

36.2.1 Is this patient fit for anesthesia?

The patient has spinal cord compression with slowly progressive neurologic symptoms and requires surgery. He has no significant comorbidities and needs no preoperative medical optimization.

36.2.2 What anesthetic technique is required?

General anesthesia is required. Lung separation has been requested by the surgeon to optimize the surgical exposure.

36.2.3 How can one lung ventilation or lung separation be achieved?

Double lumen tubes (DLT) have been considered to be the gold standard for lung separation.[1-4] However, recently introduced bronchial blockers (BBs) have been shown to provide equivalent surgical exposure when compared to the DLT.[5-8] The DLT is preferred when lung isolation is required to protect the nondiseased lung from contamination with blood or pus, in the presence of a bronchopleural or bronchopleural cutaneous fistula, and to perform unilateral pulmonary lavage.[1] A contralateral DLT is preferred when a sleeve resection, or lung transplant is performed.[5,9] However, there are many clinical situations in which a DLT may not be the best primary choice.[2] The indications for the use of a bronchial blocker include the difficult airway, distorted bronchial anatomy, the presence of a tracheostomy, when a nasal intubation is required, and to avoid the need for a tube exchange. Currently available BBs include the Univent Torque Control Blocker, the Arndt Wire-Guided Endobronchial Blocker, the Cohen Flexitip Endobronchial Blocker, the Fuji Uniblocker, the HS Endoblocker, and the Coopdech Endobronchial Blocker.[3,5,10-13]

One lung ventilation using a DLT is planned in the operating room (OR), basic monitors are applied and a left radial arterial catheter is placed under local anesthesia. Following denitrogenation, general anesthesia is induced with propofol 175 mg, sufentanil 15 ug, and rocuronium 50 mg. Bag-mask-ventilation is easily performed. Direct laryngoscopy (DL) with a #4 Macintosh blade reveals a Grade 4 Cormack/Lehane view (soft palate only). Cystic tissue is noted to be present at the posterior aspect of the tongue.

36.3   AIRWAY MANAGEMENT

36.3.1   Is this a difficult airway?

The term "difficult airway" has been used when conventional direct laryngoscopy reveals a Cormack/Lehane (C/L) Grade 3 (epiglottis only) or Grade 4 (soft palate only) view.[9,14-16] Certainly, tracheal intubation can be more difficult in this clinical setting. The ASA Task Force on Management of the Difficult Airway defines difficult airway as "the clinical situation in which a conventionally trained anesthesiologist experiences difficulty with face mask ventilation, endotracheal intubation, or both."[17] The other dimensions of airway management (ventilation by extraglottic device and surgical access to the airway) as outlined by Murphy et al must also be considered when estimating the magnitude of airway difficulty.[18] DLTs and the Univent tube have been termed "difficult tubes" as they can be more difficult to insert due to their increased outside diameter (OD) and increased overall rigidity which impedes optimal shaping of the tubes.[14,16] The criteria for difficult DLT insertion have not been well defined.[1,2] However, difficulty can be encountered in the presence of a Cormack/Lehane II (partial glottis) view.[9]

36.3.2   What are the options for airway management in this patient?

Mask ventilation has been demonstrated to be easy but direct laryngoscopy is difficult. The patient's position should have been optimal before induction. If not, then it should be optimized. Head lift and external laryngeal manipulation should be considered part of the best direct laryngoscopy technique. A blade change can be considered if it is anticipated that a specific anatomic problem can be overcome. Placement of a DLT is best accomplished with a curved blade as it leaves more space in the pharynx through which to pass the relatively bulky DLT.[9] An Eschmann tracheal introducer (bougie) is unlikely to succeed in the presence of a CL Grade 4 view and may produce trauma.

In the patient who has a difficult direct laryngoscopy and who requires lung separation, the airway management options include placement of a single tube (SLT) and utilization of a bronchial blocker, placement of a Univent tube, or placement of a DLT. The decision to use an SLT as opposed to a Univent or a DLT is based on the degree of difficulty anticipated with the more difficult tube, which is a function of the available airway management equipment (eg, video laryngoscope), the airway anatomy/geometry, and the expertise of the airway practitioner, as well

as the anticipated postoperative clinical course. If postoperative ventilation is possible or probable based on the length and extent or type of surgery, anticipated fluid shifts and transfusion requirements, hemodynamic stability, or marginal respiratory reserve, then placement of a DLT may require a tube change at the end of the case.[1,2,9] Exchange of a DLT for an SLT at the end of the case is not without risk.[2] Edema, secretions, and trauma from the initial intubation[1-3,9,16] may make reintubation at the end of surgery more difficult. Optimal positioning for intubation at the end of surgery may also be more difficult to achieve. Reintubation at the end of surgery may be extremely difficult and can be a highly dangerous maneuver[3] with potential loss of airway control.[1] Aspiration and airway trauma can also occur.[1]

The decision to proceed with intubation with an SLT, a Univent, or a DLT is a matter of clinical judgment, taking into consideration the technical and airway anatomical issues as well as the anticipated clinical course. The requirement for lung separation must also be evaluated. The absolute indications for lung separation include massive bleeding or abscess in which the non-diseased lung must be protected from contamination, unilateral air leak from bronchopleural or bronchopleural cutaneous fistula, or unilateral pulmonary lavage for alveolar proteinosis or cystic fibrosis.[1,3,9,16] Video-assisted thoracoscopic surgery (VATS) has also been included as an absolute indication for lung separation.[1,16] Other indications for lung separation are relative and are to improve surgical exposure.[3,16] Although many surgical procedures are more easily performed with the lung collapsed, if placement of a DLT or BB is problematic, the need for lung separation as well as the safety of the technique must be considered.[9]

Intubation techniques that can be used as an alternative to DL include flexible bronchoscopic intubation under general anesthesia, intubation using a video laryngoscope (Glidescope, McGrath, Pentax AirwayScope, Bullard, or Stortz VMAC), or intubation through an LMA or ILMA.

Intubation of the unconscious patient using the flexible bronchoscope is a widely accepted technique. Jaw thrust and tongue traction can be used to open the hypopharynx and facilitate passage of the scope. Minimizing the discrepancy between the OD of the bronchoscope and the internal diameter (ID) of the ensleeved endotracheal tube (ETT) will minimize the risk that the tube will meet obstruction as it is passed through the larynx into the trachea over the scope.

In the setting of *predicted* difficult DL, awake flexible bronchoscopic intubation has historically been considered to be the safest means to secure the airway[9], and in the elective, predicted difficult airway, is still recommended as the preferred technique.[3] However, with the introduction of devices that are proving to be useful in the difficult intubation, protocols are changing[9] and video laryngoscopes are challenging bronchoscopy as the first choice for accessing the difficult airway.[9,19-21]

Flexible bronchoscopic intubation using a Univent tube can be more difficult than with a conventional ETT due to the fixed concavity of the Univent as well as its larger OD.[1,22] When performing a flexible bronchoscopic intubation with a DLT, the length of the tube relative to the length of the shaft of the scope limits the maneuverability of the scope.[16,23] The rigidity of the DLT also makes it harder to advance the tube over the scope.[16]

Intubation with an SLT utilizing the Glidescope is widely practiced and is associated with a high degree of success.[24] Hernandez and Wong have reported the successful placement of a DLT using the Glidescope.[25] Shulman and Connelly used the Bullard laryngoscope in a group of 29 patients scheduled for general anesthesia and lung separation.[26] A DLT was successfully passed into the trachea in 28 of the 29 patients using the Bullard laryngoscope. Hirabayashi and Norimasa used the Airtraq laryngoscope to place #35 or #37 DLTs in 10 patients.[27] Nine of the 10 patients had a CL Grade 1 to 2 view on DL with a Macintosh blade. Suzuki et al reported the successful intubation of a patient with a #39 DLT using the Pentax AirwayScope with a modified blade.[28] Poon and Liu used the AirwayScope to place an Airway Exchange Catheter (AEC) into the trachea and then railroaded a #37 DLT over the catheter under visual control using the scope.[29] Intubation with a DLT using the Bonfils intubation fiberscope[30] and Wu scope[31] have also been reported.

Retrograde intubation is an option in the clinical scenario presented here if the equipment and expertise are available.[32,33]

Intubation with an SLT or AEC through an LMA or ILMA is also an option.[34] Intubation by transillumination utilizing a lighted stylet is a nonvisual technique and is not recommended in the presence of pharyngeal masses or anatomic abnormalities of the upper airway.[35,36] However, placement of DLTs using a lighted stylet under general anesthesia in patients with predictors of difficult DL but without airway pathology has been reported.[22,37,38]

In the case presented here, a flexible bronchoscopic intubation under general anesthesia was attempted but the vocal cords could not be visualized. The glottis was visualized with the Glidescope but the larynx was noted to be extremely anterior and neither a bougie nor an ETT could be passed through the glottis because of the acute angle that needed to be negotiated up into the larynx. An ILMA was placed and satisfactory ventilation was achieved. The flexible bronchoscope was passed through the ILMA but the vocal cords could not be identified. The patient was ventilated through the ILMA until the muscle relaxation could be reversed and then awakened.

36.3.3 What should be the next steps in this patient's management?

The patient requires urgent surgery. He was transported to the post anesthesia care unit (PACU) for a period of observation. An explanation of the airway difficulty was provided to the patient, an antisialogogue was administered, and the patient was returned to the OR about 2 hours later for an awake flexible bronchoscopic intubation.

Awake flexible bronchoscopic intubation using an adult bronchoscope and an 8.5-mm ID SLT was performed under topical anesthesia (see Chapter 3). A remifentanil infusion was used to attenuate airway reflexes. The awake intubation was uneventful and was followed by the controlled induction of general anesthesia.

36.3.4 Can awake flexible bronchoscopic intubation be done with a DLT?

Successful awake flexible bronchoscopic intubation with a DLT has been reported by Patane et al.[23] The laryngeal and carinal stimulation produced by the DLT requires profound anesthesia of

the airway.[23] When the DLT has been placed in the trachea, general anesthesia can also be induced before advancing the DLT into the mainstem bronchus under flexible bronchoscopic control.

36.3.5 What are the options for lung separation in this case now that an SLT has been placed?

The options for one lung ventilation include use of a bronchial blocker passed through the SLT or exchange of the SLT for either a Univent tube or a DLT using an AEC and under visual control utilizing a video laryngoscope.[2,9,15,39,40]

In the case presented here, it was decided to proceed with the placement of a bronchial blocker and not to exchange the SLT for a DLT. This decision was based on the degree of difficulty anticipated with the tube change and the risk associated with this maneuver, as well as the possibility of the requirement for post-op ventilation. An Arndt WEB was chosen and placed uneventfully.

The surgical procedure required 8 hours to complete. The estimated blood loss was 8000 mL. Eleven units of packed red blood cells, 1500 mL of plasma, 8 units of platelets, 6000 mL of crystalloid, and 1500 mL of colloid were administered. At the end of the case, edema of the face and tongue was evident.

36.4 POSTOPERATIVE AIRWAY CONSIDERATIONS

36.4.1 Should this patient be extubated?

The presence of airway edema will almost certainly make reintubation conditions even less favorable than they were at the beginning of the case. In addition, the patient has undergone an extensive surgical procedure, and the risk of respiratory failure in the immediate postoperative period is significant.

The BB was deflated and removed but the ETT was left in place. The patient was transported to the intensive care unit (ICU) in stable condition and electively ventilated. Twenty-four hours after the surgery the patient was awake and no longer required ventilatory support.

36.4.2 How should the patient be extubated at this point in time?

Whether the patient should be extubated in the ICU or in the OR is a matter of clinical judgment and to some extent dependent on the expertise and equipment available. Nasopharyngoscopy can be performed to determine the extent, if any, of airway edema, and the presence of an air leak around the tube may be reassuring.

Given the degree of difficulty experienced with the intubation, the patient was transported to the OR for extubation. Extubation was performed over an AEC, being careful to match the numbers on the catheter with the numbers on the SLT. A surgeon skilled in the performance of a surgical airway was present in the room and the equipment required was immediately available. Extubation was uneventful.

36.5   OTHER CONSIDERATIONS

36.5.1   If the SLT had been exchanged for a DLT after induction, how should this be done?

Tube exchange should be done utilizing an AEC and under visual control.[2,3,15,41] If the glottis cannot be visualized by DL, then a video laryngoscope such as the Glidescope, McGrath, Pentax, or Stortz VMAC can be used.[2,15] The AEC should be introduced no further than 24 to 26 cm from the teeth or lips in order to minimize the risk of trauma to the distal trachea and bronchi.[3,9,15] The AEC should be at least 70 cm in length in order to permit control of the proximal end of the catheter with the DLT ensleeved.[9] Utilization of an AEC at least 83 cm in length has also been recommended for a DLT exchange.[15]

36.5.2   If a DLT had been used for lung separation, what should the appropriate airway management have been at the end of the case? Can the patient go to ICU with a DLT in place?

Intubation was difficult at the start of the case. Given the extent and duration of the surgery and the evidence of airway edema, exchange of the DLT for an SLT at the end of the case could be a highly dangerous maneuver.[3] The view of the glottis was suboptimal with the Glidescope at induction and the angle into the larynx difficult to negotiate. The options then, are to leave the DLT in place, or perform a tracheotomy. If it is anticipated that the airway edema will recede in the immediate postoperative period and that prolonged ventilatory support will not be required, tracheotomy is not necessary at this time. Given the intraoperative course, placement of a BB through the SLT was a good decision and avoided the consideration of a potentially risky tube change at the end of the case.

A DLT can be used in the critical care setting for one lung ventilation or for postoperative two lung ventilation, if tube change to an SLT is considered to be too risky.[9] However, ICU staff are generally less experienced in the management of a DLT[16] and most ICU nurses are not comfortable with DLTs.[1] If the DLT is left in an endobronchial position, malposition can occur and it has been recommended that in this setting neuromuscular blockade be employed.[16] Alternatively, the DLT can be withdrawn such that the endobronchial lumen is above the carina and both lungs ventilated with both lumens with the bronchial cuff deflated.[9] Suction is also more difficult through a DLT and secretions can be problematic.[16]

In the postoperative setting, extubation directly from the DLT can be performed when the condition of the upper airway and ventilatory function are satisfactory. If more prolonged but short-term ventilatory support is anticipated, tube exchange to an SLT can be performed when the upper airway is favorable. If longer-term ventilation is anticipated, tracheotomy without a tube change may be more appropriate.

36.5.3   What would have been appropriate airway management if the surgery had been an emergency and could not be postponed?

Intubation had failed by DL, Glidescope, flexible bronchoscope, and via the ILMA. The expertise to perform a retrograde intubation was not available and the likelihood of success was uncertain given the airway pathology. If the neurologic deficit had been acute, then a tracheotomy could have been performed under general anesthesia with the patient ventilated via the ILMA. A bronchial blocker could then be passed through an armored ETT or conventional tracheotomy cannula inserted into the tracheotomy stoma.[9,15,42,43] If a wire-reinforced ETT is used, this can be changed for a tracheotomy cannula at the end of the case. A conventional DLT can be inserted through a tracheotomy stoma, or a DLT modified for use in tracheostomized patients (eg, Tracheopart or Naruke tube) can also be used.[3,15,43-47] A conventional DLT placed through a tracheotomy stoma has been said to be prone to malposition[15] as it is too long relative to the shortened upper airway and the tracheal cuff may be proximal to the stoma.[16] Cohen has recommended that a rigid large diameter DLT not be passed through an old tracheotomy stoma.[1] The Univent tube has also been inserted through a tracheotomy stoma to achieve one lung ventilation.[48,49]

35.5.4   If a "cannot intubate, cannot ventilate" situation had occurred at induction, what would have been the appropriate management?

If ventilation by mask or extraglottic device had become impossible during the failed intubation attempts, emergency cricothyrotomy would have been indicated.[3]

The patient made an uneventful recovery. The diagnosis of lingual tonsillar hyperplasia (see Chapter 37) was subsequently confirmed by an ear, nose, and throat consultant. No treatment was required.

36.6   SUMMARY

Lung separation can be achieved using a DLT, the Univent tube, or a bronchial blocker placed through an SLT. In the setting of a difficult airway, the decision to use a particular device must take into consideration the airway anatomy and geometry, the expertise and equipment available, and the anticipated postoperative clinical course. Airway management decisions will depend on whether the difficulty is predicted or unpredicted and whether the surgery is elective or emergency. In the management of the difficult airway, the first priority is to ensure adequate oxygenation and ventilation; one lung ventilation becomes a secondary objective.[3]

REFERENCES

1. Cohen E. Pro: the new bronchial blockers are preferable to double-lumen tubes for lung isolation. *J Cardiothorac Vasc Anesth.* 2008;22:920-924.

2. Cohen E. Recommendations for airway control and difficult airway management in thoracic anesthesia and lung separation procedures. Are we ready for the challenge? *Minerva Anestesiol.* 2009;75:3-5.

3. Merli G, Guarino A, Della Rocca G, et al. Recommendations for airway control and difficult airway management in thoracic anesthesia and lung separation procedures. *Minerva Anestesiol.* 2009;75:59-78;79-96.

4. Satya-Krishna R, Popat M. Insertion of the double lumen tube in the difficult airway. *Anaesthesia.* 2006;61:896-898.

5. Campos JH. Which device should be considered the best for lung isolation: double-lumen endotracheal tube versus bronchial blockers. *Curr Opin Anaesthesiol.* 2007;20:27-31.

6. Campos JH, Kernstine KH. A comparison of a left-sided Broncho-Cath with the torque control blocker univent and the wire-guided blocker. *Anesth Analg.* 2003;96:283-289, table of contents.

7. Campos JH, Massa FC. Is there a better right-sided tube for one-lung ventilation? A comparison of the right-sided double-lumen tube with the single-lumen tube with right-sided enclosed bronchial blocker. *Anesth Analg.* 1998;86:696-700.

8. Narayanaswamy M, McRae K, Slinger P, et al. Choosing a lung isolation device for thoracic surgery: a randomized trial of three bronchial blockers versus double-lumen tubes. *Anesth Analg.* 2009;108:1097-1101.

9. Brodsky JB. Lung separation and the difficult airway. *Br J Anaesth.* 2009;103(Suppl 1):i66-i75.

10. Arndt GA, Buchika S, Kranner PW, DeLessio ST. Wire-guided endobronchial blockade in a patient with a limited mouth opening. *Can J Anaesth.* 1999;46:87-89.

11. Arndt GA, DeLessio ST, Kranner PW, Orzepowski W, Ceranski B, Valtysson B. One-lung ventilation when intubation is difficult—presentation of a new endobronchial blocker. *Acta Anaesthesiol Scand.* 1999;43:356-358.

12. Arndt GA, Kranner PW, Rusy DA, Love R. Single-lung ventilation in a critically ill patient using a fiberoptically directed wire-guided endobronchial blocker. *Anesthesiology.* 1999;90:1484-1486.

13. Cohen E. The Cohen flexitip endobronchial blocker: an alternative to a double lumen tube. *Anesth Analg.* 2005;101:1877-1879.

14. Benumof JL. Difficult tubes and difficult airways. *J Cardiothorac Vasc Anesth.* 1998;12:131-132.

15. Campos JH. Lung isolation techniques for patients with difficult airway. *Curr Opin Anaesthesiol.* 2010;23:12-17.

16. Cohen E, Benumof JL. Lung separation in the patient with a difficult airway. *Curr Opin Anaesthesiol.* 1999;12:29-35.

17. American Society of Anesthesiologists Task Force on Management of the Difficult Airway. Practice guidelines for management of the difficult airway: an updated report by the American Society of Anesthesiologists Task Force on Management of the Difficult Airway. *Anesthesiology.* 2003;98:1269-1277.

18. Murphy M, Hung O, Launcelott G, Law JA, Morris I. Predicting the difficult laryngoscopic intubation: are we on the right track? *Can J Anaesth.* 2005;52:231-235.

19. Marco CA, Marco AP. Airway adjuncts. *Emerg Med Clin North Am.* 2008;26:1015-1027, x.

20. Pott LM, Murray WB. Review of video laryngoscopy and rigid fiberoptic laryngoscopy. *Curr Opin Anaesthesiol.* 2008;21:750-758.

21. Thong SY, Lim Y. Video and optic laryngoscopy assisted tracheal intubation—the new era. *Anaesth Intensive Care.* 2009;37:219-233.

22. O'Connor CJ, O'Connor TA. Use of lighted stylets to facilitate insertion of double-lumen endobronchial tubes in patients with difficult airway anatomy. *J Clin Anesth.* 2006;18:616-619.

23. Patane PS, Sell BA, Mahla ME. Awake fiberoptic endobronchial intubation. *J Cardiothorac Anesth.* 1990;4:229-231.

24. Cooper RM, Pacey JA, Bishop MJ, McCluskey SA. Early clinical experience with a new videolaryngoscope (GlideScope) in 728 patients. *Can J Anaesth.* 2005;52:191-198.

25. Hernandez AA, Wong DH. Using a Glidescope for intubation with a double lumen endotracheal tube. *Can J Anaesth.* 2005;52:658-659.

26. Shulman GB, Connelly NR. Double lumen tube placement with the Bullard laryngoscope. *Can J Anaesth.* 1999;46:232-234.

27. Hirabayashi Y, Seo N. The Airtraq laryngoscope for placement of double-lumen endobronchial tube. *Can J Anaesth.* 2007;54:955-957.

28. Suzuki A, Kunisawa T, Iwasaki H. Double lumen tube placement with the Pentax-Airway Scope. *Can J Anaesth.* 2007;54:853-854.

29. Poon KH, Liu EH. The Airway Scope for difficult double-lumen tube intubation. *J Clin Anesth.* 2008;20:319.

30. Bein B, Caliebe D, Romer T, Scholz J, Dorges V. Using the Bonfils intubation fiberscope with a double-lumen tracheal tube. *Anesthesiology.* 2005;102:1290-1291.

31. Smith CE, Kareti M. Fiberoptic laryngoscopy (WuScope) for double-lumen endobronchial tube placement in two difficult-intubation patients. *Anesthesiology.* 2000;93:906-907.

32. Sanchez AF, Morrison DE. Retrograde intubation. In: Hagberg CA, ed. *Handbook of Difficult Management.* Philadelphia, PA: Churchill Livingstone; 2000: pp 115-148.

33. Sanchez A. Retrograde intubation technique. In: Benumof JL, ed. *Airway Management Principles and Practice.* 2nd ed. Philadelphia, PA: Mosby Elsevier; 2007: pp 439-462.

34. Perlin DI, Hannallah MS. Double-lumen tube placement in a patient with a difficult airway. *J Cardiothorac Vasc Anesth.* 1996;10:787-788.

35. Hung OR, Stewart RD. Intubating stylets. In: Benumof J, Hagberg CA, eds. *Benumof's Airway Management Principles and Practice.* 2nd ed. Philadelphia, PA: Mosby Elsevier; 2007: pp 463-475.

36. Minkowitz H. Airway gadgets. In: Hagberg CA, ed. *Handbook of Difficult Airway Management.* Philadelphia, PA: Churchill Livingstone; 2000: pp 149-169.

37. Chen KY, Tsao SL, Lin SK, Wu HS. Double-lumen endobronchial tube intubation in patients with difficult airways using Trachlight and a modified technique. *Anesth Analg.* 2007;105:1425-1426, table of contents.

38. Scanzillo MA, Shulman MS. Lighted stylet for placement of a double-lumen endobronchial tube. *Anesth Analg.* 1995;81:205-206.

39. Hagihira S, Takashina M, Mori T, Yoshiya I. One-lung ventilation in patients with difficult airways. *J Cardiothorac Vasc Anesth.* 1998;12:186-188.

40. Chen A, Lai HY, Lin PC, Chen TY, Shyr MH. GlideScope-assisted double-lumen endobronchial tube placement in a patient with an unanticipated difficult airway. *J Cardiothorac Vasc Anesth.* 2008;22:170-172.

41. Hirabayashi Y. GlideScope-assisted endotracheal tube exchange. *J Cardiothorac Vasc Anesth.* 2007;21:777.

42. Campos JH, Kernstine KH. Use of the wire-guided endobronchial blocker for one-lung anesthesia in patients with airway abnormalities. *J Cardiothorac Vasc Anesth.* 2003;17:352-354.

43. Tobias JD. Variations on one-lung ventilation. *J Clin Anesth.* 2001;13:35-39.

44. Brodsky JB, Tobler HG, Mark JB. A double-lumen endobronchial tube for tracheostomies. *Anesthesiology.* 1991;74:387-388.

45. Robinson AR, 3rd, Gravenstein N, Alomar-Melero E, Peng YG. Lung isolation using a laryngeal mask airway and a bronchial blocker in a patient with a recent tracheostomy. *J Cardiothorac Vasc Anesth.* 2008;22:883-886.

46. Saito T, Naruke T, Carney E, Yokokawa Y, Hiraga K, Carlsson C. New double intrabronchial tube (Naruke tube) for tracheostomized patients. *Anesthesiology.* 1998;89:1038-1039.

47. Yaney LL. Double-lumen endotracheal tube for one-lung ventilation through a fresh tracheostomy stoma: a case report. *AANA J.* 2007;75:411-415.

48. Andros TG, Lennon PF. One-lung ventilation in a patient with a tracheostomy and severe tracheobronchial disease. *Anesthesiology.* 1993;79:1127-1128.

49. Bellver J, Garcia-Aguado R, De Andres J, Valia JC, Bolinches R. Selective bronchial intubation with the univent system in patients with a tracheostomy. *Anesthesiology.* 1993;79:1453-1454.

SELF-EVALUATION QUESTIONS

36.1. Why have the Univent and double lumen tubes been termed "difficult tubes"?

A. increased OD

B. increased rigidity

C. increased rigidity and increased OD

D. none of the above

36.2. Changing an SLT for a double lumen tube at the end of the case can be difficult due to:

A. edema

B. previous intubation trauma

C. suboptimal head and neck position

D. secretions

E. all of the above

36.3. Exchange of an SLT for a DLT should be done:

A. under visual control

B. with an AEC

C. with an AEC and under visual control

D. none of the above

CHAPTER (37)

Airway Management of a Patient with an Unanticipated Difficult Laryngoscopy (Lingual Tonsillar Hypertrophy)

Edward Crosby

37.1   CASE PRESENTATION

An obese, diabetic 57-year-old woman presented for femorotibial bypass with vein and graft. Despite a recommendation in favor, she refused regional anesthesia. A general anesthetic with endotracheal intubation due to the prolonged nature of the operation was planned. Following induction of general anesthesia, bag-mask-ventilation (BMV) was difficult and an immediate attempt at direct laryngoscopy was made. An obstructing soft tissue mass in the vallecula at the base of the tongue was observed with the direct laryngoscope; tracheal intubation was impossible with both direct laryngoscopy and with a lighted stylet and some bleeding was observed after several attempts at intubation. A size 3 laryngeal mask airway (LMA) was placed, adequate ventilation was achieved, the procedure was abandoned, and the patient was awakened and taken to the recovery room. Following the procedure, the patient was referred to an otolaryngologist, and nasolaryngoscopy revealed lingual tonsillar hypertrophy (LTH). The lingual tonsil was observed to be occupying and filling the vallecula and obstructing the view of both the epiglottis and the laryngeal inlet. Because she derived no symptoms from the lesion, surgical excision was not felt to be indicated and she was referred back to her vascular surgeon.

In the patient described, LTH completely obstructed the view of the larynx and access to the airway.

37.2   INTRODUCTION

37.2.1   What are lingual tonsils?

The lingual tonsils are components of Waldeyer throat ring and consist of lymphoid tissue located in the posterior third of the tongue which can extend into the vallecula. Waldeyer throat ring is completed by the adenoids and the palatine tonsils. Unlike the palatine tonsils, there is no definite capsule for lingual tonsils. They are inconsistent in their presence and are most typically absent in adults. When present, they lie on either side of the median epiglottic fold, may be both variable and asymmetric in size, and can become very large (Figures 37-1 and 37-2). The natural history of lingua tonsils is not well delineated; periodic growth and regression is likely. In a manner similar to the palatine tonsils, they may become inflamed and, when swollen (as in lingual tonsillitis), the mass may fill the vallecula and press the epiglottis down toward the glottis, causing variable degrees of airway compromise. They are not readily compressible and may not permit direct viewing of

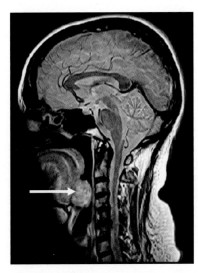

FIGURE 37-1. Magnetic resonance image of an airway with a large lingual tonsil present and identified (arrow).

the laryngeal inlet with a direct laryngoscope during the course of conventional airway management.

37.2.2 How common is lingual tonsillar hypertrophy?

Although lingual tonsillar hypertrophy or hyperplasia (LTH) was first described by Vesalius in 1543, its prevalence and relevance to clinical practice remains ill-defined.[1] Reports of airway difficulties in patients with LTH are infrequent but recurrent suggesting that patients with the condition are regularly but not commonly encountered and recognized by anesthesiologists. Whether or not LTH would always be recognized as being present and being the underlying cause of airway difficulties is a relevant question.

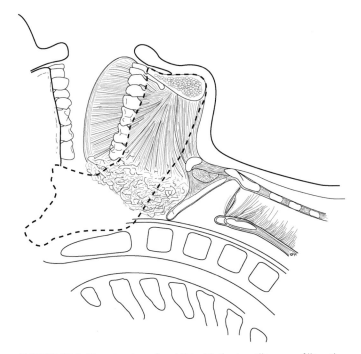

FIGURE 37-2. Line drawing of an LTH with the tonsillar mass filling the pre-epiglottic space and depressing the epiglottis toward the larynx.

Goldman and Greenland reported separately of two patients in whom airway difficulties were encountered by experienced anesthesiologists.[2,3] Postoperative assessments with video and MRI, respectively, revealed the presence of LTH which was suspected in neither case during the initial interventions.

Breitmeier et al conducted an assessment of 497 autopsy specimens to determine the incidence of LTH in an unselected population.[4] In 16 specimens (3.2%) large lingual tonsils were detected. Of the 16 specimens with LTH, 10 had normal palatine tonsils and the others had either no palatine tonsil or remnants only. Adachi et al performed fiberoptic evaluation and tracheal intubation in 105 elective adult surgical patients to determine the incidence of LTH.[5] Thirty-four patients (32%) had small lingual tonsils and seven patients (7%) had large lingual tonsils identified; there was no lingual tonsil identified in 64 (61%) patients. The correlation between the presence of a lingual tonsil and difficult intubation with a direct laryngoscope was not evaluated by these authors. Guimaraes et al evaluated the airways of 71 obese children between the ages of 13 and 21 using computed tomography to determine the frequency of LTH.[6] Forty-four (62%) of the subjects had LTH, which is greater than the frequency previously reported in both normal subjects and those with obstructive sleep apnea. Ten of the children had very large lingual tonsils. Children with previous palatine tonsillectomy had a higher prevalence of measurable lingual tonsils and large lingual tonsils compared with those who still had their palatine tonsils.

Lingual tonsils are likely more prevalent than past reports would indicate, but are still relatively uncommon and probably impact on airway care infrequently. This is because even when present, they are usually small in size. It is probable that they would present difficulties either when they become very large or combine with other factors to make airway management difficult.

37.3 PATIENT CONSIDERATIONS

37.3.1 What patient characteristics are associated with LTH?

There are no large-scale studies of populations of patients which would allow for an accurate evaluation of the etiologic and associated characteristics in patients with LTH. The literature suggests that the presence of LTH may be associated with obesity, sleep apnea, and previous palatine tonsillectomy.[1,4,6] The strength of the associations is not quantifiable and the majority of patients with these associated conditions do not have LTH. The patient described in the case was obese and, although she may have had an increased relative risk for LTH, she would have been considered to be at relatively low absolute risk due to the low population prevalence.

37.3.2 What symptoms occur in patients with LTH?

Clinical symptoms of LTH are not present in all patients with the condition and, in fact, seem absent in many, even in some who present with very large lingual tonsils. Symptoms which do occur may be subtle and are neither sensitive nor specific. Some patients report a sensation of fullness or discomfort in the throat, rarely to the extreme of dysphagia.[7] When they are inflamed, sore throat may be present. But, without knowing the presence of LTH, it is likely that the symptoms of lingual tonsillitis would often be ascribed to those of a common viral pharyngitis (simple sore throat). Very large lingual tonsils may cause obstructive sleep apnea or upper airway obstruction, but may also be associated with either mild or no symptoms.[1,8,9] Acute and complete airway obstruction as a result of inflamed lingual tonsils has been reported leading to sudden death.[10]

The patient described in the case reported no symptoms attributable to LTH and was surprised to be presented with the diagnosis. Her husband reported that she was a noisy nocturnal breather, but neither she nor her husband described any signs or symptoms suggestive of obstructive sleep apnea.

37.3.3   Is LTH detectable with preoperative airway assessment?

Most patients with characteristics associated with LTH do not have the condition and many patients who actually have LTH, including those with very large tonsils, do not have symptoms. LTH is not detectable on routine preoperative physical examination or airway assessment. It is detectable with diagnostic imaging modalities such as plain x-ray, computed tomography, and magnetic resonance imaging as well as with upper airway endoscopy. Subjecting all patients with characteristics associated with LTH to more detailed preoperative airway assessments is difficult to defend from the perspective of both evidence base and resource utilization. However, because of the association between LTH and obstructive sleep apnea (OSA), consideration should be given to diagnostic imaging or nasopharyngoscopy to rule out LTH as an underlying cause in patients newly diagnosed with OSA.

The index patient described in the case had a reassuring airway examination and would not have been considered at risk for either difficult ventilation or intubation with a conventional airway assessment. There was no indication to subject her to a more rigorous airway evaluation based on the history and airway assessment.

37.4   AIRWAY CONSIDERATIONS

37.4.1   What are the implications of LTH for anesthesiologists?

The presence of LTH has been associated with difficult airway management following the induction of anesthesia, and in most of the published reports, LTH seems to be either the only factor responsible for the difficulties with airway management, or the most important one. In many instances, the patients were asymptomatic, had a normal preoperative airway evaluation, and the difficulties were unanticipated. In the largest series published in the anesthesia literature, that of Ovassapian et al, none of the 33 patients reviewed retrospectively had an airway examination that suggested an increased potential for difficult laryngoscopy or intubation.[11] However, unanticipated difficulties were experienced

with either or both bag-mask-ventilation and direct laryngoscopy in all of them. The lungs of 12 patients were difficult to ventilate by bag and mask. In five cases, failed intubation occurred but there were no details as to the number of attempts at direct laryngoscopy; in one case two failed attempts were made; in nine cases three failed attempts were recorded; in 14 cases four failed attempts occurred; in three cases, there were five attempts; and in one case, six attempts were made before the procedure was abandoned. The tracheas of six patients were subsequently intubated using a fiberoptic bronchoscope (FOB) with the patient awake; four of these interventions were characterized as moderately difficult and two as easy. Of the remaining 27 patients who subsequently underwent FOB-assisted tracheal intubation, 4 interventions were deemed difficult, 12 were moderately difficult, and 11 were reported as easy. Difficulty was experienced passing the endotracheal tube over the FOB and into the trachea in 11 patients. All 33 patients were subsequently evaluated using fiberoptic pharyngoscopy to determine possible causes of the failure; the only finding common to all 33 patients was the presence of LTH.

Other authors have reported similar findings with either single cases or smaller series. But the themes are consistent with the report of Ovassapian et al; unanticipated difficulties were often encountered with ventilation of the lungs and intubation of the trachea.[9,12,13] These difficulties with ventilation were not always or easily overcome with the use of laryngeal mask airways nor were difficulties with tracheal intubation routinely or readily overcome with the use of adjuncts or alternatives to the direct laryngoscope. Difficulties seem common even in situations where difficulties were anticipated and experienced anesthesiologists deployed advanced alternatives for airway management. It is fortunately the case that, in many of the reports, it was possible for the anesthesiologist to maintain sufficient oxygenation through a variety of interventions to safely abandon further attempts at intubation and awaken the patient. However, Jones and Cohle reported a death due to failed airway management in a 24-year-old patient presenting with probable appendicitis.[14] Following induction of anesthesia, bag-mask-ventilation was impossible and tracheal intubation failed despite repeated attempts with both a direct laryngoscope and a fiberoptic bronchoscope. A tracheotomy was performed but the patient never regained consciousness and died 8 hours postoperatively. At autopsy, a large lingual tonsil was discovered.

In the patient described in the case, moderate difficulties were experienced with bag-mask-ventilation although it was possible to maintain her oxygen saturation in a clinically acceptable range. However tracheal intubation was unsuccessful with both direct laryngoscopy and with a lighted stylet. Because of the difficulties with ventilation, a decision was made to attempt placement of a laryngeal mask airway, which was successful and resulted in an effective airway.

37.4.2   How do lingual tonsils interfere with bag-mask-ventilation and direct laryngoscopy?

If the lingual tonsils are large enough, the airway is obstructed at the base of the tongue and elevation of the tongue may be inadequate to relieve the obstruction. Placement of an oral airway may result in the distal aperture of the airway being directly opposed by the tonsillar mass and obstructed as well. It is possible that a nasal airway may better bypass the obstruction caused by LTH than an oral airway, but this is by no means certain. In the patient described in the case, an oral airway did not seem to reduce the difficulties with bag-mask-ventilation and no attempt was made to place a nasal airway.

Successful laryngoscopy is dependent on the development of a line-of-sight from the eye to the larynx. Most difficulties with direct laryngoscopy can be grouped into a limited number of categories: mouth opening is inadequate to admit the blade adequately; airway angles are sharp and irreducible; soft tissues are either overabundant and compromising or noncompliant and unyielding; there are obstructing masses present; or blood and secretions interfere with light reflection. Horton et al demonstrated the importance during laryngoscopy of control of the hyoid bone with the tip of the laryngoscope blade reporting that the body of the hyoid was drawn forward and tilted downward.[15] This tip placement resulted in tensioning of the hyoepiglottic ligament, elevation of the epiglottis, and exposure of the laryngeal structures. Tripathi and Pandey similarly reported that placement of the tip of a curved Macintosh blade in the pre-epiglottic space (vallecula) proximal to the hyoid bone achieved elevation and tilting of the hyoid bone, tensioning of the hyoepiglottic ligaments, and an optimal glottic view.[16] The presence of the LTH at the base of the tongue, in the pre-epiglottic space, will prevent proper placement of the laryngoscope blade thus interfering with the basic mechanisms of laryngoscopy. The obstruction of the airway lumen by the LTH is the second factor that will interfere with the direct laryngoscopy.

The presence of the lingual tonsil may completely obstruct the line-of-sight necessary for successful laryngoscopy. Many of the alternatives to the direct laryngoscope, such as the indirect fiberoptic and video-optic laryngoscopes, also depend on the development of a line-of-sight from the instrument tip and this requirement may render them ineffective for the task of airway salvage if direct laryngoscopy proves to be impossible due to LTH. The use of blind techniques, such as the lightwand, in the presence of a known soft tissue mass in the airway is controversial and some would consider such techniques to be contraindicated due to the risk of tissue trauma and bleeding.

37.4.3 What airway management practices have been employed in patients with LTH?

In the majority of reports, airway management difficulties were unanticipated and included both difficult or failed ventilation and intubation. The use of laryngeal mask airways is a common feature in the reports; the outcomes of LMA deployments ranged across the spectrum from successful ventilation and intubation using the LMA as a conduit for tracheal intubation, to no improvement in ventilation and continued failed intubation. With respect to difficulties encountered with intubation, in those scenarios that were unanticipated, the most common response was persistent attempt at direct laryngoscopy without success. The use of flexible bronchoscopes, Eschmann tracheal introducers (bougies) and intubation catheters, straight blades, and an anterior commissure blade by an otolaryngologist have all been reported with variable results.

The most common technology reported as being deployed in anticipated difficult situations (interventions made subsequent to the diagnosis of LTH being made) has been the flexible bronchoscope (FB), typically in an awake patient. Although usually successful, difficulties with both accessing the airway with the FB and subsequently with advancing the endotracheal tube into the trachea are common. These difficulties likely result not only from the obstruction of the airway lumen by the LTH but also from the requirement to pass deep to the LTH with the FB along the posterior pharyngeal wall, then to turn sharply in the opposite direction to access the laryngeal inlet, and finally to turn one more time to pass into the tracheal lumen. The turning radius of the FB is likely an issue when multiple turns have to be executed over a short distance.

The Bullard laryngoscope was employed in this case as it was thought that it would be capable of lifting the epiglottis and the tonsil to allow access to the laryngeal inlet. By performing the laryngoscopy in an awake patient, it was presumed that if a laryngeal view could not be obtained, the procedure could be safely abandoned and an alternative technique attempted.

37.4.4 What is the role of extraglottic airways in the management of LTH?

The most commonly deployed extraglottic airway reportedly being used has been the laryngeal mask airway (LMA), in one form or another. These have been placed to facilitate both ventilation and intubation with varying results. In some reports, difficult ventilation was improved after the placement of the LMA, but intubation through the device was not possible.[9,13,17] In other reports, placement of an LMA resulted in both a resolution of difficult ventilation and provided a conduit for successful tracheal intubation.[2,18] Finally, some authors report little apparent improvement in difficult ventilation after placement of an LMA and failed attempts at intubation using the LMA as a conduit.[12,19] The success of the LMA in reducing the severity of difficult ventilation and providing an intubation conduit in the setting of LTH is likely impacted both by the size of the tonsil, the position of the LMA orifice in relation to the laryngeal inlet, and the degree of airway obstruction resulting from the tonsillar hypertrophy. In most reports, placement of an LMA has resulted in some reduction in the ventilation difficulties being encountered. The available reports support a recommendation that placement of an LMA be considered early if difficulty with ventilation is being experienced in the setting of an LTH. Whether a smaller than usual LMA may provide equal or greater benefit in this setting is speculative.

A laryngeal mask airway was placed easily in the case described and resulted in a much improved airway. A size 3 LMA was used, although it would have been conventional local practice to use a size 4 in this patient.

37.4.5 Which of the available airway technologies should be most effective in the setting of LTH?

There are two anatomic issues relevant to airway management which must be considered in a patient with LTH. The first issue is the angles to be negotiated between the mouth and the glottic inlet and the second is the degree of obstruction of the airway lumen by the tonsil. As discussed, if the tonsils are very large, then to either access the laryngeal inlet or obtain a view of the larynx, the airway instrument must pass deep to the base of the tongue and behind the tonsil along the posterior pharyngeal wall. To get a view of the larynx, it must then move sharply anteriorly and away from the posterior pharyngeal wall to develop the line-of-sight. To access the laryngeal inlet it also must pass anteriorly and over the posterior commissure, and then turn once again to move down through the cords, and into the tracheal lumen. If the instrument is dependent for its success on the development of a line-of-sight from its tip to the laryngeal inlet from a point in the airway above the larynx, this line-of-sight is likely to be obstructed by the presence of large tonsils.

A rigid device such as the Bullard™ laryngoscope (BL) is possibly the ideal instrument for the management of the airway in a patient with LTH, both in the anticipated and unanticipated scenario.[18, 20] It is capable of negotiating the angles described and its robust construction permits gentle manipulation of airway tissues, allowing it to create the necessary endoscopic airspace. It may be used to gently elevate the lingual tonsil to reduce the degree of obstruction and, when placed in its final position, the tip of the BL rests beyond the lingual tonsil in the laryngeal inlet, bypassing the lumenal obstruction caused by the tonsil. Although the BL does require a line-of-sight from blade tip to target, typically the blade tip should be placed beyond the tonsil when positioned. Because it can carry the tracheal tube mounted on its dedicated stylet, no second working channel is needed for tube placement—an obvious advantage in the patient with a lingual tonsil and a relatively noncompliant airway. As well, in the scenario of an airway mass, the BL can be fitted with a standard surgical camera, allowing for visualization of the entire intervention and reducing the potential for trauma to the tonsil. Despite the theoretic advantages of an instrument, such as the BL for the management of the airway in a patient with LTH, it would be imprudent to conclude that it would always be effective.

The FB may also be used to successfully negotiate the angles described and is also capable of bypassing the obstructed lumen. Whereas a rigid instrument may be used to elevate tissues and reduce the angles which must be negotiated, the FB must negotiate them as it finds them. It may be very difficult to traverse the airway due to the repeated turns which must be executed over a relatively short distance. As well, it may be difficult to avoid soiling the bronchoscope on the tonsil or cause bleeding by contacting the tonsil if there is a high degree of obstruction of the lumen. Finally, passing the tube over the FB may prove difficult as well as the tube must negotiate the same angles previously negotiated by the FB. Warming the endotracheal tube and the use of a Parker-type tube and ensuring a close match between tube and FB diameters may all increase the likelihood of successful tube passage. As well, combining a rigid blade with the FB and using the blade to elevate the soft tissues to permit passage of the FB may be an effective salvage strategy.

Ultimately, it may not be possible to secure the airway from a supraglottic approach and either a retrograde or an infraglottic surgical approach may be necessary. A wire inserted through a cricothyroid membrane puncture could be used to facilitate either a retrograde intubation or to guide a supraglottic technique (eg, threading an FB loaded with an endotracheal tube). Cricothyrotomy or tracheotomy may be performed either electively or urgently if a "cannot intubate-cannot ventilate" situation is encountered.

As previously noted, and for the reasons already outlined, awake tracheal intubation was attempted with a Bullard™ laryngoscope. The Bullard™ blade was placed under the epiglottis and used to gently elevate both the epiglottis and the tonsil affording a full view of the larynx. Intubation of the trachea was readily achieved using a tube mounted on the dedicated stylet.

37.4.6 How should the algorithms of Chapter 2 be applied to the care of the patient with LTH?

If LTH is recognized before the induction of anesthesia, the airway assessment would be considered non-reassuring and concerns would be raised regarding both bag-mask-ventilation and tracheal intubation. Given that assessment, management would be directed by Panel A of the ASA Difficult Airway Management Algorithm in Figures 2-1 and 2-2, or the Emergency Difficult Airway Algorithm in Figure 2-5 and an awake intubation would be recommended; consideration should also be given to a surgical airway in some instances. If LTH was unanticipated and difficulties are experienced with ventilation and/or intubation, management would be directed by Panel B of the ASA Difficult Airway Management Algorithm in Figures 2-1 and 2-2 or the Failed Airway Algorithm in Figure 2-6.

37.4.7 What is optimal elective airway management in a patient known to have LTH?

Although bag-mask-ventilation has usually been possible in situations where LTH was unanticipated and encountered, both difficult and failed ventilation have been reported. As well, difficult and failed intubation using either direct laryngoscopy, and adjuncts and alternatives to the direct laryngoscope are common. It is the author's opinion that the airway assessment in a patient known to have LTH is non-reassuring with respect to both bag-mask-ventilation and tracheal intubation and an awake intubation is both the most prudent and optimal approach to airway management as dictated by the ASA Difficult Airway Management Algorithm (Figure 2-2).

37.5   PATIENT MANAGEMENT

37.5.1 How was this patient managed?

When rescheduled for surgery, she again refused regional anesthesia but agreed to awake tracheal intubation. Preoperatively, she received glycopyrrolate 0.6 mg subcutaneously to dry oral-pharyngeal secretions. She was provided with supplemental oxygen by nasal prongs, incremental sedation, and topical anesthesia of the airway. A Bullard™ laryngoscope (BL) fitted with oxygen tubing (8 L·min⁻¹), a dedicated stylet with a 7.0 mm ID endotracheal tube, and a surgical camera were introduced into the airway. Under video guidance, the laryngoscope was passed to the base of the tongue and used to gently elevate the lingual tonsil, allowing the laryngoscope to move beyond and into the laryngeal inlet, whereupon the vocal cords were visualized. The trachea was intubated and the surgery then proceeded uneventfully. At the end of the procedure, the patient was allowed to awaken and once fully and cognitively responsive, her trachea was extubated. She was observed in a high-surveillance nursing unit overnight and then discharged to a ward bed.

37.5.2 Are there special considerations for tracheal extubation in patients with LTH?

It may be impossible to reestablish an airway in a patient with LTH following extubation of the trachea. The combination of the residual effects of the anesthetics, the anatomic sequela of the airway interventions, and the stress of managing a lost airway, superimposed on the preexistent pathology will likely combine to create the nightmare airway experience. Extubation of the trachea in a patient with LTH should only occur when there is clear evidence that the anesthetic effects are fully reversed, and that the patient is awake and cognitively responsive. The management of tracheal extubation in a patient with LTH would be directed by Figure 2-7, the Difficult Airway Extubation Algorithm and consideration should also be given to the routine placement of an airway exchange catheter before extubation of the trachea in these patients. As well, the anesthesia practitioner must have made preparations for a surgical airway if extubation leads to loss of the airway and it cannot be immediately reestablished.

37.6 OTHER CONSIDERATIONS

37.6.1 Do other conditions similar to LTH occur with airway implications?

Laryngeal, epiglottic, and vallecular cysts have been cited in case reports as having been associated with both difficult and failed ventilation and intubation.[21-23] They are relatively common and usually small but may become very large; most are asymptomatic with symptoms becoming more common as they become larger. Very large cysts may cause dysphagia and occasionally symptoms of airway obstruction. About half originate from the epiglottis and most of these are found on the lingual surface of the epiglottis.[24,25] In adults, they are presumed to largely originate from obstructed ducts of submucosal glands with eventual dilation of the glands causing a retention cyst. As they increase in size, they may fill the vallecula and distort the epiglottis in a manner similar to that of lingual tonsils (Figure 37-3). They may occur at any age although they seem most common in the fifth and sixth decades. Routine preoperative airway evaluation is unlikely to reveal the presence of the cyst in the absence of symptoms. If suspicions are present,

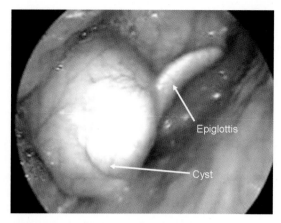

FIGURE 37-3. Photograph of a large left-sided epiglottic cyst taken during upper airway endoscopy.

multiple diagnostic imaging modalities may be used to identify large cysts and nasolaryngoscopy is also useful. In many of the available reports, difficulties with bag-mask-ventilation were not encountered. However, difficult ventilation is more likely to be a potential issue with very large cysts and failed ventilation and death has been reported at induction of anesthesia. Aspiration of the cysts to facilitate airway management has also been reported by a number of authors and has been successful in reducing the degree of obstruction caused by the cyst.[26] If large cysts have been identified on preoperative assessments, they should be more fully evaluated using diagnostic imaging and airway endoscopy to assess their size and the degree of airway compromise. Aspiration of very large cysts before the induction of anesthesia has been reported.[27] An awake intubation is probably the most prudent course of care.

37.6.2 What information should be provided to the patient once LTH is diagnosed?

The patient should be informed of the presence and implications of LTH and airway cysts and be provided with a difficult airway letter for future practitioners, stating the findings and recommendations. It has been our practice to refer these patients to an otolaryngologist for follow-up although management has been typically conservative in patients with asymptomatic lesions. Lingual tonsillectomy and excision, marsupialization, or de-roofing of cysts may be considered if the lesions are symptomatic.

37.7 SUMMARY

LTH is a relatively uncommon disorder in adults defined by overgrowth of lymphoid tissues at the base of the tongue and in the vallecula. Most lingual tonsils, even if enlarged, are small enough so as to not interfere with airway management. But some may be so large as to completely obstruct access to the airway and be life threatening. LTH may be associated with obesity, sleep apnea, and previous palatine tonsillectomy, but the majority of patients with these conditions do not have LTH. Symptoms are not common, although, if present, are obstructive in nature and some patients provide histories of sleep apnea. Routine preoperative airway assessment is not likely to reveal the presence of underlying LTH, although imaging modalities such as radiography, computed tomography, and magnetic resonance imaging and endoscopy are all effective evaluation and diagnostic strategies. If significant LTH is recognized preinduction, consideration should be given to awake intubation. The flexible bronchoscope has been the most frequently described and the most effective technique for managing such patients. If LTH is not recognized preinduction, difficult or failed ventilation and laryngoscopy/intubation may be experienced. Varying success has been reported with the use of extraglottic devices to improve ventilation. If difficult laryngoscopy is experienced, persistent efforts at laryngoscopy are not likely to be successful. Early consideration should be given to salvage attempts with the flexible bronchoscope, rigid fiberoptic devices, subglottic airways, or abandonment of the anesthetic if that can be safely achieved. Patients who are newly diagnosed with LTH should be counseled as to its implications and offered consultation with an otolaryngologist.

REFERENCES

1. Dündar A, Özüntü A, Sahan M, Özgen F. Lingual tonsil hypertrophy producing obstructive sleep apnea. *Laryngoscope*. 1996;106:1167-1169.
2. Goldman AJ, Rosenblatt WH. Use of the fiberoptic intubating LMA-CTrach in two patients with difficult airways. *Anesthesia*. 2006;61:601-603.
3. Greenland KB, Cumpston PH, Huang J. Magnetic resonance scanning of the upper airway following difficult intubation reveals an unexpected lingual tonsil. *Anaesth Intensiv Care*. 2009;37:171-174.
4. Breitmeier D, Wilke N, Schulz Y, et al. The lingual tonsillar hyperplasia in relation to unanticipated difficult intubation. *Am J Forens Med Pathol*. 2005;26:131-135.
5. Adachi YU, Satamoto M, Higuchi H, et al. Assessment of the lingual tonsil and vallecula during fiberoptic intubation. *J Anesth*. 2002;16:345-348.
6. Guimaraes CVA, Kalra M, Donnelly LF, et al. The frequency of lingual tonsil enlargement in obese children. *AJR*. 2008;190:973-975.
7. Fitzgerald P, O'Connell D. Massive hypertrophy of the lingual tonsils: an unusual cause of dysphagia. *Br J Radiol*. 1987;60:505-506.
8. Guarisco JL, Littlewood SC, Butcher RB III. Severe upper airway obstruction in children secondary to lingual tonsil hypertrophy. *Ann Oto Rhinol Laryngol*. 1990;99:621-624.
9. Davies S, Ananthanarayan C, Castro C. Asymptomatic lingual tonsillar hypertrophy and difficult airway management: a report of three cases. *Can J Anesth*. 2001;48:1020-1024.
10. Johnson CP, Burns J. Papillary hyperplasia of the lingual tonsil and sudden death in epilepsy. *Am J Med Pathol*. 1992;13:335-337.
11. Ovassapian A, Glassenberg R, Randel GI, Klock A, Mesnick. P, Klafta J. The unexpected difficult airway and lingual tonsil hyperplasia. *Anesthesiology*. 2002;97:124-132.
12. Asai T, Hirose T, Shingu K. Failed tracheal intubation using a laryngoscope and intubating laryngeal mask. *Can J Anesth*. 2000;47:325-328.
13. Asbjørnsen H, Kuwelker M, Søfteland E. A case of unexpected difficult airway due to lingual tonsil hypertrophy. *Acta Anaesthesiol Scand*. 2008;52:310-312.
14. Jones DH, Cohle SD. Unanticipated difficult airway secondary to lingual tonsillar hyperplasia. *Anesth Analg*. 1993;77:1285-1288.
15. Horton WA, Fahy L, Charters P. Disposition of the cervical vertebrae, atlantoaxial joint, hyoid and mandible during x-ray laryngoscopy. *Br J Anaesth*. 1989;63:435-438.
16. Tripathi M, Pandey M. Short thyromental distance: a predictor of difficult intubation or an indication for small blade selection. *Anesthesiology*. 2006;104:1131-1136.
17. Ojeda A, López AM, Borrat X, Valero R. Failed tracheal intubation with the LMA-CTrach in two patients with lingual tonsil hyperplasia. *Anesth Analg*. 2008;107:601-602.
18. Biro P, Shahinian H. Management of difficult intubation caused by lingual tonsillar hyperplasia. *Anesth Analg*. 1994;79:389.
19. Fundinglsand BW, Benumof JL. Difficulty using a laryngeal mask airway in a patient with lingual tonsil hyperplasia. *Anesthesiology*. 1996;84:1265-1266.
20. Crosby E, Skene D. More on lingual tonsillar hypertrophy. *Can J Anesth*. 2002;49:758.
21. Agrawal S, Asthana V, Sharma JP, Sharma UC, Meher R, Varshney S. Alternative intubation technique in valecular cyst. *J Anaesth Clin Pharmacol*. 2006;4:425-427.
22. Mason DG, Wark KJ. Unexpected difficult intubation. Asymptomatic epiglottic cysts as a cause of upper airway obstruction during anesthesia. *Anaesthesia*. 1987;42:407-410.
23. Rivo J, Matot I. Asymptomatic vallecular cyst: airway management considerations. *J Clin Anesth*. 2001;13:383-386.
24. Arens C, Glanz H, Kleinasser O. Clinical and morphological aspects of laryngeal cysts. *Eur Arch Otorhinolaryngol*. 1997;254:430-436.
25. DeSanto LW, Devine KD, Weiland LH. Cyst of the larynx: classification. *Laryngoscope*. 1970;80:145-176.
26. Shenoy P, Malik SA, Al Duwillah R. A new approach for the treatment of larger epiglottic cysts using nanoendoscopes. *Kuwait Med J*. 2007;39:59-61.
27. Keenleyside HB, Greenway RE. Management of pre-epiglottic cysts: a report of nine cases. *Can Med Assoc J*. 1968;99:645-649.

SELF-EVALUATION QUESTIONS

37.1. The presence of LTH is associated with which of the following patient characteristics?

A. obesity

B. frequent throat infections

C. male gender

D. patients >75 years old

E. Mallampati Class III or IV

37.2. The presence of LTH may be best evaluated by which of the following assessments?

A. a sleep study for obstructive sleep apnea

B. conventional preoperative airway physical examination

C. pulmonary function test: flow-volume loop

D. nasolaryngoscopy of the upper airway

E. a review of previous anesthetic records

37.3. LTH interferes with the performance of direct laryngoscopy by:

A. preventing placement of the blade tip in the vallecula

B. interfering external laryngeal manipulation

C. preventing alignment of the oral and pharyngeal axes

D. preventing alignment of the pharyngeal and tracheal axes

E. obstructing passage of the laryngoscope blade through the oral airspace

CHAPTER (38)

Airway Management of a Patient with Superior Vena Cava Obstruction Syndrome

Gordon O. Launcelott

38.1 CASE PRESENTATION

A 55-year-old male patient with superior vena caval (SVC) obstruction secondary to a mediastinal mass is scheduled for bronchoscopy and mediastinoscopy. The patient weighs 120 kg (250 lb) and has obvious swelling of the face, neck, and upper extremities. The tongue is large (Mallampati Classification IV) and the oral mucosa is plethoric. He is unable to lie flat, but is not dyspneic in the sitting position.

38.2 INTRODUCTION

38.2.1 What is the pertinent pathophysiology in SVC syndrome?

The left and right subclavian and internal jugular veins join to form the brachiocephalic (innominate) veins, which in turn join to form the SVC. Venous drainage from the head and upper extremities then finds its final conduit to the heart in this large, but easily compressible, vessel. Extensive collaterals with the SVC include the azygos, the mammary, vertebral, lateral thoracic, paraspinous, and esophageal veins. The largest of these, the azygos vein, is formed from the junction of the right subcostal and the right ascending lumbar veins. It ascends in the posterior mediastinum and then passes anteriorly over the right main stem bronchus to join the SVC as the latter enters into the right atrium. Here, the area is anatomically crowded with lymph nodes, the pulmonary artery, and the tracheobronchial structures hemmed in by the sternum anteriorly. The low-pressure SVC can be obstructed, either indirectly by external compression from vascular structures, tumor, or enlarged lymph nodes or directly by primary or secondary intraluminal thrombus or tumor (Figures 38-1 and 38-2).

Obstruction of the SVC will result in upper body venous hypertension, which forces blood to seek an alternate pathway to the heart via the previously described collateral vessels and the inferior vena cava. This upper body venous hypertension results in the classic clinical signs and symptoms of the syndrome. These include facial, neck, and arm swelling, as well as engorgement of the mucous membranes, including those of the upper airway. In some patients, it may result in laryngeal or cerebral edema, predisposing to an increased risk of surgical bleeding.

Most cases of SVC syndrome are due to extrinsic tumor compression from bronchogenic carcinoma or non-Hodgkin lymphoma occurring in the right paratracheal space or right pulmonary hilum.[1] From even a cursory glance at the anatomy, it is clear that the disease process may also compromise other major structures in the area, such as the pulmonary arteries, the right heart, and the tracheobronchial tree. With these factors in mind, the practitioner will want to determine the degree to which major structures are involved prior to embarking on induction of general anesthesia (GA).

38.3 PATIENT EVALUATION

38.3.1 What evidence of airway compromise may be apparent on history and physical examination?

Airway compression may be heralded by cough, dyspnea, hemoptysis, and a history of recurrent pulmonary infection. A change in voice may be due to recurrent laryngeal nerve involvement or vocal

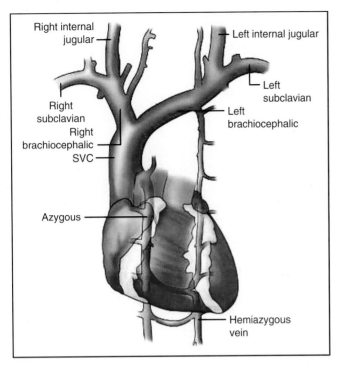

FIGURE 38-1. This diagram illustrates the venous drainage into the heart. (From Abeloff MD. *Clinical Oncology*. 3rd ed. Philadelphia, PA: Elsevier Churchill Livingston; 2004: 1048.)

cord edema. Dyspnea, often with a history of syncope, may not necessarily be due to airway compromise but secondary to right ventricular outflow tract or right heart compression.[1]

In this patient, the tongue is large, perhaps as a result of upper body venous hypertension, and the mucous membranes are plethoric, suggesting that the mucous membranes of the larynx in general, and glottis in particular, may also be engorged, edematous, and friable.

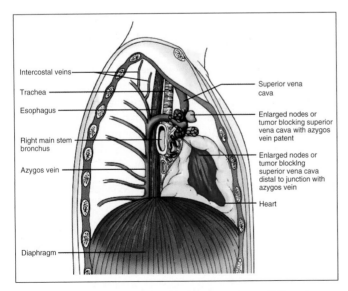

FIGURE 38-2. This diagram shows that the low-pressure SVC can be obstructed, either indirectly by external compression of vascular structures, tumor, or enlarged lymph nodes, or directly by primary or secondary intraluminal thrombus or tumor. (From Abeloff MD. *Clinical Oncology*. 3rd ed. Philadelphia, PA: Elsevier Churchill Livingston; 2004: 1048.)

38.3.2   What investigations should be done to assess the airway of the patient?

Smaller precarinal and left paratracheal tumors may not be evident, but information about the size and location of the majority of mediastinal tumors can be obtained from chest radiography. Pulmonary function tests may be useful in predicting postoperative respiratory complications. In a recent prospective study, Bechard et al[2] found a 10-fold increase in postoperative respiratory complications (pneumonia, airway edema, atelectasis) in patients with a preoperative peak expiratory flow rate (PEFR) of less than 40% of predicted. In the same study, however, PEFR was not predictive of airway collapse. Flow-volume loops, in the supine and upright position, have been advocated to assess the degree of airway obstruction as it relates to body position and to distinguish variable from fixed intrathoracic lesions.[3] However, Narang et al documented that the respiratory embarrassment caused by mediastinal masses tends to be characteristic of a fixed lesion causing predominantly inspiratory impairment.[1]

Recent contrast-enhanced CT or MRI imaging is the most useful of all investigations in defining the relation of the mass to the other mediastinal structures. The CT or MRI can provide the practitioner with the necessary information with regard to the presence of pericardial effusion, the degree of anatomic compression of the airway, and the degree to which structures, such as the pulmonary arteries, right ventricular outflow tract, and the heart, may be compromised (Figures 38-3 and 38-4A). Transthoracic echocardiography (TTE) is useful in assessing the presence of pericardial effusion and the dynamic effects of tumor mass on the heart and great vessels. Significant pericardial effusion can result in cardiovascular collapse on induction of general anesthesia and positive pressure ventilation.

In this patient, chest CT findings were consistent with SVC obstruction. There was no evidence of pulmonary artery, right ventricular outflow tract, and myocardial or tracheobronchial compromise, and no evidence of pericardial effusion.

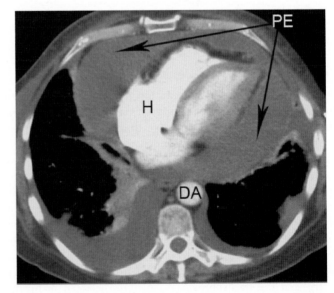

FIGURE 38-3. CT scan of the thorax of the patient with a pericardial effusion: This CT scan of the chest shows a large pericardial effusion (PE) surrounding the heart (H), anterior to the descending aorta (DA).

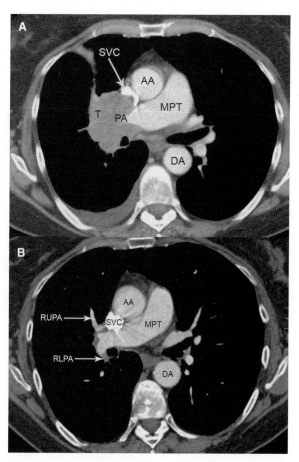

FIGURE 38-4. (A) CT scan of the thorax of the patient with a large mediastinal mass prior to chemotherapy: This CT scan of the chest shows a large right mediastinal tumor (T) encroaching the pulmonary artery (PA) and the superior vena cava (SVC). Also shown in this scan are the ascending aorta (AA), the descending aorta (DA), and the main pulmonary trunk (MPT). (B) CT scan of the thorax of the patient with a mediastinal mass after chemotherapy: This CT scan of the chest shows the normal pulmonary vasculature after chemotherapy with the disappearance of the mediastinal tumor. The superior vena cava (SVC), the anterior segmental right upper lobe pulmonary artery (RUPA), the proximal aspect of the right lower lobe pulmonary artery (RLPA), the ascending aorta (AA), the descending aorta (DA), and the main pulmonary trunk (MPT) are shown clearly without obstruction.

38.4   SPECIFIC CONCERNS FOR THIS PATIENT

38.4.1   What complications are associated with mediastinal masses and general anesthesia?

Most practitioners have a heightened sense of awareness when they are confronted with the patient with a mediastinal mass scheduled for surgery. We have all heard of the reports of airway obstruction or cardiovascular collapse.[4,5] We may even be familiar with the anesthesia management dogmas associated with these cases. Much of the literature documenting these catastrophic scenarios, however, involves pediatric populations.[6] Furthermore, it is clear that one cannot extrapolate what may happen in the adult patient

from the pediatric literature. The situation is further complicated by the fact that many of the sickest patients, like those with SVC syndrome, are managed with chemotherapy or radiation to shrink their tumors prior to presenting for surgery and general anesthesia (GA) (Figure 38-4A and B), or they are managed with less invasive surgical techniques not requiring GA. Confusing the picture even more is the fact that some series include small or posterior mediastinal masses that are unlikely to be associated with significant cardiorespiratory compromise.[2]

The only studies that have evaluated the incidence of life-threatening cardiorespiratory compromise are those by Azarow et al[6] and Bechard et al.[2] Azarow et al[6] noted that there was a significant difference in anesthetic risk between adults and children with mediastinal masses undergoing GA. The authors noted that although the mortality in both groups was similar, mortality in the pediatric group is primarily related to perioperative respiratory complications whereas mortality in the adult group is due to the malignancy itself.[7] Total airway obstruction in pediatric patients during GA has been associated with preoperative tracheal compression of more than 50%.[7] This, however, does not seem to be the case in adults. In Bechard's prospective study of 98 adult patients,[2] there was no intraoperative airway obstruction in any of the eight patients with preoperative airway compression greater than 50%. Furthermore, there has only been a single case report in the literature, reporting a parturient patient with a severe airway obstruction during anesthesia.[8] Tracheal compression greater than 50% in the adult population was, however, associated with a sevenfold increase in respiratory complications, but these were related to pneumonia, airway edema, and atelectasis in the first 48 hours postoperatively.[2]

Whether the patient exhibits signs and symptoms related to the mediastinal mass effect seems to be important. A study by Hnatiuk et al[9] suggested that symptomatic patients were more likely to experience complications, and Bechard[2] identified stridor, orthopnea, cyanosis, jugular distension, and SVC syndrome as factors associated with perioperative complications. In Bechard's study,[2] 3 of 105 anesthetics were complicated by severe cardiovascular compromise; 2 of which were associated with pericardial effusion. There have been reports of severe airway obstruction occurring in asymptomatic patients, but again this seems limited to the pediatric population.[2]

38.4.2   What are the airway concerns for this patient?

First of all, ventilation using a bag-mask may be difficult in this patient because he is obese, with a large tongue and edematous airway (see MOANS in Section 1.6.1).

Although the literature suggests that obesity,[10-12] per se, is not a predictor of difficult oxygenation/ventilation with an extraglottic device (EGD), this patient with a large tongue in addition to an edematous upper airway should cause the wise practitioner to exercise caution when considering the EGD as a rescue technique should the airway be lost. (See RODS in Section 1.6.3.)

There are several airway characteristics of this patient that would suggest a difficult direct laryngoscopy. He has a Mallampati Class IV pharyngeal view, in spite of the fact that he may have adequate mouth opening and thyromental distance. He is likely to have some reduction in neck mobility. In addition, he does have significant venous congestion that involves the mucous membranes of the mouth, probably the tongue and likely the larynx. Therefore, in all likelihood direct laryngoscopy will be difficult.

Certainly, he is obese with swelling of his neck and evidence of upper body venous hypertension, all of which would make emergency cricothyrotomy a challenge.

38.4.3   What are the major concerns with the circulation?

The major concern, from a circulatory standpoint in the patient with a mediastinal mass, is circulatory collapse on induction of anesthesia and initiation of positive pressure ventilation. This is a possibility when the mediastinal pathology results in right ventricular outflow obstruction or direct heart compression by the tumor mass, or pericardial effusion compromising cardiac output. Again, in Bechard's study, 3 of 105 patients experienced life-threatening intraoperative cardiovascular events; 2 of whom had pericardial effusions.[2]

Patients with preoperative cardiovascular compromise may have symptoms, such as dyspnea, orthopnea, and a history of syncope. The structural abnormalities, whether they be right ventricular outflow obstruction or direct heart compromise, can often be appreciated on chest CT scan (Figure 38.4A and B). Dynamic factors associated with these structural abnormalities can be further assessed with transthoracic echocardiography (TTE). Significant pericardial effusions should be drained prior to presenting to the operating room for surgery. If there is significant right ventricular outflow obstruction, or direct heart compromise, as evidenced by clinical symptoms and/or CT and TTE findings, consideration should be given to planning for elective femoral-femoral cardiopulmonary bypass (CPB). Attempting to catheterize femoral vessels to initiate CPB following cardiovascular collapse is unlikely to be successful. Therefore, it is imperative that everything be in place prior to induction of anesthesia. A Japanese center recommended the use of a temporary extracorporeal axillofemoral venous bypass as a life-saving and auxiliary device in urgent operations for acute progressive SVC syndrome with symptoms of cerebral edema and upper airway obstruction due to intrathoracic malignancies.[13]

In patients with significant cardiovascular compromise, most surgery will be directed to obtaining a diagnosis to plan future therapy. Intrathoracic surgery under general anesthesia is a risky proposition in this group of patients. Every effort should be made to obtain a tissue sample from peripheral sites under local anesthesia. It is said that the practitioner who wishes to grow old slowly should palpate the neck and axillae of all such patients before considering GA and surgery.[1]

38.4.4   Are there any other important considerations?

In patients with SVC syndrome, there is the possibility of increased intracranial pressure due to obstructed cerebral venous drainage.

Efforts to avoid the cerebral dilating effects of vapor anesthetics, such as hyperventilation and total intravenous anesthesia, may be considerations in this regard.

In the patient with SVC syndrome, large-bore IV catheters should be placed in the lower extremities as injected medications will make their way to the heart more quickly than through the obstructed route via the subclavian vein and SVC. Adequate intravascular volume is important, as is the immediate availability of inotropes and vasopressors.

38.5   AIRWAY MANAGEMENT

38.5.1   What is the most appropriate airway management option for this patient?

As a result of the factors discussed earlier, it is prudent to secure the airway awake using the flexible bronchoscope (FB). Successful topical anesthesia of the airway is improved by using a drying agent. This should be given subcutaneously (SC) or intravenously (IV) 20 minutes to 1 hour prior to bringing the patient to the induction area.[14] Following FB intubation, the ventilation of patients with mediastinal masses can be managed in a variety of ways. In Bechard's study, only 15 out of 97 patients were induced using spontaneous ventilation and in only 3 was spontaneous ventilation used throughout.[2]

The textbook dogma of maintaining spontaneous ventilation throughout in the patients with mediastinal vascular and tracheobronchial compromise is based mostly on anecdotal information. Patients with an obstructive airway component, as may be the case in patients with mediastinal tumors, are potentially susceptible to so-called dynamic hyperinflation, or auto-PEEP, following initiation of positive pressure ventilation. This can increase global intrathoracic pressure contributing to decreased venous return and increased cardiovascular compromise.[15]

From a strictly respiratory perspective, it is a common belief that patients with airway compromise secondary to mediastinal mass effect are less likely to have an airflow obstruction with maintenance of spontaneous ventilation. This is based on the erroneous belief that mediastinal tumors behave more like *variable* rather than *fixed* intrathoracic lesions. Flow-volume loops in patients with variable intrathoracic lesions show a restricted expiratory flow but a largely unaffected inspiratory flow. Fixed lesions, in contrast, have an equal reduction in both inspiratory and expiratory flows compared to normal subjects.[16] Vander Els et al[3] studied patients with intrathoracic Hodgkin disease. They found that these intrathoracic masses behave more like fixed than like variable lesions with equal inspiratory/expiratory flow impairment or a predominant inspiratory flow reduction. As a result, maintenance of spontaneous ventilation in these patients would appear to be of little benefit.[3]

In this patient with no evidence of tracheobronchial compression or significant cardiovascular compromise, it is unlikely that there would be any advantage in maintaining spontaneous ventilation. Following awake bronchoscopic intubation, the patient can be induced breathing spontaneously followed by neuromuscular block and controlled ventilation, or neuromuscular block and controlled ventilation can be initiated immediately upon induction. Spontaneous, assisted ventilation throughout may be a consideration in patients with CT or echocardiographic evidence of significant cardiovascular compromise.

38.5.2   What actually happened in this case?

The patient had no evidence of tracheobronchial, pulmonary artery, right ventricular outflow tract, or direct myocardial compromise. He received 0.4 mg glycopyrrolate subcutaneously 1 hour prior to transfer to the operating room in the sitting position. Two units of blood were immediately available. He was transferred to the operating table and was maintained in the semi-Fowler position. Standard monitors, including ECG and pulse oximetry, were applied. A 14-gauge venous catheter was placed in his left greater saphenous vein at the ankle and a #20 arterial catheter placed in the left radial artery. A 1.5-L bolus of saline was given in preparation for anesthetic induction. Increased inspired oxygen via nasal cannula at the rate of 3 L·min^{-1} was applied. The airway was anesthetized with a gargle of aqueous 4% lidocaine followed by nebulized 4% lidocaine using a DeVilbiss atomizer. The trachea was intubated with an 8.5 mm ID endotracheal tube over an adult FB. Breathing 100% oxygen, the patient received 150 mg of propofol and 30 mg of rocuronium. Following loss of consciousness, controlled manual ventilation was initiated and sevoflurane was introduced. Cardiovascular and respiratory parameters remained stable and the patient was placed on the ventilator. Once cardiovascular stability was assured, morphine 7.5 mg was given in divided doses. The surgical procedure lasted 50 minutes and was uneventful from a surgical and anesthetic standpoint. Neuromuscular block was reversed with neostigmine and glycopyrrolate. The patient was allowed to emerge from general anesthesia and extubated awake in the sitting position. The immediate post-extubation period was uneventful and he was transported, in the sitting position, to the post-anesthesia care unit (PACU) in stable condition breathing supplemental oxygen from a Venturi mask. The subsequent postoperative course was also uneventful.

38.5.3   What is a reasonable approach for extubation following emergence from general anesthesia?

For all the reasons that this patient should have his airway secured awake, tracheal extubation should also be done when the patient is fully awake. In addition, worsening of airway edema can occur following endotracheal intubation and mediastinal surgery. Consideration may even be given to leaving an airway exchange catheter in the airway following extubation.[17] The catheter can be removed when the practitioner is confident that the patient has an acceptable airway, with effective gas exchange.

38.6   SUMMARY

In adult patients with SVC syndrome, the major considerations are with the edematous, congested mucous membranes that are prone to bleed and can make direct laryngoscopy and endotracheal intubation technically difficult and extubation potentially hazardous. It appears that life-threatening intraoperative airway obstruction in the adult is less of a problem than it is in the pediatric population. Life-threatening airway obstruction is unlikely to occur in adult patients with significantly compromised airways but pneumonia, airway edema, and atelectasis are more frequent in the first 48 hours postoperatively. The threat of post-induction cardiovascular collapse is limited to those patients with pericardial effusions, direct heart compromise by the tumor mass, and/or the potential for right ventricular outflow obstruction. These patients can be identified with careful preoperative assessment, including history, physical examination, CT scan, and echocardiography.

REFERENCES

1. Narang S, Harte BH, Body SC. Anesthesia for patients with a mediastinal mass. *Anesthesiol Clin North America*. 2001;19:559-579.
2. Bechard P, Letourneau L, Lacasse Y, et al. Perioperative cardiorespiratory complications in adults with mediastinal mass: incidence and risk factors. *Anesthesiology*. 2004;100:826-834; discussion 5A.
3. Vander Els NJ, Sorhage F, Bach AM, Straus DJ, White DA. Abnormal flow volume loops in patients with intrathoracic Hodgkin's disease. *Chest*. 2000;117:1256-1261.
4. Keon TP. Death on induction of anesthesia for cervical node biopsy. *Anesthesiology*. 1981;55:471-472.
5. Levin H, Bursztein S, Heifetz M. Cardiac arrest in a child with an anterior mediastinal mass. *Anesth Analg*. 1985;64:1129-1130.
6. Azarow KS, Pearl RH, Zurcher R, Edwards FH, Cohen AJ. Primary mediastinal masses. A comparison of adult and pediatric populations. *J Thorac Cardiovasc Surg*. 1993;106:67-72.
7. Azizkhan RG, Dudgeon DL, Buck JR, et al. Life-threatening airway obstruction as a complication to the management of mediastinal masses in children. *J Pediatr Surg*. 1985;20:816-822.
8. Lai YY, Ho HC. Total airway occlusion in a parturient with a mediastinal mass after anesthetic induction—a case report. *Acta Anaesthesiol Taiwan*. 2006;44:127-130.
9. Hnatiuk OW, Corcoran PC, Sierra A. Spirometry in surgery for anterior mediastinal masses. *Chest*. 2001;120:1152-1156.
10. Combes X, Sauvat S, Leroux B, et al. Intubating laryngeal mask airway in morbidly obese and lean patients: a comparative study. *Anesthesiology*. 2005;102:1106-1109; discussion 5A.
11. Frappier J, Guenoun T, Journois D, et al. Airway management using the intubating laryngeal mask airway for the morbidly obese patient. *Anesth Analg*. 2003;96:1510-1515, table of contents.
12. Natalini G, Franceschetti ME, Pantelidi MT, Rosano A, Lanza G, Bernardini A. Comparison of the standard laryngeal mask airway and the ProSeal laryngeal mask airway in obese patients. *Br J Anaesth*. 2003;90:323-326.
13. Shimokawa S, Yamashita T, Kinjyo T, et al. Temporary extracorporeal axillofemoral venous bypass—a beneficial device in operation for superior vena caval syndrome due to intrathoracic malignancies. *Nippon Kyobu Geka Gakkai Zasshi*. 1997;45:1827-1832.
14. Watanabe H, Lindgren L, Rosenberg P, Randell T. Glycopyrronium prolongs topical anaesthesia of oral mucosa and enhances absorption of lignocaine. *Br J Anaesth*. 1993;70:94-95.
15. Pepe PE, Marini JJ. Occult positive end-expiratory pressure in mechanically ventilated patients with airflow obstruction: the auto-PEEP effect. *Am Rev Respir Dis*. 1982;126:166-170.
16. Burrows B, Knudson RJ, Quan SF et al. *Respiratory Disorders: A Pathophysiologic Approach*. 2nd ed. Chicago: Mosby; 1983.

17. American Society of Anesthesiologists Task Force on Management of the Difficult Airway. Practice guidelines for management of the difficult airway. A report by the American Society of Anesthesiologists Task Force on Management of the Difficult Airway. *Anesthesiology*. 1993;78: 597-602.

SELF-EVALUATION QUESTIONS

38.1. Which of the following is NOT a known classic clinical sign and symptom of patients with superior vena cava obstruction syndrome?

A. facial, neck, and arm swelling

B. hemoptysis

C. laryngeal edema

D. cerebral edema

E. engorgement of the mucous membranes

38.2. Which of the following airway management strategies may be difficult in patients with a large mediastinal mass and superior vena cava obstruction syndrome?

A. face-mask ventilation

B. ventilation using extraglottic devices

C. laryngoscopic intubation

D. surgical airway

E. all of the above

38.3. Which of the following is a known complication associated with mediastinal masses and general anesthesia?

A. cardiovascular collapse

B. tracheal obstruction

C. pneumonia

D. pericardial effusion

E. all of the above

CHAPTER 39

Airway Management of a Patient with History of Difficult Airway Who Refuses to Have Awake Tracheal Intubation

Dmitry Portnoy and Carin Hagberg

39.1 CASE PRESENTATION

A 46-year-old ASA III man is scheduled to have a total knee replacement. His past medical history is remarkable for severe rheumatoid arthritis (RA) with cervical spine involvement. He was recently diagnosed with atlanto-axial subluxation, but he has no neurological signs. He has a history of gastroesophageal reflux disease (GERD), but it is well controlled with proton pump inhibitors. His other medications are an NSAID and low-dose glucocorticosteroid therapy.

On physical examination, he weighs 67 kg (148 lb) and is 167 cm (5 ft 6 in) tall, his BMI is 23.9 kg·m^{-2}. Examination of his airway reveals that he has a full beard and small chin, no teeth, 3.0 cm of mouth opening, and that his neck is fixed in moderate flexion. This same surgery was previously cancelled as the patient refused to complete an awake bronchoscopic intubation. The patient now emphatically refuses to consent for awake bronchoscopic intubation.

39.2 PREOPERATIVE ANESTHETIC ASSESSMENT

39.2.1 What is rheumatoid arthritis? What are the anesthetic implications of this illness?

Rheumatoid arthritis (RA) is a lifelong (chronic) multisystem illness, which represents the most common form of chronic inflammatory arthritis and affects approximately 1% of adults (range 0.3%-2.1%) in the United States and Europe. Women are typically affected two to three times more often than men and the prevalence increases with age. The etiology of RA remains unknown, but it is evident that complex interaction between environmental factors (including infectious agents) and the immune system in genetically susceptible individuals plays an essential role.[1] The class II major histocompatibility complex allele HLA-DR4 has been found to be a major genetic risk factor. The onset of RA is typically gradual between the age of 35 and 50, and may be of nonspecific nature.[2,3] Synovial inflammation, cartilage damage, and bone erosion with subsequent destruction of joint integrity are the hallmarks of this illness. The course is characterized by symmetrical polyarthropathy and variably, considerable systemic involvement. As the disease progresses, cervical spine involvement becomes common, second only to involvement of the metatarsophalangeal joint.[1]

Extraarticular manifestations of RA are widespread and can affect as many as 40% of patients, 15% of whom appear to be severely affected.[1,2] Many of these manifestations have a serious impact on anesthesia care. *Cardiac manifestations* most commonly present as pericarditis with effusion (in one-half of patients), but may also include cardiac conduction abnormality, granulomatous myocarditis, and valvular pathology. *Rheumatoid vasculitis* can affect almost any organ system and may produce coronary artery arteritis contributing to coronary syndrome. *Pleuropulmonary* pathology, which occurs more commonly in men, includes pleural disease, effusion, pleuropulmonary nodules, interstitial fibrosis, obliterative bronchiolitis, and pneumonitis. The prevalence of airflow obstruction in rheumatoid patients is remarkably high, suggesting it might be the commonest form of pulmonary involvement.[4] Rheumatoid nodules and osteoporosis may develop in up to 30% of patients with RA. *Neurologic manifestations* may result from cervical spine subluxation and nerve entrapment secondary to proliferative synovitis or joint deformities which can produce various neuropathies.

Other important extraarticular manifestations include *ocular* involvement, which occurs in 25% of individuals with RA, such as keratoconjunctivitis sicca, and *hematologic* changes—chronic anemia and thrombocytosis.[1,2]

39.2.2   How does rheumatoid arthritis affect the airway?

Airway management is one of the most critical aspects of anesthesia care of RA patients. There are several important elements implicated in how RA progression affects the airway of these patients:

1. *Cervical spine.* (Figure 39-1) Progression of RA of the cervical spine affects 15% to 86% of these patients, eventually leading to disintegration of cervical spine joints. Twenty-five percent of hospitalized RA patients have cervical pathology. Pain (40%-88%), neurologic deficiencies (7%-34%), and even sudden death from brain stem compression (10%)[5] are possible manifestations of cervical spine involvement.[1] The three most commonly observed forms of cervical pathology in RA include: (1) anterior or rarely posterior atlanto-axial subluxation (AAS); (2) vertical subluxation or atlanto-axial impaction; and (3) subaxial subluxation. Anterior AAS, the most common of these abnormalities occurring in 43% to 86% of patients, is associated with a greater than expected mortality in this group.[1,6,7]

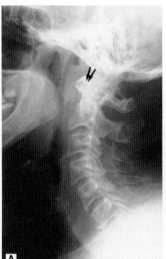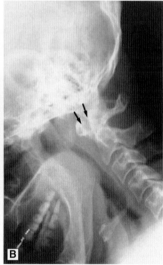

FIGURE 39-1. A lateral view of the cervical spine of a patient with rheumatoid arthritis: (A) with the neck extended, there is very little space (which is normal) between the posterior aspect of the arch of C1 and the anterior portion of the odontoid (arrows); (B) with flexion, this space markedly widens, and the odontoid is free to compress the spinal cord, which is posterior to it. (Permission obtained from Mettler FA, Jr. *Essentials of Radiology.* 2nd ed. Saunders, an Imprint of Elsevier: 2005.)

AAS is commonly associated with spinal cord compression and neurological deficits. However, absence of preoperative neurological symptoms may not assure perioperative safety, particularly under general anesthesia when neurological symptoms may not be detectable.[7] Thus, specific precautions are warranted during airway manipulation and intraoperative positioning to avoid spinal cord injury. In addition, RA-related cervical spine rigidity and flexion deformity will present further complexity in airway management.[7,8]

2. *Temporomandibular joints (TMJs) and mandible abnormalities.* Up to 31% of RA patients report TMJ dysfunction. The severe form of this abnormality can lead to TMJ ankylosis and can significantly reduce the patient's ability to open the mouth. It has also been associated with high incidence of upper airway obstruction.[9,10] In a study of 218 RA patients, a positive correlation was reported between the severity of RA and the range of motion of the jaw.[10]

3. *Micrognathia.* Hypoplastic mandible, another airway hazard, is found to be associated predominantly with a juvenile form of RA, in some cases as a congenital association, in others—due to affection of TMJ arthritis.[11]

4. *Cricoarytenoid arthritis.* This is reported in 30% to 50% of RA patients, and between 45% and 88% in postmortem studies.[12] The prevalence of this potentially life-threatening condition seems to be much higher than expected. There are numerous reports of severe and even fatal airway obstruction in any period of the perioperative course, frequently unanticipated.[12-15]

5. *Rheumatoid nodules.* These nodules of the larynx and laryngeal deformity related to RA have been occasionally reported as a cause of airway complications that contribute to difficulties in airway management of RA patients.[9,15,16]

In summary, RA patients may frequently confront the anesthesia practitioner with multiple challenges in airway management throughout the perioperative course. This may be due to a severe form of a single airway–related pathology or any combination of pathologic changes such as cervical spine problems (rigidity, AAS, low cervical subluxation), TMJ ankylosis, micrognathia, cricoarytenoid arthritis, and laryngeal tissue damage. When approaching these patients' airways, the anesthesia practitioner should bear in mind that there are two separate facets of the problem: high incidence of difficult direct laryngoscopy requiring an alternative technique(s) and a danger of neurological complications as a consequence of airway manipulation. Tests of RA activity and the duration of the disease did not show direct correlation with the incidence of difficult intubation.[17] Thus, meticulous preoperative airway assessment in these patients is warranted regardless of the severity and duration of disease.

39.2.3   What is informed consent? What are the elements of informed consent?

Legal and moral basis of informed consent is established on the ethical principle of respect for patient autonomy and self-determination. In the United States, this is also rooted in constitutional guarantees of privacy and noninterference. In 1914, the case of *Schloendorff v. Society of New York Hospital* established that it was the right of "every human being of adult years and sound mind to determine what shall happen to his own body."[18,19] The term "informed consent" came into common use in 1957 as a result of the case of *Salgo v. Trustees of Leland Stanford Hospital*, when it was postulated that physicians have a duty to inform patients about the risks and alternatives to treatment, in addition to the procedures themselves and their consequences.[19] This gave the concept of informed consent its modern interpretation, which was directed to maximize the ability of the patient to make substantially autonomous informed decisions. In other words, informed consent is the process by which a fully informed patient can participate in the decisions about his or her health in a meaningful way. It is generally accepted that in order to complete a modern informed consent properly, the following seven components and principles must be established.[19]

1. *Decision-making capacity.* Decision-making capacity is a reasonable ability to understand discussed issues and make a particular decision at a specific time as well as the ability to express a preference based on rational, internally consistent reasoning.

2. *Voluntariness.* The voluntariness principle is based on the notion that physicians should perform procedures only on competent patients who participate willingly. Anesthesiologists may potentially compromise voluntariness through manipulation and coercion when they physically or pharmacologically restrain patients who have sufficient decision-making capacity.

3. *Disclosure.* The goal of disclosure is to provide comprehensive information to the patient relevant for her/his decision-making. The exact nature of the procedure must be discussed. Reasonable alternatives to the proposed procedure must be discussed revealing pros and cons of those options.

4. *Recommendation.* Anesthesiologists should present an expert opinion regarding advantages and disadvantages of each option. Patients can then participate in decision-making to determine the best option which suits their priorities.

5. *Understanding.* Considerable efforts should be made to confirm that patients understand the risks and benefits of the proposed procedures, and why those recommendations were made. Pain and distress in various patients' groups, including parturients, do not appear to impair comprehension or preclude obtaining a legally sufficient informed consent.

6. *Decision.* After the comprehensive information, including the anesthesiologist's recommendation, the patient takes part in the choice of the appropriate anesthetic technique. Patients may vary in their preferences for decision-making participation; therefore, anesthesiologists should thoughtfully attempt to tailor the extent of patient and physician decision-making to the individual patient and the situation.

7. *Autonomous authorization.* Finally, the informed consent process concludes with the patient intentionally authorizing the anesthesiologist to perform a specific procedure or intervention, and this will constitute the patient's self-determination and the basis of informed consent.

39.2.4 What is informed refusal of treatment or a procedure? What are the options for the anesthesia practitioner in this case?

Informed consent would be meaningless if the patient cannot also decline medical intervention based on his/her reasoning.[20-22] It is essential, in recognition of patient autonomy, to show recognition and respect for different individual values that may be reflected in the patient decision-making process.[23] However, if a patient rejects an anesthesiologist's advice, or requests a technique that the anesthesiologist believes is inappropriate, the focus of discussion turns from informed consent to *informed refusal*. In this case, in addition to all requirements similar to informed consent, the patient should be substantially well versed about the risks and benefits of refusal and, importantly—about reasonable alternatives. Despite full disclosure and proper consent procedure, some patients may occasionally demand or reject an intervention that is extremely unreasonable, and predictably associated with inappropriately high risk. Determination of an appropriate choice of anesthesia is difficult and should not be made lightly or out of convenience. The conscientious physician cannot be forced by anyone, including a patient, to practice negligently.[19] It is important to remember that just as the patient can refuse to have an awake intubation, the anesthesia practitioner may also decline to provide care to a patient, unless it is an emergency. In this case, an anesthesiologist who chooses to withdraw from the patient's care is obligated to make a reasonable effort to find a competent and willing replacement.[19]

In this case, in which the patient refuses an awake intubation, a complete discussion and description of the process of awake intubation must take place and an assessment must be made to determine that the patient fully understands the procedure. Efforts should be put forth to assure that patient refusal is not a result of false beliefs based on misinformation, misunderstanding, or atypical and inappropriate previous experience.[20,23] Other alternatives to awake intubation must then be discussed with the patient, as well as the associated risks and benefits associated with these alternatives. Finally, the patient and the airway practitioner need to be in agreement with the proposed airway management plan, especially as the patient's cooperation is required.

In an emergency situation in which the patient requires a life- or limb-saving procedure and no other anesthesia care provider is available, the anesthesia practitioner is obliged to proceed under emergency conditions and honor the refusal of the patient to have a particular technique. In this situation, complete documentation should be performed, including a disclosure note on the chart that all inherent risks of the treatment options were described to the patient. The anesthesia practitioner must convey to the patient what procedure(s) is in the patient's best interest. If the patient denies consent, it may be helpful for the surgeon and/ or family members to become involved in the decision-making. If the anesthesia practitioner ultimately fails to obtain consent for a procedure and nonetheless proceeds with that procedure, he/she assumes the risk that a charge of physical assault may ensue.[24]

39.3   ANESTHETIC MANAGEMENT OPTIONS

39.3.1   What are the general principles of decision-making with regard to airway management options?

When confronted with a difficult airway, either anticipated or unanticipated, the anesthesia practitioner should keep in mind practical recommendations shaped by the ASA Difficult Airway Management Guidelines.[25] A number of different factors must be considered when making specific decisions while following guidelines recommendations. These factors include: the mechanism (cause) of the difficult airway, preexisting comorbidity, type of surgery, urgency of the procedure, the patient's position during surgery, the patient's mental status and degree of cooperation, availability of equipment, as well as the technical skills and the experience of the airway practitioner. A few essential conclusions can be drawn from these guidelines: (1) considerable efforts should be made to predict the possibility of difficult airway management by performing a methodical and comprehensive preoperative airway assessment; (2) thorough airway assessment may substantially reduce the occurrence of unanticipated difficult airway, however, it cannot completely eliminate it and the anesthesia practitioner always has to be prepared, mentally and physically, to deal with an unforeseen difficult airway; (3) if difficult airway is predicted, especially in patients with anticipated difficult ventilation, the airway should be secured while preserving uninterrupted spontaneous breathing until complete control of the airway has been achieved; and (4) always have a back-up plan(s) if the initial plan to secure the airway fails.[25]

39.3.2   What would be the *best* technique for this patient?

This patient with long-standing RA presents with multiple signs of a potentially difficult airway—rigid neck, limited mouth opening, micrognathia, and a full beard. The neck deformity and the atlanto-axial subluxation will complicate positioning for airway management. On the other hand, appropriate positioning of patients with instability of the occipito-atlanto-axial complex is still poorly understood.[7,26,27] Minimizing movements of the cervical spine is the best way to avoid exacerbation of AAS with neurological consequences. To achieve this goal, the most commonly recognized and recommended technique is awake bronchoscopic intubation which is considered the safest technique for securing a difficult airway in patients with RA complicated by AAS.[8,26,28,29] In our case, this method serves dual purposes: protecting the spinal cord by minimizing neck movements and solving the problem of an already known difficult airway. However, this patient refuses an awake tracheal intubation, thus it is necessary to develop an alternative anesthesia plan. Bearing in mind the peripheral location of the anticipated surgery, regional anesthesia may be considered and offered as a safe and practical alternative technique.

39.3.3   How does the ability to perform mask ventilation influence your anesthesia plan? How do you predict and manage difficult and impossible bag-mask-ventilation?

The ability to perform effective bag-mask-ventilation (BMV) is a quintessential element of anesthesia care. All types of anesthesia may require BMV: after induction of general anesthesia, following a respiratory arrest from a complication of regional anesthesia or as a result of excessive sedation. Failure to effectively provide BMV may have fatal consequences unless an emergency airway can be immediately established.

The incidence of difficult BMV has been reported to be 5% to 7.8% in patients presenting for general surgery.[30-32] Five independent risk factors have been identified: a history of snoring; a BMI greater than 26 kg·m^{-2}; lack of teeth; age greater than 55 years; and the presence of a beard.[31] Other authors have also included Mallampati Class 4 and male gender as independent variables.[32] Impossible BMV was found to be much less frequent—0.15%, with neck radiation changes as the most significant clinical predictor in addition to male gender, sleep apnea, Mallampati III-IV classification, and presence of a beard.[33] A considerable proportion of those patients, close to 25%, were also found to be difficult to intubate.[33] The patient in this case is edentulous, and has a full beard. He thus has two of the five risk factors and is considered to be at risk for difficult and potentially impossible BMV. The importance of this determination is a deliberate reinforcement of immediately available back-up plans, including performance of a surgical airway. Having pointed out the importance of preparation to anticipated difficult BMV; it is noteworthy to mention that there are a number of rescue techniques described to improve difficult BMV depending on contributing factors. For example, in a hairy situation (beard), as presented in our case, the use of a clear intravenous site dressing (Tegaderm™), a cut defibrillator pad over bearded area, or plastic kitchen wrap around the entire head has been proposed to reduce gas leaks from the face mask.[34-36] Use of a small mask placed between the lower lip and nostrils or an infant mask covering only the nostrils has also been suggested.[37] The last maneuver has also been described as beneficial in cases in which BMV difficulty was related to an edentulous status. It is also possible to keep a patient's dentures in place while performing BMV and then remove them just prior to intubation. Other options include using an oropharyngeal airway as early as feasible, placing gauze rolls inside the cheeks to prevent the oral cavity from collapsing. Nasal airways can also be used.

In recent years, there have been multiple reports suggesting that the laryngeal mask airway (LMA) may be an effective airway rescue device in the management of both difficult intubation and difficult BMV.[38,39] However, there are instances in which the LMA insertion (on its own) may turn out to be difficult or even impossible.[38,40,41]

In fact, there are some reports of impossible LMA insertion in patients with diseases which limit neck movement.[40,42] There are two special concerns when considering the use of an LMA in RA patients. First, extra caution should be taken during the insertion and inflation of an LMA to avoid movements in the head and neck and to avoid excessive soft tissue pressure as it may produce posterior displacement of the upper cervical spine and worsen atlanto-axial subluxation in susceptible patients.[43] Second, care is necessary to minimize mucosal trauma in the supraglottic area to reduce the chance of aggravation of any cricoarytenoid arthritis. There are several reports of acute upper airway obstruction caused by this disease manifestation in association with LMA use.[13,41,44]

39.3.4 What are some additional preoperative considerations that may influence the choice of anesthetic management?

1. Because of the high prevalence of cervical abnormality in RA, particularly AAS,[6] with associated severe morbidity and mortality,[5] preoperative imaging has been strongly recommended to determine the specific cervical spine pathology and possible instability[45] (Figure 39-1). It has been shown that flexion and extension views in addition to frontal views of the odontoid are essential in complete x-ray examination of the cervical spine to detect AAS.[45] The detection of cervical spine instability can significantly affect anesthetic management, favoring techniques that avoid unprotected manipulations of the neck under anesthesia. This valuable information could help to avoid neurological consequences during positioning.[27,45,46] In addition, the lateral neck x-ray, obtained as part of a preoperative assessment to evaluate patients with cervical deformity, may help to estimate the angle between the oral and pharyngeal axes at the base of the tongue. If this angle is less than 90°, LMA insertion may be difficult or impossible.[27,40]

2. Intraoperative patient *positioning* can play an important role in the success of many procedures, yet caution should be used as positioning may also cause postoperative complications. Cervical involvement in RA can significantly complicate head and neck positioning. In addition, it is important to determine if the patient is able to assume the specific positioning required to perform regional anesthesia and to be awake during surgery. Special care should be taken in intraoperative positioning of RA patients due to the presence of multiple joint deformities (Figure 39-2), rheumatoid subcutaneous nodules, and possible peripheral neuropathies.[47] The optimal intraoperative head position to minimize atlanto-axial subluxation in patients with RA has been reported as the protrusion position (head positioned on a flat pillow combined with a donut-shaped pillow) with support of the upper cervical spine and some extension at the craniocervical junction.[7] However, another investigator has reported a case of a rheumatoid patient with anterior AAS who was markedly worsened by the sniffing position,[27] which is similar to the above mentioned protrusion position; the only apparent difference being the degree of extension of the head at the occipito-atlanto-axial complex.

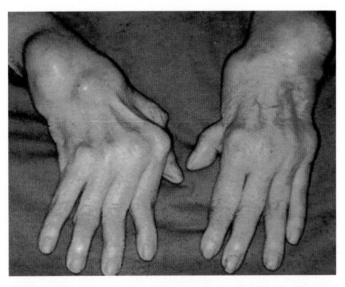

FIGURE 39-2. Severe advanced rheumatoid arthritis of the hands. There is massive tendon swelling over the dorsal surface of both wrists, severe muscle wasting, ulnar deviation of the metacarpophalangeal joints, and swan-neck deformity of the fingers. (Permission obtained from Forbes CD, Jackson WF. *Color Atlas and Text of Clinical Medicine.* 3rd ed. London: Mosby; 2003.)

3. Although this patient does not indicate severe gastroesophageal reflux disease (well controlled with proton pump inhibitors), LMA insertion may be contraindicated in those patients with untreated and symptomatic GERD.[38,42] These patients should be treated preoperatively with a histamine (H$_2$) receptor blocker, metoclopramide, and a nonparticulate antacid regardless of the type of proposed anesthesia.

4. The effects of drug therapy in RA may require certain considerations in preparing for anesthesia care. In our case, long-term NSAID use may cause gastrointestinal disturbances and chronic anemia and may also cause abnormal platelet function. As far as corticosteroid therapy is concerned, contemporary recommendations are based on the drug regimen and intensity of surgical stress. Patients receiving low therapeutic doses of corticosteroids who undergo a surgical procedure do not routinely require standard stress doses of corticosteroids if they continue to receive their usual daily dose of corticosteroid.[47,48]

5. Another prudent element of difficult airway management is planning of extubation and the post-extubation strategy ahead of time.[25] Special consideration should be given to RA patients in preparation for the post-extubation period due to the high prevalence of laryngeal involvement. Extra care should be taken to avoid post-extubation complications, for example, laryngospasm, since rescue maneuvers such as positive pressure bag-mask-ventilation will predictably be difficult, if not impossible. Laryngeal trauma during airway instrumentation, including the use of extraglottic devices, should be minimized to avoid postoperative acute upper airway obstruction caused by cricoarytenoid arthritis.[12-16] Extubation over an airway exchange catheter may be an option in these patients.

39.4   GENERAL ANESTHESIA AND TRACHEAL INTUBATION

39.4.1   What anesthetic agents should be used for induction?

If the ability to perform adequate BMV or successfully place an extraglottic device is predicted to be problematic, then uninterrupted spontaneous ventilation should be maintained during induction until the airway is secured. An inhalational induction with sevoflurane may be performed to minimize the risk of sudden loss of airway control.[49-51] However, maintenance of a patent airway without cervical spine movement may be difficult. Intravenous drugs with minimal effect on the respiratory drive, such as low-dose midazolam, ketamine, or dexmedetomidine, can be titrated in combination with an inhalational agent. Administration of opioids should be minimized, as they depress respiratory drive. Muscle relaxants should be avoided unless BMV or LMA ventilation has been established. Although not considered conventionally as safe, there are reports of induction of anesthesia without maintaining spontaneous ventilation, followed by successful LMA or other extraglottic device placement in patients with limited neck mobility.[39,52,53] However, this should only be performed if there is a high level of certainty in the ability to provide adequate BMV or LMA ventilation following the induction of GA. Only short-acting drugs, such as propofol, should be used. Particularly thorough denitrogenation is essential in this case as it will delay oxygen desaturation in the event that there are difficulties in obtaining control of the airway.

39.4.2   Following induction of general anesthesia, how should this patient's airway be secured?

Another prudent recommendation in the ASA Difficult Airway Management Guidelines regarding technique choices is: Do what you do best.[25] In general, anesthesia practitioners are familiar with both the LMA-Classic™ or LMA-Unique™ and the Intubating LMA (ILMA). These devices can be inserted with relative ease and can provide adequate positive pressure ventilation, without tracheal intubation. Additionally, these devices can serve as conduits for tracheal intubation. A 6.0-mm inner diameter (ID) endotracheal tube (ETT) can be passed through a #4 LMA-Classic™, and a 7.0 mm ID ETT through a #5. ETTs have been designed for use with the ILMA or disposable ILMA, which have special shaped tips to allow easier and less traumatic passage through the glottis (up to size 8.0 mm ID) and can be passed through the #3, #4, and #5 ILMAs. Despite the reports that LMA use in RA patients may be associated with aggravation of laryngeal rheumatoid arthritis and acute upper airway obstruction,[13,41,44] the literature has demonstrated that the LMA or ILMA are useful and effective devices in airway management in anesthetized patients with RA.[49,54-56]

The ILMA may offer potential advantages over the LMA in patients with RA, as it may be easier to insert in patients with a rigid neck[57] and is a better conduit for intubation, although the LMA-Classic™ and LMA-Unique™ may be more advantageous in patients with limited mouth opening.[39] This patient's airway may be secured with an ILMA following an inhalational induction with sevoflurane or an intravenous agent while maintaining spontaneous ventilation. Once good positioning of the ILMA is ascertained, a muscle relaxant can be administered. If the ETT designed for use with the ILMA is unavailable, a flexible bronchoscope (FB) can be used to guide a regular ETT into the trachea. Tracheal placement of the ETT can be confirmed bronchoscopically as well as by auscultation and capnography. The ILMA can then be removed using a special stabilizing device. If an FB is not available, a prewarmed, softened ETT can be inserted blindly through the ILMA by feeling for a loss of resistance, with good success (88%-98%).[58,59] However, given the airway pathology in this patient, it would not be prudent to proceed without an FB. Compared to blind insertion of an ETT, FB assistance may provide less traumatic tracheal intubation which is beneficial to RA patients to avoid exacerbation of laryngeal arthritis. Additionally, a Cook Airway Exchange Catheter (using the Rapi-fit connector, attached to the capnograph monitor to detect $EtCO_2$) or an Eschmann Introducer can be used to guide an ETT. If all these methods fail, the ILMA (or LMA) can be used alone for positive pressure ventilation throughout the case.

39.4.3   What is the role of manual in-line stabilization of the cervical spine if DL is necessary? Are there additional methods to improve stability of the cervical spine during airway instrumentation in RA patients?

The traditional standard recommendation that manual in-line stabilization (MILS) should always be applied during airway instrumentation in patients with cervical spine instability has recently been challenged. Some recent studies have indicated that direct laryngoscopy (DL) and intubation with MILS in the presence of cervical instability may worsen glottic visualization, contribute to an increased rate of intubation failure, and potentially increase pathologic cranio-cervical motion.[60-62]

In addition to awake bronchoscopic intubation, conventionally known as a proven technique of securing the airway in patients with cervical spine instability, there are a number of alternative methods that may be used with success in this patient population. Takenaka et al recently reported that use of the Airway Scope (Pentax) and the Eschmann Introducer in combination resulted in significantly reduced movements in cervical spine during endotracheal intubation.[26] Ueshima et al have also reported the successful use of the Eschmann Introducer with the Pentax Airway Scope in patients with difficult airways.[63] Other studies have used fluoroscopy to demonstrate a reduction of upper cervical spine movements during intubation using a variety of contemporary videoscopic devices.[55,64] Takenaka et al employed fluoroscopic monitoring during airway manipulation to avoid excessive AAS subluxation in a patient with severe RA.[26]

39.5   ALTERNATIVE AIRWAY TECHNIQUES

39.5.1   What other methods can be used to secure the airway after induction?

It is essential that the prudent anesthesia practitioner should always have a back-up plan(s). In a nonemergency situation, in which the patient has received a short-acting induction agent and has not been paralyzed, he/she may be allowed to awaken. Alternative techniques to secure the airway or a regional anesthetic technique may be considered.

Although a complete list of all airway management devices and techniques is beyond the scope of this chapter, a few of the more commonly used devices and techniques will be discussed. A relatively new group of airway management devices, the video laryngoscopes, have been shown to be very effective for intubation in patients with a difficult airway.[65] Both the Macintosh Video Laryngoscope (Karl Storz Endoscopy) and the Glidescope® (see Chapter 10) have been shown to be useful in facilitating intubation in patients with cervical spine immobilization.[66] The use of a styletted ETT is recommended. The advantage of the Macintosh Video Laryngoscope is that either the direct view (naked eye) or the indirect view (monitor) can be used for tracheal intubation. As with traditional laryngoscopy, intubating guides can also be utilized, if necessary.

Rigid fiberoptic laryngoscopes such as the Bullard Scope (ACMI), the Upsher Scope (Mercury Medical), and the Wu Scope (Achi Corp) also have been shown to be useful in patients with limited mouth opening and neck extension,[67] but they require a measure of experience to achieve proficiency. Similarly, the lighted stylets, such as the Trachlight™ (Laerdal Medical Corp), the Bonfils Retromolar Intubation Fiberscope (Karl Storz Endoscopy), and the Shikani Optical Stylet (Clarus Medical), are useful in patients with limited cervical spine mobility.[68-70] Finally, retrograde intubation is a useful technique, especially when visualization of the larynx from above is impossible.[71] However, since this technique is more invasive, it should be reserved as a Plan C in most hands, when the ability to ventilate is maintained (spontaneous or via bag-mask).

39.5.2   What alternative extraglottic devices can be used?

The Esophageal Tracheal Combitube™ is an alternative to the LMA in a difficult airway situation[52,72] that requires minimal mouth opening and neck mobility for its insertion. It has been shown to be useful in providing a patent airway in a patient whose neck was immobilized in the neutral position with a halo jacket.[73] Theoretically, the Combitube™ protects against aspiration since its distal cuff seals the esophagus and the tracheal lumen can be used to suction the stomach when positioned in the esophagus, yet the incidence of aspiration with the Combitube™ has been found to be similar to the LMA.[74]

Another new extraglottic device which could be used is the King Laryngeal Tube (LT) (Figure 39-3). This is a single-lumen tube with a ventral ventilation aperture. The LT is designed for blind esophageal insertion. It has both esophageal and pharyngeal cuffs that are connected to the same inflation line which create a seal above and below the ventilation aperture. Once the LT is inserted, ventilation with the cuffs inflated should be confirmed. An Aintree Extubation Catheter (Aintree, Cook Critical Care) mounted onto an FB (4 mm or smaller in diameter) can then be passed into the trachea using the LT as a conduit. Once the FB and the Aintree are in the trachea, the FB is removed, and a 15 mm Rapi-Fit Adapter can be attached to the Aintree to aid in ventilation and reconfirm tracheal placement by end-tidal CO_2 detection. By removing the Rapi-Fit connector, the LT can then be removed and the Aintree can be used as a guide over which to advance an ETT into the trachea.[75] A specially designed LT is being developed to better accommodate the passage of this catheter. Although the LT has been shown to be an effective airway device with a high rate of successful insertion,[75] its use in patients with rheumatoid cervical spine has not been sufficiently studied.

A modified nasal trumpet, which is a nasal-pharyngeal airway with an additional distal hole and an attached tracheal tube adaptor, has been useful in patients with difficult airways who are anesthetized and breathing spontaneously.[51,76] It can provide supplemental oxygen and anesthetic gas delivery to facilitate a flexible bronchoscopic intubation via the mouth or opposite nostril in patients in whom LMA placement has failed or was deemed to be impossible. The patient's entire upper airway (nostrils, oral cavity, pharynx, larynx, and trachea) should be adequately anesthetized. As a primary airway device, however, the modified nasal trumpet has not been shown to be effective.[76]

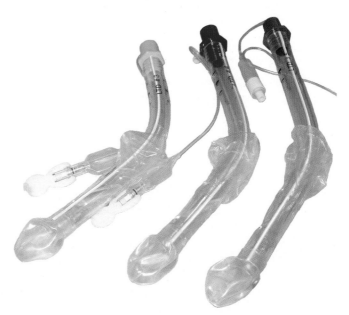

FIGURE 39-3. Laryngeal tube: Three different sizes of laryngeal tubes are shown.

39.5.3   What is your airway management plan if mask ventilation is inadequate and tracheal intubation is unsuccessful?

If both BMV and LMA ventilation are inadequate and intubation is unsuccessful, the emergency pathway of the ASA Difficult Airway Management Algorithm should be followed.[25] A call for help should be made. Following determination of the "cannot ventilate, cannot intubate" situation, the practitioner should proceed directly to an emergency surgical or percutaneous cricothyrotomy.[25] An attempt to pass the Combitube can be made while preparing to perform a surgical airway.

39.6   REGIONAL ANESTHESIA

39.6.1   What is the possible role of regional anesthesia for this patient?

In patients with RA and a predicted difficult airway, awake bronchoscopic intubation is considered to be the safest and the most recommended method to establish a secure airway for general anesthesia. If this plan fails or the patient refuses an awake intubation, regional anesthesia should be strongly considered as a safe alternative approach. However, not all regional techniques are 100% effective, and any type of regional anesthesia may lead to disastrous complications requiring emergency airway management.

Although these complications are inherent to all regional anesthetic procedures, the risks vary and are based on several factors, including the type of nerve block; needle insertion; type, concentration, and volume of drug administered; and patient comorbidity. Therefore, risks and benefits of regional versus general anesthesia should be considered individually for each patient. Chelly[77] provides a list of important factors that should be considered in making this decision (Table 39-1).

Contraindications to regional anesthesia should be excluded. These include infection at the site of needle insertion, systemic infection, bleeding abnormalities, allergy to local anesthetics, and lack of patient cooperation.[77,78] In the case of neuraxial blocks, severe hypovolemic shock, severe aortic stenosis, and high intracranial pressure should also be excluded.

Additionally, possible complications of regional anesthesia must be considered. The risk of serious complications is approximately 0.1%.[79] Local anesthetic toxicity can present either with neurological or cardiovascular symptoms, such as seizures, hypotension, and cardiac arrest.

A high spinal block, as a complication of neuraxial or major plexus blockade, can result in apnea and cardiovascular collapse. These complications may require emergency airway management. Furthermore, the possibility of hemodynamic instability during the case (eg, from significant blood loss) should be considered, as this may also require emergency airway management.

It is very important as well to determine if the patient can tolerate being awake during the procedure and communicate with the anesthesia practitioner. The patient's medical condition also influences

---

TABLE 39-1

Factors Influencing the Choice of Regional Anesthesia versus Control of the Airway in Patients with Established Difficult Airways[77,87]

Patient	• Informed consent • Cooperative and calm • Hemodynamically stable • Ability to tolerate sedation, if required • Ability to communicate with anesthesia practitioner throughout procedure • No history of claustrophobia • Adequate IV access
Anesthesia practitioner	• Expertise in both regional anesthesia and difficult airway (DA) management • Enough preoperative time to perform regional technique • Appropriate regional technique for surgical procedure • Prepared for alternative plans for DA
Surgeon	• Dependable and reliable • Willing and able to supplement regional technique with local anesthetics, if necessary • Cooperative with primary and alternative plans for DA management
Types of surgery	• Nonemergency (exception c-section) • Short duration • Patient position allows easy airway access • Can be interrupted for DA management • Limited or moderate blood loss
Support	• Availability of appropriate equipment for regional anesthesia and DA management • Staff (anesthesia practitioners/OR nurses)

this decision. For example, if the patient has severe untreated GERD, a regional anesthetic with the patient awake may be preferable to securing the airway after induction of anesthesia. If however, diseases such as severe chronic obstructive pulmonary disease or severe corrosive RA with spinal involvement prohibit the patient from lying comfortably flat, the airway should be secured.

One of the most important factors requiring consideration is the expertise of the anesthesia practitioner. This includes the appropriate experience in the chosen regional technique, as well as adequate experience in managing the patient's airway in the event of a complication. The anesthesia practitioner must know which nerves to block for both the surgery and possible tourniquet pain. The anticipated duration of the surgical procedure should also be considered and the anesthesia practitioner must ensure that the regional anesthetic will last at least that long, if not longer should delays occur.

All of the appropriate equipment for the performance of the nerve block(s) and possible emergency airway management must be available. Additional factors to consider include the site and type of surgery. A short toe procedure requiring an ankle block will have a lower risk of complications than a revision of a total hip replacement under regional anesthesia. There must also be adequate communication and cooperation between the surgeon and the anesthesia practitioner, and both must agree on the appropriateness of regional anesthesia. Expert help should be immediately available should complications occur. If GA becomes necessary, a predetermined strategy to manage the airway should be in place, including back-up plans should the primary plan fail. The landmarks for a surgical airway should be identified before induction of GA and the necessary personnel and equipment should be immediately available.

39.6.2   Is neuraxial anesthesia appropriate for this patient?

When considering neuraxial blocks in patients with RA, spinal deformity may make the technique challenging; however, the prevalence of lumbar spine involvement in RA patients has not been found to be excessive.[80] Indeed, a number of reports confirm successful use of spinal and epidural blocks for lower limb surgeries in these patients.[47,81,82] Recently, there was an interesting report by Leino et al which stated that the mean spread of sensory block after the injection of plain bupivacaine was 1.5 segments higher in patients with RA than in those without this disease.[81] Keeping in mind that the patient in our case has a well-known difficult airway, maximum efforts should be made to avoid excessive cephalad spread of spinal anesthetic which can cause respiratory arrest and cardiovascular collapse. To keep control over the spread of neuraxial anesthetic, special attention should be given to the details of the technique, including baricity of local anesthetic, total dose and patient position. Furthermore, a catheter-based neuraxial technique should be considered as it can offer even better control over the extension of the block as compared to the single-injection technique.

This patient is on an NSAID. However, a recent Consensus Conference on Neuraxial Anesthesia and Anticoagulation[78,83] concluded that NSAIDs appear to represent no added significant

risk for the development of spinal hematoma in patients having epidural or spinal anesthesia.

39.6.3   Which regional anesthetic technique would be most suitable for this patient?

A better choice for this patient may be the performance of peripheral nerve block(s), if appropriate for the surgery. Peripheral nerve blocks used as a main mode of anesthesia for RA patients have been reported by many authors.[84,85] Since the patient is scheduled for knee surgery, an anterior-approach femoral nerve block, combined with sciatic nerve block would be most appropriate. A local anesthetic mixture of mepivicaine 1.5% and ropivicaine 0.5%, using a total volume of 25 to 30 mL for each nerve block will provide superb anesthesia for a total knee replacement and possible tourniquet pain.[86] Additional obturator and lateral femoral cutaneous nerve blocks may be required, depending on the patient's response. Although a lumbar plexus block could be considered, spinal deformities may make this approach more difficult and this block has a higher risk of complications, including those requiring emergency airway management. A catheter-based technique can also be used.

39.7   SUMMARY

This case presentation of a surgical patient with a known difficult airway who refuses to have an awake tracheal intubation presents the anesthesia practitioner with a number of challenges. In addition to resolving ethical and medico-legal issues related to patient refusal of a medically indicated intervention, the anesthesia practitioner has to come forward with practical options that can be offered and accepted by the patient and surgical team. In the management of the anticipated difficult airway, the anesthesia practitioner must be familiar with a number of alternative techniques to secure the patient's airway regardless of the anesthesia plan selected. The ASA Difficult Airway Guidelines form the basis for deciding which technique is most appropriate for each individual patient. The anesthesia practitioner should perform the technique with which he/she is most comfortable and skilled, and should always have several alternative techniques available in the event the primary technique fails. Regional anesthesia may be an appropriate option for patients with a recognized difficult airway, if certain conditions are met, and the patient, surgeon, and anesthesia practitioner are prepared to overcome the failure or complications of this technique.

REFERENCES

1. St. Clair W, Pisetsky DS, Haynes BF. *Rheumatoid Arthritis*. Philadelphia, PA: Lippincott Williams & Wilkins; 2004.
2. Fauci AS, Fauci AS, Kasper KL, et al. *Harrison's Principles of Internal Medicine*. 17th ed. New York: McGraw-Hill; 2008.
3. Hines RL, Marschall KE. *Stoelting's Anesthesia and Coexisting Disease*. 5th ed. Philadelphia, PA: Elsevier Inc.; 2008.
4. Geddes DM, Webley M, Emerson PA. Airways obstruction in rheumatoid arthritis. *Ann Rheum Dis*. 1979;38:222-225.

5. Yaszemski MJ, Shepler TR. Sudden death from cord compression associated with atlanto-axial instability in rheumatoid arthritis. A case report. *Spine (Phila Pa 1976)*. 1990;15:338-341.

6. Riise T, Jacobsen BK, Gran JT. High mortality in patients with rheumatoid arthritis and atlantoaxial subluxation. *J Rheumatol*. 2001;28:2425-2429.

7. Tokunaga D, Hase H, Mikami Y, et al. Atlantoaxial subluxation in different intraoperative head positions in patients with rheumatoid arthritis. *Anesthesiology*. 2006;104:675-679.

8. Hakala P, Randell T. Intubation difficulties in patients with rheumatoid arthritis. A retrospective analysis. *Acta Anaesthesiol Scand*. 1998;42:195-198.

9. Bandi V, Munnur U, Braman SS. Airway problems in patients with rheumatologic disorders. *Crit Care Clin*. 2002;18:749-765.

10. Yoshida A, Higuchi Y, Kondo M, et al. Range of motion of the temporomandibular joint in rheumatoid arthritis: relationship to the severity of disease. *Cranio*. 1998;16:162-167.

11. Sairanen E. On the etiology of growth disturbance of the mandible in juvenile rheumatoid arthritis. *Scand J Rheumatol*. 1987;16:136-143.

12. Bengtsson M, Bengtsson A. Cricoarytenoid arthritis—a cause of upper airway obstruction in the rheumatoid arthritis patient. *Intensive Care Med*. 1998;24:643.

13. Hayashi I, Komeichi Y, Morinaga N, Mizoguchi H, Takakuwa R, Fujiwara M. A case report of severe laryngeal edema which occured before removal of a laryngeal mask airway. *Masui*. 2004;53:679-681.

14. Kolman J, Morris I. Cricoarytenoid arthritis: a cause of acute upper airway obstruction in rheumatoid arthritis. *Can J Anaesth*. 2002;49:729-732.

15. Segebarth PB, Limbird TJ. Perioperative acute upper airway obstruction secondary to severe rheumatoid arthritis. *J Arthroplasty*. 2007;22:916-919.

16. Wattenmaker I, Concepcion M, Hibberd P, Lipson S. Upper-airway obstruction and perioperative management of the airway in patients managed with posterior operations on the cervical spine for rheumatoid arthritis. *J Bone Joint Surg Am*. 1994;76:360-365.

17. Cagla Ozbakis Akkurt B, Guler H, Inanoglu K, et al. Disease activity in rheumatoid arthritis as a predictor of difficult intubation? *Eur J Anaesthesiol*. 2008;25:800-804.

18. McCullough LB, Chervenak FA. Informed consent. *Clin Perinatol*. 2007;34:275-285, vi.

19. Waisel DB. Legal aspects of anesthesia care. In: Miller R, et al, eds. *Miller's Anesthesia*. Philadelphia, PA: Churchill Livingstone; 2009.

20. Faden R, Faden A. False belief and the refusal of medical treatment. *J Med Ethics*. 1977;3:133-136.

21. Kleinman I. The right to refuse treatment: ethical considerations for the competent patient. *CMAJ*. 1991;144:1219-1222.

22. Sullivan MD, Youngner SJ. Depression, competence, and the right to refuse lifesaving medical treatment. *Am J Psychiatry*. 1994;151:971-978.

23. Ward M, Savulescu J. Patients who challenge. *Best Pract Res Clin Anaesthesiol*. 2006;20:545-563.

24. Van Norman G. Informed consent in the operating room. *Ethics in Medicine*. Washington DC: University of Washington.

25. American Society of Anesthesiologists Task Force on Management of the Difficult Airway. Practice guidelines for management of the difficult airway: an updated report by the American Society of Anesthesiologists Task Force on Management of the Difficult Airway. *Anesthesiology*. 2003;98:1269-1277.

26. Takenaka I, Aoyama K, Iwagaki T, Ishimura H, Kadoya T. Fluoroscopic observation of the occipitoatlantoaxial complex during intubation attempt in a rheumatoid patient with severe atlantoaxial subluxation. *Anesthesiology*. 2009;111:917-919.

27. Takenaka I, Urakami Y, Aoyama K, Nakamura M, Fukuyama H, Kadoya T. Severe subluxation in the sniffing position in a rheumatoid patient with anterior atlantoaxial subluxation. *Anesthesiology*. 2004;101:1235-1237.

28. Popat MT, Chippa JH, Russell R. Awake fibreoptic intubation following failed regional anaesthesia for caesarean section in a parturient with Still's disease. *Eur J Anaesthesiol*. 2000;17:211-214.

29. Skues MA, Welchew EA. Anaesthesia and rheumatoid arthritis. *Anaesthesia*. 1993;48:989-997.

30. Kheterpal S, Han R, Tremper KK, et al. Incidence and predictors of difficult and impossible mask ventilation. *Anesthesiology*. 2006;105:885-891.

31. Langeron O, Masso E, Huraux C, et al. Prediction of difficult mask ventilation. *Anesthesiology*. 2000;92:1229-1236.

32. Yildiz TS, Solak M, Toker K. The incidence and risk factors of difficult mask ventilation. *J Anesth*. 2005;19:7-11.

33. Kheterpal S, Martin L, Shanks AM, Tremper KK. Prediction and outcomes of impossible mask ventilation: a review of 50,000 anesthetics. *Anesthesiology*. 2009;110:891-897.

34. Dalgleish DJ. A hairy situation. *Anesthesiology*. 2000;92:1199.

35. Jaeger K, Ruschulte H, Heine J. Management of the beard problem. *Resuscitation*. 2000;45:146-147.

36. Johnson JO, Bradway JA, Blood T. A hairy situation. *Anesthesiology*. 1999; 91:595.

37. Garewal DS. Difficult mask ventilation. *Anesthesiology*. 2000;92:1199.

38. Pennant JH, White PF. The laryngeal mask airway. Its uses in anesthesiology. *Anesthesiology*. 1993;79:144-163.

39. Pothmann W, Eckert S, Fullekrug B. Use of laryngeal mask in difficult intubation. *Anaesthesist*. 1993;42:644-647.

40. Ishimura H, Minami K, Sata T, et al. Impossible insertion of the laryngeal mask airway and oropharyngeal axes. *Anesthesiology*. 1995;83:867-869.

41. Takakura K, Hirakawa S, Kudo K, et al. Cricoarytenoid arthritis diagnosed after tracheostomy in a rheumatoid arthritis patient. *Masui*. 2005;54:690-693.

42. Takenaka I, Kadoya T, Aoyama K. Is awake intubation necessary when the laryngeal mask airway is feasible? *Anesth Analg*. 2000;91:246-247.

43. Crosby ET. Airway management in adults after cervical spine trauma. *Anesthesiology*. 2006;104:1293-1318.

44. Miyanohara T, Igarashi T, Suzuki H, et al. Aggravation of laryngeal rheumatoid arthritis after use of a laryngeal mask airway. *J Clin Rheumatol*. 2006; 12:142-144.

45. Kwek TK, Lew TW, Thoo FL. The role of preoperative cervical spine X-rays in rheumatoid arthritis. *Anaesth Intensive Care*. 1998;26:636-641.

46. Macarthur A, Kleiman S. Rheumatoid cervical joint disease—a challenge to the anaesthetist. *Can J Anaesth*. 1993;40:154-159.

47. Khanam T. Anaesthetic risks in rheumatoid arthritis. *Br J Hosp Med*. 1994; 52:320-325.

48. Marik PE, Varon J. Requirement of perioperative stress doses of corticosteroids: a systematic review of the literature. *Arch Surg*. 2008;143:1222-1226.

49. Inagaki Y, Watanabe T, Ishibe Y, et al. Vital capacity rapid inhalation induction (VCRII) technique with sevoflurane for a rheumatoid patient with difficult airway. *Masui*. 2002;51:411-413.

50. Lu PP, Brimacombe J, Ho AC, et al. The intubating laryngeal mask airway in severe ankylosing spondylitis. *Can J Anaesth*. 2001;48:1015-1019.

51. Metz S, Beattie C. A modified nasal trumpet to facilitate fibreoptic intubation. *Br J Anaesth*. 2003;90:388-391.

52. Agro F, Frass M, Benumof J, et al. The esophageal tracheal combitube as a non-invasive alternative to endotracheal intubation. A review. *Minerva Anestesiol*. 2001;67:863-874.

53. Hsin ST, Chen CH, Juan CH, et al. A modified method for intubation of a patient with ankylosing spondylitis using intubating laryngeal mask airway (LMA-Fastrach)—a case report. *Acta Anaesthesiol Sin*. 2001;39:179-182.

54. Bilgin H, Bozkurt M. Tracheal intubation using the ILMA, C-Trach or McCoy laryngoscope in patients with simulated cervical spine injury. *Anaesthesia*. 2006;61:685-691.

55. Malik MA, Maharaj CH, Harte BH, Laffey JG. Comparison of Macintosh, Truview EVO$_2$, Glidescope, and Airwayscope laryngoscope use in patients with cervical spine immobilization. *Br J Anaesth*. 2008;101:723-730.

56. Mashio H, Kojima T, Goda Y, et al. Intubation of a patient with rheumatoid arthritis with a 7.5-mm-ID armored endotracheal tube using a laryngeal mask airway. *Masui*. 1997;46:1639-1643.

57. Asai T, Wagle AU, Stacey M. Placement of the intubating laryngeal mask is easier than the laryngeal mask during manual in-line neck stabilization. *Br J Anaesth*. 1999;82:712-714.

58. Caponas G. Intubating laryngeal mask airway. *Anaesth Intensive Care*. 2002;30:551-569.

59. Joo HS, Rose DK. The intubating laryngeal mask airway with and without fiberoptic guidance. *Anesth Analg*. 1999;88:662-666.

60. Crosby ET, Lui A. The adult cervical spine: implications for airway management. *Can J Anaesth*. 1990;37:77-93.

61. Santoni BG, Hindman BJ, Puttlitz CM, et al. Manual in-line stabilization increases pressures applied by the laryngoscope blade during direct laryngoscopy and orotracheal intubation. *Anesthesiology*. 2009;110:24-31.

62. Thiboutot F, Nicole PC, Trepanier CA, et al. Effect of manual in-line stabilization of the cervical spine in adults on the rate of difficult orotracheal intubation by direct laryngoscopy: a randomized controlled trial. *Can J Anaesth*. 2009;56:412-418.

63. Ueshima H, Asai T, Shingu K, et al. Use of a gum elastic bougie for tracheal intubation with Pentax-AWS airway scope. *Masui*. 2008;57:82-84.

64. Malik MA, Subramaniam R, Churasia S, et al. Tracheal intubation in patients with cervical spine immobilization: a comparison of the Airwayscope, LMA CTrach, and the Macintosh laryngoscopes. *Br J Anaesth*. 2009;102:654-661.

65. Cooper RM. Use of a new videolaryngoscope (GlideScope) in the management of a difficult airway. *Can J Anaesth*. 2003;50:611-613.

66. Agro F, Barzoi G, Montecchia F. Tracheal intubation using a Macintosh laryngoscope or a GlideScope in 15 patients with cervical spine immobilization. *Br J Anaesth*. 2003;90:705-706.

67. Gorback MS: Management of the challenging airway with the Bullard laryngoscope. *J Clin Anesth*. 1991;3:473-477.

68. Abramson SI, Holmes AA, Hagberg CA. Awake insertion of the Bonfils Retromolar Intubation Fiberscope in five patients with anticipated difficult airways. *Anesth Analg*. 2008;106:1215-1217.

69. Davis L, Cook-Sather SD, Schreiner MS. Lighted stylet tracheal intubation: a review. *Anesth Analg*. 2000;90:745-756.

70. Turkstra TP, Pelz DM, Shaikh AA, Craen RA. Cervical spine motion: a fluoroscopic comparison of Shikani Optical Stylet vs Macintosh laryngoscope. *Can J Anaesth*. 2007;54:441-447.

71. Slots P, Vegger PB, Bettger H, Reinstrup P. Retrograde intubation with a Mini-Trach II kit. *Acta Anaesthesiol Scand*. 2003;47:274-277.

72. Frass M, Frenzer R, Zahler J, et al. Ventilation via the esophageal tracheal combitube in a case of difficult intubation. *J Cardiothorac Anesth*. 1987;1:565-568.

73. Mercer M. Respiratory failure after tracheal extubation in a patient with halo frame cervical spine immobilization—rescue therapy using the Combitube airway. *Br J Anaesth*. 2001;86:886-891.

74. Hagberg CA, Vartazarian TN, Chelly JE, Ovassapian A. The incidence of gastroesophageal reflux and tracheal aspiration detected with pH electrodes is similar with the Laryngeal Mask Airway and Esophageal Tracheal Combitube—a pilot study. *Can J Anaesth*. 2004;51:243-249.

75. Genzwuerker HV, Vollmer T, Ellinger K. Fibreoptic tracheal intubation after placement of the laryngeal tube. *Br J Anaesth*. 2002;89:733-738.

76. Metz S. Perioperative use of the modified nasal trumpet in 346 patients. *Br J Anaesth*. 2004;92:694-696.

77. Chelly JE. Regional anesthesia and the difficult airway. In: Hagberg CA, ed. *Airway Management: Principles and Practice*. 2nd ed. St. Louis: Mosby; 2007.

78. Horlocker TT, Wedel DJ, Benzon H, et al. Regional anesthesia in the anticoagulated patient: defining the risks (the second ASRA Consensus Conference on Neuraxial Anesthesia and Anticoagulation). *Reg Anesth Pain Med*. 2003;28:172-197.

79. Auroy Y, Narchi P, Messiah A, et al. Serious complications related to regional anesthesia: results of a prospective survey in France. *Anesthesiology*. 1997;87:479-486.

80. Harzy T, Allali F, Bennani-Othmani M, Hajjaj-Hassouni N. Radiological characteristics of the lumbar spine in patients with rheumatoid arthritis. *Presse Med*. 2007;36:1385-1389.

81. Leino KA, Kuusniemi KS, Palve HK, et al. Spread of spinal block in patients with rheumatoid arthritis. *Acta Anaesthesiol Scand*. 2010;54:65-69.

82. Scott RD. Total hip and knee arthroplasty in juvenile rheumatoid arthritis. *Clin Orthop Relat Res*. 1990;83-91.

83. Broadman LM. Non-steroidal anti-inflammatory drugs, antiplatelet medications and spinal axis anesthesia. *Best Pract Res Clin Anaesthesiol*. 2005;19:47-58.

84. Jenkins LC, McGraw RW. Anaesthetic management of the patient with rheumatoid arthritis. *Can Anaesth Soc J*. 1969;16:407-415.

85. Mathies B, Sjostrom K, Raunio P. Evaluation of 350 sciatic blocks in rheumatoid foot surgery. *Arch Orthop Unfallchir*. 1977;87:171-175.

86. Lau HP, Yip KM, Jiang CC. Regional nerve block for total knee arthroplasty. *J Formos Med Assoc*. 1998;97:428-430.

87. Benumof JL. Management of the difficult airway. *Ann Acad Med Singapore*. 1994;23:589-591.

SELF-EVALUATION QUESTIONS

39.1. Patients with rheumatoid arthritis:

A. may have cervical spine rigidity and upper cervical subluxation

B. are found with high prevalence of airflow obstruction, especially in men

C. may report TMJ dysfunction in up to 31% of cases

D. have the same incidence of lumbar spine involvement as in the general population, thus suitable for spinal block

E. all of the above

39.2. If a patient refuses an indicated procedure as part of anesthesia care

A. The anesthesiologist is not obligated to provide anesthesia care under any circumstances.

B. Psychiatric consultation is mandatory to determine the patient's competency.

C. The anesthesiologist has to comply with patient's wishes and proceed with the patient's selected type of anesthesia.

D. It must be determined that the patient has a reasonable understanding of the issues being discussed and her/or his judgment is not based on inaccurate information.

E. None of the above.

39.3. Impossible mask ventilation:

A. occurs approximately in 5% of patients presented for general surgery

B. can be predicted in the presence of neck radiation changes

C. is rarely associated with difficult intubation

D. is reported more in women than in men

E. none of the above

CHAPTER (40)

Airway Management in the Operating Room of a Morbidly Obese Patient in a "Cannot Intubate, Cannot Ventilate" Situation due to a Suspected Infectious Etiology

David T. Wong

40.1 CASE PRESENTATION

A 68-year-old man is scheduled for an elective anterior cervical decompression and fusion due to a progressive cervical radiculopathy with numbness and pain in the C6 distribution bilaterally. He has stable coronary artery disease with Class II angina and well-controlled type 2 diabetes mellitus. He is a nonsmoker and has no history of sleep apnea. He has no allergies and he is taking metoprolol, amlodipine, glyburide, and is on a nitroglycerine patch.

His chest is clear and heart sounds are normal. His airway examination reveals that he is edentulous with a full beard. He has a Mallampati Class II pharyngeal view, a 6.0 cm thyromental distance, and 4.0 cm of mouth opening. There is a slight reduction of neck extension (approximately 30 degrees). He is 170 cm tall (5 ft 7 in), and weighs 110 kg (242 lb) with a BMI 38 kg·m^{-2}. His vital signs are: blood pressure (BP) 140/95 mm Hg, heart rate (HR) 64 beats per minute (bpm), respiratory rate (RR) 20 breaths per minute, SpO$_2$ 95% on room air.

Laboratory investigations reveal normal CBC, electrolytes, and creatinine. The random blood glucose is 7.1 mmol·L^{-1}. He has a normal ECG. An MRI of the cervical spine shows disc protrusion at the C4-5 and C5-6 levels causing nerve root compression at the C6 level bilaterally and CSF effacement in front of C4-5 and C5-6 levels without signal changes in the spinal cord.

A diagnosis of cervical radiculopathy has been made.

40.2 PATIENT CONSIDERATIONS

40.2.1 What are the anesthetic considerations for a morbidly obese patient with a BMI of 38?

Morbid obesity is associated with a number of anatomic, physiologic, and biochemical changes (see also Chapter 18).[1] The cardiovascular system of obese patients is characterized by increased cardiac output, increased circulatory blood volume, and an increased incidence of systemic hypertension and coronary artery disease. In the respiratory system, they have increased oxygen consumption, increased carbon dioxide production, reduced functional residual capacity, increased premature airway closure and shunt, decreased chest wall compliance, and increased work of breathing. There is an increased incidence of pulmonary hypertension and obstructive sleep apnea. There is also a higher incidence of hiatus hernia, gastroesophageal reflux, glucose intolerance, and diabetes mellitus. Airway considerations are detailed later.

40.2.2 Is this patient at an increased risk of having a perioperative cardiac event?

Yes. This patient has several risk factors and is at a higher risk of having a perioperative cardiac event. There are several well-established perioperative cardiac risk assessment tools. He has diabetes and stable, functional Class II angina which according to the 2007 ACC/AHA guidelines[2,3] are two clinical risk factors. Utilizing the Lee cardiac risk score,[4] he has two (CAD and diabetes) of six risk factors and is predicted to have a perioperative cardiac event rate of approximately 5%. Utilization of perioperative beta-blockade may be useful in reducing his risk of cardiac events.

40.2.3 Some patients with cervical spine pathology scheduled for anterior decompression and fusion undergo awake intubations. Does our patient need one?

It is the opinion of the author that three categories of patients may require awake endotracheal intubation:

- The first group has signs and symptoms of cervical myelopathy. Clinically, this may manifest itself as bilateral upper extremity numbness, pain or weakness, or long track signs such as bilateral leg symptoms. These symptoms may worsen with certain neck movements. Radiologically, cerebral spinal fluid effacement, deformation of spinal cord contour, and particularly signal changes within the spinal cord are suggestive of myelopathy. Although there are no studies which show that patients with spinal cord pathology or injury have improved outcome when intubated awake versus asleep.[5-8] The author believes that patients with clinically evident myelopathy should have an awake endotracheal intubation to avoid the possibility of further spinal cord compromise with neck movement encountered during asleep intubation.

- Second, patients with cervical spine ligamentous or bony instability constitute another potential indication for awake intubation. Examples include C1-2 subluxation from rheumatoid arthritis or traumatic cervical spine instability.

- Third, patients with proven or suspected difficult airways should be considered for awake intubation.

40.2.4 Should this patient be admitted to the ICU postoperatively to monitor for airway swelling and compromise?

It is possible that patients undergoing anterior cervical decompression and fusion are at a slightly increased risk of postoperative airway obstruction. However, it is reasonably safe to observe these patients in the PACU for 4 to 6 hours postoperatively, and if they have an uneventful course, discharge them to the floor. We have used the above protocol for management of postoperative anterior cervical spine fusion patients for more than 6 years in our institution and have not encountered any significant airway problems on the first day postoperatively. Patients who undergo prolonged surgery, multiple segmental fusion, corpectomy, difficult surgical exposure with excessive traction, massive fluid shifts, or those who have received large amounts of intravenous (IV) fluids should be admitted directly to the ICU.

Postoperatively, it is crucial that the patient be followed closely for the onset of stridor, increasing difficulty in swallowing or breathing, or signs of increasing external neck swelling. Airway obstruction can occur rapidly in the face of a neck hematoma, edema, lymphatic obstruction, or nerve palsies. Patients exhibiting any of the above signs or symptoms in the immediate postoperative period should immediately have an examination of the airway awake under topical anesthesia using a flexible nasopharyngoscope. Should the airway look normal and intubation is deemed to be unnecessary, close and continuous observation is indicated. If the airway is narrowed or partially obstructed, it should be secured using an awake endotracheal intubation technique. Life-threatening airway obstruction can rapidly ensue either spontaneously, with airway topicalization, or upon airway instrumentation.[9-11] It is imperative to have immediate availability of equipment and personnel skilled in insertion of an infraglottic airway in anticipation of complete airway obstruction.

40.3 AIRWAY CONSIDERATIONS

40.3.1 How often does difficult intubation occur in clinical practice? How is difficult intubation defined?

The incidence of difficult intubation depends on its definition. In 1993, the ASA task force[12] defined difficult intubation as occurring when "proper insertion of the tracheal tube with conventional laryngoscopy requires more than three attempts or more than 10 minutes." In 1998, the Canadian Airway Focus Group[13] used the following definition: "when an experienced laryngoscopist using direct laryngoscopy, requires: (1) more than two attempts with the same blade or; (2) a change in the blade or an adjunct to a direct laryngoscope or; (3) use of an alternative device or technique following failed intubation with direct laryngoscopy." The incidence of difficult intubation reported in the literature ranges from 1.15% to 3.8%.[13]

40.3.2 Is the patient predicted to have a difficult airway? How accurate are our predictions for difficult intubation?

The ASA Task Force on Management of the Difficult Airway outlined 11 criteria for preoperative airway assessment.[14] No single airway test has perfect sensitivity or specificity in predicting difficult intubation. In general, many single airway predictors share a common set of characteristics: low sensitivity, high specificity, and low positive predictive value. Combinations of several airway predictors tend to improve the positive predictive value for difficult intubation. (See Chapter 1.)

Our patient had a Mallampati II score, a thyromental distance of 6.0 cm, mouth opening of 4.0 cm, slightly reduced cervical extension, and a full set of dentures. In combination, these characteristics place this patient at low risk of difficult laryngoscopic intubation.

40.3.3   Is there a concern about difficult bag-mask-ventilation in our patient? How is difficult mask ventilation defined?

The ASA Task Force on Management of the Difficult Airway defined difficult bag-mask-ventilation as: "it is not possible for the anesthesia practitioner to provide adequate face mask ventilation due to one or more of the following problems: inadequate mask seal, excessive gas leak, or excessive resistance to the ingress or egress of gas."[14] The incidence of difficult bag-mask-ventilation is in the range of 5%[15] while failed bag-mask-ventilation is in the range of 0.01% to 0.08%.[13]

Langeron identified five risk factors for difficult mask ventilation: beard, obese (BMI >26), age greater than 55, lack of teeth, and history of snoring (MOANS, see Section 1.6.1).[15] Our patient has four of the five risk factors and is at a moderately increased risk of difficult mask ventilation. More recently, Kheterpal et al identified independent predictors for difficult or impossible mask ventilation: obese (BMI >30), beard, Mallampati III or IV, age = 57, limited jaw protrusion, snoring, neck radiation, male gender, and obstructive sleep apnea.[16,17]

40.3.4   How often does the "cannot intubate, cannot ventilate" situation arise in clinical practice?

"Cannot intubate, cannot ventilate" (CICV) situations are life threatening. In 1991, the incidence of CICV was estimated to be 0.01 to 2 per 10,000 patient cases.[18] The LMA has since been shown to be effective in providing rescue ventilation in the majority of CICV situations.[19] The current incidence of CICV requiring emergency infraglottic airway insertion may be lower than 2:10,000 patients. Anesthesia practitioners need to be fully prepared to insert an infraglottic airway in this rare but deadly situation.

40.4   PREPARATION AND PLANS

40.4.1   How do you plan to intubate the trachea of this patient?

The patient is undergoing an anterior cervical fusion and will require general anesthesia with endotracheal intubation. As he does not have cervical myelopathy, instability, or prediction of a difficult intubation, the plan is to proceed with endotracheal intubation after IV induction of general anesthesia.

40.4.2   Are you concerned about difficulties in mask ventilation?

Yes. The patient is at an increased risk for difficult mask ventilation but is not predicted to have a difficult laryngoscopic intubation or difficulty in using an extraglottic device. Therefore, a variety of airway devices are prepared including face masks, nasopharyngeal airways, oropharyngeal airways, Eschmann Tracheal Introducer (bougie), Laryngeal Mask Airways, and the Combitube™. Operating room personnel are alerted to the possible need to perform two-person bag-mask-ventilation.

40.4.3   What are your plans if after the induction of general anesthesia, intubation with a direct laryngoscope is unsuccessful but ventilation is easy using bag-mask technique?

This unsuccessful intubation, but adequate ventilation clinical setting places us in the second tier of The Failed Airway Algorithm (see Chapter 2) and in the middle of the ASA Difficult Airway Algorithm nonemergency pathway.[14] If all six factors defining an optimal laryngoscopic attempt (see Section 1.6.2) have been met, it makes no sense to persist with further attempts with direct laryngoscopy. Instead, since one has time, alternative approaches such as use of the flexible bronchoscope, intubating laryngeal mask airway, lighted stylet, or the GlideScope® may be attempted.[20,21] It is important to impose a time or number of attempts limit when using these alternative techniques such that a CICV situation following repeated airway instrumentation does not occur. In the event that intubation is unsuccessful after multiple attempts with alternative techniques in a nonemergency scenario, the patient should be awakened and an awake intubation performed.

40.4.4   Should this evolve into a CICV situation after the induction of general anesthesia, what should one do? (Table 40-1)

CICV is an absolute medical emergency. Hypoxic brain damage and death can ensue unless successful corrective measures are undertaken immediately. CICV may occur immediately after induction of anesthesia or during the course of repeated airway instrumentation. The Failed Airway Algorithm directs one to immediately prepare to perform a cricothyrotomy, although while preparations are underway one may attempt to place an extraglottic device (EGD, [LMA or Combitube™]). This differs from the ASA Difficult Airway Algorithm,[14] in that these interventions occur concurrently rather than sequentially. If ventilation and oxygenation become adequate with an EGD, time becomes available to attempt alternative techniques.

40.4.5   A CICV situation wherein the patient becomes progressively hypoxemic necessitates an immediate surgical airway. What is your preferred technique and instrument? (Table 40-1)

The most common techniques employed to secure an infraglottic airway include percutaneous IV catheter cricothyrotomy; percutaneous dilational cricothyrotomy; open surgical cricothyrotomy; and surgical tracheotomy (see Chapter 13). In a Canada-wide anesthesiologist survey,[22] respondents preferred using cricothyrotomy by intravenous catheter (51%), followed by percutaneous dilational cricothyrotomy (28%) and tracheotomy by surgeon (7%).

TABLE 40-1

Cannot Intubate, Cannot Ventilate Management Options

>Optimization of lung ventilation	• Reposition the head, apply jaw lift • Optimize mask: change face mask, adjust the amount of air in the face mask • Insert oropharyngeal and two nasopharyngeal airways (appropriately sized) • Use a two-person, BMV technique: one operator applies a two-hand mask hold and the second operator provides manual bag ventilation • Insert an LMA (appropriately sized) • Consider shaving the beard to improve mask seal
Insertion of an infraglottic airway: options	• IV catheter: nonkinkable • Percutaneous dilational cricothyrotomy kit • Open surgical cricothyrotomy • Open surgical tracheotomy by surgeon
Adjuncts for infraglottic airway	• Hand-held transtracheal jet ventilator with pressure reduction to 20 psi • Saline-soaked ribbon gauze throat pack

40.4.6 What are the advantages and disadvantages of these infraglottic airway techniques?

Although cricothyrotomy by IV catheter is the simplest to perform, it is difficult to fixate the catheter, is difficult to maintain patency, offers no airway protection, provides variable amounts of ventilation, lacks a conduit for suction, is associated with significant risks of barotraumas, and requires a special attachment for jet ventilation.[22] Scrase et al[23] concluded in a review article that jet ventilation does not provide adequate ventilation via an IV catheter and is potentially dangerous. Anesthesia practitioners are generally uncomfortable performing an open cricothyrotomy. The percutaneous dilational cricothyrotomy technique incorporates many advantages of the open cricothyrotomy. It is more stable, offers airway protection, provides a conduit for suctioning, and can be readily connected to a ventilation bag with a 15-mm connector. Furthermore, the percutaneous Seldinger dilational technique is familiar to most airway practitioners who perform central venous cannulation. Most anesthesiologists in the above survey were unfamiliar with the methodology and instruments involved in open tracheotomy or cricothyrotomy.[22]

40.4.7 Is there evidence in the literature to indicate which cricothyrotomy technique is superior to others in terms of speed of insertion and success rates?

Review of the literature reveals few randomized controlled trials using infraglottic airway techniques and none in actual patients in CICV situations.[24,25] Eisenburger et al[26] compared the performance of percutaneous wire-guided and surgical cricothyrotomy by intensive care trainees on cadavers. The cricothyrotomy times

were 100 seconds and 102 seconds, respectively. Chan et al[27] did a similar comparative study for emergency medicine attending physicians and residents. He found similar times (75 vs 73 seconds) for the percutaneous and surgical cricothyrotomy groups. Schaumann et al compared the performance of percutaneous and surgical cricothyrotomy on cadavers by emergency physicians.[28] The cricothyrotomy times were significantly shorter in the percutaneous compared to the surgical group (108.6 vs 136.6 seconds). In contrast, Dimitriadis et al[29] and Sulaiman et al[30] showed that surgical cricothyrotomy insertion times were significantly shorter than percutaneous wire-guided technique in a mannequin model.

40.4.8 Many airway practitioners have never performed a cricothyrotomy or encountered a CICV situation. How can one acquire proficiency in the performance of infraglottic airway insertion?

To optimize the success rate of surgical cricothyrotomy, it is necessary to commit to memory all the sequential steps and to acquire experience in a simulated setting. Bainton reported that the time taken to perform a cricothyrotomy on dogs improved significantly after practicing on cricothyrotomy simulator models.[31] Wong et al[32] showed that procedure times and success rates improved significantly in 102 subjects, each performing 10 consecutive cricothyrotomies on mannequins. From the first to tenth attempt, procedure times improved from 41.2 seconds to 24.4 seconds (41% change) and success rate went from 62% to 99% (37% change). Knowing the cricothyrotomy equipment, familiarity with a cricothyrotomy procedure algorithm, and practical experience with using such devices on mannequins provide the practitioner the best chance of success when called upon to perform a cricothyrotomy in an emergency, such as a CICV airway.

40.4.9   How do you plan to denitrogenate this patient prior to anesthesia induction?

There are many reasons to ensure adequate oxygenation prior to induction. First, the patient is morbidly obese which is associated with reduced functional residual capacity, increased airway closure and shunt, decreased chest wall compliance, and increased work of breathing. He will desaturate much faster than a normal individual with hypoventilation. Second, he is potentially difficult to bag-mask-ventilate. Provision of supranormal denitrogenation will provide the patient and anesthesia practitioner a wider margin of safety on induction. Third, he has significant coronary artery disease. With his increased cardiac oxygen requirement due to obesity and reduced coronary reserve, he may not be able to tolerate arterial hypoxemia. Therefore, the goal should be to provide denitrogenation for at least 3 minutes and end-tidal O_2 ≥90%, similar to that in rapid-sequence induction.

40.5   ACTUAL CONDUCT OF TRACHEAL INTUBATION

40.5.1   How was the induction and airway management approached?

Anesthesia equipment and drugs were fully prepared prior to induction. The patient was denitrogenated for 5 minutes, pretreated with fentanyl, induced with propofol, and paralyzed with rocuronium. After 2 minutes, direct laryngoscopy with a MAC #3 blade was attempted. Only the epiglottis was visible. A MAC #4 blade was tried with the application of anterior laryngeal pressure with no improvement of laryngeal view. A blind insertion of a styletted endotracheal tube behind the epiglottis was performed, but no CO_2 waveform was detected and the endotracheal tube was removed. Bag-mask-ventilation was performed but due to a large mask leak the SpO_2 decreased to 88%.

We now have a failed intubation coupled with borderline bag-mask-ventilation. A 9.0 mm oral-pharyngeal airway and two nasal airways were inserted. The anesthesia practitioner then performed a two-hand mask hold while ventilation was provided by the operating room nurse. Despite these measures, the SpO_2 continued to decline to 80%.

40.5.2   Confronted with a "cannot intubate, cannot ventilate" situation, what ought to happen next?

Cricothyrotomy! In the meantime, as the cricothyrotomy equipment is being set up, one may attempt an intubating LMA or other EGD. This should not be a *sequential* step, as indicated in the ASA Difficult Airway Algorithm; it is *concurrent* with preparation to perform a surgical airway as in The Failed Airway Algorithm (Chapter 2). If the EGD rescue is successful and adequate ventilation is restored, then intubation attempts with

alternative intubation equipment, such as a flexible bronchoscope and GlideScope® are appropriate. However, in the CICV situation, attempts to intubate with alternative techniques, such as the flexible bronchoscope and GlideScope® are not appropriate and waste valuable time.

In this case scenario, the patient was hypoxemic and deteriorating in a CICV situation. A decision was made to insert an infraglottic airway immediately. Concurrently, an LMA was inserted, but ventilation via the LMA was not successful. The anesthesia practitioner decided to use a percutaneous dilational cricothyrotomy technique.

40.5.3   Describe the actual steps taken to insert the percutaneous dilational cricothyrotomy

The instrument used to perform cricothyrotomy was a preassembled Melker Emergency Percutaneous Dilational Set (Cook Critical Care) which consisted of a needle, syringe, guide wire, scalpel, dilator, and airway, which in the newer sets is cuffed. (See Chapter 31 for details.) The cricothyroid membrane was located and punctured with an 18-gauge needle directed caudally. Correct intraluminal location of the needle in the airway was confirmed by the aspiration of air (Figure 40-1). The 0.038-in guide wire was inserted via the needle into the airway (Figure 40-2) and the needle was removed over the wire. The puncture site was enlarged by a stab with a #15 scalpel blade, and a cuffed tracheotomy tube or airway catheter (5.0 mm ID) with the dilator (18 FR) (Figure 40-3) inserted into the trachea over the wire (Figure 40-4). The dilator and the wire were removed, ventilation was performed, and correct

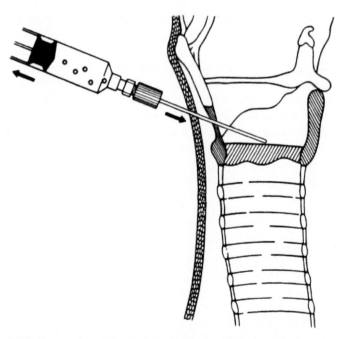

FIGURE 40-1. Cricothyroid membrane puncture: The cricothyroid membrane is punctured with an 18-gauge needle directed caudally and correct intraluminal location is confirmed by the aspiration of air. (Courtesy of Cook Incorporated, Bloomington, Indiana.)

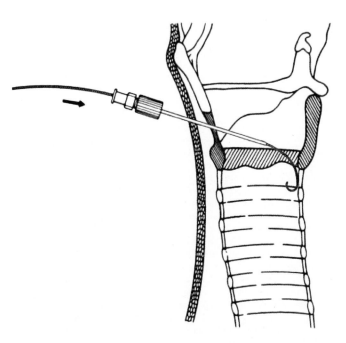

FIGURE 40-2. Insertion of the guide wire: A guide wire is inserted via the needle into the trachea. (Courtesy of Cook Incorporated, Bloomington, Indiana.)

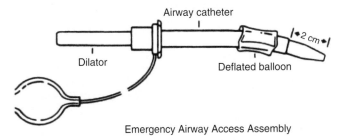

FIGURE 40-3. Cuffed tracheotomy tube: This figure depicts a cuffed airway catheter or tracheotomy tube with the dilator. (Courtesy of Cook Incorporated, Bloomington, Indiana.)

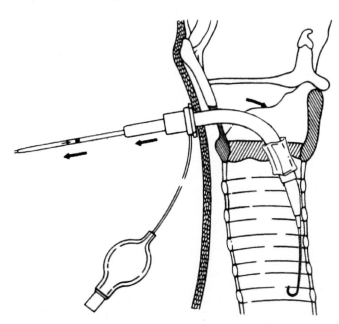

FIGURE 40-4. Insertion of tracheotomy tube: With the dilator in place, the cuffed tracheotomy tube is inserted into the trachea over the guidewire. (Courtesy of Cook Incorporated, Bloomington, Indiana.)

placement was confirmed using capnography and auscultation. A CO_2 waveform was obtained and the SpO_2 improved to greater than 90% 2 minutes after establishment of ventilation via the cricothyrotomy.

40.5.4 Is it feasible to perform an open surgical cricothyrotomy instead of the percutaneous dilational approach?

Yes, it is a feasible option. Most anesthesia practitioners are not comfortable with a surgical cricothyrotomy; but many surgeons and emergency room physicians are.[22] The technique consists of locating the cricothyroid membrane; making a midline longitudinal incision through skin; followed by a transverse incision through the cricothyroid membrane using a scalpel; insertion of a tracheotomy hook placed beneath the inferior border of the thyroid cartilage; applying traction in an anterior/cephalad direction to expose the airway lumen; placement of an endotracheal or cricothyrotomy tube; and confirmation of positioning using capnography and auscultation (see Section 13.2.1). Open cricothyrotomy kits are commercially available. Alternatively, the necessary equipment can be assembled by the individual institution and potential practitioners made aware of the contents.

40.6 POSTINTUBATION MANAGEMENT

40.6.1 At present, oxygenation and ventilation are satisfactory. What is your next step?

Although there is some controversy, most consider a cricothyrotomy to be a temporary life-saving airway which should not be maintained for prolong periods (see Chapters 13 and 31). Therefore, a surgeon was requested to perform a tracheotomy. A size 8.0 mm ID cuffed tracheotomy tube was inserted and the temporary cricothyrotomy was removed.

40.6.2 Now that the airway is secured, the neurosurgeon is anxious to proceed with the anterior cervical fusion. Should we go ahead?

No. The surgery is elective. The patient almost died due to a failed intubation and was subjected to repeated airway instrumentation before a surgical airway was secured. There are three reasons for not performing the surgery at this time. First, anterior cervical fusion involves traction and manipulation in the neck. Should the tracheotomy tube be dislodged, it may be very difficult to reinsert through the track of a newly created tracheotomy. Second, cervical surgery in addition to the intubation attempts will increase the risk of postoperative airway edema. Third, having a tracheotomy tube in the immediate vicinity of a fresh surgical incision increases the potential for surgical site infection.

40.6.3   As a decision has been made not to proceed with cervical surgery, what do we do next?

The patient was brought to the ICU. He was ventilated and allowed to awaken. Once awake and adequate spontaneous ventilation was reestablished, he was removed from the ventilator and placed on a tracheotomy mask. The patient was discharged to the surgical floor after overnight observation.

40.6.4   When can we bring him back for his cervical fusion?

A reasonable course of action is to remove his tracheotomy tube 24 hours post ICU discharge and allow the track and skin to close. He will be brought back for his surgery in 1 to 2 months. An awake intubation could then be performed before induction of general anesthesia.

40.7   SUMMARY

In summary, CICV is a rare but life-threatening situation that all anesthesia practitioners should be prepared to manage. If intubation fails and oxygenation cannot be maintained by bag-mask-ventilation despite a two-person technique, oropharyngeal, nasopharyngeal airways, and an EGD, an immediate decision should be made to perform a cricothyrotomy. Time and again, patients suffer hypoxic brain damage or death from a delayed decision to proceed with an infraglottic airway.

Every airway practitioner must be familiar with the cricothyrotomy equipment available locally and must acquire the necessary skills by performing cricothyrotomy on mannequins or cadavers so that emergency cricothyrotomy can be rapidly performed if required in the clinical setting.

It is better to have a live patient with a neck incision than a dead patient with a nice looking neck.

REFERENCES

1. Buckley FP, Martay K. Anesthesia, obesity and gastrointestinal disorders. In: Barash PG, Cullen BF, Calkins H, eds. *Clinical Anesthesia.* 4th ed. Philadelphia, PA: Lippincott Williams & Wilkins; 2001:1035-1041.
2. Eagle KA, Berger PB, Calkins H, et al. ACC/AHA guideline update for perioperative cardiovascular evaluation for noncardiac surgery—executive summary: a report of the American College of Cardiology/American Heart Association Task Force on Practice Guidelines (Committee to Update the 1996 Guidelines on Perioperative Cardiovascular Evaluation for Noncardiac Surgery). *J Am Coll Cardiol.* 2002;39:542-553.
3. Fleisher LA, Beckman JA, Brown KA, et al. ACC/AHA 2007 Guidelines on Perioperative Cardiovascular Evaluation and Care for Noncardiac Surgery: Executive Summary: A Report of the American College of Cardiology/American Heart Association Task Force on Practice Guidelines (Writing Committee to Revise the 2002 Guidelines on Perioperative Cardiovascular Evaluation for Noncardiac Surgery): Developed in Collaboration With the American Society of Echocardiography, American Society of Nuclear Cardiology, Heart Rhythm Society, Society of Cardiovascular Anesthesiologists, Society for Cardiovascular Angiography and Interventions, Society for Vascular Medicine and Biology, and Society for Vascular Surgery. *Circulation.* 2007;116:1971-1996.
4. Lee TH, Marcantonio ER, Mangione CM, et al. Derivation and prospective validation of a simple index for prediction of cardiac risk of major noncardiac surgery. *Circulation.* 1999;100:1043-1049.
5. Criswell JC, Parr MJ, Nolan JP. Emergency airway management in patients with cervical spine injuries. *Anaesthesia.* 1994;49:900-903.
6. Crosby ET. Airway management in adults after cervical spine trauma. *Anesthesiology.* 2006;104:1293-1318.
7. Meschino A, Devitt JH, Koch JP, et al. The safety of awake tracheal intubation in cervical spine injury. *Can J Anaesth.* 1992;39:114-117.
8. Suderman VS, Crosby ET, Lui A. Elective oral tracheal intubation in cervical spine-injured adults. *Can J Anaesth.* 1991;38:785-789.
9. Ho AM, Chung DC, To EW, Karmakar MK. Total airway obstruction during local anesthesia in a non-sedated patient with a compromised airway. *Can J Anaesth.* 2004;51:838-841.
10. McGuire G, el-Beheiry H. Complete upper airway obstruction during awake fibreoptic intubation in patients with unstable cervical spine fractures. *Can J Anaesth.* 1999;46:176-178.
11. Shaw IC, Welchew EA, Harrison BJ, Michael S. Complete airway obstruction during awake fibreoptic intubation. *Anaesthesia.* 1997;52:582-585.
12. Caplan RA, Benumof JL, Berry FA, et al. Practice guidelines for management of the difficult airway: a report by the American Society of Anesthesiologists Task Force on Management of the Difficult Airway. *Anesthesiology.* 1993;78: 597-602.
13. Crosby ET, Cooper RM, Douglas MJ, et al. The unanticipated difficult airway with recommendations for management. *Can J Anaesth.* 1998;45:757-776.
14. Caplan RA, Benumof JL, Berry FA, et al. Practice guidelines for management of the difficult airway: an updated report by the American Society of Anesthesiologists Task Force on Management of the Difficult Airway. *Anesthesiology.* 2003;98:1269-1277.
15. Langeron O, Masso E, Huraux C, et al. Prediction of difficult mask ventilation. *Anesthesiology.* 2000;92:1229-1236.
16. Kheterpal S, Han R, Tremper KK, et al. Incidence and predictors of difficult and impossible mask ventilation. *Anesthesiology.* 2006;105:885-891.
17. Kheterpal S, Martin L, Shanks AM, Tremper KK. Prediction and outcomes of impossible mask ventilation: a review of 50,000 anesthetics. *Anesthesiology.* 2009;110:891-897.
18. Benumof JL. Management of the difficult adult airway. With special emphasis on awake tracheal intubation. *Anesthesiology.* 1991;75:1087-1110.
19. Parmet JL, Colonna-Romano P, Horrow JC, Miller F, Gonzales J, Rosenberg H. The laryngeal mask airway reliably provides rescue ventilation in cases of unanticipated difficult tracheal intubation along with difficult mask ventilation. *Anesth Analg.* 1998;87:661-665.
20. Jenkins K, Wong DT, Correa R. Management choices for the difficult airway by anesthesiologists in Canada. *Can J Anaesth.* 2002;49:850-856.
21. Rosenblatt WH, Wagner PJ, Ovassapian A, Kain ZN. Practice patterns in managing the difficult airway by anesthesiologists in the United States. *Anesth Analg.* 1998;87:153-157.
22. Wong DT, Lai K, Chung FF, Ho RY. Cannot intubate-cannot ventilate and difficult intubation strategies: results of a Canadian national survey. *Anesth Analg.* 2005;100:1439-1446.
23. Scrase I, Woollard M. Needle vs surgical cricothyroidotomy: a short cut to effective ventilation. *Anaesthesia.* 2006;61:962-974.
24. Chang RS, Hamilton RJ, Carter WA. Declining rate of cricothyrotomy in trauma patients with an emergency medicine residency: implications for skills training. *Acad Emerg Med.* 1998;5:247-251.
25. Erlandson MJ, Clinton JE, Ruiz E, Cohen J. Cricothyrotomy in the emergency department revisited. *J Emerg Med.* 1989;7:115-118.
26. Eisenburger P, Laczika K, List M, et al. Comparison of conventional surgical versus Seldinger technique emergency cricothyrotomy performed by inexperienced clinicians. *Anesthesiology.* 2000;92:687-690.
27. Chan TC, Vilke GM, Bramwell KJ, Davis DR, Hamilton RS, Rosen P. Comparison of wire-guided cricothyrotomy versus standard surgical cricothyrotomy technique. *J Emerg Med.* 1999;17:957-962.
28. Schaumann N, Lorenz V, Schellongowski P, et al. Evaluation of Seldinger technique emergency cricothyroidotomy versus standard surgical cricothyroidotomy in 200 cadavers. *Anesthesiology.* 2005;102:7-11.
29. Dimitriadis JC, Paoloni R. Emergency cricothyroidotomy: a randomised crossover study of four methods. *Anaesthesia.* 2008;63:1204-1208.
30. Sulaiman L, Tighe SQ, Nelson RA. Surgical vs wire-guided cricothyroidotomy: a randomised crossover study of cuffed and uncuffed tracheal tube insertion. *Anaesthesia.* 2006;61:565-570.
31. Bainton CR. Cricothyrotomy. *Int Anesthesiol Clin.* 1994;32:95-108.
32. Wong DT, Prabhu AJ, Coloma M, et al. What is the minimum training required for successful cricothyroidotomy? A study in mannequins. *Anesthesiology.* 2003;98:349-353.

SELF-EVALUATION QUESTIONS

40.1. The major difference between the ASA Difficult Airway Algorithm and The Failed Airway Algorithm in Chapter 2 of this text is:

A. The definition of the failed airway is different.

B. The ASA algorithm recommends that LMAs and cricothyrotomy be performed sequentially; this text recommends that they be performed concurrently.

C. The ASA algorithm recommends that LMAs and cricothyrotomy be performed concurrently; this text recommends that they be performed sequentially.

D. The role of video laryngoscopes is different.

E. The ASA algorithm recommends canceling the case; this text makes no mention of canceling the case.

40.2. The evidence with respect to cricothyrotomy suggests:

A. that practice on improves performance

B. that anesthesia practitioners do not like to perform it

C. that, on average, anesthesia practitioners do not know how to perform one

D. two of A, B, C

E. all of A, B, C

40.3. Difficult mask ventilation:

A. may be mitigated by the use of an oral airway and two nasal airways

B. is associated with an age greater than 65

C. is less common with the use of transparent masks

D. is less common in the elderly with no teeth

E. is associated with failed laryngoscopy and intubation

CHAPTER (41)

Airway Management in a Patient with Epidermolysis Bullosa for Peripheral Procedure

Sarah H. Wiser and Wendy Howard

41.1 CASE PRESENTATION

A 14-year-old adolescent girl with a history of dystrophic epidermolysis bullosa (DEB) presents to the operating room for surgical correction of pseudosyndactyly of her right hand.

The patient was diagnosed with DEB shortly after birth. She has had repeated episodes of blister formation that have resulted in scarring and fusion of the fingers, leading to pseudosyndactyly, has contractures of the arms and legs, and periods of dysphagia that have required esophageal dilations in the past. She currently has no dysphagia. Her medications include minocycline 100 mg po BID, and prednisone 10 mg po QD.

On physical examination, the patient is notably anxious. Her vital signs are: blood pressure (BP) 105/65 mm Hg, heart rate (HR) 95 beats per minute, respiratory rate (RR) 16 breaths per minutes. She weighs 85 lb (38.6 kg) and is 5 ft (152.4 cm) tall. Her BMI is 16.6 kg·m^{-2}. Cardiac and pulmonary examinations are normal. She has contractures of both the upper and lower extremities, and several erosions on the extensor surfaces of her legs.

Airway examination reveals a small mouth with limited opening due to perioral scarring. Despite being unable to protrude her tongue, she has a Mallampati II Classification. She has full dentition which is in poor condition. Thyromental distance is normal (5 cm). Neck extension is significantly limited due to scaring around the neck.

Laboratory data reveal normal electrolytes and renal function. Her hematocrit is 32% and albumin is 3.0 g/dL. Echocardiogram was normal.

The patient was consulted regarding the use of regional anesthesia, but she adamantly refused.

41.2 PATIENT CONSIDERATIONS

41.2.1 What is epidermolysis bullosa?

Epidermolysis bullosa (EB) is a group of hereditary mechanobullous diseases that were first described in 1879 by Fox.[1] The primary pathophysiologic abnormality is thought to be due to either: (1) mutations in the gene coding for type VII collagen with disturbances in the anchoring fibrils in stratified squamous epithelium; or (2) an increase in collagenase activity causing breakdown of the periepidermal-dermal junction of the skin and mucous membranes.[2-4] There are more than 20 types of EB, each transmitted by various modes of autosomal inheritance, with three main subtypes: simplex, junctional, and dystrophic. The exact layer of skin injury, and resultant degree of severity, is dependent on the disease type. Diagnosis of EB is made early in the life of a child and can be lethal in infancy with some types of EB, but most survive until the third or fourth decade of life.[5,6]

The type of EB most relevant to the practice of anesthesiology is dystrophic epidermolysis bullosa (DEB) of the autosomal recessive type. The incidence is 1 in 300,000 live births.[4] The focus of injury is at the dermo-epidermal junction, below the level of the lamina densa. Injury at this level heals in the form of scarring, where chronic repeated injury results in contractures.[5]

Patients affected with DEB experience severe blistering due to any mechanical *shearing* or *friction* of the skin and mucous membranes. In fact, these patients are often referred to as having *cotton wool* skin.[4] Bullae can occur anywhere on the body and mucous membranes, but the areas most affected are those that require frequent use, such as the hands. The bullae produced are large, fluid filled, flaccid, and are easily ruptured and bleed. These lesions are very painful and pruritus is common during healing. Scratching leads to further bullae formation.

Patients often exhibit various stages of healing as well as significant degrees of scarring. Due to the healing-scaring process, the patients develop pseudosyndactyly, classically *mitten type*, flexion contractures of the arms and legs, and contractures around the eyes and mouth. Mucous membrane involvement causes painful feeding and defecation, and leads to scarring of the mouth (microstomia), fixation of the tongue to the floor of the mouth, esophageal strictures or webs, and chronic constipation.[5,7] Abnormal enamel development, recurrent oral infections, and painful oral hygiene frequently lead to poor dentition and gums.[5] Abnormalities of the cornea of the eye, hair, and nails are also associated with the disorder.[5,8]

Of note, the mucous membranes of the larynx and trachea are rarely involved, as these areas are lined with ciliated columnar epithelium, not stratified squamous epithelium.[9]

41.2.2 Are there any medical conditions associated with DEB?

Due to chronic blister formation, hemorrhagic rupture, the healing process, and difficult feeding because of pain or esophageal strictures, patients with DEB are chronically malnourished with growth retardation. Protein deficiency, iron deficiency anemia, and electrolyte disturbances are key features.[8] Patients with severe DEB are at increased risk of developing dilated cardiomyopathy, thought to be secondary to carnitine deficiency.[10]

Exposed denuded skin makes supra-infection and sepsis frequent, especially with *Staphylococcus aureus* and *beta-hemolytic streptococci* and acquisition of nosocomial multidrug-resistant pathogens is a concern. Patients with DEB also have a higher incidence of postinfectious glomerulonephritis due to chronic streptococcal skin infections.[5] The chronic inflammatory response and renal amyloid deposition may also be associated with renal insufficiency or failure.[7,11-13]

There is concern that some neuromuscular junction diseases, such as myasthenia gravis and muscular dystrophy, may coexist with DEB, but the exact association has not been determined.[5]

Long-term DEB patients are at significantly increased risk for cutaneous neoplasms.[4,6,11] Squamous cell carcinoma is the major cause of death in patients who survive to adulthood.[5]

Some early reports indicated an association between porphyria cunea tarda (PCT) and DEB due to similar cutaneous manifestations. However, when DEB patients have been tested for PCT, the results have been consistently negative.[4] Currently, with the advent of electron microscopy and immunofluorescence evaluation of skin biopsies, a definitive diagnosis can be obtained.[11]

41.2.3 What is the treatment for DEB?

There is no cure for DEB. Management requires a multimodal approach. Central to management is prevention of bullae formation, nutrition, and proper wound care. Patients are often given a trial of phenytoin to reduce collagenase activity or synthesis,

however not all patients respond. Minocycline has also been useful in uncontrolled studies.[11,14] Systemic and local steroids are used to reduce the severity of scaring and pruritus associated with healing. Pain management is essential as these patients often experience significant pain from blisters and wound care. Physical therapy helps to maintain mobility and minimize contractures, but surgical intervention is often necessary.[5]

Corrective surgeries, including the release of contractures, are required when the patient loses mobility of the hands, arms, or legs. Esophageal dilations are indicated for dysphagia secondary to esophageal strictures. Unfortunately, surgical correction is only a temporary solution, as the deformity invariably recurs.[3]

41.3 SURGICAL CONSIDERATIONS

Patients with DEB may present for a number of surgical procedures beyond those listed above, including surgical excision of skin neoplasms, dental surgery, whirlpool treatments for skin debridement, percutaneous endoscopic gastrostomy (PEG) or open gastrostomy, gastrointestinal (GI) endoscopy, central lines and dressing changes, as well as for procedures unrelated to their dermatologic disease. Appropriate perioperative antibiotics need to be considered. The common adhesive surgical electrocautery pad cannot be placed for the reasons detailed later (see Section 41.4.1) and the surgical site cannot be prepped with a rubbing motion. The prep must be dabbed on and gently blotted to remove excess solution.

41.4 ANESTHETIC CONSIDERATIONS

41.4.1 Does the patient require special handling/monitoring?

Caring for the patient with DEB is challenging. Since the skin is extremely fragile, a *no touch* premise must be instituted.[15] Absolutely no tape or adhesive should be applied to the patient, as this can result in significant blistering when removed.

Intravenous (IV) access can be difficult to obtain due to scaring. The skin site can be cleaned by dabbing (do not rub) the area with an alcohol wipe, and the IV should be protected with Vaseline gauze (Xeroform®) placed underneath the hub of the angiocatheter, then wrapped with cotton gauze or Koban® wrap.

All monitoring should be performed with utmost care. Noninvasive blood pressure cuffs are safe to use, provided the location for the cuff is properly protected with cotton gauze before placing the cuff. The primary cause of injury is frictional in nature, not perpendicular pressure as occurs with NIBP or tourniquet usage.[4,11] Both should only be used after the skin has been protected with cotton gauze (Webril®). Pulse oximetry should be performed with the use of a clip-style ear or finger probe, as opposed to adhesive probes. Electrocardiogram (ECG) monitoring can be preformed either through the use of needle electrodes or, more commonly, by removing the adhesive area of the pad, leaving only the gel sphere. The pads can then be put on the patient and held into place with the use of cotton gauze wrapped around the thorax or positioned underneath the patient, allowing the patient's weight to hold them in place. There are also reports of adhering the ECG leads to an x-ray film that has had holes cut out in the desired position for the ECG leads. This allows for the gel sphere of the lead be in contact with the patient when he/she lies supine on the film, without the adhesive touching the patient.[13,15] A temperature probe should not be placed in the patient's mouth, nose, or anus, but rather be well lubricated and placed in the axilla.

Ideally, the patient should be awake enough to move him/herself from the bed to the operating room table to prevent injury. If the patient is unable to move, he or she should be lifted up and transferred. A surgical lifting system provides a safe method for transfer. All surfaces the patient lies on should be well cushioned with egg crate or sheep skin, and care taken to ensure there are no folds or wrinkles in the sheets.

The patient's eyes should not be secured closed with any adhesive. Due to scarring around the eyes, eye closure may be hindered. To properly protect the eyes, an eye lubricant should be used and damp gauze can be placed over the eyes.

All of the needed supplies should be gathered and prepared ahead of time and the operating room should be warmed.

41.4.2 Are there any special considerations with regard to medications or route of administration?

Hypoproteinemia can affect the volume and distribution of many protein-bound drugs and may affect the duration of action, especially with the nondepolarizing muscle relaxants (NDMR).[8] One may consider the use of cisatracurium, the NMDR of choice, given its mechanism of degradation with no reliance on the renal or hepatic systems for clearance. Several reports recommend caution in the use of succinylcholine in patients with contractures and muscle wasting due to concern about a hyperkalemic response.[4,8] However, Griffin and Mayou, in a major case series, reported the use of succinylcholine 76 times without incident, and consider it safe to use.[11,14] Other case reports have also demonstrated the safety of succinylcholine in this patient group.[12,15] In patients with coexisting neuromuscular diseases, succinylcholine should be avoided.[5]

Intravenous injection is the preferred route of parenteral medication administration. Intramuscular administration has, however, been used without the formation of new bullae.[15] Intravenous access is notoriously difficult in these patients, especially in the pediatric population, thus inhalation induction is often utilized, with IV access subsequently achieved.

41.4.3 What are the airway considerations in patients with DEB?

The greatest concern for the anesthesia practitioners in caring for patients with DEB is management of the airway. Controversy exists with regard to the ideal anesthetic technique due to the extreme fragility of the skin and mucosa, in addition to coexisting oral deformities. Some prefer to intubate the trachea and secure the airway, whereas others prefer to use mask-ventilation, and yet others prefer regional anesthesia if at all possible.[6,9,16]

Patients with DEB often have chronic bullae and scarring around and in the mouth leading to microstomia (Figure 41-1).

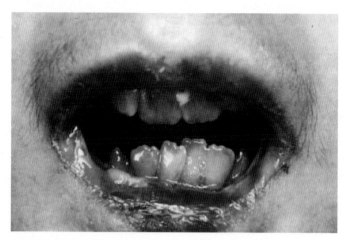

FIGURE 41-1. Microstomia in a patient with dystrophic epidermolysis bullosa. (Reproduced from Ames WA, Mayou BJ, Williams K. Anaesthetic management of epidermolysis bullosa. *Br J Anaesthesia*. 1999;82:76-51. Used with permission.)

Restricted mouth opening and tongue movement can occur as well as poor dentition and restricted neck mobility. Some patients develop ankylosis of the temporomandibular joint which further limits mouth opening. Instrumentation of the oral mucosa with laryngoscopes, flexible bronchoscope, and LMAs pose a risk of oropharyngeal and laryngeal blister formation. All of these factors add to the anxiety of the airway management.

Numerous practitioners have reviewed their experience with the anesthetic management of patients with DEB, and have shown that airway management can be safely performed, provided special precautions and preparations are taken.

Ames et al[15] reported that 2 of 51 patients had difficult airways and required flexible bronchoscopic intubation. Iohom and Lyons[17] reported that 2 of 10 children requiring general anesthesia had difficult tracheal intubation. Griffin and Mayou[11] reported difficult tracheal intubation in 10 of 44 (23%) of patients in their case series. Intubation was ultimately successful via a blind nasal technique, flexible bronchoscopic intubation, or laryngeal mask airway.

James and Wark[9] reported 73 patients with DEB who underwent 309 anesthetics. None of whom developed laryngeal bullae, postoperative stridor, or airway obstruction. One hundred and thirteen tracheal intubations were performed. Seventeen of 33 patients (51%) had restricted mouth opening or gross dental problems interfering with intubation, and the trachea of 2 patients could not be intubated. Intraoral bullae formation could be directly attributed to intubation as the cause in only three cases, none of which resulted in postoperative problems. There are no reports of tracheal bullae occurring during or following anesthesia, likely due to the columnar epithelium of the trachea versus the squamous epithelium of the oral cavity and pharynx.

There is only one report of laryngeal stenosis due to an epiglottic abnormality necessitating tracheotomy.[18] There are a few reports of tracheal stenosis in patients who have a rarer junctional DEB, albeit unrelated to intubation.[19,20]

Lin and Golianu[21] reviewed 25 patients who underwent 121 anesthetics with no deaths or major perioperative complications: 48% were intubated and three cases required bronchoscopic intubation with intravenous sedation due to restricted mouth opening.

Twenty one percent had mask anesthesia and 31% had intravenous sedation (six with nerve block).

Venous access is often difficult and therefore inhalation induction may be required.[15] Sevoflurane is the most commonly used agent.

Mask ventilation is often easier than expected due to the scaring in the oral cavity that causes the tongue to be fixed to the floor of the mouth. The tissues are often stiff and less likely to collapse with loss of consciousness. Oral and nasal airways are to be avoided as they may cause new bullae formation, but if needed, should be well lubricated. The mask should also be well lubricated and care taken not to apply shear force on the face with the fingers and hand holding the mask.

When performing tracheal intubation with a laryngoscope, the blade and endotracheal tube should be well lubricated before insertion into the mouth. The laryngoscope blade may cause new bullae formation if not properly handled. The tube, ideally a smaller size than normal, should be secured with care. Traction on the corners of the mouth may cause bullae. Movement of the tube in the oral cavity and pharynx may also cause new bullae. Suction of the oral cavity prior to extubation can cause life-threatening bullae and should either not be preformed, or performed only carefully if absolutely necessary. If the patient has copious secretions, an antisialagogue may be administered.

Patients with DEB often require frequent anesthetics and become opinionated about what techniques best suit them. Anesthesia practitioners should be reasonably sensitive to their desires.

41.4.4   Is it safe to use an LMA™ in patients with DEB?

The literature historically has not reported the use of laryngeal mask airway (LMA) in patients with DEB. However, more recently the device has been used with increasing frequency. The primary concern is the development of new intraoral bullae. Ames[15] used the LMA in 57 cases (20% of anesthetics) with only one new lingual bulla. No airway compromise occurred in this series. Griffin[11] also described the use of the LMA. As anesthesia practitioners become more comfortable with the use of LMAs in DEB patients, it seems that the LMA is an acceptable technique for airway management. Some even feel it is superior to endotracheal intubation.

When choosing to use an LMA, a smaller size than normally selected should be chosen and the tube and cuff should be well lubricated. The cuff should be inflated to maintain shape, but not overinflated, and may even allow a leak. Care should be taken in securing the device, if at all. Gentle LMA removal is imperative to avoid the development of bullae. The possibility of removal of the device prior to awaking should be considered. The LMA can be an extremely useful device in the airway management of the patient with DEB who needs a general anesthetic.

41.4.5   What are the benefits of regional anesthesia in a patient with DEB?

Regional anesthesia is an excellent option when possible. It has become the technique of choice for many centers since it adheres more closely to the *no touch* technique, and minimizes dermal trauma and airway manipulation.[12,16,22-24] Regional anesthesia also provides postoperative pain relief, decreasing discomfort and thrashing on recovery. Historically, regional techniques were avoided due to fears of local infiltration causing new bullae and increased risks of infection. However, this has not been reported and more regional techniques are being performed safely.

As a group, patients with DEB tend to be underdeveloped and malnourished, thus the landmarks for regional anesthesia are easily identified. However, many of the patients are young, exceedingly anxious, and may not tolerate the procedure. Mask inhalation induction may be necessary to facilitate the injection of local anesthesia.[16,24] Sedation often cannot be avoided, and airway support may be needed during the procedure or operation.

Chevaleraud[16] reported 22 patients who underwent 160 operative procedures on their hands. One hundred and forty two cases were performed under regional anesthesia (140 axillary blocks). General anesthesia was only required in 20 cases, either alone or in conjunction with a block. Ninety eight percent of blocks were successful. For children younger than 10 years of age, a parent was present throughout the operative course to decrease anxiety.

Kelly[12] reported inadequate axillary blocks and the need for additional injections to block the musculocutaneous and the thoracobrachialis nerves in order to complete the procedure and permit the patient to tolerate the use of the tourniquet. Ankle, penile, caudal, subarachnoid, and epidural blocks have also been described.[15,23-25]

Contraindications to regional anesthesia include language barriers and children too young to comply with long procedures. Limitations also include erosion or infected blisters at the site of the block.

41.4.6   Are there any special techniques that should be used to avoid injury during regional anesthesia in a patient with DEB?

The skin cannot be rubbed so the antiseptic should either be dabbed or poured on the skin and then dabbed off gently. Theoretically, chlorohexidine prep should be avoided because it requires rubbing. If a continuous catheter is placed (a consideration for patients undergoing staged procedures of the upper extremity, or epidural), the method of securing the catheter cannot include tape to the skin. The regional block site must be inspected for local bullae and/or infection. A skin wheal injection should be avoided, but deep infiltration is safe.

41.4.7   Is it safe to perform a regional anesthetic on a DEB patient with a suspected difficult airway?

Regional anesthetic techniques are ideal for patients with DEB since airway manipulation is minimized or unnecessary. New facial and oropharyngeal bullae are well-documented complications of general anesthesia with airway manipulation. The decision to use regional techniques also depends upon the expertise of the anesthesia practitioner in both regional anesthesia and airway management. Patient position and the duration of the procedure must also be considered. If a regional technique is planned, then back-up plans must be in place to provide adequate anesthesia should the regional anesthesia be inadequate or fail. These back up plans include repeating the block or supplementation at the surgical site, intravenous sedation (propofol or ketamine), and general anesthesia.

If the patient has a known or predicted difficult airway, then the necessary airway equipment should be immediately available (flexible bronchoscope, extraglottic devices, video laryngoscopes, etc), as well as the equipment and expertise required to perform a surgical airway should it become necessary. As with any suspected difficult airway, a number of back up plans should be considered and helpful hands readily available prior to proceeding with the block. Blind nasal intubations have been reported[9,11,15] as an option for the difficult airway in the DEB patient.

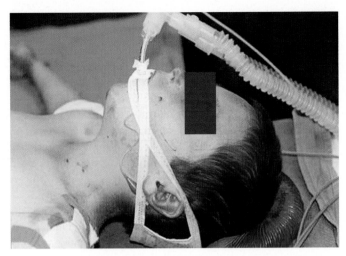

FIGURE 41-2. Technique to secure an ETT with the use of a surgical face mask. (Reproduced from Guidelines from the Anesthetic Management of Epidermolysis Bullosa (EB). http://pedsanesthesia. stanford.edu/downloads/guideline-eb.pdf, (c) Elliot Krane, MD, with permission of author.)

41.5   AIRWAY MANAGEMENT

41.5.1   How should this patient's airway be approached?

This patient has refused regional anesthesia, however an effort should be made to fully explain the benefits of regional and postoperative pain management versus the risks of airway management to her. Airway management options for general anesthesia include bag-mask-ventilation, extraglottic airway, or endotracheal intubation. Mask anesthesia is an option; however this procedure may last several hours and does carry the risk of trauma to the facial skin from prolonged exposure to the mask. An LMA would be a viable option, but with the patient's limited mouth opening, insertion of the LMA could prove difficult. She has significant risk factors for a difficult laryngoscopic intubation, small mouth with limited opening, and limited neck extension, but no risk factors for difficult mask ventilation, so an asleep flexible bronchoscopic intubation was planned.

A difficult airway cart was brought into the operating room. Midazolam 1 mg IM was administered preoperatively to help ease her anxiety, yet allow her to position herself on the operative table in a comfortable manner and participate fully in skin padding and protection. A 22-gauge intravenous peripheral line was placed in the nonoperative arm and protected with Vaseline gauze and secured with Koban® wrap. A clip-style pulse oximeter and well-padded blood pressure cuff were applied to the same arm. ECG monitoring was accomplished by removing the adhesive from the pads and placed on the patient. Webril® was wrapped around the patient's thorax to maintain lead position. A well-lubricated mask was gently held to her face and denitrogenation was performed for 5 minutes. Induction was accomplished with IV 50 ug of fentanyl, 40 mg of lidocaine, and 100 mg of propofol. Had we not been able to start an intravenous line, we would have used an inhalation induction and started a peripheral line after loss of consciousness. Upon loss of consciousness, she was easily ventilated with bag-mask. Cisatracurium 10 mg was administered and mask ventilation was continued with sevoflurane and oxygen. Her trachea was intubated with a pediatric flexible bronchoscope using a 6.0 mm ID cuffed endotracheal tube. The tube was secured using

a surgical face mask that was placed across the back of her neck with the ties gently securing the tube (Figure 41-2). Eye lubricant was placed in her conjunctival sacs and her eyelids were covered with moist gauze pads.

41.6   POSTINTUBATION CONSIDERATIONS

41.6.1   What is your extubation plan for this patient?

The prevention of new bullae formation extends throughout the emergency and postoperative period. Oropharyngeal suctioning should not be performed since it can lead to severe bullae formation in the mouth and pharynx. If necessary, suction gently with a well-lubricated catheter. Postoperative nausea and vomiting prophylaxis should be given to prevent retching and vomiting, which can lead to esophageal rupture. Adequate postoperative analgesia should be obtained to prevent thrashing and movement.

Ideally, the patient is extubated awake and face mask use minimized, but one must weigh face mask use with the risks of the patient bucking and moving around on the operative table.

41.6.2   Discuss other postoperative care of this patient

Supplemental oxygenation should be avoided via face mask as the sharp edges are traumatic. Blow-by oxygen is a good option. The patient's family or familiar caregivers should be available to the PACU to calm the patient and prevent thrashing in the bed. Pruritus should be avoided and, if occurs, should be treated immediately. Patients with DEB often require unusually large doses of benzodiazepines and opioids to achieve restful states in the PACU. New skin lesions should be evaluated and dressed.

41.7 SUMMARY

Patients with dystrophic epidermolysis bullosa present a significant challenge to the anesthesia practitioner and surgical team. These patients may have challenging IV access, difficult airways, and are fragile to handle. Furthermore, the need for repetitive surgeries and resultant psychological trauma often requires delicate handling emotionally, as well as physically. It is imperative that adequate preparation and consultation is performed prior to anesthetizing patients with this disease. With this preparation, DEB patients can be safely cared for.

REFERENCES

1. Fox T. On unusual or rare forms of skin disease, no. 4. Congenital ulceration of the skin (two cases) with pemphigus eruption and arrest of development generally. *Lancet*. 1897;1:766-767.
2. Cakmakkaya OS, Altindas F, Kaya G, Baghaki S. Anesthesia in children with epidermolysis bullosa. *Plast Reconstr Surg*. 2008;122:34e-35e.
3. Ciccarelli AO, Rothaus KO, Carter DM, Lin AN. Plastic and reconstructive surgery in epidermolysis bullosa: clinical experience with 110 procedures in 25 patients. *Ann Plast Surg*. 1995;35:254-261.
4. Culpepper TL. Anesthetic implications in epidermolysis bullosa dystrophica. *AANA J*. 2001;69:114-118.
5. Herod J, Denyer J, Goldman A, Howard R. Epidermolysis bullosa in children: pathophysiology, anaesthesia and pain management. *Paediatr Anaesth*. 2002;12:388-397.
6. Lin AN, Carter DM. Epidermolysis bullosa. *Annu Rev Med*. 1993;44:189-199.
7. Smith GB, Shribman AJ. Anaesthesia and severe skin disease. *Anaesthesia*. 1984;39:443-455.
8. Hagen R, Langenberg C. Anaesthetic management in patients with epidermolysis bullosa dystrophica. *Anaesthesia*. 1988;43:482-485.
9. James I, Wark H. Airway management during anesthesia in patients with epidermolysis bullosa dystrophica. *Anesthesiology*. 1982;56:323-326.
10. Sidwell RU, Yates R, Atherton D. Dilated cardiomyopathy in dystrophic epidermolysis bullosa. *Arch Dis Child*. 2000;83:59-63.
11. Griffin RP, Mayou BJ. The anaesthetic management of patients with dystrophic epidermolysis bullosa. A review of 44 patients over a 10 year period. *Anaesthesia*. 1993;48:810-815.
12. Kelly RE, Koff HD, Rothaus KO, et al. Brachial plexus anesthesia in eight patients with recessive dystrophic epidermolysis bullosa. *Anesth Analg*. 1987;66:1318-1320.
13. Patch MR, Woodey RD. Spinal anaesthesia in a patient with epidermolysis bullosa dystrophica. *Anaesth Intensive Care*. 2000;28: 446-448.
14. White JE. Minocycline for dystrophic epidermolysis bullosa. *Lancet*. 1989;1:966.
15. Ames WA, Mayou BJ, Williams KN. Anaesthetic management of epidermolysis bullosa. *Br J Anaesth*. 1999;82:746-751.
16. Chevaleraud E, Ragot JM, Glicenstein J. Anesthesia for hand surgery in patients with epidermolysis bullosa. *Ann Fr Anesth Reanim*. 1995;14: 399-405.
17. Iohom G, Lyons B. Anaesthesia for children with epidermolysis bullosa: a review of 20 years' experience. *Eur J Anaesthesiol*. 2001;18:745-754.
18. Haruyama T, Furukawa M, Matsumoto F, et al. Laryngeal stenosis in epidermolysis bullosa dystrophica. *Auris Nasus Larynx*. 2009;36:106-109.
19. Fine JD, Johnson LB, Weiner M, Suchindran C. Tracheolaryngeal complications of inherited epidermolysis bullosa: cumulative experience of the national epidermolysis bullosa registry. *Laryngoscope*. 2007;117:1652-1660.
20. Holzman RS, Worthen HM, Johnson KL. Anaesthesia for children with junctional epidermolysis bullosa (letalis). *Can J Anaesth*. 1987;34:395-399.
21. Lin YC, Golianu B. Anesthesia and pain management for pediatric patients with dystrophic epidermolysis bullosa. *J Clin Anesth*. 2006;18:268-271.
22. Boughton R, Crawford MR, Vonwiller JB. Epidermolysis bullosa—a review of 15 years' experience, including experience with combined general and regional anaesthetic techniques. *Anaesth Intensive Care*. 1988;16:260-264.
23. Farber NE, Troshynski TJ, Turco G. Spinal anesthesia in an infant with epidermolysis bullosa. *Anesthesiology*. 1995;83:1364-1367.
24. Lin AN, Lateef F, Kelly R, et al. Anesthetic management in epidermolysis bullosa: review of 129 anesthetic episodes in 32 patients. *J Am Acad Dermatol*. 1994;30:412-416.
25. Spielman FJ, Mann ES. Subarachnoid and epidural anaesthesia for patients with epidermolysis bullosa. *Can Anaesth Soc J*. 1984;31:549-551.

SELF-EVALUATION QUESTIONS

41.1. Which medication has been proven to be unsafe to use in patients with dystrophic epidermolysis bullosa (DEB)?

A. thiopental

B. propofol

C. cisatracurium

D. succinylcholine

E. none of above

41.2. What laboratory evaluation should be performed in patients with DEB?

A. electrolyte panel

B. CBC

C. renal function testes

D. albumin

E. all the above

41.3. Which of the following is true with regards to airway management in patients with DEB?

A. Intubation should be avoided due to the risk of laryngeal bullae formation.

B. A higher risk of difficult airway is present in this patient population.

C. Difficult bag-mask-ventilation due to airway obstruction is more frequent.

D. LMA use is contraindicated.

E. The tracheal tube should be secured by suturing it to the skin.

CHAPTER (42)

Unique Airway Issues in the Pediatric Population

Laura V. Duggan and Narasimhan Jagannathan

42.1 CASE PRESENTATION

A full-term 2-day-old newborn has been persistently vomiting and has been in the neonatal intensive care unit since birth. After delivery, the baby was vigorous, and had APGAR scores of 9/9. The neonatologists order an abdominal x-ray which reveals multiple air-fluid levels indicative of small bowel obstruction. The surgeons are worried about potential intestinal perforation. They want to proceed to the operating room for an exploratory laporotomy as soon as possible. You are on call and immediately attend to the baby for assessment. You notice severe micrognathia, obvious signs of respiratory distress including tachypnea with indrawing of the chest, and a distended tender abdomen. The baby's oxygen saturation on 2 L·min⁻¹ of oxygen via nasal cannula is 93%. What are your concerns and how would you manage this child's airway?

42.2 THE BASICS

42.2.1 Why is a separate chapter on pediatrics important?

The Pediatric Perioperative Cardiac Arrest (POCA) Registry is a subdivision of the ASA Closed Claims Registry specifically dedicated to pediatrics. According to the POCA Registry during the 1970s and 1980s, 50% of all cardiac arrests were due to respiratory causes. Hypoxia quickly led to bradycardia and cardiac arrest.[1]

Thanks to the advent of pulse oximetry and better monitoring, and perhaps better medications and equipment, respiratory causes are now the second most common reason for death and brain damage, although inadequate oxygenation continues to account for approximately 25% of all pediatric cardiac arrests. *Currently, the number one reason for death and brain damage is cardiovascular causes, such as unrecognized hypovolemia.[1]*

Ironically, even though children with ASA Physical Status 3 to 5 are at higher individual risk, two-thirds of children suffering perioperative death or permanent brain damage are ASA Physical Status 1 and 2.

Most pediatric anesthesia practitioners are not pediatric specialists; over 80% of all pediatric anesthesia care in the United States is provided in nonpediatric centers as part of a mixed practice, usually for ASA Physical Status 1 and 2 pediatric patients.

Fortunately, there are more similarities between the pediatric and the adult airway than there are differences. The traditional emphasis on the differences between adults and children is unfortunate and likely impairs the performance of a practitioner that deals mostly or exclusively with adults when faced with an ill child for fear that they will do something wrong. *The biggest differences are found in the child under 2 years of age.* For this reason, this age group will be emphasized. The purpose of this chapter is to provide essential information and recommendations regarding pediatric airway management that is evidence based and practical in such settings.

4.2.2 What is unique about pediatric airway management?

Variability in equipment sizes, drug dosages, and the propensity of children to be both uncooperative and quickly desaturate make even the most-experienced practitioner wary. A crisis situation is also no time to be calculating drug doses or discovering inadequate or inappropriate equipment. Calculating medication doses and equipment sizes is not algorithmic, does not translate into a reflexive skill, and will invariably increase cognitive load. Errors happen: the POCA database estimates 18% of children received wrong drug doses that contributed to their morbidity and mortality.[2]

Immediate access to such information in any clinical scenario including planned and unplanned difficult airway situations will allow the practitioner the mental space to focus on critical decision-making. The authors enthusiastically support the use of pre-calculated systems for both drug dosages and equipment sizes. This can be done in a number of ways, such as based on the actual weight, or the length of the child, using a system such as the Broselow-Luten® tape[3,4] (Armstrong Medical, Lincolnshire, IL, USA). Other settings have taken the approach of including drug doses in the front of every child's chart. However, this assumes both the creation and presence of a chart.

In other words, having a system that provides information on drug dosages and equipment sizes during a resuscitation situation decreases cognitive load,[5] allowing the practitioner to focus on what is essential clinical decision-making.

42.2.3 What is the incidence of difficult laryngoscopic intubation in children?

The Children's Hospital of Philadelphia reported a difficult laryngoscopic intubation rate of 0.25% (16/6524 patients) over a 5-month period.[6] Notably, the majority or 14 of the 16 were anticipated. The rate of unanticipated difficult intubation rate is therefore 0.03%, with no patients being unable to be oxygenated with bag-mask-ventilation (BVM). A laryngeal mask airway (LMA) was inserted in 44% of patients as a bridge to intubation. The most common physical signs in this group were narrow inter-incisor distance (93.8%) and mandibular hypoplasia (87.5%). Akpek reported a difficult intubation rate of 1.25% or 16 of 1278 pediatric cardiac patients, again in a pediatric center.[7] Half of the difficult intubation patients were syndromic and the other half had an extreme anterior airway and micrognathia. For comparison, the incidence of unanticipated difficult intubation in adults is approximately 5.8%.[8]

Unanticipated difficult intubation in children is less common than in adults, but can occur. Fortunately, most difficult airway situations in children are syndromic, rarely unanticipated, and allow for planning prior to induction. A few examples of both congenital and acquired syndromes that can lead to difficult laryngoscopy or intubation in children are listed in Table 42-1.

42.2.4 How common is the "cannot intubate cannot ventilate" scenario in children?

While the exact incidence in unknown, this is a rare event. Children with a potentially difficult tracheal intubation are often easy to mask ventilate, and difficulty in intubation is usually anticipated. There are always exceptions to this generalization. A child with a difficult airway is often detected prenatally and has an associated craniofacial syndrome[9] (Pierre-Robin, Goldenhaar, Treacher Collins, Cystic Hygroma, also see Figures 42-1 and 42-2 and Table 42-1). At birth, if the newborn is unable to maintain their airway, a tracheotomy is placed or ex-utero intrapartum

---

> ### TABLE 42-1

Examples of Commonly Encountered Pediatric Syndromes with Airway Implications and Possible Management Techniques

Pierre-Robin Syndrome

1:8000 newborns, variable micrognathia and cleft palate; improves with age

- Prone positioning, LMA, elective prone intubation, intubation through an LMA (Figure 42-1)

Mucopolysaccharidoses

A group of glycosaminoglycan storage diseases; can get worse with age

- Elective tracheotomy, nasal intubation, surgical backup

Down Syndrome

Possible cervical spine instability, large tongue, gastroesophageal reflux, and pharyngeal hypotonia

- Straight blade, Eschmann Introducer, video device, LMA-assisted flexible bronchoscopic intubation

Cystic Hygroma

Large tumor of the lymph system of the neck causing pressure on the upper airway and generalized swelling. The tongue protrudes in an attempt to keep the airway open (Figure 42-2)

- Awake nasal intubation

Juvenile Rheumatoid Arthritis

Temporomandibular ankylosis, atlanto-axial and low cervical-spine instability, mandibular hypoplasia, and possible vocal cord fixation

- Awake bronchoscopic intubation; consider nasal intubation

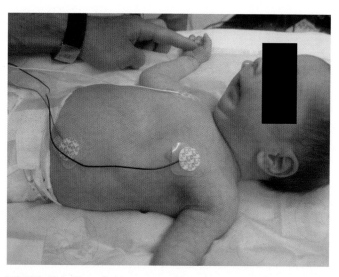

FIGURE 42-1. Pierre-Robin neonate. Note the micrognathia and resultant sternal retraction.

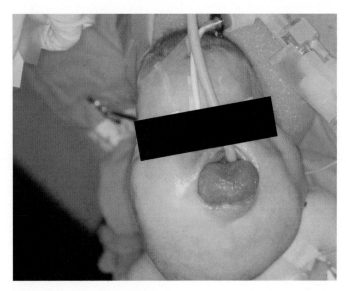

FIGURE 42-2. Congenital cystic hygroma.

treatment (EXIT) procedure is performed by an otorhinolaryngologist.[10] If obstruction is mild to moderate, they may undergo procedures to advance their mandible or improve mouth opening during the first few days of life. This is the population that may be at higher risk for CICV scenario.

42.2.5   Is there an airway algorithm that specifically addresses pediatric patients?

No. The principles of difficult and failed airway management are no different in children than they are in adults: oxygenation not intubation saves lives. Although the ASA Difficult Airway Algorithm was designed for use in adults, the general principle is applicable to the pediatric population.[11]

42.3   ANATOMICAL AND PHYSIOLOGIC DIFFERENCES

42.3.1   What are the main anatomic differences in the pediatric airway?

The pediatric upper airway consists of the nose and mouth leading to the nasopharynx and oropharynx, respectively. These structures are contiguous. The ala of the nose leads to two separate nasal compartments separated by the nasal septum. The lateral wall of each nasal compartment has three scroll-like conchae or turbinate bones. The major air passage lies below the inferior turbinate and is the preferred route for nasal intubation.

The posterior nasal aperture leading to the nasopharynx is called the "choanae." Choanal atresia occurs in approximately 1:7000 births but only approximately 50% of these babies will have respiratory distress. Although it was once thought infants are obligatory nose breathers, it is now thought infants are more accurately described as "preferential nasal breathers."[12] If infants have

respiratory distress, they will usually cry, raise their soft palate, and instantly become mouth breathers. This is borne out by the observation that when infants get a stuffy nose, they do not suffer hypoxic brain damage but are more likely to appear uncomfortable because of the energy required to contract their soft tissues in order to mouth breath.[13]

From infancy until approximately 2 years of age, the tongue is relatively large surrounded by a small jaw. There is simply not enough space to sweep the tongue to the left of the oral cavity as occurs with direct laryngoscopy employing a curved Macintosh blade in an adult. For this reason, and a few others that will follow, *a straight or Miller blade is generally preferred in this age group.*

42.3.2   What is the narrowest portion of the infant's airway?

Traditionally, the airway of a child under 2 years has been described as "cone shaped" with the narrowest part being at the level of the cricoid cartilage, the only complete cartilaginous ring of the respiratory tract. Recent studies however question whether this is actually true. Cadaveric studies originally described the narrowest part of the pediatric airway being the cricoid ring, but this may be inaccurate. *Recent studies using bronchoscopy*[14] *and MRI imaging*[15] *show the narrowest part of the pediatric airway to be at the level of the vocal cords, the same as an adult.* These studies were performed on children under general anesthesia without NMB and therefore preserved muscle tone. Studies in paralyzed children are still required. This may help to explain why cuffed endotracheal tubes in children even in infancy are very well tolerated without an increase in complication rates both in the intensive care[16] and operative settings.[17]

42.3.3   Why do children desaturate so quickly?

As with the anatomy of the airway, the major physiologic differences between adults and children occur in the first 2 years of life.

Young children consume oxygen at two to three times the adult rate (6 mL·kg⁻¹·min⁻¹ vs 2 mL·kg⁻¹·min⁻¹), and have a smaller FRC under general anesthetic relative to adults (10-15 mL·kg⁻¹ vs 30 mL·kg⁻¹, respectively). The result is that young children consume their oxygen reserve and desaturate much more quickly than adults.

Although children have a tidal volume that is similar to adults (7 mL·kg⁻¹), their dead space to tidal volume ratio is larger, leading to proportionately less alveolar ventilation per breath. But, in children, an increase in demand in ventilation is primarily achieved by increasing the respiratory rate rather than the depth of each breath. Taken together, this means that respiratory distress in an infant may be subtle and heralded by tachypnea. In turn, because infants and small children have more type 2 respiratory muscle fibers, they are prone to fatigue. By 2 years of age, children have developed a rich supply of type 1 respiratory muscle fibers, which do not fatigue as easily.

Additionally, because the rib cage of young children is highly compliant due to its cartilaginous nature, increased work of breathing does not necessarily translate into better alveolar ventilation as the chest wall collapses or indraws, as seen in the case presented. The diaphragm is also very compliant leading to a cephalad shift in the face of abdominal distension, such as with a bowel obstruction and distension (as in this case) or gastric distension due to overzealous noninvasive bag-mask-ventilation. This limits reserve and achievable tidal volume while increasing the work of breathing. The ideal maneuver is to decrease the amount of gut distension by decompression with a nasogastric tube if possible.

42.3.4   I know I have to worry about hypoxia, but do I have to worry about respiratory acidosis as well?

Unlike metabolic acidosis, respiratory acidosis is exceptionally well tolerated in children. Goldstein reported a case series of five young children aged 1 day to 6 months in an intensive care setting who underwent permissive hypercapnia for a period of 35 minutes to 2 days.[18] Arterial carbon dioxide values ranged between 155 and 269 mm Hg with accompanying pH values of 6.76 to 7.10. The only acute change was generalized slowing of their EEG tracing. All five infants made a complete neurologic recovery. Although only a small study, it does beg the question whether carbon dioxide values in an acute difficult airway situation really matter.

Perhaps it is time, as some have suggested,[19] to change our description in difficult airway literature from "cannot intubate cannot ventilate" to the more accurate "cannot intubate cannot oxygenate."

42.4   HOW DO I ASSESS FOR A DIFFICULT AIRWAY IN PEDIATRICS?

The mnemonics presented earlier (Chapter 1) with respect to the evaluation of the adult airway for difficulties are: MOANS for difficult bag-mask-ventilation (BMV); RODS for difficult use of extraglottic device (EGD); LEMON for difficult direct laryngoscopy and intubation; and SHORT for a difficult surgical airway.

These mnemonics do not translate directly to small children. The classification system suggested by Hall[20] (discussed later) provides a framework that prepares the practitioner with limited pediatric airway management experience to anticipate airway management difficulty and formulate Plans B and C accordingly.

42.4.1   Does a classification system for the anticipated difficult airway in pediatrics exist?

Hall[18] described four types of a pediatric difficult airway:

1. Congenital abnormality resulting in chronic upper airway obstruction (eg, Pierre-Robin [also known as Robin sequence], see Chapter 46).
2. Congenital or acquired abnormalities resulting in difficult direct laryngoscopy (eg, retrolingual tonsil or tonsillar tissue in the vallecula).

3. Infectious, tending to be progressive (rapidly or slowly depending on the type and degree of infection). All fascial layers in the neck are contiguous meaning that infections can spread to adjacent facial planes.
4. Foreign body, which can suddenly lead to a complete obstruction.

Although this is helpful when thinking of the types of various difficult airways, the classification per se does not immediately lead to an airway plan. Additionally, some children may have overlap categories (eg, a child with Down syndrome with a postoperative tonsillar bleed). Furthermore, difficult direct laryngoscopy in Group 2 does not necessarily mean difficult airway. Given the explosion of available alternatives to direct laryngoscopy, such as video laryngoscopy or flexible bronchoscopic intubation through an extraglottic device, intubation may be relatively straightforward using alternative devices or a combination of devices.

42.4.2   Does this classification help me manage the anticipated difficult airway?

The first question when managing a difficult airway is whether a child should be awake or asleep. If the child will be put to sleep, the second question is whether the child be paralyzed. As a general rule, if a child is dependent on his/her own intrinsic muscle tone to keep an airway open, *don't paralyze*. For example in infectious[21] or foreign body scenarios,[22] the practitioner should seriously consider maintaining spontaneous ventilation.

In a 2005 survey of Canadian pediatric anesthesiologists, the majority favored spontaneous ventilation for all difficult airway scenarios except when the airway was shared with a surgeon. Most preferred an inhalational technique while maintaining spontaneous ventilation.[23]

42.4.3   How do I plan for a difficult airway in children? How does my planning change depending on whether it is an anticipated or unanticipated difficult airway?

Children need exactly what their adult counterparts do: effective oxygenation. A paradigm shift, where oxygenation, not intubation is the gold standard in airway management prevents task fixation (ie, repeated attempts at intubation in the setting of poor oxygenation). Research performed in an urban Emergency Medical System has shown that there is no difference in survival or neurologic outcome between bag-mask-ventilation and endotracheal intubation by paramedics in the field.[24]

Planning for the anticipated difficult airway includes communication with all members of the health-care team including parents and the child if appropriate. The airway plan must be clearly documented and followed. In particular, the parents and child (if appropriate for that child) should know what the bottom-line plan is, particularly if a surgical airway is a possibility (Table 42-2).

TABLE 42-2

Management of Anticipated versus Unanticipated Pediatric Difficult Airway

Anticipated
- Parents aware
- Child aware if appropriate age
- Surgeon in room scrubbed and ready with all equipment checked and assembled
- All health-care providers aware
- Maintenance and extubation plan in place
- Plan well documented and discussed

Unanticipated
- Can I BMV this patient?
- If not, call for help, two-handed BMV technique
- Consider atropine now
- Consider succinylcholine if appropriate
- Insert an extraglottic device while preparing for surgical airway

42.5   AIRWAY DEVICES AND EQUIPMENT

42.5.1   What size endotracheal tube should I use in a child?

Tube sizes are measured in millimeter of internal diameter (ID) with the external diameter (OD) dependent on the material used and the manufacturer. The smallest uncuffed tube is 2.0 mm ID. The smallest cuffed tube is 3.0 mm ID. Sizes increase by 0.5 mm increments and the OD can vary greatly for the same ID.[25] Because of the large tracheal diameter of the adult airway (20-25 mm), this factor may not be of significance. However, in children with much smaller tracheal diameters depending on age,[26] the size of the ETT wall may be a significant consideration. Pediatric ETTs also vary with respect to their beveled end and the presence of a Murphy eye. Some ETTs have a flexible *beaked* tip that may help in advancing the ETT over a flexible bronchoscope (eg, Parker ETT, [see Section 9.3.3]), although it has also been shown that this beak potentially obstruct the distal opening of the ETT.

The location and material of the cuff on cuffed ETTs will also vary with the manufacturer. Most cuffs are made of polyvinylchloride (PVC) but can also be made of thinner polyurethane. Polyurethane, such as the one seen in the pediatric Microcuff (Kimberly-Clark, Atlanta, USA), has a lower sealing pressure than PVC.[27] An excellent review regarding the various types of pediatric tubes has recently been published by Leong and Black.[25]

The exact size of tube that ought to be selected for a particular patient can be estimated by several means. Perhaps the best method is to use the length of the patient, such as used in the Broselow-Luten® tape. Patient age is also commonly used. The Cole formula[28] originally published in 1957 based on age has been modified to:

$$Age/4 \text{ plus } 4$$

The modified Cole formula was designed to be used for uncuffed tubes. If anything, it underestimates uncuffed tube size. It is recommended that the formula be modified for cuffed tubes to:

$$(Age/4 \text{ plus } 4) \text{ minus } 0.5$$

Neither the size of the smallest finger of a child nor the size of the external nares estimates ETT size accurately.

In any case, the cautious practitioner has the size predicted (determined by whatever means) and both a half size larger and smaller immediately available.

42.5.2   Can I use cuffed ETTs in children? Is this a safe practice?

Cadaveric studies originally described the narrowest part of the pediatric airway being the cricoid ring. This led to a tradition of using uncuffed tubes in children because the cricoid ring was thought to provide a snug seal for the tube without the need for a cuff. Practitioners also preferred uncuffed tubes because older pediatric cuffed ETTs possessed high-pressure low-volume cuffs that were associated with ischemic airway mucosal damage and subsequent subglottic stenosis.

Recently, a prospective randomized controlled multicenter trial[17] studied the use of uncuffed tubes from various manufacturers and compared them to Microcuff tubes (Kimberly-Clark, Atlanta, USA) in children under 5 years of age. This study randomized over 2000 children and found the incidence of postoperative croup to be similar. The authors of the study, however, emphasized that cuff pressures need to be monitored. The average cuff pressure was 10.6 cm H_2O, well under the threshold pressure of 25 cm H_2O that has been shown in past studies using uncuffed tubes to increase morbidity.[29] It should also be noted that the conclusions drawn from this study might not be valid for cuffed ETTs from other manufacturers with thicker cuff walls and perhaps higher cuff pressures needed to achieve a similar seal.

A most significant finding of this large study was that uncuffed tubes needed to be switched to an alternative size in 30% of patients. Cuffed tubes were switched out for another tube size only 2% of the time. Estimation of appropriate sizing for all ETTs was done as per each center's guidelines.

Preventing the need to switch ETT sizes in a difficult airway situation obviously offers tremendous benefit; emphasizing the recommendation that cuffed tubes be considered in this setting. This is a pivotal study and, with the accompanying editorial stating "Thus, the 'uncuffed camp' will now have to prove, based on prospectively gathered data, that the use of adequately designed cuffed tracheal tubes is in fact harmful to the pediatric airway."[30]

There is no question that damage to the airway can occur with both cuffed and uncuffed tubes.[31,32] The practitioner needs to reflect on the specifics of the ETTs they use (eg, different manufacturers have the cuffs in different positions, and some can herniate onto the vocal cords), as well as the sizing. Finally, it has been shown that movement of the child increases the incidence of airway damage.

42.5.3 What are the new devices available in pediatric sizes for the management of the difficult airway?

Over the past 5 years, a number of new devices have been made available in pediatric sizes for routine, difficult, and failed airway management. These devices can be divided into two groups: optical devices that are similar to the traditional laryngoscope and the optical stylets. The video/optical laryngoscopes include the GlideScope® (Verathon, Bothwell, Washington), the STORZ Video Laryngoscope™ (Karl Storz Endoscopy, Tuttlingen, Germany), and the Truview EVO2™ (Truphatek, Netanya, Israel). These devices combine and incorporate video technology into the tip of the laryngoscope blade. This allows images from beyond the tip of the blade to be displayed on video monitors, permitting one to place the ETT into the trachea. The GlideScope® incorporates a 60-degree angulated distal tip. (See Section 10.4.4 and Figures 10-18A and 10-18B). The Truview EVO2™ is a rigid laryngoscope with an angulated tip that uses a series of prisms to transmit the image from the distal tip to an eyepiece. The tip is angulated 46 degrees anteriorly from the direct line of sight, and the device provides a wide-angle magnified view. A new version of this device called the Truview PCD has a video camera and screen that is mounted to a proximal eyepiece converting it to a video laryngoscope (see Section 10.3.2.6 and Figure 10-13).

The Airtraq™ (Prodol Meditec SA, Vizcaya, Spain) is a novel device that combines a video image with a tube delivery capability. The image provided to the practitioner is a magnified wide-angle view transmitted via a series of mirrors similar to that of a submarine periscope. Once the glottis is viewed, an ETT that has been preloaded into the ETT delivery channel is advanced into the trachea. This is a single-use device with antifogging capability at the distal tip of the blade. There is no need for an external monitor. (See Section 10.4.2.2 and Figure 10-16.)

The optical stylets combine the optics of a flexible bronchoscope with the features of a lightwand. Those available for pediatric use include the Shikani Optical Stylet (Clarus Medical, Minneapolis, Minnesota), a malleable stainless steel sheath housing a fiberoptic bundle connected to a distal light source with a fixed eyepiece (see Section 10.2.3.2 and Figure 10-2); and the Bonfils (Karl Storz Endoscopy, Tuttlingen, Germany), a rigid optical stylet with a swiveling eyepiece (see Section 10.2.3.1 and Figure 10-1).

All of the above devices have been used to manage the pediatric difficult airway in case series and case reports.[33-43] Larger pediatric studies regarding these devices are ongoing. Many of the prospective studies involving the GlideScope[36,44,45] and video laryngoscope[46,47] compared to direct laryngoscopy show that both these devices provide an improved view of the glottis in children with normal airway anatomy, but require a longer time for intubation. This longer time is probably not significant in clinical practice, and the benefit offered by an improved view probably outweighs the minimal increase in time for tracheal intubation.

42.5.4 Is there a difference between a pediatric flexible bronchoscope compared to the adult bronchoscope?

With the exception of bronchoscope diameter, the answer is "NO". There is no material difference between a flexible pediatric bronchoscope and an adult bronchoscope. Generally, a bronchoscope (50-60 cm in length) that is less than 4.0 mm in tip diameter is called a pediatric bronchoscope. Those larger than 4.0 mm in tip diameter tend to be called adult bronchoscopes.

The flexible bronchoscope remains the cornerstone of pediatric difficult airway management. Fiberoptic image transmission is being replaced by CMOS camera technology providing exceptionally high-quality images. These high-definition scopes with a working channel are limited in size, the smallest being approximately 2.8 mm in tip diameter. Ultrathin bronchoscopes without a suction channel have a tip diameter of 2.2 to 2.5 mm and are generally used as nasoendoscopes used by our ENT colleagues. Bronchoscopes with a suction channel have an outer diameter of at least 2.8 mm. The smallest flexible bronchoscope with a suction channel (2.8 mm) has poorer optical quality than the 2.5 mm scope without the suction channel because the channel takes up considerable space at the expense of light and optical fibers.

42.5.5 What extraglottic devices are used in children?

Extraglottic devices (EGDs) that are available for use in the pediatric population (below age 2 and <30 kg) include the following (see Chapter 12):

- The LMA family of devices including the LMA-Classic™, the LMA-Proseal™, and the LMA-Unique™ (LMA North America, San Diego, CA, USA)
- The Air-Q Intubating Laryngeal Airway™ (Air-Q ILA) (Cookgas LLC, St. Louis, Mo, USA)
- The Cobra Perilaryngeal Airway™ (CobraPLA) (Engineered Medical Systems, Indianapolis, Indiana)
- The King LT™ family of devices (King Systems, Noblesville, Indiana), also known as the Laryngeal Tube in Europe

The Combitube™ and the Easy Tube™ are available in small adult sizes making them potentially useful for children older than 10 to 12 years as rescue devices.

42.5.6 What rescue devices are available for pediatric patients? Is there an intubating extraglottic device for pediatric patients?

The above-named EGDs constitute the mainstay of nonsurgical rescue airway devices for infants and children less than 10 years of age. The most commonly used EGD used in children is the LMA-Classic™. The LMA-Proseal™ provides a better laryngeal seal pressure than the LMA-Classic™,[48,49] and incorporates an esophageal

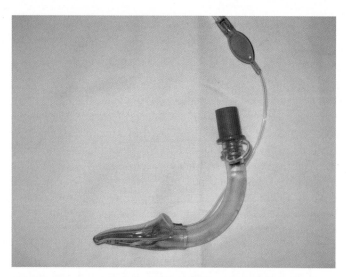

FIGURE 42-3. Size 1.5 Air-Q ILA. A total of four pediatric sizes available: 1, 1.5, 2, 2.5. Note the shorter, wider, curved airway tube which is similar in design to the adult ILMA. This allows for placement of a cuffed ETT with the ability to easily remove the Air-Q ILA after successful tracheal intubation.

drain tube and a bite block. This device has been used with greater success when positive pressure ventilation is desired.[50] Other devices used include the CobraPLA™, the King LT™/Laryngeal Tube.

There is no LMA-Fastrach™ (Intubating LMA) for pediatric patients. The smallest of these devices is a size 3 which has been used successfully in children greater than 12. For smaller children and infants, the family of Air-Q® ILA devices has shown promise and (Figure 42-3) may overcome some of the limitations that have been associated with LMA-Classic™-guided intubation.[51]

A summary of the devices available along with the clinical advantages and limitations for the management of the difficult pediatric airway is shown in Table 42-3.

42.6   AIRWAY MANAGEMENT ISSUES IN CHILDREN

42.6.1   Can rapid-sequence intubation be employed in children? If so, how is it done and is it safe?

When emergency intubation is indicated, RSI is the technique of choice in children, as it is in adults.[52] Although there are no randomized prospective studies, large series from multiple centers support the use of RSI in children and document its safety and apparent superiority to other methods.[52,53] The sequence of events and drug selection for RSI are no different in children than it is in adults.

42.6.2   Is cricoid pressure useful in children?

Sellick originally described the maneuver applying external pressure to the cricoid ring in order to occlude the esophagus to prevent passive regurgitation of stomach contents during rapid-sequence intubation.[54] Its success rate in preventing aspiration in adults and children has not been proven. In 2001, a survey of British pediatric anesthetists showed perceived benefit of the Sellick maneuver to be quite variable; only 49% would use cricoid pressure in an emergency case even with known risk factors (hiatus hernia, known reflux etc).[55] Cricoid pressure was used more often by general anesthetists during an emergency case, 60% in infants and 96% in school-age children.[56] Obviously, the question as to the efficacy of cricoid pressure remains unresolved.[57]

What has been shown in children, however, is that the Sellick maneuver is very effective in decreasing gastric insufflation during BMV even with ventilation pressures exceeding 40 cm H_2O.[55,58] This is especially important in infants, in whom gastric distention may lead to decreased diaphragmatic excursion, decreased ability to ventilate, and increase the risk of aspiration. For this reason, it may be reasonable to apply cricoid pressure during prolonged BMV ventilation, recognizing that it may hinder the view of the larynx on direct laryngoscopy.[59]

42.6.3   What neuromuscular blocking agents should be used in children?

The ideal neuromuscular blocking agents (NMBA) varies depending on the clinical situation. Speed of onset, duration of action, and side-effect profile need to be weighed in order to chose the appropriate drug.

In elective cases, with adequate denitrogenation and when the onset of action does not need to be less than 60 seconds, a drug with the fewest side effects can be chosen, for example, rocuronium in standard doses (0.3-0.6 mg·kg⁻¹) depending on how fast the practitioner wishes for onset time.

In emergency cases, the ideal drug is one that has a very rapid onset of effect. A short duration of action may also be of benefit in the event one needs to revert to spontaneous ventilation. Succinylcholine is the only depolarizing NMBA agent on the market today. It has been on the market for over 50 years. Succinylcholine (1.5 mg·kg⁻¹) compared to rocuronium (0.9 mg·kg⁻¹) in healthy children showed that both drugs produced good intubating conditions in less than 60 seconds.[60] Sixty seconds of apnea after effective denitrogenation for 2 minutes may be very well tolerated in children of various ages, including infants undergoing elective intubation,[61] but this may not be the case in an emergency where denitrogenation is suboptimal.[62]

Whether high-dose rocuronium (1.2 mg·kg⁻¹) has a similar onset as succinylcholine (1.5-2 mg·kg⁻¹) in children remains unclear. A 2007 Cochrane review of the literature evaluating rocuronium versus succinylcholine in rapid-sequence intubation, primarily in adult studies, found that succinylcholine (1.5-2 mg·kg⁻¹ on average) created superior intubation conditions versus rocuronium at any dose less than 1.2 mg·kg⁻¹. It was concluded that succinylcholine was clinically superior as it has a shorter duration of action.[63] Perhaps with the introduction of sugammadex as a reversal agent for rocuronium, succinylcholine may not play as pivotal a role in emergency situations. However, at present succinylcholine will continue to play a central role in pediatric emergency airway management.

TABLE 42-3

Devices Available Along with Clinical Advantages and Limitations for the Management of the Difficult Pediatric Airway

DEVICE	ADVANTAGES	LIMITATIONS
GlideScope	• Wide magnified view • Portable • Antifog camera	• May be difficult to overcome the curve of the blade when placing endotracheal tube • May have a suboptimal view in the bleeding airway • Requires moderate degree of mouth opening
Video laryngoscope	• Similar in use to direct laryngoscopy • Panoramic view of laryngeal structures	• May have a suboptimal view in the bleeding airway • Requires some degree of mouth opening
Airtraq	• Portable/disposable • Wide magnified view of laryngeal structures • Antifog camera	• May have a suboptimal view in the bleeding airway • Requires some degree of mouth opening
Flexible bronchoscope	• Use in limited mouth opening: nasal or oral • Can use in conjunction with extraglottic devices	• Learning curve • Expensive to clean • Less portable • May have a suboptimal view in the bleeding airway
Shikani optical stylet bonfils	• Use in limited mouth opening • Shikani is somewhat malleable; can use with an extraglottic device and tailor to patient's anatomy	• May have a suboptimal view in the bleeding airway • Short optical depth of field • No antifog capability
LMA-Classic™	• Long history of reliability • Portable • Airway rescue • Conduit for tracheal intubation	• May require use of another visualization device, for example, flexible bronchoscope • Requires some degree of mouth opening • Cannot drain the stomach
LMA-Proseal™	• Same as above • Able to place a drain tube • Can ventilate at higher seal pressures	• May be more difficult to insert than the LMA-Classic™ • Endotracheal intubation through this device more difficult than the LMA-Classic™ or Air-Q ILA • Requires some degree of mouth opening
Air-Q ILA	• Portable • Airway rescue • Conduit for tracheal intubation • Designed for tracheal intubation	• May require use of another visualization device, for example, flexible bronchoscope • Requires some degree of mouth opening • Cannot drain the stomach

42.6.4 Can I use succinylcholine (suxamethonium) in children?

Arguably, the drug that has received the most attention in the pediatric anesthesia literature is succinylcholine. In order to understand the indications and concerns about its use, it is important to understand its history.

In December 1993, one of the manufacturers of the drug identified 36 deaths in young children and adolescents secondary to cardiac arrhythmias/arrest being reported with the use of the drug, and recommended that the drug should not be used in children. The cardiac arrests and arrhythmias carried a mortality rate that exceeded 50% and were thought to be due to undiagnosed muscular dystrophies, the most common being undiagnosed Duchenne muscular dystrophy in boys below the age of 8.[64]

The FDA in the United States initially recommended that a warning be added to the label cautioning the practitioner to be aware that rare hyperkalemic arrest can occur, especially in boys under the age of 8 years. The FDA went on to meet with representatives of the pharmaceutical industry and this warning was then upgraded to a *relative contraindication* in children under the age of 16 years. The response from the pediatric anesthesia community in the United States was swift and bold: Succinylcholine was too important a drug in emergency situations to be taken away altogether. The argument was made that more deaths would occur by *not* giving succinylcholine in situations where securing an airway was a life-saving maneuver than would ever be prevented in rare cases of undiagnosed muscular dystrophies. The FDA reversed its decision and downgraded their recommendation to a *warning* in 1994.[65]

In a recent pro-con debate regarding the use of succinylcholine in pediatrics, both debaters agreed that when neuromuscular blockade (NMB) is indicated, *succinylcholine should be reserved for those emergency situations where the airway needs to be secured in the fastest means possible*. The debaters also agreed that succinylcholine should not be used in elective pediatric patients.[66]

42.6.5 Should NMB ever be used in pediatrics when a difficult airway is predicted?

It depends on why the airway is predicted to be difficult. If the patency of the airway is reliant on the patient's muscle tone, NMB is contraindicated. However, if the child's muscle tone is the problem, such as in the case of laryngospasm, NMB can be quite helpful. In the POCA Registry, laryngospasm is the most common reason for airway obstruction.[1]

NMB may decrease the risk of difficult tracheal intubation.[67] In those clinical situations where the airway needs to be secured quickly, such as in the case of pyloric stenosis or postoperative tonsillar bleed, NMB may help decrease the time required to intubate the trachea by improving the laryngeal view. Obviously, the practitioner in these cases will want to use the NMBA with the most rapid onset.

42.7 AIRWAY MANAGEMENT AT VARIOUS AGES

With regards to airway development, children can be thought of in three general age groups:

1. Young (0-2 years)
2. Middle aged (2-8 years)
3. Older (8-16 years)

The major difference in airway anatomy, and therefore equipment, is in the child under 2 years of age.

42.7.1 How do I manage the airway of a small child?

The most notable differences between the pediatric and adult airway occurs in the birth to age 2 groups. The young pediatric airway is set up for one task: breastfeeding. The nose is small and upturned to allow breathing intermittently during feeding. The tongue is large to allow for less effort during latching, and the epiglottis is relatively large and redundant in order to protect the glottic opening from liquids.

During BMV in the child less than 2, the practitioner must recognize that the occiput is much larger than in the adult, causing

the cervical spine to flex when a child is placed supine. Flexion of the cervical spine can lead to significant partial airway obstruction. A shoulder roll is very useful allowing the cervical spine to stay in neutral position[68] aiding BMV, as it does for *all* other airway interventions, such as placement of an extraglottic device, intubation, and very rarely, a surgical airway (Figure 42-4).

The most important feature of BMV in this age group is gentleness. Mask seal is usually not an issue, but attempting a forceful jaw thrust may compress the submandibular soft tissues and easily obstruct the airway. The solution is not to be more forceful, but to reposition, reapply the mask on the face from the bridge of the nose to the mentum of the chin while adding a slight chin lift.

42.7.2 How do I intubate the trachea of a child less than 2 years old using direct laryngoscopy?

The larynx is in a more cephalad position being at the level of the third cervical vertebrae instead of the fifth cervical vertebrae in the adult. Lying over the laryngeal inlet is a large floppy omega-shaped epiglottis. During direct laryngoscopy it is much easier to lift the epiglottis along with the tongue with a straight or Miller blade than it is to have the tongue follow the blade when compressing the hyoepiglottic ligament in the vallecula with a curved or Macintosh blade. Usually, the posterior third of the tongue will obscure the view of the glottis with a curved blade in the vallecula. Although many authors describe the larynx as anterior in the young child, it is actually cephalad, tucked up under the tongue at the angle of the mandible.

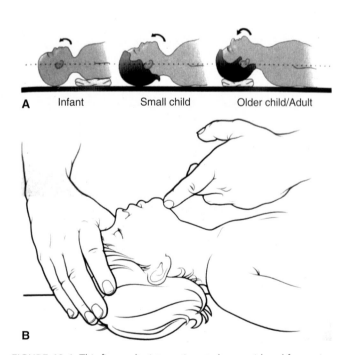

| A | Infant | Small child | Older child/Adult |

FIGURE 42-4. This figure depicts options to be considered for positioning children of various age groups for BMV and tracheal intubation. (Reproduced with permission from Luten R, Godwin S. Pediatric airway techniques. In: Walls RM, Murphy MF, Luten R, Schneider R, eds. *Manual of Emergency Airway Management*. Philadelphia, PA: Lippincott, Williams & Wilkins; 2004:228-235, Figure 20-1.)

Given the acute angle between the oropharynx and the laryngeal inlet, styletted tubes are very helpful in this age group. Infant endotracheal intubating (EI) stylets are also manufactured (eg, Cook Medical, Bloomington, IN, USA) and, as in adults, can be useful for Grade 3 laryngeal views.

42.7.3 Why are micrognathic infants difficult to intubate by direct laryngoscopy?

An extreme situation of anterior airway is in the setting of micrognathia, such as Pierre-Robin syndrome (Figure 42-1), also known as Robin sequence. In this setting, the tongue lies against the posterior oropharyngeal wall, causing upper airway obstruction. It is nearly impossible to compress the tongue into the mandibular space, because there is not any space. A straight or Miller-type blade can be used in a paraglossal manner by placing the blade along the buccal mucosa, lifting the epiglottis from the side of the mouth and avoiding the tongue altogether. Since this is not the normal orientation of structures, practice with this technique during elective intubations is encouraged.

42.7.4 Are there other alternatives to direct laryngoscopy in this age group?

Infant and pediatric sizes of the Airtraq, GlideScope, and the Storz Video Laryngoscope are available (approximating a Miller #1 blade in size). A very good alternative to direct laryngoscopy is flexible bronchoscopic intubation through an extraglottic device. The extraglottic device serves as a conduit to direct the bronchoscope to the laryngeal inlet. Further details are provided in Sections 42.5.3 to 42.5.6.

42.7.5 Why use an extraglottic device as a conduit for tracheal intubation in infants?

These devices are usually easy to place, provide the ability to oxygenate and ventilate, have a long history of clinical reliability,[69] and allow for excellent glottic isolation.[70-73] Due to greater oxygen consumption and a decreased oxygen reserve, infants and neonates generally do not tolerate a long period of apnea. These devices are ideal for this patient population, thereby allowing the practitioner to minimize the disconnect time from the breathing circuit while providing a conduit for successful tracheal intubation. Asai has described a technique in which an extraglottic device is placed in the awake state in neonates to help overcome an upper airway obstruction; then it is used as a conduit for flexible bronchoscopic intubation.[74]

42.7.6 Can I intubate the trachea blindly through an extraglottic device in small children?

In adult patients, this is commonly done, especially when using the LMA-Fastrach™. In children, particularly in neonates and infants, the incidence of epiglottic downfolding by an inserted LMA is higher than the adult population. Studies of glottic views through the LMA and CobraPLA using a flexible bronchoscope have shown that the degree to which the glottis is visualized is reduced in smaller children (<10 kg).[75-77] As a result, the use of hybrid techniques, such as a flexible bronchoscope combined with an LMA, is likely to yield a more successful result.

42.7.7 Is blind nasotracheal intubation an option in children?

Two combined anatomic variations conspire against *blind* nasotracheal intubation in children less than 8 to 10 years of age: the presence of nasopharyngeal adenoidal tissue that is frequently enlarged; and the acute angle of the higher riding upper airway in the nasopharynx in the child as opposed to the adult.[78]

Adenoidal tissue is often dissected by and lodges in the lumen of the nasotracheal tube in children. The injury leads to bleeding, hindered visualization, and the inability to use a flexible bronchoscope. The dissected adenoid tissue, if not recognized and removed from the ETT, can be forced into the lung leading to tracheal obstruction.

While blind techniques are fraught with hazard, video-assisted techniques may be more successful and safer and include:

- An indirect visualization technique using a fiberoptic bronchoscope in small infants and children with small mouth openings.[79]
- A nasotracheal tube passed to the oropharynx and placed into the airway with Magill forceps under oral laryngoscopic view using a GlideScope or Storz video laryngoscope.

42.7.8 I am planning on extubating this infant with a difficult airway. Will I be able to extubate over an airway exchange catheter?

The ASA Difficult Airway Algorithm recommends the use of an airway exchange catheter upon tracheal extubation in adult patient with a difficult airway.[11] This should also apply to the pediatric population. Cook Critical Care supplies airway exchange catheters made for ETT greater than 3 mm ID.

42.8 THE SURGICAL AIRWAY IN CHILDREN

42.8.1 How do I perform a surgical airway in a child less than 2 years of age?

The need for an emergency surgical airway in a child of this age is very rare, particularly since the introduction of extraglottic devices. *Cricothyrotomy is not an option in patients under approximately 8 years of age.* Cricothyrotomy is only an option in children over the age of approximately 8 years, when the cricothyroid membrane is large enough to accommodate the smallest available cricothyrotomy device. Table 42-4 and Figure 42-5 show the relative sizes

TABLE 42-4

Relative Sizes of the Cricothyroid Membrane According to Age

AGE	<2 YEARS	2-8 YEARS	ADULT
Cricothyroid membrane	3 mm × 2.5 mm	10 mm × 8-10 mm	25 mm × 20 mm

and anatomic differences between the adult and infant cricothyroid membranes, respectively.

There are two options for a surgical airway in children under 8 years of age: needle tracheotomy and formal tracheotomy. Formal tracheotomy takes over 10 minutes to perform even in the most-skilled pediatric otolaryngologist's hands. Therefore, in a crisis, the alternative is more likely to be a needle tracheotomy.

An alternative to a surgical airway may be rigid laryngoscopy or bronchoscopy, although few nonsurgically trained practitioners have experience with this technique. Rigid techniques usually are immediately available in the operating room setting for anticipated difficult airway scenarios, such as foreign body removal or post-tonsillectomy bleed. This calls for planning with the surgical team and preparation of all necessary equipment.

42.8.2   How often is needle tracheotomy used in children?

An exhaustive literature search revealed only six cases of emergency needle tracheotomy reported since 1950. This is a very rare occurrence. Because emergency pediatric needle tracheotomy is such

a rare event, there is a dearth of literature about the technique and very little equipment development. As a result, many pieces of equipment have been suggested as *possibly* being useful in this situation in the form of letters to the editor in many anesthesia journals without ever being evaluated in humans, animals, or even experimental lung models. Central and hemodialysis lines, nasal prongs, ends of various sizes of ETTs attached to various syringe barrels, just to name a few, have been suggested. Such literature without evidence perpetuates and makes murkier an already confusing area. The use of commercially available, purpose-specific equipment is to be encouraged. Improvisation in the face of a deadly emergency is to be discouraged.

42.8.3   How do I perform a needle tracheotomy (see also Section 13.2)?

1. A specific needle cricothyrotomy device is connected to a 3-mL saline-filled syringe.
2. The cricothyroid membrane is palpated.
3. Air is aspirated via the device into the syringe.
4. The needle from the device is withdrawn.

42.8.4   Can I use an intravenous catheter as a needle cricothyrotomy device?

The use of an intravenous catheter is not recommended due to a much higher rate of kinking at the skin with resultant obstruction.

42.8.5   What commercially manufactured needle cricothyrotomy devices are available for children?

Catheters manufactured for this specific task[80] in a baby (16 gauge) and child (14 gauge) sizes (VBM Laboratories, Germany) can be seen in Figure 42-6. These are Teflon-coated catheters and have

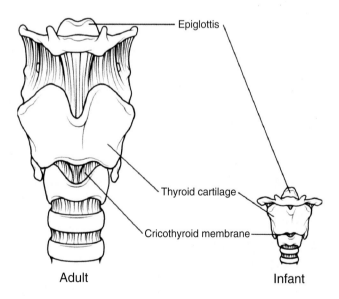

Epiglottis

Thyroid cartilage

Cricothyroid membrane

Adult   Infant

FIGURE 42-5. Adult larynx (left) versus infant larynx (right). Note the difference in size of the cricothyroid membrane. Also see Table 42-4 for dimensions of the cricothyroid membrane in various age groups. (Reproduced with permission from Luten R, Godwin SA. Pediatric airway techniques. In: Walls RM, Murphy MF, Luten R, Schinder R, eds. *Manual of Emergency Airway Management*. Philadelphia, PA: Lippincott, Williams & Wilkins; 2004:228-235, Figure 20-2.)

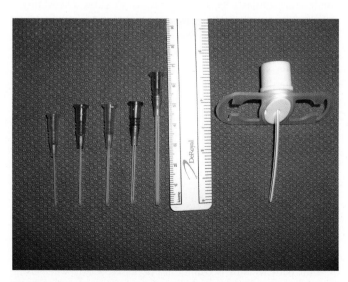

FIGURE 42-6. Ravussin needle tracheostomy catheter.

been used electively in case series for laryngeal surgery, including some in children. Another option is the Arndt Emergency Cricothyrotomy Set (Cook Medical, Bloomington, IN, USA) that can also be placed transtracheally. It has a 3-mm internal diameter, 18-gauge outer diameter, and is long for a small child at 6 cm.

42.8.6 What oxygen source should I be using?

Terminology surrounding the use of oxygen in clinical practice is confusing. Various terms are used depending on whether pressure or flow is being measured.

"Jet ventilation" refers to the use of high-pressure oxygen, usually measured in pound per square inch (psi), in a range of 5 to 50 psi. Hospital oxygen pipeline pressure is 50 psi.

"High-flow" oxygen is completely different. It is a flow rate of 15 to 18 L·min^{-1} under low pressure, usually less than 1 psi. It is delivered through the flow meters available at the bedside in most hospitals and is also known as wall oxygen.

Because the terms are confusing and conversion among pressure units is not easily performed, equivalents between flow and pressure are described below:

- *Pipeline oxygen* has a pressure of 50 psi = 160 L·min^{-1} oxygen flow = 2.7 L·sec^{-1}.
- *Standard wall oxygen* provides 1 psi, or approximately 70 cm H$_2$O.
- *Oxygen flush valve* on the modern anesthesia machines deliver oxygen at 7 to 15 psi, depending on the manufacturer.

42.8.7 If needle tracheotomy is so rare in children, what has been proven to work in children?

To date, there is very little literature available. The best evidence is in the pig animal model. Adequate oxygenation has been demonstrated in the pig model using a low-pressure oxygen supply (ie, wall oxygen at 1-15 L·min^{-1}) attached to an Enk Oxygen Flow Regulator (Cook Medical, [Figure 42-7]). This technique has been

shown to provide effective oxygenation for at least 15 minutes.[81,82] Unfortunately, these experiments were halted at 15 minutes because of experimental protocol. The authors state in their conclusions that since oxygen saturation was sustained at 97%, even in a large 40-kg pig, throughout the experimental time period, there was no reason to think that this could not have continued. To date, there are no pediatric case reports or series in the literature using this device.

42.8.8 Are there any recommendations about how much oxygen flow to attach to my catheter?

Yes, but they are more consensus than evidence based because there is little information in this area. The Pediatric Advanced Life Support (PALS course)[11] recommends 100 mL·kg^{-1}·min^{-1}. The Advanced Pediatric Life Support (APLS) course recommends 1 L·min^{-1}·y^{-1} of age. No recommendation is given, however, regarding the setting of any ventilation parameters such as tidal volume, the I:E ratio, and so on.

42.8.9 Shouldn't I be using transtracheal jet ventilation (high-pressure oxygen) according to the ASA Difficult Airway Algorithm?

Gaughan published tidal volumes using a mechanical lung model with various lung compliances and tracheal diameters.[83] Table 42-5 shows the tidal volumes generated with normal pediatric lung compliance and tracheal size. Normal tidal volume in children is the same as in adults, approximately 7 mL·kg^{-1}. Therefore, *high-pressure jet ventilation is not required in children to generate normal tidal volumes up to 30 to 50 kg.* The average 8-year-old in the United States is 40 kg. *Therefore transtracheal jet ventilation is never required in children because after the age of 8 years, formal cricothyrotomy can be performed.*

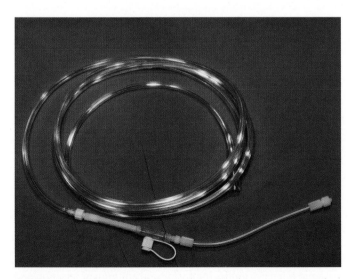

FIGURE 42-7. Enk Oxygen Flow Regulator. Used in conjunction with an emergency transtracheal catheter when conventional ventilation by mask or ETT cannot be performed.

TABLE 42-5

Tidal Volumes Generated in a Mechanical Lung Model with Normal Pediatric Lung Compliance and Tracheal Diameter

PRESSURE	VOLUME[a]
15 L·min^{-1} (<1 psi)	220-350 mL
5 psi	250-400 mL
25 psi	650-900 mL
50 psi	1600-2200 mL

[a]*1 second inspiratory time through a 16-gauge catheter.*
(Adapted from Gaughan SD, Ozaki GT, Benumof JL. A comparison in a lung model of low- and high-flow regulators for transtracheal jet ventilation. Anesthesiology. 1992;77:189-199.)[83]

TABLE 42-6

Summary of Airway Management Options in Older Age Groups

AGE (YEARS)	2-8	8-16
Airway changes	Muscle tone increases, as does the caliber of the aerodigestive tract. The epiglottis becomes firmer and less wide and floppy	Similar configuration to the adult airway
BVM	Sizing of the mask is the same as in adults	Sizing of the mask is the same as in adults
EGD	LMA-Classic™ LMA-Proseal™ Air-Q ILA	Above 30 kg more options available such as ILMA, Combitube, SLIPA
Direct laryngoscopy	The curved or Macintosh blade becomes more useful	Analogous to the adult
Beyond Laryngoscopy	GlideScope Video laryngoscope Airtraq Flexible bronchoscope	All airway devices available, just as in adults
Surgical options	Formal tracheotomy or needle tracheotomy	Formal cricothyrotomy, as in adults

42.8.10   What are the disadvantages of transtracheal jet ventilation?

The ASA Difficult Airway Algorithm was originally published in 1993 when both extraglottic and cricothyrotomy devices in adults were limited. Jet ventilation with high-pressure oxygen was seen as a means of providing adult tidal volumes. It is defined as a noninvasive airway (vs a surgical airway).

Unfortunately, jet ventilation has not been without consequences. The catheter provides a conduit for pushing oxygen into lungs, but does not provide a pathway for expiration. As a result, in the setting of upper airway obstruction, transtracheal or transcricoid membrane jet ventilation can quickly lead to barotrauma and cardiovascular collapse.

In analyzing the ASA Closed Claims database, Peterson[84] found nine adults in whom jet ventilation was attempted from 1985 to 1999. Eight out of nine patients sustained pneumothorax, subcutaneous emphysema, or pneumomediastinum.

The incidence and successful emergency transtracheal ventilation in children is unknown. In an elective case series of 16 infants and children undergoing 28 upper airway endoscopic procedures using transtracheal jet ventilation at a pressure of 4.3 psi, $FiO_2 = 0.30$, I:E =1:3 and rate of 100 per minute, Depierraz found a complication rate of 10.7%.[85] These three cases included cardiovascular collapse, bilateral pneumothorax, and extensive subcutaneous emphysema.

42.8.11   What other measures should I be taking during transtracheal ventilation?

Although the transtracheal catheter provides a means to allow oxygen into the lungs, it is too small to allow for adequate expiration.

Therefore, continued attempts at opening the upper airway by jaw thrust, EGD, or tracheal intubation are essential. Transtracheal ventilation may aid in attempts to intubate a patient. Chandradeva reported two cases of severe upper airway swelling in which intubation was successful after the institution of transtracheal ventilation because the high intrathoracic pressure caused the glottis to open.[86] This is the equivalent of asking an assistant to press on the chest during laryngoscopy in order to identify escape of air through the glottis when the larynx is unidentifiable.

48.8.12   What about airway management in children above age 2?

As stated earlier, once the child has reached the age of 2, airway management with the exception of size, is less different than it is before the age of 2. Table 42-6 summarizes airway management issues in older age groups.

42.9   SUMMARY

Pediatric airway management engenders fear in most who do not manage children on a daily basis, particularly when the difficult or failed airway is encountered. This fear is compounded by the need to rapidly adjust drug dosages for size and weight, the limited availability of age- and size-specific equipment and the mystery surrounding surgical airway management in the young child. This chapter is meant to assist such practitioners in accessing rapid reference guides for dosing and equipment selection and demystifying the management of the difficult and failed pediatric airway.

REFERENCES

1. Jimenez N, Posner KL, Cheney FW, Caplan RA, Lee LA, Domino KB. An update on pediatric anesthesia liability: a closed claims analysis. *Anesth Analg.* 2007;104:147-153.

2. Bhananker SM, Ramamoorthy C, Geiduschek JM, et al. Anesthesia-related cardiac arrest in children: update from the Pediatric Perioperative Cardiac Arrest Registry. *Anesth Analg.* 2007;105:344-350.

3. Lubitz DS, Seidel JS, Chameides L, Luten RC, Zaritsky AL, Campbell FW. A rapid method for estimating weight and resuscitation drug dosages from length in the pediatric age group. *Ann Emerg Med.* 1988;17:576-581.

4. Luten RC, Wears RL, Broselow J, et al. Length-based endotracheal tube and emergency equipment in pediatrics. *Ann Emerg Med.* 1992;21:900-904.

5. Croskerry P. Human factors in airway management. In: Kovacs G, Law, JA, eds. *Airway Managment in Emergencies.* New York: McGraw-Hill; 2008: 283-290.

6. Tong D, Litman R. The Children's Hospital of Philadelphia Difficult Intubation Registry. Winter Society of Pediatric Anesthesia Meeting. 2007:P43.

7. Akpek EA, Mutlu H, Kayhan Z. Difficult intubation in pediatric cardiac anesthesia. *J Cardiothorac Vasc Anesth.* 2004;18:610-612.

8. Shiga T, Wajima Z, Inoue T, Sakamoto A. Predicting difficult intubation in apparently normal patients: a meta-analysis of bedside screening test performance. *Anesthesiology.* 2005;103:429-437.

9. Nargozian C. The airway in patients with craniofacial abnormalities. *Paediatric Anaesthesia.* 2004;14:53-59.

10. Marwan A, Crombleholme TM. The EXIT procedure: principles, pitfalls, and progress. *Semin Pediatr Surg.* 2006;15:107-115.

11. American Society of Anesthesiologists. Practice guidelines for management of the difficult airway: an updated report by the American Society of Anesthesiologists Task Force on Management of the Difficult Airway. *Anesthesiology.* 2003;98:1269-1277.

12. Bergeson PS, Shaw JC. Are infants really obligatory nasal breathers? *Clin Pediatr (Phila).* 2001;40:567-569.

13. Santillanes G, Gausche-Hill M. Pediatric airway management. *Emerg Med Clin North Am.* 2008;26:961-975, ix.

14. Litman RS, Weissend EE, Shibata D, Westesson PL. Developmental changes of laryngeal dimensions in unparalyzed, sedated children. *Anesthesiology.* 2003;98:41-45.

15. Dalal PG, Murray D, Messner AH, Feng A, McAllister J, Molter D. Pediatric laryngeal dimensions: an age-based analysis. *Anesth Analg.* 2009;108: 1475-1479.

16. Newth CJ, Rachman B, Patel N, Hammer J. The use of cuffed versus uncuffed endotracheal tubes in pediatric intensive care. *J Pediatr.* 2004;144:333-337.

17. Weiss M, Dullenkopf A, Fischer JE, Keller C, Gerber AC. Prospective randomized controlled multi-centre trial of cuffed or uncuffed endotracheal tubes in small children. *Brit J Anaesth.* 2009;103:867-873.

18. Goldstein B, Shannon DC, Todres ID. Supercarbia in children: clinical course and outcome. *Crit Care Med.* 1990;18:166-168.

19. Walls R. *The Decision to Intubate.* 3rd ed. Philedelphia, PA: Lippincott, Williams and Wilkins; 2008.

20. Hall SC. The difficult pediatric airway—recognition, evaluation, and management. *Can J Anesth.* 2001;48:R1-R5.

21. Jenkins IA, Saunders M. Infections of the airway. *Paediatr Anaesth.* 2009;19(Suppl 1):118-130.

22. Zur KB, Litman RS. Pediatric airway foreign body retrieval: surgical and anesthetic perspectives. *Paediatr Anaesth.* 2009;19(Suppl 1):109-117.

23. Brooks P, Ree R, Rosen D, Ansermino M. Canadian pediatric anesthesiologists prefer inhalational anesthesia to manage difficult airways. *Can J Anaesth.* 2005;52:285-290.

24. Gausche M, Lewis RJ, Stratton SJ, et al. Effect of out-of-hospital pediatric endotracheal intubation on survival and neurological outcome: a controlled clinical trial. *JAMA.* 2000;283:783-790.

25. Leong L, Black AE. The design of pediatric tracheal tubes. *Paediatr Anaesth.* 2009;19(Suppl 1):38-45.

26. Dullenkopf A, Kretschmar O, Knirsch W, et al. Comparison of tracheal tube cuff diameters with internal transverse diameters of the trachea in children. *Acta Anaesthesiol Scand.* 2006;50:201-205.

27. Dullenkopf A, Schmitz A, Gerber AC, Weiss M. Tracheal sealing characteristics of pediatric cuffed tracheal tubes. *Paediatr Anaesth.* 2004;14:825-830.

28. Cole F. Pediatric formulas for the anesthesiologist. *AMA J Dis Child.* 1957;94:672-673.

29. Suominen P, Taivainen T, Tuominen N, et al. Optimally fitted tracheal tubes decrease the probability of postextubation adverse events in children undergoing general anesthesia. *Paediatr Anaesth.* 2006;16:641-647.

30. Lonnqvist PA. Cuffed or uncuffed tracheal tubes during anaesthesia in infants and small children: time to put the eternal discussion to rest? *Br J Anaesth.* 2009;103:783-785.

31. Holzki J, Laschat M, Puder C. Stridor is not a scientifically valid outcome measure for assessing airway injury. *Paediatr Anaesth.* 2009;19(Suppl 1):180-197.

32. Holzki J, Laschat M, Puder C. Iatrogenic damage to the pediatric airway. Mechanisms and scar development. *Paediatr Anaesth.* 2009;19(Suppl 1): 131-146.

33. Aucoin S, Vlatten A, Hackmann T. Difficult airway management with the Bonfils fiberscope in a child with Hurler syndrome. *Paediatr Anaesth.* 2009;19:421-422.

34. Bishop S, Clements P, Kale K, Tremlett MR. Use of GlideScope Ranger in the management of a child with Treacher Collins syndrome in a developing world setting. *Paediatr Anaesth.* 2009;19:695-696.

35. Caruselli M, Zannini R, Giretti R, Camilletti G. Difficult intubation in a small for gestational age newborn by Bonfils fiberscope. *Paediatr Anaesth.* 2008;18:990-991.

36. Kim JT, Na HS, Bae JY, et al. GlideScope video laryngoscope: a randomized clinical trial in 203 paediatric patients. *Br J Anaesth.* 2008;101:531-534.

37. Milne AD, Dower AM, Hackmann T. Airway management using the pediatric GlideScope in a child with Goldenhar syndrome and atypical plasma cholinesterase. *Paediatr Anaesth.* 2007;17:484-487.

38. Pfitzner L, Cooper MG, Ho D. The Shikani Seeing Stylet for difficult intubation in children: initial experience. *Anaesth Intensive Care.* 2002;30:462-466.

39. Shukry M, Hanson RD, Koveleskie JR, Ramadhyani U. Management of the difficult pediatric airway with Shikani Optical Stylet. *Paediatr Anaesth.* 2005;15:342-345.

40. Vlatten A, Aucoin S, Gray A, Soder C. Difficult airway management with the STORZ video laryngoscope in a child with Robin sequence. *Paediatr Anaesth.* 2009;19:700-701.

41. Vlatten A, Soder C. Airtraq optical laryngoscope intubation in a 5-month-old infant with a difficult airway because of Robin sequence. *Paediatr Anaesth.* 2009;19:699-700.

42. Xue FS, Liao X, Zhang YM, Luo MP. More maneuvers to facilitate endotracheal intubation using the Bonfils fiberscope in children with difficult airways. *Paediatr Anaesth.* 2009;19:418-419.

43. Xue FS, Zhang YM, Liao X, Xu YC. Measures to decrease failed intubation with the pediatric Bonfils fiberscope by the obscure vision. *Paediatr Anaesth.* 2009;19:419-421.

44. Redel A, Karademir F, Schlitterlau A, et al. Validation of the GlideScope video laryngoscope in pediatric patients. *Paediatr Anaesth.* 2009;19:667-671.

45. White M, Weale N, Nolan J, Sale S, Bayley G. Comparison of the Cobalt Glidescope video laryngoscope with conventional laryngoscopy in simulated normal and difficult infant airways. *Paediatr Anaesth.* 2009;19:1108-1112.

46. Fiadjoe JE, Stricker PA, Hackell RS, et al. The efficacy of the Storz Miller 1 video laryngoscope in a simulated infant difficult intubation. *Anesth Analg.* 2009;108:1783-1786.

47. Vlatten A, Aucoin S, Litz S, Macmanus B, Soder C. A comparison of the STORZ video laryngoscope and standard direct laryngoscopy for intubation in the pediatric airway—a randomized clinical trial. *Paediatr Anaesth.* 2009;19:1102-1107.

48. Lardner DR, Cox RG, Ewen A, Dickinson D. Comparison of laryngeal mask airway (LMA)—Proseal and the LMA-Classic in ventilated children receiving neuromuscular blockade. *Can J Anaesth.* 2008;55:29-35.

49. Lu PP, Brimacombe J, Yang C, Shyr M. ProSeal versus the Classic Laryngeal Mask airway for positive pressure ventilation during laparoscopic cholecystectomy. *Br J Anaesth.* 2002;88:824-827.

50. Goldmann K, Roettger C, Wulf H. Use of the ProSeal laryngeal mask airway for pressure-controlled ventilation with and without positive end-expiratory pressure in paediatric patients: a randomized, controlled study. *Br J Anaesth.* 2005;95:831-834.

51. Jagannathan N, Roth AG, Sohn LE, Pak TY, Amin S, Suresh S. The new Air-Q intubating laryngeal airway for tracheal intubation in children with anticipated difficult airway: a case series. *Paediatr Anaesth.* 2009;19:618-622.

52. Bledsoe GH, Schexnayder SM. Pediatric rapid sequence intubation: a review. *Pediatr Emerg Care.* 2004;20:339-344.

53. Sakles JC, Laurin EG, Rantapaa AA, Panacek EA. Airway management in the emergency department: a one-year study of 610 tracheal intubations. *Ann Emerg Med.* 1998;31:325-332.

54. Sellick BA. Cricoid pressure to control regurgitation of stomach contents during induction of anaesthesia. *Lancet.* 1961;2:404-406.

55. Engelhardt T, Strachan L, Johnston G. Aspiration and regurgitation prophylaxis in paediatric anaesthesia. *Paediatr Anaesth.* 2001;11:147-150.

56. Stedeford J, Stoddart P. RSI in pediatric anesthesia—is it used by nonpediatric anesthetists? A survey from south-west England. *Paediatr Anaesth.* 2007;17:235-242.

57. Lerman J. On cricoid pressure: "may the force be with you." *Anesth Analg.* 2009;109:1363-1366.

58. Moynihan RJ, Brock-Utne JG, Archer JH, Feld LH, Kreitzman TR. The effect of cricoid pressure on preventing gastric insufflation in infants and children. *Anesthesiology.* 1993;78:652-656.

59. Brock-Utne JG. Is cricoid pressure necessary? *Paediatr Anaesth.* 2002;12:1-4.

60. Cheng CA, Aun CS, Gin T. Comparison of rocuronium and suxamethonium for rapid tracheal intubation in children. *Paediatr Anaesth.* 2002;12:140-145.

61. Xue FS, Huang YG, Tong SY, et al. A comparative study of early postoperative hypoxemia in infants, children, and adults undergoing elective plastic surgery. *Anesth Analg.* 1996;83:709-715.

62. Weiss M, Gerber AC. Rapid sequence induction in children—it's not a matter of time! *Paediatr Anaesth.* 2008;18:97-99.

63. Perry JJ, Lee JS, Sillberg V. Comparison of two muscle relaxants, rocuronium and succinylcholine, to facilitate rapid sequence induction and intubation. In: *Cochrane Database of Systematic Reviews.* 2007 ed. 2007.

64. Goudsouzian NG. Recent changes in the package insert for succinylcholine chloride: should this drug be contraindicated for routine use in children and adolescents? (Summary of the discussions of the anesthetic and life support drug advisory meeting of the Food and Drug Administration, FDA building, Rockville, MD, June 9, 1994). *Anesth Analg.* 1995;80:207-208.

65. Morell RC, Berman JM, Royster RI, Petrozza PH, Kelly JS, Colonna DM. Revised label regarding use of succinylcholine in children and adolescents. *Anesthesiology.* 1994;80:242-245.

66. Rawicz M, Brandom BW, Wolf A. The place of suxamethonium in pediatric anesthesia. *Paediatr Anaesth.* 2009;19:561-570.

67. Lundstrom LH, Moller AM, Rosenstock C, et al. Avoidance of neuromuscular blocking agents may increase the risk of difficult tracheal intubation: a cohort study of 103,812 consecutive adult patients recorded in the Danish Anaesthesia Database. *Br J Anaesth.* 2009;103:283-290.

68. Bingham RM, Proctor LT. Airway management. *Pediatr Clin North Am.* 2008;55:873-886, ix-x.

69. White MC, Cook TM, Stoddart PA. A critique of elective pediatric supraglottic airway devices. *Paediatr Anaesth.* 2009;19(Suppl 1):55-65.

70. Brain AI, Verghese C, Addy EV, Kapila A. The intubating laryngeal mask. I: Development of a new device for intubation of the trachea. *Br J Anaesth.* 1997;79:699-703.

71. Brain AI, Verghese C, Addy EV, Kapila A, Brimacombe J. The intubating laryngeal mask. II: a preliminary clinical report of a new means of intubating the trachea. *Br J Anaesth.* 1997;79:704-709.

72. Lopez-Gil M, Brimacombe J. The ProSeal laryngeal mask airway in children. *Paediatr Anaesth.* 2005;15:229-234.

73. Lopez-Gil M, Brimacombe J, Alvarez M. Safety and efficacy of the laryngeal mask airway. A prospective survey of 1400 children. *Anaesthesia.* 1996;51:969-972.

74. Asai T, Nagata A, Shingu K. Awake tracheal intubation through the laryngeal mask in neonates with upper airway obstruction. *Paediatr Anaesth.* 2008;18:77-80.

75. Park C, Bahk JH, Ahn WS, Do SH, Lee KH. The laryngeal mask airway in infants and children. *Can J Anaesth.* 2001;48:413-417.

76. Polaner DM, Ahuja D, Zuk J, Pan Z. Video assessment of supraglottic airway orientation through the perilaryngeal airway in pediatric patients. *Anesth Analg.* 2006;102:1685-1688.

77. Tsujimura Y. Downfolding of the epiglottis induced by the laryngeal mask airway in children: a comparison between two insertion techniques. *Paediatr Anaesth.* 2001;11:651-655.

78. Luten RC MJ. Approach to the pediatric airway. In: Walls Ron, Murphy M, ed. *Manual of Emergency Airway Management.* Philadelphia, PA: Lippincott, Williams and Wilkins; 2008:263-281.

79. Holm-Knudsen R, Eriksen K, Rasmussen LS. Using a nasopharyngeal airway during fiberoptic intubation in small children with a difficult airway. *Paediatr Anaesth.* 2005;15:839-845.

80. Ravussin P, Freeman J. A new transtracheal catheter for ventilation and resuscitation. *Can Anaesth Soc J.* 1985;32:60-64.

81. Preussler NP, Schreiber T, Huter L, et al. Percutaneous transtracheal ventilation: effects of a new oxygen flow modulator on oxygenation and ventilation in pigs compared with a hand triggered emergency jet injector. *Resuscitation.* 2003;56:329-333.

82. Schaefer R, Hueter L, Preussler NP, Schreiber T, Schwarzkopf K. Percutaneous transtracheal emergency ventilation with a self-made device in an animal model. *Paediatr Anaesth.* 2007;17:972-976.

83. Gaughan SD, Ozaki GT, Benumof JL. A comparison in a lung model of low- and high-flow regulators for transtracheal jet ventilation. *Anesthesiology.* 1992;77:189-199.

84. Peterson GN, Domino KB, Caplan RA, Posner KL, Lee LA, Cheney FW. Management of the difficult airway: a closed claims analysis. *Anesthesiology.* 2005;103:33-39.

85. Depierraz B, Ravussin P, Brossard E, Monnier P. Percutaneous transtracheal jet ventilation for paediatric endoscopic laser treatment of laryngeal and subglottic lesions. *Can J Anaesth.* 1994;41:1200-1207.

86. Chandradeva K, Palin C, Ghosh SM, Pinches SC. Percutaneous transtracheal jet ventilation as a guide to tracheal intubation in severe upper airway obstruction from supraglottic oedema. *Br J Anaesth.* 2005;94:683-686.

SELF-EVALUATION QUESTIONS

42.1. Regarding succinylcholine (suxamethonium) use in children less than 16 years of age:

A. The FDA defines it as relatively contraindicated.

B. The FDA defines it as contraindicated.

C. The FDA has approved it only in emergency situations.

D. The FDA has warned against its use in various settings.

E. The FDA has never issued any warning regarding its use.

42.2. Cuffed endotracheal tubes:

A. are associated with increase in airway injury compared to uncuffed tubes in children less than 2 years

B. have not been associated with increased airway injury in children less than 2 years compared to uncuffed tubes

C. their cuff pressure must be measured and maintained at less than 30 cm H_2O

D. are not available for children less than 2 years

E. should not be used for infants

42.4. Which of the following is true regarding rapid-sequence intubation (RSI) in children?

A. Rocuronium is the drug of choice.

B. Cricoid pressure improves laryngoscopic grade upon direct laryngoscopy.

C. It is safer in adults versus infants.

D. Cricoid pressure is effective in decreasing gastric insufflation even with ventilation pressures greater than 40 cm H_2O.

E. RSI is contraindicated in neonates.

CHAPTER (43)

Airway Management of a Child with Supraglottitis

Christian M. Soder and Liane B. Johnson

43.1 CASE PRESENTATION

A previously healthy 4-year-old boy is en route to the children's hospital via helicopter. He was well until 8 hours ago when he began to complain of sore throat and pain on swallowing. His mother brought him to the local emergency department (ED). The emergency physician on duty met a sick, flushed, aphonic, and fearful boy who sat very still and reluctantly swallowed his saliva with visible effort and discomfort. He had no visible respiratory distress or stridor. He was able to lie down on request but preferred to sit. His temperature was 39.6°C, BP 142/75 mm Hg, and HR 145 bpm. Examination of the chest revealed no signs of distress, but coarse ronchi were audible on auscultation. The throat was not examined and the remainder of the general physical examination was negative. On direct questioning, the mother admitted that she did not believe in vaccinations and that their children had not received the hemophilus influenza B (HIB) vaccine. The ED physician suspected supraglottitis and called for an emergency transfer to the nearest children's hospital. While waiting for the helicopter to arrive, the physician started an IV, administered 0.6 mg·kg^{-1} of dexamethasone, 25 mg·kg^{-1} of ceftriaxone, and started oxygen 40% by face mask. During transport, the air medical crew administered epinephrine aerosols every 20 minutes. The transport was uneventful but it was noted that the boy was developing moderate indrawing and was insisting on sitting up. His pulse oximeter read 100% on oxygen 4.0 L·min^{-1} flow, by non-rebreathing face mask, throughout the flight. He arrived in the ED at the children's hospital after a 25-minute flight. On examination, the physical findings were as before but the boy had now adopted the classic *tripod sniffing position*. His breath sounds were muted, he was visibly drooling, and he maintained a

posture of fearful rigidity. When made to speak, he had a muffled *hot potato in the mouth* voice. Chest examination revealed mild intercostal and sternal notch indrawing. Without supplementary oxygen his oxygen saturation by pulse oximeter dropped to 89%. After preliminary assessment, he was transferred immediately to the operating room for airway management. No lateral neck airway radiographs were taken.

43.2 INTRODUCTION

43.2.1 What is supraglottitis and what is its pathophysiology? How does supraglottitis in a child usually present?

Supraglottitis is characterized by inflammation of the structures above the insertion point of the glottis. These include the epiglottis, aryepiglottic folds, arytenoid soft tissue, and the uvula. It is quite common for the terms *supraglottitis* and *epiglottitis* to be used interchangeably.[1] While traditionally the term *epiglottitis* was more widely used, the more recently used term *supraglottitis* is perhaps anatomically more correct, and hence will be used throughout this narrative.

Now a rarity, supraglottitis was once the most common pediatric airway emergency faced by anesthesia practitioners and ENT surgeons. Most cases were caused by infection with an invasive strain of HIB. While the widespread introduction of conjugated HIB vaccine in the early 1990s caused a 100-fold reduction in the incidence of supraglottitis in the United States, Western Europe,

Canada, and Australia,[2] the annual incidence of adult supraglottitis has been increasing from a rate of 0.79 cases/100,000 in 1986[3] to a documented rate of 2.1 cases/100,000 in 2005.[4] Despite vaccination however, HIB remains the primary culprit in children. Interestingly, over the past decade, acute supraglottitis in children has seen a resurgence in the United Kingdom, while the cause still remains undetermined.[4]

While some cases may represent failure or refusal of vaccination, others are due to other bacteria known to cause the disease: *Hemophilus parainfluenzae* and other *Hemophilus* strains; *Streptococcus pneumoniae*; *Staphylococcus aureus*; and beta-hemolytic streptococcus. Some viruses have been implicated as possible causes and fungi, or unusual bacteria, may cause supraglottitis in the immunocompromised host. Smoke inhalation and flash burns may cause a thermal supraglottitis, with many features of the infectious disease.

The pathophysiology of non-HIB supraglottitis is similar to that of the classical form of the disease. The infection causes a local cellulitis of the epiglottis, the aryepiglottic folds (false cords), and the mucosa covering the arytenoid cartilages. In the HIB form of the disease, positive blood cultures are common, while most non-HIB cases have negative blood cultures. Culture of direct swabs of the epiglottis may be positive for the responsible pathogen.

The natural history of the disease is progressive glottic inlet swelling that can progress to complete upper airway obstruction causing death. Classic supraglottitis is most common between the ages of 2 and 5, but cases have been reported at all ages. Some believe that the first US President, George Washington, died of the disease at age 67.

Current treatment for all forms of bacterial supraglottitis consists of emergency placement of an artificial airway and a 10-day course of intravenous antibiotics. More recently, some centers have reported successful conservative ICU management without airway instrumentation, using humidified oxygen, inhaled nebulized epinephrine, and intravenous steroids.[5] These measures, especially when started early, may reduce the rate of progression and prevent complete airway occlusion.

43.2.2   What is the differential diagnosis?

While supraglottitis is now rare, croup (or laryngotracheobronchitis) is still the most common cause of upper airway obstruction in preschool children. It is usually caused by a viral infection of the upper airway. Since children have small-caliber tracheas, and because the cricoid ring is rigid, minor degrees of subglottic mucosal swelling produce major degrees of airway obstruction.

Despite the often dramatic symptoms, croup is normally a self-limited illness that rarely progresses to complete airway obstruction. It is almost always treated conservatively with *masterful inactivity*. More severe cases are treated in hospital with humidified oxygen, steroids, and inhaled vasoconstrictors such as phenylephrine, or epinephrine. Very rarely, croup may progress to severe airway obstruction and require emergency airway management.

Croup is easily differentiated from supraglottitis in most cases, but correct diagnosis is extremely important because the two illnesses run profoundly different courses. Children with croup tend to be younger, afebrile, and noisy; they have the classic *barking* cough, hoarse stridor, and vocal agitation of the unhappy toddler. Respiratory effort is often pronounced and dysphagia is not present. Occasionally, the inflammation of croup may extend to the glottic structures and present with some clinical features of supraglottitis.

Other cases suspected to be supraglottitis are actually peritonsillar and retropharyngeal abscesses. These conditions usually present with gradual onset of fever, pain, and dysphagia. Airway obstruction is a late finding in advanced severe cases. Clinical differentiation of these conditions from croup and supraglottitis is usually based on the slow rate of progression, the absence of respiratory distress, and the clinical or radiological detection of a mass.

43.3   PATIENT EVALUATION

43.3.1   How do you assess the patient's airway?

The case of the 4-year-old boy presented earlier is a classic presentation for supraglottitis. The diagnosis is made on history and physical observation from a safe, nonthreatening distance. The patient should not be touched, or disturbed, and imaging studies should not be performed. Agitation of the patient may incite crying which is associated with increased inspiratory airflow velocity which in turn increases turbulent air flow and resistance leading to *dynamic* airway obstruction that may be fatal. Blood cultures and routine blood work can be drawn after the airway is secure. He should be moved to the operating room without delay.

The definitive diagnosis of supraglottitis is usually made in the operating room during laryngoscopy for intubation. In the current era, many patients do not present with classic features. If airway obstruction is not severe, physical examination and diagnostic imaging may be appropriate with the caveat that, as long as supraglottitis remains on the differential diagnosis, direct or optical examinations of the throat should be avoided. While some have advocated flexible endoscopy for adult patients suspected of having supraglottitis, this practice is still considered dangerous in children. The fear is that the procedure may trigger life-threatening dynamic airflow obstruction or laryngospasm.

If it is deemed appropriate to undertake investigation before intervention, the first investigation should be a lateral airway radiograph, often performed with the parent or guardian holding the child. The appearance of the classic *thumb sign* (Figure 43-1), caused by the obliteration of the vallecula by the swollen epiglottis, confirms the diagnosis of supraglottitis. In contrast, if the epiglottis has its normal *pencil-like* appearance and the rest of the radiographic appearance is normal, the patient probably has croup. Radiology texts describe the subglottic region in croup as *blurred* on lateral view, with a *church steeple appearance* on anterior view, but these are subtle findings that may be hard to differentiate. If a peritonsillar or retropharyngeal mass is detected on clinical examination, or suspected on a plain neck radiograph, a CT scan is usually recommended to map out the location, size, and density of the lesion.[6]

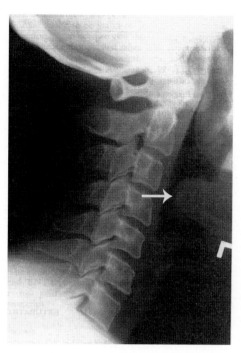

FIGURE 43-1. Lateral radiographic view of the head and neck of the patient with supraglottitis shows the typical swollen epiglottis (the *thumb sign* [arrow]). (Permission for use obtained from Cambridge.)

43.3.2 Do you have any other medical concerns for this patient? Should you do any laboratory investigations?

Patients with supraglottitis are usually septic, toxic, dehydrated, and very afraid (high sympathetic state). In advanced states, they may be hypercarbic, hypoxemic, hypocalcemic, and hyperkalemic. Their airways are reactive, inflamed, overflowing with secretions, and obstructed. Induction of inhalational anesthesia may be complicated by complete airway obstruction, laryngospasm, hypotension, cardiac arrhythmias, and cardiac arrest.

43.4 AIRWAY MANAGEMENT

43.4.1 What are the options in airway management for this patient?

Prior to the 1980s, recommended approaches to the airway were tracheal intubations while awake, perhaps with rigid bronchoscopy, followed by general anesthesia.

In the 1980s, nasotracheal intubation under inhalational halothane anesthesia became the treatment of choice. More recently, some authors have described the use of sevoflurane[7] or intravenous induction and rapid-sequence intubation. The following is the airway management plan currently used by most pediatric centers:

Plan A: Inhalation induction and endotracheal intubation

Plan B: Failed intubation—proceed to rigid bronchoscopy

Plan C: Failed airway—proceed to surgical airway

Supraglottitis and croup in children represent departures from the normal algorithms for difficult airway management. Despite the increasing availability of new pediatric airway tools, there is little or no evidence or experience to support the use of extraglottic devices, alternate intubation devices, or flexible bronchoscopic intubation, in the management of supraglottitis and croup. This probably reflects the paucity of cases and the fact that the airway challenge is not in exposure and visualization of the glottic opening, but rather, in recognition of landmarks (supraglottitis) and intubation of anatomy grossly distorted by inflammation (croup and supraglottitis). It is unlikely that modern airway devices will prove to be of benefit.

Bag-mask-ventilation (BMV) and direct laryngoscopy (DL), with rigid bronchoscopy and ENT as backup, are the state of the art. Based on the skill and experience of the anesthesia practitioner and ENT surgeon, the optically enhanced telescopic rigid bronchoscope may indeed succeed when direct laryngoscopy intubation fails. The enhancement of visualization coupled with the ability to directly advance a rigid tube through the swollen structures may help explain the long and successful history of rigid bronchoscopy in supraglottitis.

43.4.2 Discuss the preparations necessary in managing the airway of this patient?

The OR team should include two experienced health care providers: at minimum an anesthesia practitioner and otolaryngologist (or other qualified rigid bronchoscopist). Necessary airway equipment includes: a functional suction device; different size face masks; two laryngoscope handles with straight and curved blades of varying length and width; and 4.0, 4.5, and 5.0 mm ID tracheal tubes, preloaded with well-lubricated intubating stylets; two appropriate-sized, lubricated, tested rigid telescope-bronchoscopes connected to light source and suction; a tracheotomy tray; and a #1 Melker uncuffed cricothyrotomy set for percutaneous tracheotomy.

Succinylcholine 20 mg (for laryngospasm), atropine 0.4 mg (to treat bradycardia), and epinephrine 100 μg ([1 mL 1/10,000] to respond to hypoxemia-induced myocardial depression) are drawn up. Other standard resuscitation drugs and equipment are at hand.

43.4.3 How do you perform tracheal intubation under inhalational anesthesia?

The child is brought into the OR. Parental attendance is often forgone in this scenario, to minimize distraction, unless it is clear that the parents will help to calm the child (and the anesthesia practitioner!) during induction. If not already present, an IV is inserted immediately after induction of anesthesia. Atropine 0.1 mg IV may be administered to reduce secretions and mitigate vagal responses (bradycardia). Pulse oximeter, BP cuff, and ECG monitors are applied.

Inhalation inductions in the presence of supraglottitis require patience and excellent BMV technique. It is important to remember that supraglottitis produces obstruction of the glottic inlet but leaves oral, pharyngeal, glottic, and subglottic anatomy unchanged.

There is an ever-present risk of acute life-threatening events during induction. Laryngospasm, complete glottic inlet occlusion, hypoxic seizures, and obstructive pulmonary edema have all been described. Accumulated secretions above and below the vocal cords are usually present, may contribute to airway obstruction, and can trigger laryngospasm.

Induction of anesthesia starts with incremental levels; sevoflurane (5%-8%) blended with 100% oxygen at 6.0 L·min^{-1} flow. BMV with applied-mask continuous positive airway pressure (CPAP) 5 to 10 cm of H$_{2O}$ is applied to deal with increased airway obstruction during the excitement phase. While only marginally effective at overcoming anatomic glottic inlet obstruction, mask CPAP is useful in treating pharyngeal obstruction and laryngospasm. The maneuver plays a vital role in managing inhalational induction of anesthesia. There is an ever-present risk of, and need to avoid, gastric distension.

Induction is usually prolonged by the reduced alveolar ventilation and high cardiac output commonly present in supraglottitis. It is important to be patient and to persist until there is evidence of deep anesthesia, as indicated by falling heart rate and blood pressure. When the patient is judged to be deeply anesthetized, the laryngoscope blade is gently introduced. It is immediately withdrawn if the patient responds by moving, swallowing, coughing, or closing the vocal cords. In this case, anesthesia must be deepened by continuing with mask inhalation.

When laryngoscopy is fully tolerated, the blade is advanced along the lateral tongue margin until the glottic structures are identified. Direct laryngoscopy itself is not usually difficult but visual recognition of structures at the glottic opening can be extremely difficult. Early in the course of the illness, glottic inlet structures are red and swollen, but recognizable, and the vocal cords (or at least the false cords) can be seen during direct laryngoscopy. Such patients are easily intubated with a normal-sized endotracheal tube for age. With progression of the inflammation, the swollen tissues begin to obscure normal anatomy. The epiglottis, aryepiglottic folds, and the loose areolar tissue overlying the arytenoid cartilages become reddened and swollen. Visually, these structures merge to form the famous *red cherry* at the base of the tongue. It is important to realize that the glottic inlet lies roughly at the center of the *cherry*, not posterior to it (Figure 43-2). In the most severe cases, all recognizable structures are effaced and the laryngoscopic appearance is that of a frightening, featureless, red mass.

Spontaneous breathing, or a stroke of chest compression, may help in identifying the glottic opening by creating bubbles of air streaming through saliva and secretions. In cases with significant distortion of normal anatomy, it is usually recommended that a tube one-half size smaller than usual (in this case a 4.5 mm ID tube), fortified by an intubating stylet, be inserted through the tiny orifice. If the appearance is that of a *cherry-like* structure, the endotracheal tube is gently advanced, with the bevel aligned to the axis of the glottic opening (ie, the tube is sideways) toward the center of the *cherry*. Often a dimple is noticed at the center of the cherry: this marks the opening, and air may be seen bubbling through it. Experienced pediatric anesthesia practitioners have often pointed out to their colleagues that the appearance of the glottis in supraglottitis is similar to that of the cervix, as visualized during

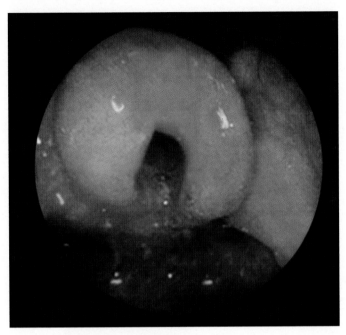

FIGURE 43-2. The flexible fiberscope view of the red and swollen epiglottis (the *red cherry*) in a patient with supraglottitis.

gynecologic speculum examination—the os cervix represents the glottic aperture. Intubation of the trachea with supraglottitis is visually analogous to the insertion of an intrauterine device. The good news about supraglottitis intubation is that while the glottic inlet structures may be massively swollen, they are soft, not firm. Therefore, once the glottic aperture is identified, it should not be difficult to pass the endotracheal tube through the larynx.

If the diagnosis in this case unexpectedly turns out to be severe atypical croup, the glottic inlet will appear normal and airway obstruction will be isolated to the subglottic area. In this case, laryngeal visualization will be easy, but passing the endotracheal tube will be difficult. A significantly smaller than normal endotracheal tube, fortified by a straight intubating stylet, or a rigid bronchoscope, is usually required to pass through the obstruction.

In supraglottitis, repeat laryngoscopy following a failed attempt is acceptable, if the BMV airway and oxygen saturation can be restored and maintained between attempts. Second-attempt laryngoscopy may include blade change, position change, and personnel change. Although it is not reported in the literature, it seems logical that external laryngeal manipulation might be helpful. There is minimal experience with the use of the Eschmann Tracheal Introducer (bougie) or alternate intubation devices in this condition.[8,9] Since the problem is one of anatomic obliteration of normal structures, it is improbable that indirect intubation techniques will prove to be useful.

43.4.4 If laryngoscopic intubation is not possible, what would you do next?

If intubation fails after two or three attempts with the laryngoscope, the rigid bronchoscope should be employed. It can be inserted directly, or with the assistance of a laryngoscope. Bronchoscopy is complicated by the same factors that make intubation difficult; but the optically enhanced visualization, and rigid construction of the bronchoscope, may lead to success where laryngoscopy failed. If the bronchoscope is successfully inserted, the patient should be suctioned and ventilated through the scope and anesthesia should be deepened. A long-acting muscle relaxant may be given at this stage to facilitate intubation. An endotracheal tube can then be inserted directly, or an appropriately sized bougie can be passed through the bronchoscope. The bronchoscope can then be removed, a laryngoscope positioned, and a bougie-assisted intubation completed. The process of tube change is not as intimidating as it might seem; once the airway has been opened by the passage of a bronchoscope, the glottis usually holds its shape and remains patent, and visible, for several minutes after removal of the bronchoscope. This temporary stenting effect makes reinsertion significantly less difficult than primary intubation.

43.4.5 At what stage would you consider tracheotomy appropriate for this patient?

If airway patency, oxygenation, or ventilation cannot be maintained (or recovered) by BMV at any time; or if intubation is unsuccessful after three attempts, the failed airway plan is activated. Depending on the skill and experience of the anesthesia practitioners and surgeons present, either a surgical tracheotomy is performed, or a #1 Melker percutaneous tracheotomy tube is inserted using Seldinger technique. The surgical airway is a useful option of last resort in supraglottitis, because subglottic anatomy is normal. The usual pediatric limitation applies: the cricothyroid membrane is too small to be useful. A trans-tracheal approach is necessary for either surgical or percutaneous tracheotomy tube insertion.[10]

In contrast, tracheotomy is less likely to be successful in croup, because the obstruction occurs at the level of the proximal trachea. Unless the trachea is entered below the level of maximum swelling, it may be no easier to insert a tracheotomy tube than an endotracheal tube.

43.4.6 How do you manage the airway of this patient if he has a strong family history of malignant hyperthermia?

In early cases with minimal evidence of airway obstruction, denitrogenation followed by a rapid-sequence induction using sodium pentothal, propofol, or midazolam, in combination with pancuronium or rocuronium, is recommended. In cases of severe airway obstruction, awake laryngoscopy, possibly facilitated by topical anesthesia, and/or anxiolytic doses of midazolam, should be attempted. If the laryngeal inlet is found to have recognizable anatomy, the awake attempt can be aborted and a rapid-sequence induction performed. If the laryngeal inlet remains obscured, awake intubation, or awake rigid bronchoscopy, is recommended. Postintubation sedation with non-triggering agents should proceed, as described in the next section.

43.5 OTHER CONSIDERATIONS

43.5.1 Discuss the appropriate postintubation management

Endotracheal placement must be confirmed initially by CO_2 detection. Since inadvertent endobronchial intubation of children is common (especially under stressful circumstances), radiographic confirmation is required to confirm tube tip location. The endotracheal tube must be well secured using a commercial fixation device, or by highly adherent adhesive tape fixed to the skin of the upper lip. Tincture of benzoin (Friars' Balsam) may be used to dry and degrease the skin. The patient should be sedated and restrained in the ICU to minimize the risk of accidental extubation. Fortunately, accidental extubation is not necessarily catastrophic. Because the glottis holds its shape for some time after removal of the ETT, re-intubation is usually accomplished far more easily than the original intubation. Experience has shown that extubation can be safely performed upon defervescence—as early as 6 hours after initiation of antibiotics. The average duration of intubation is approximately 24 hours.[10] Twelve hours after extubation, once it is clear that the airway will remain free from obstruction, the child may be transferred from the ICU to a regular ward (and later, home) to complete his course of antibiotics.

43.5.2 Is it necessary to have tracheal intubation for all supraglottitis?

Conservative management of supraglottitis has been described in adult and pediatric patients with some success, especially in early cases with mild airway obstruction. Patients are admitted to intensive care, monitored closely, and treated with intravenous antibiotics, dexamethasone, and inhaled catecholamines such as epinephrine or phenylephrine. This approach is still considered experimental, especially in children, and it is essential that the personnel and equipment necessary for tracheal intubation be immediately available in case of failure.

43.5.3 If orotracheal intubation is successful during laryngoscopy, is it necessary to change it to a nasal route?

The use of orotracheal versus nasotracheal tubes reflects local practice: there is no compelling evidence to favor one technique over the other. Nasotracheal intubation is considered by some to carry a lower risk of accidental extubation, but orotracheal intubation is less likely to be complicated by otitis media, or nasopharyngeal hemorrhage. The recognition that duration of intubation in supraglottitis need not be prolonged, and the observation that re-intubation after accidental extubation is usually not difficult, has made orotracheal intubation combined with deep sedation a popular approach in many centers.

43.5.4   How does adult supraglottitis (acute supraglottitis) differ from the childhood illness?

Acute supraglottitis (AS) in an adult is more likely to be encountered in one's clinical practice than is supraglottitis in a child. This infectious process can lead to significant, sudden airway obstruction and is potentially fatal. Historically, supraglottitis was an adult disease until the 1960s when it shifted primarily to a pediatric process.

While there is no predominant organism isolated in AS, bacterial, viral, or a combination thereof have all been documented. There is a very low yield from reported throat cultures in the adult patient population. However, the most commonly isolated organisms include *H. influenzae, S. pneumoniae, Staphylococcus aureus, Moraxella catarrhalis, Pseudomonas* spp, *Candida albicans, Kelbsiella pneumoniae, Pasteurella multocida,* as well as herpes simplex, parainfluenzae, varicella zoster, and Epstein-Barr viruses.[11,12] Noninfectious causes such as trauma, thermal injury, and posttransplant lymphoproliferative disorder have been reported by Rosbe et al.[13]

Clinical presentation of AS is also more variable than in children. AS presents primarily (90%-100%) with sore throat or odynophagia, while at least half of such patients will be drooling, and approximately one-third will have stridor or other symptoms of respiratory compromise.[1] Patients may also present with a muffled voice, neck pain, or foreign body sensation. The inflammation seen is not limited to the epiglottis, but rather often encompasses all of the supraglottic tissues, namely the epiglottis, the aryepiglottic folds, the arytenoid mucosa, and the false cords. The typical cherry red epiglottis is not seen, but rather encompassing diffusely edematous and erythematous supraglottic tissues. Generally the oral cavity and oropharynx are devoid of clinical findings.

Patient assessment must be performed cautiously and with care as manipulation of the airway can lead to acute airway obstruction. The use of tongue depressors may trigger laryngospasm either by inciting a gag reflex or by displacing the soft tissues. Oral cavity examination is best done with good lighting and without any manipulation. Flexible endoscopy of the larynx is the mainstay of diagnosis and airway assessment, but some practitioners prefer to secure the airway first and rely on their clinical judgment and experience to make the diagnosis. A lateral neck soft tissue radiograph has a high false-negative rate (as high as 56%),[14] thus transporting a potentially unstable airway to the imaging department for a relatively unreliable test is probably best be avoided, unless the diagnosis is uncertain, the patient's airway is stable, and/or flexible endoscopy is not available or feasible.

Overall consensus on airway management is quite difficult as practitioners' clinical judgment and experience are quite variable. Unfortunately, the cardinal signs of airway obstruction in children which mandate intervention (ie, stertor, stridor, dyspnea, intercostal and suprasternal retraction, tachypnea, and cyanosis) are rarely present until AS is in its advanced stages.[15] Many measurable indicators have been studied as an adjunct to clinical acumen and to assist in determining the need for and timing of intervention. Two measures are commonly used: Friedman's staging system for AS (Table 43-1) and the time between onset of symptoms to the time of presentation. Friedman's staging system for AS is increasingly used and recognized as a tool to facilitate decision-making when faced with a compromised airway. Madhotra et al[14] reported that adult AS patients who presented within less than 24 hours of symptom onset with stridor and respiratory distress (Friedman stage III) were most likely to require airway stabilization with endotracheal intubation and monitoring in an intensive care unit. Patients with lesser Friedman stage or with Friedman stage III whose symptom onset was slower (>24 hours) were more likely to improve with conservative management (antibiotics, intravenous rehydration, and frequently, systemic corticosteroids) and close monitoring.

Delayed airway obstruction has been reported to occur days after symptom onset. Daily endoscopic examination of the larynx has been suggested as a means of tracking progression or resolution of airway obstruction.[16]

Although rare, AS in adults is a serious infection that can become life-threatening in a fairly short period of time. Visualization of the larynx is the prime modality for diagnosis, although in times of critical airway symptomatology, airway stabilization is at the forefront of patient care. Clinical judgment and approaching the patient sensibly and with caution while ensuring good communication between the patient, family, and surgical and anesthesia practitioners will ensure the best possible outcome for the patient.

TABLE 43-1

Friedman's Staging of Adult Supraglottitis

	STAGE I	STAGE II	STAGE III	STAGE IV
Respiratory distress	None	Subjective	Moderate	Severe
Respiratory rate	≤20/minute	>20/minute	>30/minute	>30/minute
Other symptoms			Stridor, retractions, perioral cyanosis, P_{CO_2} >45 mm Hg	Severe stridor, retractions, cyanosis, delirium, hypoxia, respiratory arrest

43.6   SUMMARY

The successful treatment of supraglottitis using tracheal intubation under general anesthesia became a world-wide standard of care in the 1980s and mortality from this condition fell to near zero. The massive reduction in the incidence of this disease by widespread vaccination against HIB, while obviously a desirable outcome, has raised new concerns. Post vaccine-era cases are more likely to be atypical in presentation, more delayed in recognition, and less likely to be well managed as clinicians experienced in the diagnosis and treatment of the condition become less prevalent. As a result, it is possible that mortality in this now rare but still life-threatening condition will again rise. It is important that education in airway management continues to include supraglottitis as an area of focus.

REFERENCES

1. Glynn F, Fenton JE. Diagnosis and management of supraglottitis (epiglottitis). *Curr Infect Dis Rep.* 2008;10:200-204.
2. McEwan J, Giridharan W, Clarke RW, Shears P. Paediatric acute epiglottitis: not a disappearing entity. *Int J Pediatr Otorhinolaryngol.* 2003;67:317-321.
3. Mayo-Smith MF, Spinale JW, Donskey CJ, Yukawa M, Li RH. Acute epiglottitis. An 18-year experience in Rhode Island. *Chest.* 1995;108:1640-1647.
4. Guldfred LA, Lyhne D, Becker BC. Acute epiglottitis: epidemiology, clinical presentation, management and outcome. *J Laryngol Otol.* 2008;122:818-823.
5. Damm M, Eckel HE, Jungehulsing M, Roth B. Airway endoscopy in the interdisciplinary management of acute epiglottitis. *Int J Pediatr Otorhinolaryngol.* 1996;38:41-51.
6. Verghese ST, Hannallah RS. Pediatric otolaryngologic emergencies. *Anesthesiol Clin North America.* 2001;19:237-256, vi.
7. Spalding MB, Ala-Kokko TI. The use of inhaled sevoflurane for endotracheal intubation in epiglottitis. *Anesthesiology.* 1998;89:1025-1026.
8. Santer DM, D'Alessandro P. Acute Epiglottitis. Virtual Pediatric Hospital, TM. http://www.virtualpediatrichospital.org/providers/ElectricAirway/Text/Epiglottitis.shtml. Accessed July 18, 2011.
9. Rucklidge MW, Patel A. Failure of the single-use bougie in acute epiglottitis. *Anaesthesia.* 2004;59:925-926.
10. Navsa N, Tossel G, Boon JM. Dimensions of the neonatal cricothyroid membrane—how feasible is a surgical cricothyroidotomy? *Paediatr Anaesth.* 2005;15:402-406.
11. Senior BA, Radkowski D, MacArthur C, et al. Changing patterns in pediatric supraglottitis: a multi-institutional review, 1980 to 1992. *Laryngoscope.* 1994;104:1314-1322.
12. Ward MA. Emergency department management of acute respiratory infections. *Semin Respir Infect.* 2002;17:65-71.
13. Rosbe KW, Perez-Atayde AR, Roberson DW, Kenna M. Pathology forum: quiz case 1. Diagnosis: posttransplant lymphoproliferative disease (PTLD) of the epiglottis. *Arch Otolaryngol Head Neck Surg.* 2000;126:1153.
14. Madhotra D, Fenton JE, Makura ZG, Charters P, Roland NJ. Airway intervention in adult supraglottitis. *Ir J Med Sci.* 2004;173:197-199.
15. Kilham H, Gillis J, Benjamin B. Severe upper airway obstruction. *Pediatr Clin North Am.* 1987;34:1-14.
16. Berger G, Landau T, Berger S, Finkelstein Y, Bernheim J, Ophir D. The rising incidence of adult acute epiglottitis and epiglottic abscess. *Am J Otolaryngol.* 2003;24:374-383.

SELF-EVALUATION QUESTIONS

43.1   Croup is distinguished from supraglottitis by all of the following **EXCEPT**:

  A. age of onset

  B. rapidity of onset

  C. presence of a fever

  D. cough

  E. dysphagia

43.2   Management of significantly symptomatic pediatric supraglottitis may include all of the following **EXCEPT**:

  A. airway inspection by laryngoscopy or endoscopy

  B. inhalational induction of anesthesia

  C. expedient transfer to the operating room for airway securement

  D. rigid bronchoscopy

  E. surgical airway

43.3   Intubation sequences for pediatric supraglottitis may include all of the following **EXCEPT**:

  A. bag-mask-ventilation

  B. CPAP

  C. atropine

  D. extraglottic airway adjuvants

  E. tracheal tube half size smaller than normal, with intubating stylet

CHAPTER 44

Management of a 12-Year-Old Child with a Foreign Body in the Bronchus

Liane B. Johnson

44.1 CASE PRESENTATION

An 88-lb (40 kg), 12-year-old-boy with a history of cervical spine fusion due to syringomyelia presents to the hospital following the accidental inhalation of a pushpin during sneezing. There is no associated thoracic scoliosis or any neuromuscular deficit. He is otherwise healthy, takes no medications, and has no known drug allergies.

44.2 PATIENT ASSESSMENT

44.2.1 What are the initial clinical steps in patient management?

Initial management when presented with a definitive history of aspiration of a foreign body begins with the ABCs. An awake, alert patient without overt airway distress will permit a more complete workup, while a severely distressed patient with stridor and desaturation will mandate acute stabilization prior to transfer to the operating room for surgical removal. All patients should have pulse oximetry. Supplemental oxygen may be provided to maximize oxygenation. To optimize patient care and potentially minimize the need for emergency intervention, a member of the anesthesia or surgical team should accompany the patient during airway stabilization and transportation to the operating room.

Respiratory distress or the presence of stridor implies compromise of the airway and reduced airflow. Heliox 70/30 (70% helium and 30% oxygen) will improve oxygenation by maximizing laminar airflow and reducing airflow resistance. The use of Heliox serves as a temporizing measure in the setting of foreign body aspiration in young children as it decreases the work of breathing and the associated anxiety.[1] Intravenous dexamethasone at a dose of 0.5 mg·kg^{-1} may be beneficial in reducing the mucosal edema which partly contributes to the airway obstruction.[2] Aerosolized epinephrine may be an additional means of reducing airway edema. The use of bronchodilators is considered to be relatively contraindicated until the foreign body is removed from the airway, as its use may predispose to dislodgement and distal migration of the foreign body due to an increase in airway caliber. Bronchodilators, however, are important adjuncts to pulmonary toilet following foreign body removal.[3]

44.2.2 What are the appropriate investigations for a foreign body in the trachea?

Radiologic studies are used as an adjunct to the physical examination in diagnosing suspected aerodigestive foreign bodies. Anteroposterior and lateral chest radiographs with inspiratory and expiratory views are helpful tools if the foreign body is opaque, or if there is evidence of bronchial obstruction. Typical findings will reveal a foreign body shadow, air trapping, segmental or lobar collapse, or consolidation. Unfortunately, the false-negative rate (ie, normal chest x-ray) ranges between 24% and 33% when compared to bronchoscopic findings.[4]

Spiral CT has shown some benefit when faced with persistent symptoms in a pediatric patient in the setting of an atypical history and normal chest x-ray. Fluoroscopy and cine CT are of little added benefit when a timely workup is of essence, especially if a plain radiograph or spiral CT has already confirmed the presence of a foreign body.[4] Ultimately, the gold standard for diagnosing an aspirated foreign body is rigid bronchoscopy under general anesthesia.[3,5]

44.2.3 Do different types of foreign bodies (organics, metals, plastics) influence patient management and outcomes?

Organic matter (nuts, corn, seeds, etc) and plastics are radiolucent items that are not commonly visualized on x-ray. Organics must be removed as soon as possible as the diameter of the object will increase over time due to the absorption of secretions and moisture. This may convert a stable, partial obstruction to an acute, complete obstruction, or obliterate the available space around the foreign body complicating removal with forceps. Furthermore, over time the organic matter will become more friable, potentially breaking into multiple pieces, making complete removal very difficult. This enhances the risk of obstruction and infection in the distal, smaller generation bronchi.

44.2.4 What are the pathophysiologic changes in the presence of an aspirated foreign body?

Determining the site of airway obstruction, the size and shape of the aspirated object, and the timeline since obstruction are crucial to patient outcomes and guide the plan for removal. Airway obstruction following foreign body aspiration may be total or partial, depending on all of the above factors. The incidence of foreign body aspiration is not dependent on socioeconomic status or geographic location. However, there is a relationship in the type of aspirated object, particularly if it is a food substance that is dependent on the age of the patient and the country in which the patient resides.

Toddlers, under 3 years, are at highest risk of foreign body aspiration as they explore their environment by placing encountered objects in their mouths, are more likely to talk, laugh, and run while eating, have relatively immature laryngeal protective reflexes,[5] and incomplete dentition. The most commonly aspirated organics are nuts (peanut, sunflower seed), meat (chicken, hot dog), popcorn, and carrots. Fatalities are most frequent with hot dogs and other meats, candies, grapes, and peanuts.[6]

A foreign body lodged in the lower airway may manifest with different pulmonary findings depending on the type of impaction. Four lower airway obstructive mechanisms have been described: check valve, ball valve, bypass valve, and stop valve.[7] Check valve implies air can be inhaled but not exhaled, creating alveolar air trapping and flattening of the ipsilateral diaphragm. This is in contrast to a ball valve which allows expiration but not inspiration of air, creating segmental bronchopulmonary collapse. A bypass valve obstruction allows partial airflow on both inspiration and expiration around the foreign body and may not exhibit specific clinical findings. A stop valve creates complete obstruction to airflow, causing airway collapse and consolidation distal to the obstruction.[7]

The ability to correctly ascertain the type of obstruction and object aspirated may help determine the stability of the patient's airway and the requisite acuity of intervention. This key point is of utmost importance when the patient is not distressed, possibly lulling the practitioner into a false sense of (airway) security.

44.3 AIRWAY CONSIDERATIONS

44.3.1 What are the usual clinical presentations of a foreign body in the airway with or without airway obstruction and air trapping? What are the specific airway concerns in this patient?

Presenting symptoms following foreign body aspiration are related to the type of object aspirated, location of the object within the airway, and the overall duration of the obstructive event. Airway obstruction may be complete or partial. Complete obstruction of the trachea or large airway is an emergency situation usually associated with hypoxemia, cardiovascular compromise, and subsequent collapse. In contrast, partial obstruction can often present with more subtle symptoms such as coughing, focal or diffuse wheezing, and decreased air entry on the affected side.[3,8] These may progress over time to drooling, dyspnea, stridor, and respiratory distress.

It is critical to appreciate that to produce symptoms a foreign body must encroach on 75% of the airway lumen to create turbulent airflow. This degree of obstruction may occur acutely, due primarily to the foreign body itself or secondarily, due to the local tissue reaction. Aspiration of organic matter will promote, over time, local airway swelling and the production of granulation tissue. Thus even a small foreign body can produce significant obstructive symptoms when left in the airway for as little as 5 to 7 days. This generally necessitates immediate intervention to avoid a disastrous outcome.[8]

In this patient, the aspirated foreign body may be found anywhere in the upper airway, down to the level of the carina, and occasionally in the mainstem bronchi. Sharp objects, like pins, will generally be found with the sharp end embedded in the mucosa proximally, while the larger, blunt end is distal. It is unlikely that a pushpin, in and of itself, would cause obstruction of the larger airways. However, the associated mucosal edema, and/or displacement into the smaller generation bronchi, may create airway obstruction.

Our patient is able to provide an accurate history of aspiration and subsequent, persistent cough. His airway is currently stable. However, his previous cervical fusion may provide a challenge for both the anesthesia practitioner and endoscopist. The following sections will further delve into anesthetic management and the surgical options presented by this challenging scenario.

A key principle in managing the airways of children is to ensure communication between the anesthesia practitioner and the surgeon prior to the patient's arrival in the operating room. It is essential that the surgical setup be ready prior to the induction of anesthesia, that a backup plan has been discussed and agreed upon, and that the equipment for performing a surgical airway is available.

44.4   ANESTHESIA CONSIDERATIONS

44.4.1   What are the anesthetic options if the patient is uncooperative? How would you approach the induction of this patient?

Children with airway obstruction pose a challenge to the anesthesia practitioner. Physiologically, children have a limited functional residual capacity (FRC), reduced respiratory reserve, increased shunting, and a propensity for airway closure (laryngospasm and bronchospasm). In the setting of a relative increase in oxygen consumption and suboptimal ventilation, the anesthesia practitioner is faced with a patient who will likely develop hypoxemia rapidly. An inhalation induction may be prolonged if there is reduced alveolar ventilation due to airway obstruction.

Anesthetic management in the setting of foreign body aspiration is predicated on providing a safe anesthetic for the patient, while maintaining control of the airway and preventing the undesirable physiologic responses associated with airway manipulation. Inhalational agents may provide an optimal technique to maintain control of the airway.[8] Halothane and sevoflurane provide the most rapid and uneventful induction in this scenario. Sevoflurane may be the preferred inhalational agent because it allows for a smooth and rapid induction of general anesthesia. In addition, sevoflurane has antitussive properties and far greater cardiorespiratory stability than halothane.[9] The other fluorinated inhalational agents, such as isoflurane, enflurane, and desflurane, are more likely to produce airway irritation on induction and are commonly avoided. However, they may be used following induction to maintain a deep plane of anesthesia.[8]

Anticholinergics (atropine and glycopyrrolate) block vagally mediated airway responses, such as excessive production of airway secretions, bradycardia, and bronchoconstriction.[8] Topical lidocaine works synergistically with the inhalational agent decreasing the physiologic response to laryngoscopy and bronchoscopy. Intravenous opioids, such as remifentanil and fentanyl, are also helpful in suppressing airway reflexes and may be used as an adjunct to the anesthetic, ensuring that the airway is already secured, as there may be associated respiratory depression.[8,10] Total intravenous anesthesia with propofol infusion is also a feasible option, as long as spontaneous respiration is maintained. Similarly, small doses of short-acting muscle relaxants provide short-term neuromuscular blockade, inhibit coughing, facilitate oxygenation, and minimize atelectasis.[10] The use of muscle relaxants, once again, mandates prior stabilization and control of the airway.[10,11]

It is generally felt that positive pressure ventilation (PPV) is to be avoided as this may lead to dislodgement and distal displacement of the foreign body.[8,10] However, in a retrospective review of 94 children with tracheal and bronchial foreign body, Litman et al found that neither spontaneous nor controlled ventilation was associated with an increased incidence of adverse events.[10] Nitrous oxide should also be avoided because it decreases the percentage of delivered oxygen, encourages atelectasis, and expands cavities containing trapped air. Indeed, augmentation of air that is trapped may be of sufficient magnitude to severely compromise pulmonary compliance and generate a pneumothorax.[8] Although some might consider awake-intubation to be an option, in this patient, it is likely to be stormy with the potential to dislodge the pushpin and create a more hazardous situation.

When faced with an uncooperative patient or a precarious airway, an intramuscular agent, such as ketamine, may provide a window of opportunity for an inhalation induction, without significant depression of the respiratory drive.[12]

Although the patient with a foreign body in the airway is considered at high risk for aspiration, the urgency of the airway status takes precedence. If immediate intervention is not indicated, some advocate a waiting period for the patient with a full stomach, while others believe that the stress associated with foreign body aspiration is likely to inhibit gastric emptying and advise against waiting. Likewise, some advocate a rapid-sequence induction to protect the airway, although most believe that a slow inhalation induction with spontaneous ventilation is associated with minimal risk of aspiration and maximizes control. If, however, bag-mask-ventilation is required to maintain or regain control of the airway, then the risk of aspiration increases, mandating early control of the airway.[8-11]

In this case, our patient provides an interesting twist, as the complexity of the challenge is enhanced by limited neck extension. This case also reflects the importance of communication among the team of caregivers and highlights the need for an alternate plan should the initial approach fail. The inability to predict whether the airway will be easily accessed provides a strong argument for a slow, spontaneous ventilation induction, with topicalization of the airway using lidocaine. Should the airway not be visualized on laryngoscopy, or with a rigid bronchoscope, other modalities may be attempted (McGrath video laryngoscope, lightwand, laryngeal mask airway, etc) provided one has ascertained that blind techniques will not lead to dislodgement or impaction of the foreign body. The specifics of airway management for our patient scenario will be discussed in depth in the next section.

44.5   AIRWAY MANAGEMENT

44.5.1   How do you perform rigid bronchoscopy for foreign body removal?

A complete airway assessment is fundamental to planning the approach to remove the foreign body and preparing for difficulties that might be encountered. Our patient has had a cervical fusion potentially limiting neck extension, making laryngoscopy and rigid bronchoscopy challenging, if not impossible. The safest means of removing a sharp foreign body requires that under direct vision it be grasped, released from its hold on the mucosa by advancing it more distally, and then sheathing it within the rigid bronchoscope for removal when the bronchoscope is withdrawn. Large tracheal foreign bodies that cannot be ensheathed within the bronchoscope are likely to become impacted at the level of the glottis during removal, potentially leading to complete airway obstruction. In situations where obstruction is, or becomes, complete, the object may need to be rapidly pushed distally, usually into the right mainstem bronchus.

It is important to note that the entire airway, trachea, and first- and second-generation bronchi must be visualized following removal of the foreign body to ensure the absence of trauma or a second airway foreign body, which may be present in up to 5% of foreign body aspirations.[13]

44.5.2   How do you provide oxygenation during rigid bronchoscopy?

Provided that an appropriately sized bronchoscope is used, rigid bronchoscopy allows for oxygenation through side ports. Newer endoscopic technology allows visualization of the airway on a monitor. The advent of endoscopic foreign body forceps allows spontaneous ventilation through the bronchoscope, with minimal loss of anesthetic gases into the operating room and better mainte- nance of the depth of anesthesia. Depending on the type and shape of the object to be retrieved, a selection of endoscopic foreign body forceps should be available.

44.5.3   What are the potential complications and limitations of rigid bronchoscopy?

Complications of rigid bronchoscopy include: dental injury, cervical spine injury (due to aggressive patient positioning or underlying patient disorder), glottic or arytenoid injury, and posterior tracheal wall tear which may occasionally lead to the formation of a tracheoesophageal fistula. Hemodynamic instabil- ity, hypercapnia, or hypoxemia may also occur in association with hypoventilation, dislodgement of the foreign body, or the use of an inappropriately large bronchoscope limiting insufflation and efflux of gases. Rigid bronchoscopes in the tracheobronchial tree have limited maneuverability and cannot access secondary bronchi and smaller airways.

44.5.4   What is the role of flexible bronchoscopy in the management of foreign bodies in the airway?

The use of flexible bronchoscopy (FB) as a primary tool for foreign body removal is not widely practiced. Some advocate its use to evaluate the airway prior to foreign body removal by rigid

bronchoscopy to allow for localization and planning.[14] It may also be used following retrieval to ensure that the foreign body has been removed in its entirety and no other foreign bodies exist. A group in Mexico is currently using FB in approximately 40% of their pediatric airway foreign body cases, with a 93% success rate.[15]

The risks of using FB for foreign body removal are multifaceted. It is customary to secure the airway with an endotracheal tube prior to endoscopy, as there are no ventilation ports. There is a limited selection of grasping forceps that may be passed through the channel of the FB. The foreign body cannot be ensheathed within the FB to protect the airway during its removal, potentially increasing the risk of injury to the airway if the object is sharp. It also increases the risk of complete airway obstruction, if the object is dropped as it is retracted proximally.

44.5.5   What is the incidence of an open surgical procedure to remove foreign bodies from the airway?

Open surgical procedures are seldom required to remove foreign bodies from the airway. Such an approach is generally required in a setting where rigid bronchoscopy has failed or in the following situations: (1) if the foreign body is found in a small, inaccessible peripheral bronchus; (2) if the foreign body is sharp, pointed, and embedded in the tracheal or bronchial wall; (3) if it has been present for a prolonged period of time, often for several years; and (4) if there is significant difficulty in maintaining control of the airway following rigid bronchoscope insertion and manipulation. Interestingly, aspirated plastic pen caps more often require open surgical procedures due to a high rate of bronchoscopic extrac- tion failure secondary to their size, shape, and position in the airway.[16,17]

44.5.6   How do you remove the foreign body from this patient?

Because of the limitation of cervical spine movement and the anticipated difficulty in performing a rigid bronchoscopy in this patient, once the airway was controlled, a temporary tracheotomy was performed through which a rigid bronchoscope was passed to retrieve the pushpin.

In cases such as this, the tracheotomy may be closed primarily provided that there is minimal airway edema compromising the lumen, and recognizing that there is a small risk of air leak into the neck with primary closure. If the patient is expected to cough or strain, or require ventilatory assistance, then primary closure may not be the best option.

If an object still cannot be removed, an open thoracotomy is required. In such cases, a bronchotomy or partial lung paren- chymal resection may be necessary to remove the object. The latter is more commonly seen when the diagnosis of foreign body aspiration is delayed and secondary complications, such as bron- chiectasis, empyema, segmental collapse, or recurrent pneumonia have occurred.[3]

44.6   POSTOPERATIVE MANAGEMENT

44.6.1   Is there a role for steroids, aerosolized epinephrine, bronchodilators, and antibiotics in the postoperative care of this patient?

The use of steroids in the postoperative period may be beneficial if mucosal edema and granulation tissue were present in the vicinity of the airway foreign body. Aerosolized epinephrine is unlikely to be needed unless faced with postoperative stridor following traumatic foreign body removal. Bronchodilators are used infrequently, but may be helpful in the presence of persistent segmental atelectasis, more commonly seen if the foreign body has been present for a prolonged period of time. Similarly, antibiotics are not used routinely, unless there is evidence of perforation, granulation tissue or suppuration around the foreign body, or in the distal airways.[3]

44.6.2   What investigative modalities are warranted postoperatively? What is the appropriate management of this patient if the immediate postoperative chest radiograph shows the presence of pneumomediastinum?

Postoperatively, the patient should be observed upon emergence from anesthesia to ensure that there are no sequelae, such as airway compromise or respiratory distress, following foreign body retrieval. If the object was small and completely removed, with minimal underlying airway edema, the patient may be discharged following a brief period of observation. Difficult retrievals or instability in the operating or recovery rooms definitely mandate overnight-monitored observation.

If the patient exhibits pneumomediastinum on postoperative chest x-ray, clinical symptomatology must be correlated to determine whether further investigation or invasive therapies are warranted. Most commonly, there are few signs or symptoms associated with pneumomediastinum, precordial crepitus and voice change being the most common. Ideally, PPV should be avoided if possible as this may exacerbate the situation. Generally, such patients are monitored in an intensive care setting and are subject to serial chest radiographs to monitor regression or progression. Usually there is slow resolution over a few days, without significant sequelae.

44.7   SUMMARY

Airway foreign bodies in children can pose multiple challenges. The task of removing the object requires a team approach for the best possible patient outcome. Gathering as much information as possible prior to entering the operating room will enable better planning for foreign body retrieval, while keeping the patient's safety at the forefront. The size and nature of the aspirated object, its location in the airway, the time elapsed since aspiration, and patient factors such as age, and other associated comorbidities, all weigh into the planning of retrieval. Communication, preparation, and practice are the means by which successful outcomes are achieved.

REFERENCES

1. Brown L, Sherwin T, Perez JE, Perez DU. Heliox as a temporizing measure for pediatric foreign body aspiration. *Acad Emerg Med.* Apr 2002;9(4): 346-347.
2. Thomas GR, Dave S, Furze A, et al. Managing common otolaryngologic emergencies. *Emerg Med.* 2005;37(5):18-47.
3. Rovin JD, Rodgers BM. Pediatric foreign body aspiration. *Pediatr Rev.* Mar 2000;21(3):86-90.
4. Hong SJ, Goo HW, Roh JL. Utility of spiral and cine CT scans in pediatric patients suspected of aspirating radiolucent foreign bodies. *Otolaryngol Head Neck Surg.* May 2008;138(5):576-580.
5. Gibson SE, Shot SR. Foreign bodies of the upper aerodigestive tract. *The Pediatric Airway—An Interdisciplinary Approach.* Philadelphia, PA: JB Lippincott Co.; 1995.
6. Altkorn R, Chen X, Milkovich S, et al. Fatal and non-fatal food injuries among children (aged 0-14 years). *Int J Pediatr Otorhinolaryngol.* Jul 2008; 72(7):1041-1046.
7. Chatterji S, Chatterji P. The management of foreign bodies in air passages. *Anaesthesia.* Oct 1972;27(4):390-395.
8. Tan HK, Tan SS. Inhaled foreign bodies in children—anaesthetic considerations. *Singapore Med J.* Oct 2000;41(10):506-510.
9. Kumra VP. Anaesthetic considerations for specialized surgeries peculiar to paediatric age group. *Indian J Anaesth.* 2004;48:376-386.
10. Litman RS, Ponnuri J, Trogan I. Anesthesia for tracheal or bronchial foreign body removal in children: an analysis of ninety-four cases. *Anesth Analg.* Dec 2000;91(6):1389-1391.
11. Holzman RS. Spontaneous for suspected airway foreign body removal. *Society for Pediatric Anesthesia. Summer Newsletter.* 2001.
12. Paterson NA. Management of an unusual pediatric difficult airway using ketamine as a sole agent. *Paediatr Anaesth.* Aug 2008;18(8):785-788.
13. McGuirt WF, Holmes KD, Feehs R, Browne JD. Tracheobronchial foreign bodies. *Laryngoscope.* Jun 1988;98(6 Pt 1):615-618.
14. Midulla F, de Blic J, Barbato A, et al. Flexible endoscopy of paediatric airways. *Eur Respir J.* Oct 2003;22(4):698-708.
15. Ramirez-Figueroa JL, Gochicoa-Rangel LG, Ramirez-San Juan DH, Vargas MH. Foreign body removal by flexible fiberoptic bronchoscopy in infants and children. *Pediatr Pulmonol.* Nov 2005;40(5):392-397.
16. Marks SC, Marsh BR, Dudgeon DL. Indications for open surgical removal of airway foreign bodies. *Ann Otol Rhinol Laryngol.* Sep 1993;102(9):690-694.
17. Ulku R, Onen A, Onat S, Ozcelik C. The value of open surgical approaches for aspirated pen caps. *J Pediatr Surg.* Nov 2005;40(11):1780-1783.

SELF-EVALUATION QUESTIONS

44.1. Which of the following is **NOT** recommended for, nor to facilitate, the inhalational induction of anesthesia to remove a foreign body from the trachea?

A. desflurane

B. atropine

C. midazolam

D. sevoflurane

E. halothane

44.2. All of the following aids are generally considered to be reasonable in the removal of an airway foreign body **EXCEPT**:

A. LMA

B. flexible bronchoscope for object removal

C. avoidance of the use of nitrous oxide

D. avoidance of IPPV

E. removal of the foreign body through a rigid bronchoscope

44.3. Surgical removal of an airway foreign body is recommended under all of the following circumstances **EXCEPT**:

A. if the foreign body is sharp, pointed, and embedded in the tracheal or bronchial wall

B. if the foreign body is found in a small inaccessible peripheral bronchus

C. if the foreign body has been present for a prolonged period often for several years

D. if there is significant instability in maintaining control of the airway upon insertion and manipulation with the bronchoscope

E. if the foreign body is lodged at the carina

CHAPTER (45)

Management of a Child with a History of Difficult Intubation and Post-tonsillectomy Bleed

Arnim Vlatten

45.1 CASE PRESENTATION

A 6-year-old-boy with Down syndrome is on his way to the children's hospital by ambulance with post-tonsillectomy bleeding.

He underwent adenotonsillectomy because of recurrent tonsillitis and enlarged adenoids under general anesthesia the day before, some 22 hours ago. Despite being overweight at 37 kg and enlarged adenoids he did not suffer from sleep apnea. Prior to his original surgery, the child was uncooperative necessitating an inhalation induction with some struggling. Venous access was difficult even post-induction requiring several attempts, and finally being achieved in the left saphenous vein at the ankle. Because of possible atlanto-occipital instability associated with Down syndrome, laryngoscopy was performed with cervical spine (C-spine) precautions. Direct laryngoscopy presented a Grade 3 view due to an enlarged tongue. Bag-mask-ventilation with an oropharyngeal airway was easy throughout the preintubation phase. Indirect laryngoscopy using the GlideScope® revealed a Grade 1 view followed by the placement of a styletted, uncuffed 5-mm ID oral RAE tube. Adenotonsillectomy was performed in the usual fashion and the child was discharged home after an uneventful 20 hour overnight observation period.

Apparently, while momentarily unattended at home, the boy ate a hard tea biscuit. The child immediately experienced a sharp pain and an intra-oral bleeding started.

The emergency physician on duty is confronted with an overweight boy, sitting on a stretcher and spitting blood frequently into a kidney basin. The child is in moderate distress with the following vital signs (HR 152 bpm, BP 97/57 mm Hg). The child will not tolerate nasal prong oxygen and the pulse oximeter reading is 94%

on room air. Auscultation of the chest is clear. Examination of the mouth reveals brisk bleeding in the right tonsillar bed. An attempt to start an intravenous line in the right saphenous vein is not successful, but blood is obtained for a CBC, coagulation parameters, and cross match for blood. The child is then transferred to the operating room (OR).

45.2 INTRODUCTION

45.2.1 What is the incidence, morbidity, and mortality of pediatric post-tonsillectomy bleeding?

Tonsillectomy is one of the most frequently performed surgical procedures in children. Rates in children aged 0 to 14 vary considerably within and between countries. In 1998, they varied from 19 per 10,000 children in Canada to 118 per 10,000 in Northern Ireland, so a very common procedure in both countries.[1]

The most common post-tonsillectomy complications include postoperative nausea and vomiting and pain. Dehydration may occur in children due to delayed and poor oral intake, nausea, and fever. Delayed postoperative bleeding is the most significant complication and though uncommon, is not rare.[2] Many estimates of the incidence of post-tonsillectomy bleeding exist in the literature varying widely from 0% to 11.5%.[3] Typically, however, the rate ranges between 2.9% and 3.4%.[4] Mortality rates are rarely reported in the literature. Two large studies reported 0 out of 15,996 and 1 out of 16,381 tonsillectomies in 1979 and 1970, respectively.[5] On the other hand, there are many published case reports.

Sixty-seven percent of post-adenotonsillectomy bleeding originates in the tonsillar fossa and 27% in the nasopharynx. There are two major time frames for postoperative bleeding. Most often, the bleeding occurs within the first 24 hours after surgery (primary bleeding).[5] Primary bleeding is generally related to surgical technique, and incidence is declining. Twenty five percent of all post-tonsillectomy hemorrhage occurs after 24 hours. This secondary bleeding is not related to surgical technique, is rare and of unchanged prevalence over the years.[5] It is mainly observed between the 5th and 10th postoperative day, although it may occur at any time.[6] Infection of the tonsillar bed with clot sloughing is believed to be the major cause of secondary bleeding. It tends to occur more commonly in older pediatric patients, because the indication for tonsillectomy in this age group is usually related to recurrent infections rather than airway obstruction, the most common indication in the younger pediatric age group.[5]

Since tonsillectomy is usually performed to improve the quality of life in otherwise healthy, young children, any death is unacceptable.

45.3   PATIENT EVALUATION

45.3.1   What are the initial clinical steps one should take in the patient with post-tonsillectomy bleeding?

The diagnosis of post-tonsillectomy bleeding is usually made by a quick history. Parents or patients will mention right away the previous surgery. Differential diagnosis is blunt or sharp trauma to the oropharynx. Rare cases are bleeding tumors of the oropharynx, like hemangiomas.

The child will present with fresh blood in the mouth and frequent swallowing of blood. Nausea with or without emesis of fresh blood is common. Newer and more potent antiemetic medications may mask or suppress vomiting. Therefore, the amount of blood swallowed may be underestimated. It is not uncommon for children to have been bleeding silently for a prolonged period of time with extensive blood loss.

The child is often restless, diaphoretic, and pale. The vital signs may show an increased heart rate, because of pain and hypovolemia. In awake children, hypotension following blood loss is a very late sign and then indicates significant hypovolemia. Intravenous access must be established as soon as possible followed by initial volume resuscitation with crystalloid or colloid solution. A blood sample for baseline hematocrit or hemoglobin is necessary as well as for blood type and cross match.

An intra-oral examination will show blood and blood clots. A bleeding source may be seen in the tonsillar bed.

Bleeding from the tonsillar bed may initially be controlled using pharyngeal packs and cautery. But children with post-tonsillectomy bleeding should be taken back to the operating room for exploration and surgical hemostasis. Repeated attempts to stop bleeding on the ward or in the emergency department should be avoided, except if exsanguination is imminent.

A questionnaire of children undergoing tonsillectomy with or without postoperative bleeding showed an increased incidence of posttraumatic stress disorder if the children with bleeding were treated on the ward compared to children without bleeding or if the bleeding was treated in the operating room.[7]

45.4   AIRWAY MANAGEMENT

45.4.1   How is the airway usually managed in post-tonsillectomy bleeding?

Large volumes of blood may be swallowed, and blood or blood clots are often present in the oral cavity of these children. Despite the fact that the aspiration of blood is not similar in severity to aspiration of gastric acid, it remains an undesirable occurrence.

In addition to hypovolemia, patients with post-tonsillectomy bleeding present two major problems:

- Aspiration: These patients must be considered to have a full stomach and are at an increased risk of aspiration.
- Difficult airway: Blood and blood clots may impair visualization to the vocal cords. In addition swelling of the oropharynx may have occurred because of surgery or infection. This may lead to a changed laryngeal anatomy.

Because of the risk of aspiration, a mask induction maintaining spontaneous breathing is not desirable and a rapid-sequence induction should be considered. The efficacy and use of cricoid pressure, especially in children, is currently controversial. It is noteworthy that cricoid pressure can distort the laryngeal anatomy and worsen the view of the larynx. In addition, it can induce vomiting in the partially anesthetized patient.

The blood and blood clots in the oropharynx can impair vision during laryngoscopy or cause plugging of the endotracheal tube. A working suction apparatus is lifesaving and must be prepared in duplicate. One should be a large-bore, rigid surgical suction and the other mounted with a flexible endotracheal suction catheter. If one becomes blocked with a blood clot, another is readily available. If large amounts of clot are present, it may be necessary during the initial laryngoscopy to manually remove them with a finger or gauze. Magill forceps should be available to grab clots deeper in the pharynx, recognizing that these clots may be too fragile to be grasped and removed from the oral cavity using the forceps.

Awareness of a past history of difficult laryngoscopy is helpful, although this never precludes preparations for a difficult and failed airway. Different-sized curved and straight blades as well as a flex tip blade (McCoy laryngoscope) should be readily available. Different-sized cuffed endotracheal tubes, with one size up and down of the calculated size must be prepared. They should be preloaded with a well-lubricated intubating stylet, as is standard for a rapid-sequence induction.

An Eschmann Tracheal Introducer may be helpful in the presence of a Grade 3 view. If the epiglottis is visible, but no laryngeal entrance can be appreciated, a stroke of chest compression may help find the glottic opening by creating air bubbles.

The pediatric lightwand represents an elegant technique for intubation in the case of a glottic view obscured by secretions or blood. The extremely bright light can shine easily through blood and blood clots. However, experience is necessary when using this device.

Indirect laryngoscopy using the video laryngoscope (GlideScope® or the Airtraq®) can be difficult. Blood and secretions may block the optical lenses and impair the view to the vocal cords. The lens in the Airtraq® with its position between the lightsource on one side and the guide channel for the endotracheal tube on the other side might be more protected than the lens of the GlideScope®. Case reports or studies, however, have not been published in this regard.

The laryngeal mask plays an accepted role as an alternative airway device in managing the difficult pediatric airway (see Chapter 42). It is used frequently in primary adenotonsillectomies. It can be placed quickly and can be used as a conduit for a flexible bronchoscope to guide intubation if required. On the positive side, a laryngeal mask may briefly tamponade the bleeding site, and therefore protect the airway and the optical lens of the bronchoscope. Though, on the other hand, it may not provide sufficient airway protection in situations with increased risk of aspiration like post-tonsillectomy bleeding. A case report recently described the successful use of a laryngeal mask for a failed intubation in a post-tonsillectomy bleed.[8]

The use of a flexible bronchoscope alone is not recommended in cases of oropharyngeal bleeding. Experts recommend that the practitioner should rely on the alternative techniques with which they have the most experience and skill.

Preparation for the unexpected is essential. An experienced otolaryngologist or other qualified rigid laryngoscopist/bronchoscopist should be in the OR for all of these cases. If direct laryngoscopy fails, a rigid device wielded by the otolaryngologist may just be successful. An appropriately sized, lubricated, and tested rigid laryngoscope/bronchoscope connected to a light source and suction must be readily available at the head of the child. Preparation for a surgical airway is also essential (eg, tracheotomy tray opened and ready).

To reduce the risk of postoperative nausea and vomiting the stomach content of the child should be suctioned using an orogastric tube at the end of the procedure, recognizing that this does not guarantee an empty stomach as much of the blood may be clotted.

45.4.2   What are the airway management options for this patient?

This patient presents several issues regarding anesthesia induction and airway management:

- Uncooperative
- High risk of aspiration
- Difficult intravenous access
- Suspected atlanto-occipital instability
- Known difficult direct laryngoscopy with easy face mask ventilation
- Expected difficult view of the larynx due to blood and secretions

Several options for the anesthetic and airway management of this child need to be weighed and considered in light of their risks and benefits.

45.4.2.1   Intravenous Induction versus Inhalation Induction without IV Access

This child is undergoing a second surgical procedure within 24 hours. Due to the frightening emergency situation, pain, bleeding, and his mental impairment, he is distressed and uncooperative. While a smooth inhalation induction with a face mask was preferred for his first surgery, a stomach potentially full of blood mitigates against this approach and for a rapid-sequence induction to minimize the duration of an unprotected airway. One might even hope for a rapid venous access following a mask induction to permit medication administration but we know in this case that is not likely.

45.4.2.2   Anesthesia Induction with C-spine Precautions versus no C-spine Precautions

Down syndrome is associated with atlanto-occipital instability in up to 20% of cases. It can occur in children as young as 4 years of age. The atlanto-occipital instability of this child with Down syndrome places him at increased risk for C-spine injury during anesthetic induction. Radiographic findings of C-spine instability in Down syndrome remain controversial. Lateral radiographs of the neck in flexion and extension do not reliably detect atlanto-occipital instability. Due to impaired cognition and anxiety, positioning of the patient can be difficult. Old lateral neck radiographs are not available for this child. Due to the emergency situation, a current neck radiograph is not possible. Therefore C-spine precautions should be performed. Extreme neck extension should be avoided in this child.

45.4.2.3   Awake Tracheotomy versus Anesthesia Induction with Attempted Laryngoscopy

The fact that this child has a known difficult direct laryngoscopy together with a documented Grade 3 view favors an awake tracheotomy under local anesthesia. This approach would maintain a protected airway at all times. Awake tracheotomy in adults and children are challenging. Optimal surgical positioning with neck extension is crucial for successful procedure. It is not expected that this child will tolerate this procedure. This fact, together with the required C-spine precautions would exclude an awake tracheotomy as an option for this child.

The plan is to perform an intravenous rapid-sequence induction employing indirect laryngoscopy to place an endotracheal tube. Preparations for rigid laryngoscopy are in place and the surgeon is prepared to embark immediately with a surgical airway (in this case a triple setup).

45.4.3   How should you prepare for this case?

Following the failed attempt to start an intravenous line in the emergency department, the child was brought to the operating room. As previously outlined, venous access is crucial for induction and fluid resuscitation. Placement of a central line in the awake child is a possible option. For internal jugular vein access, the head may need to be rotated with increased risk associated with the presumed atlanto-occipital instability. The subclavian approach has the risk of a pneumothorax. An ultrasound-guided femoral vein approach is an alternative.

On the other hand, several studies have shown that an intraosseous cannula can be placed within 60 seconds and that this line provides an excellent access for the administration of medications and fluids. Because of the risks associated with central line placement, the child was prepared for an intraosseous cannula. The right leg was prepped with antiseptic solution, and local anesthetic injected at the tibial plateau. An intraosseous cannula was placed without incident. A normal saline solution flowed freely, permitting the administration of 20 mL·kg^{-1} body weight.

Atropine 0.1 mg IV was administered to reduce additional secretions and mitigate vagal responses secondary to laryngoscopy. The usual monitors were applied (pulse oximetry, noninvasive blood pressure, and ECG).

The surgeon was prepared as was his equipment; the rescue airway cart was in the room.

45.4.4   Management of this child

Concurrent with the placement of the intraosseous cannula, the child was prepared for a rapid-sequence induction. The lungs of the child were denitrogenated with 100% F$_{IO_2}$ for 3 minutes employing a facemask that was reasonably tolerated with much cajoling. Considering the possibility of significant hypovolemia a 50-50 mix of ketamine and propofol (ketofol) was selected for induction and succinylcholine for neuromuscular blockade. Cricoid pressure during induction was not applied to avoid stimulating vomiting in the already agitated child. It was applied after the child was deeply anesthetized. As soon as the child was deeply asleep and paralyzed, the mouth was suctioned easily and several clots were removed with the Magill forceps. The brisk bleeding from the right tonsillar bed was noted.

Since the previous direct laryngoscopy showed a Grade 3 view, a repeated direct laryngoscopy was not attempted. Because the oral cavity seemed to be free of clot, it was decided to proceed with indirect laryngoscopy with the GlideScope®. Unfortunately, blood obscured the lens and following a prolonged laryngoscopy the attempt to intubate was abandoned. Oxygen saturations fell from 100% to 94% and despite the risk of aspiration, bag-mask-ventilation was begun and cricoid pressure was maintained. Oxygen saturations recovered nicely.

At this point, faced with a failed intubation, rather than a failed airway it was decided to insert an LMA-Proseal™. The oral cavity was once again suctioned with a rigid catheter under direct laryngoscopy and a number 3.0 LMA-Proseal™ was easily placed. No air leak was noted and pressure-controlled ventilation with a pressure limit of 15 cm H$_2$O was started. A 5.5-mm ID uncuffed endotracheal tube was loaded on a pediatric flexible bronchoscope. Using the LMA-Proseal™ as a conduit, the bronchoscope was advanced into the trachea. Blood and secretions were

present in the LMA and in the trachea but did not obscure the view through the bronchoscope. The ETT was advanced easily over the bronchoscope into the trachea. With a small air leak at 20 cm H$_2$O airway pressure, it was decided not to change the ETT over a pediatric Cook airway exchanger to a cuffed ETT. Since the LMA-Proseal™ did not obscure the surgeons view, it was decided to leave the LMA-Proseal™ in place and remove it together with the ETT at the conclusion of the procedure and anesthesia.

With a secured airway, the ENT surgeon cauterized the tonsillar bed, and the bleeding artery could be ligated.

At the end of the procedure, a nasogastric tube was placed through the suction port of the LMA-Proseal™ and the stomach suctioned. The child was taken to the pediatric ICU where the ETT and LMA-Proseal™ were removed together an hour later.

45.5   OTHER CONSIDERATIONS

45.5.1   What is the current thinking with respect to the surgical management of post-tonsillectomy bleeding?

Life-threatening post-tonsillectomy bleeding requires an aggressive approach to surgical management. Initially, pressure on the bleeding tonsillar fossa with a clamped gauze or the index finger may give sufficient time to start an intravenous line for blood work and cross match, and to provide for fluid resuscitation or blood transfusion if indicated.

If intraoperative localization of the bleeding source is time consuming and local treatment is ineffective, ligation of the external carotid artery at an early stage may be required. Aberrant arterial blood supply to the tonsillar region deriving from the internal carotid artery or the carotid bulb may be present. In cases such as these, packing of the pharynx and angiographic embolization of the feeding artery may be necessary.[9]

45.5.2   Are there specific measures that one ought to employ to reduce the postoperative morbidity and mortality of patients following tonsillectomy?

The focus on post-tonsillectomy bleeding is on preventive measures, both by the surgeon and the anesthesia practitioner.

45.5.2.1   Tonsillectomy Technique

In comparison to the cold knife technique, hot techniques employing bipolar diathermy or coblation tonsillectomy are associated with an increased rate of secondary bleeding.[4,9] The duration, frequency, and surgical extent of these techniques are linked to the amount of damage to the surrounding tissue. This damage leads to deeper zones of local necrosis which is vulnerable to bacteria- and enzyme-containing saliva, and therefore at increased risk of secondary bleeding.[4,5]

45.5.2.2 Effects of Postoperative, Nonsteroidal, Anti-inflammatory Drugs

Nonsteroidal anti-inflammatory drugs (NSAIDs) inhibit platelet cyclo-oxygenase (COX). A recent meta-analysis showed an increased risk of reoperation for hemostasis post-tonsillectomy if conventional NSAIDs such as ketorolac, ibuprofen, or ketoprofen were used for postoperative pain control in children.[2] On the other hand ketorolac has been proven to be an effective treatment for post-tonsillectomy pain, and as a non-opioid delivers an intraoperative opioid-sparing effect and leads to a reduction in postoperative respiratory depression, nausea, and vomiting. A most recent meta-analysis did not find an altered number of perioperative bleeding events in patients given an NSAID.[10] Still, the use of these drugs should be discussed with the surgeon and used with caution.

45.5.2.3 Effects of Dexamethasone for Postoperative Nausea and Vomiting

Postoperative nausea and vomiting (PONV) increases the risk of primary hemorrhage and unexpected postoperative hospital admission. Dexamethasone has antiemetic properties in the perioperative setting. However, dexamethasone may inhibit wound healing, attenuate the inflammatory response to local infection, and as a result perhaps increase the risk of postoperative bleeding. A recent study in children undergoing tonsillectomy and administered dexamethasone was prematurely terminated because of an increased bleeding rate.[11] Similar to NSAIDs, the use of dexamethasone should be discussed with the surgeon and used with caution.

45.5.2.4 Tonsillectomy As Outpatient Surgery

Traditionally, tonsillectomy has been associated with a hospital inpatient admission. Economic imperatives have pushed hospitals to perform tonsillectomies as outpatient day surgery procedures.

The evidence has shown that this can be safely performed with the following exceptions:

- Age under 3 years
- Medical disorders that increase anesthetic and surgical risk
- Craniofacial abnormalities
- Abnormal coagulation, with or without an identifiable bleeding disorder
- Obstructive sleep apnea
- Acute peritonsillar abscess
- Family conditions that prevent easy and rapid return to a medical facility

Patients should always be observed for a minimum of 6 hours. They should be able to tolerate oral fluids and be pain tolerant prior to discharge. As an alternative to hospital admission, a 23-hour overnight observation period can be considered.

45.6 SUMMARY

Post-tonsillectomy bleeding is a rare event, which occurs most often within 24 hours following tonsillectomy. However, it may be delayed for up to 14 days postoperatively. The amount and severity of bleeding along with the need to ensure patient comfort and a still surgical field most often make operative revision under general anesthesia necessary. The insidious and continuous nature of the bleeding may lead to significant hypovolemia which is often difficult to assess. Blood work and cross match as well as preoperative intravenous access with fluid resuscitation are crucial in the management of these children.

Aspiration and a difficult airway are ever-present risks during the induction of anesthesia in patients with post-tonsillectomy bleed. Rapid-sequence induction with direct laryngoscopy and endotracheal intubation is the accepted first choice in the management of these children.

An array of pediatric airway management devices need to be immediately available. Blood and secretions can obscure the laryngeal view and can make some devices more useful than others. A surgeon experienced in rigid bronchoscopy and establishment of a surgical airway must be present during anesthesia induction. Cautious use of nonsteroidal inflammatory drugs and steroids is advocated.

REFERENCES

1. Van Den Akker EH, Hoes AW, Burton MJ, Schilder AG. Large international differences in (adeno)tonsillectomy rates. *Clin Otolaryngol Allied Sci.* 2004;29:161-164.
2. Marret E, Flahault A, Samama CM, Bonnet F. Effects of postoperative, nonsteroidal, antiinflammatory drugs on bleeding risk after tonsillectomy: meta-analysis of randomized, controlled trials. *Anesthesiology.* 2003;98:1497-1502.
3. Windfuhr JP. Coblation tonsillectomy: a review of the literature. *HNO.* 2007;55:337-348.
4. Lowe D, van der Meulen J. Tonsillectomy technique as a risk factor for postoperative haemorrhage. *Lancet.* 2004;364:697-702.
5. Windfuhr JP, Schloendorff G, Sesterhenn AM, et al. A devastating outcome after adenoidectomy and tonsillectomy: ideas for improved prevention and management. *Otolaryngol Head Neck Surg.* 2009;140:191-196.
6. Peterson J, Losek JD. Post-tonsillectomy hemorrhage and pediatric emergency care. *Clin Pediatr (Phila).* 2004;43:445-448.
7. Bissonnette B, Dalens BJ. *Pediatric Anesthesia: Principles and Practice.* New York: McGraw-Hill; 2002.
8. Lim NL. The use of the laryngeal mask airway in post-tonsillectomy haemorrhage—a case report. *Ann Acad Med Singapore.* 2000;29:764-765.
9. Windfuhr JP, Schloendorff G, Baburi D, Kremer B. Life-threatening post-tonsillectomy hemorrhage. *Laryngoscope.* 2008;118:1389-1394.
10. Cardwell M, Siviter G, Smith A. Non-steroidal anti-inflammatory drugs and perioperative bleeding in paediatric tonsillectomy. *Cochrane Database Syst Rev.* 2005:CD003591.
11. Czarnetzki C, Elia N, Lysakowski C, et al. Dexamethasone and risk of nausea and vomiting and postoperative bleeding after tonsillectomy in children: a randomized trial. *JAMA.* 2008;300:2621-2630.

SELF-EVALUATION QUESTIONS

45.1. All of the following airway devices are acceptable in the management of post-tonsillectomy bleeding **EXCEPT**:

   A. direct laryngoscopy

   B. indirect laryngoscopy

   C. Trachlight

   D. awake bronchoscopy

   E. LMA with subsequent bronchoscopy-guided endotracheal intubation

45.2. What is the generally accepted perioperative management in severe post-tonsillectomy bleeding:

A. history and physical, followed by rapid IV access with fluid resuscitation and operative revision under general anesthesia with endotracheal intubation

B. history and physical, followed by IV access with fluid resuscitation and operative revision under sedation without endotracheal intubation, to avoid laryngospasm

C. endotracheal intubation in the emergency room as soon as possible because of the risk of rapid swelling of the oropharynx

D. no operative intervention, as chance of spontaneous stop of bleeding outweighs the anesthesia risk (aspiration, difficult airway, etc)

E. history and physical, IV access and blood work, and elective operative revision as soon as the 6 hours NPO timeframe is reached because of the risk of aspiration

45.3. All of the following medications should be used with caution during post-tonsillectomy bleeding **EXCEPT**:

A. ketorolac

B dexamethasone

C. ibuprofen

D. morphine

E. hetastarch

CHAPTER (46)

Airway Management in a 1-Year-Old with Pierre Robin Syndrome for Myringotomy and Tubes

Christian M. Soder

46.1 CASE PRESENTATION

A 1-year-old-infant known to have Robin sequence (synonym: Pierre Robin syndrome or Pierre Robin sequence) presents with chronic otitis media and significant conductive hearing loss. The pediatric otolaryngologist has booked him for bilateral myringotomy and tube insertion. An operating room time of 20 minutes has been scheduled. The patient has been evaluated in the outpatient clinic by an anesthesia colleague. Her consultation report states that the infant was hospitalized for the first 3 months of his life for severe airway obstruction and feeding difficulties. Mandibular distraction osteogenesis surgery is not performed at this center, so the airway was managed by *glossopexy* (tongue sutured to lip) during the first month of life. The anesthesia record for this procedure indicates that the infant was intubated awake with great difficulty by a team of pediatric anesthesia practitioners, employing an unorthodox combination of the infant-size Trachlight™ and direct straight-blade laryngoscopy. It is noted that the infant currently still sleeps on his stomach without apparent apnea or airway obstruction, but develops stridor and apnea if placed on his back.

46.2 INTRODUCTION

46.2.1 What is Robin sequence?

Robin sequence (named for the eminent French dentist, Pierre Robin, who first described it) has become synonymous with the pediatric anesthesia practitioner's worst airway nightmare. The condition is believed to be the result of primary failure in fetal mandibular development. The resulting micrognathia leads to rostral displacement of the tongue, termed *glossoptosis*. In 50% of cases the displacement of the normal-sized tongue into the roof of the mouth leads to failure of fusion of the maxillary arches and a resultant cleft palate. The combination of cleft palate and malposition of the tongue leads to airway obstruction, recurrent episodes of hypoxemia and hypercapnia, pulmonary hypertension, sleep apnea, swallowing difficulties, failure to thrive, and chronic ear disease.[1] Although the Robin sequence is an isolated anomaly in two-thirds of cases, similar features are found in multiple malformation patterns, including Treacher Collins syndrome, Stickler syndrome, and Velocardiofacial syndrome. Accurate diagnosis of multiple anomaly syndromes is important in formulating the airway plan because of the possible presence of associated major malformations, such as congenital heart disease.

Older texts quote a mortality of 50% for this anomaly. Good positioning (nursing in prone position), tube feeding, glossopexy (suturing the tongue to the lip to pull it forward), mandibular distraction osteogenesis surgery,[2,3] prevention or treatment of aspiration pneumonia, and reduced incidence of pulmonary hypertension (less exposure to hypoxemia and hypercarbia) have combined to reduce mortality to below 5%. After birth, growth of the mandible proceeds normally, and surgical closure of the cleft palate eventually allows for the development of near-normal airway anatomy, normal swallowing, normal growth, and full physical and intellectual development.

The anesthesia practitioner respects this malformation because the trachea of these patients is notoriously difficult to intubate and BMV is often difficult, which is unfortunate because they frequently need surgery. To compound the matter, the currently recommended treatment is long-term conservative management that does not usually include tracheotomy. The challenge for the anesthesia team is to safely provide repeated general anesthetics to a child with a terrible airway. The good news is that the long-term prognosis for the syndrome is excellent, if the patient survives the repeated general anesthetics.

46.3   PATIENT CONSIDERATION

46.3.1   How do you assess the airway of this patient?

Robin sequence poses the classic *small chin conundrum*: difficult BMV and difficult direct laryngoscopy (DL).[4,5] The lack of a well-developed mentum creates significant problems with mask fit (no seal below the lower lip), making BMV difficult or impossible. The glossoptosis places the tongue posteriorly and superiorly into apposition with the roof of the mouth. If Mallampati scores could be performed on these infants, they would score a IV! With loss of consciousness, airway obstruction often becomes complete, and its correction by an oropharyngeal airway is difficult unless a perfect fit is achieved. These patients are usually at their best in the prone position, because gravity helps keep the tongue off the roof of the mouth. They may develop varying degrees of obstruction when placed supine.

On the positive side, extraglottic devices, such as the laryngeal mask airway (LMA), have been reported to be effective in providing ventilation and oxygenation.[6,7,8] An appropriately sized oropharyngeal airway (OPA), nasopharyngeal airway (NPA), or laryngeal mask airway (LMA), can often be placed easily and will usually maintain the airway. The LMA may well prove to be the airway of choice for some surgical procedures in Robin sequence, particularly minor procedures not involving or near the airway.

Glossoptosis and mandibular hypoplasia combine to make direct laryngoscopy very difficult. The glottic opening is angled away from the oral axis more than the usual 90 degrees, and the virtual absence of a submental space means that the laryngoscope blade cannot displace the tongue into this area. Fortunately, the cleft palate in Robin sequence is not accompanied by a cleft lip, and therefore does not interfere with laryngoscopy. In extreme cases, the mandibular hypoplasia is so severe that the tongue completely obstructs direct visualization of the larynx, despite optimal direct laryngoscopic technique, delivering a true Cormack/Lehane (C/L) Grade 4 view of the larynx.

Until recently, many alternate intubation devices were not available in pediatric sizes. However, there is now growing experience with newer alternate pediatric intubation techniques. The author and his colleagues have successfully intubated infants with Robin sequence using the infant Airtraq optical laryngoscope™, Trachlight™, STORZ video laryngoscope™, GlideScope®, and Bonfils intubation fiberscope™. Others have reported successful use of the Bullard™ laryngoscope, Shikani optical stylet™,[9] and flexible bronchoscopic intubation, with or without the use of an LMA guide.[10]

Subglottic anatomy is normal but these patients are usually too young to have an identifiable cricothyroid membrane: This precludes surgical or percutaneous cricothyrotomy. However, open or percutaneous tracheotomy is possible and increased familiarity,

and experience, with percutaneous tracheal access may bring this approach within the skill set of most pediatric anesthesia practitioners. Tracheal catheter jet ventilation using the Enk™ adaptor is still considered a feasible emergency pediatric option, although experience is extremely limited. Surgical backup and even full double setup is advisable for severe cases.

How do we recognize such a severe case? Risk factors include hyomental distance less than 1 cm (ie, severe mandibular hypoplasia), inability to maintain airway when awake and supine (severe glossoptosis), oxygen dependence, history of significant pulmonary disease, and prior episodes of failed airway in competent hands.

46.3.2   Do you have any medical concerns for this patient?

Isolated Robin sequence is not associated with major cardiac or other malformations. However, these patients usually require anesthetics during their first year of life—a time when their anatomic challenges are complicated by the normal physiologic limitations of infancy, such as reduced effectiveness of denitrogenation increasing the risk and speed of onset of desaturation. In addition, some of these infants have problems with recurrent aspiration and pulmonary hypertension further reducing cardiopulmonary reserve. In Robin sequence infants airway obstruction is followed almost immediately by desaturation and bradycardia. Planning steps A, B, and C is vital as there is precious little time to think once the airway is lost.

46.4   AIRWAY MANAGEMENT

46.4.1   What are the alternatives in managing the airway of this patient under general anesthesia?

At age 1, this patient is no longer at maximum risk: He has survived to discharge, has lived safely at home, does not need home oxygen, and has no history of serious pulmonary disease. However, the history of a previously failed airway with the need for glossopexy in the newborn period, and persistent airway obstruction when supine, are evidence of significant on-going glossoptosis. These issues indicate an increased risk for difficult DL and BMV. The airway management plan for Robin sequence must reflect these risks.

46.4.1.1   Plan A: Attempt to Maintain an Extraglottic Airway

After the placement of an intravenous catheter, and the application of appropriate monitors, anesthesia is induced with oxygen-sevoflurane. Under deep anesthesia, an extraglottic device is placed. This will be followed by myringotomy and tube insertion surgery.

46.4.1.2   Plan B: Failed Extraglottic Airway

Should an extraglottic airway fail, additional assistance should immediately be summoned. It is reasonable to attempt a return to BMV, but if this fails then intubation with DL using a straight blade should be attempted. Should intubation by DL fail, it may nonetheless be possible to effect gas exchange by maintaining an open airway with the laryngoscope in position, employing the patient's own spontaneous respiratory efforts to maintain saturations and anesthesia. This is followed by the implementation of a planned sequence of alternate intubation techniques. Alternately, it is reasonable to bypass DL and proceed directly to an alternate airway management technique.

46.4.1.3   Plan C: Failed Ventilation and Intubation

If ventilation and intubation fail (cannot intubate, cannot ventilate [CICV]), one should proceed to either percutaneous tracheostomy or surgical tracheostomy, depending on the available resources. Concurrent or nearly concurrent actions may be indicated depending on the ability to maintain oxygen saturation.

The airway management plan for the infant with an inadequate submandibular space due to Robin sequence presents some unusual features. The airway of choice for bilateral myringotomy and tube in Robin sequence is the OPA or LMA (Plan A). The anatomy is suitable for supraglottic device placement and experience has shown that it usually works. The anatomy is unfavorable for laryngoscopy and an endotracheal tube is not necessary for the surgery. However if a supraglottic airway does fail and the airway cannot be restored promptly by BMV, the next maneuver should be the insertion of a laryngoscope blade or an alternate intubation device (Plan B). Many pediatric anesthesia practitioners have observed that displacing the glossoptotic tongue with a device can open the obstructed Robin sequence airway, permitting spontaneous ventilation to continue. This technique can buy time to optimize laryngoscopy, manipulate the airway, deploy airway adjuncts, and attempt alternate intubation techniques. If the airway cannot be maintained by an extraglottic device, cannot be obtained by laryngoscopy or alternate technique, and cannot be awakened, the failed airway procedure becomes necessary (Plan C).

46.4.2   How do you prepare to manage the anesthesia and airway of this patient?

Even though the procedure is scheduled for less than 1 hour and is, therefore, a minor procedure, it is a major anesthetic, and this paradox must be discussed with the surgeon, staff, and family. In addition to the usual pre-anesthetic routine, airway equipment preparations ought to include several potentially useful masks and OPAs, and two laryngoscope handles with straight blades of varying length and width. The Flagg or Wisconsin designs have the advantage of being completely straight (maximum optical path efficiency) and having circular cross-sections (more room to see and pass the tube). Multiple 3.0, 3.5, and 4.0 mm ID endotracheal tubes, with well-lubricated hockey-stick-shaped intubating stylets preloaded on one tube of each size, are prepared, as are number 0 to 2 LMAs, tested, and lubricated. A lubricated pediatric-size Eschmann tracheal tube introducer should be prepared. The anesthesia practitioner, based on familiarity with the techniques, should also set up one or more alternate intubating devices connected to light source, loaded, defogged, lubricated, and

tested as appropriate for the device. Options include but are not limited to a rigid laryngoscope; Bullard™ laryngoscope; Trachlight™; Air-Traq Optical Laryngoscope™; Storz Video Laryngoscope™; GlideScope®; Bonfils Intubation Fibrescope™; and Shikani Optical Stylet™.

Surgical equipment available should include a surgical tracheotomy tray, a #1 Melker™ uncuffed cricothyrotomy set, or an 18/16 gauge IV cannula and Enk adaptor. If the patient presented with more threatening risk factors (eg, severe pulmonary disease), the surgeon should be gowned and gloved, the tray would be opened, the tracheotomy tube selected, and the skin prepared prior to induction of anesthesia. In this case, a second anesthesia practitioner should be on stand-by in the room.

Succinylcholine 20 mg (for laryngospasm on BMV or LMA), atropine 0.4 mg (to mitigate bradycardia), and epinephrine 1 cc 1/10,000 (to respond to hypoxemia-induced myocardial depression) are drawn up. Other standard resuscitation drugs should be available on the cart.

46.4.3   Discuss the conduct of anesthesia for this patient

The child is brought into the operating room (OR). Parental attendance is usually forgone in this scenario, to minimize distraction. An IV is inserted prior to induction of anesthesia. Atropine 0.1 mg IV is administered to reduce secretions and mitigate vagal responses (bradycardia). Pulse oximeter, BP cuff, and ECG monitors are applied. Mask fitting and denitrogenation proceed for 2 to 3 minutes. Induction starts with 8% sevoflurane and 100% oxygen at 2 L·min^{-1} flow. The OPA or LMA is inserted after the sevoflurane excitement phase passes.

Position is confirmed by CO_2 detection, and anesthetic depth is optimized. When sustained regular spontaneous respirations, normal pulse oximetry readings, and appropriate heart rate and blood pressure for age are achieved, the surgical procedure may begin. If the airway is lost and cannot be regained at any stage of the proceedings, a laryngoscope (#2 straight blade) is inserted using a paraglossal approach to displace the tongue laterally. If the airway is opened by this maneuver and if spontaneous breathing continues, endotracheal intubation is attempted when anesthetic depth is adequate. Laryngoscopy can be optimized by external laryngeal manipulation and placement of the endotracheal tube can be facilitated by the traditional hockey-stick-shaped intubating stylet, or the infant Eschmann tracheal tube introducer. The endotracheal tube can also be mounted on a hockey-stick-shaped Trachlight™, to improve visualization and confirm location.

If a C/L Grade 3 view can be obtained intubation by DL, using a stylet, is almost always possible. However, if the C/L Grade is 4, and/or intubation is unsuccessful, alternate intubation techniques may be helpful. The laryngoscope blade is left in situ for tongue control while oxygen and anesthetic agent, normally sevoflurane, are blown toward the airway. This can be achieved by inserting a 3.0 mm ETT into the oropharynx or nostril, and connecting it to the anesthesia circuit. Fresh gas flow of 6 to 10 L usually permits insufflation of sufficient oxygen and agent to maintain normoxemia and anesthesia. The following maneuvers are then considered in the order most familiar to the anesthesia practitioner: repeat laryngoscopy with blade or technique change; apply tongue traction using forceps or gauze to pull the tongue out of the mouth toward the left; attempt an alternate intubation technique; or attempt bronchoscopic intubation, with or without an LMA.

If, at any time, the airway or ventilation are lost and cannot be recovered by laryngoscopy, or alternate extraglottic techniques, the failed airway Plan C is activated. Depending on the skill and experience of the anesthesia practitioners and surgeons, a surgical tracheotomy is performed, a #1 Melker™ percutaneous tracheal tube is inserted, or a #16 or #18 gauge IV catheter is inserted into the trachea and connected to an Enk adaptor and oxygen source.

46.5   OTHER CONSIDERATIONS

46.5.1   Discuss postintubation management of this patient

Accurate endotracheal placement must be confirmed by end-tidal CO_2 detection. Although the published rate of inadvertent endobronchial intubation in a general pediatric intensive care population has been reported to be 2% to 3%, it is widely believed to be much more common in infants. Asymmetry of chest movement and persistent hypoxemia may follow endobronchial intubation in some cases, but there are no clinical signs with high specificity and reliability. Chest auscultation can be highly misleading due to ready transmission of breath sounds through the small infant chest cavity. Well-described adult techniques, including lightwand-assisted placement and flexible bronchoscopy, should theoretically be useful in pediatrics, but have not been assessed. Radiographic confirmation remains the definitive test and may be required if there is any doubt about tube tip location. It is obvious that, following a difficult intubation, the endotracheal tube must be well secured using a commercial fixation device, or by highly adherent adhesive tape fixed to the skin of the upper lip. Tincture of benzoin (Friars Balsam), or similar skin preparation agents, are recommended to dry and degrease the skin. At the end of the procedure, awake extubation is mandatory. Extubation in the prone position may be helpful. Complications of traumatic intubation, including subglottic edema, bleeding, and laryngeal injury, should be anticipated and planned for.

46.5.2   What is the extubation plan if the tracheal intubation was traumatic with significant airway edema?

Patients who have been intubated with difficulty are at risk for the development of post-extubation stridor, usually caused by subglottic edema or laryngeal inlet trauma. The symptoms usually appear within 4 hours of the inciting intubation and may persist for several days. Following a difficult intubation, there may well be a reluctance to remove the endotracheal tube because of the potential need for reintubation. In cases where trauma to the airway appears to have been minimal and a leak around the tube is present at the end of the case, awake extubation in the recovery room can be performed. If stridor develops, it is treated with epinephrine or phenylephrine aerosols and intravenous dexamethasone 0.5 to 1.0 mg·kg⁻¹. If available, heliox may be useful, although the reduction in work of breathing must be weighed against the reduction in F_{IO_2}. Pulse oximetry is essential. In obviously traumatic cases, or where there is no audible tube leak, the patient should be transferred to ICU for delayed extubation. Treatment there should include sedation, ventilation, and intravenous dexamethasone for 12 to 48 hours. When an audible leak around the tube is present, extubation should be considered. Flexible nasopharyngoscope or direct laryngoscopy should be considered to assess the state of the laryngeal inlet prior to extubation.

46.6   SUMMARY

Robin sequence is the pediatric model for difficult airway: the ultimate anterior larynx. Many congenital anomalies include Robin sequence or some of its features. There is no doubt that the severe glossoptosis in Robin sequence is intimidating, but the basic issues involved should be familiar ground for anesthesia practitioners. The approach is very similar to that used for the adult case that presents a C/L Grade 3 or 4 view on laryngoscopy. Face or laryngeal mask fit is the essential prerequisite to a basic airway (and to reduced practitioner stress!). The first attempts at intubation usually include maneuvers such as blade change (eg, straight blade), approach change (eg, paraglossal), position change (eg, flexion, head elevation), external laryngeal and/or tongue manipulation, and use of an Eschmann tracheal tube introducer or intubating stylet. Failing successful DL alternate intubation techniques using the Bullard™ Laryngoscope, Airtraq optical laryngoscope™, STORZ video laryngoscope™, Glidescope®, Bonfils intubation fiberscope™, and other devices, may be successful. Rescue can be accomplished with an LMA, and direct tracheal cannulation offers a final option. With anticipation and a good airway management plan, most patients with Robin sequence can be successfully managed and tracheotomy is rarely required.

REFERENCES

1. van den Elzen AP, Semmekrot BA, Bongers EM, Huygen PL, Marres HA. Diagnosis and treatment of the Pierre Robin sequence: results of a retrospective clinical study and review of the literature. *Eur J Pediatr.* 2001 Jan; 160(1):47-53.

2. Genecov DG, Barceló CR, Steinberg D, Trone T, Sperry E. Clinical experience with the application of distraction osteogenesis for airway obstruction. *J Craniofac Surg.* 2009 Sep; 20(Supp 2):1817-18213;

3. Nargozian C: The airway in patients with craniofacial abnormalities. *Paediatr Anaesth.* 2004 Jan;14(1):53-59.

4. Schaefer RB, Gosain AK. Airway management in patients with isolated Pierre Robin sequence during the first year of life. *J Craniofac Surg.* 2003 Jul;14(4):462-467.

5. Baraka A. Laryngeal mask airway for resuscitation of a newborn with Pierre-Robin syndrome. *Anaesthesiology.* 1996;83:645-646.

6. Selim M, Mowafi H, Al-Ghamdi A, Adu-Gyamfi Y. Intubation via LMA in pediatric patients with difficult airways. *Can J Anaesth.* 1999;46(9):891-893.

7. Ofer R, Dworzak H. The laryngeal mask—a valuable instrument for cases of difficult intubation in children. Anesthesiologic management in the presence of Pierre-Robin syndrome. *Der Anaesthesist.* 1996;45(3):268-270.

8. Baraka A, Muallem M. Bullard laryngoscopy for tracheal intubation in a neonate with Pierre-Robin syndrome. *Paediatr Anaesth*. 1994;4:111-113.

9. Schelle JG, Schulman SR. Fiberoptic bronchoscopic guidance for intubation of a neonate with Pierre Robin syndrome. *Anaesth Analg*. 1992;75:822-824.

10. Rasch DK, Browder F, Barr M, et al. Anaesthesia for Treacher Collins and Pierre Robin syndromes: a report of three cases. *Can Anaesth Soc J*. 1986 May; 33(3 Pt 1):364-370.

SELF-ASSESSMENT QUESTIONS

46.1 Patients with Robin sequence present challenges in airway management because of all of the following **EXCEPT**:

A. small mouth opening

B. mandibular hypoplasia

C. glossoptosis (apposition of tongue to palate)

D. high incidence of C/L Grade 3 or 4 views of the larynx

E. poor mask fit

46.2 Airway rescue techniques for the CICV situation that are possible in infants less than 1 year of age include all of the following **EXCEPT**:

A. tracheal cannulation with IV catheter and Enk adaptor

B. surgical tracheotomy

C. percutaneous cricothyroidotomy

D. insertion of Melker percutaneous tracheostomy tube

E. tracheal intubation using a flexible bronchoscope

46.3 All of the following findings in a patient with Robin sequence indicate increased risk of difficult airway management **EXCEPT**:

A. hyomental distance less than 1 cm

B. airway obstruction when prone

C. oxygen dependence

D. prior history of difficult intubation by qualified practitioners

E. presence of cleft palate

CHAPTER 47

Airway Management of a 6-Year-Old with a History of Difficult Airway for Bilateral Inguinal Hernia Repair

David C. Abramson

47.1 CASE PRESENTATION

A 6-year-old child with Crouzon syndrome (CS) presents with bilateral inguinal hernia for repair. His parents report that a previous craniosynostosis repair, at the age of 9 months, and a LeFort III osteotomy, at the age of 4 years, were both associated with a difficult airway and that the anesthesia practitioners had told them to pass this information onto the next practitioner. The child is otherwise well and of normal intelligence.

47.2 INTRODUCTION

47.2.1 What is Crouzon syndrome?

Crouzon and Apert syndromes are the most common of the craniosynostosis syndromes. In addition to craniosynostosis, these children also have fusion of the bony sutures in the cranial base and midface, and shallow eye sockets. This gives the appearance of a flat midface and eyes which protrude. Children with Apert syndrome (AS) also have syndactaly (webbing) of the hands and feet. The infant's shallow midface and/or small or partially obstructed nasal passages can cause airway compromise and airway management difficulties, as in this case. Evaluation by ENT specialists is important and a tracheotomy may be necessary to relieve chronic airway obstruction.[1]

CS occurs in approximately one in 25,000 births. It may be transmitted as an autosomal dominant genetic condition or appear as a fresh mutation (no affected parents). The appearance of an infant with CS can vary in severity from a mild presentation with subtle midface characteristics to severe forms with multiple fused cranial sutures and marked midface and eye problems. The incidence of AS is approximately one in 100,000 births and most cases are fresh mutations. The general features of a child with AS are similar to those in CS. However, there is not as much variability between cases and the degree of presentation is more severe.

47.2.2 Why is the team approach so important in cases like this?

Essential to the handling of this patient on an elective surgery basis is communication and preparation. The surgeon, on scheduling the case, should contact the anesthesia practitioner to advise them of the potential difficult airway management to prevent surprises and case cancellation. Should prior notification not occur, it is perfectly reasonable to delay this elective surgical procedure until information regarding the patient's past medical history is obtained.

The situation in an emergency is obviously much different with teamwork taking a *responsive* as opposed to a *proactive* posture, although many of the same specialists are usually involved in the care of these patients.

47.3 AIRWAY ASSESSMENT AND PREPARATION

47.3.1 How do you assess the airway of this child? What if he is uncooperative?

As 2 years have passed since the last surgery, one can expect some growth changes in the airway (see Chapter 42). This patient ought to be approached as a *new* difficult airway. It is incumbent upon the anesthesia practitioner to take a good history, paying particular attention as to whether this child has difficulty in breathing with different body positions, and whether there are symptoms of *upper-airway resistance syndrome*[2-8] or *sleep apnea* and, if present, whether these conditions have been formally evaluated. Typically, CS (proptosis, craniosynostosis, and maxillary hypoplasia) patients do not present with significant obstructive airway symptoms.

While the airway assessment (MOANS, LEMON, RODS, and SHORT) discussed in Chapter 1 is helpful to predict a difficult and failed airway in adults, it may not be applicable in the pediatric population. Examination of the airway should then focus on the ability of the patient to flex and extend the neck, open the mouth, and, most importantly, the capacity of the submandibular space to accommodate the tongue on direct laryngoscopy. Even if all these measurements are normal, a difficult airway under anesthesia should be anticipated and preparations made. In addition, an accurate weight and height should be recorded, as should a hematocrit.

47.3.2   What are the airway management options for this patient?

Several anesthesia options exist for this patient and all have been employed in children younger than 6 years:

1. Local/regional anesthesia without airway intervention
2. General and local/regional anesthesia with airway intervention
3. General anesthesia with intubation
   a. Direct laryngoscopy and intubation
   b. Flexible bronchoscopic intubation both with and without a guide
   c. Videolaryngoscopic intubation
4. Awake intubation prior to the induction of general anesthesia

From a pragmatic perspective, one is faced with a 6-year-old child requiring a bilateral inguinal hernia repair that does not require muscle relaxation and who is unlikely to cooperate with a procedure under local anesthesia.

47.3.3   What preparations for airway management are required?

If airway intervention is contemplated, IV access is mandatory and can be achieved either under sedation or awake. If awake, this may be facilitated by the use of either EMLA® (AstraZeneca) or LMX4® (ELA-Max) (Ferndale Laboratories, Inc., MI) applied topically to the skin 60 to 90 minutes prior to the IV start.[9] Similarly, if one is considering regional anesthesia (caudal or spinal) without airway intervention, application of these agents to the relevant anatomical area can easily be achieved and relatively painless regional anesthesia can be accomplished.

As usual, all anesthetic and emergency drugs should be prepared in advance. In addition, a difficult airway cart with appropriate equipment should be available in the operating room and checked (see Chapter 59). Experienced airway assistants should also be available, including a surgical staff who can perform a surgical airway, should it become necessary.

47.4   ANESTHESIA AND AIRWAY MANAGEMENT

47.4.1   How exactly should the airway of this patient be managed?

Most children will require some form of sedation prior to a procedure, particularly children with multiple prior contacts with health care providers as these children harbor a healthy suspicion of these providers! Midazolam is a reasonable anxiolytic, either as commercially available syrup or the concentrated IV form suspended in flavored syrup (although this concoction is usually unpleasantly bitter). A dose of 0.5 mg·kg⁻¹ (maximum 10 mg) is administered orally at least 15 minutes before attempting any separation from caretakers.[10] At this dose, respiratory depression has not been reported. Once IV access is obtained, further small incremental doses of midazolam can be titrated to effect, should a sedation technique be employed.

Most anesthesia practitioners would employ a combined general and regional anesthesia technique using a Laryngeal Mask Airway (LMA) or another of the increasingly available extraglottic devices (EGDs). Inhalation induction is the most common approach in these patients. This takes advantage of the fact that this technique maintains spontaneous ventilation and the ability of reversing the anesthetic at any point should airway maintenance become questionable. This technique is generally considered to be safe, particularly since neuromuscular-blocking agents (NMBA) are not being employed.

While many consider sevoflurane to be the preferred anesthetic agent for induction and maintenance of pediatric anesthesia, it does have several limitations:

1. Much higher incidence of emergence delirium.[11]
2. Marked depression of respiration in high concentration.
3. Too rapid a change in the level of consciousness.

If an IV is in place, some practitioners advise the administration of glycopyrrolate, 5 to 10 µg·kg⁻¹, as an antisialagogue. Atropine is less desirable as it has less drying action and more tachycardia associated with its use.

IV induction may be easily achieved with a number of agents, but, in the case of potential airway manipulation, propofol is often the drug of choice as it blunts airway responses to manipulation and is easily titratable.

Once anesthetized, an LMA or other EGD should be placed.[12] The insertion method for the LMA is described in Chapters 12 and 42. Correct placement is confirmed by hearing breath sounds and can be further validated by successful ventilation with positive pressure as well as a good end-tidal CO_2 tracing.

47.4.2   If one wants to perform a caudal block, how may that be done, especially if an LMA is in place?

Once the LMA/EGD is placed and secured, the child is turned into the left lateral decubitus position (for a right-handed practitioner) to perform the caudal block and then returned to the supine position for surgery. Attention to securing the LMA/EGD during any positioning procedure is vital as the seal is easily lost. This is particularly important in the smaller child (<10 kg), where initial placement tends to be more difficult.[13]

A detailed discussion of caudal block technique is beyond the scope of this chapter. Briefly, an agent with a rapid onset is preferred to avoid potential laryngospasm with surgical incision. An equal mixture of 2% lidocaine and 0.25% levobupivacaine (or 0.2% ropivacaine) 1 mL·kg⁻¹ will achieve this goal and produce a block of long duration as well. The addition of clonidine 1 to 2 $\mu g \cdot kg^{-1}$ [14] or neostigmine 2 to 4 $\mu g \cdot kg^{-1}$ [15] has been suggested to prolong the duration of the block. The caudal block can reduce the requirement of the anesthetic vapor and avoid respiratory depression associated with the use of opioid. If airway difficulty is encountered at any stage during the induction, simply turning off the inhalational agent and administering 100% oxygen will result in rapid awakening and recovery of airway reflexes.

47.4.3   How would one perform a flexible bronchoscopic intubation in this child?

If Plan A is unsuccessful or not practically feasible, Plans B and C should be prepared before bringing the patient to the operating room.

Flexible bronchoscopic intubation is ordinarily one of those plans. This can be done awake or asleep in this age group with patience and careful planning. These children can be very challenging, particularly if they have had previous negative interactions with health care personnel. It is difficult to employ logic and reasoning with a 6-year-old child. For this reason, moderate to heavy sedation is usually required. Oral midazolam 0.5 mg·kg⁻¹ (maximum 10 mg) is often effective as an initial sedating agent as one begins the process of preparing for the flexible bronchoscopic intubation.

Initially, both nasal passages are anesthetized with 4% aqueous lidocaine and vasoconstriction achieved with topical oxymetazoline. Nebulization of lidocaine is an effective airway anesthetic. The 4% solution commonly available can be diluted (with water, not saline because saline changes its pH) to 2% to give greater volume. Not more than 5 mg·kg⁻¹ should be placed in the nebulizing chamber and allowed to be slowly inhaled either in the holding area or on the way to the operating room. The finely nebulized particles will anesthetize the glottis and trachea to varying degrees.

Once in the operating room, IV access is mandatory before proceeding further, and, once secured, 5 µg·kg⁻¹ glycopyrrolate IV should immediately be given. Monitoring should be instituted (pulse oximetry, noninvasive blood pressure, and ECG at a minimum); suction, oxygen, emergency drugs, and airway equipment should be checked as discussed earlier. An experienced assistant will be required to help. If there is a failed airway and ventilation is not possible at any point during the intubating attempt, a surgeon should be immediately available to perform a rigid bronchoscopy or a surgical technique.

It is prudent to avoid the use of bolus doses of sedatives. For sedation, incremental doses of IV midazolam and propofol administered via an infusion pump should be done slowly. Importantly, one must allow time for the onset of drug effect to occur after titrating dosages. Haste is strongly discouraged as it increases the risk of losing the airway of a spontaneously breathing patient. If the patient becomes unconscious and apneic with the propofol infusion, it can be turned off and return of spontaneous ventilation should occur rapidly. It is a matter of personal preference to employ drug infusions instead of volatile agents for sedation or anesthesia for this procedure. Generally, infusions are easier to control than volatile agents, which can pollute the operating room environment. Additionally, it may be difficult to achieve a constant anesthetic concentration during the intubation procedure.

Flexible bronchoscopic intubation through the mouth without a guide to maintain the pediatric flexible bronchoscope (FB) in the midline is difficult to achieve without practice. Some practitioners use an LMA/EGD to keep the FB in the midline position. However, most find the nasal route much easier, since the tip of the bronchoscope usually emerges in the pharynx in the midline just above the glottis. The nasal passages may be dilated by passing increasingly larger diameter nasal trumpets, well lubricated with lidocaine jelly, every few minutes. The aim is to pass a trumpet slightly bigger than the proposed nasotracheal tube. As there is no contraindication to use cuffed tubes in pediatric patients, a smaller cuffed tube should be used to secure the airway of this patient.[16] Gentleness cannot be over emphasized; bleeding from the nasal passages can turn an elective controlled procedure very rapidly into an emergency disaster. Blood in the airway may render the FB nasal intubation technique difficult or impossible.

Some manufacturers (eg, Karl Storz Endoscopy, CA) stiffen neonatal and pediatric bronchoscopes that are intended for intubation. Although bronchoscopes as small as 2.3 mm in diameter are available, the procedure is usually performed with device that has a 3.0- to 3.5-mm tip diameter. The major disadvantage of pediatric and neonatal bronchoscopes is the small ineffective working channel for suctioning. Generally, the insufflation of high-flow oxygen through the working channel is discouraged due to the risk of gastric insufflation, perforation, and death.[17,18] However, some practitioners adopt a low-flow oxygen insufflation technique through the working channel at about ½ L·min⁻¹ to blow secretions out of the way while being extremely careful to regulate the flow of oxygen and never advance the bronchoscope unless under vision.

Before using the bronchoscope, it is important to confirm the correct functioning of the light source and the controls and to ensure that it is in focus. In the event one plans to inject local anesthetic through the working channel, 2 to 3 mL air flush is needed to flush the drug out of the distal lumen.

Once the nasal passages are dilated and anesthetized and the patient is adequately sedated, the appropriately sized and softened (hot water works well), and externally lubricated endotracheal tube (ETT) is passed into the chosen nares (the larger of the two) and advanced until the tip passes beyond the nasopharynx into the upper oropharynx. This point is generally appreciated as an abrupt loss of resistance associated with advancing the ETT. Any adenoidal tissue dissected by the tube tip and lodging in the distal ETT must be evacuated usually by gently pulling the ETT into the oral cavity with Magill forceps and blowing it out. The bronchoscope is inserted through the lumen of the ETT (previously lubricated with a silicon-based solution) to emerge just above the larynx in the oropharynx and then maneuvered into the trachea and advanced to the carina. Then, the ETT can be advanced over the bronchoscope into the trachea and positioned in midtrachea with the bronchoscope.

The process of repeated nasal trumpet insertion can be quite stimulating, and therefore, once the final nasal trumpet has been passed and the patient is comfortable with it in place, the need for deeper sedation ought to be minimal.

With a spontaneously breathing patient, regular movement of the airway may help to guide the bronchoscope to the right direction. If the patient is cooperative, one can ask the patient to stick out their tongue, or ask an assistant to gently pull the tongue forward with a gauze swab. This serves to open the hypopharynx, which often will help expose the cords. Alternatively, a gentle jaw thrust in a drowsy patient will also help to elevate the tongue and epiglottis.[19-24]

At this point, 0.5 to 1.0 mL of 1% or 2% lidocaine can be instilled through the working channel onto the cords to allow easy passage of the FB between the cords, followed by the nasotracheal tube. In some situations, particularly if violent coughing occurs, a small bolus of propofol can be administered rapidly by an assistant to facilitate the advancement of the ETT. The FB is then removed and general anesthesia is induced.

The nasal route is not always available, either due to anatomical difficulties or surgical considerations. In this case, the oral route may be used. While the nebulized lidocaine often adequately anesthetizes the nasal passages of children, oral topical anesthesia is often inadequate using this technique. Persuading a 6-year-old child to gargle lidocaine may work in selected patients. Attention to the cumulative dose of local anesthetic is important. Applying lidocaine jelly to the tongue slowly and progressively with a tongue depressor may also be effective. In an awake child, eliminating the gag reflex may be achieved by one quick squirt of local anesthetic on the uvula, which can be achieved with patience.

Passing an appropriately sized LMA/EGD has been shown to facilitate oral flexible bronchoscopic intubation.[25-31] Prior to starting the procedure, lubricate the inside of the LMA/EGD shaft with a silicon spray. Find an ETT that fits the lumen of the LMA. Because there are a number of manufacturers, it is difficult in a chapter such as this to publish size guidelines since outer diameters of ETTs vary from manufacturer to manufacturer.

A standard ETT may be of insufficient length. In this event, the following work-around is advised. Obtain a second, identical tube. Take the tube connector of one of the tubes and cut the shaft off the connector as close as possible to the hub. This short (about 1-2 cm) connector can be used to join the two ETTs together back to back, giving you one long ETT (Figure 47-1).[32] Since it is very slightly thickened at the joint, make sure that this new tube will fit through the LMA/FB combination. Alternatively, a long Microlaryngeal Tube (MLT, Rusch Inc., Duluth, GA) can be used.

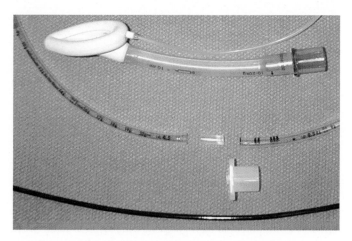

FIGURE 47-1. The equipment needed to perform a flexible bronchoscope-guided intubation through an LMA. A tube connector is created by cutting the shaft off the connector from a similar size ETT. This short connector can then be used to join the two endotracheal tubes together back to back, thus providing a sufficiently long endotracheal tube to pass through the LMA. (Reproduced with permission, from Muraika L, Heyman JS, Shevchenko Y. Fiberoptic tracheal intubation through a laryngeal mask airway in a child with Treacher Collins syndrome. *Anesth Analg.* 2003;97:1298-1299.)

It is also a reasonable technique to advance the ETT blindly into the trachea through the LMA and then use the FB to confirm placement. Once the ETT is in place, the LMA may be withdrawn over the elongated tube without extubating the patient. This works for both regular tubes and RAE (Ring, Adair, and Elwyn) preformed tubes, and can even be done with a cuffed tube, provided that the LMA is loaded from the distal end with the balloon and pilot tube of the cuff protruding from the distal end of the LMA.

Cobra manufactures a disposable perilaryngeal airway that comes in pediatric sizes. It is placed in a similar fashion to, and functions similarly to the LMA-Classic™. Its major advantage as a guide for oral flexible bronchoscopic intubation is that the bore of the shaft is larger than that of the LMA, allowing the easier passage of the FB and accompanying ETT. Similarly, the air-Q™ airway (Mercury Medical, Clearwater, FL) is a disposable EGD designed to facilitate blind intubation. The reuseable variant is called the Cook-ILA. It functions similarly to the Intubating LMA (LMA-Fastrach™, LMA North America, San Diego CA) in adults, but is available in sizes appropriate for infants and small children (see Chapter 42).[33]

47.4.4 What about the use of a video laryngoscope?

Video laryngoscopes have the advantage of being able to *see around corners* and possessing a wide field of view. While initially developed for adult patients, many manufacturers have made models available for pediatric practice. Manufacturers include Verathon (GlideScope®, Bothwell, WA) and Storz (Tuttlingen, Germany). A novel disposable video device possessing an ETT delivery channel and supplied in sizes appropriate for infants and small children is the Airtraq™.[34]

47.4.5 What if a flexible bronchoscopic intubation or the use of a video laryngoscope is unsuccessful?

In the event that the flexible bronchoscopic intubation cannot be achieved in a child with a difficult airway, or the use of the video laryngoscope is unsuccessful, a tracheotomy in a spontaneously breathing anesthetized patient may be the best course of action, and is quite commonly done.[35]

47.5 SUMMARY

Congenital anomalies associated with CS often present a difficult airway for anesthesia practitioners. In patients with a known difficult airway, the relationship between surgeon and anesthesia practitioner is important from the communication and patient-management perspective. In this particular case, the patient was known to have a difficult intubation and the practitioner was prepared to manage the airway with sedation, topical anesthesia, and flexible bronchoscopic intubation through the nose. Reassurance, adequate sedation, adequate topical anesthesia, and a gentle technique are crucial attributes to success. The use of an extraglottic device, such as LMA, as a conduit to flexible bronchoscopic intubation is an important adjunct as oral flexible bronchoscopic intubation guides used in adults may not be suitable for children.

Finally, the prominent role of the EGD as a rescue technique in infants and small children cannot be over emphasized.

REFERENCES

1. Crouzon and Aprert Syndrome. Available at: http://www.kidsplastsurg.com/skull.cfm#crouzons.
2. Ng DK, Chow PY, Chan CH, Kwok KL, Cheung JM, Kong FY. An update on childhood snoring. *Acta Paediatr.* 2006 Sep;95(9):1029-1035.
3. Guilleminault C, Khramtsov A. Upper airway resistance syndrome in children: a clinical review. *Semin Pediatr Neurol.* 2001;8:207-215.
4. Guilleminault C, Pelayo R. Sleep-disordered breathing in children. *Ann Med.* 1998;30:350-356.
5. Guilleminault C, Pelayo R, Leger D, Clerk A, Bocian RC. Recognition of sleep-disordered breathing in children. *Pediatrics.* 1996;98:871-882.
6. Dreimane D. Obstructive sleep apnea in children. *Tex Med.* 2009;105(2):47-50.
7. Hasan N, Fletcher EC. Upper airway resistance syndrome. *J Ky Med Assoc.* 1998;96:261-263.
8. Marcus CL, Katz ES, Lutz J, Black CA, Galster P, Carson KA. Upper airway dynamic responses in children with the obstructive sleep apnea syndrome. *Pediatr Res.* 2005;57:99-107.
9. Koh JL, Harrison D, Myers R, et al. A randomized, double-blind comparison study of EMLA and ELA-Max for topical anesthesia in children undergoing intravenous insertion. *Paediatr Anaesth.* 2004;14:977-982.
10. Khalil SN, Vije HN, Kee SS, et al. A paediatric trial comparing midazolam/Syrpalta mixture with premixed midazolam syrup (Roche). *Paediatr Anaesth.* 2003;13:205-209.
11. Cravero JP, Beach M, Dodge CP, Whalen K. Emergence characteristics of sevoflurane compared to halothane in pediatric patients undergoing bilateral pressure equalization tube insertion. *J Clin Anesth.* 2000;12:397-401.
12. Soh CR, Ng AS. Laryngeal mask airway insertion in paediatric anaesthesia: comparison between the reverse and standard techniques. *Anaesth Intensive Care.* 2001;29:515-519.
13. Bagshaw O. The size 1.5 laryngeal mask airway (LMA) in paediatric anaesthetic practice. *Paediatr Anaesth.* 2002;12:420-423.
14. Klimscha W, Chiari A, Michalek-Sauberer A, et al. The efficacy and safety of a clonidine/bupivacaine combination in caudal blockade for pediatric hernia repair. *Anesth Analg.* 1998;86:54-61.
15. Karaaslam K, Gulcu N, Ozturk H, Sarpkaya A, Colak C, Kocoglu H. Two different doses of caudal neostigmine co-administered with levobupivacaine produces analgesia in children. *Pediatr Anesth.* 2009;19:487-493.
16. Newth CJ, Rachman B, Patel N, Hammer J. The use of cuffed versus uncuffed endotracheal tubes in pediatric intensive care. *J Pediatr.* 2004;144:333-337.
17. Hershey MD, Hannenberg AA. Gastric distention and rupture from oxygen insufflation during flexible endoscopic intubation. *Anesthesiology.* 1996;85:1479-1480.
18. Ovassapian A, Mesnick PS. Oxygen insufflation through the fiberscope to assist intubation is not recommended. *Anesthesiology.* 1997;87:183-184.
19. Aoyama K, Takenaka I, Nagaoka E, Kadoya T. Jaw thrust maneuver for endotracheal intubation using a fiberoptic stylet. Anesth Analg. 2000;90:1457-1458.
20. Durga VK, Millns JP, Smith JE. Maneuvers used to clear the airway during fibreoptic intubation. *Br J Anaesth.* 2001;87:207-211.
21. Schwartz D, Johnson C, Roberts J. A maneuver to facilitate flexible fiberoptic intubation. *Anesthesiology.* 1989;71:470-471.
22. Stacey MR, Rassam S, Sivasankar R, Hall JE, Latto IP. A comparison of direct laryngoscopy and jaw thrust to aid fibreoptic intubation. *Anaesthesia.* 2005;60:445-448.
23. Stella JP, Kageler WV, Epker BN. Fiberoptic endotracheal intubation in oral and maxillofacial surgery. *J Oral Maxillofac Surg.* 1986;44:923-925.
24. Uzun L, Ugur MB, Altunkaya H, et al. Effectiveness of the jaw-thrust maneuver in opening the airway: a flexible fiberoptic endoscopic study. *ORL J Otorhinolaryngol Relat Spec.* 2005;67:39-44.
25. Benumof JL. A new technique of fiberoptic intubation through a standard LMA. *Anesthesiology.* 2001;95:1541.
26. Choi JE, Leal YR, Johnson MD. Fiberoptic intubation through the laryngeal mask airway. *J Clin Anesth.* 1996;8:687-688.
27. Ianchulev SA. Through-the-LMA fiberoptic intubation of the trachea in a patient with an unexpected difficult airway. *Anesth Analg.* 2005;101:1882-1883.
28. Johr M, Berger TM. Fiberoptic intubation through the laryngeal mask airway (LMA) as a standardized procedure. *Paediatr Anaesth.* 2004;14:614.
29. Talke PO, Nguyen H. Concept for easy fiberoptic intubation via a laryngeal airway mask. *Anesth Analg.* 1999;88:228-229.
30. Weiss M, Gerber AC, Schmitz A. Continuous ventilation technique for laryngeal mask airway (LMA) removal after fiberoptic intubation in children. *Paediatr Anaesth.* 2004;14:936-940.
31. Yilmaz AS, Gurkan Y, Toker K, Solak M. Laryngeal mask airway-guided fiberoptic tracheal intubation in a 1,200-g infant with difficult airway. *Paediatr Anaesth.* 2005;15:1147-1148.
32. Muraika L, Heyman JS, Shevchenko Y. Fiberoptic tracheal intubation through a laryngeal mask airway in a child with Treacher Collins syndrome. *Anesth Analg.* 2003;97:1298-1299.
33. Jagannathan N, Roth AG, Sohn LE, Pak TY, Amin S, Suresh S. The new air-Q™ intubating laryngeal airway for tracheal intubation in children with anticipated difficult airway: a case series. *Pediatr Anesth.* 2009;19:618-622.
34. Redel A, Krademir F, Schlitterlau AF, et al. Validation of the Glidescope video laryngoscope in pediatric patients. *Pediatr Anesth.* 2009;19:667-671.
35. Sculerati N, Gottlieb MD, Zimbler MS, Chibbaro PD, McCarthy JG. Airway management in children with major craniofacial anomalies. *Laryngoscope.* 1998;108:1806-1812.

SELF-EVALUATION QUESTIONS

47.1. All of the following statements regarding flexible bronchoscopic intubation of the child are true **EXCEPT**:

A. The nasal route is usually easier than the oral route.

B. General anesthesia is not usually successful.

C. Inhaled anesthetic agents for sedation are preferred over IV agents in a child because starting an IV is so difficult.

D. An extraglottic airway (EGD) may be used as a conduit for intubation.

E. Extreme caution needs to be taken if oxygen is to be insufflated down the scope to blow secretions away.

47.2. Pediatric flexible bronchoscopes—all of the following are true **EXCEPT**:

A. are generally between 2.3 and 3.5 mm tip diameter

B. are often stiffened to permit intubation

C. have working channels that are very effective

D. are generally 500 to 600 mm in length

E. are more easily damaged than adult scopes because they are so small

47.3. When using an LMA as a guide to flexible bronchoscopic intubation, the most significant problem one encounters in a child is:

A. It is difficult to seal LMAs in children.

B. The upper airway is too difficult to anesthetize to accept an LMA.

C. The LMA flips the epiglottis down, and therefore you cannot get under it with a flexible bronchoscope.

D. The lumen of the LMA is too small to pass a cuffed ETT through.

E. Standard ETTs are too short for this technique.

CHAPTER (48)

Pediatric Patient with a Closed Head Injury

Joshua Nagler and Robert C. Luten

48.1 CASE PRESENTATION

A 7-year-old boy is brought to the emergency department (ED) by ambulance following a bicycle accident. The paramedic team reports that the child was not wearing a helmet when he struck a pole while travelling at a high speed. The patient was found minimally responsive on the sidewalk, beside his bicycle. There was immediate concern for head and chest trauma. The patient was immobilized for possible C-spine injury. No other information is available.

Upon arrival at the ED, his vital signs are: temperature 36°C, heart rate 115 beats per minute (bpm), noisy breathing with a respiratory rate of 24 breaths per minute, and a blood pressure of 106/86 mm Hg. His oxygen saturation is 89% on a non-rebreather oxygen face mask. The Glasgow coma scale (GCS) score is 6. The patient is estimated to be 110 cm tall and weighs approximately 30 kg.

48.2 INITIAL MANAGEMENT

48.2.1 How should the airway of this child be managed in the field?

Airway management in the field is discussed in detail in Chapter 14.

Establishing and maintaining an airway in a trauma patient is the first priority of prehospital providers. Maintaining oxygenation and avoiding hypercarbia are particularly important in those in whom traumatic brain injury is suspected. Intuitively, establishing a definitive airway early in the course seems favorable. However, many studies have demonstrated increased morbidity

and mortality with prehospital advanced airway management in head-injured adults.[1-4] Pediatric data also fail to demonstrate benefit of prehospital intubation. A retrospective review of a large pediatric trauma registry showed no improvement in survival with prehospital endotracheal intubation over bag-mask-ventilation.[5] Similarly, a prospective, randomized trial in pediatric patients found no improvement in survival for those who underwent prehospital intubation, although the subset of patients in the study with head injuries was relatively small.[6] While local protocols may vary, it is generally recommended that in an urban setting head-injured children who can be adequately oxygenated and ventilated by bag-mask-ventilation be transported as rapidly as possible to the local trauma center for definitive airway management and further evaluation and care. The use of oral or nasopharyngeal airways to assist in airway patency is encouraged, when contraindications, such as severe facial injuries, do not exist.

48.2.2 What are the evaluation and management priorities in this patient and where does airway fit?

Airway is the first priority in any trauma patient, as identified by the airway, breathing, and circulation (ABCs) schema. While the cervical spine is immobilized, an adequate airway must be established to allow for effective oxygenation and ventilation. When appropriate resources are available, concurrent efforts should be aimed at obtaining vascular access to address circulatory compromise, as well as recognition and stabilization of other life-threatening injuries.

Airway management is particularly urgent in patients with head trauma. Failure to maintain oxygenation has been linked to secondary brain injury. Many pediatric studies have demonstrated poor outcomes and increased mortality in hypoxemic head-injured patients.[7-9]

Importantly, several other issues emerge as concurrent and perhaps complicating priorities in considering airway management in head-injured pediatric patients:

- The risk of cervical spine injury is approximately 5% in head-injured pediatric and adult patients, and higher for those with more severe injuries.[10-12] However, maintenance of in-line stabilization before, during, and after airway management in those with cervical spine injuries prevents neurologic injury.[13-16]

- Although children have resilient cardiovascular systems, hemodynamic instability in the face of multisystem injuries can occur.[17-20] Hypotension is a late sign of shock in pediatric patients, and tachycardia alone may herald significant hypovolemia. This may influence later decisions regarding fluid resuscitation, as well as the pharmacotherapy for rapid-sequence intubation (eg, avoiding fentanyl and propofol).

- Acutely injured patients are assumed to have a full stomach and gastric dilation. This is a significant risk factor for regurgitation and aspiration, and may also inhibit diaphragmatic excursion, effectively reducing lung compliance (a restrictive lung defect).[20,21]

- Rapidly obtaining vascular access in children can be challenging, although this is more common in younger infants and children. Inability to gain access constrains the pharmacologic options available for the airway practitioner, although intraosseous access is a viable alternative in trauma resuscitations.

- The issue of "cognitive load" (mental burden experienced by the airway practitioner) is unique to pediatric resuscitations where drug dosing and equipment selection are not as *automatic* as in adult patients.[22]

- There is an *angst in the room* factor that attends all pediatric resuscitations. This additional stress has the potential to lead to performance deterioration.[23]

48.3 AIRWAY MANAGEMENT

48.3.1 Is active airway intervention required in this case?

The first question to be answered is whether or not this patient requires intubation. For the following reasons, the answer is "yes":

- Hypoxemia, as demonstrated by persistent low oxygen saturation in spite of maximum supplemental oxygen, contributes to secondary brain injury.

- A GCS score of less than or equal to 8 is commonly regarded as an indication for intubation to ensure adequate airway protection.[24-26]

- A depressed level of consciousness frequently results in hypoventilation or apnea, and resultant hypercarbia can contribute to secondary brain injury and increased intracranial pressure.

- This patient will require multisystem evaluation including potentially prolonged diagnostic imaging of both plain radiography and computed tomography (CT), and airway patency must be assured throughout.

- Depending on local policies, this patient may require transfer to a pediatric trauma center. The ability to protect the airway and provide oxygenation and ventilation is facilitated by endotracheal intubation.

In practice, this means that the airway practitioner physically positions themselves at the head of the patient and begins the process of denitrogenation. In a patient with adequate, spontaneous respirations, this may be done with a nonbreather face mask over 3 minutes. However, for this patient with persistent hypoxemia, despite maximum supplemental oxygen, 1 minute of positive pressure ventilation with a bag-mask has been shown to be an effective and more rapid alternative.[27] For the spontaneously breathing child, the airway practitioner should coordinate gentle assisted breaths with the child's respiratory efforts, to avoid inflation of the stomach.

A methodical evaluation of the airway, including the potential for *difficult airway* may now be carried out.

48.3.2 What challenges do we face in managing this child's airway?

This patient does not have a *crash airway* (see Chapter 2, Figure 2.3) therefore immediate intubation is not indicated. The next priority is evaluating the patient for a potentially difficult airway and the suitability of rapid-sequence induction (RSI). The algorithms and mnemonics introduced in Chapters 1 and 2 are designed to guide the evaluation of the airway in such a way that important features known to predict a difficult airway are not overlooked. Although specific elements of the mnemonics may not be applicable in children, the principles remain the same. Employing the strategies for evaluating the airway for difficulty presented in Chapter 1:

- Will bag-mask-ventilation (BMV) of this patient be difficult (MOANS, see Section 1.6.1)? Mask seal is not anticipated to be difficult. This child is described as having noisy breathing which may signify some degree of upper airway obstruction. Given the depressed mental status, this is likely a result of an obstructing tongue which can be easily overcome with a simple jaw thrust or using oral or nasal airways. Obviously, this patient is not aged (older than 65), is not edentulous, and is not stiff (increased resistance or reduced compliance). However, the potential for acute gastric dilation to compromise thoracic compliance exists and must be addressed as indicated. So, evaluation using MOANS does not indicate any likely difficulties with bag-mask-ventilation.

- Will the insertion of an extraglottic device (EGD) be difficult (RODS, see Section 1.6.3)? Mouth opening can be limited by neck immobilization. However, this can be easily addressed by opening the front of the hard collar and maintaining in-line stabilization. Airway obstruction at or above the glottis is not suspected. There is no airway distortion to prevent a seal with an EGD, although the inability to move the neck may hinder seal characteristics of an LMA. Stiffness was evaluated with MOANS.

- Will a surgical airway be difficult (SHORT, see Section 1.6.4)? A 7-year-old has a small cricothyroid membrane. Therefore, a surgical cricothyrotomy will rarely be successful and should not be attempted in most circumstances. The surgical procedure of choice will be a transtracheal cannula. (see also Chapter 42). Ventilation through the transtracheal catheter may be performed manually with a bag-mask unit, with a jet ventilation device attached to a wall outlet with the initial pressure reduced to 20 lb per square inch (PSI), or with an Enk Flow Modulator (Cook Critical Care, see Chapter 59 for contact information) attached to a wall flow-meter at 7 L·min⁻¹ (1 L·min⁻¹ for each year of age).[28] This particular patient would not be expected to have any other potential problems with a surgical airway, that is, no prior neck surgery, no hematoma or infection over the anterior neck, no obesity, no radiation therapy, and has no tumor in the airway.

- Will it be difficult to perform laryngoscopy or intubation in this patient (LEMON, see Section 1.6.2)? Looking at the patient reveals no gross features that might predict a difficult laryngoscopy or intubation. The evaluation (3-3-2) of the geometry of his mandible and the position of his larynx (using the patient's own fingers) is normal. Mouth opening is adequate, although one is unable to evaluate a Mallampati score in this obtunded patient. There is no significant upper airway obstruction. The neck (cervical spine) is treated as if there could be a potential injury and therefore in-line stabilization is maintained. However, this is not of sufficient concern that an awake intubation is indicated.

Thus, in the absence of a difficult airway, the decision is made to proceed with a rapid-sequence intubation (RSI) as per Figure 2.3 in Chapter 2. Plan A is routine RSI. Plan B is an EGD such as an LMA. The use of the Combitube™ for this patient would not be appropriate as the patient has yet to reach 48 in (approximately 120 cm) in height. Plan C is a transtracheal cannula approach.

48.3.3 How exactly does one proceed with an RSI in this patient?

Reflecting the previous discussion, several factors will influence how RSI is accomplished:

- This patient has an acute severe head injury with the potential for elevated intracranial pressure (ICP).

- Prior to clearing the cervical spine with appropriate radiologic procedures, in-line stabilization is provided by a trained individual dedicated entirely to this task.

- A full stomach and acute gastric dilation are assumed.

- Hemodynamic compromise is possible, as indicated by persistent tachycardia.

48.3.3.1 Preparation

Equipment for Plans A, B, and C are assembled and tested. Drugs are drawn up as per the Broselow-Luten System (Vital Signs, Inc.,

Totowa, NJ). A functioning suction with a Yankauer catheter should be readily available given the potential for blood or secretions in the hypopharynx, and the risk of regurgitation of gastric contents.

48.3.3.2 Denitrogenation

Bag-mask-assisted ventilation is already underway.

48.3.3.3 Pretreatment

The efficacy of lidocaine in attenuating the rise in ICP during laryngoscopy and intubation is controversial.[29-32] However, if it is to be effective, it should be given a minimum of 2 to 3 minutes prior to intubation and at a dose of 1.5 mg·kg⁻¹ or 45 mg for this patient.[33,34] Fentanyl has not been shown to effectively blunt increases in ICP during intubation in children, and is specifically omitted as hemodynamic instability is suspected. Reduced muscle mass in children translates to less concern for fasciculations affecting ICP; therefore defasiculating doses with nondepolarizing neuromuscular-blocking (NMB) agent are not needed. Atropine has historically been used to prevent bradycardia related to succinylcholine use. However, recent studies have suggested this may be unnecessary.[35] Atropine use is considered optional in children less than 1 year of age who are at increased risk of bradycardia related to laryngoscopy. For older children such as this patient, it is recommended that atropine be available for rapid administration if bradycardia develops during intubation.

48.3.3.4 Potential Cervical Spine Injury

In-line stabilization is maintained throughout.

48.3.3.5 Induction and Paralysis

Since hemodynamic instability is suspected, a reduced dose of etomidate from 0.3 to 0.2 mg·kg⁻¹ or 6.0 mg is selected as the induction agent and is administered rapidly. Ketamine 1.0 to 2.0 mg·kg⁻¹ is an effective induction agent that has recently gained favor in hemodynamically compromised patients because of resultant release of endogenous catecholamines. However, this pressor response has raised questions about worsening ICP in head-injured patients. Recent suggestions are that ketamine can safely be used in head-injured patients who do not exhibit obvious hypertension.[36] Succinylcholine 1.5 mg·kg⁻¹ or 45 mg for this patient is administered rapidly after the induction agent is injected. Unlike the induction agent, the dose of the NMB agent is never tailored to the hemodynamic status.

48.3.3.6 Protection against Aspiration

Cricoid pressure is applied with care taken to:

- Avoid stimulation of gag during induction
- Avoid cervical spinal motion
- Not obstruct or deform the relatively compliant airway of the child

Although artificial ventilation in this child is risky due to the potential for gastric insufflation and regurgitation, there is little choice but to perform careful BMV in order to maintain normal arterial carbon dioxide levels and mitigate increases in ICP. In addition, appropriately applied cricoid pressure decreases the risk of further gastric insufflation.[37,38]

48.3.3.7   Placement of the Endotracheal Tube

The placement of the endotracheal tube is performed under direct laryngoscopy as delicately and atraumatically as possible to attenuate any increase in blood pressure, heart rate, and ICP. Tracheal tube placement is confirmed with end-tidal CO_2 detection and a complete clinical evaluation, including auscultation. Immediately after intubation, the blood pressure is assessed. If the child is hypertensive for age, this can be managed with appropriate sedation and analgesia with opioids and benzodiazepines or with small bolus doses of propofol. Conversely, if hypotension is noted, volume infusion, up to 20 mL·kg^{-1} of balanced salt solution should be rapidly administered.

If the endotracheal tube is inadvertently placed in the esophagus, the tube may be immediately removed and intubation reattempted. Alternatively, one of the following two maneuvers may be employed, depending on the oxygen saturation:

- Oxygen saturation greater than 90%: Move the incorrectly positioned tube to the left corner of the mouth and reattempt intubation with a second tube, with careful attention to the relative position of the known esophageal tube.

- Oxygen saturation less than 90%: Quickly inflate the balloon of the ETT with as much air as it will accommodate without breaking (ordinarily 5.0-15 mL depending on the size of the ETT). Compress the epigastrum to empty as much air and liquid stomach contents as possible. Deflate the balloon and remove the ETT while suctioning the hypopharynx. Perform BMV to recover the oxygen saturations and reattempt orotracheal intubation.

If at any point oxygen saturation becomes unacceptable and cannot be corrected, a failed airway has supervened and the appropriate algorithm should be followed.

48.3.3.8   Postintubation Management

Maintaining hemodynamic stability with acceptable blood gases ($Paco_2$ 35-40 mm Hg) should become a priority after successful tracheal intubation. Routine hyperventilation is no longer advised due to decreased cerebral blood flow and resultant ischemia.[39] Neuromuscular blockade should be continued using longer-acting nondepolarizing agents such as rocuromium (0.6-1.2 mg·kg^{-1}), vecuronium (0.1 mg·kg^{-1}), or pancuronium (0.1 mg·kg^{-1}) provided repeated neurological examinations are not essential. Sedation with bolus doses of midazolam 0.5 to 1.0 mg per dose may be required from time to time, the need dictated by a rising heart rate and/or blood pressure. Opioids such as fentanyl 1.0 μg·kg^{-1} may be necessary if pain is suspected. One must pay particular attention to the effect of small doses of sedative hypnotics and opioids on the hemodynamic stability of the patient. Gastric decompression using an orogastric or nasogastric tube is indicated.

48.3.4   What if the trachea cannot be intubated after three attempts?

Failure to successfully intubate after three attempts constitutes a failed airway. There are two types of failed airways:

- Cannot intubate, can ventilate—A situation in which three attempts at conventional intubation have failed but gas exchange is possible and saturations acceptable (eg, BMV, or EGD such as an LMA). In this situation, there is time to use alternative nonsurgical techniques, such as video laryngoscopy or flexible bronchoscopy, recognizing the ongoing risk of regurgitation and aspiration.

- Cannot intubate, cannot ventilate—A situation in which neither intubation nor ventilation is possible. In such a case, there is no time for further intubation attempts and a surgical airway must be performed. In this case, an LMA may be attempted as preparations are made to insert a transtracheal catheter, but not *instead of preparing* to insert one, that is, these activities are concurrent not sequential.

48.4   SUMMARY

Acute severe head injury is a common indication for emergency tracheal intubation in children. While airway protection and appropriate oxygenation and ventilation are the top priorities, many other factors impact decisions about airway management. These include the potential for concomitant cervical spine injury; elevated intracranial pressure; hemodynamic stability; and the presence of an acute gastric dilation. Since there is often a need to manage multiple problems in these patients, attention to detail is crucial.

Given the emotionally charged atmosphere that can surround the resuscitation of a child, there is a risk of practitioners getting sidetracked by concurrent confounding issues. Therefore, a planned, methodical, and disciplined approach to airway evaluation and management in the injured child is important. This chapter attempts to reinforce that crucial principle.

REFERENCES

1. Murray JA, Demetriades D, Berne TV, et al. Prehospital intubation in patients with severe head injury. *J Trauma.* 2000;49:1065-1070.
2. Sloane C, Vilke GM, Chan TC, et al. Rapid sequence intubation in the field versus hospital in trauma patients. *J Emerg Med.* 2000;19:259-264.
3. Wang HE, Peitzman AB, Cassidy LD, Adelson PD, Yealy DM. Out-of-hospital endotracheal intubation and outcome after traumatic brain injury. *Ann Emerg Med.* 2004;44:439-450.
4. Stiell IG, Nesbitt LP, Pickett W, et al. The OPALS Major Trauma Study: impact of advanced life-support on survival and morbidity. *CMAJ.* 2008;178:1141-1152.
5. Cooper A, DiScala C, Foltin G, Tunik M, Markenson D, Welborn C. Prehospital endotracheal intubation for severe head injury in children: a reappraisal. *Semin Pediatr Surg.* 2001;10:3-6.
6. Gausche M, Lewis RJ, Stratton SJ, et al. Effect of out-of-hospital pediatric endotracheal intubation on survival and neurological outcome: a controlled clinical trial. *JAMA.* 2000;283:783-790.
7. Michaud LJ, Rivara FP, Grady MS, Reay DT. Predictors of survival and severity of disability after severe brain injury in children. *Neurosurgery.* 1992; 31:254-264.

8. Mayer TA, Walker ML. Pediatric head injury: the critical role of the emergency physician. *Ann Emerg Med.* 1985;14:1178-1184.

9. Ong L, Selladurai BM, Dhillon MK, Atan M, Lye MS. The prognostic value of the Glasgow Coma Scale, hypoxia and computerised tomography in outcome prediction of pediatric head injury. *Pediatr Neurosurg.* 1996;24:285-291.

10. Hills MW, Deane SA. Head injury and facial injury: is there an increased risk of cervical spine injury? *J Trauma.* 1993;34:549-553; discussion 553-554.

11. Michael DB, Guyot DR, Darmody WR. Coincidence of head and cervical spine injury. *J Neurotrauma.* 1989;6:177-189.

12. Holly LT, Kelly DF, Counelis GJ, Blinman T, McArthur DL, Cryer HG. Cervical spine trauma associated with moderate and severe head injury: incidence, risk factors, and injury characteristics. *J Neurosurg.* 2002;96:285-291.

13. Holley J, Jorden R. Airway management in patients with unstable cervical spine fractures. *Ann Emerg Med.* 1989;18:1237-1239.

14. Ghafoor AU, Martin TW, Gopalakrishnan S, Viswamitra S. Caring for the patients with cervical spine injuries: what have we learned? *J Clin Anesth.* 2005;17:640-649.

15. Ollerton JE, Parr MJ, Harrison K, Hanrahan B, Sugrue M. Potential cervical spine injury and difficult airway management for emergency intubation of trauma adults in the emergency department—a systematic review. *Emerg Med J.* 2006;23:3-11.

16. Crosby E. Airway management after upper cervical spine injury: what have we learned? *Can J Anaesth.* 2002;49:733-744.

17. Schiff JS, Moore B, Louie J. Pediatric trauma—unique considerations in evaluating and treating children. *Minn Med.* 2005;88:46-51.

18. Morgan WM, 3rd, O'Neill JA, Jr. Hemorrhagic and obstructive shock in pediatric patients. *New Horiz.* 1998;6:150-154.

19. Kirk JA. Pediatric trauma. *CRNA.* 1997;8:135-143.

20. Jambor CR, Steedman DJ. Acute gastric dilation after trauma. *J R Coll Surg Edinb.* 1991;36:29-31.

21. Cogbill TH, Bintz M, Johnson JA, Strutt PJ. Acute gastric dilatation after trauma. *J Trauma.* 1987;27:1113-1117.

22. Luten R, Wears RL, Broselow J, et al. Managing the unique size-related issues of pediatric resuscitation: reducing cognitive load with resuscitation aids. *Acad Emerg Med.* 2002;9:840-847.

23. Lawton L. Paediatric trauma—the care of anthony. *Accid Emerg Nurs.* 1995;3:172-176.

24. Gentleman D, Dearden M, Midgley S, Maclean D. Guidelines for resuscitation and transfer of patients with serious head injury. *BMJ.* 1993;307:547-552.

25. American College of Surgeons Committee on Trauma. *Advanced Trauma Life Support for Doctors: ATLS Student Course Manual.* 8th ed. Chicago: American College of Surgeons; 2008.

26. Gabriel EJ, Ghajar J, Jagoda A, Pons PT, Scalea T, Walters BC. Guidelines for prehospital management of traumatic brain injury. *J Neurotrauma.* 2002;19:111-174.

27. Chiron B, Mas C, Ferrandiere M, et al. Standard preoxygenation vs two techniques in children. *Paediatr Anaesth.* 2007;17:963-967.

28. Baker PA, Brown AJ. Experimental adaptation of the Enk oxygen flow modulator for potential pediatric use. *Paediatr Anaesth.* 2009;19:458-463.

29. Nakayama DK, Waggoner T, Venkataraman ST, Gardner M, Lynch JM, Orr RA. The use of drugs in emergency airway management in pediatric trauma. *Ann Surg.* 1992;216:205-211.

30. Bozeman WP, Idris AH. Intracranial pressure changes during rapid sequence intubation: a swine model. *J Trauma.* 2005;58:278-283.

31. Yano M, Nishiyama H, Yokota H, et al. Effect of lidocaine on ICP response to endotracheal suctioning. *Anesthesiology.* 1986;64:651-653.

32. Robinson N, Clancy M. In patients with head injury undergoing rapid sequence intubation, does pretreatment with intravenous lignocaine/lidocaine lead to an improved neurological outcome? A review of the literature. *Emerg Med J.* 2001;18:453-457.

33. Lev R, Rosen P. Prophylactic lidocaine use preintubation: a review. *J Emerg Med.* 1994;12:499-506.

34. Grover VK, Reddy GM, Kak VK, Singh S. Intracranial pressure changes with different doses of lignocaine under general anaesthesia. *Neurol India.* 1999;47:118-121.

35. McAuliffe G, Bissonnette B, Boutin C. Should the routine use of atropine before succinylcholine in children be reconsidered? *Can J Anaesth.* 1995;42:724-729.

36. Filanovsky Y, Miller P, Kao J. Myth: ketamine should not be used as an induction agent for intubation in patients with head injury. *CJEM.* 12:154-157.

37. Salem MR, Wong AY, Mani M, Sellick BA. Efficacy of cricoid pressure in preventing gastric inflation during bag-mask ventilation in pediatric patients. *Anesthesiology.* 1974;40:96-98.

38. Moynihan RJ, Brock-Utne JG, Archer JH, Feld LH, Kreitzman TR. The effect of cricoid pressure on preventing gastric insufflation in infants and children. *Anesthesiology.* 1993;78:652-656.

39. Skippen P, Seear M, Poskitt K, et al. Effect of hyperventilation on regional cerebral blood flow in head-injured children. *Crit Care Med.* 1997;25:1402-1409.

SELF-EVALUATION QUESTIONS

48.1 Airway management in a child with acute severe head injury needs to respect all of the following **EXCEPT**:

A. The potential for raised ICP.

B. The potential for unrecognized hemodynamic instability.

C. That managing hypotension takes precedence over intubation.

D. In-line stabilization of the cervical spine before, during, and after intubation is crucial.

E. Acute gastric dilation is common in injured children.

48.2 Rapid-sequence intubation (RSI) in a 70-year-old with an acute severe head injury should include all the following **EXCEPT**:

A. lower dose etomidate, if the patient is hemodynamically compromised

B. pretreatment with fentanyl

C. cricoid pressure

D. augmented ventilation through the process

E. succinylcholine 1.5 mg·kg^{-1}

48.3 You have attempted an RSI on a 7-year-old with an acute severe head injury and have failed to intubate on the first attempt. The oxygen saturations have fallen to the mid 80s and BMV is not helping. What is the next most appropriate thing to do?

A. Attempt intubation two more times.

B. Quickly attempt a nasal endoscopic intubation.

C. Attempt to insert a Combitube™.

D. Move directly to a transtracheal approach.

E. Try an LMA, and if oxygenation is successful, move to an alternative technique, such as a video laryngoscope (GlideScope®).

CHAPTER (49)

What Is Unique about the Obstetrical Airway?

Brian K. Ross and Dolores M. McKeen

49.1 INTRODUCTION

The ability to maintain a patent airway, provide adequate ventilation, and place an endotracheal tube remains a major concern for airway practitioners. There is no location that produces more anxiety in this regard than labor and delivery. Obstetrical anesthesia is a high-risk practice that is replete with medicolegal liability and laden with clinical challenges. On the obstetric service, the practitioner is required to provide safe anesthesia care to two patients, mother and baby, both of whom have unique and demanding anatomical and physiological requirements. The purpose of this chapter is to briefly review the status of maternal morbidity/mortality, highlight the principal reasons that airways of parturients might be difficult to manage, and propose an algorithm for the management of the obstetrical airway.

Underpinning all discussion is the critical importance of being prepared cognitively for the unexpected occurrence and being facile with appropriate emergency airway equipment. Early consultation for anesthesia intervention, and airway assessment of obstetric patients at high risk for operative intervention, particularly parturients who may be obese or have advanced maternal age, remain a key preventative pillar of care. Of equal importance is teamwork between the anesthesia practitioner, the labor and delivery nurses, and the obstetrician. Improved perioperative training of labor and delivery unit support staff (including anesthesia resources for airway management during and after general anesthesia) are important clinical care considerations. Practicing difficult airway scenarios is invaluable. Being unprepared will certainly guarantee failure.

49.2 MATERNAL MORBIDITY AND MORTALITY

49.2.1 Discuss the anesthetic-related morbidity and mortality of parturients

Women continue to experience preventable pregnancy-related deaths, and anesthesia is the seventh leading cause of such mortality in the United States.[1] These anesthesia-related deaths are particularly catastrophic, because many of these anesthetics are elective and are administered to young, otherwise well, mothers.

Hawkins and her colleagues characterized obstetrical anesthesia deaths in the United States by specific cause, relationship to type of anesthetic, and type of obstetrical procedure.[2] Most women who died from anesthesia complications were undergoing cesarean section delivery (82%), whereas only about 5% of the deaths were associated with vaginal deliveries. Women who died of complications of general anesthesia (52% of all maternal deaths) primarily died as a result of airway management problems which included aspiration, intubation difficulties, and inadequate ventilation.

In 1985, a unique perspective on anesthesia morbidity and mortality was unveiled with the institution of the American Society of Anesthesiologists Committee on Professional Liability Closed Claims Project. The data from this project are an accumulation of personal damage insurance claims filed against anesthesiologists and subsequently settled.[3] Of the nearly 6500 cases in the database, 12% have been associated with obstetrical anesthesia care and nearly three-fourths of these claims have been associated with cesarean section. Critical events involving the respiratory system were the most common precipitating events in the obstetrical files. Trauma from repeated attempts at intubation was recognized as an issue of particular hazard.

Obstetrical airway catastrophes occur most frequently during emergency cesarean sections. It is in these settings that regional anesthesia may not be possible because of either maternal condition or severe fetal distress. It is also in these settings that airway evaluation may be particularly hurried and harassed. Overall incidences of obstetrical airway problems are low (7.9%)[4] but appear to be greater than in the non-obstetric patient (2.5%).[5] Mask-ventilation can be difficult or impossible in approximately 0.02% of parturients, an incidence not dissimilar to other surgical patients.[6]

There is little prospective evidence and the literature is unclear as to the actual incidence of failed intubation under general anesthesia in obstetrical patients. While ranges have been given from 1 in 283 to 1 in 2130, a composite incidence of about 0.2%[7] to 0.4%[8] has been suggested. However, in a 2005 systematic review, Goldszmidt challenged the conventional wisdom and examined the evidence as to whether the obstetric airway is truly more difficult to intubate.[9] In his review, difficult and failed intubation in the obstetric population was found to be rare, and there was no difference in the occurrence of difficult (1%-6%) or failed intubation (0%-0.7%) compared to general surgical populations.

While the incidence of a difficult airway in the obstetrical population remains unclear, there are concerns that the rates of failed intubation in the obstetric population will increase with declining numbers of women requiring general anesthetics, and the potential loss of skills in managing the airway of an obstetric patient.[8,10-15]

49.3   THE PARTURIENT AIRWAY

49.3.1   Why do parturients have more airway complications compared to the general population?

The parturient is at significantly greater risk for airway complications and difficult intubations than her nonpregnant counterpart.[16] A wide range of both anatomical and physiological changes occur during pregnancy and many of these may impact the airway directly, or indirectly (Table 49-1). Many of the changes are hormonally driven and the gravid uterus has a significant impact on the respiratory, cardiovascular, and gastrointestinal systems. Finally, there are a number of abnormal pregnancy-related processes that impact heavily on the parturient airway.

49.3.2   How do the physiological changes associated with pregnancy impact the airway of parturients?

The difficulties in airway management for obstetrical patients may be related to a number of factors as discussed in the following sections.

TABLE 49-1

Factors Affecting Management of the Parturient Airway

Weight gain (12-20 kg)	• Enlarging gravid uterus • Increasing total body water and interstitial fluid • Increasing blood volume • Deposition of new fat • Enlargement of the breasts
Respiratory system	• Decrease in respirator reserve volume • Decrease in functional residual capacity (20%-30%) • Increased oxygen consumption • More rapid desaturation
Airway	• Increased oral, nasal, pharyngeal, and tracheal mucosal edema • Vascular engorgement of oral, pharyngeal, and nasal capillaries • Edema of face and neck • Advancement of Mallampati classification with pregnancy • Advancement of Mallampati classification with bearing down during labor
Cardiovascular system	• Inferior caval syndrome (supine hypotensive syndrome) requiring left uterine tilt
Gastrointestinal system	• Steadily increasing intragastric pressure as pregnancy progresses • Decreased lower esophageal sphincter tone due to increasing progesterone • Symptomatic gastroesophageal reflux • Distortion of gastric anatomy • Increased gastric acidity

49.3.3.1 Weight Gain

During pregnancy, average weight gain can be 12 to 20 kg over the parturient prepregnant weight. This weight gain is related to increases in total body water, interstitial fluid (generalized body edema), blood volume, deposition of new fat and protein, uterine size and contents, and enlargement of the breasts.

Obesity (BMI >30) has become much more frequently encountered in the general population over the past decade. Mask ventilation is often difficult in obese patients because of reduced chest compliance and increased intra-abdominal pressure. The incidence of partially obliterated oropharyngeal structures in obese parturients is double that of non-obese parturients.[4] In addition, weight gain may create a short neck, a large tongue, and large breasts, all of which contribute to difficult laryngoscopy. In the morbidly obese parturient (>140 kg or approximately 300 lb, BMI ≥40), the risks for diabetes, hypertension, preeclampsia, and primary cesarean delivery are all increased. There is also a higher incidence of difficult labor resulting in instrumental deliveries, postpartum hemorrhage, or other conditions that require anesthetic intervention.[17]

Morbidly obese parturients are at increased risks for anesthesia-related complications during cesarean delivery, and increased risks for failed intubation and gastric aspiration if general anesthesia is required.[18] The cesarean section rate in these patients can exceed 50%, with one-third of attempted tracheal intubations being difficult and 6% being failures.[19] In the ASA closed claims obstetrical files, damaging events related to the respiratory system were significantly more common among obese (32%) than non-obese (7%) parturients.[20]

49.3.3.2 Respiratory Changes

Respiratory changes during pregnancy are of special significance to the anesthesia practitioner. Over the course of a normal gestation, the parturient experiences a 30% to 60% increase in oxygen consumption, because of the metabolic demands of the growing fetus, uterus, and placenta. This, in combination with a reduction in functional residual capacity (FRC), which begins to decline as early as the fifth month and is reduced to 80% of nonpregnant values by term, invites exceedingly rapid desaturation with apnea. The tendency toward rapid desaturation is further aggravated by the supine position.

Displacement of abdominal contents toward the chest, as a result of the enlarged uterus, causes a reduction in FRC and premature airway closure, with widening of the alveolar-arterial oxygen gradient. As a result of these changes, oxygenation of the mother and fetus are easily compromised.[21]

49.3.3.3 Airway Changes

Generalized edema may affect the oropharynx, nasopharynx, and trachea. These changes are aggravated by elevated estrogen levels that stimulate the development of mucosal edema and hypervascularity in the upper airways. Capillary engorgement of the nasal and oropharyngeal mucosa begins early in the first trimester and increases progressively throughout pregnancy. Accordingly, the parturient frequently appears to have symptoms of upper respiratory infection and laryngitis, with nasal congestion and voice changes due to swelling of the false vocal cords and arytenoids. Nasal obstruction from vascularity and edema may complicate bag-mask-ventilation (BMV).[22]

Numerous case reports suggest that edema of the pharyngeal and laryngeal structures, and vocal cords, may hinder visualization of the cords and passage of an endotracheal tube.[23,24] Tongue edema may make retraction of the tongue into the mandibular space during laryngoscopy difficult. The increased engorgement and vascularity present special challenges in manipulating the nasopharynx (nasal trumpets, nasogastric tubes) or when considering repeated attempts at intubation. An endotracheal tube one size smaller than might be usual (ie, 6.0-7.0 mm ID) should be routinely used.

Excessive weight gain, even mild upper respiratory tract infections, preeclampsia, fluid overload, and bearing down, can all exacerbate airway edema potentially leading to a severely compromised airway. The classical Mallampati classification (Samsoon and Young modification) of mouth opening has been reported to advance by one or two classes during pregnancy.[15] This may change even further as a consequence of bearing down, the score may not return to the pre-labor state for a further 12 hours postpartum.[25,26] Acoustic reflectometry, which measures oropharyngeal volumes, and is likely a surrogate marker for ease of intubation, revealed decreased volumes both in women after delivery, and in women whose pregnancy was complicated by preeclampsia.[22,26,27]

49.3.3.4 Cardiovascular Changes

The supine position may result in compression of the aorta, the inferior vena cava, or both by the enlarged pregnant uterus. Compression of the aorta decreases uterine blood flow, impairing fetal oxygenation. Vena caval compression decreases venous return, cardiac output, and ultimately uterine blood flow. A combination of respiratory desaturation and compromised cardiac output is particularly lethal for the pregnant mother. It is therefore imperative that the parturient be positioned with a wedge under the right hip, creating left lateral displacement of the uterus, away from the great vessels. Unfortunately, such displacement may hinder adequate preoperative airway evaluation and the creation of an optimum position for intubation.

49.3.3.5 Gastrointestinal Changes

The risk of aspiration in the parturient impacts how the anesthesia practitioner approaches and manages the parturient's airway. Several factors increase the risk of aspiration in these patients. While intragastric pressure increases steadily during pregnancy, as the gravid uterus enlarges, a concomitant decrease in lower esophageal tone occurs as circulating levels of progesterone increase.

The enlarging uterus distorts esophageal and gastric anatomy. The cephalad pressure of the abdominal uterus decreases the obliquity with which the esophagus contacts the stomach, permitting reflux of gastric contents at lower than usual trans-sphincter pressures. Gastric emptying appears to be unaffected by pregnancy, though intestinal transit time and gastric acidity are increased. With the onset of labor, gastric emptying slows and may be further aggravated by the administration of opioids for labor pain management. Taken together, these gastrointestinal changes mandate that precautions be taken when a parturient undergoes general anesthesia.

49.3.3.6   Obstetrical Factors

There are a number of comorbid obstetrical factors that may put the parturient at risk for airway management difficulties and related complications. Gestational hypertension, eclampsia, and preeclampsia aggravate mucosal and interstitial edema.[22] Concomitant proteinuria, with reduced intravascular plasma protein levels, leads to increased edema of the upper airway, an enlarged and less mobile tongue, and soft tissue deposition in the neck.

Preeclampsia is frequently accompanied by coagulopathy and edema, both of which may exaggerate bleeding with repeated attempts at direct laryngoscopy. Airway and laryngeal edema can develop exceedingly rapidly in preeclamptic patients and neck and face edema, and dysphonia from uvular edema, should alert the practitioner to the possibility of difficult intubation.[28] In these patients, extreme caution should be exercised not only at intubation, but at the time of extubation as well.

Maternal knee-chest and left lateral positioning, as part of intrauterine fetal resuscitation for non-reassuring fetal heart tracings, may also limit ability to conduct adequate preoperative airway evaluation. The impact that this maternal positioning has on the validity, and the positive and negative predictive value of the preoperative airway assessment, is unknown.

Massive peripartum hemorrhage (eg, placenta previa, accreta, abruption) and acute fetal distress (eg, abruption, cord prolapse) are frequently encountered obstetrical emergencies occurring acutely and unannounced. The visual impact of profuse vaginal bleeding, or the slow ominous sound of the tocodynamometer with fetal distress, frequently pushes obstetricians and anesthesia practitioners to urgently proceed to general anesthesia, without taking the time to adequately assess the patient's airway. General anesthesia in the obstetric population is most frequently conducted for emergency clinical indications.[29,30] Most airway catastrophes occur when the difficult airway is not recognized before the induction of anesthesia. Indeed, retrospective publications have reported poor ability to predict difficulty in the obstetrical population, and poor documentation of preoperative airway evaluation.[8,13] Endler et al found that emergency surgery was implicated in up to 80% of maternal deaths with general anesthesia, and difficult or failed intubation was associated with 4 of 15 deaths.[18]

49.4   AIRWAY EVALUATION

49.4.1   Why is it important to assess the airway of each parturient?

Every pregnant patient admitted to the labor and delivery service must have a thorough preanesthetic evaluation. With the always-present risk of acute-onset fetal distress, an essential and critical part of airway management is an accurate assessment of the patient's airway.

A detailed discussion of the airway examination and those predictors associated with management difficulties is found in Chapter 1. Most predictive studies have been conducted on general surgical populations, not parturients. Some 20 factors predicting difficult laryngoscopic intubation have been identified. The obstetrical patient presents unique assessment challenges, often the most important being a pressure of time.

49.4.2   How do you assess the airway of a parturient? What are the predictors or risk factors of a difficult airway for a parturient?

The increasing use of regional anesthetic techniques for delivery has significantly decreased opportunity for research in patients undergoing general anesthesia. While parturients pose many unique airway challenges to anesthesia practitioners, assessment of the pillars of airway management (bag-mask-ventilation, the use of extraglottic devices, tracheal intubation, and establishment of a surgical airway) should not differ from the non-obstetrical population.

49.4.2.1   Difficult Bag-Mask-Ventilation

As discussed, difficult bag-mask-ventilation (BMV) can be difficult to impossible in approximately 0.02% of parturients. However, this incidence is comparable to the general surgical patient.[6] While the mnemonic MOANS (see Section 1.6.1) is a helpful reminder of the five patient characteristics associated with difficult BMV,[31] many of these characteristics do not apply to the obstetrical population. For example, young and healthy pregnant women are typically not older than 55 years of age, or edentulous, and they do not generally have facial hair. Obesity, however, is an important consideration and is becoming increasingly more prevalent amongst pregnant women. It is noteworthy that, 28% of pregnant patients and 75% of preeclamptic women reported snoring compared to 14% of nonpregnant women.[22]

49.4.2.2   Difficult Laryngoscopy and Tracheal Intubation

Section 1.6.2 discusses in detail the current evidence in assessing the predictors of difficult laryngoscopy and intubation (LEMON). Dupont and colleagues conducted one of the early airway studies in the obstetrical population[32] and reported that the risk of difficult laryngoscopic intubation was eight times greater than in the general surgical population.

The literature suggests a variety of clinical signs that can help determine the degree of difficult laryngoscopic intubation (Table 49-2); however, none of these has a high positive predictive value as a single tool, particularly in the obstetrical patient. A number of studies suggest that, although the presence of risk factors was

---

▶ TABLE 49-2

Features of the Airway Examination Useful in Predicting Difficult Laryngoscopy

In the parturient	• Mallampati Class III or IV • Limited thyromental distance • Short thick neck • Limited mouth opening • Prominent incisors

useful, they were not as reliable as the Mallampati examination. Benumof has frequently suggested that a patient's relative tongue/pharyngeal size (Mallampati), degree of atlanto-occipital joint extension, and adequacy of the mandibular space provide the clinician with three easy to perform and accurate predictors of difficulty in laryngoscopic intubation.[33]

Rocke et al conducted one of the sentinel studies specifically looking at the obstetrical population and difficult airway predictors.[4] They prospectively evaluated the airways of 1500 parturients presenting for elective and emergency intubations, and found that a highly predictive sign for a difficult airway was a neutral to extension sterno-mental distance variation of less than 5 cm. In addition, the authors built a scale of predictive factors showing clearly that the greater the number of abnormal findings, the higher the prediction accuracy for a difficult intubation (Figure 49-1). The associated risk factors included short neck (SN), protruding maxillary incisors (PMI), receding mandible (RM), and Mallampati Class III and IV. The relative risk of experiencing a difficult intubation in comparison to an uncomplicated Class I airway assessment was as follows: Class II, 3.23; Class III, 7.58; Class IV, 11.3; SN 5.01; RM, 9.71; and PMI, 8.0. Using the probability index, or combination of risk factors, Roche et al showed that a combination of either Class III or IV, plus PMI, SN, and RM, correlated with a probability of difficult laryngoscopy of greater than 90%. It was interesting that neither facial edema nor swollen tongue was associated with difficult laryngoscopic intubation. This may further support the concept that previously published increased rates of difficult and failed intubation in the parturient may in fact be related to anatomic abnormalities unrelated to pregnancy but rather emergency conditions, lack of preoperative airway assessment, or differences in intubation experience and expertise.[9]

Overall, the mnemonic LEMON (see Section 1.6.2) examines almost all of the difficult laryngoscopic intubation characteristics (with the exception of the protruding maxillary incisors) and remains a useful guide for the obstetrical population.

In the obstetrical patient, obesity and large pendulous breasts often compound airway problems. It is important that the parturient be assessed in the recumbent position with left uterine displacement. Adjustments in the patient's position should be made before induction of anesthesia, to make intubating conditions easier, but there are limits to the extent that these adjustments can be employed, because of the positioning required to reduce aortocaval compression. In the morbidly obese parturient, elevations (ie, ramping) (Figure 49-2 and Chapter 17) of the thorax, shoulders, and head may be necessary to bring the anatomical axes of the oral, pharyngeal, and laryngeal structures into alignment. Positioning on a ramp may also mitigate the problem of the laryngoscope handle abutting on the patient's chest.

49.4.2.3   Difficulty in Use of Extraglottic Device

The use of an extraglottic device (EGD) is an important backup maneuver (Plan B) and serves as a bridging attempt to reestablish gas exchange in a "cannot intubate, cannot ventilate (CICV) setting, while one prepares to perform a cricothyrotomy in parturients. RODS (see Section 1.6.3) is a mnemonic that is intended to identify patients where the use of an EGD may be difficult.

49.4.2.4   Difficult Surgical Airway

While the necessity to perform a surgical airway, or cricothyrotomy, in an obstetrical population is exceedingly rare, all parturients requiring a general anesthetic ought to have an assessment of the feasibility

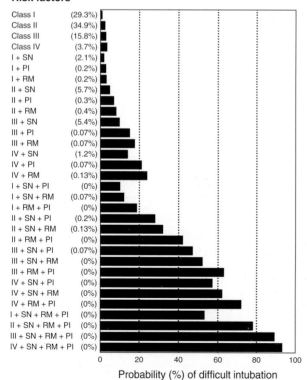

Risk factors

Class I	(29.3%)	
Class II	(34.9%)	
Class III	(15.8%)	
Class IV	(3.7%)	
I + SN	(2.1%)	
I + PI	(0.2%)	
I + RM	(0.2%)	
II + SN	(5.7%)	
II + PI	(0.3%)	
II + RM	(0.4%)	
III + SN	(5.4%)	
III + PI	(0.07%)	
III + RM	(0.07%)	
IV + SN	(1.2%)	
IV + PI	(0.07%)	
IV + RM	(0.13%)	
I + SN + PI	(0%)	
I + SN + RM	(0.07%)	
I + RM + PI	(0%)	
II + SN + PI	(0.2%)	
II + SN + RM	(0.13%)	
II + RM + PI	(0%)	
III + SN + PI	(0.07%)	
III + SN + RM	(0%)	
III + RM + PI	(0%)	
IV + SN + PI	(0%)	
IV + SN + RM	(0%)	
IV + RM + PI	(0%)	
I + SN + RM + PI	(0%)	
II + SN + RM + PI	(0%)	
III + SN + RM + PI	(0%)	
IV + SN + RM + PI	(0%)	

Probability (%) of difficult intubation

FIGURE 49-1. The probability of experiencing a difficult laryngoscopic intubation for the varying combinations of risk factors and the observed incidence of these combinations. (From Rocke D, Murray W, Rout C, et al. Relative risk factors associated with difficult intubation in obstetric anesthesia. *Anesthesiology.* 1992;77:67-73, with permission.)

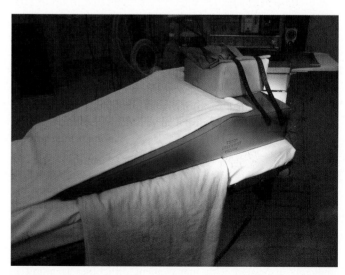

FIGURE 49-2. The Troop Elevation Pillow®: The pillow can help to raise the head and neck above the patient's chest and abdomen. The goal is to position the earlobes at the level of the Angle of Louis. (Courtesy from Mercury Medical.)

of this maneuver. The mnemonic SHORT (see Section 1.6.4) can be used to quickly assess the patient for features that may indicate a difficult cricothyrotomy. Most obstetricians do not have experience in performing a surgical airway, and it is incumbent upon the anesthesia practitioner to maintain capacity in this regard. Nonetheless, it may be prudent to consult with an experienced surgical colleague for assistance when the need for surgical airway is likely.

49.4.3 When a difficult laryngoscopy is anticipated in a parturient, is it useful to perform an awake direct laryngoscopy (an awake look)?

Awake direct laryngoscopy with a topically anesthetized airway (ie, awake look) has been suggested as useful assessment tool of the potentially difficult airway prior to induction of anesthesia. However, one must recognize that the airway as it appears with the patient awake and unparalyzed might look quite different with the patient under general anesthesia and with muscle paralysis.[34]

49.5 CONDUCT OF ANESTHESIA AND TRACHEAL INTUBATION

49.5.1 What are necessary preparations for general anesthesia for a parturient?

There are several preparations that must be made on the labor and delivery suite to ensure safe and expeditious care of the parturient should general anesthesia be required.

The operating room bed should have a ramp on it at all times (Figure 49-2 and Chapter 18). This will prove to be an invaluable aid in optimizing head position and will help align the oral, pharyngeal, and laryngeal axes in the obese parturient. Furthermore, it will not be problematic in the patient with easy tracheal intubation.

It is important to have all difficult airway equipment in the operating room. It is also important to recognize the importance of having well-trained assistants to help with all aspects of airway management, including rescue devices, as well as application of cricoid pressure. Because time is often of the essence, and resources often limited, the practitioner must carefully choose devices with which they are familiar and comfortable, and techniques that can be practiced regularly.

Table 49-3 details some of the suggested equipment necessary to manage the difficult airway on the labor floor. A short laryngoscope handle (stubby) can be particularly helpful.

All obstetrical patients requiring general anesthesia must receive aspiration prophylaxis (nonparticulate antacid and H_2 blocker). Induction must be in rapid-sequence fashion including the application of cricoid pressure. Recent work has shown that, even when correctly applied, cricoid pressure may not always be completely effective.[35] Nevertheless, it has the potential to convert a flood into a trickle.

Because the pregnant patient is at increased risk for hypoxemia, even during short periods of apnea, it is especially important that adequate denitrogenation with 100% oxygen prior to the induction of general anesthesia is performed. Various techniques for denitrogenation have been advocated. Norris and Dewan observed that 3 minutes of denitrogenation, and the four-breath denitrogenation technique, resulted in similar measurements of Pao_2 in pregnant women undergoing rapid-sequence induction of general anesthesia for cesarean section.[21] If the tidal volume is large, and the respiratory rate is high, denitrogenation may need to be only 1 minute in duration. However, this 1 minute can be one of the most important minutes of the induction and should not be further abbreviated.

TABLE 49-3

Equipment Required for Management of Difficult OB Airway

Bed ramp	Troop pillow (Figure 49-2)
Oral airway	Three sizes
Intubation guides	• Eschmann Tracheal Introducer (Portex Limited, Hythe, UK) • Frova intubation introducer (Cook Inc., Bloomington, IN, USA) • Lightwand
Endotracheal tubes	At least three different sized (6.0, 6.5, 7.0)
Laryngoscope	• MAC #3, 4 • Miller #2, 3 *Stubby* short handle
LMA	• Classic #3, #4 • ProSeal #3, #4 • Fastrach #3 ILA (intubating laryngeal airway)
Flexible bronchoscope	
Percutaneous cricothyrotomy kit	

49.5.2 Describe an appropriate algorithm for a difficult/failed intubation in a parturient

The difficult airway algorithm in the parturient is significantly different from that used in the operating room for non-obstetrical surgical patients. In general, the differences focus on the presence or absence of fetal distress.

Frequently, general anesthetics on the labor and delivery service are required in patients with whom the anesthesia practitioner has little or no foreknowledge. In addition, the environment is often volatile, with considerable pressure to proceed with an emergency induction, because fetal viability is in question and fetal rescue is required. In such an event, it is imperative that the practitioner has a simple, clear algorithm to follow when a difficult airway is encountered. Equally important is that the practitioner regularly practices this algorithm with the labor and delivery personnel, and that they are familiar with the airway devices that might be employed in an emergency.

49.5.2.1 Anticipated Difficult Airway

When the anesthesia practitioner anticipates a difficult airway, a regional anesthetic technique may be preferable (Table 49-4). However, there are numerous conditions that may preclude the use of regional anesthesia. When regional anesthesia is not possible, one of the first things that must occur is a thorough discussion with the obstetrician, the patient, the patient's family, and nurses, pointing out any airway management concerns that the anesthesia practitioner has. In some circumstances, the anesthesia practitioner ought to make it clear that the patient's airway management cannot be hurried, implying that a decision to go to surgery may need to be made earlier rather than later. The hope is that one is not pushed into a general anesthetic when more deliberate planning may have permitted a regional technique.

In those instances when regional anesthesia is contraindicated, an anticipated difficult airway is recognized, and time permits, an awake intubation technique should be employed. Flexible bronchoscopy (FB) has become the method most frequently used. The specifics of this technique are found in Chapter 9. However, there are several points that should be reiterated for the obstetrical patient. Because the parturient airway is often edematous,

and engorged, topicalization of the upper airway can frequently be difficult and requires considerable patience. A drying agent is necessary and aspiration prophylaxis must be initiated before topical anesthesia begins. One should not hesitate to sedate the mother as needed.

Blind nasal intubation is an option that must be approached with caution. Any attempt at nasal instrumentation incurs the risk of nasal and pharyngeal bleeding that can compromise subsequent efforts at direct laryngoscopy or bronchoscopic intubation.

Retrograde intubation techniques have been shown to be valuable in the management of the difficult airway in the past, but have little, if any, value today in the care of the obstetrical patient.

There are a host of specialized fiberoptic or video laryngoscope blades and handles (eg, Bullard, GlideScope®, UpsherScope™, Storz Videoscope), each with individualized bulbs, light sources, or fiberoptic bundles ending at various distances into the oral pharynx (see Chapter 10). Considerable effort is needed to maintain these and considerable practice is necessary to become skilled in their use. Certainly, for the anticipated difficult airway in which time and technical assistance will be available, these devices may be useful. However, in general, time and assistance are perpetually in short supply on labor and delivery services.

49.5.2.2 Unanticipated Difficult Airway

Table 49-5 lists several important points to remember in managing an unanticipated difficult obstetrical airway. Figures 49-3 and 49-4 are algorithms one might choose to use in the event of an unanticipated failed tracheal intubation in the obstetrical patient. Figure 49-3 outlines the critical breakpoints in the management of an obstetrical patient requiring general anesthesia: anticipated versus not anticipated; adequate ventilation versus inadequate ventilation; fetal distress versus no fetal distress.

If ventilation is possible, the decision to continue hinges on the presence or absence of fetal distress. If there is no fetal distress, the patient should be awakened and an alternative anesthetic technique chosen. If, on the other hand, fetal distress is present, one may elect to continue with the case using mask ventilation or an EGD. The patient continues to be at risk of aspiration and cricoid pressure should be continued.

If ventilation is impossible, the patient should be allowed to wake up regardless of the presence of fetal distress. In the interim, rescue

---

( ) TABLE 49-4

Important Points for Managing the Anticipated Difficult Obstetrical Airway

Identify parturients at high risk for operative intervention	• Obesity • Advanced maternal age • Non-reassuring fetal or maternal conditions
Detailed discussions with the obstetrician concerning delivery plan	• Crash induction is not an option • Speak to patient and family early in labor • Persist with regional techniques • Awake intubation if necessary—using a flexible bronchoscope • Wishful thinking is a poor anesthetic plan—*know* that your regional technique is working

TABLE 49-5

Important Points for Managing the Unanticipated Difficult Obstetrical Airway

Thorough and careful airway evaluations	• Know your predictors—which ones work for you
Strategy for intubating the difficult airway	• Pick your algorithm ahead of time
Make basic preparations for the difficult airway	• Pick your equipment ahead of time (LMA, LMA-Proseal™, LMA-Fastrach™, Eschmann, Combitube™, jet ventilator, cricothyrotomy kit) • Keep it simple—get real with your gadgets • Practice, practice, practice

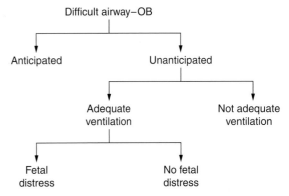

FIGURE 49-3. Basic decision points for the Difficult Airway Algorithm in the obstetrical patient.

techniques may be necessary. Placing the LMA-Classic™, LMA-Fastrach™, or LMA-Proseal™ could be lifesaving in this instance. If, during the awakening process, ventilation is reestablished, one may then elect to continue with the case, if fetal distress is present. A more critical situation is one where, in addition to fetal distress, obstetrical hemorrhage or some other life-threatening condition for the mother exists. Most situations of antepartum hemorrhage do not improve until delivery of the fetus and placenta. The LMA-Fastrach™ may be an excellent choice in this setting.

Several alternative methods to mask ventilation have been described which, of necessity, can be instituted quickly; insertion of the Esophageal Tracheal Combitube™; or insertion of an LMA (Classic, ProSeal, and Fastrach ILMA). If these fail, one may institute trans-tracheal jet ventilation, or perform an emergency cricothyrotomy, or tracheotomy.

The Combitube™ is a plastic twin-lumen tube that can be placed blindly and, when properly positioned, serves to seal the esophagus and ventilate the trachea (see Section 12.6). The Combitube™ has been employed in diverse clinical circumstances to provide adequate ventilation and oxygenation. There is only one report of its use in the parturient.[36] A major drawback of the Combitube™ is that it is a disposable device that one would not use electively and, therefore, not something one can easily practice with in nonemergency situations.

The laryngeal mask airway (LMA) is a well-established device in the ASA difficult airway algorithm and must be part of every difficult airway cart on the labor and delivery floor. The LMA has rapidly become a mainstay in difficult airway management because it is used on a daily basis and practitioners are comfortable with its use. The LMA has been used effectively and safely in selected healthy non-obese parturients, although this is not a practice that the authors would support, other than as a rescue maneuver.[37]

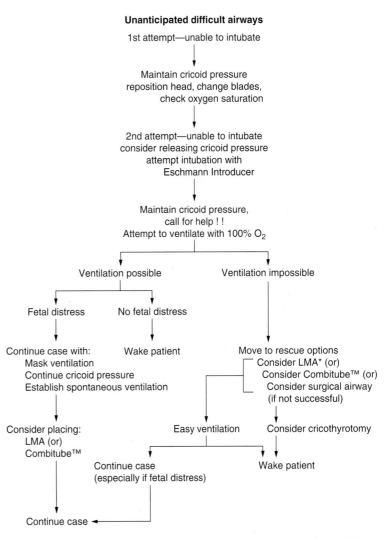

*May consider placing an endotracheal tube through the LMA, this maneuver must be practiced ahead of time.

FIGURE 49-4. Difficult Airway Algorithm in the obstetrical patient.

When the LMA is placed in the failed intubation/failed ventilation scenario, cricoid pressure should be continued.

The LMA-Proseal™ is a redesigned LMA that may offer a degree of protection against aspiration to the parturient, in comparison with the LMA-Classic™. The LMA-Proseal™, designed to facilitate controlled ventilation and to mitigate the potential for reflux, has been used successfully in failed intubation emergency cesarean section.[38]

Finally, the LMA-Fastrach™ may have a significant advantage over the LMA-Classic™, or the LMA-Proseal™, in the obstetrical patient. Following placement of the LMA-Fastrach™, an endotracheal tube can be placed through the LMA to secure the airway.

While transtracheal jet ventilation (TTJV) is said to be simple, quick, and relatively safe, it is technically difficult to perform in obstetrical patients. As reports of catastrophes have surfaced with TTJV during emergency situations, this technique has slowly lost favor and is seldom used in favor of using the LMA, or a surgical cricothyrotomy.

A surgical airway is indicated when one is confronted with a failed airway. Percutaneous surgical cricothyrotomy is a viable alternative to open surgical cricothyrotomy. Several kits have become commercially available. These kits appear to be simple, rapid, and safe to use. There is increasing enthusiasm that anesthesia practitioners learn this technique, instead of TTJV.

49.6   SUMMARY

Difficult or failed intubation is a major contributor to maternal morbidity and mortality during obstetrical emergencies. Careful preanesthetic evaluation focusing on the parturient's airway should identify patients at risk for difficult airway management. Early communication with the obstetricians, regular review and practice of a formal Difficult Airway Algorithm, and facility with current difficult airway devices should mitigate some of the risk of injuries to parturients when a failed intubation does occur.

REFERENCES

1. Whitehead SJ, Berg CJ, Chang J. Pregnancy-related mortality due to cardiomyopathy: United States, 1991-1997. *Obstet Gynecol.* 2003;102:1326-1331.
2. Hawkins JL, Koonin LM, Palmer SK, Gibbs CP. Anesthesia-related deaths during obstetric delivery in the United States, 1979-1990. *Anesthesiology.* 1997;86:277-284.
3. Ross BK. ASA closed claims in obstetrics: lessons learned. *Anesthesiol Clin North Am.* 2003;21:183-197.
4. Rocke DA, Murray WB, Rout CC, Gouws E. Relative risk analysis of factors associated with difficult intubation in obstetric anesthesia. *Anesthesiology.* 1992;77:67-73.
5. Rose DK, Cohen MM. The airway: problems and predictions in 18,500 patients. *Can J Anaesth.* 1994;41:372-383.
6. Benumof JL. Difficult laryngoscopy: obtaining the best view. *Can J Anaesth.* 1994;41:361-365.
7. Davies JM, Weeks S, Crone LA, Pavlin E. Difficult intubation in the parturient. *Can J Anaesth.* 1989;36:668-674.
8. Hawthorne L, Wilson R, Lyons G, Dresner M. Failed intubation revisited: 17-yr experience in a teaching maternity unit. *Br J Anaesth.* 1996;76:680-684.
9. Goldszmidt E. Principles and practices of obstetric airway management. *Anesthesiol Clin.* 2008;26:109-125, vii.
10. Cook TM. Failed intubation in obstetric anaesthesia. *Anaesthesia.* 2006;61:605-606; author reply 606-607.
11. Cooper G, Reynolds F. The drive for regional anaesthesia for elective caesarean section has gone too far. *Int J Obstet Anesth.* 2002;11:289-295.
12. Cormack RS. Failed intubation in obstetric anaesthesia. *Anaesthesia.* 2006;61:505-506.
13. Jenkins JG. Failed intubation during obstetric anaesthesia. *Br J Anaesth.* 1996;77:698.
14. Lipman S, Carvalho B, Brock-Utne J. The demise of general anesthesia in obstetrics revisited: prescription for a cure. *Int J Obstet Anesth.* 2005;14:2-4.
15. Saravanakumar K, Cooper GM. Failed intubation in obstetrics: has the incidence changed recently? *Br J Anaesth.* 2005;94:690.
16. Munnur U, Suresh MS. Airway problems in pregnancy. *Crit Care Clin.* 2004;20:617-642.
17. Cedergren MI. Maternal morbid obesity and the risk of adverse pregnancy outcome. *Obstet Gynecol.* 2004;103:219-224.
18. Endler GC, Mariona FG, Sokol RJ, Stevenson LB. Anesthesia-related maternal mortality in Michigan, 1972 to 1984. *Am J Obstet Gynecol.* 1988;159:187-193.
19. Hood DD, Dewan DM. Anesthetic and obstetric outcome in morbidly obese parturients. *Anesthesiology.* 1993;79:1210-1218.
20. Chadwick HS. Obstetric anesthesia closed claims update II. *Anesthesiol Newslet.* 1999;1-6.
21. Norris MC, Dewan DM. Preoxygenation for cesarean section: a comparison of two techniques. *Anesthesiology.* 1985;62:827-829.
22. Izci B, Riha RL, Martin SE, et al. The upper airway in pregnancy and preeclampsia. *Am J Respir Crit Care Med.* 2003;167:137-140.
23. Dobb G. Laryngeal oedema complicating obstetric anaesthesia. *Anaesthesia.* 1978;33:839-840.
24. Jouppila R, Jouppila P, Hollmen A. Laryngeal oedema as an obstetric anaesthesia complication: case reports. *Acta Anaesthesiol Scand.* 1980;24:97-98.
25. Farcon EL, Kim MH, Marx GF. Changing Mallampati score during labour. *Can J Anaesth.* 1994;41:50-51.
26. Kodali BS, Chandrasekhar S, Bulich LN, et al. Airway changes during labor and delivery. *Anesthesiology.* 2008;108:357-362.
27. Bhavani-Shankar K, Bulich L, Kafiluddir R, et al. Does labor and delivery induce airway changes? *Anesthesiology.* 2001;93:A1035.
28. Perlow JH, Kirz DS. Severe preeclampsia presenting as dysphonia secondary to uvular edema. A case report. *J Reprod Med.* 1990;35:1059-1062.
29. McDonnell NJ, Paech MJ, Clavisi OM, Scott KL. Difficult and failed intubation in obstetric anaesthesia: an observational study of airway management and complications associated with general anaesthesia for caesarean section. *Int J Obstet Anesth.* 2008;17:292-297.
30. Tsen LC, Pitner R, Camann WR. General anesthesia for cesarean section at a tertiary care hospital 1990-1995: indications and implications. *Int J Obstet Anesth.* 1998;7:147-152.
31. Langeron O, Masso E, Huraux C, et al. Prediction of difficult mask ventilation. *Anesthesiology.* 2000;92:1229-1236.
32. Dupont X, Hamza J, Jullien P, Narchi P. Risk factors associated with difficult airway in normotensive parturients. *Anesthesiology.* 1990;73:A999.
33. Benumof JL. Management of the difficult adult airway. With special emphasis on awake tracheal intubation. *Anesthesiology.* 1991;75:1087-1110.
34. Sivarajan M, Fink BR. The position and the state of the larynx during general anesthesia and muscle paralysis. *Anesthesiology.* 1990;72:439-442.
35. Brimacombe JR, Berry AM. Cricoid pressure. *Can J Anaesth.* 1997;44:414-425.
36. Wissler RN. The esophageal-tracheal Combitube. *Anesthesiol Rev.* 1993;20:147-152.
37. Han TH, Brimacombe J, Lee EJ, Yang HS. The laryngeal mask airway is effective (and probably safe) in selected healthy parturients for elective Cesarean section: a prospective study of 1067 cases. *Can J Anaesth.* 2001;48:1117-1121.
38. Awan R, Nolan JP, Cook TM. Use of a ProSeal laryngeal mask airway for airway maintenance during emergency Caesarean section after failed tracheal intubation. *Br J Anaesth.* 2004;92:144-146.

SELF-EVALUATION QUESTIONS

49.1 Which of the following combination of patient characteristics have been shown to have a high prediction accuracy for a difficult laryngoscopy and intubation in obstetrical population?

    A. high Mallampati grade, plus short neck (SN), plus protruding maxillary incisors (PMI), and receding mandible (RM)

    B. SN, plus PMI, and RM

C. PMI plus RM

D. high Mallampati grade alone

E. none of the above

49.2 Which of the following gastrointestinal changes associated with pregnancy is **NOT** true?

A. A decrease in lower esophageal tone.

B. An intragastric pressure increases steadily during pregnancy, as the gravid uterus enlarges.

C. Gastric emptying appears to be delayed during pregnancy.

D. There is an increased risk of gastric aspiration.

E. Gastric acidity is increased during pregnancy.

49.3 All of the following are known airway changes associated with pregnancy **EXCEPT**:

A. Generalized edema of the oropharynx, nasopharynx, and trachea.

B. Voice changes are common due to swelling of the false vocal cords and arytenoids.

C. Capillary engorgement of the nasal increases progressively throughout pregnancy.

D. Mallampati classification of the oropharyngeal space has been reported to advance by one or two classes during labor.

E. All the airway changes return to pre-labor state within 12 hours postpartum.

CHAPTER (50)

Airway Management of the Obstetrical Patient with an Anticipated Difficult Airway

Brian K. Ross

50.1 CASE PRESENTATION

The patient is a 32-year-old black woman G1P0 at 31-weeks gestation. Her medical history is notable for mild obesity (102 kg; BMI 39), a suggestion of sleep apnea (a report of significant snoring and periods of apnea while she sleeps), and treatment for chronic hypertension for the past 6 years.

Five days prior to admission, the patient's hypertension and peripheral edema worsened, and she developed new-onset proteinuria. A 3.0 kg weight gain during the 7 days prior to admission was also noted. At the time of admission, the patient had a blood pressure of 168/102 mm Hg, a heart rate of 85 beats per minute (bpm), a short neck, large breasts, an airway classified as Mallampati Class IV, a 3 cm mouth opening with prominent incisor teeth, a thyromental distance of 2.0 cm, and a limited range of motion of her neck. She was placed on strict bed rest and treated aggressively with atenolol and furosemide.

Twenty-four hours prior to delivery, a non-stress test demonstrated little or no reactivity and late decelerations with the few contractions she was having. The decision was made to induce labor and deliver the fetus. In the 8 hours preceding her induction, her hematocrit rose from 32% to 41% and her platelet count fell from 178K to 75K × 10⁹/L. The patient was placed on a magnesium sulfate intravenous infusion. She was noted to become increasingly edematous and somnolent.

With induction of labor, the patient has developed regular contractions of appropriate strength for some 12 hours. She has progressed to 10 cm cervical dilation and has been pushing for 3 hours. The baby has remained at –1 station and does not appear to be descending. Because of the risk of inadequate coagulation, the patient has been managed throughout labor with a systemic opioid. A decision has been made to perform a cesarean section. The fetus is stable at the present time.

50.2 PATIENT CONSIDERATIONS

50.2.1 What are the physiological changes of pregnancy that impact on the airway management of this patient?

This patient is at considerable risk of rapid oxygen desaturation because of her pregnancy-associated increase in oxygen consumption, decrease in FRC, increase in closing volume, and increase in alveolar-arterial oxygen gradient. She is also at risk for aspiration because of pregnancy-related decreased gastroesophageal sphincter tone, increased gastric acid production, and decreased gastrointestinal motility. Therefore, this patient must be pretreated with a nonparticulate antacid and perhaps an H_2 receptor blocker. If the patient is rendered unconscious before her airway is secured, a rapid-sequence induction with cricoid pressure must be employed to minimize the risk of gastric content reflux and aspiration.

50.2.2 What is the most likely diagnosis for this patient?

This patient has chronic hypertension, with superimposed severe preeclampsia, that is, severe hypertension, edema, and proteinuria. She has been given magnesium sulfate for both seizure prophylaxis and blood pressure control. In addition, she has developed thrombocytopenia and a likely associated platelet dysfunction. Regional anesthesia, while preferred, is considered contraindicated under these circumstances.

50.2.3   What is preeclampsia?

Preeclampsia is a term that describes a subset of pregnancy-induced hypertension accompanied by proteinuria, low plasma oncotic pressure, generalized capillary leakage, and edema, including the airway, after the 20th week of gestation. While edema is commonly present, it is no longer a required criterion for diagnosis of preeclampsia.[1] Preeclampsia is more dangerous if onset is prior to 34 weeks.

Preeclampsia can be mild or severe. Severe preeclampsia is defined by the presence of at least one of the following: blood pressures ≥160 mm Hg systolic or 110 mm Hg diastolic; proteinuria ≥5 g/24 h; headache; blurred vision; epigastric or right upper quadrant pain; and pulmonary edema.

Because thrombocytopenic coagulopathy frequently complicates preeclampsia, general anesthesia is usually employed, if an operative delivery is required.

50.2.4   What are the consequences of preeclampsia on the parturient airway?

The possibility of severe upper airway edema constitutes a major concern with preeclampsia.[2] Any suggestion of stridor or dyspnea should particularly alert the practitioner to the possible hazards of a difficult airway. However, extreme difficulty may be encountered in preeclamptic patients who are asymptomatic. The airway of a preeclamptic patient will be edematous and friable, and thus very unforgiving if multiple attempts at intubation are required. In addition, there have been observations of pharyngeal narrowing that could contribute to difficulty in blind intubating procedures.

50.2.5   What is the impact of weight gain and obesity on the parturient?

Weight gain is a natural consequence of pregnancy, however in recent years the proportion of women gaining greater than the recommended weight has increased.[3] This patient has experienced a rapid weight gain of greater than 3.0 kg in the week prior to intervention, primarily as a result of generalized edema. This patient is of particular concern because her preeclampsia was preceded by significant obesity.

Obesity places the parturient at greater risk for hypertension, diabetes, preeclampsia, difficult labor, increased likelihood of instrumental delivery, and postpartum hemorrhage. All of these conditions frequently require surgical intervention.[4-6] Difficult mask ventilation, as well as increased volume and acidity of gastric contents, are also associated with obesity. Indeed, there is a documented association of obesity with airway difficulty and maternal mortality.[7-10]

50.2.6   Does labor have any effect on the parturient airway?

The incidence of Mallampati Class IV airways increases by as much as 34 % as pregnancy progresses from 12 to 34 weeks' gestation.[11]

In addition, airway status can deteriorate significantly as labor proceeds.[12,13] This suggests that the dynamic airway status should be examined repeatedly throughout labor, particularly in those patients where initial concerns of a possible difficult airway exist.[14]

50.2.7   Does this patient have a worrisome airway?

The patient, as described, is likely to be difficult at laryngoscopy and intubation. While no single measurement is sufficient to predict a difficult laryngoscopy, this patient certainly has more than two of the usual predictors. The Mallampati Class IV assessment indicates that oral structures are large in relation to mandibular size. The short thyromental distance and prominent incisors correlate with difficulty in placing a laryngoscope blade.[15] All of these, in association with a short thick neck, limited range of motion of the neck, and large pendulous breasts, suggest that laryngoscopic intubation would be very difficult.

In addition to an unfavorable anatomical presentation, the patient's obesity and potential sleep apnea would suggest potential difficulties with mask ventilation.[16] The combination of potential difficult mask ventilation and difficult laryngoscopic intubation drastically limit the options available for oxygenating this patient. If this patient's fetus was experiencing a significant distress, management of her airway would be even more problematic.

50.3   AIRWAY MANAGEMENT FOR A PARTURIENT WITH AN ANTICIPATED DIFFICULT AIRWAY

50.3.1   What initial preparations should be made with the obstetricians as induction of labor is undertaken?

One of the most important things that an anesthesia practitioner must do is to communicate with the obstetricians, the nurses, the patient, and the patient's family. The health care team and the patient/family must understand that every effort would be made to avoid the necessity for an urgent induction of general anesthesia. The reasons underlying this plan must be clearly and frankly explained. Nevertheless, all equipment must be readied for urgent induction, and obstetrically relevant protocols should be reviewed by all caregivers. Algorithms used on the obstetrical floor are quite different from the ones used in the general operating room (see Chapter 49).

50.3.2   What anesthetic technique would be most appropriate for a surgical delivery of a parturient with an anticipated difficult airway?

Some form of regional anesthesia (epidural, spinal, continuous spinal, or combined spinal/epidural) would be the preferred management technique for a parturient with an anticipated difficult airway. However, this patient's developing coagulopathy precludes the use of a regional technique. While it is very unusual for a successful regional technique to require conversion to general anesthesia, there are reports of failed regional techniques, and circumstances may arise, necessitating induction of general anesthesia. Therefore, backup plans for induction of general anesthesia, should the need arise, must be formulated in advance.

50.3.3 What specific equipment should be available in caring for this patient: a parturient with an anticipated difficult airway, short thick neck with anatomy distorted by edema and obesity, and at considerable risk for bleeding and excessive secretions?

The operating room (OR) should be readied—the OR bed should be ramped (see Section 18.3.2) and the difficult airway cart (see Chapter 59) should be immediately available at the induction site.

While there are a number of alternative intubating techniques under general anesthesia, the authors believe they all have limitations. Rapid-sequence induction with direct laryngoscopy, under any circumstance, is dangerous. Techniques requiring transillumination are technically very difficult in obese patients with a short neck, or excessive neck tissue and edema. Poor neck anatomy greatly hinders rescue techniques such as transtracheal jet ventilation, cricothyrotomy, or tracheotomy. Blind nasotracheal tube placement will inevitably lead to considerable bleeding in a pregnant preeclamptic patient; and blind placement of the endotracheal tube using an Eschmann tracheal introducer, or its equivalent, requires at least some visualization of the epiglottis. There is some enthusiasm for the elective utilization of an LMA in a pregnant patient at term,[17] but such advocacy is usually limited to healthy non-obese patients and is very rarely used in North America. Laryngeal mask airways such as the LMA-ProSeal™ (LMAP), or the disposable LMA-Supreme™, with incorporated esophageal vents, have the potential advantage over the LMA-Classic™ of providing some protection against the aspiration of gastric contents. Unfortunately, there are case reports of gastric regurgitation and aspiration during their use,[18,19] particularly if the LMAP is not properly placed in the hypopharynx. An intubating LMA (ILMA or LMA-Fastrach™) might also be considered; however failure with these devices is not unknown.

In recent years there has been a profusion of video laryngoscopic devices introduced on the market. Numerous studies, in non-obstetric patients with difficult airways, report improved laryngoscopic views and intubation success rates compared with direct laryngoscopy.[20-22] There are also some published reports of improved laryngoscopic views, and intubation success rates, in morbidly obese patients using video laryngoscopes. However, the results are inconsistent and vary according to particular devices and skill set of the anesthesia practitioner.[23-25] There are no published reports of the success rates of these devices in obstetric patients.

An awake technique is probably most appropriate for this patient. A number of practitioners employ an *awake look* technique. That is, the airway is topicalized, or anesthetized using laryngeal nerve blocks, and then examined under direct vision using a laryngoscope. However, evidence exists of poor correlation between airway visualization in an awake patient and patients who are subsequently anesthetized and paralyzed.[26]

For this patient, the authors would choose awake intubation using a flexible bronchoscope. Sedatives and hypnotics will usually be required to facilitate an awake intubation and consideration will be required in regard to unusual sensitivity to these agents in pregnant patients, and patients with sleep apnea. In addition, potential impact of drugs and techniques on the newborn will require consideration. Pharyngeal and laryngeal structures must be anesthetized adequately for awake bronchoscopic intubation to be successful, and topicalization of the airway in edematous airways is usually difficult and requires patience. Some practitioners advocate laryngeal nerve blocks in this instance. However, in the edematous obese neck, nerve blocks are both difficult and frequently not successful.

50.4 POSTINTUBATION CARE OF THE PARTURIENT WITH A DIFFICULT AIRWAY

50.4.1 What precautions must be taken when the case ends?

The difficult airway case does not end with intubation. One must be equally cautious with the extubation. There are certainly many occasions in which one might consider leaving the obese preeclamptic patient intubated for several hours after surgery, to allow time to remobilize some of the edema fluid, and improve airway conditions. The preeclamptic patient is invariably on magnesium for seizure prophylaxis and if non-depolarizing neuromuscular blocking agents have been used, complete reversal of these agents must be ensured. Prior to extubation, the patient must be fully awake and capable of protecting her airway from aspiration. In many instances, one might consider checking for an air leak (a leak test) around the deflated cuff of the endotracheal tube, to further ensure that the patient's airway will be patent after extubation. Consideration should also be given to extubation over an airway exchange catheter which may be left in situ and be used as a conduit for reintubation.[27]

50.5 SUMMARY

The obese preeclamptic patients with an anticipated difficult airway can be exceedingly challenging to manage and are best cared for in a team effort. Thorough understanding of the pathophysiology of preeclampsia is critical in providing the optimal anesthetic care for these patients. Their care cannot be rushed, and decisions must be made in a logical and methodical manner. In addition, the practitioner must continue to review the difficult airway algorithm and make a concerted effort to remain facile with those devices that may be needed in difficult airway scenarios.

REFERENCES

1. Brown MA, Lindheimer MD, de Swiet M, Van Assche A, Moutquin JM. The classification and diagnosis of the hypertensive disorders of pregnancy: statement from the International Society for the Study of Hypertension in Pregnancy (ISSHP). *Hypertens Pregnancy.* 2001;20:IX-XIV.

2. Izci B, Riha RL, Martin SE, et al. The upper airway in pregnancy and pre-eclampsia. *Am J Respir Crit Care Med.* 2003;167:137-140.

3. Institute of Medicine and National Research Council. *Weight Gain During Pregnancy: Reexamining the Guidelines.* Washington, DC: The National Academies Press; 2009.

4. Callaway LK, Prins JB, Chang AM, McIntyre HD. The prevalence and impact of overweight and obesity in an Australian obstetric population. *Med J Aust.* 2006;184:56-59.

5. Crane JM, White J, Murphy P, et al. The effect of gestational weight gain by body mass index on maternal and neonatal outcomes. *J Obstet Gynaecol Can.* 2009;31:28-35.

6. Yogev Y, Catalano PM. Pregnancy and obesity. *Obstet Gynecol Clin North Am.* 2009;36:285-300, viii.

7. Endler GC, Mariona FG, Sokol RJ, Stevenson LB. Anesthesia-related maternal mortality in Michigan, 1972 to 1984. *Am J Obstet Gynecol.* 1988;159: 187-193.

8. Lewis G. The confidential enquiry into maternal and child health (CEMACH). Why Mothers Die 2000-2002. The sixth report on confidential enquiries into maternal death in the United Kingdom. London: RCOG; 2004

9. Lewis G. The confidential enquiry into maternal and child health (CEMACH). Saving mother's lives: reviewing maternal deaths to make motherhood safer: 2003-2005. The seventh report on confidential enquiries into maternal deaths in the United Kingdom. London: CEMACH; 2007.

10. Ross BK. ASA closed claims in obstetrics: lessons learned. *Anesthesiol Clin North Am.* 2003;21:183-197.

11. Pilkington S, Carli F, Dakin MJ, et al. Increase in Mallampati score during pregnancy. *Br J Anaesth.* 1995;74:638-642.

12. Farcon EL, Kim MH, Marx GF. Changing Mallampati score during labour. *Can J Anaesth.* 1994;41:50-51.

13. Kodali BS, Chandrasekhar S, Bulich LN, Topulos GP, Datta S. Airway changes during labor and delivery. *Anesthesiology.* 2008;108:357-362.

14. Lewin SB, Cheek TG, Deutschman CS. Airway management in the obstetric patient. *Crit Care Clin.* 2000;16:505-513.

15. Rocke DA, Murray WB, Rout CC, Gouws E. Relative risk analysis of factors associated with difficult intubation in obstetric anesthesia. *Anesthesiology.* 1992;77:67-73.

16. Kheterpal S, Han R, Tremper KK, et al. Incidence and predictors of difficult and impossible mask ventilation. *Anesthesiology.* 2006;105:885-891.

17. Han TH, Brimacombe J, Lee EJ, Yang HS. The laryngeal mask airway is effective (and probably safe) in selected healthy parturients for elective Cesarean section: a prospective study of 1067 cases. *Can J Anaesth.* 2001;48: 1117-1121.

18. Brimacombe J, Keller C. Aspiration of gastric contents during use of a ProSeal laryngeal mask airway secondary to unidentified foldover malposition. *Anesth Analg.* 2003;97:1192-1194.

19. Koay CK. A case of aspiration using the proseal LMA. *Anaesth Intensive Care.* 2003;31:123.

20. Jungbauer A, Schumann M, Brunkhorst V, Börgers A, Groeben H. Expected difficult tracheal intubation: a prospective comparison of direct laryngoscopy and video laryngoscopy in 200 patients. *Br J Anaesth.* 2009;102:546-550.

21. Serocki G, Bein B, Scholz J, Dorges V. Management of the predicted difficult airway: a comparison of conventional blade laryngoscopy with video-assisted blade laryngoscopy and the GlideScope. *Eur J Anaesthesiol.* 2010;27:24-30.

22. Stroumpoulis K, Pagoulatou A, Violari M, et al. Videolaryngoscopy in the management of the difficult airway: a comparison with the Macintosh blade. *Eur J Anaesthesiol.* 2009;26:218-222.

23. Dhonneur G, Abdi W, Ndoko SK, et al. Video-assisted versus conventional tracheal intubation in morbidly obese patients. *Obes Surg.* 2009;19:1096-1101.

24. Maassen R, Lee R, Hermans B, et al. A comparison of three videolaryngoscopes: the Macintosh laryngoscope blade reduces, but does not replace, routine stylet use for intubation in morbidly obese patients. *Anesth Analg.* 2009;109:1560-1565.

25. Marrel J, Blanc C, Frascarolo P, Magnusson L. Videolaryngoscopy improves intubation condition in morbidly obese patients. *Eur J Anaesthesiol.* 2007;24: 1045-1049.

26. Sivarajan M, Fink BR. The position and the state of the larynx during general anesthesia and muscle paralysis. *Anesthesiology.* 1990;72:439-442.

27. Mort TC. Continuous airway access for the difficult extubation: the efficacy of the airway exchange catheter. *Anesth Analg.* 2007;105:1357-1362.

SELF-EVALUATION QUESTIONS

50.1 Which of the following is **NOT** a physiological change of pregnancy that would impact on the airway management of the patient?

   A. increase in oxygen consumption

   B. decrease in FRC

   C. increase risk of aspiration

   D. decrease in alveolar-arterial oxygen gradient

   E. increase in closing volume

50.2 All of the following are potential problems of preeclampsia on the parturient airway **EXCEPT**?

   A. Severe upper airway edema.

   B. Friable airway and thus very unforgiving if multiple attempts at intubation are required.

   C. Pharyngeal narrowing that could contribute to difficulty in blind intubating techniques.

   D. Bronchoscopic intubation under indirect vision is contraindicated because of the potential airway bleeding.

   E. Blind nasotracheal intubation will inevitably lead to considerable bleeding.

50.3 Which of the following is a reasonable intubating technique for an obese parturient with severe preeclampsia and a history of difficult laryngoscopic intubation?

   A. awake bronchoscopic intubation

   B. laryngoscopic intubation following a rapid-sequence induction

   C. awake intubation using a lightwand

   D. awake blind nasal intubation

   E. intubation through an intubating LMA under general anesthesia

CHAPTER (51)

Unanticipated Difficult Airway in an Obstetrical Patient Requiring an Emergency Cesarean Section

Adeyemi J. Olufolabi and Holly A. Muir

51.1 CASE PRESENTATION

A 25-year-old primigravida at 39-week gestational age presents to the case room with ruptured membranes and frequent uterine contractions. She does not want to have epidural analgesia because of a story she heard about an epidural complication suffered by one of her distant relatives. After 14 hours of labor, augmented with oxytocin, and now 2 hours of pushing, she is urgently taken to the operating room for emergency cesarean section, for prolonged late decelerations. She weighs 253 lb (115 kg) and is 5 ft 3 in (160 cm) tall, giving her a BMI of approximately 45. Airway examination reveals a Mallampati Class III and a thyromental distance of 5 cm. She has a full neck extension with normal dentition and a normal mouth opening. She has large gravid breasts. Her blood pressure is 128/68 mm Hg, heart rate 100 beats per minute (bpm), respiration rate 20 breaths per minute, and SaO_2 of 99% on a 100% O_2 rebreathing face mask. On arrival in the operating room, the fetal heart rate is 80 bpm.

51.2 ANESTHETIC CONSIDERATIONS

51.2.1 What are the anesthetic options for cesarean section in this patient?

An emergency cesarean section is mandated to deliver the fetus with persistent bradycardia (late deceleration), while minimizing potential/preventable risk to the mother. Anesthesia risk factors for airway management in this patient include her BMI (45 kg·m^{-2}) and enlarged breasts. Although regional anesthetic techniques have become the standard of anesthetic care for operative delivery in obstetrics,[1] this patient has refused the regional approach.

The concerns for emergency cesarean section under general anesthesia include securing the airway, reducing the sympathetic response to laryngoscopy and intubation, adequate fluid resuscitation, and the potential of blood loss due to volatile-agent-induced uterine atony. With respect to the first of these concerns, all labor and delivery facilities must have a difficult airway cart and contingency plans for failed laryngoscopic intubation.[1]

51.3 AIRWAY CONSIDERATIONS

51.3.1 What are the airway considerations in pregnant women?

Pregnancy is associated with fluid retention and weight gain.[2] Mallampati Class III and IV seem to be more prevalent in parturients at the beginning of labor (28%) than in the general adult population (7%-17%), suggesting that tongue volume increase maybe one of the physiologic changes of a normal pregnancy.[3] Structurally, the pharyngeal airway is surrounded by soft tissues, such as the tongue and soft palate, which are enclosed by bony structures, such as the mandible and spine. Size of the airway space is determined by the balance between the bony enclosure space and soft tissue volume, when pharyngeal muscles are inactivated by general anesthetics and muscle relaxants. Pharyngeal edema, presumably due to fluid retention during pregnancy, and pharyngeal swelling acutely developed during labor, increases the soft tissue volume surrounding the airway, narrowing the pharyngeal airway in parturients.[2] Many have hypothesized on predictors of this event including weight gain during the pregnancy, fluid administration during labor, and the length of the first and second stage of labor. A recent study from France by Boutonnet et al demonstrated an increase in the incidence of Mallampati Class III and IV from the eighth month of pregnancy to the beginning of labor, and during labor, and this incidence was not fully reversed up to 48 hours after delivery.[4]

Moreover, these changes occurred irrespective of any increase in body weight, duration of first and second stages of labor, or volume of IV fluid administered. In their study, they made observation at four time points: at 8 months of gestation (not in labor); when the epidural was placed; 20 minutes after delivery; and finally at 48 hours after delivery. They found no changes in score in 38.8% of their patients, however, in the remaining women, significant changes were observed both in the interval between the first nonlaboring assessment, and at placement of the epidural, and between placing the epidural and delivery. As illustrated in Figure 51-1, a progressive increase in Mallampati Class III and IV airway was seen.

Similar results were observed by Kodali et al.[5] As with the Boutonnet study,[4] no correlation was observed between airway changes during labor and duration of labor, or fluids administered during labor.

Recent extensive research on the pathophysiology of upper airway obstruction revealed a significant role of lung volume reduction in pharyngeal narrowing.[6] Obese parturients, a high-risk group for perioperative airway catastrophe, are prone to develop progressively narrower pharyngeal airways due to increase of soft tissue volume surrounding the pharyngeal airway, and decrease of lung volume during pregnancy. Lung volume reduction during general anesthesia is known to be more prominent and prolonged in obese patients.

The assessment of the pregnant patient must specifically address features that increase the risk of difficult laryngoscopic intubation, including receding mandible, limited mouth opening, short neck, limited neck movement, and high Mallampati Grade (III and IV). Taken together, these features are known to increase the likelihood of a difficult laryngoscopic intubation.[7] Using the airway assessment strategies as described in Chapter 1 (MOANS, LEMON, RODS, and SHORT), this patient's airway assessment suggests possible difficult bag-mask-ventilation (BMV), possible difficult use of extraglottic device (EGD), and possible difficult surgical airway. But there are no other predictors of a difficult laryngoscopy and intubation.[8,9]

The standard of care in obstetrical anesthesia demands that the airway of this patient be secured in such a manner that the risk of aspiration is minimized, leaving the airway practitioner with two choices in this case: rapid-sequence induction (RSI) or an awake technique. An awake technique reduces the risk of a failed airway in an anesthetized and paralyzed patient. The decision to perform an awake intubation technique, rather than an RSI, should be based on clinical findings and the experience of the practitioner. In either case, contingency plans (Plans B and C) must be in place in the event that these techniques fail. One of the contingency plans must be a surgical airway, or cricothyrotomy.

51.4 CONDUCT OF ANESTHESIA

51.4.1 How should the anesthetic be conducted in this patient?

Reflux/aspiration prophylaxis using oral 0.3 M sodium citrate (30 mL) and intravenous ranitidine 50 mg (± metoclopramide 10 mg) should be given, following the placement of an intravenous catheter. Appropriate intravenous anesthesia induction agents (propofol 2 mg·kg⁻¹, or thiopentone 3-4 mg·kg⁻¹, and succinylcholine 1.5 mg·kg⁻¹) are prepared. A designated assistant with experience in applying cricoid pressure during the RSI must be available.

The patient is placed in a left tilt (at least 15 degrees) to minimize the threat of aortocaval compression syndrome (or supine hypotensive syndrome). In addition, the thorax, shoulders, neck, and head of this morbidly obese parturient should be elevated (ramping) to bring the anatomical axes of the oral, pharyngeal, and laryngeal structures into alignment (see Figures 18-2 and 49-2). A polio-handle (short handle) laryngoscope may be required during intubation to facilitate laryngoscope blade insertion, in the face of large breasts. Alternatively, an assistant may be designated to retract the breasts caudally during laryngoscopy. A difficult airway cart with appropriate airway devices must be immediately available. Denitrogenation is achieved. It should be noted that modified shorter duration denitrogenation techniques may suffice and have been shown to be effective.[10,11]

Following an RSI with cricoid pressure, direct laryngoscopy, using a #3 Macintosh blade, reveals a Cormack/Lehane (C/L) Grade IV view (only the hard palate is visible). A second attempt at laryngoscopy using a #3 Miller blade also fails to reveal any identifiable glottic structures, despite laryngeal manipulation. Following the second attempt at laryngoscopic intubation, the patient's O_2 saturation falls to 85%, her heart rate is 120 bpm, and her BP is 180/120 mm Hg.

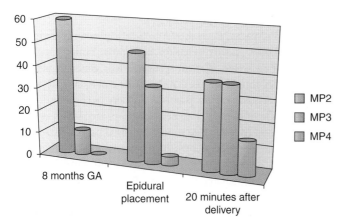

FIGURE 51-1. Progression of Mallampati changes seen from late pregnancy to delivery in a study by Boutonnet et al.[4]

51.4.2   What does one do if one cannot visualize the cords on second attempt of laryngoscopy?

There should be no delay in summoning additional assistance and informing all team members of the gravity of the situation. It is necessary to analyze why the attempts were unsuccessful by recalling the six factors that affect the success of the attempt: the practitioner, optimum head and neck position, optimum paralysis, best external laryngeal manipulation, type of blade, and length of blade (see Section 1.6.2).

Various laryngoscope blades, rigid fiberoptic laryngoscopes, and video laryngoscopes (with modified curved and straight blades) can be considered, if the practitioner possesses a degree of expertise in their use. These include the McCoy, Shikani, Bullard, GlideScope, and McGrath laryngoscopes. Improperly applied cricoid pressure can make visualization of the glottic opening more difficult, necessitating guidance by the practitioner. Backward, upward, and right-side pressure (BURP) on the thyroid cartilage can also be guided by the practitioner, and may help to improve the laryngeal view. An Eschmann Tracheal Introducer is useful if the epiglottis can be visualized, otherwise it has a limited role. In the environment of a rapidly developing crisis, and a glottis that is difficult to visualize, a flexible bronchoscopic intubation would likely be inappropriate.

51.4.3   How does one apply the failed airway algorithm in this situation?

The rapid desaturation after the second intubation attempt is likely related to the decrease in functional residual capacity (FRC) and increase in O_2 consumption (basal metabolic rate) seen in the gravid state.[12] This patient's respiratory reserve is further compromised by her obesity, and by being placed in the supine position. In addition, repeated attempts at intubation are likely to lead to upper airway trauma, particularly in the parturient, where the airway is edematous and the submucosal capillaries are fragile.

Because of these factors, and in the face of unacceptable oxygen saturations after the second attempt, it is imprudent to proceed to a third laryngoscopic attempt, without first attempting BMV while maintaining cricoid pressure. Adopting a Failed Airway Algorithm approach at this point must be considered. If BMV is successful, provided the fetal distress has resolved, awakening the patient ought to be considered, followed by an awake technique to secure the airway (see Chapter 49, Figure 49-4).

In the presence of fetal distress, if BMV is possible with cricoid pressure, a decision should be made about proceeding. Factors to be considered in this decision include: the availability of extra hands, the expected duration of the surgery, the skill of the obstetrician, the availability of equipment and skill to execute a definitive plan for securing the airway, and an assessment of the potential intraoperative complication this patient may pose (such as hemorrhage). A plan must be in place for securing the airway if a decision is made to proceed. If BMV is unsuccessful, even by easing the cricoid pressure, a rescue device should be inserted.

The ASA Difficult Airway Algorithm recommends that a laryngeal mask airway (LMA) should be inserted as a rescue device for ventilation and oxygenation in a *cannot ventilate, cannot intubate* (CICV) situation.[9] Failing that, the ASA algorithm recommends a surgical approach. It is the opinion of the authors and editors that this sequential approach in an airway emergency is imprudent, and a concurrent approach should be advocated (see Failed Airway Algorithm, Chapter 2).

As the parturient has an increased aspiration risk, an LMA-ProSeal™ or a disposable LMA-Supreme™ with an esophageal vent may be a more appropriate rescue device, as long as the practitioner is familiar with its placement. Anecdotal reports have demonstrated success with its use in similar circumstances, with better seating and ventilation, and a reduced risk of aspiration related to the venting of contents through the gastric port.[13,14] On the other hand, an intubating LMA (ILMA) has the advantage of serving as a conduit to secure the airway with an endotracheal tube. Placement of the tracheal tube can be achieved blindly through the ILMA device,[15] or can be facilitated using a flexible bronchoscope (FB),[16] or a lightwand device.[17] The use of an FB allows visualization of the cords, facilitating the placement of the endotracheal tube under indirect vision and avoiding potential trauma from a blind technique.

Placement of the LMA, LMA-ProSeal™, or ILMA may be hindered by cricoid pressure. It has been suggested that relaxing cricoid pressure, briefly, may allow higher placement success rates.[18,19] Cricoid pressure has also been shown to reduce tidal volumes and increase airway pressures.[20] These difficulties have served to highlight recent studies, questioning the efficacy of cricoid pressure in the prevention aspiration and its hindrance in airway management.[21,22] Others, however, have not demonstrated such disadvantages.[23]

51.4.4   If one is successful in providing ventilation and oxygenation with an LMA, should one proceed with the cesarean section?

When an airway cannot be secured with an endotracheal tube, devices, such as the LMA are effective rescue aids. Following the insertion of the LMA, proper placement should be confirmed by end-tidal CO_2 ($ETCO_2$) detection, an unobstructed $ETCO_2$ trace pattern (if capnography is employed), and adequate chest and abdominal excursion during ventilation.

While the LMA has been shown to be effective and safe in providing ventilation and oxygenation to healthy, non-obese, fasted parturients for elective cesarean section,[24] it is generally accepted that the LMA should be used only as an emergency device for airway management in the parturient when tracheal intubation is unexpectedly difficult.[25] The decision to proceed with cesarean section with an LMA in place should be based on the risk–benefit assessment on the effectiveness of oxygenation with the LMA, the condition of the fetus, the ability to expedite the delivery of the fetus, and ultimately, the safety of the parturient (context sensitive).

Actions that may lead to regurgitation and aspiration must be minimized if one proceeds with an LMA as the airway. Coughing related to light anesthesia may lead to regurgitation and must be avoided. High intragastric pressure, and incompetence of the lower esophageal sphincter, likewise predispose to regurgitation. There is evidence that gastric insufflation leading to elevated intragastric pressure is reduced by the application of cricoid pressure,[26,27] and the avoidance of increased intragastric pressure may permit ventilation of the patient at a lower peak airway pressure.[28] Finally, the obstetrician should be advised to minimize fundal pressure, if possible, during delivery of the baby.[29]

Should there be a serious doubt with regards to the safety of the mother in regard to difficult airway scenario options, the parturient should be awakened despite the presence of fetal distress. An alternative means of intubation (such as a flexible bronchoscopic technique), or of anesthesia (regional or local anesthesia), should then be undertaken.

51.4.5 If a Combitube™ is used to secure the airway, what other management issues should be considered?

The Combitube™ is an alternative, double-lumen airway device that is designed to be inserted blindly into the esophagus with over 80% success on the first attempt. It is commonly used among emergency medical services personnel with limited intubation experience.[30] It may also be employed as a rescue airway device. If placed properly, it permits gas exchange and probably provides a measure of protection against aspiration (see The Combitube™, Section 12.6, for a detailed description of the device and how it is used). Little information on the use of this device in the obstetric population exists. A theoretical disadvantage may be the potential for trauma (bleeding) in an already engorged airway during its insertion.

51.4.6 When should one proceed with a surgical airway? Who should do it? What equipment should be immediately available on the labor unit?

A surgical airway in a parturient is performed when the patient's airway can neither be intubated nor ventilated (CICV airway). Clinically, the oxygen saturation declines rapidly due to increased metabolic rate and diminished FRC in the pregnant woman. Delay in recognizing a CICV failed airway contributes to adverse outcomes and increased maternal mortality.[31] Surgical and nursing support must be immediately available to assist as necessary.

Commercially available cuffed cricothyrotomy kits are standard tools that must be available in all maternal suites, and their use should be regularly reviewed. Chapter 13 provides a detailed description of the commercial kit recommended, and the techniques of surgical airway management.

It should be emphasized that the recognition of the potential difficult airway, avoiding delay in recognizing the CICV situation, and regular practice of a failed intubation drill will contribute toward improving the outcome. Although both surgical and anesthesia practitioners should be conversant with this procedure, the onus is on the anesthesia practitioner to perform the procedure if indicated. With the risk of the failed airway being 10 times more common in the parturient than in the general surgical population, it is mandatory that those who provide anesthesia care in the labor ward be trained in the use of these devices and techniques.[32]

51.5 POSTOPERATIVE CONSIDERATIONS

51.5.1 Having secured the airway, how does one manage this patient postoperatively?

The likelihood of successful extubation is based on several factors, and guided by the condition of the patient's airway, but must err on the side of caution. In situations in which airway edema is anticipated to increase, such as significant fluid resuscitation, or an already edematous airway having suffered trauma during intubation attempts, the prudent course is to ventilate the patient for 12 to 24 hours postoperatively in a 15 to 30-degree head-up position.

Consideration should also be given to the effect of residual sedatives, or the likely need for further sedatives or analgesics, in the postoperative period. The pharyngeal airway is a collapsible tube and its patency is regulated by upper airway dilating muscles. Increase in the dilating muscle activity acts to maintain the narrowed pharyngeal airway in awake patients with obstructive sleep apnea, and similar neural mechanisms, presumably compensate the progressive upper airway narrowing in parturients. Preservation of these neural regulatory mechanisms is, therefore, crucial for parturients with a high Mallampati class. The neural compensatory mechanisms become weaker during general anesthesia, sedation, and sleep with residual anesthetics. It is important to stress that the size of the airway space is determined by the balance between the bony enclosure size and soft tissue volume (anatomical balance), when pharyngeal muscles are inactivated by general anesthetics and muscle relaxants.[3] General anesthesia for emergency cesarean delivery in obese parturients, during or immediately after labor, may tend to exaggerate upper airway swelling and lung volume dependence. This is in addition to impairment of neural compensatory mechanisms, and is, therefore, a potential worst-case scenario for upper airway maintenance.

A trial of extubation may only be attempted if the patient is fully awake, muscle relaxation fully reversed, and preparations are in place for immediate reintubation. The Frova Introducer, or other tracheal tube exchanger (see Section 11.2.2), may be placed through the tracheal tube, prior to its removal, to serve as a reintubation guide should it be required. The patient usually tolerates these small diameter devices reasonably well, if local anesthetic is instilled down the endotracheal tube prior to placement. These devices have a hollow lumen, providing limited gas insufflation capacity if reintubation over the guide proves difficult or impossible. Employing a laryngoscope to straighten the angle of approach aids tracheal placement over a guide, as do smaller tracheal tubes that are less likely to become impinged on the laryngeal structures. Increasing obstruction, significant respiratory effort, or increasing acidosis are early indications of extubation failure.

51.6 SUMMARY

The incidence of the CICV failed airway is more than 10-fold in the parturient at term, compared to a general surgical population. The obstetrical anesthesia practitioner must be prepared to manage the difficult and failed airway. Regular rehearsal of a failed airway plan of action along with the obstetric team, maintaining skills in the use of a rescue device (eg, the intubating LMA), and ensuring that surgical airway devices are immediately available are essential components of that preparation.

REFERENCES

1. Kuczkowski KM, Reisner LS, Benumof JL. Airway problems and new solutions for the obstetric patient. *J Clin Anesth*. 2003;15:552-563.
2. Pilkington S, Carli F, Dakin MJ, et al. Increase in Mallampati score during pregnancy. *Br J Anaesth*. 1995;74:638-642.
3. Watanabe T, Isono S, Tanaka A, Tanzawa H, Nishino T. Contribution of body habitus and craniofacial characteristics to segmental closing pressures of the passive pharynx in patients with sleep-disordered breathing. *Am J Respir Crit Care Med*. 2002;165:260-265.
4. Boutonnet M, Faitot V, Katz A, Salomon L, Keita H. Mallampati class changes during pregnancy, labour, and after delivery: can these be predicted? *Br J Anaesth*. 2010;104:67-70.
5. Kodali BS, Chandrasekhar S, Bulich LN, Topulos GP, Datta S. Airway changes during labor and delivery. *Anesthesiology*. 2008;108:357-362.
6. Tagaito Y, Isono S, Remmers JE, Tanaka A, Nishino T. Lung volume and collapsibility of the passive pharynx in patients with sleep-disordered breathing. *J Appl Physiol*. 2007;103:1379-1385.
7. Rocke DA, Murray WB, Rout CC, Gouws E. Relative risk analysis of factors associated with difficult intubation in obstetric anesthesia. *Anesthesiology*. 1992;77:67-73.
8. Mallampati SR, Gatt SP, Gugino LD. A clinical sign to predict difficult tracheal intubation: a prospective study. *Can Anaesth Soc J*. 1985;32:429-434.
9. Rose DK, Cohen MM. The airway: problems and predictions in 18,500 patients. *Can J Anaesth*. 1994;41:372-383.
10. Baraka A, Haroun-Bizri S, Khoury S, Chehab IR. Single vital capacity breath for preoxygenation. *Can J Anaesth*. 2000;47:1144-1146.
11. Nimmagadda U, Chiravuri SD, Salem MR, et al. Preoxygenation with tidal volume and deep breathing techniques: the impact of duration of breathing and fresh gas flow. *Anesth Analg*. 2001;92:1337-1341.
12. Russell IF, Chambers WA. Closing volume in normal pregnancy. *Br J Anaesth*. 1981;53:1043-1047.
13. Awan R, Nolan JP, Cook TM. Use of a ProSeal laryngeal mask airway for airway maintenance during emergency caesarean section after failed tracheal intubation. *Br J Anaesth*. 2004;92:144-146.
14. Keller C, Brimacombe J, Lirk P, Puhringer F. Failed obstetric tracheal intubation and postoperative respiratory support with the ProSeal laryngeal mask airway. *Anesth Analg*. 2004;98:1467-1470.
15. Minville V, N'Guyen L, Coustet B, Fourcade O, Samii K. Difficult airway in obstetric using Ilma-Fastrach. *Anesth Analg*. 2004;99:1873.
16. Joo HS, Rose DK. The intubating laryngeal mask airway with and without fiberoptic guidance. *Anesth Analg*. 1999;88:662-666.
17. Fan KH, Hung OR, Agro F. A comparative study of tracheal intubation using an intubating laryngeal mask (Fastrach) alone or together with a lightwand (Trachlight). *J Clin Anesth*. 2000;12:581-585.
18. Aoyama K, Takenaka I, Sata T, Shigematsu A. Cricoid pressure impedes positioning and ventilation through the laryngeal mask airway. *Can J Anaesth*. 1996;43:1035-1040.
19. Harry RM, Nolan JP. The use of cricoid pressure with the intubating laryngeal mask. *Anaesthesia*. 1999;54:656-659.
20. Hocking G, Roberts FL, Thew ME. Airway obstruction with cricoid pressure and lateral tilt. *Anaesthesia*. 2001;56:825-828.
21. Jackson SH. Efficacy and safety of cricoid pressure needs scientific validation. *Anesthesiology*. 1996;84:751-752.
22. Janda M, Vagts DA, Noldge-Schomburg GF. Cricoid pressure—safety necessity or unnecessary risk? *Anaesthesiol Reanim*. 2004;29:4-7.
23. Brimacombe JR, Berry AM. Cricoid pressure. *Can J Anaesth*. 1997;44:414-425.
24. Han TH, Brimacombe J, Lee EJ, Yang HS. The laryngeal mask airway is effective (and probably safe) in selected healthy parturients for elective cesarean section: a prospective study of 1067 cases. *Can J Anaesth*. 2001;48:1117-1121.
25. Preston R. The evolving role of the laryngeal mask airway in obstetrics. *Can J Anaesth*. 2001;48:1061-1065.
26. Asai T, Barclay K, McBeth C, Vaughan RS. Cricoid pressure applied after placement of the laryngeal mask prevents gastric insufflation but inhibits ventilation. *Br J Anaesth*. 1996;76:772-776.
27. Lawes EG, Campbell I, Mercer D. Inflation pressure, gastric insufflation and rapid sequence induction. *Br J Anaesth*. 1987;59:315-318.
28. Moynihan RJ, Brock-Utne JG, Archer JH, Feld LH, Kreitzman TR. The effect of cricoid pressure on preventing gastric insufflation in infants and children. *Anesthesiology*. 1993;78:652-656.
29. Hartsilver EL, Vanner RG, Bewley J, Clayton T. Gastric pressure during emergency caesarean section under general anaesthesia. *Br J Anaesth*. 1999;82:752-754.
30. Davis DP, Valentine C, Ochs M, Vilke GM, Hoyt DB. The Combitube as a salvage airway device for paramedic rapid sequence intubation. *Ann Emerg Med*. 2003;42:697-704.
31. Walls RM. Management of the difficult airway in the trauma patient. *Emerg Med Clin North Am*. 1998;16:45-61.
32. Samsoon GL, Young JR. Difficult tracheal intubation: a retrospective study. *Anaesthesia*. 1987;42:487-490.

SELF-EVALUATION QUESTIONS

51.1. Which of the following is true with regard to the use of an LMA for the parturient undergoing the cesarean section under general anesthesia?

A. LMA can be used as a rescue device in a parturient with a failed airway undergoing emergency cesarean section.

B. LMA has been shown to be effective and safe in providing ventilation for all parturients undergoing cesarean section.

C. There are no data to support the use of LMA for any parturient undergoing cesarean section.

D. The LMA has been shown to be effective and safe in providing ventilation for obese parturients undergoing cesarean section.

E. Use of LMA is associated with a reduced risk of aspiration for parturients undergoing cesarean section.

51.2. What should the anesthesia practitioner do if the vocal cords cannot be seen after two attempts at laryngoscopy in a parturient requiring an emergency cesarean section for placenta previa associated with exsanguinating hemorrhage?

A. Awaken the patient and perform an awake bronchoscopic intubation.

B. Awaken the patient and perform the cesarean section under regional anesthesia.

C. Immediate cricothyrotomy.

D. Ventilation using BMV or an EGD while maintaining cricoid pressure and if oxygenation is unsatisfactory proceed with the emergency surgical airway.

E. Reposition the head and neck of the parturient to facilitate further attempts of laryngoscopy.

51.3. Which of the following is a reasonable approach to minimize the risk of regurgitation and aspiration in a healthy parturient undergoing emergency cesarean section?

A. preoperative oral administration of 0.3 M sodium citrate (30 mL)

B. preoperative IV administration of ranitidine

C. preoperative IV administration of metoclopramide

D. a designated assistant with experience in applying cricoid pressure during the rapid-sequence intubation

E. all of the above

CHAPTER (52)

Airway Management in the Pregnant Trauma Victim

Adeyemi J. Olufolabi and Holly A. Muir

52.1 CASE PRESENTATION

A 35-year-old pregnant woman, at approximately 36 weeks gesta-tion, is admitted to the emergency department (ED) following a motor vehicle crash. She has a closed head injury, bilateral femoral fractures, and possible abdominal trauma. Her Glasgow coma score (GCS) is 5; she does not open her eyes (1); there is no audible vocalization (2); and she is showing decorticate rigidity (3). Her heart rate is 135 beats per minute (bpm), blood pressure 85/40 mm Hg, and respiratory rate is 40 breaths per minute and shallow. Fetal heart rate (FHR) is 110 bpm. The oxygen saturation (SaO_2) is 90% on a non-rebreathing oxygen mask. A cervical collar is in place and Thomas splints are being applied to the legs.

52.2 INITIAL ASSESSMENT OF THE PATIENT

52.2.1 What are the immediate evaluation and management priorities in this patient?

Initial evaluation and management priorities for the near-term parturient are no different than any trauma victim—assessment of airway, breathing, and circulation (ABCs), followed by a secondary survey, including assessment of the abdomen and fetus.

Unique considerations related to the pregnancy, such as supine hypotensive syndrome and the significant capillary engorgement of the nasal and oropharyngeal mucosa, may impact positioning, hemodynamics, and airway management.[1]

Immediate attention is directed toward the airway. Her GCS and oxygen saturations mandate endotracheal intubation and

ventilation. She is not a crash airway, and therefore an evaluation for difficulty is performed employing the MOANS, LEMON, RODS, and SHORT mnemonics (see Sections 1.6.1, 1.6.2, 1.6.3, and 1.6.4). In this particular patient, difficulty should be anticipated and an approach as suggested in the Difficult Airway Algorithm (see Chapter 2) adopted, recognizing that parturients at term have a substantially elevated risk of aspiration, particularly in this circumstance where protective airway reflexes are compromised.

Following airway management, attention is directed to an assess-ment of breathing. Her lung fields must be evaluated for presence, equality, and quality of breath sounds. This evaluation, coupled with a stat portable chest x-ray, may uncover a pneumothorax and/ or hemothorax that could require treatment.

In pregnancy, minute ventilation is normally increased by approx-imately 45%, largely through an increase in tidal volume. This increased minute ventilation results in a fall in P_aCO_2 to approxi-mately 30 mm Hg. Therefore, one should initially moderately hyperventilate this patient empirically. Ventilation may be guided by arterial blood gases, once resuscitation has been established.

During pregnancy, an increase in gastric acid production results not only in an increased volume but a decrease in the pH. Coupled with a decrease in the competency of the lower esophageal sphinc-ter, a greatly enhanced risk of reflux is present. The most effective protection against aspiration in this situation is the presence of a cuffed endotracheal tube in the trachea.

The final step of the primary survey is directed to the evaluation and management of the circulation. This patient is hypotensive. Positioning to minimize supine hypotensive syndrome (or aorto-caval compression syndrome) and volume resuscitation should be undertaken. A wedge should be placed under the right hip to create 30 degrees of left uterine displacement. This will reduce aortocaval compression and improve systemic and placental perfusion.[2]

Large-bore IV cannula and fluids must be initiated as the parturient can lose 30% of her blood volume before demonstrating cardiovascular changes.[3] There is a strong correlation between hypotension and negative outcome for both an injured brain, and a fetus in utero.

Relative anemia (approximately 11 g/dL or 6.9 mmol·L⁻¹), related to an enhanced blood volume, is a physiologic response to pregnancy. In a healthy near-term parturient, blood pressure may remain at near-normal values until greater than 1000 mL of blood loss occurs. In addition to the usual sources of blood loss in a trauma victim, the uterus can be a source of significant hemorrhage, for example, both placental and uterine abruption may be associated with blunt abdominal trauma, such as lap belt injury.

Now the attention can be turned to the secondary survey focusing on her head injury, the abdomen, and the stabilization of her fractures. Her GCS of less than 7 indicates a significant head injury at risk of further decompensation at any time. Securing an airway in a timely fashion may be critical in limiting hypoxic brain injury and avoiding surges in intracranial pressure (ICP) related to elevations of P_aCO_2.[4]

52.3   AIRWAY CONSIDERATIONS

52.3.1   What is unique about managing the airway urgently in the traumatic brain-injured patient who also happens to be a near-term parturient?

As discussed earlier, the practitioner must deal with competing priorities: the patient has features suggestive of difficult intubation, specifically, difficult bag-mask-ventilation (BMV) and difficult extraglottic device (EGD) use—secondary to the suspicion of blunt trauma injury to the thorax. Additionally, she needs to have her airway managed atraumatically and quickly in the presence of traumatic brain injury, and a greatly increased aspiration risk. Adherence to the Difficult Airway Algorithm (see Chapter 2) may result in some delay, while resorting to rapid-sequence induction (RSI) runs the risk of inducing and paralyzing a patient at high risk for aspiration and difficult airway.

The practitioner has time to call for help and a difficult airway cart, as the SaO₂ is acceptable, while borderline, and the FHR is normal. The airway practitioner should begin denitrogenation quickly using a mask with a rebreathing bag, and 15 L·min⁻¹ of flesh gas flow with oxygen.

Assisted ventilation may be required, taking care to avoid inflating the stomach, and the rapid respiratory rate makes this a challenge. If the practitioner is not confident of tracheal intubation, or his/her capacity to provide gas exchange using BMV or EGD, an awake look with a laryngoscope may help with the decision to move to a surgical airway, or to embark on an RSI pathway. As the status of the cervical spine (C-spine) stability is unclear, the collar is gently removed and airway evaluation and management is performed while maintaining in-line stabilization.

Should RSI be selected in the setting of a patient with acute severe head injury, the patient ought to be pretreated with an opioid, lidocaine, and defasciculating agent, although some would argue that pretreatment with an opioid, or even lidocaine, will further compromise respiration in a patient who does not have a secured tracheal tube. The selection of an induction agent and the dose employed will be guided by the degree of hemodynamic stability, and in this case, is likely to be etomidate at a reduced dose (eg, 0.2 mg·kg⁻¹). The dose of the neuromuscular blocker, such as succinylcholine, is never modified and is 1.5 mg·kg⁻¹.

Alternatively, an awake look to determine *intubatability* may be performed. This patient has a GCS of 5 and may not require sedation (eg, etomidate titration). However, patients with acute severe head injury may present with a clenched jaw, prohibiting an awake look. If this occurs, the only options are RSI and cricothyrotomy.

Induction and neuromuscular blocking agents must be prepared prior to securing the airway. A selection of intubation and rescue airway devices familiar to the airway practitioner must also be prepared. In this case, laryngoscopic intubation is judged to be highly likely (Plan A). Plan B is to use an intubating LMA (ILMA), and Plan C is a surgical airway should both fail. Following denitrogenation with 100% oxygen, pretreatment, induction, paralysis, and the application of cricoid pressure by an experienced assistant are undertaken. A third person maintains manual in-line stabilization of the neck, and the trachea is successfully intubated. After carbon dioxide detection confirms tracheal placement, the endotracheal tube is secured. An orogastric tube may be placed to reduce the risk of aspiration.

As a cautionary note, despite the advances that are continuously made in airway management, the incidence of the failed or difficult airway in an obstetrical population remains higher than that seen in the general population. A recent Australian multi-institution audit conducted to assess practice of general anesthesia for cesarean section confirmed an incidence of failed intubation of 1:274, and difficult intubation of 1:30.[5] These numbers are generally quoted in the literature.

It is recognized that the concept of difficult intubation in pregnancy is not without controversy. Some have argued that the difficulty is self-imposed: by anxiety with the urgency of situation; use of junior anesthesia practitioners on labor units; and the lack of opportunity to practice skills; and as a consequence of the high use of regional anesthesia in obstetrics.[6,7] This reservation notwithstanding, the possible loss of an airway, with a resulting period of hypoxia, and the increased possibility of acid aspiration, put both the mother's and her fetus' life in peril. Furthermore, her status of an unclear C-spine carries additional risk of injury, if a difficult intubation is encountered.

If, on assessment of this mother, there is any element of doubt about one's ability to efficiently and safely place a tracheal tube, a strong argument could be made for a surgical airway (without paralysis or sedation), by a skilled practitioner. She may well need a tracheotomy for prolonged ventilation at any rate.

52.3.2   How would you secure the airway if three attempts at laryngoscopic intubation failed despite laryngeal manipulation?

While maintaining cricoid pressure, ventilation should be provided by BMV with 100% oxygen. Gradual relaxation of cricoid pressure may be indicated if it is felt to hinder the ability to ventilate. If, at any point, the ability to maintain oxygen saturation is lost, an immediate surgical airway is indicated. As preparations for the surgical airway are underway, an ILMA can be inserted. Should this reestablish adequate ventilation, tracheal intubation through the ILMA can be considered.

Oxygen desaturation and hypotension are associated with poor outcomes in patients with acute severe head injury.

52.3.3 What specific concerns related to the airway do you have if this patient needs to be transported to the radiology suite for diagnostic imaging?

This patient will require ongoing sedation, paralysis, and mechanical ventilation during transport to diagnostic imaging to maintain oxygenation and to keep her P_aCO_2 within her physiologic range (between 30 and 32 mm Hg). Although hypocapnia has traditionally been considered an important part of the management of head injury in pregnancy, a reduction in P_aCO_2 below 30 mm Hg can be associated with a harmful reduction in uterine and cerebral blood flow with compromise to fetal perfusion.[8] Following the acute resuscitation phase, P_aCO_2 levels should be monitored continuously by capnometry/capnography, or periodically by arterial blood gas sampling.

The endotracheal tube should be properly secured, as movement from stretchers to radiology tables increases the risk of accidental extubation. In addition, appropriate equipment and personnel to manage reintubation should be immediately available, including drugs (both induction agents and neuromuscular blocking drugs), laryngoscopes, endotracheal tubes, and rescue devices (including an Eschmann Tracheal Introducer and an LMA).

52.3.4 Are sedating drugs and muscle relaxants safe in pregnancy?

The duration of action of agents, such as vecuronium and rocuronium, may be prolonged in the pregnant state, and therefore, in non-resuscitation situations, dosing should be titrated using a neuromuscular block monitor.[9] Although small amounts of non-depolarizing muscle relaxants are known to cross the placenta to the fetus when administered as a bolus, there are no reports of adverse fetal effects. The effects of prolonged (>24 hours) neuromuscular blocking drug administration on a fetus are unknown. It has been shown, however, that the fetal-maternal ratio of vecuronium increases significantly with prolonged induction to delivery times.[10] In a scenario such as this, personnel should be available to ventilate or intubate the trachea of a neonate should the need arise.

All patients intubated as part of an emergency resuscitation effort ought to receive sufficient sedation and muscle relaxation to facilitate mechanical ventilation and attenuate the stress responses (increased airways resistance, ICP, blood pressure, and heart rate). This is particularly important in patients with poorly controlled elevated ICP, such as in this patient. Drug selection in pregnancy is somewhat problematic, as few of the available drugs are approved for use in parturients. The US Federal Drug Administration has created a classification structure for drugs administered to women during pregnancy.[11] This five-level system of classification categorizes agents from safe to use, with well-controlled studies (category A—no risk to the fetus), to those which are clearly contraindicated (category X).

Most anesthetic and sedating agents fall into the category C group, in which risks cannot be ruled out (often due to the lack of controlled studies). It is recommended that category C agents be used only if the potential benefit to the mother justifies the potential risk to the fetus. Although the key teratogenic period is from 31 to 71 days postconception, fetal brain and organ development continues throughout gestation, rendering them susceptible to the adverse affects of agents administered to the mother.

The prevailing wisdom in the decision-making process is to bear in mind that the general health and well-being of the fetus is *entirely* dependent on the survival and well-being of the mother. As a general principle, drugs with a known safe history of use in pregnancy, such as thiopental and fentanyl, can be used. There is a growing body of evidence that propofol is also safe, although the experience is substantially less than those for thiopental and fentanyl. The fact that propofol is commonly used in the care of adult patients with neurotrauma would suggest its favorable application in this case. Despite traditional cautions in regard to possible teratogenic effects of benzodiazepines, recent evidence indicates that these agents are not proven human teratogens.[12] The safety of etomidate in pregnancy has not been established. The drug crosses the placenta and has been shown to produce a fall in serum cortisol in the fetus lasting for about 6 hours. The significance of this finding is unclear. The selection of etomidate in this case was driven by the considerable hemodynamic instability noted in the mother.

By and large, there is little evidence that a single dose of any currently available IV induction agents is harmful to the fetus.

52.4 OTHER CONSIDERATIONS

52.4.1 What fetal monitoring is required in this situation?

Fetal monitoring during trauma resuscitation is often challenging because of limited access to the abdomen. Continuous fetal monitoring is possible from about 18 weeks gestational age, although it is technically difficult to perform transabdominally early in gestation. FHR variability as an indicator of fetal well-being is usually not established until 25 to 27 weeks of gestation. Additionally, sedating agents affect FHR variability, further limiting its usefulness.[13] Therefore, persistent and marked fetal bradycardia may be the only true indicator of fetal distress in early pregnancy or in pregnant patients receiving sedating medications.

Blunt or perforating abdominal trauma place the fetus directly at risk due to the potential for placental abruption, or uterine hypoperfusion, related to maternal hemodynamic instability.

As indicated earlier, it is reasonable, therefore, to use continuous fetal monitoring in a pregnant trauma victim if it is physically possible. This assumes that personnel skilled in fetal heart trace reading are available, and a plan to deliver the fetus if there is evidence of fetal compromise. The American College of Obstetricians and Gynecologists supports a position of individualizing the use of monitoring in these situations as a team approach, so as to optimize the safety of both the mother and the fetus.[14] After 35 weeks gestation, delivery results in minimal morbidity to the fetus.

52.4.2   What findings would lead to a decision to expedite the delivery of the fetus?

Evaluation of the pregnant trauma victim involves the evaluation of two patients, the mother and the fetus. Assessment and stabilization of the mother is always the first priority. Occasionally, the resuscitation of the mother requires the delivery of the fetus. The classic example is during maternal cardiac arrest. If the fetus is older than 24 weeks, and if it has not been possible to resuscitate the mother after 4 minutes of cardiopulmonary resuscitation (CPR), the fetus should be delivered by emergency cesarean section. This is done to improve both fetal outcome and the effectiveness of maternal CPR, by removing any aortocaval obstruction.

In cases where the mother is hemodynamically unstable secondary to hemorrhage and possible placental abruption, delivery of the fetus may be necessary as part of maternal resuscitation. Immediate induction of anesthesia with airway management is mandated.

A more common scenario is that of a hemodynamically stable mother, with a fetus demonstrating signs of terminal fetal distress (severe fetal bradycardia). This situation parallels any other emergency cesarean section for fetal distress. As in all situations where anesthesia induction agents and muscle relaxants are used, a strategic plan (Plans A, B, and C) must be in place for management of the failed intubation.

52.5   SUMMARY

The management of trauma in a parturient often provides significant challenges to practitioners. The physiologic changes of pregnancy must be considered when one interprets vital signs, response to resuscitative maneuvers, and laboratory investigations in these trauma victims. The fetus adds a second dimension to the resuscitation, although maternal well-being and safety should remain the primary concern.

The benefit of left uterine displacement as part of the resuscitation must be recognized. Airway protection is a critical part of management, as these patients are at higher risk of aspiration due to the physiologic and mechanical changes of pregnancy. The value of Airway Management Algorithms in crisis situations, such as the resuscitation of the parturient, cannot be overemphasized.

REFERENCES

1. Leontic EA. Respiratory disease in pregnancy. *Med Clin North Am.* 1977;61:111-128.
2. Camann WR, Ostheimer GW. Physiological adaptations during pregnancy. *Int Anesthesiol Clin.* 1990;28:2-10.
3. ACOG Educational Bulletin. Obstetric aspects of trauma management. Number 251, September 1998 (replaces number 151, January 1991, and number 161, November 1991). American College of Obstetricians and Gynecologists. *Int J Gynaecol Obstet.* 1999;64:87-94.
4. Gelb AW, Manninen PH, Mezon BJ, Lee RJ, Durward QJ. The anaesthetist and the head-injured patient. *Can Anaesth Soc J.* 1984;31:98-108.
5. McDonnell NJ, Paech MJ, Clavisi OM, Scott KL. Difficult and failed intubation in obstetric anaesthesia: an observational study of airway management and complications associated with general anaesthesia for caesarean section. *Int J Obstet Anesth.* 2008;17:292-297.
6. Djabatey EA, Barclay PM: Difficult and failed intubation in 3430 obstetric general anaesthetics. *Anaesthesia.* 2009;64:1168-1171.
7. Goldszmidt E. Principles and practices of obstetric airway management. *Anesthesiol Clin.* 2008;26:109-125, vii.
8. Morishima HO, Daniel SS, Adamsons K, Jr., James LS. Effects of positive pressure ventilation of the mother upon the acid-base state of the fetus. *Am J Obstet Gynecol.* 1965;93:269-273.
9. Khuenl-Brady KS, Koller J, Mair P, Puhringer F, Mitterschiffthaler G. Comparison of vecuronium- and atracurium-induced neuromuscular blockade in postpartum and nonpregnant patients. *Anesth Analg.* 1991;72:110-113.
10. Iwama H, Kaneko T, Tobishima S, Komatsu T, Watanabe K, Akutsu H. Time dependency of the ratio of umbilical vein/maternal artery concentrations of vecuronium in caesarean section. *Acta Anaesthesiol Scand.* 1999;43:9-12.
11. Teratology Society Public Affairs Committee. FDA classification of drugs for teratogenic risk. *Teratology.* 1994;49:446-447.
12. Sheppard T. *Catalog of Teratogenic Agents.* 7th ed. Baltimore, MD: John Hopkins University Press; 1992.
13. Immer-Bansi A, Immer FF, Henle S, Sporri S, Petersen-Felix S. Unnecessary emergency caesarean section due to silent CTG during anaesthesia? *Br J Anaesth.* 2001;87:791-793.
14. ACOG Committee. Nonobstetric surgery in pregnancy (opinion number 284, August 2003). *Obstet Gynecol.* 2003;102:431.

SELF-EVALUATION QUESTIONS

52.1. Which of the following anesthetic induction agents has been shown in clinical trials to be safe for a pregnant patient?

A. etomidate

B. propofol

C. thiopental

D. ketamine

E. none of the above

52.2. During a rapid-sequence induction for an emergency cesarean section, you are neither able to intubate nor ventilate the patient. Which of the following is **NOT** an appropriate course of action?

A. repeat laryngoscopy and intubation

B. ventilation using Combitube™

C. immediate preparations for cricothyrotomy

D. ventilation using an LMA

E. relaxing cricoid pressure to determine if BMV can be improved

52.3. Which of the following is **NOT** an indication to deliver the fetus in a trauma victim who is 37 weeks pregnant?

A. To aid in the resuscitation of the mother, the fetus must be delivered in an expeditious fashion.

B. Maternal cardiac arrest.

C. Hemodynamically stable mother and the fetus is showing signs of terminal fetal distress with severe fetal bradycardia.

D. The mother is hemodynamically unstable secondary to hemorrhage and placental abruption.

E. Maternal respiratory arrest.

CHAPTER (53)

Appendicitis in Pregnancy

Narendra Vakharia and Ronald B. George

53.1 CASE PRESENTATION

A 20-year-old woman, G_1P_0 at 17 weeks' gestation, presented to the emergency department (ED) 10 hours ago complaining of right-sided abdominal pain accompanied by nausea and two episodes of vomiting. She is afebrile at present, blood pressure is 130/72 mm Hg, heart rate is 86 beats per minute (bpm), and respiratory rate is 20 breaths per minute. She weighs 198 lb (90 kg) and is 5 ft 7 in (169 cm) in height, with a body mass index (BMI) of 31 kg·m^{-2}. She admits to right-sided tenderness to palpation localized to the inguinal region. She underwent an ultrasound evaluation by an obstetrician who did not find any cause for the pain related to her pregnancy. The general surgery service was consulted, and it is their opinion that the patient has appendicitis and will require a laparoscopic appendectomy.

Her pregnancy has been unremarkable up to this point and is otherwise healthy. She has had no previous anesthetics and no family history of anesthesia-related problems. She takes prenatal vitamins, denies any allergies, does not smoke or drink alcohol, and takes no drugs. Physical examination of her heart and lungs is normal. Her airway examination reveals a Mallampati Class IV airway with limited mouth opening, normal range of motion of head and neck, full dentition, and minimal mandibular protrusion. The thyromental distance is 5 cm and the hyomental distance is 3 cm. There are no other abnormalities in her history or physical examination.

53.2 INTRODUCTION

53.2.1 What is the incidence of appendicitis in pregnancy?

Appendicitis has an incidence of approximately 1 in 1500 pregnancies, with appendectomy being the most common non-obstetric surgical procedure during pregnancy.[1,2] The relative incidence is estimated to be 30% in the first trimester, 45% in the second trimester, and 25% in the third trimester[3]; and the most common predictor of fetal-maternal mortality is appendiceal perforation, with an estimated risk of 43%, and the risk of perforation increases with increasing gestation and delay in diagnosis.[4,5] The estimated risk of fetal loss with appendiceal perforation is 36%.[6]

53.2.2 How is appendicitis diagnosed during pregnancy?

Anatomic and physiologic changes accompanying pregnancy make diagnosis of appendicitis challenging, therefore a careful history and physical examination, combined with a high index of suspicion, is required. The appendix is pushed superiorly and laterally with advancing gestation. However, according to studies, 84% of pregnant patients present with right lower quadrant pain.[3,5] The usual clinical signs and diagnostic tests may be confounded by the physiologic and anatomic changes accompanying pregnancy.

Ultrasound examination may be useful to identify a normal appendix and rule out other causes of abdominal pain in this patient population. However, due to the size of the uterus, it may be difficult to localize the appendix during the third trimester.[4] Diagnostic imaging using helical CT scanning has been reported to have a sensitivity and specificity of 92% to 98% and 99% to 100%, respectively.[7,8] Fetal radiation exposure with the helical CT scan approximates 300 milliradian (mrad) which is well below the 5 rad considered the maximal safe level of fetal exposure.[9]

53.2.3 What are the surgical options for appendectomy in pregnancy?

There are two surgical options for performing an appendectomy. Appendectomy can be performed via either an exploratory laparotomy (open technique) or laparoscopic technique. The advantages of the open technique are thought to include possibly better direct visualization, decreased operating room costs, and reduced fetal exposure to carbon dioxide. The advantages of the laparoscopic technique include fewer wound infections, reduced postoperative pain and opioid use, reduced uterine handling, early return of GI function, reduced risk of ileus, earlier ambulation, and shorter hospital stay. The disadvantages of laparoscopic technique include potential uterine or fetal injury, reduced cardiac output and uterine blood flow, preterm labor, and fetal acidosis.[9-11] Laparoscopic appendectomy is considered to be safe during any trimester.[9] but pregnant patients should receive venous thromboembolism prophylaxis due to a risk of venous stasis secondary to carbon dioxide pneumoperitoneum.[9]

53.2.4 How does laparoscopy impact physiology in the pregnant patient?

The physiologic changes accompanying the pregnant state are reviewed in detail in standard obstetric anesthesia texts.[12] Under normal circumstances, the creation of the pneumoperitoneum will impact cardiovascular and respiratory physiology. Carbon dioxide insufflation of the peritoneal cavity will initially result in an increase in venous return as intravascular blood volume is augmented by compression of the splanchnic vasculature. This results in an increase in cardiac output and arterial blood pressure. Sympathetic nervous system activation due to carbon dioxide absorption results in an increase in systemic vascular resistance.[13] As intra-abdominal pressure increases beyond 15 mm Hg, venous return will decrease due to compression of the vena cava leading to a reduction in cardiac output and hypotension. Intra-abdominal pressures should be limited to 10 to 15 mm Hg.[9] Insufflation may also result in bradyarrhythmias due to vagal effects from peritoneal stretching, or tachyarrhythmia due to sympathetic activation and hypercarbia. Aortocaval compression secondary to pregnancy may be exacerbated by the elevated intra-abdominal pressure and may compromise uterine and placental perfusion. Patients should be positioned with left uterine displacement to maximize uterine perfusion. Respiratory system changes due to the pneumoperitoneum will decrease pulmonary and thoracic compliance and increase peak inspiratory pressures. Elevation of the diaphragm will further reduce the functional residual capacity, possibly leading to

hypoxemia. Carbon dioxide absorption may produce respiratory acidosis. These changes may lead to fetal compromise as a result of hypotension, hypoxemia, and fetal acidosis. Other sources of respiratory complications include subcutaneous emphysema, pneumothorax, endobronchial intubation, and gas embolism.[14]

53.3 ANESTHETIC MANAGEMENT

53.3.1 What are the anesthetic options for laparoscopic appendectomy?

Laparoscopic procedures can and have been carried out under general anesthesia and regional anesthesia.[13] While regional anesthesia, such as epidural or spinal techniques, may be used for the laparoscopic procedure, they are not recommended in the pregnant patient, as the pneumoperitoneum, increased intra-abdominal pressures, and gravid uterus will compromise spontaneous ventilation causing hypercarbia and hypoxemia.[10] In addition, diaphragmatic irritation due to carbon dioxide insufflation will produce shoulder tip pain, necessitating supplementation with sedatives and analgesics. Increased intra-abdominal pressure will also increase the risk of regurgitation and aspiration. Therefore, general anesthesia with endotracheal intubation may be a better choice to provide a secure airway. In addition, general anesthesia also permits controlled ventilation to avoid hypercarbia and hypoxemia and allows the use of muscle relaxants.

53.3.2 What are your concerns in giving a general anesthetic to a 17-week pregnant patient?

Cohen-Kerem et al conducted an extensive systematic review (with a patient population of 12,452) to evaluate the effects of non-obstetric surgical procedures (under both regional and general anesthesia) on maternal and fetal outcome.[15] The rate of premature labor induced by non-obstetric surgical intervention was 3.5%. Sub-analysis of studies reporting on appendectomy during pregnancy revealed a high rate or premature labor (4.6%). Fetal loss associated with appendectomy was 2.6%, and this rate was quadrupled (10.9%) when peritonitis was present. These findings suggest that acute appendicitis has significantly more adverse effects on the maternal and fetal outcome, particularly if peritonitis develops when compared to other acute surgical conditions during pregnancy.

In other words, apart from the anesthetic care of this patient, special considerations must be given to the well-being and the safety of the fetus. The anesthetic agents and other drugs administered perioperatively may be potentially harmful to the fetus. To address the concern of drugs administered to females during pregnancy, the US Federal Drug Administration (FDA) published the classification of drugs for teratogenic risk in 1994[16] (see Section 52.3.4). In general, anesthetic drugs and muscle relaxants fall into the category C group, in which risks cannot be ruled out. However, in the clinical doses that are commonly administered, most anesthetic agents, including the volatile agents, nitrous oxide, propofol, thiopental, opioids, benzodiazepines, and muscle relaxants, are not considered teratogenic and are likely to be safe to use.[17]

53.3.3   Should fetal monitoring be used during the procedure for this patient?

Fetal monitoring practices will vary based on institutional protocols but is usually performed intraoperatively provided it does not interfere with surgical access for the procedure and does not impact the management of the case. This is particularly true in cases where the fetus is considered to be previable. According to the 2009 American Society of Anesthesiologists and the American College of Obstetricians and Gynecologists Joint Statement on Nonobstetric Surgery During Pregnancy, physicians should "obtain obstetric consultation before performing non-obstetric surgery and some invasive procedures (eg, cardiac catheterization, colonoscopy) because obstetricians are uniquely qualified to discuss aspects of maternal physiology and anatomy that may affect intraoperative maternal-fetal well-being" and "if the fetus is considered previable, it is generally sufficient to ascertain the fetal heart rate by Doppler before and after the procedure."[18] The definition of fetal viability is problematic. However, the majority of consensus statements on the topic as well as clinical practice consider 24 weeks' gestational age to be the standard limit.[19,20] In this case, 17 weeks is considered previable and it would be sufficient to check fetal heart rates before and after the surgical procedure.

53.4   AIRWAY MANAGEMENT

53.4.1   How do you assess the airway of this patient?

Airway evaluation should focus on identifying patient characteristics predictive of difficulty in bag-mask-ventilation, use of extraglottic devices, performance of direct laryngoscopy and endotracheal intubation, and ease of achievement of a surgical airway.

The mnemonic MOANS (see Section 1.6.1) is used to identify predictors of ease of ventilation. This patient has at least two predictors of difficulty in ventilation. She is obese and she has a Mallampati Class IV airway.

Of the four predictors of difficulty in use of an extraglottic device identified by the mnemonic RODS (see Section 1.6.3), this patient has two predictors of difficulties. She has restricted mouth opening and decreased thoracic compliance due to her obesity and the gravid uterus.

The mnemonic LEMON (see Section 1.6.2) is used to identify features which would make direct laryngoscopy and intubation difficult. This patient demonstrates a limited mouth opening and a Mallampati Class IV airway. Restricted mouth opening may also limit the ability to utilize rigid and semirigid fiberoptic devices and video laryngoscopy for tracheal intubation.

The mnemonic SHORT (see Section 1.6.4) describes features that might make a surgical airway a challenge. Apart from obesity, this patient has no other features suggesting difficulty with a surgical airway if needed.

53.4.2   What preparations should be made prior to surgery?

The operating room should be prepared and anesthesia equipment checked. In light of the patient's obesity, limited mouth opening and a Mallampati Class IV airway, a difficult airway situation should be anticipated. Furthermore, the patient is at risk for gastrointestinal stasis, reflux, and aspiration. A difficult airway cart should be brought into the room and appropriately trained assistance should be available.

Prior to proceeding to the operating room, a thorough history and physical examination of the patient must be completed. Specific information regarding previous anesthesia experiences and airway management-related issues should be elicited and previous anesthesia records procured. In this case, the patient has limited mouth opening. The inter-incisor distance should be assessed to determine the potential utility of various devices and techniques available to the anesthesia practitioner.

The patient should be maintained NPO and have intravenous access established. She should receive acid aspiration prophylaxis in the form of metoclopramide 10 mg IV, ranitidine 50 mg IV, and 30 mL of 0.3 N sodium citrate by mouth.

The operating table should be prepared with a ramp to position the patient in anticipation of a difficult airway (see Figure 49-2). In addition, care should be taken to ensure that the patient is positioned appropriately on the operating table with left uterine displacement.

53.4.3   How should the airway of this patient be managed?

The specific technique and devices used for airway management under any circumstances should be predicated on the results of the patient's airway assessment and the anesthesia practitioner's skill, proficiency, and confidence with various devices and techniques to secure the airway.

In light of this patient's airway assessment, a rapid-sequence induction followed by direct laryngoscopy would likely be a poor choice. The patient's airway should be secured prior to induction of general anesthesia. The patient should be treated with an antisialogogue in preparation for awake airway management. The patient's airway will need to be anesthetized with topical anesthetics. Specific details regarding the technique of topicalization of the airway may be found in Chapter 3.

While flexible bronchoscopic intubation will be the usual technique of choice for this patient, there are numerous alternative techniques and devices which may be used to secure the airway awake in this patient. The decision will be based on availability of equipment and the inter-incisor distance. For example, the patient can undergo a retrograde intubation with mild sedation. This technique has been used numerous times in patients with very limited mouth opening.[14,21] In this patient however, it may be difficult to adequately locate the landmarks for a cricothyroid membrane puncture as a result of her obesity. However, with meticulous technique and adequate experience with the technique, it is possible to secure the airway. This technique has been thoroughly reviewed recently (see Section 11.6).[22,23]

There are a number of fiberoptic intubating stylets available (see Chapter 10). Shikani performed five awake intubations using the Shikani Optical Scope® during his initial report.[24] The Bonfils retromolar fiberscope was used by Corbanese et al[25] to successfully carry out awake intubation in 29 or 30 patients with difficult airway. These can be used with either direct laryngoscopy or with a jaw thrust to improve visualization. Most of these devices vary in diameter between 5 mm and 6 mm and can accommodate 5.5 mm ID and larger endotracheal tubes. A number of them have been used successfully to carry out awake intubations in patients with difficult airways or small mouth opening.[26-29]

Rigid fiberoptic laryngoscopes and video laryngoscopes, such as the Bullard laryngoscope, UpsherScope®, WuScope® and GlideScope®, may be useful in this patient. Cohn[30] performed awake intubations using the Bullard laryngoscope in eight patients at risk for neurological injury and requiring awake intubation. However, none of the patients were specifically reported to have limited mouth opening. The Bullard has a spatula-like blade which may be useful in patients with limited mouth opening. Due to its profile, it may be possible to carry out laryngoscopy with an inter-incisor distance of as little as 6 mm. However, it may prove to be difficult to insert or manipulate an endotracheal tube of 6 mm ID or larger size. The WuScope®, due to its design, requires an inter-incisor distance of at least 20 mm to adequately accommodate the scope and endotracheal tube combination.[31] The use of the GlideScope® for difficult airway management has increased in recent years. It has been used for awake intubation in patients with a difficult airway,[32] and as an adjunct for awake bronchoscopic intubation.[33] The GlideScope® provides an improved view of the laryngeal inlet and has been shown to have a high rate of intubation success. The newer model has a 14.5 mm blade flange profile which may be useful in this patient. It must be remembered that all of the optical stylets and video laryngoscopes share the disadvantage of fogging and require some antifogging maneuver prior to their use. In addition, as any blood or secretions in the airway will obscure the view, it is highly recommended that the oropharynx be suctioned prior to the insertion of these devices.

While numerous options to secure the airway of patients with an anticipated difficult laryngoscopic intubation have been discussed, the use of these devices in obstetrical patients is limited. However, it is the author's preference to perform an awake bronchoscopic intubation in this patient. Successful awake intubation will depend upon satisfactory topical anesthesia of pharyngeal and laryngeal structures. Airway edema which accompanies the pregnant state may pose a challenge to topicalization and considerable patience may be required.

Specific details of the techniques of topicalization and bronchoscopic intubation are discussed in Chapters 3 and 9.

53.4.4 What is the plan for extubation of this patient following appendectomy?

No difficult airway management plan is considered complete without a predefined strategy for the safe and successful extubation of the patient following the completion of the procedure. In this case, one must assure that all muscle relaxants have been reversed and the patient is fully awake, following commands, and able to protect her airway prior to extubation. All equipment required for reintubation should be ready and available at the time of extubation. The patient should be extubated in the operating room where access to equipment and medications is assured.

53.5 SUMMARY

Although the use of general anesthesia in obstetric patients has been declining, it may still be required in specific situations. Patients presenting for non-obstetric surgery may have potential difficult airways. Airway management plans must be designed and formulated based upon a thorough airway examination and familiarity, and skill with various airway devices and techniques. Familiarity with devices and techniques is gained through regular review and practice, and anesthesia practitioners must become facile with a number of options for airway management. Patients with limited mouth opening present numerous challenges and there are various options for securing the airway. The final management plan should depend on the airway evaluation of the patient, the available resources, and the skill set of the anesthesia practitioner.

REFERENCES

1. Andersen B, Nielsen TF. Appendicitis in pregnancy: diagnosis, management and complications. *Acta Obstet Gynecol Scand*. 1999;78:758-762.
2. Guttman R, Goldman RD, Koren G. Appendicitis during pregnancy. *Can Fam Physician*. 2004;50:355-357.
3. Mourad J, Elliott JP, Erickson L, Lisboa L. Appendicitis in pregnancy: new information that contradicts long-held clinical beliefs. *Am J Obstet Gynecol*. 2000;182:1027-1029.
4. Borst AR. Acute appendicitis: pregnancy complicates this diagnosis. *JAAPA*. 2007;20:36-38,41.
5. Melnick DM, Wahl WL, Dalton VK. Management of general surgical problems in the pregnant patient. *Am J Surg*. 2004;187:170-180.
6. Fallon WF, Jr, Newman JS, Fallon GL, Malangoni MA. The surgical management of intra-abdominal inflammatory conditions during pregnancy. *Surg Clin North Am*. 1995;75:15-31.
7. Ames Castro M, Shipp TD, Castro EE, Ouzounian J, Rao P. The use of helical computed tomography in pregnancy for the diagnosis of acute appendicitis. *Am J Obstet Gynecol*. 2001;184:954-957.
8. Lazarus E, Mayo-Smith WW, Mainiero MB, Spencer PK. CT in the evaluation of nontraumatic abdominal pain in pregnant women. *Radiology*. 2007;244:784-790.
9. Society of American Gastrointestinal Endoscopic Surgeons (SAGES). Guidelines for diagnosis, treatment and use of laparoscopy for surgical problems during pregnancy. *Surg Endosc*. 2008;22:849-861.
10. Kirshtein B, Perry ZH, Avinoach E, et al. Safety of laparoscopic appendectomy during pregnancy. *World J Surg*. 2009;33:475-480.
11. Kuczkowski KM. Laparoscopic procedures during pregnancy and the risks of anesthesia: what does an obstetrician need to know? *Arch Gynecol Obstet*. 2007;276:201-209.
12. Chestnut DH, Polley LS, Tsen LC, Wong CA, eds. *Chestnut's Obstetric Anesthesia: Principles and Practice*. 4th ed. Philadelphia, PA: Mosby-Elsevier; 2009.
13. Gerges FJ, Kanazi GE, Jabbour-Khoury SI. Anesthesia for laparoscopy: a review. *J Clin Anesth*. 2006;18:67-78.
14. Biswas BK, Bhattacharyya P, Joshi S, Tuladhar UR, Baniwal S. Fluoroscope-aided retrograde placement of guide wire for tracheal intubation in patients with limited mouth opening. *Br J Anaesth*. 2005;94:128-131.
15. Cohen-Kerem R, Railton C, Oren D, Lishner M, Koren G. Pregnancy outcome following non-obstetric surgical intervention. *Am J Surg*. 2005;190:467-473.

16. Teratology Society Public Affairs Committee. FDA classification of drugs for teratogenic risk. *Teratology*. 1994;49:446-447.

17. Rosen MA. Anesthesia for the pregnant patient undergoing surgery. ASA Refresher Course; 2009.

18. American Society of Anesthesiologists (ASA) and the American College of Obstetricians and Gynecologists (ACOG). Statement on nonobstetric surgery during pregnancy. http://www.asahq.org/publicationsandservices/standards/51.pdf. Accessed September 28, 2010.

19. Morgan MA, Goldenberg RL, Schulkin J. Obstetrician-gynecologists' practices regarding preterm birth at the limit of viability. *J Matern Fetal Neonatal Med*. 2008;21:115-121.

20. Vavasseur C, Foran A, Murphy JF. Consensus statements on the borderlands of neonatal viability: from uncertainty to grey areas. *Ir Med J*. 2007;100:561-564.

21. Bhattacharya P, Biswas BK, Baniwal S. Retrieval of a retrograde catheter using suction, in patients who cannot open their mouths. *Br J Anaesth*. 2004;92:888-901.

22. Burbulys D, Kiai K. Retrograde intubation. *Emerg Med Clin North Am*. 2008;26:1029-1041, x.

23. Dhara SS. Retrograde tracheal intubation. *Anaesthesia*. 2009;64:1094-1104.

24. Shikani AH. New "seeing" stylet-scope and method for the management of the difficult airway. *Otolaryngol Head Neck Surg*. 1999;120:113-116.

25. Corbanese U, Possamai C. Awake intubation with the Bonfils fibrescope in patients with difficult airway. *Eur J Anaesthesiol*. 2009;26:837-841.

26. Abramson SI, Holmes AA, Hagberg CA. Awake insertion of the Bonfils Retromolar Intubation Fiberscope in five patients with anticipated difficult airways. *Anesth Analg*. 2008;106:1215-1217, table of contents.

27. Hamada T, Morokura N, Suzuki Y, Katori K, Yamamoto S, Higa K. Orotracheal intubation using a styletscope in a patient to avoid neck recurvation. *Masui*. 2001;50:519-520.

28. He N, Xue FS, Xu YC, Liao X, Xu XZ. Awake orotracheal intubation under airway topical anesthesia using the Bonfils in patients with a predicted difficult airway. *Can J Anaesth*. 2008;55:881-882.

29. Nagashima M, Saito T, Takahata O, et al. Orotracheal intubation using a Styletscope in a patient with restricted opening of the mouth. *Masui*. 2002;51:775-776.

30. Cohn AI, Zornow MH. Awake endotracheal intubation in patients with cervical spine disease: a comparison of the Bullard laryngoscope and the fiberoptic bronchoscope. *Anesth Analg*. 1995;81:1283-1286.

31. Smith CE, Sidhu TS, Lever J, Pinchak AB. The complexity of tracheal intubation using rigid fiberoptic laryngoscopy (WuScope). *Anesth Analg*. 1999;89:236-239.

32. Doyle DJ. Awake intubation using the GlideScope video laryngoscope: initial experience in four cases. *Can J Anaesth*. 2004;51:520-521.

33. Xue FS, Li CW, Zhang GH, et al. GlideScope-assisted awake fibreoptic intubation: initial experience in 13 patients. *Anaesthesia*. 2006;61:1014-1015.

SELF-EVALUATION QUESTIONS

53.1. Which of the following is true about appendicitis in pregnancy?

A. It occurs rarely during pregnancy.

B. It is predominantly a condition of the first trimester.

C. Delay in diagnosis increases risk of morbidity and mortality.

D. Laparoscopic procedures are contraindicated during pregnancy.

53.2. The most important factor in successful airway management is:

A. performing a rapid-sequence induction to secure the airway rapidly

B. performing a thorough evaluation of the airway to formulate an appropriate plan

C. using novel devices to secure the airway

D. convincing the patient to have regional anesthesia

53.3. Which is true in managing patients with limited mouth opening?

A. Patients with limited mouth opening can usually be intubated via direct laryngoscopy post-induction of general anesthesia.

B. Degree of mouth opening will determine which device or technique may be useful in securing the airway.

C. Any device can be used for this patient population.

D. Awake fiberoptic intubation is the only technique to secure the airway in this patient population.

CHAPTER (54)

Unique Challenges of Ectopic Airway Management

Michael F. Murphy

54.1 CASE PRESENTATION

A 42-year-old obese man is undergoing renal dialysis in a hospital dialysis unit when he suddenly suffers a cardiac arrest. He is diabetic with a history of cerebrovascular disease, peripheral vascular disease, and angina. He is a nonsmoker. He had no premonitory symptoms.

You are called to manage his airway. When you arrive on the scene from your unit, you see a cyanotic male looking older than his stated age, reclining at 45 degrees in a dialysis chair. He is still connected to a dialysis machine via a vascular shunt in his left arm. The head of the chair, which is not on wheels, is against the wall. A dialysis technician is straddling the patient performing cardiopulmonary resuscitation and a nurse is delivering ineffective bag-mask-ventilation (BMV) from the right side of the patient. You are informed that he receives dialysis three times a week. His *dry weight* is 414 lb (188 kg).

The crash cart has arrived, containing both oral and nasal airways, endotracheal tubes, a laryngoscope handle, and #3 and #4 Macintosh blades. There is an intubating stylet as well. This is the third time this year you have been called to this unit. Unfortunately, the equipment you prefer to use for airway management is *never* available in the dialysis unit, despite continuous reminders that you prefer a Miller blade.

54.2 INTRODUCTION

54.2.1 What is meant by the term "ectopic airway management"?

Anesthesia practitioners, emergency physicians, intensivists, hospitalists, and other health care providers with airway management

expertise often become involved in emergency and urgent airway management outside of their usual operating milieu. This is referred to as "ectopic" airway management.

54.2.2 What are the common examples of ectopic venues?

There are several areas of a hospital where it should be *anticipated* that emergency airway management will be required occasionally, or even perhaps regularly. These include but are not exclusive to:

- Post-anesthetic care unit (PACU)
- Diagnostic imaging locations where emergency and intensive care unit (ICU) patients are taken; particularly CT, MRI, ultrasound, and angiography units
- Units where procedural sedation is undertaken:
  - Endoscopy
  - Invasive cardiology
  - Interventional imaging
  - Pediatric clinics, such as dentistry, ophthalmology, EEG, ENT, and others
  - Lithotripsy
  - Cardiac stress testing facilities
  - Medical and surgical inpatient units
  - Obstetrical delivery suites

Outpatient clinics, medical offices, and non-patient care areas (eg, cafeterias, residences, waiting rooms, administrative offices, and the areas immediately external to the health care facility) are occasionally the site of an airway emergency.

54.3   AIRWAY MANAGEMENT CHALLENGES

54.3.1   What issues are the unique challenges of ectopic airway management?

Managing a difficult airway is always anxiety provoking and somewhat dysphoric. Most ectopic airway management is difficult for a variety of reasons: some are related to the patient's airway anatomy; others to the patient's condition; and some are unique to the situation. The result is performance anxiety that may lead to less than optimal performance. Consider the following unique challenges inherent in managing the ectopic airway:

- Medicolegal risk
- Consistency of airway kits/carts
- Unfamiliar environment
- Unknown patient medical conditions
- Assistants unfamiliar with airway management
- Emotionally charged environment; stressed response
- Postintubation management

54.3.2   What are the medicolegal risks associated with ectopic airway management?

Ectopic airway management is associated with an element of medicolegal risk in the event of a poor outcome. Peterson et al published an update of the *Management of the Difficult Airway: A Closed Claims Analysis* in 2005. Out of 179 claims for difficult airway management, 86 (48%) were from events occurring from 1985 to 1992 and 93 (52%) were from events occurring from 1993 to 1999. The majority of claims for difficult airway management (156 out of 179 or 87%) involved perioperative care and 23 claims (13%) involved ectopic locations. Out of these 23 cases of airway management *misadventures* outside the operating room environment, 25% involved endotracheal tube change, and nearly half were not related to surgical procedures. Reintubation on the ward or ICU some time after a surgical procedure was related to neck swelling with respiratory distress. The procedures included cervical fusion (n = 3), total thyroidectomy (n = 1), intraoral/pharyngeal procedures (n = 2), and fluid extravasation from a central catheter (n = 1).[1]

The typical scenario coming to litigation has the following features:

- The patient is unknown to the airway practitioner.
- It is an emergency situation:
  - Which is emotionally charged and chaotic
  - In which events preceding the airway emergency are unclear
  - In which the amount of information about the patient is limited
  - In which action is needed immediately
  - With a difficult airway (eg, post-thyroidectomy in PACU; patient in a halo jacket)
  - In which evaluation of the airway for difficulty is inadequate
  - In which paralytic agents are inappropriately given
  - In which the management strategy is poorly thought out and executed, leading to a failed airway

The fact that the airway practitioner is thrust into an emotionally charged and unfamiliar environment provides little if any legal protection or indemnification. Furthermore, the defense of *lack of familiarity* or *lack of desired equipment* may be discredited. This is particularly so if it can be established that emergency airway management is *expected* to occur from time to time in that unit *and* that the individual charged with airway management in such situations (ie, you) *knew or ought to have known* that they might be summoned to do so.

Part of the solution to this problem is to *prevent* failure by establishing policies and procedures with respect to the availability of airway management equipment and its maintenance in areas where it is predictable that emergency or urgent airway intervention will occasionally be required. This requires that the disciplines involved take ownership of this issue and communicate with each other, and among themselves, about the specifics of such policies that will ensure safe, and hopefully litigation free, ectopic airway management.

54.3.3   What airway equipment or carts should be available in these ectopic facilities?

Airways are managed virtually every day in the operating rooms, emergency departments, and ICUs of most hospitals. These units ordinarily assemble routine and rescue airway management equipment into varying configurations of storage units where they are checked regularly (eg, daily or with shift change) for availability and function, and are easily accessed in an emergency. Routine and difficult/failed airway equipment may be arranged in separate drawers in the storage areas of the same cart (eg, emergency departments and ICUs); or sometimes in different carts (eg, the operating room's difficult airway cart, see Chapter 59 for details). The literature, albeit limited, provides little guidance as to what ought to be stocked in these *carts*, or alternatively in a *carry out* kit that the practitioner takes along to an airway management event.[2-6]

The equipment on the carts is typically determined by the consensus among the practitioners or staff who respond to manage an airway emergency in these units. The equipment should be arranged in a consistent fashion such that the drawers always contain the same airway equipment. This site-to-site consistency is particularly important when large specialty groups cover several facilities. Such consistency will likely avoid wasting valuable time to find the proper airway equipment in an emergency situation. Chapter 59 addresses the policy and content aspects of difficult airway carts in operating suites, emergency departments, and ICUs. It also serves as a resource for contacting equipment manufacturers and suppliers.

In areas of the hospital where airway management may be required on a regular basis, or patients are placed at risk for respiratory failure (see discussed earlier), it is recommended that routine and rescue airway management equipment be immediately available. Furthermore, the storage of this equipment should be consistent from area to area, and the equipment should be checked for inventory and function daily.

Carry out emergency airway satchels that can be quickly retrieved and carried to the site of an airway emergency are used by some practitioners and departments. The same issues arise with these kits as with permanent on-site carts, including:

- It is in a location that is less than familiar to the airway practitioner.
- The same issues arise with these kits as with permanent on-site carts such as:
  - Consistent location of kits to permit rapid retrieval
  - Contain both routine and rescue devices
  - Organized consistently to permit rapid access to the desired equipment
  - Regular inspections to ensure that the kits are complete and replenished after each use
  - Daily inspections of each kit to ensure proper function of all devices

Some areas may have unique needs that require special equipment. The most common example is an area serving pediatric patients. Some areas of a health care facility may see this population from time to time, while others may not.

54.3.4 What are the challenges associated with managing the airway in the ectopic environment?

Leaving the comfort of one's usual environment and venturing into unfamiliar territory should not hinder appropriate airway management. Practitioners who may be summoned to ectopic areas to manage airways should familiarize themselves with the staff, the equipment, and the storage systems *before* the emergency arises. Participating in the decisions as to what is stored, where it is stored, and how it is maintained (ie, policy) is only reasonable.

The scene on arrival is generally chaotic, emotionally charged, and boisterous. As there are substantial expectations placed on the responding airway practitioner, it is critical that the airway practitioner does not participate in or inflame the chaos, which fosters bad airway management decisions.

54.3.5 Why is airway management in an ectopic location more challenging?

Patients requiring airway management in these ectopic locations are generally not known to the airway practitioners. Most of these patients are not prepared for airway management (eg, often have a full stomach with a higher risk of gastric regurgitation and aspiration). Furthermore, airway assessment is often hurried and incomplete. Thus, the formulation of a rational and well thought out airway management plan is unlikely. As indicated previously, the single most important factor leading to a failed airway is failure

to properly assess a patient and predict a difficult airway.[1,7,8] Consequently, it is more common to encounter a *difficult airway* in an ectopic environment.

54.3.6 What are the challenges faced by the practitioners managing these patients' airways in ectopic locations?

Emergency airway management presenting in PACU (eg, post-thyroidectomy bleed) may be quite different from those occurring in the CT scanner (eg, pediatric patients). Airway practitioners have varying skills and few are expert at managing all types of situations.

In addition, unlike the situation in the operating room, PACU, ICU, or emergency department, airway management assistants in these ectopic locations may be unfamiliar with even the basic needs of the airway practitioner. Maneuvers, such as cricoid pressure, external laryngeal manipulation (BURP), head lift, or even passing the endotracheal tube correctly to the airway practitioner, may not be fully understood.

To minimize these difficulties, institutions should provide basic training to both airway practitioners and assistants to manage the airways of patients that present in various ectopic locations.

54.3.7 How should the airway be managed in ectopic locations?

The following simple rules of engagement may be helpful:

- Remain calm and take control of the scene.
- Speak firmly and give clear instructions to assistants without shouting.
- Consider titration of intravenous haloperidol and/or ketamine (*not* succinylcholine) if the patient's behavior hinders adequate management of ventilation and oxygenation.
- If patient behavior management is not an issue, managing oxygenation and ventilation or gas exchange must be achieved quickly:
  - Move to the head of the patient and establish ventilation and oxygenation.
  - Establish airway patency.
  - Take over BMV and avoid aggressive ventilation (ie, avoid high-frequency, large tidal volume, and high airway pressure).
  - Insert an oral airway and two nasal trumpets if needed.
  - If this fails, inserting an LMA is reasonable.
  - Gather your wits and composure as you establish adequate gas exchange.
- While maintaining gas exchange, it is important to evaluate the airway and formulate a plan.
  - Formally evaluate the airway using the mnemonics described in Chapter 1 (eg, with MOANS, LEMON, RODS, SHORT).
  - Identify Plans A, B, and C; assemble the required equipment and drugs.

○ Avoid muscle paralysis if the ability to maintain ventilation or gas exchange is uncertain.

○ Optimize conditions—invest time to properly position the patient at the head of the bed, elevate the bed to the proper height, and place the patient's head and neck in the appropriate (eg, *sniffing*) position.

○ Execute the plan in a deliberate and a controlled manner.

When faced with inadequate equipment (or skills) in an ectopic location, it is important to think of alternatives:

• Call for assistance if available. A colleague or an assistant can contribute with suggestions, expertise, and more importantly, moral support.

• Does the patient really need tracheal intubation *right now* or will a BMV or an extraglottic device (eg, LMA) suffice until additional equipment or expertise arrives?

• Are there any other options (eg, blind nasal intubation)?

Finally, Mort compared the outcomes of patients undergoing emergency tracheal intubation in his institution before and after the application of the American Society of Anesthesiologists (ASA) guidelines.[9] The rate of cardiac arrest during emergency intubation was reduced by 50%.

54.4   POSTINTUBATION CONSIDERATION

54.4.1   What should be done following tracheal intubation in ectopic locations?

While confirmation of tracheal intubation is critical following intubation, proper equipment (capnography or an esophageal detection device [EDD] self-inflating bulb) may not be available. This important equipment, together with hemodynamic monitors such as a BP cuff and pulse oximetry, should be called for if they are not available. Ensure that the airway device (eg, ETT, LMA) is secured properly. Longer-term neuromuscular blockade may be necessary to facilitate mechanical ventilation and ensure that the patient does not self-extubate. Ensure that appropriate mechanical ventilation parameters are established if indicated.

Following airway management in these unusual environments, it is essential to document the following elements:

• Any evaluation that indicates that the airway might be difficult

• Ensure that the resuscitation record or nurses' notes accurately record the time you were summoned, arrived, completed key interventions, etc.

• Ensure that drug doses are accurately recorded

• Document the airway management, and the intratracheal verification methods employed (end-tidal carbon dioxide detection is the standard of care)

54.5   SUMMARY

To minimize the risk, adverse outcome, and the anxiety associated with airway management of patients in an ectopic environment, it is important to:

• Participate in crafting hospital and departmental policies regarding airway management equipment in areas where you are called to manage them (see Chapter 59).

• Familiarize yourself with different hospital units and their staff

• Minimize the chaos

• Assess the airway and formulate airway strategies quickly

• Call for assistance early

• Avoid paralyzing the patient if the ability to artificially maintain post-paralysis gas exchange is uncertain

• Document the airway management episode

REFERENCES

1. Peterson GN, Domino KB, Caplan RA, Posner KL, Lee LA, Cheney FW. Management of the difficult airway: a closed claims analysis. *Anesthesiology.* 2005;103:33-39.
2. Murphy MF. The difficult airway cart. In: Walls RM, Murphy MF, Luten RC, Schneider R, eds. *Manual of Emergency Airway Management for PDA.* 2nd ed., Philadelphia, PA: Lippincott Williams and Wilkins; 2004.
3. McGuire GP, Wong DT. Airway management: contents of a difficult intubation cart. *Can J Anesth.* 1999;46:190-191.
4. Practice guidelines for the management of the difficult airway. A report by the ASA task force on management of the difficult airway. *Anesthesiology.* 1993;78:597-602.
5. Practice guidelines for management of the difficult airway: an updated report by the American Society of Anesthesiologists Task Force on management of the difficult airway. *Anesthesiology.* 2003;98:1269-1277.
6. Crosby ET, Cooper RM, Douglas MJ, et al. The unanticipated difficult airway with recommendations for management. *Can J Anaesth.* 1998;45:757-776.
7. Mort TC. Emergency tracheal intubation: complications associated with repeated laryngoscopic attempts. *Anesth Analg.* 2004;99:607-613.
8. Cheney FW, Posner KL, Caplan RA. Adverse respiratory events infrequently leading to malpractice suits. A closed claims analysis. *Anesthesiology.* 1991;75:932-939.
9. Mort TC. The incidence and risk factors for cardiac arrest during emergency tracheal intubation: a justification for incorporating the ASA Guidelines in the remote location. *J Clin Anesth.* 2004;16:508-516.

SELF-EVALUATION QUESTIONS

54.1. Ectopic airway management is associated with measurable medicolegal risk. Of the closed claims related to difficult airway management in the ASA Closed Claims Database between 1985 and 1999, the approximate percentage of those occurring at an ectopic location is:

A. 2%

B. 5%

C. 15%

D. 25%

E. 43%

54.2. The most important factor related to successfully managing an airway in an ectopic location is:

A. Getting there quickly.

B. Making it clear that you are the most skilled airway practitioner at the scene.

C. You have familiarized yourself with the equipment that will be available to you beforehand.

D. That you speak in a low voice to avoid fanning the flames of anxiety.

E. That you paralyze the patient quickly to enhance your success rate.

54.3. All of the following are associated with ectopic airway management **EXCEPT**:

A. Chaos is the norm.

B. Failure rates are higher in locations where you usually work.

C. Policies with respect to airway management equipment maintenance are the norm.

D. Good help is usually present at the scene.

E. The person who performs the intubation is responsible to see that it is secured in place.

CHAPTER 55

Management of the Patient with a Neck Hematoma

J. Adam Law

55.1 CASE PRESENTATION

A 69-year-old man has been in the post-anesthetic recovery unit (PACU) for 6 hours with a slowly expanding neck hematoma following an uneventful left carotid endarterectomy under general anesthesia. Over the last 45 minutes he has become symptomatically short of breath. Neurosurgery has booked him to return to the operating room (OR) for wound exploration and evacuation of hematoma. Preoperatively, he was otherwise healthy, taking no medications, and was noted to have normal-looking airway anatomy. Post-induction at the original surgery, he was documented to have been easy to ventilate using a bag-mask, presented a Cormack/Lehane (C/L)[1] Grade 1 view at direct laryngoscopy using a Macintosh #3 blade, and the trachea was easily intubated with an 8.5-mm internal diameter (ID) endotracheal tube (ETT).

In the PACU he is sitting upright, breathing oxygen at 10 L·min^{-1} via a non-rebreathing facemask. Although restless, he is rational, complaining of dyspnea, dysphagia, and neck pain. Blood pressure is 180/95 mm Hg, heart rate 100 beats per minute (bpm), respiratory rate 30 breaths per minute, and his SpO$_2$ is 95%. He is audibly stridulous. Under a blood-stained dressing, the left side of his neck looks visibly enlarged and discolored (Figure 55-1). The patient is 5 ft 10 in (178 cm) in height and weighs 230 lb (105 kg). He has vascular access. An OR is being prepared for his return.

55.2 PATIENT EVALUATION AND MANAGEMENT OPTIONS

55.2.1 In what ways might this patient present difficulty with airway management? What are key aspects of the airway examination in this situation?

This is an urgent situation. The patient must be quickly assessed and decisions made. Although some patients with neck hematomas are simply observed, case reports attest to difficulty in predicting if or when these individuals will go on to sudden and catastrophic airway obstruction.[2-4] As part of the patient's evaluation, a formal airway examination should be performed, seeking predictors of difficulty in all aspects of airway management.[5] Even though the patient's anatomy presented no difficulty with airway management earlier that day, the presence of a neck hematoma changes everything. With evidence of obstructing pathology in the airway—as manifested by stridor, neck swelling, and the patient's dyspnea and agitation—difficulty can now be anticipated with both bag-mask-ventilation (BMV) and use of an extraglottic device (EGD). Similarly, direct laryngoscopy in the presence of pathological obstruction may also be difficult as anatomic

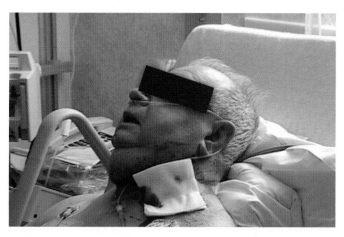

FIGURE 55-1. The patient. A dressing is covering the site of the surgical incision.

landmarks become distorted, displaced, or obscured. Finally, cricothyrotomy by percutaneous or open surgical routes may also be difficult as landmarks are shifted or become indistinct.

If time and patient cooperation permit, any patient with obstructing airway pathology can be considered for further assessment by nasopharyngoscopy. This is generally well tolerated and can give information about any displacement of the larynx to left or right; the degree of perilaryngeal edema, and vocal cord function.

55.2.2   What other patient factors may be relevant in this situation?

With predicted difficulty in all aspects of airway management limiting options in this patient, an awake approach at securing the airway is preferable. However, for awake airway interventions, substantial patient *cooperation* is generally needed. Patient cooperation may be lost (a) as hypoxemia occurs and/or (b) the patient panics as dyspnea worsens with progressive airway lumen narrowing. This speaks to the need for early identification of the patient requiring re-intubation, while cooperation can still be counted upon. Although sedative medications may help to render a patient more cooperative, sedating a patient with a tenuous airway is hazardous and may itself precipitate complete airway obstruction.[6,7] Other patient comorbidities will assume secondary importance compared to the gravity of threatened loss of the airway.

55.2.3   What are the causes of airway obstruction in a patient with a postsurgical neck hematoma?

Neck hematomas originate from venous or capillary oozing more often than arterial bleeding.[8-10] Although arterial bleeds may present earlier,[8] neck hematomas arising from a venous or capillary source can be insidious and just as devastating in their ability to cause obstruction. The following mechanisms may contribute to the development of symptomatic airway obstruction in the patient with a neck hematoma:

1. *Physical pressure effect*: The presence of a hematoma in the neck can mechanically *displace* the laryngeal inlet dramatically away from the midline position[4,8,11,12] in addition to physically *compressing* the lumen of the pharynx, laryngeal inlet, or tracheal airway. Some authors consider significant compression of the larynx and trachea unlikely due to their rigid cartilaginous structures.[13,14] Carr and colleagues performed a bench study with pig tracheas and observed that with applied pressures of just over 250 mm Hg (ie, equivalent to maximal systolic blood pressure), they were unable to demonstrate more than a 20% loss of the original anterior-posterior tracheal diameter.[14] However, as other authors have pointed out, the posterior, membranous portion of the trachea may still be significantly compressed by a hematoma.[15] Indeed, there are published case reports showing CT scan images of impressive tracheal compression by hematomas.[16,17] Bukht described a case[18] in which an adult patient with a neck hematoma was intubated with difficulty with a 5 mm ETT. No leak was apparent even with the cuff deflated, however upon subsequent release of the hematoma, a large leak immediately developed, suggesting that tracheal or laryngeal compression can indeed occur with neck hematomas.

2. *The development of peri-laryngeal edema*: This is a consistent feature in case reports of patients with neck hematomas[2-4,8,12,16,18-20] and is often out of proportion to any degree of externally visible neck swelling or discoloration. Most authors agree that this is due to interference with normal venous and/or lymphatic[21] drainage by both the neck hematoma itself as well as blood tracking into tissue planes away from the hematoma.[4,13,16,20,22] Release of tissue inflammatory mediators may also contribute to it.[22,23] At direct laryngoscopy, the resulting edema is variously described as "swollen supraglottic mucosal folds"[4,8] or a "watery, pale swelling of the mucosa"[13,20] (Figure 55-2) which in many cases completely obscures the glottic opening. Interestingly, some case reports document the development of similar perilaryngeal edema after neck surgery even without an obvious hematoma.[8,24]

3. *Blood dissection along tissue planes in the neck*: The parapharyngeal space is contiguous medially with the retropharyngeal space,[15] which in turn extends from the skull base to the upper mediastinum.[25] The parapharyngeal space also communicates anteriorly with pretracheal and submandibular spaces as well as subcutaneous tissues.[25] Blood from a neck hematoma in any of these areas can thus spread remotely from its initial location to further compromise the airway. Retropharyngeal collections of blood are often manifested symptomatically with neck pain and dysphagia or odynophagia in addition to hoarseness and dyspnea. Retropharyngeal hematomas can cause airway obstruction by compression of the arytenoid cartilages, which may in turn adduct the vocal cords.[26] In addition, retropharyngeal swelling can render direct laryngoscopy more difficult by (a) shifting the laryngeal inlet anteriorly;[27] (b) apposing the posterior pharyngeal wall to the epiglottis; and (c) as it is a large, dark mass, a retropharyngeal hematoma can absorb light from the laryngoscope, worsening visibility.[27]

It should be noted that of the causes of airway compromise mentioned earlier, edema and remotely tracking blood will not remit immediately upon evacuation of a neck hematoma, accounting for the variable success of urgently reopening a surgical incision in alleviating respiratory extremis in these patients.

Three other factors can also potentially contribute to postoperative airway compromise in patients undergoing routine head and neck surgery:

1. Large volumes of fluid administered intraoperatively can exacerbate airway edema.

2. Simply undergoing certain operations in the head and neck region may transiently cause narrowing of the upper airway, even in the absence of a neck hematoma. Carmichael and colleagues[28,29] demonstrated a significant loss (up to 32%) of airway volume after routine carotid endarterectomy, greatest in the region of the hyoid but also present at the level of the arytenoids and cricoid ring.

3. Neck surgery can result in transient palsies to cranial nerves (IX-XII)[30,31] due to direct injury during dissection, retractor pressure, or other causes.[32] If unilateral, such palsies may be asymptomatic; however, particularly in patients with a history of previous neck surgery or presenting for staged bilateral procedures, (eg, carotid endarterectomies), bilateral nerve damage can result in complete airway obstruction. Vocal cord palsy can result from damage to the vagal trunk or its recurrent laryngeal branches, while bilateral hypoglossal nerve palsies can result in airway obstruction from loss of innervation to the intrinsic muscles of the tongue and pharyngeal musculature.[30] One final point to note in the patient undergoing staged bilateral carotid endarterectomies is that ablation of the carotid bodies bilaterally will result in loss of the ventilatory response to hypoxia.[33]

55.3   MANAGING THE AIRWAY

55.3.1   Pending the decision of whether and where to re-intubate, how can the patient be symptomatically temporized?

It should be reiterated that patients with partial airway obstruction are unpredictable in when, where, and if they will go on to complete airway obstruction. Indeed, some case reports document a decision to conservatively manage neck hematoma patients by observation, only to be confronted with sudden and catastrophic complete airway obstruction some hours later.[3,4] In addition, patients going on to complete airway obstruction in this setting can do so without first developing the physical sign of stridor.[2,3,8] It follows that nursing staff and airway managers must be educated to recognize the early signs of impending obstruction from a possible neck hematoma, including subtle voice changes and hoarseness, with later progression to agitation, dyspnea, and eventually stridor. Stridor, a late sign of airway compromise, is variously considered to be a sign of an extrathoracic airway narrowed by 50%[34] or to

a diameter of 4 mm or less.[35] The patient in the presented case should be assumed to be in respiratory extremis. Once a compromising neck hematoma is suspected, plans should be undertaken for immediate definitive care: release and reexploration of the neck wound, and securing of the airway.

For temporizing a case such as this on the short term, (eg, while organizing a return to the OR, or while obtaining equipment for re-intubation), a number of maneuvers can be undertaken:

1. The head of the bed should be elevated, anywhere from 30 degrees to fully sitting, to promote venous drainage and improve the mechanics of breathing. The patient with significant airway compromise will most likely naturally wish to assume the sitting position.

2. Heliox can be administered. Heliox, a mixture of helium gas with oxygen, is less dense than air or pure oxygen. With its lower density, a helium-oxygen mixture minimizes the work of breathing by converting some or all of the turbulent flow through a critically narrowed airway to laminar flow.[36,37] Heliox is available in different oxygen-helium dilutions from 20/80 to 40/60: to maximize its clinical effect, the mixture with the highest concentration of helium should be used that is consistent with adequate oxygenation. Improved flow with heliox can lead to larger tidal volumes and less alveolar shunting, sometimes with improved oxygenation.[36,38,39] In addition, as a patient breathes more easily with alleviation of dyspnea-associated anxiety, the lessened negative inspiratory pressure applied to the obstructed area may result in less airway collapse, thus actually improving the degree of obstruction.[36] Heliox use in the patient with a critically narrowed airway can provide dramatic symptomatic relief, in turn potentially improving patient cooperation. In the setting of a neck hematoma, however, it should be assumed that heliox has no definitive therapeutic effect and is strictly a temporizing agent.

3. Early consideration should be given to *reopening the neck wound* when a postsurgical neck hematoma is causing airway compromise. Some,[18,40] although certainly not all[8,20,41] case reports document rapid clinical improvement following this maneuver. While a significant hematoma mass may be decompressed immediately, associated laryngeal edema and/or blood tracking remotely from the hematoma site will resolve more slowly. Clinical judgment dictates where and when to open the neck wound: the patient in respiratory extremis should have it opened immediately, while others may be safely managed upon returning to the more controlled conditions of the OR. However, any attempt at tracheal intubation should generally be preceded by release of the neck wound, whether in or out of the OR. It should be noted that this directive contrasts with the management of the patient with penetrating neck trauma, in whom the possible presence of damaged major vessels mandates securing the airway by intubation prior to neck exploration.

4. The use of epinephrine aerosols[42] and systemic steroids has been described for upper airway edema; however, there is no published evidence of their short-term efficacy in the setting of neck hematoma-induced airway compromise.

55.3.2 Should the trachea of this patient be intubated in the PACU or in the operating room? How do you decide?

The short answer is that the patient with a neck hematoma is ideally re-intubated in the controlled conditions of the OR. The OR has the advantage of a more sterile environment, with availability of surgical equipment and staff for an *airway double setup* (Table 55-1) together with easier access to difficult airway equipment and expert help. In addition, the OR offers the option of an inhalational induction if desired. Ultimately the decision about re-intubation on the spot versus a return to the OR will be tempered by the following factors:

1. Is the patient *in extremis*? If so, the airway should be secured on the spot.

2. If the patient is becoming increasingly dyspneic, is the rate of decline such that a return to the OR may be safely undertaken?

3. How far is the OR from the patient's present location and is the OR located on the same floor as the PACU?

4. If the patient obstructs during transport to the OR, will one be able to bag-mask ventilate the patient? The extensive upper airway edema accompanying most neck hematomas may make BMV impossible once the patient has fully obstructed.

55.3.3 How should such an airway be approached, and why?

Patients with significant narrowing of the airway due to pathological processes are in a dangerous situation. Onset of dyspnea, and then stridor, suggests critical airway narrowing, and in the setting of a neck hematoma should generally be regarded as signs of impending complete obstruction. Our airway assessment has suggested the potential for difficulty with BMV, laryngoscopic intubation, EGD rescue ventilation, and surgical airway. Careful consideration must therefore be given as to how best to proceed. A number of options exist:

1. *Local or regional anesthesia.* One published case series in the surgical literature documents hematoma evacuation in eight patients under local anesthesia with no morbidity, which contrasted significantly with the 57% complication rate in seven other patients done under general anesthesia.[9] Hematoma evacuation and exploration using local or regional anesthesia may be feasible before the patient is significantly short of breath and is still able to lie flat and cooperate. However, regional anesthesia, (eg, superficial cervical blockade) may be difficult to perform if an enlarging hematoma obscures anatomic landmarks.[8]

◖ TABLE 55-1

The Airway Double Setup

Definition:
The presence of equipment and personnel for the purpose of moving rapidly to cricothyrotomy should an attempted tracheal intubation from above result in a failed airway situation.
Rationale:
Attempted oral or nasal tracheal intubation in the patient with an advanced degree of pathologic airway obstruction can result in complete loss of the airway during the attempt. If the patient cannot be oxygenated with BMV, and intubation with direct laryngoscopy fails, rapid cricothyrotomy is needed to avoid a hypoxemic arrest.
Preparation:
The following conditions should be met:
Personnel: scrubbed/gowned scrub nurse; circulating nurse; scrubbed/gowned ENT, plastic, neuro, or general surgeon in addition to anesthesia staff;
Equipment: surgical instruments for an open surgical cricothyrotomy. A percutaneous cricothyrotomy kit may be available;
Patient: in position of comfort; cricothyroid membrane identified; overlying skin marked, prepped, and possibly infiltrated with local anesthetic.
Execution:
Cricothyrotomy commences as soon as a failed airway, cannot intubate, cannot ventilate/oxygenate is declared. Generally, a single attempt at EGD placement is warranted before putting knife to skin.
Consider this!
Some patients with obstructing pathology may have marked submandibular swelling as part of their disease process that extends down to and obscures landmarks of the cricothyroid membrane. As this may preclude easy and rapid cricothyrotomy, the safety margin provided by the airway double setup is diminished. As such, it may be an indication that the primary technique of choice should be awake tracheotomy under local anesthesia, rather than attempted intubation from above.

2. *Awake cricothyrotomy or tracheotomy under local anesthesia.* Some authorities suggest that patients with advanced degrees of obstructing airway pathology, particularly those with lesions of sufficient size to preclude passage of even a small ETT, should have their airways secured with awake tracheotomy under local anesthesia.[34,43] In expert hands and with patient cooperation, this is a procedure that can be done relatively quickly and painlessly. Technical difficulty can be encountered if midline landmarks are shifted or obscured by an expanding hematoma. In addition, airway edema can also occur internally at the level of the cricoid ring, potentially impacting ease of cricothyrotomy.[23]

3. *Awake oral or nasal (trans-laryngeal) intubation.* Awake trans-laryngeal intubation (via oral or nasal routes) confers the advantage of having a breathing patient who is maintaining and protecting the airway, and would be judged the method of choice by many experts in this situation. In the setting of a neck hematoma, grossly distorted anatomy can be anticipated, (see Section 55.2.3 earlier), yet in the awake patient, movement of swollen mucosal folds (and possibly, bubbles) may help locate the laryngeal inlet (Figure 55-2). An attempted awake intubation from above must, however, confer a high probability of success in order to outweigh the risk of loss of the airway during the attempt[25] (which can happen even in expert hands[6]). Attention to topical airway anesthesia (see Section 3.3.4 as well as Section 55.3.11 later), good flexible bronchoscopic equipment, and the expertise to use it will be necessary.[8,44] Alternatively, direct laryngoscopy has also been described for awake intubations in the setting of neck hematomas.[10]

4. *Inhalational induction.* An inhalational induction has been espoused in a number of reports as an option to facilitate intubation of a patient with a neck hematoma.[8,21,25,34] However, during an inhalational induction, while spontaneous ventilatory efforts are generally maintained, it must be appreciated that volatile anesthetics have deleterious effects on upper airway tone and patency similar to those of intravenously administered sedatives.[45] While the inhalational induction may be considered for the patient unable to cooperate with an awake intubation or tracheotomy, an airway double setup should be arranged, the neck wound should be opened before beginning, and close attention should be paid to maximizing airway patency as the patient loses consciousness (Table 55-2). Inhalational inductions in the setting of neck hematomas in published case reports have generally been successful although in some cases prolonged or difficult.[4,8,18,25]

5. *Intravenous (IV) induction.* Unless the patient is asymptomatic and a nasopharyngoscopic assessment has ruled out significant edema or laryngeal displacement, this route *cannot be recommended* as the method of choice for the patient with obstructing airway pathology due to a neck hematoma. IV induction of anesthesia with or without muscle relaxant administration is fraught with hazard in this setting with case reports attesting to the lack of any identifiable landmarks at direct laryngoscopy,[4,46] *often in conjunction with the inability to bag-mask ventilate* the patient.[8,46]

55.3.4   How should we proceed in this case?

Our Plan A here is for an awake intubation under topical airway anesthesia, a viable option if good equipment and expertise are available with the flexible bronchoscope, and if patient cooperation can be enlisted. In the event of an uncooperative patient, an inhalational induction could be considered. Plan B, in the event of loss of the airway during the attempt at awake intubation or inhalational induction, would be rapid conversion to a cricothyrotomy.

55.3.5   How will you prepare for the awake intubation?

In the OR, an airway double setup should be readied (Table 55-1), with scrubbed surgical staff and equipment available for urgent cricothyrotomy. The difficult airway cart should be in the room. IV access should be assured, monitors applied, and the patient positioned in his position of comfort (often sitting). The cricothyroid membrane should be identified, marked, and prepped. If not already done, all layers[47,48] of the surgical incision should be opened, any easily accessible clot removed, and covered with a sterile dressing. Psychological preparation should be undertaken with confident reassurance that successful intubation will totally alleviate the patient's dyspnea, while at the same time explaining the gravity of the situation and emphasizing the need for cooperation. If heliox had been applied, it should be interrupted for only brief periods during application of topical airway anesthesia. Topical airway anesthetic agents and techniques have been addressed elsewhere (see Chapter 3). Ideally, systemic sedation should be omitted. An adult flexible bronchoscope (eg, 6.2-mm OD) should be loaded with a small (eg, 7 mm ID) ETT. An assistant should apply gentle tongue traction.

TABLE 55-2

Strategies to Help Maximize Upper Airway Patency during Difficult Inhalational Inductions

1. Maintain the patient in a sitting or semi-sitting position

2. Keep the head and upper C-spine extended and lower C-spine flexed, to maintain longitudinal traction on the upper airway, thus decreasing its collapsibility[45]

3. Apply a jaw thrust to increase retropalatal and retrolingual airway caliber[45]

4. Through a nostril already topically anesthetized, insert a nasopharyngeal airway to help overcome approximation of the soft palate to the posterior pharyngeal wall, while the patient is still too light to tolerate an oropharyngeal airway[34]

5. Application of PEEP during the inhalational induction may help to splint open collapsible supraglottic structures

55.3.6 What can you expect during the awake flexible bronchoscopic intubation?

Awake flexible bronchoscopic intubation of the patient with extensive upper airway edema due to a neck hematoma differs substantially from that done in a patient without obstructing pathology. In the patient with no obstructing pathology, navigation of the bronchoscope can proceed from landmark to landmark in the upper airway, for example, from uvula to base of tongue, to epiglottis, then to and through cords. In the patient with upper airway edema, both the epiglottis and glottic opening may be obscured by *clouds* of edematous tissue (Figure 55-2). Often this leaves tissue movement and the suggestion of an opening as the only indication of the path to the vocal cords. As the patient exhales, the edematous tissues will *abduct* somewhat, giving an impression of an opening (Figure 55-2A/B). Small bubbles may also appear during this phase of respiration. As this happens, the bronchoscope is advanced in a slow and controlled fashion toward the opening or bubbles (Figure 55-2C). During inspiration, the tissue may *adduct* somewhat and the view will likely become obscured (Figure 55-2D).

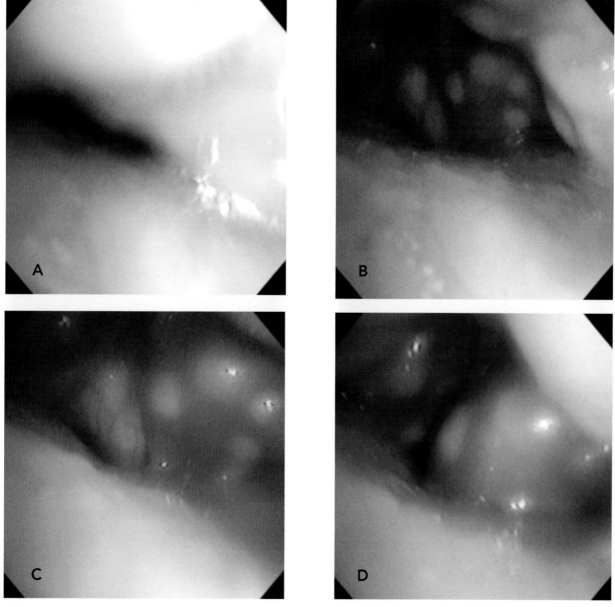

FIGURE 55-2. Typical findings seen during bronchoscopic intubation of a patient with a neck hematoma. A. As the bronchoscopic intubation begins, the practitioner simply advances the scope toward the opening appearing with expiration. B. With usual landmarks such as the epiglottis obscured, bizarre, edematous tissue appear in the distance. C. The scope is further advanced toward movement. D. With inspiration, swollen and edematous supraglottic tissues adduct to almost meet in the midline. E. With the next expiration, edematous tissues again move aside, allowing further advancement of the bronchoscope. F. The yellow tissue is a posteriorly located corniculate cartilage, with the entrance to the esophagus beneath, and a suggestion of glottic opening above, although still largely obscured by edematous tissue. G. Now beyond the edematous supraglottic tissue, the piriform sinus comes into view on the left, with an edematous, pale aryepiglottic fold in the middle of the view, and a suggestion of glottic opening on the right. H. Navigation of the bronchoscope to the right enables access to the glottic inlet.

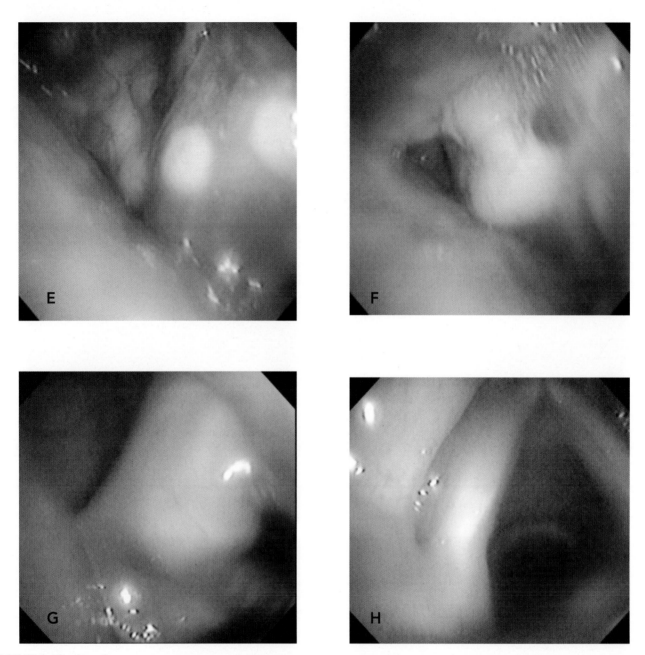

FIGURE 55-2. (Continued)

It is important to have the bronchoscope remain motionless in the airway during this phase, simply waiting for the view to reappear during the next expiration (Figure 55-2E), prior to resuming scope advancement. Often in this setting, one simply continues navigating toward the opening suggested by movement until the cords suddenly appear just in front of the scope (Figures 55-2F-H).

As the only landmarks leading to the airway after the uvula, presence of both movement and bubbles on expiration are crucial clues—this is one reason why it is critical to avoid ablation of spontaneous respirations in these patients.

It should also be noted that a neck hematoma can significantly push the larynx to the left or right of its expected location—this can be anticipated before beginning the bronchoscopic intubation by examining the front of the neck, looking or feeling for the location of the thyroid cartilage.

55.3.7 During application of topical airway anesthesia, the patient obstructs. What should you do now?

If the patient obstructs, common sense should prevail. You should do what you would always do to ventilate the apneic patient: attempt an airway-opening maneuver and perform BMV, using a two-person technique. An oropharyngeal or nasopharyngeal airway may be used, depending on the level of consciousness of the patient. PEEP should be applied during bag-mask-ventilation to help splint open collapsed tissues and ease any laryngospasm.[45,49]

55.3.8   What if the BMV fails? Should a surgical airway be performed?

A failed airway situation can be defined as the inability to maintain adequate O_2 saturation with BMV *and* failure to intubate on at least one occasion (see Section 2.5.5). Despite the failure to bag-mask ventilate the patient, failed airway criteria are only met if the patient also cannot be intubated. A single attempt at direct laryngoscopic intubation should be made. If this is unsuccessful, a failed airway is declared, and the default response becomes cricothyrotomy.

55.3.9   At direct laryngoscopy, only extensive edematous mucosa is seen, along with the tip of the epiglottis, deviated to the right

If the patient is already unconscious from hypoxemia, it may be worth performing a single chest compression to see if a bubble is produced, indicating the entrance to the airway. With or without a bubble, a tracheal tube introducer or small tube can be blindly placed where the glottic opening would be expected to be, beneath the epiglottis. If this single attempt fails, however, the default maneuver is to directly proceed to cricothyrotomy in order to maximize the chances of salvaging a bad situation. Often, the decision to proceed with cricothyrotomy is made too late to salvage the patient.

55.3.10   What is the role, if any, for an EGD such as a laryngeal mask airway?

An EGD such as a laryngeal mask airway (LMA) may fail to oxygenate the patient in this setting as (a) correct seating in the pharynx may be difficult due to a displaced laryngeal inlet and (b) extensive edema at or above the level of the cords may preclude effective ventilation. However, several centers have reported successful oxygenation of patients with LMAs in failed airway situations due to neck hematomas[41,46,50] or other obstructing pathology.[51,52] This may occur as the EGD bypasses more proximal edematous and obstructing soft tissues, allowing positive pressure ventilation from a position immediately in front of the laryngeal inlet. While the correct response in the failed airway (cannot intubate/cannot ventilate) situation is a cricothyrotomy, it is worth a single attempt at EGD insertion while obtaining and opening cricothyrotomy equipment.

55.3.11   I thought that awake bronchoscopic intubation was the foolproof gold standard for difficult airway. Why did the patient obstruct during application of topical airway anesthesia?

Loss of the airway during application of topical airway anesthesia[49,52,53] or awake bronchoscopic intubation[6,41,54] from above in the patient with a neck hematoma or other obstructing pathology is well described. Apart from the natural progression of the disease process, this may occur for a number of reasons:

1. *Systemically administered sedative agents.* These may have adverse effects on airway patency.[6,45]

2. *Laryngospasm.* This may occur during the airway topicalization process,[34,52,55] particularly in the patient with heavier degrees of sedation.

3. *Patient panic.* As the dyspneic patient desperately tries to inspire, the high negative inspiratory pressure applied to an already narrowed, collapsible upper airway may contribute to complete collapse.[55,56]

4. *Direct effect of local anesthetic agents on upper airway mechanoreceptors.* The existence of laryngeal and supra-laryngeal pressure and stretch receptors has been hypothesized, responsible for maintaining airway patency by responding to negative intra-luminal airway pressure via increasing neural and muscular activity.[57,58] The activity of such receptors can be affected or abolished by application of topical airway anesthesia.[57,58] This in turn can significantly affect inspiratory flow, even in normal individuals. Pulmonary function studies in volunteers have demonstrated a significant reduction in maximal,[59] peak, and forced[60] inspiratory flow rates following topical airway anesthesia. Studies of the sleep-apnea population in whom topical airway anesthesia has been applied have also shown worsening of obstructive parameters. This is an underappreciated side effect of topical airway anesthesia and in the patient with a tenuous airway may be an important phenomenon to consider (see Section 3.3.4). It does not preclude choosing awake intubation with topical airway anesthesia, but does underscore the need for planning and an airway double setup.

55.4   OTHER CONSIDERATIONS

55.4.1   What should be the postoperative disposition of a patient re-intubated for a neck hematoma?

Although the immediate mechanical compression of the airway caused by the hematoma may be relieved after surgical reexploration and blood evacuation, other mechanisms of airway compromise, for example, laryngeal inlet edema and blood dissection along tissue planes may take longer to resolve. Caution must prevail and strong consideration should be given to keeping the patient intubated and ventilated for a period of time, (eg, 24 hours) in an intensive-care setting. The patient should be nursed head-up to promote venous drainage, and consideration can be given to administering steroids. Admittedly, many randomized controlled trials looking at the effect of steroid administration on upper airway[29] and laryngeal edema[61] or post-extubation stridor[62] in adults have failed to demonstrate a beneficial effect. Results of studies in the pediatric setting have been mixed.[63,64] Future studies looking at alternative doses, dosing intervals, or specific subpopulations may yet identify a beneficial effect of steroid administration.

55.4.2   What criteria should be met prior to extubation?

In addition to usual extubation criteria, prior to extubation of the patient intubated for airway pathology, such as a neck hematoma, an attempt should be made to evaluate both the caliber of the subglottic airway and the condition of the laryngeal inlet. Traditionally, presence of a cuff leak has been sought as a reassuring sign of an airway patent enough to withstand extubation. Clinically, testing for a cuff leak has been described in a number of ways:

1. In the spontaneously breathing patient, simply deflating the ETT cuff, briefly manually occluding the end of the ETT, and evaluating the patient's ability to breath around the tube.[65,66]

2. With the cuff deflated, delivering a positive pressure volume, with a satisfactory result being the presence of a leak at a delivered peak pressure of 15 cm H_2O or less.[4,8]

3. A more objective evaluation has been described by having a ventilator deliver a set volume (eg, 10 mL·kg^{-1}) with the ETT cuff deflated, then measuring the expired volume in milliliters[67,68] or as a percentage of the delivered inspiratory volume.[69,70]

Most[65,67,70,71] but not all[68] studies on the subject agree that the presence of a leak (present qualitatively or measured quantitatively[69]) is predictive of successful extubation (ie, absence of stridor post-extubation and/or no need for re-intubation). Conversely, many studies also showed that the absence of a leak did not necessarily preclude successful extubation.[66,69,70,72] This latter group of patients, however, would be particularly good candidates for further evaluation of the upper airway prior to extubation, for example, through direct or indirect (eg, with a nasopharyngoscope or oral video laryngoscope such as a GlideScope®) laryngoscopic assessment, looking for three parameters:

1. An appropriate midline location of the laryngeal inlet

2. The lack of significant perilaryngeal edema

3. Appropriate bilateral vocal cord movement[32]

If extubation is elected in this group, consideration should be given to extubating over an airway exchange catheter. In worrisome cases, extubation can be done in the OR as this may facilitate inspection of the laryngeal inlet with direct or indirect laryngoscopy,

in addition to permitting easier access to equipment for a difficult re-intubation.

55.4.3   What other situations or types of surgery incur the risk of neck hematomas? Are there any risk factors or preventive measures that can be undertaken?

Any surgery of the head, neck, and thorax can lead to airway-compromising hematomas. Common examples include carotid endarterectomies,[8,73] parathyroid and thyroid surgery,[13,20] and anterior cervical discectomy/fusion,[40] with most reported series suggesting a neck hematoma incidence of 1% to 5%.[10,74-80] Case reports have also documented central line insertion attempts[2,3,11,12,16,81] and stellate ganglion blocks[82] in the development of life-threatening neck hematomas. Spontaneous bleeds resulting in neck hematomas have also occurred, in both anticoagulated and non-anticoagulated patients.[25,83-87] Blunt trauma has been contributory in some.[88,89]

At least for carotid artery surgery, risk factors for the development of post-op hematomas include antiplatelet agents;[4,8] the nonreversal of intraoperatively administered heparin;[22,73,90,91] use of a vein graft,[92] shunt,[91] and experiencing significant intraoperative hypotension[91] or postoperative hypertension (eg, systolic blood pressure of >200 mm Hg).[4,8,22,73] This latter underscores the importance of aggressive control of hemodynamics in a high-dependency care environment postoperatively. Surgical drains have not demonstrated a benefit in the prevention of post-op neck hematomas in the setting of thyroidectomy[47,74] or carotid endarterectomy.[93]

55.4.4   How does a neck hematoma affect the patient's prognosis?

The occurrence of a postsurgical neck hematoma in the patient undergoing carotid endarterectomy increases the risk of stroke or death 2.5 to 4-fold.[77,94] At least part of this morbidity and mortality may be related to the significant airway compromise that can accompany this complication.

55.5   SUMMARY

Once a postsurgical neck hematoma has been identified, the patient should be observed in a high-dependency nursing unit until a decision is made on definitive care. If re-intubation is required for worsening respiratory distress, it should occur early, while patient cooperation allows the option of awake intubation. Even with awake intubation or an inhalational induction in the patient with a postsurgical neck hematoma, the risk of complete loss of the airway is always present during the procedure. Primary awake tracheotomy will avoid this eventuality in the patient with severe airway compromise, or, if intubation from above is attempted, it should be with prior release of the neck wound, and must always be with the *airway double setup* availability of equipment and personnel to allow an emergency cricothyrotomy, should it become necessary.

REFERENCES

1. Cormack RS, Lehane J. Difficult tracheal intubation in obstetrics. *Anaesthesia.* 1984;39:1105-1111.
2. Randalls B, Toomey PJ. Laryngeal oedema from a neck haematoma. A complication of internal jugular vein cannulation. *Anaesthesia.* 1990;45:850-852.
3. Digby S. Fatal respiratory obstruction following insertion of a central venous line. *Anaesthesia.* 1994;49:1013-1014.
4. Munro FJ, Makin AP, Reid J. Airway problems after carotid endarterectomy. *Br J Anaesth.* 1996;76:156-159.
5. Murphy M, Hung O, Launcelott G, Law JA, Morris I. Predicting the difficult laryngoscopic intubation: are we on the right track? *Can J Anaesth.* 2005;52:231-235.
6. McGuire G, el-Beheiry H. Complete upper airway obstruction during awake fibreoptic intubation in patients with unstable cervical spine fractures. *Can J Anaesth.* 1999;46:176-178.
7. Byard RW, Gilbert JD. Narcotic administration and stenosing lesions of the upper airway—a potentially lethal combination. *J Clin Forensic Med.* 2005;12:29-31.
8. O'Sullivan JC, Wells DG, Wells GR. Difficult airway management with neck swelling after carotid endarterectomy. *Anaesth Intensive Care.* 1986;14: 460-464.
9. Kunkel JM, Gomez ER, Spebar MJ, Delgado RJ, Jarstfer. BS, Collins GJ. Wound hematomas after carotid endarterectomy. *Am J Surg.* 1984;148:844-847.
10. Shakespeare WA, Lanier WL, Perkins WJ, Pasternak JJ. Airway management in patients who develop neck hematomas after carotid endarterectomy. *Anesth Analg.* 2010;110:588-593.
11. Smurthwaite GJ, Letheren MJ. Airway obstruction after trans-jugular liver biopsy: anaesthetic management. *Br J Anaesth.* 1995;75:102-104.
12. Lo WK, Chong JL. Neck haematoma and airway obstruction in a pre-eclamptic patient: a complication of internal jugular vein cannulation. *Anaesth Intensive Care.* 1997;25:423-425.
13. Hare R. Respiratory obstruction after thyroidectomy. *Anaesthesia.* 1982;37:1136.
14. Carr ER, Benjamin E. In vitro study investigating post neck surgery haematoma airway obstruction. *J Laryngol Otol.* 2009;123:662-665.
15. Paleri V, Maroju RS, Ali MS, Ruckley RW. Spontaneous retro- and parapharyngeal haematoma caused by intrathyroid bleed. *J Laryngol Otol.* 2002;116:854-858.
16. Kua JS, Tan IK. Airway obstruction following internal jugular vein cannulation. *Anaesthesia.* 1997;52:776-780.
17. Thomas MD, Torres A, Garcia-Polo J, Gavilan C. Life-threatening cervicomediastinal haematoma after carotid sinus massage. *J Laryngol Otol.* 1991;105:381-383.
18. Bukht D, Langford RM. Airway obstruction after surgery in the neck. *Anaesthesia.* 1983;38:389-390.
19. Knoblanche GE. Respiratory obstruction due to haematoma following internal jugular vein cannulation. *Anaesth Intensive Care.* 1979;7:286.
20. Bexton MD, Radford R. An unusual cause of respiratory obstruction after thyroidectomy. *Anaesthesia.* 1982;37:596.
21. Wells DG, Zelcer J, Wells GR, Sherman GP. A theoretical mechanism for massive supraglottic swelling following carotid endarterectomy. *Aust N Z J Surg.* 1988;58:979-981.
22. Holdsworth RJ, McCollum PT. Acute laryngeal oedema following carotid endarterectomy. *J Cardiovasc Surg (Torino).* 1994;35:249-251.
23. Carmichael FJ, McGuire GP, Wong DT, Crofts S, Sharma S, Montanera W. Computed tomographic analysis of airway dimensions after carotid endarterectomy. *Anesth Analg.* 1996;83:12-17.
24. Wade JS. Cecil Joll Lecture, 1979. Respiratory obstruction in thyroid surgery. *Ann R Coll Surg Engl.* 1980;62:15-24.
25. Ahmed J, Philpott J, Lew-Gor S, Blunt D. Airway obstruction: a rare complication of thrombolytic therapy. *J Laryngol Otol.* 2005;119:819-821.
26. Field JR, DeSaussure RL. Retropharyngeal hemorrhage with respiratory obstruction following angiography. *J Neurosurg.* 1965;22:610-611.
27. Myssiorek D, Shalmi C. Traumatic retropharyngeal hematoma. *Arch Otolaryngol Head Neck Surg.* 1989;115:1130-1132.
28. Carmichael F, McGuire G, Wong D, et al. Computed Tomographic analysis of airway dimensions after carotid endarterectomy. *Anesth Analg.* 1996;83:12-17.
29. Hughes R, McGuire G, Montanera W, Wong D, Carmichael FJ. Upper airway edema after carotid endarterectomy: the effect of steroid administration. *Anesth Analg.* 1997;84:475-458.
30. Spiekermann BF, Stone DJ, Bogdonoff DL, Yemen TA. Airway management in neuroanaesthesia. *Can J Anaesth.* 1996;43:820-834.
31. Itobi E, Sutherland AD, Whinney D, Davies JN. Acute airway obstruction complicating unilateral carotid endarterectomy. *Eur J Vasc Endovasc Surg.* 2005;30:152-153.
32. Tyers MR, Cronin K. Airway obstruction following second operation for carotid endarterectomy. *Anaesth Intensive Care.* 1986;14:314-316.
33. Wade JG, Larson CP, Jr., Hickey RF, Ehrenfeld WK, Severinghaus JW. Effect of carotid endarterectomy on carotid chemoreceptor and baroreceptor function in man. *N Engl J Med.* 1970;282:823-829.
34. Mason RA, Fielder CP. The obstructed airway in head and neck surgery. *Anaesthesia.* 1999;54:625-628.
35. Donlon J, Jr. *Anesthetic and Airway Management of Laryngoscopy and Bronchoscopy.* St. Louis: Mosby; 1996.
36. Ho AM, Dion PW, Karmakar MK, Chung DC, Tay BA. Use of heliox in critical upper airway obstruction. Physical and physiologic considerations in choosing the optimal helium:oxygen mix. *Resuscitation.* 2002;52:297-300.
37. Hessan H, Houck J, Harvey H. Airway obstruction due to lymphoma of the larynx and trachea. *Laryngoscope.* 1988;98:176-180.
38. Khanlou H, Eiger G. Safety and efficacy of heliox as a treatment for upper airway obstruction due to radiation-induced laryngeal dysfunction. *Heart Lung.* 2001;30:146-147.
39. Riley RH, Raper GD, Newman MA. Helium-oxygen and cardiopulmonary bypass standby in anaesthesia for tracheal stenosis. *Anaesth Intensive Care* 1994;22:710-713.
40. Roy SP. Acute postoperative neck hematoma. *Am J Emerg Med.* 1999;17:308-309.
41. Martin R, Girouard Y, Cote DJ. Use of a laryngeal mask in acute airway obstruction after carotid endarterectomy. *Can J Anaesth.* 2002;49:890.
42. MacDonnell SP, Timmins AC, Watson JD. Adrenaline administered via a nebulizer in adult patients with upper airway obstruction. *Anaesthesia.* 1995;50:35-36.
43. Goldberg D, Bhatti N. Management of the impaired airway in the adult. In: Cummings CW, Flint PW, Haughey BH, et al, eds. *Otolaryngology, Head and Neck Surgery.* 4th ed. Philadelphia, PA: Elsevier, Mosby; 2005: 2441-2453.
44. Ovassapian A, Tuncbilek M, Weitzel EK, Joshi CW. Airway management in adult patients with deep neck infections: a case series and review of the literature. *Anesth Analg.* 2005;100:585-589.
45. Hillman DR, Platt PR, Eastwood PR. The upper airway during anaesthesia. *Br J Anaesth.* 2003;91:31-39.
46. Augoustides JG, Groff BE, Mann DG, Johansson JS. Difficult airway management after carotid endarterectomy: utility and limitations of the Laryngeal Mask Airway. *J Clin Anesth.* 2007;19:218-221.
47. Shandilya M, Kieran S, Walshe P, Timon C. Cervical haematoma after thyroid surgery: management and prevention. *Ir Med J.* 2006;99:266-268.
48. Pelizzo MR, Toniato A, Piotto A, et al. Prevention and treatment of intra- and post-operative complications in thyroid surgery. *Ann Ital Chir.* 2001;72:273-276.
49. Calder I, Koh K. Cervical haematoma and airway obstruction. *Br J Anaesth.* 1996;76:888-889.
50. Jones DA, Geraghty IF. Emergency management of upper airway obstruction due to a rapidly expanding haematoma in the neck. *Br J Hosp Med.* 1995;53:589-590.
51. King CJ, Davey AJ, Chandradeva K. Emergency use of the laryngeal mask airway in severe upper airway obstruction caused by supraglottic oedema. *Br J Anaesth.* 1995;75:785-786.
52. Shaw IC, Welchew EA, Harrison BJ, Michael S. Complete airway obstruction during awake fibreoptic intubation. *Anaesthesia.* 1997;52:582-585.
53. White MC, Reynolds F. Sudden airway obstruction following inhalation drug abuse. *Br J Anaesth.* 1999;82:808.
54. Wulf H, Brinkmann G, Rautenberg M. Management of the difficult airway. A case of failed fiberoptic intubation. *Acta Anaesthesiol Scand.* 1997;41:1080-1082.
55. Ho AM, Chung DC, To EW, Karmakar MK. Total airway obstruction during local anesthesia in a non-sedated patient with a compromised airway. *Can J Anaesth.* 2004;51:838-841.

56. Shiratori T, Hara K, Ando N. Acute airway obstruction secondary to retropharyngeal hematoma. *J Anesth*. 2003;17:46-48.

57. Horner RL, Innes JA, Holden HB, Guz A. Afferent pathway(s) for pharyngeal dilator reflex to negative pressure in man: a study using upper airway anesthesia. *J Physiol*. 1991;436:31-44.

58. Berry RB, McNellis MI, Kouchi K, Light RW. Upper airway anesthesia reduces phasic genioglossus activity during sleep apnea. *Am J Respir Crit Care Med*. 1997;156:127-132.

59. Liistro G, Stanescu DC, Veriter C, Rodenstein DO, D'Odemont JP. Upper airway anesthesia induces airflow limitation in awake humans. *Am Rev Respir Dis*. 1992;146:581-585.

60. Kuna ST, Woodson GE, Sant'Ambrogio G. Effect of laryngeal anesthesia on pulmonary function testing in normal subjects. *Am Rev Respir Dis*. 1988;137:656-661.

61. Darmon JY, Rauss A, Dreyfuss D, et al. Evaluation of risk factors for laryngeal edema after tracheal extubation in adults and its prevention by dexamethasone. A placebo-controlled, double-blind, multicenter study. *Anesthesiology*. 1992;77:245-251.

62. Ho LI, Harn HJ, Lien TC, et al. Postextubation laryngeal edema in adults. Risk factor evaluation and prevention by hydrocortisone. *Intensive Care Med*. 1996;22:933-936.

63. Anene O, Meert KL, Uy H, et al. Dexamethasone for the prevention of postextubation airway obstruction: a prospective, randomized, double-blind, placebo-controlled trial. *Crit Care Med*, 1996;24:1666-1669.

64. Tellez DW, Galvis AG, Storgion SA, Amer HN, Hoseyni M, Deakers TW. Dexamethasone in the prevention of postextubation stridor in children. *J Pediatr*. 1991;118:289-294.

65. Potgieter PD, Hammond JM. "Cuff" test for safe extubation following laryngeal edema. *Crit Care Med*. 1988;16:818.

66. Marik PE. The cuff-leak test as a predictor of postextubation stridor: a prospective study. *Respiratory Care*. 1996;41:509-511.

67. Miller RL, Cole RP. Association between reduced cuff leak volume and postextubation stridor. *Chest*. 1996;110:1035-1040.

68. Engoren M. Evaluation of the cuff-leak test in a cardiac surgery population. *Chest*. 1999;116:1029-1031.

69. Sandhu RS, Pasquale MD, Miller K, Wasser TE. Measurement of endotracheal tube cuff leak to predict postextubation stridor and need for reintubation. *J Am Coll Surg*. 2000;190:682-687.

70. Jaber S, Chanques G, Matecki S, et al. Post-extubation stridor in intensive care unit patients. Risk factors evaluation and importance of the cuff-leak test. *Intensive Care Med*. 2003;29:69-74.

71. De Bast Y, De Backer D, Moraine JJ, et al. The cuff leak test to predict failure of tracheal extubation for laryngeal edema. *Intensive Care Med*. 2002;28:1267-1272.

72. Fisher MM, Raper RF. The "cuff-leak" test for extubation. *Anaesthesia*. 1992;47:10-12.

73. Nunn DB. Carotid endarterectomy: an analysis of 234 operative cases. *Ann Surg*. 1975;182:733-738.

74. Sanabria A, Carvalho AL, Silver CE, et al. Routine drainage after thyroid surgery—a meta-analysis. *J Surg Oncol*. 2007;96:273-280.

75. Fountas KN, Kapsalaki EZ, Nikolakakos LG, et al. Anterior cervical discectomy and fusion associated complications. *Spine* (Phila Pa 1976). 2007;32:2310-2317.

76. Assadian A, Knobl P, Hubl W, et al. Safety and efficacy of intravenous enoxaparin for carotid endarterectomy: a prospective randomized pilot trial. *J Vasc Surg*. 2008;47:537-542.

77. Greenstein AJ, Chassin MR, Wang J, et al. Association between minor and major surgical complications after carotid endarterectomy: results of the New York Carotid Artery Surgery study. *J Vasc Surg*. 2007;46:1138-1144; discussion 1145-1146.

78. Bertalanffy H, Eggert HR. Complications of anterior cervical discectomy without fusion in 450 consecutive patients. *Acta Neurochir* (Wien). 1989;99:41-50.

79. Lee HS, Lee BJ, Kim SW, et al. Patterns of post-thyroidectomy hemorrhage. *Clin Exp Otorhinolaryngol*. 2009;2:72-77.

80. Liu JT, Briner RP, Friedman JA. Comparison of inpatient vs. outpatient anterior cervical discectomy and fusion: a retrospective case series. *BMC Surg*. 2009;9:3.

81. Guilbert MC, Elkouri S, Bracco D, et al. Arterial trauma during central venous catheter insertion: case series, review and proposed algorithm. *J Vasc Surg*. 2008;48:918-925; discussion 925.

82. Higa K, Hirata K, Hirota K, et al. Retropharyngeal hematoma after stellate ganglion block: analysis of 27 patients reported in the literature. *Anesthesiology*. 2006;105:1238-1245; discussion 5A-6A.

83. Pazardzhikliev DD, Yovchev IP, Zhelev DD. Neck hematoma caused by spontaneous common carotid artery rupture. *Laryngoscope*. 2008;118:684-686.

84. Getnick GS, Lin SJ, Raviv JR, et al. Lingual hematoma and heparin-induced thrombocytopenia: a case report. *Ear Nose Throat J*. 2008;87:163-165.

85. Kirkham L, Homewood J, Brook P. Case of the month: a case of airway obstruction following tenecteplase administration. *Emerg Med J*. 2006;23:815-816.

86. Akoglu E, Seyfeli E, Akoglu S, Karazincir S, Okuyucu E, Dagli AS. Retropharyngeal hematoma as a complication of anticoagulation therapy. *Ear Nose Throat J*. 2008;87:156-159.

87. Stenner M, Helmstaedter V, Spuentrup E, Quante G, Huettenbrink KB. Cervical hemorrhage due to spontaneous rupture of the superior thyroid artery: case report and review of the literature. *Head Neck*. 2010;32(9):1277-1281.

88. Lin JY, Wang CH, Huang TW. Traumatic retropharyngeal hematoma: case report. *Auris Nasus Larynx*. 2007;34:423-425.

89. Keogh IJ, Rowley H, Russell J. Critical airway compromise caused by neck haematoma. *Clin Otolaryngol Allied Sci*. 2002;27:244-245.

90. Dellagrammaticas D, Lewis SC, Gough MJ. Is heparin reversal with protamine after carotid endarterectomy dangerous? *Eur J Vasc Endovasc Surg*. 2008;36:41-44.

91. Self DD, Bryson GL, Sullivan PJ. Risk factors for post-carotid endarterectomy hematoma formation. *Can J Anaesth*. 1999;46:635-640.

92. Tawes RL, Jr, Treiman RL. Vein patch rupture after carotid endarterectomy: a survey of the Western Vascular Society members. *Ann Vasc Surg*. 1991;5:71-73.

93. Youssef F, Jenkins MP, Dawson KJ, Berger L, Myint F, Hamilton G. The value of suction wound drain after carotid and femoral artery surgery: a randomised trial using duplex assessment of the volume of post-operative haematoma. *Eur J Vasc Endovasc Surg*. 2005;29:162-166.

94. Ferguson GG, Eliasziw M, Barr HW, et al. The North American Symptomatic Carotid Endarterectomy Trial: surgical results in 1415 patients. *Stroke*. 1999;30:1751-1758.

SELF-EVALUATION QUESTIONS

55.1. Recognizing that no method of intubation can be guaranteed 100% complication free, which of the following approaches to securing the airway is **LEAST** safe in the patient with a neck hematoma?

A. awake intubation with topical airway anesthesia

B. rapid-sequence intubation with induction agent and muscle relaxant

C. local or regional anesthesia for evacuation of hematoma and no intubation

D. inhalational induction

E. awake tracheostomy under local anesthesia

55.2. In the patient with obstructing airway pathology such as a neck hematoma, which of the following is the **LEAST** safe option to help symptomatically temporize the patient while preparing for intubation?

A. Use sedative agents to alleviate patient anxiety.

B. If patient oxygenation permits, use heliox to help the work of breathing.

C. Have the patient in the sitting or semi-sitting position.

D. Administer racemic epinephrine via aerosol.

E. Give intravenous steroids to help counteract any inflammatory component.

55.3. In the patient with obstructing airway pathology such as a neck hematoma, which of the following airway management techniques would be (at least relatively) contraindicated?

A. direct laryngoscopy and intubation

B. placement of a laryngeal mask airway

C. blind tube passage through an intubating (Fastrach™) laryngeal mask airway

D. awake intubation with a flexible bronchoscope

E. bag-mask-ventilation with an oropharyngeal airway

CHAPTER 56

Airway Management in Austere Environments

Thomas J. Coonan, Phil Blum, and J. Adam Law

56.1 CASE PRESENTATION

As an anesthesia practitioner, you were in a developing country on a short-term, 2-week mission with a team of plastic and maxillofacial surgeons. The team's mandate was to operate on patients with unrepaired cleft lips and palates. As word spread in the area of the team's successes, on the final day of the mission a 12-year-old boy was brought to the clinic. One year before, the boy had sustained significant burns to his lower face, neck, and chest. No surgical remediation had been undertaken and he now had severe burn contractures (Figure 56-1).

56.2 INTRODUCTION

In the developed world, about 1:50 general anesthesia cases will present with difficult tracheal intubation; 1:75 will result in a failed intubation; and a failure to intubate and to ventilate occurs in 1:1000 to 1:12,000. Obstetrical anesthesia is particularly challenging in this regard, as the airway may be complicated by edema related to toxemia or prolonged labor (see Section 1.2.1). Although the principles of airway management are similar worldwide, the anesthesia practitioner in the developing world can expect to face challenges both unrelated, and related, to difficult airway anatomy (Table 56-1). A variety of difficult conditions will be encountered, often in later stages of evolution, presenting greater challenges with higher airway acuity. Pathology less familiar to the average practitioner can also be expected. A higher proportion of anesthesia practice appears to be made up of pediatric and obstetrical patients.

56.2.1 What are the risks inherent in airway management in austere environments?

Forty years of intense commitment has greatly reduced avoidable anesthesia-related mortality in wealthy countries to a rate of about 1/56,000 anesthetics (1/180,000 when anesthesia is the sole cause of mortality and morbidity), and airway misadventure is no longer the primary reason for seriously adverse outcome.[1] Training in airway management has advanced, guidelines and standards have been introduced, technology has evolved immensely, and a culture of safety is in place.[2,3] Sadly, such benefits have been largely restricted to the few who live in relatively privileged societies. Published mortality due to airway misadventure in less resourced areas can vary from 100 to 1000 times that in affluent societies.[4-7] Indeed, in one report, the avoidable mortality from airway-related causes was 1/183 anesthetics.[7] Obstetric anesthesia is a particular risk in this regard.[8]

The challenges facing developing countries are far more profound than the unavailability of the latest aids for tracheal intubation. The greatest barrier is the inability through lack of resources to provide adequate training, adequate supervision, essential monitoring techniques, sustainable organizational structure, and a modern system of quality review. One major priority, universal pulse oximetry, is lacking, but so too are vigorous educational support, mentorship, and team building.

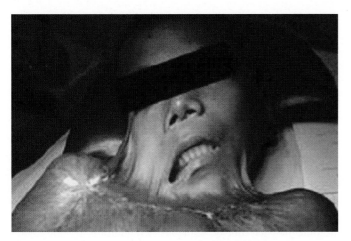

FIGURE 56-1. A 12-year-old boy with severe burn contractures.

TABLE 56-1

Expected Developing Country Conditions with the Potential for Difficult Airway Management

- Familiar conditions, but more advanced:
  - Obstetrics—preeclampsia, placenta previa, placenta accreta
  - Goiter

- Upper airway infections and tumors
- Less familiar conditions:
  - Severe uncorrected head/neck burn contractures
  - Uncorrected congenital defects
  - Cancrum oris (*Noma*)
  - Late presentations of obstructing tumors
  - Temporomandibular ankylosis

- Higher proportion of pediatric and obstetric anesthesia practice

56.3 AIRWAY EQUIPMENT IN AUSTERE ENVIRONMENT

56.3.1 What are the equipment considerations for difficult airway management in the developing world?

Aggressive attention to the needs of the developing world has been undertaken by the international anesthesia community since 1989,[2] and a series of standards have evolved, most recently the WHO Guidelines for Safe Surgery.[9] These guidelines are sensitive to an immense global variation in resources and capacities, and standards are stratified to reflect what is possible for most regions.

TABLE 56-2

Medications Available in Level 1 Facilities

- Ketamine
- Lidocaine
- Diazepam or midazolam
- Morphine
- Pethidine
- Epinephrine
- Atropine
- Perhaps a volatile anesthetic agent

WHO 2009.[9]

56.3.1.1 Equipment Recommended for Level 1 Facilities: Small Hospitals or Health Centers

Such facilities provide minor surgery, normal obstetric delivery, and stabilization of emergencies. Level 1 facilities are staffed by paramedical staff, anesthetic officers, nurses, and midwives. In many environments, the supply of compressed gases is unreliable and expensive, meaning that oxygen concentrators, and draw-over anesthesia offer significant advantages.[10] If only a single laryngoscope blade can be made available, it perhaps should be a Macintosh #4, as the tip of the blade can be used for neonates and children. WHO guidelines for medication and equipment availability in Level 1 facilities appear in Table 56-2 and 56-3.

56.3.1.2 Equipment Recommended for Level 2 Facilities: District or Provincial Hospitals

Level 2 facilities undertake procedures such as caesarean section, laparotomy, and internal fixation of fractures that do not require a high level of specialization and technology. Such facilities have at least one trained anesthesiologist, with district medical officers, senior clinical officers, nurses, and midwives.

TABLE 56-3

Equipment Available in Level 1 Facilities

- Adult and pediatric self-inflating bags with mask
- Foot-powered suction
- Stethoscope, sphygmomanometer, thermometer
- Pulse oximeter
- Oxygen concentrator, or tank oxygen
- Draw-over vaporizer with hoses (at times)
- Laryngoscopes
- Tracheal tube introducers (bougies)
- Airways
- Tracheal tubes

WHO 2009.[9]

TABLE 56-4

Additional Medication Available at Level 2 Facilities

- Thiopental
- Suxamethonium bromide
- Pancuronium
- Neostigmine
- Ether, halothane, or other vapors

WHO 2009.[9]

TABLE 56-5

Additional Equipment Available at Level 2 Facilities

- Pediatric anesthesia systems
- Pulse oximetry—adult and pediatric probes
- Face masks size 00-5
- Oxygen analyzers, oxygen supply failure alarms
- Capnography
- Laryngoscopes, Macintosh blades 1-3 (4)
- Magills forceps, adult and child
- Oral airways, size 000-4
- Tracheal tubes size with ID 3-8 mm

WHO 2009.[9]

There are one or more resident surgeons and obstetricians, and there are visiting specialists. Additional drugs and equipment are available to supplement those found in Level 1 facilities (Tables 56-4 and 56-5).

56.3.1.3   Equipment Recommended for Level 3 Facilities: Referral Hospital

Such facilities usually have the capacity to undertake facial surgery, intracranial surgery, bowel resection surgery, pediatric and neonatal surgery, thoracic surgery, major eye surgery, major gynecological surgery, and the management of critically ill patients. Personnel include surgical, anesthesia, and critical care subspecialists. Available recommended medications and equipment (in addition to those available at Level 1 and 2 facilities) appear in Tables 56-6 and 56-7.

TABLE 56-6

Additional Medication Available at Level 3 Facilities

- Propofol
- Various modern neuromuscular blocking agents
- Various modern inhalational agents

TABLE 56-7

Additional Equipment Available at Level 3 Facilities

- Laryngeal mask airways, size 2, 3, 4
- Tracheal tube introducers, adult and child

These guidelines provide a useful measure of the resources which will likely be encountered in developing countries. At times, resources available may exceed those recommended in the WHO guidelines. Not infrequently, however, material support suggested in guidelines may not be available.[11] In addition, teaching clinicians can expect to encounter local practitioners with less airway management experience due to the extensive use of local and regional anesthesia for surgical procedures.

56.3.2   What are portable equipment considerations for volunteers on missions?

There is a dichotomy in the needs for difficult airway equipment in austere environment practice, depending on the nature of the mission. Longer-term teaching missions generally involve teaching local practitioners to use equipment already present (or easily obtained) and maintained in the environment. In general, equipment inventory will reflect WHO standards. In contrast, with short-term service missions, a traveling team arrives to directly provide medical care, and airway equipment is generally transported in and out with the team.[12]

56.3.2.1   Airway Equipment Considerations for Longer-Term/Teaching Missions

In general, a fundamental premise of longer-term teaching missions is to teach and use airway equipment that is locally sustainable. A "locally sustainable" device is defined as one that is already present in the environment, or can readily be obtained from that location (Tables 56-3, 56-5, and 56-7). In addition, it must be easily disinfected and should be simple to maintain or repair if broken. If electronically powered, the device should have a reliable power source, batteries or otherwise, and in this context, it must be stressed that electrical power (and compressed gases), are often unreliable in disadvantaged countries. Generally, equipment must be reusable, and it must be assumed that any single-use items will be reused.

Even if a device can be obtained and maintained, other factors must be considered. Introducing devices with unfavorable learning curves, or complex storage or disinfection needs, should be discouraged. Donation of equipment that is fragile or requires frequent servicing (eg, a flexible bronchoscope with a video tower), while well-meaning, can be futile and counterproductive in an austere environment. If such a device is presented, it helps to designate one local practitioner as champion for the product, charged with responsibility for ensuring it is used, cleaned, and stored appropriately.

TABLE 56-8

Sample Airway Equipment for a Short-Term Service Mission

Basic equipment
- Portable pulse oximeter/capnograph
- Draw-over circuit and vaporizer
- Laryngoscopes with spare blades, bulbs, and batteries
- Face masks
- Complete set of tracheal tubes and stylets
- Oxygen tubing
- Tracheal tube introducers (Eschmann Tracheal Introducers) adult and child
- Precordial stethoscope

Difficult airway equipment
- Alternative intubation devices, eg, one or more of:
  - Trachlight™
  - LMA-Fastrach™
  - Rigid fiberoptic, eg, Bullard, optical stylets
  - Optical devices, eg, Airtraq
  - Flexible bronchoscope, battery powered
- Extraglottic devices
- Seldinger cricothyrotomy device
- Colorimetric CO_2 detection devices[19]

TABLE 56-9

Recommended Equipment Management in Austere Environments

1. Single-use bacterial filters are now standard issue for many missions.
2. Rubber reusable and plastic single-use tubing should be decontaminated and cleaned. After drying, rubber tubing can be autoclaved. Plastic tubing cannot be autoclaved and should be disinfected.
3. Ambu or Heidbrink valves must be decontaminated, cleaned, and disinfected after each patient when a filter is not used. Ambu valves can be autoclaved.
4. Face masks, Guedel airways, laryngoscope blades, Yankauer suctions are decontaminated, cleaned, and sterilized (metal) or disinfected (plastic).

TABLE 56-10

Management of Consumable Anesthetic Equipment in Austere Environments

1. Single-use tubes are to be used as single use if supplies are sufficient. If in short supply they can be decontaminated, cleaned, and disinfected. Great care is required to ensure that disinfectant solution is removed.
2. Reusable rubber tubes are to be decontaminated, cleaned, and autoclaved.
3. Reusable laryngeal mask airways (LMA-Classic™) are to be decontaminated, cleaned, and autoclaved between each patient.

56.3.2.2 Equipment Considerations for Short-Term/Service Missions

Airway equipment considerations differ for a short-term service mission (Table 56-8). Under these conditions, routine and difficult airway equipment is transported by the team, such equipment being limited only by its portability and robustness. The equipment should ideally be available in adult and pediatric versions, given the high occurrence of pediatric cases. If battery powered, sufficient batteries should also accompany the equipment, and disinfection requirements should be straightforward. It should be noted in this context that many practitioners consider the use of outdated medications or equipment unacceptable.

56.3.3 What can be done to disinfect equipment in an austere environment?

Disinfection methodologies of the developed world are seldom possible in austere environments and a great deal of ingenuity can be found in the methods of steam/sterilization, hypochlorite (bleach), boiling, formaldehyde, and chlorhexidine/cetrimide. Balance is often required between levels of sterility assurance and the possibility of doing a greater good with surgery. High-level disinfection may have to be accepted rather than sterilization. A sampling of common practice guidelines can be found in Tables 56-9 to 56-11.

56.4 DIFFICULT AIRWAY MANAGEMENT IN AUSTERE ENVIRONMENT

56.4.1 Should a patient with a very difficult airway be managed in the austere environment at all?

There is no shortage of very difficult airway anatomy in the developing world. If presented with such a case, a methodological approach should be undertaken. For a service mission with defined objectives, a very high acuity case may fall outside the team's capabilities, for example, due to extreme airway considerations or the anticipated significant need for blood products. Even if the case may be possible from a surgical and anesthetic perspective, postoperative requirements may exceed available infrastructure, for example, the lack of an intensive-care facility with ventilators, or suction and humidification for postoperative management of a patient with a fresh tracheotomy. Careful consideration must always be given to the ultimate patient interest (eg, in an emergency

TABLE 56-11

Disinfection Options in Austere Environments

1. Items should be decontaminated and thoroughly cleaned.
2. Items should be left for 20 minutes in solution.
   Chlorhexidine/cetrimide solution is satisfactory for this purpose, but another solution (eg, gluteraldehyde, bleach) may be used if more appropriate for the program.
3. A rolling boil (100°C for 10-20 minutes) may be preferable for materials that will be reused in the airway. Must boil for longer time at altitude (water boils at 85°C at 5000 ft).
4. Rinse well with water.
5. Dry before next use.
6. Chlorhexidine/cetrimide solution:
   - 20 mL of 1.5% chlorhexidine/20% cetrimide solution is diluted into 1000 mL of water.
7. Hypochlorite (bleach) solution:
   - 1 part bleach to 49 parts water for disinfection.
   - Soak in mixture for 20 minutes.
   - Corrodes metal and may destroy adhesives with prolonged soaking.
   - Wash thoroughly.

situation) and to the reality that concepts of cause and effect can vary significantly over a breadth of environments. Especially in children, it may be possible to arrange care, through aid organizations, in a more favorable environment.

56.4.2 Can the surgical procedure be done with local or regional anesthesia?

Using regional or local anesthesia may allow a procedure to occur without airway manipulation. Equally, local anesthesia may allow a minor surgical revision of difficult airway anatomy that would then allow safer induction of general anesthesia, for example, the partial release of a burn contracture.

56.4.3 If general anesthesia is required, can the airway be safely secured post-induction?

The guiding principles of the ASA Difficult Airway Algorithm (see Section 2.4.2) are still applicable in the less developed world, despite the common absence of flexible bronchoscopy and newer airway adjuncts. Awake intubation with blind nasal techniques (see Section 11.5), retrograde catheters (see Section 11.6), manual techniques (see Section 11.4), and direct laryngoscopy are the rule for the difficult airway in austere environments—and creative approaches in these regards have been reported. For example, 14 to 16 French gauge suction catheters, or hollow ureteric dilators, can be used as anterograde guides in retrograde intubations.[13,14] It should also be emphasized that there are a number of thin flexible scopes that can be used for intubation, including ureteroscopes. An interesting report suggests that in the event of an inability to negotiate a nasotracheal tube through the larynx in children, the tube could be left in the esophagus and an Eschmann Tracheal Introducer placed in the alternative nostril. The blindly placed bougie will often find its way into the trachea.[15]

Notwithstanding such creativity, equipment challenges and a lack of patient cooperation due to language barriers as well as patient age may militate against successful awake intubation in the patient with a difficult airway. Prerequisites for anesthesia induction and pharmacologic paralysis in the patient with significant predictors of difficult direct laryngoscopy include: the absence of obstructing upper airway pathology; anticipated successful BMV and rescue oxygenation by EGD or cricothyrotomy; a reasonable chance of successful intubation by direct laryngoscopy; skills in the use of alternative intubation devices (if available); and the presence of skilled help. It also should be borne in mind that a case traditionally done with endotracheal intubation might be safely done with an extraglottic device in a patient with a difficult airway. An interesting report has described the use of the modified nasal trumpet, a #7.0 or #8.0 standard nasopharyngeal airway with an added distal fenestration and fitted with a 15 mm adaptor to permit connection to an anesthesia circuit.[16] Considerable judgment is required across the spectrum of clinical circumstances.

56.5   PATIENT MANAGEMENT

56.5.1 Are there likely to be difficulties with BMV in this patient?

This patient's contractures and facial deformity will make mask application very difficult. Burn contracture will also preclude airway-opening maneuvers, such as head extension and jaw thrust. BMV is thus predicted to be very difficult in this patient.

56.5.2 Are there likely to be difficulties in placement of an extraglottic device in this patient?

It is unlikely that sufficient mouth opening can be achieved in this patient to allow the insertion of an EGD. Furthermore, by limiting head and upper neck extension (see Section 1.6.3) and distorting the airway, the neck and upper torso contractures may create difficulty with EGD passage into the pharynx, or *seat and seal* properly once there.

56.5.3 Are there likely to be difficulties with laryngoscopy and orotracheal intubation in this patient?

Tracheal intubation of this patient by direct laryngoscopy is likely to be impossible on the basis of limited mouth opening and severely limited head and neck extension. In addition, burn contracture will make the mandibular space stiff and noncompliant, so that tongue displacement and compression will be difficult.

56.5.4 Would cricothyrotomy be feasible in this patient?

Scarring and contracture would make cricothyrotomy almost impossible in this patient.

56.5.5 What coexisting medical problems can be anticipated in this patient?

The patient's contractures are likely to have compromised nutrition and general conditioning; a chronic airway obstruction may be present, and there may be chronic reflux and aspiration. In addition, if a substantial part of the chest was involved with the burn, scarring and contracture of the chest will significantly reduce the compliance of the lungs (restrictive pulmonary dysfunction).[17]

56.5.6 What was done in this case?

A feasibility assessment was performed. Equipment for skin harvesting was available, and as the area requiring grafting was limited, the need for blood products was judged unlikely. Local medical and nursing expertise was deemed capable of taking on postoperative care. Airway assessment suggested that awake tracheal intubation would be safest for the required general anesthetic. Unfortunately, a flexible bronchoscope was not available, and patient cooperation could have been an issue.

An interpreter was obtained, the patient was taken to the operating room, and intravenous access obtained. Local anesthesia was used to enable release of some of the contractures limiting mouth opening, jaw mobility, and head extension. Thereafter, with the patient still awake, a mixture of local anesthetic jelly and a small amount of sweetener was used to anesthetize the mouth and pharynx, and a size 2.5 LMA was inserted (as previously described).[18] This was well tolerated. Good seating of the LMA was confirmed, and with the patient breathing spontaneously, draw-over inhalational anesthesia was introduced. Under general anesthesia and with unobstructed spontaneous ventilation, further contracture release with skin grafting was safely completed.

56.6 SUMMARY

Airway management in the austere environment of many developing countries can be challenging on many fronts: the advanced state of the pathology encountered; equipment availability; and possibly substandard local hospital infrastructure and staffing. The practitioner teaching or practicing in these conditions must be resourceful and sensitive to local culture and conditions. Cases presenting with difficult airway considerations should be approached bearing in mind the limitations of both intra- and postoperative resources.

REFERENCES

1. Mackay P, Cousins M. Safety in anaesthesia. *Anaesth Intensive Care.* 2006;34:303-304.
2. Eichorn JH. Prevention of intraoperative anesthesia accidents and related severe injury through safety monitoring. *Anesthesiology.* 1989;70:572-577.
3. WFSA Comité de Seguridad. *International Standard for Safe Practice of Anaesthesia.* Anaesthesiology WFoSo; 2008.
4. Hansen D, Gausi SC, Merikebu M. Anaesthesia in Malawi: complications and deaths. *Trop Doct.* 2000;30:146-149.
5. Heywood AJ, Wilson IH, Sinclair JR. Perioperative mortality in Zambia. *Ann R Coll Surg Engl.* 1989;71:354-358.
6. McKenzie AG. Mortality associated with anaesthesia at Zimbabwean teaching hospitals. *S Afr Med J.* 1996;86:338-342.
7. Ouro-Bang'na Maman AF, Tomta K, Ahouangbevi S, Chobli M. Deaths associated with anaesthesia in Togo, West Africa. *Trop Doct.* 2005;35:220-222.
8. Vasdev GM, Harrison BA, Keegan MT, Burkle CM. Management of the difficult and failed airway in obstetric anesthesia. *J Anesth.* 2008;22:38-48.
9. WHO. WHO *Guidelines for Safe Surgery.* Geneva: World Health Organization; 2009.
10. Dobson M. *Surgical Care at the District Hospital.* Geneva: World Health Organization; 2003.
11. Hodges SC, Mijumbi C, Okello M, McCormick BA, Walker IA, Wilson IH. Anaesthesia services in developing countries: defining the problems. *Anaesthesia.* 2007;62:4-11.
12. Hodges SC, Hodges AM. A protocol for safe anasthesia for cleft lip and palate surgery in developing countries. *Anaesthesia.* 2000;55:436-441.
13. Dahra SS. Aids to tracheal intubation. World Anaesthesia, Update in Anaesthesia 2003;17:8-13.
14. Wilson IH, Kopf A. Prediction and management of difficult tracheal intubation. World Anaesthesia, Update in Anaesthesia 1998;9:37-45.
15. Arora MK, Karamchandani K, Trikha A. Use of a gum elastic bougie to facilitate blind nasotracheal intubation in children: a series of three cases. *Anaesthesia.* 2006;61:291-294.
16. Metz S, Beattie C. A modified nasal trumpet to facilitate fibreoptic intubation. *Br J Anaesth.* 2003;90:388-391.
17. Mlcak R, Desai MH, Robinson E, Nichols R, Herndon DN. Lung function following thermal injury in children—an 8-year follow up. *Burns.* 1998; 24:213-216.
18. Goodly M, Reddy ARR. Use of LMA for awake intubation for Caesarean section. *Can J Anesth.* 1996;43:299-302.
19. Goldberg JS, Rawle PR, Zehnder JL, Sladen RN. Colorimetric end-tidal carbon dioxide monitoring for tracheal intubation. *Anesth Analg.* 1990;70: 191-194.

SELF-EVALUATION QUESTIONS

56.1. Which of the following is not included in WHO guidelines for district hospitals in all countries?

A. pulse oximetry

B. capnography

C. flexible fiberoscopy

D. tracheal intubating bougies

E. oxygen analyzers

56.2. In purchasing airway equipment for poorly resourced countries, which of the following is least relevant at this time?

A. cost of compressed gases

B. ease of maintenance

C. unreliability of electrical power

D. uniformity of international standards

E. cost of equipment

56.3. Which of the following is not a disinfection option for airway equipment in developing countries?

A. autoclaving

B. ethylene oxide

C. bleach

D. chlorhexidine/cetrimide

E. boiling

CHAPTER (57)

Respiratory Arrest in the Magnetic Resonance Imaging Suite

D. John Doyle

57.1 CASE PRESENTATION: PART I

Mr. S is a 52-year-old entrepreneur in the waste management industry. He weighs 262 lb (approximately 119 kg), is 5 ft 9 in (approximately 175 cm) tall, and is being investigated for dizzy spells that appear to be panic attacks. His medical problem list includes obesity, untreated hypertension, and possible obstructive sleep apnea (OSA) (based on his wife's nocturnal observation that "sometimes he just stops breathing"). When questioned, he admits to extreme claustrophobia, possibly the result of a protracted period of time spent in a car trunk as a child. A previous attempt at a magnetic resonance imaging (MRI) scan was unsuccessful because Mr. S, startled by the onset of the loud noises made by the MRI machine, panicked and tried to get out of the MRI scanner, pulling out his IV in the process.

On this occasion, the MRI team decides that Mr. S might be more cooperative with pharmacologic assistance and to this end has given him 5 mg of IV midazolam (Versed®). Unknown to the clinical team, just before entering the MRI suite, Mr. S had also taken 6 mg of sublingual lorazepam (Ativan®) to help reduce his considerable anxiety. For the scan, a pulse oximeter and nasal capnograph are used to monitor respiration. Oxygen is administered by nasal prongs at 3 L·min^{-1}.

About 10 minutes into the scan, the pulse oximeter alarm activates, drawing attention to an oxygen saturation reading of 83%. The pulse oximeter waveform quality appears to be good. However, no waveform can be obtained from the capnograph. Since Mr. S is deep inside the MRI machine, it is hard to see how well he is actually breathing. You are summoned to the MRI suite to help manage this patient.

57.2 THE MAGNETIC RESONANCE IMAGING SUITE

57.2.1 What is MRI and why is it done?

MRI has steadily increased in popularity as a noninvasive, painless diagnostic imaging procedure. MRI images are produced using a strong (typically, 1.5 tesla [15,000 gauss]) magnetic field into which radiofrequency (RF) pulses are injected. MRI is the imaging method of choice for examinations in which water content differences make it possible to differentiate tissue types.[1] It offers distinct advantages over computed tomography, both in terms of the quality of the obtained images for certain types of tissue (like brain) and the lack of exposure to ionizing radiation. MRI scans are frequently ordered by neurologists and neurosurgeons for patients of all ages with neurological disorders. In addition to intra-axial pathology, orthopedic problems such as osteomyelitis, soft tissue muscle tumors, and damaged knee menisci can be assessed using MRI techniques.[1]

57.2.2 What is unique about the MRI suite in terms of caring for a patient?

The extreme strength of the magnetic field in an MRI scanner can be hazardous. For example, patients with implanted ferromagnetic objects like aneurysm clips have had these fatally pulled out of position by the magnetic field.[2] Similarly, some authorities have expressed concerns about carrying out MRI scans in patients with pacemakers.[3] Likewise, ferromagnetic objects like wrenches, scissors, IV poles, pens, stethoscopes, and even hair barrettes can become accidental projectiles. In one case, a pillow containing metal springs, not detectable using a handheld magnet, flew into the magnet during positioning of a patient, fortunately without causing injury,[4] However, projectile oxygen and nitrous oxide tank cylinder accidents causing injuries and even death have been reported during the last decade.[5-7]

Zimmer et al[8] relate the following interesting cautionary tale. A 2-year-old boy underwent abdominal MRI scanning under general anesthesia. During the procedure, an anesthesia practitioner carried a portable sevoflurane vaporizer into the MRI suite. When the vaporizer was placed on an examination table, it was vigorously attracted toward the scanner, and it was only by the strength of two people that the vaporizer was directed to strike against the gantry, instead of flying directly into the magnet where it might have hit the child. Quenching the magnet, that is, emergency release of liquid helium from the scanner to collapse the magnetic field was initially considered, but the vaporizer could be removed with the help of a third individual. Of interest, immediately after the mishap the portable vaporizer was tested for magnetism with a strong handheld magnet, and no attraction was apparent. A review of the event revealed that the vaporizer contained ferromagnetic material in the temperature compensation module.

In addition to the attractive forces of the magnetic field on ferromagnetic objects, the strong magnetic field and associated RF pulses can interfere with the operation of ordinary anesthesia machines, as well as with patient-monitoring equipment, sometimes resulting in patient injury.[9]

It should be emphasized that some anesthesia machines and patient monitors that are alleged to be MRI compatible may still contain ferromagnetic components and may pose risks when safety precautions (often described in fine print in the user's manual) are violated.

57.2.3 Why might MRI require moderate or deep sedation, or general anesthesia?

Patients must remain motionless during MRI scans. However, the long duration (up to 20 minutes or more) of some MRI scans and the loud noise of the MRI machine may eventually lead to significant discomfort for many patients. In addition to fidgeting, many MRI patients are fearful or claustrophobic. Moderate to deep sedation, and sometimes general anesthesia, may be required to immobilize these patients sufficiently to obtain good quality scan images, particularly in children and mentally challenged patients.

57.2.4 What special precautions must clinicians take when responding to or working in the MRI suite?

Clinicians caring for patients in MRI suites must be careful to rid themselves of all objects with possible ferromagnetic components, such as pagers, mobile phones, keys, pens, and stethoscopes. In addition, credit cards and ID badges may be demagnetized by the magnetic field.

There are serious concerns regarding the clinical monitoring modalities available in an MRI unit. In order to monitor the patients undergoing general anesthesia properly, it is necessary to have MRI-compatible systems that support automatic noninvasive blood pressure monitoring, electrocardiography, pulse oximetry, capnography, and even multichannel invasive pressure monitoring. To avoid burns[10] and fires,[11] electrocardiogram electrodes must be applied at a distance from the imaging area, or (in special cases) should be replaced with special MRI-compatible carbon electrodes.

57.2.5 Where can one obtain MRI-compatible anesthesia equipment?

The list of MRI-compatible anesthesia equipment needed in an MRI suite can be extensive and includes, but is not limited to, anesthesia machines, patient monitors, oxygen cylinders, and laryngoscopes. Hospital purchasing departments should be able to provide useful information on the availability of this equipment. The author recommends getting information from the web site www. magmedix.com. Additional resources appear in Appendix 57.1.

57.3 AIRWAY MANAGEMENT CONSIDERATIONS IN AN MRI UNIT

57.3.1 What airway equipment may or may not be used in an MRI unit?

The answer to the question regarding which airway management devices are safe to use in an MRI unit can be both simple and complex. The simple answer is that devices, such as conventional laryngoscopes that contain substantial amounts of ferromagnetic materials, can easily become dangerous projectiles, while items completely free of ferromagnetic materials are completely safe. The complex answer is that most airway instruments and devices that have not been specifically designed for use in an MRI environment are likely to have at least some ferromagnetic components. Even apparently benign products, like endotracheal tubes and laryngeal mask airways (LMAs), may have small amounts of ferromagnetic materials, such as metallic springs in the cuff inflation valve. While such small ferromagnetic objects do not generally present a projectile safety hazard, they can interfere with the image quality, possibly introducing an information hole if located near the imaging area.

57.3.2 What are some other airway management issues in the MRI environment?

Since most airway devices are not specifically designed for the MRI environment, equipment like flexible bronchoscopes, rigid fiberoptic laryngoscopes (such as the Bullard laryngoscope), or video laryngoscopes (such as the GlideScope®) must be specifically tested for suitability in the MRI environment by experienced MRI personnel. The same applies to the LMA-Fastrach™

and LMA-CTrach™, though the LMA-Fastrach™ single-use device is metal free. In addition, there is a theoretical concern that armored endotracheal tubes and other airway devices with wire-reinforced elements may either interfere with image quality, or undergo self-heating from absorbed electromagnetic radiation.

It should also be pointed out that airway equipment containing electronic circuits could possibly be affected by strong magnetic fields, for example, by the mechanism of closing a normally open switch containing ferromagnetic elements. This has been alleged to sometimes occur with the Trachlight™ intubating lightwand.

57.4   MANAGEMENT OF THIS PATIENT

57.4.1   What are immediate management options for this patient?

Before we proceed with the management of the patient, for patient's safety, all health care providers, including the airway practitioners, should remove all objects containing ferromagnetic substance, before entering the MRI unit. Mr. S, who is now turning blue is likely over-sedated and has an obstructed airway. Based on the history from his wife that he sometimes "just stops breathing" while asleep, it is likely that OSA is involved. The management options available include the following:

1. If the patient is accessible, a simple jaw thrust or head tilt often suffices to restore respiration. Most of the time, however, the scan will have to be temporarily suspended to permit this to occur. (This does not, however, mean that the magnet needs to be turned off). Some practitioners have tried taping the patient's jaw to the MRI head frame to keep the airway open.

2. The patient may also benefit from a nasopharyngeal airway. An oropharyngeal airway may also be considered but these tend to be less well tolerated.

3. If a simple jaw thrust, head tilt, or artificial airway does not promptly restore effective ventilation and oxygenation, positive pressure ventilation with 100% oxygen, using bag-mask-ventilation (BMV), will be needed to restore oxygenation. Certainly, when the patient is severely hypoxemic, this should be the first step undertaken.

4. Pharmacologic reversal of the lorazepam/midazolam may be helpful to reduce the level of sedation and restore the airway. Intravenous flumazenil, administered in 100 µg increments, is a benzodiazepine antagonist that antagonizes the sedation produced by all benzodiazepines. In the case of opioids, pharmacologic reversal can be achieved using intravenous naloxone (Narcan), also using 100 µg increments. It should be emphasized that since both naloxone and flumazenil have relatively short durations of action, resedation can occur. As Mr. S is a chronic user of benzodiazepines, he may be physically dependent on them. As such, it is possible that flumazenil, administered in traditionally recommended doses, may induce seizures.[12]

5. Insertion of an LMA, or even tracheal intubation, may be necessary in the absence of ventilation. Although LMAs may compromise the MRI image, this is not a constant finding. As mentioned, ferromagnetic laryngoscopes cannot be used. Commercially available MRI-compatible laryngoscopes along with MRI-compatible batteries should be readily available in the vicinity of the MRI unit.

57.5   CASE PRESENTATION: PART II

Given that Mr. S has developed respiratory difficulties, it is decided to remove him from the scanner to allow for positive pressure ventilation, or other intervention. With the commotion of being moved about, Mr. S becomes aroused, and spontaneous respirations resume. Instead of positive pressure ventilation with a bag-mask-ventilation (BMV) unit, a non-rebreathing face mask is used and the pulse oximeter is soon providing reassuring oxygen saturation. Mr. S remains drowsy when left undisturbed and he continues to have intermittent obstruction of his airway. The radiologist is eager to have the scan completed, emphasizing that Mr. S's neurologist has called repeatedly about the results (being concerned about ruling out a brain tumor) and also pointing out that this is the second time an MRI has been attempted on Mr. S.

Your examination shows that Mr. S has a Mallampati Class II view, with good mouth opening and good jaw protrusion. However, his considerable obesity and his apparent history of OSA raise concerns regarding possible difficult BMV, difficulty with direct laryngoscopic intubation, and difficulty establishing an emergency surgical airway. In addition, there are issues regarding cooperation, possible substance abuse, and an increased potential for rapid desaturation (because of a small functional residual capacity).

57.5.1   How should we proceed (if we did proceed) with managing the airway?

With the concerns listed earlier, and the urgency to proceed, a variety of means to secure the airway can be considered. Provided that BMV is not anticipated to be difficult, the first option, Plan A, is to induce anesthesia using propofol and achieve muscle relaxation using succinylcholine. Assuming that the patient is not prone to aspiration, and expert help is readily available, induction of anesthesia could either be done in the induction area some distance from the MRI scanner or in a regular operating room. Ramped positioning should be employed. An appropriate variety of airway devices and adjuncts, like an intubating stylet, an Eschmann tracheal introducer (bougie), and an LMA must be immediately available.

If the view at laryngoscopy proves to be unsatisfactory, even with external laryngeal manipulation, and especially if the use of an Eschmann tracheal introducer is unlikely to be successful (eg, Grade 4 airway), this author recommends the use of Plan B with a GlideScope®. This instrument has proven to be especially valuable.[13] Failing that, Plan C would be to use bronchoscopic intubation, either awake (having awakened the patient) or under general anesthesia.

There are several possible options for the use of the flexible bronchoscope in the anesthetized patient. These include tracheal intubation using the flexible bronchoscope through the LMA-Classic™ (or other extraglottic device) with the aid of an Aintree catheter[14] or using the GlideScope® to facilitate bronchoscopic intubation.[15]

If one's overall clinical impression is that inducing general anesthesia is not a prudent course, a more cautious approach would likely be awake intubation under topical anesthesia, using a flexible bronchoscope or using the GlideScope®.[15]

57.5.2   Discuss postintubation management

At the end of the MRI scanning procedure, a decision should be made whether it is safe to perform tracheal extubation in the MRI suite or in the post-anesthetic care unit after a period of elective ventilation (as might be appropriate if intubation was difficult and it is suspected that the airway structures are edematous). Consideration will, at times, be given to extubation over a tube exchanger.

57.6   OTHER CONSIDERATIONS

57.6.1   How do you manage a patient with a history of difficult airway in the MRI suite?

A review of the patient's previous medical records (especially anesthesia records) can be valuable to determine why previous intubation attempts may have been difficult. Depending on what information is found in the medical records, and the results of the airway examination, options will range from maintaining spontaneous ventilation in the patient in a setting of minimal sedation, to full general anesthesia preceded by awake endotracheal intubation. In particular, patients with severe reflux may require rapid-sequence intubation, or awake intubation methods, to minimize the risk of aspiration. As most of the airway devices and intubating equipment may not be compatible in the MRI unit, if the patient requires tracheal intubation for the MRI scanning, it would perhaps be wise to secure the airway in the operating room, prior to going to the MRI suite.

57.6.2   Does the American Society of Anesthesiologists have any advice on working in the MRI suite?

In March 2009, the American Society of Anesthesiologists published a comprehensive document that should be very helpful to anesthesiologists.[16] The following are some highlights from the report:

- Anesthesiologists should work with their institutions to properly identify and label anesthesia-related equipment according to convention (safe, unsafe, or conditional) for each MRI scanner.

- For every case, the anesthesiologist should communicate with the patient, referring physician, and radiologist to determine whether the patient presents with a high-risk medical condition, requires equipment, has implanted devices (eg, pacemakers, cardioverter–defibrillators, nerve stimulators), has been screened for the presence of implanted ferromagnetic items, and imbedded foreign bodies.

- For every case, the anesthesiologist should have a plan for providing optimal anesthetic care within the MRI suite. In addition to addressing the medical needs of the patient, features of the plan should include: (1) requirements of the scan and personnel needs; (2) positioning of equipment; (3) special requirements or unique issues of the patient or imaging study; (4) positioning of the anesthesiologist and the patient; and (5) planning for emergencies.

- Unique features of airway management during an MRI scan include: (1) the limited accessibility of the patient's airway; and (2) the difficulty of conducting visual and auditory assessments of the patient. Airway providers should have a pre-formulated plan in place to deal with instrumentation of the airway and common airway problems when patients are in an MRI environment.

- If a patient presents with a high-risk medical condition, the anesthesiologist should collaborate with all participants to determine how the patient will be managed during the MRI procedure.

- For patients with acute or severe renal insufficiency, the anesthesiologist should not administer gadolinium because of the increased risk of nephrogenic systemic fibrosis.

- Cardiac pacemakers and implantable cardioverter–defibrillators generally contraindicate MRI scanning.

- Anesthesiologists should have a clear line of sight of the patient and physiologic monitors, whether by direct observation or by video camera.

- Anesthesiologists should prepare a plan for rapidly summoning additional personnel in the event of an emergency.

57.7   SUMMARY

The key message from this chapter is that the MRI suite is a potentially hostile environment for patients with a difficult airway and numerous special precautions must be taken to prevent airway-related problems in these patients. Such precautions include having an additional airway practitioner readily available, as well as having primary and secondary backup plans for airway management. It is also essential to consider in advance what equipment can or cannot be used near the MRI scanner. The unique role of the recently introduced single-use, metal-free LMA Fastrach™ is yet to be determined, although it seems uniquely suited to the MRI environment, particularly for patients with a potentially difficult airway.

Because it can be difficult to directly observe whether a patient is breathing adequately when they are deep inside the MRI scanner, other means of respiratory monitoring (such as capnography) are especially important. In some situations, tracheal intubation is necessary because of the high likelihood of airway obstruction with sedation; in such cases, consideration must be given to the possibility that tracheal intubation may be difficult, without special equipment and/or special techniques.

11. Kugel H, Bremer C, Puschel M, et al. Hazardous situation in the MR bore: induction in ECG leads causes fire. *Eur Radiol.* 2003;13:690-694.
12. Spivey WH. Flumazenil and seizures: analysis of 43 cases. *Clin Ther.* 1992;14: 292-305.
13. Cooper RM, Pacey JA, Bishop MJ, McCluskey SA. Early clinical experience with a new videolaryngoscope (GlideScope) in 728 patients. *Can J Anaesth.* 2005;52:191-198.
14. Zura A, Doyle DJ, Orlandi M. Use of the Aintree intubation catheter in a patient with an unexpected difficult airway. *Can J Anaesth.* 2005;52:646-649.
15. Doyle DJ. GlideScope-assisted fiberoptic intubation: a new airway teaching method. *Anesthesiology.* 2004;101:1252.
16. Practice advisory on anesthetic care for magnetic resonance imaging: a report by the Society of Anesthesiologists Task Force on Anesthetic Care for Magnetic Resonance Imaging. *Anesthesiology.* 2009;110:459-479.

APPENDIX 57.1

Where can I get more information on MRI safety issues?

A good place to start is on the web at www.mrisafety.com. Unfortunately, one must register to use this site. Another valuable resource is from the American College of Radiology Blue Ribbon Panel on MR Safety. This site offers a number of useful safety guidelines and clinical protocols and can be accessed at http://www.acr.org/SecondaryMainMenuCategories/quality_safety/MRSafety/safe_mr07.aspx.

An interesting report from the Institute for Safe Medication Practices (http://www.ismp.org/newsletters/acutecare/articles/20040408.asp) explains that patient burns can occur when medication patches employing an aluminized backing are used (like many of those in common use containing nicotine, nitroglycerine, scopolamine, etc.). What happens is that the RF pulses heat up the metal involved, even if the metal is not ferromagnetic. Of interest, this problem can also occur when patients have tattoos containing metal pigments.

A comprehensive list of MRI-forbidden objects is available at www.newmri.com/html/mr_safety.asp.

REFERENCES

1. Vlaardingerbroek M, den Boer J. *Magnetic Resonance Imaging: Theory and Practice.* 2nd ed. New York, NY: Springer-Verlag Telos; 1999.
2. Klucznik RP, Carrier DA, Pyka R, Haid RW. Placement of a ferromagnetic intracerebral aneurysm clip in a magnetic field with a fatal outcome. *Radiology.* 1993;187:855-856.
3. Pinski SL, Trohman RG. Interference in implanted cardiac devices, part II. *Pacing Clin Electrophysiol.* 2002;25:1496-1509.
4. Condon B, Hadley DM, Hodgson R. The ferromagnetic pillow: a potential MR hazard not detectable by a hand-held magnet. *Br J Radiol.* 2001;74:847-851.
5. Chaljub G, Kramer LA, Johnson RF, 3rd, Johnson RF, Jr, Singh H, Crow WN. Projectile cylinder accidents resulting from the presence of ferromagnetic nitrous oxide or oxygen tanks in the MR suite. *AJR Am J Roentgenol.* 2001;177:27-30.
6. Mitka M. Safety improvements urged for MRI facilities. *JAMA.* 2005;294: 2145-2148.
7. Chen DW. Boy, 6, dies of skull injury during MRI. *The New York Times.* 2001 Jul 31: Sec. B:1, 5.
8. Zimmer C, Janssen MN, Treschan TA, Peters J. Near-miss accident during magnetic resonance imaging by a "flying sevoflurane vaporizer" due to ferromagnetism undetectable by handheld magnet. *Anesthesiology.* 2004;100: 1329-1330.
9. Shellock FG, Slimp GL. Severe burn of the finger caused by using a pulse oximeter during MR imaging. *AJR Am J Roentgenol.* 1989;153:1105.
10. Jones S, Jaffe W, Alvi R. Burns associated with electrocardiographic monitoring during magnetic resonance imaging. *Burns.* 1996;22:420-421.

SELF-EVALUATION QUESTIONS

57.1. Practitioners must take all of the following precautions when managing the airway of a patient in the MRI suite **EXCEPT**:

A. Remove objects with possible ferromagnetic components before entering the MRI suite.

B. Remove credit cards and ID badges before entering the MRI suite.

C. Use special asbestos MRI-compatible ECG electrodes.

D. ECG electrodes should be placed away from the imaging area.

E. Use MRI-compatible oxygen cylinders.

57.2. What airway equipment may be used safely in an MRI unit?

A. laryngeal mask airway

B. video laryngoscopes (eg, GlideScope®)

C. flexible fiberoptic bronchoscope

D. Macintosh laryngoscope

E. Bullard laryngoscope

57.3. Which of the following is **NOT** a known hazard in the MRI suite?

A. Patients with implanted ferromagnetic objects like aneurysm clips have had these objects fatally pulled out of position by the magnetic field.

B. Patients with pacemakers.

C. The endotracheal tube.

D. Stethoscopes.

E. Portable sevoflurane vaporizer.

CHAPTER (58)

Post-obstructive Pulmonary Edema

Matthew G. Simms and J. Adam Law

58.1 CASE PRESENTATION

A 43-year-old morbidly obese woman presented for gastroplasty. Her past medical history included treated hypothyroidism and past surgical history was unremarkable. She reported functional Class II to III dyspnea on exertion. Her medications consisted of L-thyroxine, amitriptyline, codeine, and furosemide. Laboratory investigations and ECG were normal. She weighed 340 lb (150 kg) and was 5 ft 6 in (168 cm) tall. Preoperative airway examination revealed normal mouth opening with full teeth, a thyromental span of 7 cm, and good jaw protrusion. She demonstrated a modified Mallampati Score III and had slightly restricted head extension. The rest of her physical examination was unremarkable.

Following appropriate positioning and denitrogenation, a rapid-sequence induction (RSI) was performed using midazolam, fentanyl, propofol, and succinylcholine. Direct laryngoscopy using a Macintosh #3 blade revealed a Cormack/Lehane (C/L)[1] Grade 2 view. Although some difficulty with tube passage was encountered, successful tracheal intubation using a styletted 7-mm internal diameter (ID) endotracheal tube (ETT) occurred on the second attempt. General anesthesia was maintained with sevoflurane, further doses of fentanyl, and rocuronium for muscle relaxation. Two liters of Lactated Ringer were given during the 2-hour procedure. On emergence, residual neuromuscular blockade was fully reversed, and she demonstrated a regular pattern of spontaneous respiration, with good tidal volumes.

At this time, the patient vigorously bit down on the ETT. For a period of approximately 90 seconds, no gas exchange occurred, even with attempted assisted manual ventilation via the anesthetic circuit. Although respiratory efforts continued, no CO_2 trace was apparent during the episode. Oxygen saturation fell to 78% before her jaw relaxed somewhat, allowing assisted, then spontaneous

ventilation to resume. She was subsequently placed in the lateral position until her eyes opened and she was able to obey commands. At this point, she was extubated. Shortly after extubation, she began to cough up frothy, pink fluid without either retching or vomiting. Her oxygen saturation, which had been 97% on a simple oxygen face mask immediately post-extubation, dropped to 85%.

58.2 INTRODUCTION

58.2.1 What is post-obstructive pulmonary edema?

Post-obstructive pulmonary edema (POPE) is characterized by the sudden onset of pulmonary edema of varying severity following vigorous inspiratory efforts against an obstructed upper airway. It most often occurs in a patient with no intrinsic cardiac, neurologic, or pulmonary disease. POPE usually presents with dyspnea, tachypnea, hypoxemia, and a cough productive of pink, frothy sputum. After confirming that the obstruction has been relieved, treatment of POPE is usually symptomatic, and varies from simple application of supplemental oxygen, to intubation with mechanical ventilation and application of positive end-expiratory pressure (PEEP). The condition usually resolves within 24 to 48 hours and most patients suffer no long-term sequelae.

Pulmonary edema following acute upper airway obstruction was first described in children in 1973.[2] A few years later, Oswalt described a number of cases of respiratory distress and pulmonary congestion following episodes of severe acute upper airway obstruction in otherwise healthy patients.[3] Since then, numerous case reports and case series have been published on this phenomenon.

58.2.2   What synonyms have been used to refer to POPE?

Many synonyms appear in the literature to describe this process. These include the following:

- Negative pressure pulmonary edema[4-12]
- Post-laryngospasm pulmonary edema[13]
- Laryngospasm-induced pulmonary edema[7,14,15]
- Post-extubation pulmonary edema[16,17]
- Non-cardiogenic pulmonary edema[4]
- Athletic pulmonary edema[7]

58.2.3   What are the two types of POPE?

Two types of POPE have been described.[18] They present with similar clinical pictures, and most likely have similar pathophysiologies:

- *POPE type I*: This typically occurs shortly after relief of an episode of acute upper airway obstruction from any cause, for example, laryngospasm.
- *POPE type II*: POPE type II occurs after relief of a chronic upper airway obstruction, caused by conditions such as chronic tonsillar hypertrophy, laryngeal tumor, goiter, or bilateral vocal cord paralysis.[4]

The remainder of this chapter refers mainly to POPE type I, as this is most commonly encountered in anesthetic and airway management practice.

58.3   INCIDENCE, ETIOLOGY, AND PATHOPHYSIOLOGY

58.3.1   What is the incidence of POPE?

The incidence of POPE has been estimated at 0.5 to 1.0 case per thousand surgical patients.[6,19] Of patients who have experienced, or required intervention for an episode of acute upper airway obstruction, published figures suggest a 5% to 10% incidence of progression to POPE.[8,19,20] POPE occurs most often in younger adults and children, most with ASA 1 and 2 status.[5,6] Young, athletic males are strongly represented in case series,[17,21] possibly because their well-developed musculature enables them to develop stronger inspiratory efforts against the upper airway obstruction, with resultant highly negative intrathoracic pressures. Most cases occur following tracheal extubation.[6]

58.3.2   What predisposes to the occurrence of POPE?

In the adult population, the most common cause of POPE is post-extubation laryngospasm,[17,22] while in children younger than 10, most cases follow upper airway obstruction from croup, epiglottitis,[5,20] and to a lesser extent, laryngospasm. However, POPE following vigorous attempts to inspire against upper airway obstruction has been reported from many other causes, including biting down and occluding the lumen of ETTs[9,23] and laryngeal mask airways (LMAs).[11,12] POPE has also been reported following upper airway obstruction from hanging, strangulation,[3,9] foreign body aspiration,[24,25] laryngeal tumor,[5] hematoma, goiter,[9,26] obstructive sleep apnea,[27] bilateral vocal cord paralysis,[28] and direct suctioning of both ETTs[29] and chest tubes.[30] Unilateral POPE has also been described in a lung occluded by an accidental mainstem bronchus intubation of the contralateral lung.[31]

58.3.3   What is the pathophysiology of POPE?

The variable clinical and laboratory manifestations of POPE probably reflect its multifactorial pathophysiology and various degrees of severity. The two proposed mechanisms of edema formation relate to (a) consequences of the highly negative intrathoracic pressure generated during an episode of complete upper airway obstruction (the Mueller maneuver),[20,22,25] and (b) the hyperadrenergic response to airway obstruction and hypoxia[5,16,18] (Figure 58-1). The following are probable contributory mechanisms:

1. *Negative pressure transfer to the pulmonary alveoli and interstitium* affects Starling forces by creating a gradient that favors transudation of fluid out of the pulmonary capillaries to the interstitium.[4,24] Once the capacity of pulmonary lymphatics to remove fluid from the interstitium is exceeded, leakage of fluid occurs into the alveolar space.[16,32,33]

2. *Enhanced venous return to the right heart and pulmonary arteries* results from the generated negative intrathoracic pressure[4-6,22,24] and is compounded by central blood redistribution from the hyperadrenergic state caused by significant hypoxemia, anxiety, and hypercarbia.[5,9,16,22,24,32,34] Higher pulmonary arteriole and capillary bed blood volumes and hydrostatic pressures further favor fluid transudation from capillary to interstitium.[8]

3. *Impeded outflow from the pulmonary capillary bed* occurs as left-sided pressures rise from (a) decreased stroke volume resulting from increased systemic vascular resistance;[6,24,32,34] (b) decreased left ventricular diastolic compliance (from right ventricular distension); and (c) depression of myocardial contractility, from hypoxia and acidosis.[9]

4. *Hypoxic pulmonary vasoconstriction* directly contributes to increases in pulmonary capillary pressures.[5,16]

5. *Disruption of the alveolar-capillary membrane* (stress failure)[35] and its barrier function can eventually occur from damage to the capillary endothelium by increased pulmonary capillary volume and pressures. In addition, particularly with prolonged hypoxia,[24] the hyperadrenergic state can directly contribute to further membrane disruption.[4,6] Such disruption can be manifested by the leakage of both protein-rich exudative and hemorrhagic fluid.

POPE has a spectrum of clinical presentations. It is likely that in most cases, with intact pulmonary capillaries, simple alteration in Starling forces result in the transudative production of low-protein edema.[34] Fremont and his group looked retrospectively at a series of 341 patients intubated for pulmonary edema and identified 10

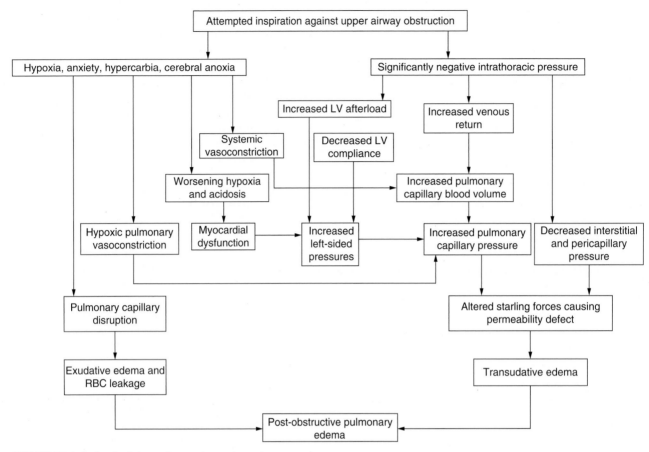

FIGURE 58-1. Pathophysiology of post-obstructive pulmonary edema.

individuals who had POPE as the etiology. Analysis of the edema fluid of this subset of patients, looking at the edema fluid-plasma protein ratio and its rate of clearance, strongly suggested a transudative, hydrostatic mechanism in most of the patients.[36]

However, higher negative intrathoracic pressures, coupled with a hyperadrenergic response, may result in ultrastructural changes in the capillary endothelial barrier, allowing the escape of exudative edema, as documented in some case reports.[28,37] Extreme cases result in breaks in the alveolar-capillary membrane, allowing red blood cell leakage, and possibly frank hemorrhage. Chest radiographs in this latter situation may show an alveolar pattern of edema, in contrast to the more interstitial pattern typical of transudative edema.[7] That case reports differ in their reporting of transudative and exudative edema, or primarily interstitial or alveolar patterns of edema on chest radiography probably reflects the varying degrees of severity of the obstructive episode causing the POPE.

58.3.4 Why does POPE appear only after the relief of upper airway obstruction?

Type I POPE generally appears shortly after the relief of an acute upper airway obstruction. In many cases, this is a fixed obstruction, such as laryngospasm or an occluded ETT. Profoundly negative intrathoracic pressures generated during attempted inspiration (Mueller maneuvers) may be balanced during attempted expiration against the same fixed obstruction (ie, a Valsalva maneuver), akin to an *auto-PEEP* phenomenon. It may be that this PEEP-like

effect during attempted expiration is somewhat protective by limiting the transcapillary pressure gradient. On relief of the obstruction, pulmonary edema becomes manifest[5,6,24] with the sudden transient drop in mean airway pressure,[8] together with the increase in venous return and pulmonary hydrostatic pressure.[7,32]

In type II POPE, chronic, usually variable obstruction favors the Mueller maneuver in that more obstruction occurs during attempted inspiration than expiration. In this situation, the generated negative intrathoracic pressure is counteracted by more modest levels of PEEP. Although still somewhat protective against the development of pulmonary edema,[38] published reports document abnormal A-a gradients and radiographic evidence of pulmonary edema *before* relief of chronic upper airway obstructions.[5,6,24] Following the relief of both type I and type II obstructions, it is likely that altered capillary permeability, previously occult interstitial edema[38] and LV dysfunction,[24] contribute to the development of POPE in spite of now-normal lung volumes and pressures.

58.4 DIAGNOSIS AND INVESTIGATIONS

58.4.1 What are the presenting symptoms and signs of POPE?

The patient with POPE often presents within minutes[5,22] after the relief of an episode of upper airway obstruction characterized by vigorous inspiratory efforts without significant air movement.[16,34] The initial presentation is often with dyspnea,[8] tachypnea,[24,39,40] agitation,[8,21,34] and cough[11,21,22] producing pink, frothy fluid.[3,4,8,9,22,34,41] In addition to hypoxemia,[7,39] the patient is also often tachycardic[14,34] and hypertensive.[34] Other patients have presented with frank hemoptysis,[9,12,19,23,42] although this is less frequent. Residual partial obstruction may be present in this population, manifested by stridor[8,11,16,21,43] or intercostal and subcostal retractions.[21,24,44] On auscultation, most patients have rales,[12,16,22,24,40,41] sometimes with associated rhonchi.[3,14,22,25,34,40]

58.4.2 What are the results of investigations typically performed on the patient with POPE?

- *Invasive monitoring* of central venous (CVP) or pulmonary artery pressures (PAP) is rarely undertaken in the patient recognized to have POPE. However, when reported, pressures, including CVP[3,22] and pulmonary capillary wedge pressures (PCWP)[5,22,45,46] have generally been normal, while PAPs have been normal or only slightly elevated.[22]

- *Chest radiographs* of the patient with POPE often show signs of edema with either an alveolar (airspace consolidation)[9,16,19,44] or interstitial (perihilar haze, perivascular or peribronchial cuffing, and Kerley lines)[3,4,6,25] pattern, or both.[7,24,39] Most often the edema distribution is predominantly central and bilateral, although asymmetrical[34] or even unilateral distributions have been reported.[7,11,19] Heart size is generally normal.[7,19,24] Vascular pedicle width in one series was found to be above normal, suggesting an increase in central blood volume.[7]

- *High-resolution CT scans* of the chest have shown findings of ground-glass opacities, peribronchial cuffing, and interlobular septal thickening, typical of interstitial pulmonary edema.[25,42] Others have shown diffuse patchy lobular airspace disease.[24]

- *Bronchoscopy* performed on patients with POPE has shown punctate bleeding lesions in both trachea and mainstem bronchi[43] or more generalized blood staining of the tracheobronchial tree.[23,34] Bronchial-alveolar lavage (BAL) in one report revealed a progressively bloody return, consistent with alveolar hemorrhage,[34] while in a second report, BAL produced clear returns.[23]

- No specific *electrocardiogram (ECG) pattern* has been reported in the POPE patient population. When reported, ECG findings have been uniformly normal.

58.4.3 Should the patient presenting with POPE be referred for echocardiography?

Most case reports and case series of patients experiencing POPE have documented rapid resolution of the episode with no long-term sequelae and no special cardiac work up performed. Echocardiograms have generally been normal.[9,16,19,25,26,34,42,47,48] One exception was a case series of six patients who had experienced POPE, all of whom had echocardiograms. In this small retrospective series, abnormalities were detected in 50% of the cases:

one patient had hypertrophic cardiomyopathy, and the other two had pulmonary and tricuspid valvular insufficiency.[4] However, in the absence of other recognized indications, the current lack of evidence does not support a recommendation for routine echocardiographic testing of all POPE patients.

58.5 CLINICAL MANAGEMENT

58.5.1 What is the usual clinical course of POPE?

Following relief of the acute upper airway obstruction, the onset of POPE is generally rapid, that is, within minutes, however a minority of case reports document delayed onset of up to 4 to 6 hours,[5,38] suggesting that following an episode of acute, severe upper airway obstruction,[18] patients should be monitored for 6 to 12 hours. The same recommendation has been made for patients who have had surgical relief of chronic upper airway obstruction.[18]

In most cases, POPE runs a benign course, with symptoms, and clinical and radiologic signs clearing within 24 to 48 hours.[4,6,17,22,38,44,48]

58.5.2 How is POPE managed?

As the name implies, most cases of POPE present *after* the upper airway obstruction has been alleviated. After confirming airway patency, supplemental oxygen should be administered, and may be all that is required.[3,6,16,22] Continuous positive airway pressure (CPAP) by face mask has also been shown to be an effective intervention,[14,19] and the use of noninvasive ventilation has been reported.[26] Hypoxemia, or patient fatigue that is unresponsive to noninvasive methods may require reintubation and positive pressure ventilation. The larger case series report re-intubation rates of between 66.5%[8] and 85%.[5,6,22] Of those patients re-intubated, about half require mechanical ventilation[5] with[3,4,34] or without PEEP, usually for less than 24 hours.[6]

Although diuretics are often used in the setting of POPE[3,5,6,14,23,24,34,44] this practice has been questioned[5,24] based on the finding of normal central filling pressures, and the equally rapid resolution of symptoms when they are not used.[9,44] The use of steroids has been reported sporadically,[3,14,44] although as with the use of diuretics, their use is controversial[18] and without proven benefit. Other case reports make mention of fluid restriction[3,18] and the administration of conventional congestive cardiac failure (CCF) medications such as morphine or digoxin.[22]

The available evidence would suggest that if the diagnosis of POPE is correct, drug therapy is unlikely to be of benefit, particularly in view of the self-limited and rapidly resolving course of the condition. With rare exceptions,[4,10] the same can be said of invasive hemodynamic monitoring.[16]

58.5.3 What is the differential diagnosis of POPE?

The primary alternate diagnosis to POPE is aspiration pneumonitis, which may lead to pulmonary edema even when frank regurgitation has not been noted.[5] The initial management of this condition is identical to that of POPE, unless of course the aspirate is suspected to be particulate or contaminated by bacteria. It is more important to rule out other causes of pulmonary edema where management differs from that of POPE, including iatrogenic volume overload, primary cardiogenic causes, or drug reactions.

58.5.4 What are risk factors and preventive strategies for the development of POPE?

A number of factors place the patient at higher risk for the development of POPE. Some are unavoidable, while some can be minimized by employing the principles of good airway management. The early recognition and management of acute, severe upper airway obstruction, and the conditions leading to it, are critical to the prevention of POPE:

- *Laryngospasm*: Most cases of POPE in adults, and many in children follow an episode of laryngospasm. Many case reports of POPE document laryngospasm following extubation during emergence from anesthesia, before the patient is fully awake.[44,49] Therefore, it is recommended that extubation be performed in patients who are either deeply anesthetized or fully awake. The prevention of intra-operative laryngospasm under mask or extraglottic device (EGD) anesthesia requires deep general anesthesia, particularly for highly stimulating surgical procedures. Prior to removing an ETT, suctioning of blood or secretions that may trigger laryngospasm is essential, particularly following upper airway surgery. Should laryngospasm occur, the initial treatment is to relieve any soft tissue obstruction together with gentle application of 10 to 20 cm H_2O CPAP by mask. However, the administration of succinylcholine 0.2 mg·kg^{-1} (or other appropriate neuromuscular blocking agent) may be indicated in patients making vigorous inspiratory efforts against a closed glottis, particularly if it persists for more than 30 seconds.[49]

- *Tube occlusion by biting down*: POPE has been described in patients who have *bitten down* to occlude ETTs[41,44] and EGDs (eg, LMA).[11,12,50] Most reports have documented this occurring on emergence from anesthesia, although it has also been described during the positioning process.[11] Use of a rolled gauze bite block alongside the lumen of an endotracheal tube[9,41] or LMA (as recommended by its inventor[50]) ought to minimize this risk. As with laryngospasm, the administration of a neuromuscular blocking agent may be indicated. Alternatively, deflation of the cuff of the ETT or EGD may permit sufficient alleviation of obstruction to prevent the marked negative intrathoracic pressure that leads to the development of POPE.

- *Other soft tissue obstruction*: POPE has been described as a complication of obstructive sleep apnea, in patients with obesity and vocal cord paralysis, and in those with other risk factors for upper airway obstruction.[16,40] The preoperative identification of patients at risk for these conditions mandates full recovery of neuromuscular function and that they be fully awake prior to extubation.

- *Type of surgery*: A retrospective study by Deepika et al showed that the majority of POPE cases (63%) occurred following surgery to the aerodigestive tract,[6] suggesting that vigilance be exercised in patients suffering from chronic tonsillar hypertrophy, goiter, and other conditions leading to chronic upper airway obstruction. In other published case series, none of the patients was undergoing aerodigestive tract surgery.[17]

- *Patient*: In adults, POPE occurs about twice as often in male patients,[4-6,8,17] and in those with an average age of 25 to 45 years.[4-6,8,17] The male preponderance may be related to well-developed musculature and their ability to generate high negative intrathoracic pressures.[21] Early and aggressive treatment of airway obstruction should occur in this population.

58.6 PROGNOSIS

POPE is an important cause of morbidity in otherwise young, healthy patients that may lead to an unplanned hospital or ICU admission. With prompt recognition and appropriate therapy, the condition generally resolves inside 24 to 48 hours without long-term sequelae.[6,19] However, deaths can occur; a recent review of published adult case series of POPE reported three deaths in 146 patients—a mortality rate of 2%.[8]

58.7 PATIENT MANAGEMENT

Following extubation in the operating room, the patient exhibited clinical evidence of developing pulmonary edema and increasing respiratory distress. Her oropharynx was suctioned and she was placed in a semi-sitting position. Oxygen, 100%, was administered via a face mask through the anesthetic circuit and CPAP was applied. This failed to improve the SpO_2 above 90%, so assisted bag-mask-ventilation (BMV) was attempted. However, agitation and reduced lung compliance made assisted ventilation increasingly difficult, and the SpO_2 could not be maintained above 90%. Therefore, the patient was re-intubated using a rapid-sequence intubation technique. Following intubation, her SpO_2 returned to 97% with 2 minutes of mechanical ventilation using an FIO_2 of 100%; suctioning yielded copious quantities of pink, frothy fluid. Sedation was maintained with midazolam and she received IV furosemide 40 mg. An arterial line was placed, and the patient was admitted to the ICU. A chest x-ray showed signs of pulmonary edema. A 12-lead ECG was normal and troponins were negative. The patient remained sedated, intubated, and ventilated overnight. By the following day, her radiographic findings and arterial blood gases had improved, and she was extubated that evening. There were no further respiratory complications.

58.8 SUMMARY

Post-obstructive pulmonary edema is an uncommon, yet potentially life-threatening condition. Occurring shortly after the relief of acute or chronic upper airway obstruction of varying cause,

POPE presents with dyspnea, cough, progressive oxygen desaturation, tachypnea, and agitation. In most cases, POPE resolves within 24 to 48 hours. Sometimes, nothing more than supportive care with supplemental oxygen administration is required. Mask-delivered CPAP or noninvasive ventilation may also be effective. However, some patients with POPE may require tracheal intubation and mechanical ventilation with PEEP to maintain adequate oxygenation. Although often used, the benefits of diuretics and steroids in managing POPE remain unproven.

Practitioners should be aware of this condition, be able to identify and where possible avoid the predisposing risk factors, and be able to manage it if it occurs. Prompt management of acute upper airway obstruction is crucial in reducing the incidence of POPE and improving outcome, particularly as deaths have been reported.

REFERENCES

1. Cormack RS, Lehane J. Difficult tracheal intubation in obstetrics. *Anaesthesia.* 1984;39:1105-1111.
2. Capitanio MA, Kirkpatrick JA. Obstructions of the upper airway in children as reflected on the chest radiograph. *Radiology.* 1973;107:159-161.
3. Oswalt CE, Gates GA, Holmstrom MG. Pulmonary edema as a complication of acute airway obstruction. *JAMA.* 1977;238:1833-1835.
4. Goldenberg JD, Portugal LG, Wenig BL, Weingarten RT. Negative-pressure pulmonary edema in the otolaryngology patient. *Otolaryngol Head Neck Surg.* 1997;117:62-66.
5. Lang SA, Duncan PG, Shephard DA, Ha HC. Pulmonary oedema associated with airway obstruction. *Can J Anaesth.* 1990;37:210-218.
6. Deepika K, Kenaan CA, Barrocas AM, Fonseca JJ, Bikazi GB. Negative pressure pulmonary edema after acute upper airway obstruction. *J Clin Anesth.* 1997;9:403-408.
7. Cascade PN, Alexander GD, Mackie DS. Negative-pressure pulmonary edema after endotracheal intubation. *Radiology.* 1993;186:671-675.
8. Westreich R, Sampson I, Shaari CM, Lawson W. Negative-pressure pulmonary edema after routine septorhinoplasty: discussion of pathophysiology, treatment, and prevention. *Arch Facial Plast Surg.* 2006;8:8-15.
9. Koh MS, Hsu AA, Eng P. Negative pressure pulmonary oedema in the medical intensive care unit. *Intensive Care Med.* 2003;29:1601-1604.
10. Louis PJ, Fernandes R. Negative pressure pulmonary edema. *Oral Surg Oral Med Oral Pathol Oral Radiol Endod.* 2002;93:4-6.
11. Sullivan M. Unilateral negative pressure pulmonary edema during anesthesia with a laryngeal mask airway. *Can J Anaesth.* 1999;46:1053-1056.
12. Devys JM, Balleau C, Jayr C, Bourgain JL. Biting the laryngeal mask: an unusual cause of negative pressure pulmonary edema. *Can J Anaesth.* 2000;47:176-178.
13. Baltimore JJ. Postlaryngospasm pulmonary edema in adults. *AORN J.* 1999;70:468-479.
14. Jackson FN, Rowland V, Corssen G. Laryngospasm-induced pulmonary edema. *Chest.* 1980;78:819-821.
15. McConkey P. Airway bleeding in negative-pressure pulmonary edema. *Anesthesiology.* 2001;95:272.
16. Lorch DG, Sahn SA. Post-extubation pulmonary edema following anesthesia induced by upper airway obstruction. Are certain patients at increased risk? *Chest.* 1986;90:802-805.
17. Mulkey Z, Yarbrough S, Guerra D, Roongsritong C, Nugent K, Phy MP. Postextubation pulmonary edema: a case series and review. *Respir Med.* 2008;102:1659-1662.
18. Guffin TN, Har-el G, Sanders A, Lucente FE, Nash M. Acute postobstructive pulmonary edema. *Otolaryngol Head Neck Surg.* 1995;112:235-237.
19. McConkey PP. Postobstructive pulmonary oedema—a case series and review. *Anaesth Intensive Care.* 2000;28:72-76.
20. Galvis AG. Pulmonary edema complicating relief of upper airway obstruction. *Am J Emerg Med.* 1987;5:294-297.
21. Holmes JR, Hensinger RN, Wojtys EW. Postoperative pulmonary edema in young, athletic adults. *Am J Sports Med.* 1991;19:365-371.
22. Willms D, Shure D. Pulmonary edema due to upper airway obstruction in adults. *Chest.* 1988;94:1090-1092.
23. Sow Nam Y, Garewal D. Pulmonary hemorrhage in association with negative pressure edema in an intubated patient. *Acta Anaesthesiol Scand.* 2001;45:911-913.
24. Ringold S, Klein EJ, Del Beccaro MA. Postobstructive pulmonary edema in children. *Pediatr Emerg Care.* 2004;20:391-395.
25. Maniwa K, Tanaka E, Inoue T, et al. Interstitial pulmonary edema revealed by high-resolution CT after relief of acute upper airway obstruction. *Radiat Med.* 2005;23:139-141.
26. Ikeda H, Asato R, Chin K, et al. Negative-pressure pulmonary edema after resection of mediastinum thyroid goiter. *Acta Otolaryngol.* 2006;126:886-888.
27. Chaudhary BA, Nadimi M, Chaudhary TK, Speir WA. Pulmonary edema due to obstructive sleep apnea. *South Med J.* 1984;77:499-501.
28. Dohi S, Okubo N, Kondo Y. Pulmonary oedema after airway obstruction due to bilateral vocal cord paralysis. *Can J Anaesth.* 1991;38:492-495.
29. Pang WW, Chang DP, Lin CH, Huang MH. Negative pressure pulmonary oedema induced by direct suctioning of endotracheal tube adapter. *Can J Anaesth.* 1998;45:785-788.
30. Memtsoudis SG, Rosenberger P, Sadovnikoff N. Chest tube suction-associated unilateral negative pressure pulmonary edema in a lung transplant patient. *Anesth Analg.* 2005;101:38-40, table of contents.
31. Goodman BT, Richardson MG. Case report: unilateral negative pressure pulmonary edema—a complication of endobronchial intubation. *Can J Anaesth.* 2008;55:691-695.
32. Ciavarro C, Kelly JP. Postobstructive pulmonary edema in an obese child after an oral surgery procedure under general anesthesia: a case report. *J Oral Maxillofac Surg.* 2002;60:1503-1505.
33. Thiagarajan RR, Laussen PC. Negative pressure pulmonary edema in children—pathogenesis and clinical management. *Paediatr Anaesth.* 2007;17:307-310.
34. Schwartz DR, Maroo A, Malhotra A, Kesselman H. Negative pressure pulmonary hemorrhage. *Chest.* 1999;115:1194-1197.
35. West JB, Tsukimoto K, Mathieu-Costello O, Prediletto R. Stress failure in pulmonary capillaries. *J Appl Physiol.* 1991;70:1731-1742.
36. Fremont RD, Kallet RH, Matthay MA, Ware LB. Postobstructive pulmonary edema: a case for hydrostatic mechanisms. *Chest.* 2007;131:1742-1746.
37. Kollef MH, Pluss J. Noncardiogenic pulmonary edema following upper airway obstruction. 7 cases and a review of the literature. *Medicine* (Baltimore). 1991;70:91-98.
38. Van Kooy MA, Gargiulo RF. Postobstructive pulmonary edema. *Am Fam Physician.* 2000;62:401-404.
39. Sofer S, Bar-Ziv J, Scharf SM. Pulmonary edema following relief of upper airway obstruction. *Chest.* 1984;86:401-403.
40. Brandom BW. Pulmonary edema after airway obstruction. *Int Anesthesiol Clin.* 1997;35:75-84.
41. Liu EH, Yih PS. Negative pressure pulmonary oedema caused by biting and endotracheal tube occlusion—a case for oropharyngeal airways. *Singapore Med J.* 1999;40:174-175.
42. Perez RO, Bresciani C, Jacob CE, et al. Negative pressure post-extubation pulmonary edema complicating appendectomy in a young patient: case report. *Curr Surg.* 2004;61:463-465.
43. Koch SM, Abramson DC, Ford M, et al. Bronchoscopic findings in post-obstructive pulmonary oedema. *Can J Anaesth.* 1996;43:73-76.
44. Herrick IA, Mahendran B, Penny FJ. Postobstructive pulmonary edema following anesthesia. *J Clin Anesth.* 1990;2:116-120.
45. Weissman C, Damask MC, Yang J. Noncardiogenic pulmonary edema following laryngeal obstruction. *Anesthesiology.* 1984;60:163-165.
46. Stradling JR, Bolton P. Upper airways obstruction as cause of pulmonary oedema. *Lancet.* 1982;1:1353-1354.
47. Silva PS, Monteiro Neto H, Andrade MM, Neves CV. Negative-pressure pulmonary edema: a rare complication of upper airway obstruction in children. *Pediatr Emerg Care.* 2005;21:751-754.
48. Mehta VM, Har-El G, Goldstein NA. Postobstructive pulmonary edema after laryngospasm in the otolaryngology patient. *Laryngoscope.* 2006;116:1693-1696.
49. Lee KW, Downes JJ. Pulmonary edema secondary to laryngospasm in children. *Anesthesiology.* 1983;59:347-349.
50. Brain AI. The laryngeal mask—a new concept in airway management. *Br J Anaesth.* 1983;55:801-805.

SELF-EVALUATION QUESTIONS

58.1. Which of the following situations would be **LEAST** likely to result in an episode of post-obstructive pulmonary edema?

A. A 25-year-old man bites and occludes the endotracheal tube for a period of less than 60 seconds on emergence from a desflurane-based anesthetic. He never desaturates below an SpO$_2$ of 90%.

B. A 25-year-old man was scheduled for appendectomy. During RSI using fentanyl, propofol, and rocuronium, tracheal intubation was achieved with a Trachlight™ following three failed intubation attempts using a Macintosh blade; difficulty with BMV was experienced between intubation attempts.

C. A 25-year-old man has been extubated *deep* following surgery for a deviated nasal septum. At the time of extubation, end-tidal desflurane was 3%.

D. A 6-year-old child has presented to the ED with acute epiglottitis, is *tripoding* with stridor, drooling, and respiratory distress. Intubation using an inhalational induction in the operating room is planned.

E. A 25-year-old man weighing 120 kg is having banding of hemorrhoids under general anesthesia with a laryngeal mask airway. Following a propofol induction, he has been given a total of 100 μg of fentanyl, is breathing a mixture of air and sevoflurane, with an end-tidal sevoflurane concentration of 1.7%.

58.2. Emerging from general anesthesia for shoulder acromioplasty and shortly after extubation, a 25-year-old man experiences an episode of laryngospasm and makes vigorous, yet futile inspiratory attempts against his closed glottis. Which of the following responses would be appropriate?

A. Suction the back of the throat with rigid tonsil suction, insert an oral airway, and perform an exaggerated jaw thrust.

B. Immediately give succinylcholine 100 mg as he is at high risk of post-obstructive pulmonary edema.

C. As the laryngospasm is probably related to pain, give a dose of parenteral narcotic such as sufentanil 5 μg.

D. Give lidocaine 100 mg intravenously.

E. Perform an airway opening maneuver and apply CPAP by mask; if this does not break the laryngospasm within 30 seconds, give succinylcholine.

58.3. Which of the following patient conditions is considered a risk factor for the development of postoperative pulmonary edema?

A. The patient with an ASA of 3 or 4.

B. The patient emerging from surgery of the aerodigestive tract.

C. The patient with a history of difficult intubation.

D. The patient with a history of severe gastroesophageal reflux.

E. The patient with a history of asthma.

SECTION 4 Practical Considerations in Difficult and Failed Airway Management

CHAPTER (59)

Difficult Airway Carts

Saul Pytka and Michael F. Murphy

59.1 INTRODUCTION

59.1.1 Why are difficult airway carts necessary?

The concept of emergency difficult airway carts is not a novel one. It has long been acknowledged that having emergency equipment readily available in a reliable location is a standard of care. The "cardiac crash cart," for example, is a mandatory addition to operating rooms (OR), emergency departments (ED), and other patient care areas where they may be required. Many labor and delivery rooms have an *emergency cart* ready for unanticipated *crash* cesarean sections, while trauma units have an emergency surgical setup for occasions when a chest or abdomen must be rapidly opened.

Although the literature is silent on the actual benefits of having an emergency airway cart available, there is strong consensus among experts that the ready access to alternative devices for airway management has the potential for reducing risks and complications in the management of the unanticipated difficult airway.[1-3] In 1993, the American Society of Anesthesiologists Task Force on Management of the Difficult Airway published their Practice Guidelines for Management of the Difficult Airway.[1] This document, subsequently updated in 2003, contained a clear statement that "at least one portable storage unit that contains specialized equipment for difficult airway management should be readily available."[2] They followed with a suggested list of specialized equipment that this storage unit, or cart, should contain.

Beyond the scope of the original ASA guidelines, Crosby and a group of consultants reviewed the pertinent literature on airway management in Canada and published recommendations for the management of the unanticipated difficult airway.[3] This group recommended that a difficult airway cart be available for emergency airway interventions in addition to the standard airway equipment available in every OR. They also suggested a minimum equipment list for such a cart.

59.1.2 Is there any evidence that airway carts are beneficial in the setting of difficult or failed airway management?

The literature is replete with the advantages of using alternative airway devices in situations where a difficult airway is encountered, both expected and unanticipated. Just as emergency drugs and the presence of a defibrillator on the *crash cart* are indispensable in the management of a cardiac emergency, the readily available rescue airway devices in an airway emergency clearly represent an improvement in patient care.

The increase in morbidity and mortality associated with difficulties in airway management is well recognized.[4,5] Both the ASA and Canadian groups recommend limiting the number of attempts at direct laryngoscopy to three and two, respectively.[1-3] Mort has shown that the increasing number of attempts at intubation by direct laryngoscopy correlates with an increased incidence of respiratory and hemodynamic complications.[6] In this study, a database was created to record complications following emergency airway interventions outside the OR. When three or more attempts were made to secure an airway by direct laryngoscopy, the incidence of hypoxemia increased from 11% to 70%, regurgitation from 2% to 22%, aspiration from 0.8% to 13%, and cardiac arrest from 0.7% to 11% (Table 59-1). One could speculate that the presence of alternate airway devices would have prevented the need for repeated attempts at direct laryngoscopy.

TABLE 59-1

Complications by Intubation Attempts[6]

	2 OR FEWER ATTEMPTS (90%)	>2 ATTEMPTS (10%)*	RELATIVE RISK FOR <2 ATTEMPTS	95% CI FOR RISK RATIO
Complication				
Hypoxemia	10.5%	70%	9×	4.20-15.92
Severe hypoxemia	1.9%	28%	14×	7.36-24.34
Esophageal intubation	4.8%	51.4%	6×	3.71-8.72
Regurgitation	1.9%	22%	7×	2.82-10.14
Aspiration	0.8%	13%	4×	1.89-7.18
Bradycardia	1.6%	18.5%	4×	1.71-6.74
Cardiac arrest	0.7%	11%	7×	2.39-9.87

*All categories p <.001 when comparing 2 or fewer attempts to >2 attempts.
Hypoxemia—SpO_2 <90%; severe hypoxemia—SpO_2 <70%.

Mort reviewed the incidence and etiology of out-of-OR cardiac arrests occurring during emergency intubation before and after the introduction of emergency airway carts.[7] In 1995, the institution, a level-one trauma center, introduced airway carts or kits containing *advanced* airway equipment and tracheal tube verifying devices. A retrospective study compared the time periods of 1990 to 1995 and 1995 to 2002 for a number of variables, the primary comparator being cardiac arrest. The compelling results showed an overall reduction of 50% in airway-related cardiac arrests between the two time periods, attributable to the presence of the carts (Figure 59-1).[7]

Although the data compiled from these papers were gathered from nonoperating room locales, the conclusions are clearly applicable to all areas that airway management may be performed, including the OR. The ready accessibility of difficult airway carts is indispensable in reducing airway-related morbidity and mortality.

59.1.3 What steps should be taken to ensure that the carts remain well stocked and contain equipment in good working order?

It is important that when an airway practitioner arrives at the scene of an airway emergency, or when the difficult airway cart is summoned, all of the equipment that is needed must be present and functional. To achieve this, departmental and hospital policies or processes must be crafted, which should identify:

- The numbers and locations of such carts.
- A process of annual review of the cart locations and how they are equipped and updated.
- A staff member (a clinician, a nurse, or a respiratory therapist) must be responsible for the cart in each assigned area as the *keeper of the cart.*
- How equipment is added to and deleted from the standard list of contents, and how such changes are suggested, vetted, implemented, and communicated to the relevant staff.
- How the drawers will be arranged and labeled.
- How equipment with maintenance schedules are to be maintained (eg, bronchoscopes).
- Time frames and responsibilities regarding replenishment after equipment is used.
- Who will check the inventory and how often it will be checked. The checklist includes the functioning of essential equipment, such as bulbs and batteries, and time-sensitive supplies such as local anesthetic agents and vasoconstrictors.
- If cleaning is to be done, who will do it, how it will be done (eg, bronchoscopes), and how long the *out of service for cleaning* interval will be.

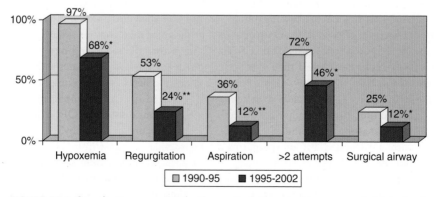

FIGURE 59-1. Complications associated with repeated attempts at laryngoscopic intubation.[6]
*p <.01
**p < .03

- An inventory of replenishment supplies to be kept immediately on hand, particularly disposables (eg, Combitube™, Melker Cricothyrotomy kit, etc).

- Where equipment manufacturers' literature will be kept.

Routine airway management equipment that one expects to use in most if not all airway management emergencies, such as laryngoscopes, airways, endotracheal tubes (ETTs), intubating stylets (eg, Eschmann Introducer or Frova), tonsil and catheter suction devices, etc, should be immediately available and not clutter the drawers of the cart. These equipment need not be on an OR cart as each anesthetizing location ought to have them available. Carts should be located in each area of the hospital where airway management might reasonably be expected to occur, such as ED, ICU, cardiac catheterization units, labor and delivery suites, endoscopy suites, diagnostic imaging unit, and other locations where sedatives will be administered. In locations where both children and adults are cared for, the pediatric cart should be distinctly separate from the adult cart (different style, and perhaps different color). An array of ETT sizes, masks, oral and nasal airways, etc, must be easily accessible in the event pediatric patients are cared for. Perhaps the best system currently available to meet this need is the Broselow-Luten System.[8] Alternatively, canvas-pocketed systems that are rolled up for storage can easily and quickly be unrolled to access the equipment.

If at all possible, airway carts should be in a consistent location (eg, with the cardiac crash cart). The cart should be secured with a plastic twist removable lock. The cart is secured after each check, signaling that the cart has been replenished and is ready for use. The absence of the lock signifies that the cart needs immediate inspection. A keyed lock may be required for drawers that contain medications. The locking mechanism for this drawer must be limited to this drawer only and should not impede access to the other drawers with airway devices.

59.2 DIFFICULT AIRWAY CART IN THE OPERATING ROOM

59.2.1 What are the guiding principles for establishing a difficult airway cart for the OR area?

Historically, the contents of the difficult airway cart in most anesthesia locations varied widely, as various practitioners demanded the addition of newer or their preferred devices. Unfortunately, items that nobody had ever used or would ever use were included. The contents would often be forgotten, and little or no maintenance would occur. Basically, they were difficult airway carts in name only.

Although a number of publications describe difficult airway cart setup, most are simply a description of the author's departmental cart.[9] However, such a list can be a good starting point for creating a useful cart, with the end users customizing the contents according to departmental needs, preferences, and available resources. A designated individual or committee should be responsible for soliciting input from users in determining what should be on the cart. The decision about the contents ought to be reviewed quarterly or semiannually to ensure that carts have the most up-to-date

and effective equipment. Deletions and additions need to be communicated to all users in a timely manner. Surprises in the midst of a failed airway are most unwelcome!

In principle, the cart should be one that is easily accessible and has equipment familiar to the users and other unit personnel. An assortment of well-arranged and quickly accessible devices should be available to handle most needs. Decisions about disposable versus reusable equipment should be made consistent with hospital policies and published evidence of equipment effectiveness (discussed later in this chapter).

In this all-inclusive difficult airway cart, all equipment needed for difficult airway situations (so-called Plan B and Plan C) should be present. Equipment on the cart need not duplicate routine airway equipment otherwise available on anesthetic carts in the ORs. This may be where an OR difficult airway cart differs from airway carts in other locations: in ICU or ED settings, airway kits or carts may contain both routine and alternative airway equipment.

Familiarity with the difficult airway cart and its contents is crucial. Using difficult airway equipment for routine intubations will add to the skills in using alternative devices and will also help the anesthesia practitioner and support personnel gain needed familiarity with cart contents and location. This in turn will lead to more effective management of an emergency unanticipated difficult and failed airway, minimizing stress for all concerned. However, with regular use of the difficult airway cart, there must be a routine to ensure that it is properly maintained: disposables must be replenished and reusable equipment disinfected and replaced as quickly as possible (see Section 59.4 later). This in turn implies that designated personnel familiar with the cart routinely check and replenish it. This is the same principle that applies to maintenance of the cardiac arrest crash cart.

59.2.2 What equipment should be available on a difficult airway cart for the OR?

The cart containing the equipment should be mobile, small enough to be safely and easily moved by one person, and should fit into the ORs through the doorways. It should be located in a central location that is familiar and visible to all. Smooth castors on the cart and the drawers are important to ensure that the cart does not become an obstacle in itself, and is safe from being overturned. Cables and cords should be neatly attached so that nothing can be snagged while the cart is being moved or people are working around it. Failure to pay attention to this could lead to damage to equipment or injury to staff. The drawers should be clearly labeled as per their contents.

The equipment included on the cart should cover the range of options that might be needed in a difficult airway scenario. This will include categories such as:

- Equipment to facilitate mechanical (bag-mask or EGD) ventilation
- Adjuncts to direct laryngoscopy
- Alternatives to direct laryngoscopy
- Equipment to facilitate transtracheal access
- Light sources, cameras, and monitors for techniques requiring, or facilitated by, this equipment

- Equipment and drugs for application of topical airway anesthesia or airway blocks
- Miscellaneous equipment as determined by each facility.

59.2.3 What equipment to facilitate mechanical (bag-mask or EGD) ventilation should be included in difficult airway cart for the OR?

At least one bag-mask device should be available for delivery of positive pressure ventilation. Nonstandard mask sizes may belong in the cart. The group or individual responsible for the airway cart should decide which extraglottic devices to stock. If classic or disposable laryngeal mask airways are routinely stocked in the OR, then the cart may contain, for example, the LMA-ProSeal™ and intubating LMA (LMA-Fastrach™). Other EGDs such as the Combitube™ or King LT™ Airway can be considered, but the devices should be the ones with which the department members have experience and have found useful.

59.2.4 What adjuncts to direct laryngoscopy should be included in a difficult airway cart for the OR?

An assortment of alternate blades designed to fit standard laryngoscope handles used in the OR should be available. For example, Miller (straight) and Macintosh (curved) blades of various sizes, as well as levering tip (McCoy/CLM) laryngoscope blades, might be kept in this section. The presence of a variety of ETTs (eg, Endotrol®, Microlaryngeal Tubes) not routinely stocked in the OR, including a range of smaller sizes, is important.

The presence of a flexible, Coudé-tipped (distal 2.5 cm and angled approximately 35 degrees) Eschmann Tracheal Tube Introducer (the gum-elastic bougie) or the single-use Cook Frova® is an essential addition to an emergency cart. It can be guided below the epiglottis when a Mallampati Class II or III view of the larynx is encountered, whereupon the ETT can be advanced over it (see Section 11.2.1). Because they should be kept straight, rather than bent to fit into a drawer, some tracheal tube introducers (eg, Portex) may be stored in their original shipping case, secured to the side of the cart (Figure 59-2). As a simple, yet useful, device most would suggest that these introducers be an integral part of standard equipment found in every room or location where anesthetics are administered.

59.2.5 What alternatives to direct laryngoscopy should be included in a difficult airway cart for the OR?

Here is where the list of objects becomes potentially extensive. Again, the principles are not to duplicate what already exists as routine airway management equipment in the OR, but to stock only those devices familiar to the anesthesia practitioner and support staff.

Options for inclusion in this section are as follows:

- *Intubating LMA (LMA Fastrach™)* in a variety of sizes (#3 - #5), their dedicated silicone-ETTs (7-8 mm ID), and the tube stabilizer to aid with subsequent LMA Fastrach™ removal.

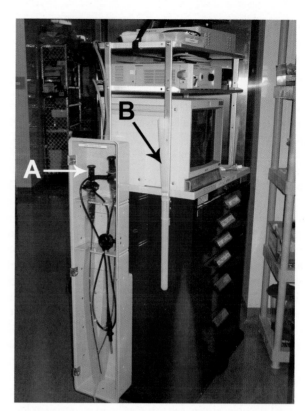

FIGURE 59-2. The proposed difficult airway cart with different drawers for different airway equipment, video monitor, flexible fiberoptic bronchoscope in a secure compartment (A), and Eschmann tracheal introducer stored in its original shipping case (B).

- *Intubating lighted stylet (eg, Trachlight™)*: There should be at least one handle, which is tested daily to ensure that the batteries are functional, as well as two or three wands. Some institutions stock the cart with one Trachlight™ loaded with a precut (26 cm) 7.5-mm ID ETT (see Chapter 11) in the cart as well.

- *Flexible bronchoscope devices*: The flexible bronchoscope (FB) should be kept in a secure compartment, where it can be stored so that it is not tightly curled (Figure 59-2). This ensures maximum protection of the fragile shaft and the motion cable that controls the scope tip. FBs ought to be handled with great care as they are fragile devices and repairs may be expensive. Discussion often arises regarding the use of pediatric versus adult scopes. In a difficult intubation, particularly where failed attempts at direct laryngoscopy have traumatized the airway, the adult scope has the advantage of having a more functional suction lumen in addition to being a more rigid (and sturdy) scope. Ideally, a scope that will allow intubation with a 6 mm ID or larger ETT should be sought. Pediatric scopes are fragile and may not have the rigidity to facilitate the insertion of a large-diameter ETT tube around tight corners, and have smaller working channels compromising their suction capacity. They are, however, indispensable in confirming the position of devices when lung isolation is required. Included in the drawer where the FB equipment is kept should be devices to protect the scope from being bitten, such as a bite block Tudor Williams (Figure 9-24), Ovassapian (Figure 9-25), or Berman

Intubating Pharyngeal airways (Figure 9-22) in an assortment of sizes.

- *Rigid fiberoptic and video laryngoscopic devices*: These devices provide indirect visualization of the larynx via fiberoptics or video display (e.g. Airtraq® Optical Laryngoscope and Pentax AirwayScope). Some devices such as the Bullard Laryngoscope, UpsherScope™, McGrath®, GlideScope and C-Mac have a blade to aid with tongue control, while others, such as the Shikani SOS™, Bonfils, and Levitan FPS, are simply fiberoptic optical stylets, enabling visualization through an ensleeved ETT. Further details on these devices appear in Chapter 10. Many of these devices can be operated with batteries, making them portable.

A recent review of the literature revealed that, although visualization of the glottic opening is improved with many of these devices, insertion of the ETT may remain problematic.[10] Indeed, some significant trauma to the pharyngeal and tracheal structures has been documented with some of these devices. Intubations under different anatomical situations are facilitated more by some of the video laryngoscopes than by others. In other words, none of the scopes is a panacea. In conclusion, although "video laryngoscopes are promising intubation devices, … their precise role in airway management remains to be established."[10]

59.2.6 What equipment to facilitate transtracheal access should be available in the difficult airway cart for the OR?

In a failed airway situation, particularly when ventilation and intubation are not possible, quick direct transtracheal access to the airway must occur (see Chapter 13 for details). For those trained in transtracheal-jet-ventilation, a nonkinking catheter should be available, together with a regulated oxygen source. The latter can be affixed directly to the cart. The substantial dangers and poor track record of success for transtracheal jet ventilation in the setting of a failed airway have led most experts to recommend that one proceed directly to open surgical or percutaneous cricothyrotomy. Commercial kits are available with equipment for one or both techniques. The percutaneous Melker cricothyrotomy kits are now available with a cuffed cannula, making this a particularly useful device. For those departments with members familiar with the technique, equipment for retrograde intubation can be considered an option in less urgent situations. Again, this is available commercially in a kit.

59.6.7 What video accessory equipment should be available in the difficult airway cart for the OR?

Many of the newer flexible bronchoscopes can run on a battery-powered light source, while visualization occurs through a traditional eyepiece. Other FBs and the newer video bronchoscopes require a separate light source that attaches to the scope via a cable. This light source is generally brighter than the battery-powered light sources. A particularly useful device is a camera with an appropriate adaptor that attaches to a bronchoscope's eyepiece to give a video feed to a monitor (Figure 59-2). This allows much better viewing of the airway, as the image is magnified and is brighter than that viewed through the eyepiece. It allows an assistant to visualize what is happening and in a teaching institution, it can be invaluable when explaining or directing a trainee what to do next. Still or video images can be recorded for documentation of the procedure as well as any pathology encountered.

59.2.8 What other miscellaneous equipment should be available in a difficult airway cart?

Ancillary equipment, such as medication cups for holding and mixing solutions, tongue depressors, tonsil forceps (eg, the Kraus or Jackson forceps) for applying gauze balls for superior laryngeal nerve blocks, as well as antifog agents for the flexible bronchoscopes, are a few other additions to the cart. The need for awake intubation is always a possibility, so appropriate types and volumes of local anesthetic agents should also be kept on the cart. These agents can be injected (eg, with transtracheal injection and/or percutaneous superior laryngeal nerve blocks) or applied topically, for example, by gargling, dripping onto the extended or tractioned tongue, or with a nebulizer or DeVilbiss atomizer. For a more detailed description of airway anesthesia techniques, see Chapter 3. Water-soluble lubricants, silicone liquid, or other antifog agents should also be available.

An array of airway exchange catheters is always appropriate for use in changing tubes in difficult situations or for the extubation of the patient whose trachea was difficult to intubate.

Availability of pediatric equipment will be dictated to an extent by the practice pattern of the hospital, although very small-for-age adults, disaster preparedness, and airway pathology situations make it advisable for adult hospitals to carry some pediatric equipment. Other equipment for inclusion on the difficult airway cart will be dictated by the department's practice environment. For instance, some institutions include rigid bronchoscopes and anterior commissure scopes on their cart.

59.3 DIFFICULT AIRWAY CART OUTSIDE THE OR

59.3.1 How might equipment requirements differ for out-of-OR locations such as the ICU or ED and why?

The processes governing airway carts in non-OR areas are no different than those described earlier. A variety of policies and practices are essential in ensuring that vital life saving equipment is available and in working order when required, including the following:

- Who should be involved to decide what the cart contains?
- How are suggestions as to contents made and how are those decisions made?
- How are cart modifications communicated effectively to all staff that may be affected?

- How often is the cart checked for contents and equipment function and by whom?
- Who is responsible to ensure that the carts are restocked routinely after use?
- How is this process documented?

Some areas are more airway intervention prone than others. EDs, ICUs, free-standing day-surgery operations, post anesthesia care units, pediatric dental clinics, nonhospital surgical facilities, and pediatric cancer care units are obvious examples. It is reasonable to expect that airway intervention may occur with some regularity in these units and that routine and difficult airway management equipment ought to be immediately available.

Others are less obvious. These include units where procedural sedation is undertaken, such as endoscopy suites, angiography and cardiac catheterization units, and others. While routine airway management equipment ought to be immediately available on these units, it may be financially prohibitive to create potentially expensive, fully equipped carts as described earlier. However, it is not unreasonable to expect that such units have relatively inexpensive, proven adjuncts, such as oral and nasal airways, and rescue devices, such as disposable LMA (LMA Unique™), LMA Fastrach™, Combitube™, and intubating stylets.

Some institutions designate that anesthesia be a part of the team that responds to declared intra-institutional airway emergencies. In response, some of these anesthesia departments have created portable airway management bags to be taken to the site of the airway emergency. Policy considerations as to contents and their working order are no different for these kits than for the cart described above.

Furthermore, and crucially important from a medicolegal perspective is the involvement of anesthesia in the design and maintenance of unit resident carts (eg, ICU, ED) if they are responsible for responding to those units (or elect to do so) to support airway management activities. It is the duty of the hospitals and unit management and anesthesia practitioners to understand and embrace this accountability.

59.4   DISPOSABLE VERSUS REUSABLE DEVICES CONSIDERATIONS FOR DIFFICULT AIRWAY CARTS

59.4.1   What is transmissible bovine spongiform encephalitis? Should airway practitioners be concerned about it?

The widespread awareness of the possibility of transmission of infections via the use of reusable medical equipment has led to adherence to standards for sterilization as a routine practice. Until recently, it was assumed that the adherence to these measures would assure that equipment was sterile and the prevention of iatrogenic disease transmission by this route.

Creutzfeldt-Jakob disease (CJD), bovine spongiform encephalitis (BSE or mad cow disease), as well as variant CJD (vCJD) are examples of the transmissible spongiform encephalopathies (TSE). All of these diseases are transmitted by malformed protein particles, referred to as prions. These infectious prion proteins attach themselves to native prion proteins in the recipient's brain, resulting in production of more of the distorted, abnormal prions, and the clinical specter of progressive neurological symptoms leading to death. Almost any symptom can present, from motor, to sensory, to cognitive dysfunction. This often makes the diagnosis difficult as the symptoms can be confused with other neurological conditions. Definitive diagnosis is made histologically by biopsy or at autopsy. The term "spongiform" refers to the spongy gross appearance of the brain caused by TSE.

The incidence of TSE in humans is extremely low. Sporadic (90% of CJD) and familial (10% of all CJD) forms of CJD occur at a frequency of 1:1,000,000 in the general population. Iatrogenic forms of CJD have occurred from the transfer of infected neural tissues (pituitary extract, cornea, or dura mater) and represent less than 1% of all cases of CJD. In 1986, the first case of BSE was reported in Britain. By 2001, it was estimated that 180,000 cattle were infected. Widespread control measures were taken at that time with the mass destruction of herds throughout the United Kingdom. There appears to be a link between BSE and vCJD. This variant has some significant differences from the sporadic form of CJD. Among the differences between the two disease entities is the notable discovery of a prion specific to vCJD in lymphoid tissues (tonsil, spleen, appendix, and lymph nodes). Prior to this, the only location of the agents responsible for BSE was felt to be neural tissue involving brain, spinal cord, dura mater, or eye. The discovery of prions in lymphoid tissue occurs very early in the disease process, before the onset of clinical symptoms. Furthermore, the tissues are very highly infectious. A mass of 1 µg of infected lymphoid tissue has the same risk of infectivity as 1 g of neural tissue from BSE-infected tissues.[11,12] This makes the tissue infected with the vCJD prion particle 1000 times more infectious than the neural tissue from sporadic CJD-infected subjects.

By the year 2002, a total of 134 cases of human TSE felt secondary to BSE had been reported worldwide.[11] The vast majority (126) were in the United Kingdom and Ireland, 6 in France, 1 in Italy, and 1 in the United States. The US (FL) resident, however, was from the United Kingdom and it was felt the disease had been acquired there. Clearly, the transmission of TSE has been documented through the use of neural tissues, both dural grafts and pituitary growth hormone. It has also been reported to have passed from patient to patient via reusable neurosurgical instruments, despite employing standard cleaning and disinfection methods. While it is difficult to assess the risk of transmission via reusable airway instruments, either surgical or anesthetic, that have come in contact with lymphoid tissue in an infected patient, the infectivity of the vCJD prion from such tissue as mentioned earlier, is approximately 1000 times that of the material from neural tissue. In spite of the above data, there have been no reported cases, to date, of vCJD transmitted via contaminated airway equipment. Furthermore, projections of the future risks of deaths from vCJD show dramatic decreases, such that the incidence of deaths from the disease will be almost negligible over the next 70 years.[13]

59.4.2 How effective is sterilization in destroying the prion particle?

Discovery of prion transmission through the use of infected surgical instruments created an alarming realization that the usual methods of sterilization were not reliable in disinfecting medical equipment.[14,15] It has been shown that the prion particles associated with TSE are extremely resistant to accepted standard sterilization procedures; particles withstanding autoclaving (120°C), ultraviolet radiation, as well as ionizing radiation.[15] The discovery that protein residue is present in medical instruments used for airway manipulation after routine cleaning procedures creates even more concern. This is particularly worrisome in light of the presence of prions in lymphoid tissues in patients later diagnosed with vCJD. Miller showed in the assessment of 20 cleaned reusable LMAs that all had residual protein deposits on them, ranging from mild (55%) to heavy staining (20%).[16] Similarly, of 61 used laryngoscope blades that had been cleaned and returned for use, 50 were contaminated. This finding was confirmed by Clery and others.[17]

The recognition that: (i) prions related to vCJD were present in tonsil tissue; (ii) the specific prion was much more virulent than the agent for vCJD; and (iii) material from patients was present on airway instruments in spite of adequate techniques of sterilization has led to the suggestion that single-use instruments be used in place of reusable varieties where the risk of cross-contamination with tonsil tissue can occur. Indeed, in 2001, the Department of Health in the United Kingdom mandated the use of disposable surgical and anesthetic instruments for use in tonsil surgery. However, within a year, the high incidence of surgical complications deemed to be secondary to the introduction of these disposable instruments led to the reversal of the directive. It was decided that the risk of complications from the disposable instruments outweighed the risk of transmission of vCJD from cross-contamination of inadequately cleaned multiple-use instruments. Although the ban on reusable anesthetic equipment was initially lifted, it was reimposed in 2002.

59.4.3 How well do single-use (disposable) airway devices work when compared to the reusable instruments?

Following the concern that reusable airway equipment could cause the transmission of vCJD, a large number of single-use instruments were introduced into the market. These included, but were not limited to, laryngoscope blades, tracheal tube introducers (eg, Eschmann Introducer), LMA, and other extraglottic devices, as well as disposable covers for laryngoscope blades. However, there are no strict testing or standards that must be met by any of these devices. Consequently, a great deal of controversy has arisen as to their effectiveness, when compared to the traditional equipment.

Twigg et al[18] compared six single-use laryngoscope blades with the standard Macintosh blade in a simulator model. Twenty experienced anesthesiologists used each device, both in an easy scenario and a simulated difficult airway. Time to intubate, need for the use of an Eschmann introducer, Cormack/Lehane (C/L) grading, and percentage of glottic opening visible (POGO) scores were recorded. Although considerable variability existed between the disposable devices, the best performer in both normal and difficult scenarios was the Macintosh blade. Not surprisingly, it was the difficult airway that brought out the greatest differences between the best and the worst performers. Some of the single-use blades performed reasonably well, the best being the Europa, which is a metal instrument. The results were so troubling that the investigators concluded, "We believe that intubation equipment that fails to match standard equipment should be avoided and is clinically unsafe. The unregulated use of single-use laryngoscopes must be questioned."[18]

Annamaneni et al[19] demonstrated a difference between single-use and disposable tracheal introducers (bougies) in simulated difficult intubations. Twenty anesthesiologists attempted intubation twice with both a reusable introducer and a single-use introducer, with success measured by tracheal as opposed to esophageal insertion. The success with first attempts was 85% versus 15% for the multiple-use and disposable devices, respectively. The results were similar for the second attempt.

Evans et al[20] compared disposable and nondisposable laryngoscopes by studying the time to intubate as well as measuring the force used to obtain an adequate laryngoscopic view, for both routine and difficult intubation in a manikin. They had 60 anesthesiologists performing intubations with five different laryngoscope blades, both routinely and with a cervical collar on the manikin. The blades included the standard Macintosh #3, a disposable metal, and three plastic blades. The time was significantly greater with the plastic blades when compared to the metal, for both the routine and "difficult" intubations. The increase ranged from 33% to 85%. Forces generated were statistically greater for the plastic blades when compared to those for the metal blades, by as much as 35%. The forces generated, even though they were not out of the range used clinically, were sufficient to cause three of the plastic blades to fracture during the study.

Anderson and Bhadal measured the effect on the illumination by placing a protective cover over a reusable Macintosh blade.[21] They showed that a predictable reduction in illumination occurred, with a mean reduction of 19%. Others have commented on their findings that disposable laryngoscope blades are inferior to reusable devices.[22,23]

One of the authors of this chapter (SP) had the experience of having been provided with a disposable plastic blade in the ICU when called to assist with a failed intubation. The blade fractured during the intubation attempt, causing a laceration on the patient's tongue and adding to an already stressful situation. Intubation was successful following the use of a reusable metal Macintosh blade.

Another area where the influx of single-use, disposable devices has flooded the marketplace is the LMA. The reasons cited are again cost as well as infection control.

The significant increase in the marketing of these devices is unfortunately devoid of studies showing their safety and reliability. The materials used differ significantly from the ones used in the original LMA-Classic™. In the LMA-Classic™ device, silicon was the chosen material. It produces a good seal due to its pliability. It is, however, more expensive than the polyvinylchloride (PVC) material used in the single-use devices. Of note, Brain rejected PVC as the materials for his LMA devices in the development stages. PVC, by its nature, is a rather rigid material, and therefore not very compliant. Plasticizers are needed to make PVC pliable and therefore produce a decent seal. These additives, however, potentially can make these products toxic, as phthalates—the most commonly used plasticizer—have been suggested as being potentially carcinogenic. Another concern regarding single-use devices is the effects on the environment with the disposal of these nonbiodegradable plastic products.

Most importantly, there is a lack of standardized guidelines for the manufacturing of disposable devices, as well as the lack of studies comparing their efficacy to the original, reusable LMA devices. Just as with the disposable laryngoscopes and bougies, studies may reveal that the performance and safety of these devices may or may not meet expectations.

59.4.4   Should reusable or disposable equipment be kept in the difficult airway carts?

The only reliable ways to avoid the transmission of vCJD is to either use disposable instruments or not perform airway manipulation on patients infected with prion agent, and thus avoid contamination of reusable equipment. Clearly, the risk of contaminating equipment depends upon the probability of caring for an infected individual. The data from the World Health Organization (WHO) show that the incidence varies worldwide and is very low, even in countries at highest risk (eg, the United Kingdom). Indeed, the risk of transmission through the use of contaminated instruments was felt to be less than the risk of complications posed by disposable surgical instruments used for tonsillectomy in 2001. Fortunately, the risks of anesthetic-related airway mishaps are lower than the risks posed by complications from our surgical colleagues. The number of failed intubations are too low to have adequate power to reveal what the increased risks posed are to patients by using disposable devices. Certainly, the risk posed by cross contamination of vCJD is unknown. However, as discussed earlier, there has not been a single reported case of transmission of vCJD via airway equipment at the time of this publication. In their editorial, Blunt and Burchett[11] discuss the hypothetical relative risks and come to the conclusion that the risk to the patient with poorly functioning airway equipment is likely greater than that of acquiring TSE through contaminated airway instruments.

The cost and reliability must be taken into account for all single-use instruments. Although Galinski et al[24] felt that the disposable instruments were acceptable, they also state that, "it may be advisable to maintain conventional laryngoscopes in reserve for difficult intubations." More effective cleansing methods would also reduce risk, albeit not eliminate it. In the final analysis, it is important to weigh the relative risks of possible contamination with vCJD prions, negligible in most areas of the world and dropping, to those of risks created during airway management with what could be, and has been shown to be, less than optimal equipment. The decision to keep reusable or disposable equipment in the difficult airway carts should be based on sound scientific evidence, relative risk, and cost-benefit assessments.

Unfortunately, a lack of studies supporting the efficacy and safety of the large number of disposable airway devices flooding the market is concerning, making informed decision difficult. Furthermore, many of the studies that have been performed show that these devices are frequently substandard when compared to their reusable counterparts. The issue of cost, discussed by Cook in an editorial in the BJA suggests that this may not be the advantage as previously thought.[25]

Finally, when dealing with the most difficult airway situation, where the emergency airway cart is required, one could argue that the best, most reliable, and proven equipment should be selected.

59.5   SUMMARY

The use of alternative airway devices has clearly improved patient care. The ready availability of these devices is markedly facilitated by the creation of an airway cart. This cart should be easy to use, well laid out, and maintained to ensure optimum functionality. The contents should encompass a range of devices as described in various publications, and should be customized to the needs of a given department and its members. Although the decision to keep reusable or disposable equipment in these airway carts is not an easy one, it should be based on relative risk, scientific evidence, and the cost-benefit assessments.

Appendix 59.1 itemizes how a difficult airway cart might be structured.

REFERENCES

1. American Society of Anesthesiologists Task Force on Management of the Difficult Airway. Practice guidelines for the difficult airway. *Anesthesiology.* 1993;78:597-602.
2. American Society of Anesthesiologists Task Force on Management of the Difficult Airway. Practice guidelines for management of the difficult airway: an updated report by the American Society of Anesthesiologists Task Force on Management of the Difficult Airway. *Anesthesiology.* 2003;98:1269-1277.
3. Crosby ET, Cooper RM, Douglas MJ, et al. The unanticipated difficult airway with recommendations for management. *Can J Anaesth.* 1998;45:757-776.
4. Rose DK, Cohen MM. The airway: problems and predictions in 18,500 patients. *Can J Anaesth.* 1994;41:372-383.
5. Schwartz DE, Matthay MA, Cohen NH. Death and other complications of emergency airway management in critically ill adults. A prospective investigation of 297 tracheal intubations. *Anesthesiology.* 1995;82:367-376.
6. Mort TC. Emergency tracheal intubation: complications associated with repeated laryngoscopic attempts. *Anesth Analg.* 2004;99:607-613, table of contents.
7. Mort TC. The incidence and risk factors for cardiac arrest during emergency tracheal intubation: a justification for incorporating the ASA Guidelines in the remote location. *J Clin Anesth.* 2004;16:508-516.
8. Luten R, Broselow J. Rainbow care: the Broselow-Luten system. Implications for pediatric patient safety. *Ambul Outreach.* 1999;Fall:14-16.
9. McGuire GP, Wong DT. Airway management: contents of a difficult intubation cart. *Can J Anaesth.* 1999;46:190-191.
10. Niforopoulou P, Pantazopoulos I, Demestiha T, Koudouna E, Xanthos T. Video-laryngoscopes in the adult airway management: a topical review of the literature. *Acta Anaesthesiol Scand.* 2010;54:1050-1061.
11. Blunt MC, Burchett KR. Variant Creutzfeldt-Jakob disease and disposable anaesthetic equipment-balancing the risks. *Br J Anaesth.* 2003;90:1-3.
12. Bruce ME, McConnell I, Will RG, Ironside JW. Detection of variant Creutzfeldt-Jakob disease infectivity in extraneural tissues. *Lancet.* 2001;358:208-209.
13. Ghani AC, Donnelly CA, Ferguson NM, Anderson RM. Updated projections of future vCJD deaths in the UK. *BMC Infect Dis.* 2003;3:4.

14. Brown P, Preece M, Brandel JP, et al. Iatrogenic Creutzfeldt-Jakob disease at the millennium. *Neurology.* 2000;55:1075-1081.
15. Zobeley E, Flechsig E, Cozzio A, Enari M, Weissmann C. Infectivity of scrapie prions bound to a stainless steel surface. *Mol Med.* 1999;5:240-243.
16. Miller DM, Youkhana I, Karunaratne WU, Pearce A. Presence of protein deposits on "cleaned" re-usable anaesthetic equipment. *Anaesthesia.* 2001;56:1069-1072.
17. Clery G, Brimacombe J, Stone T, Keller C, Curtis S. Routine cleaning and autoclaving does not remove protein deposits from reusable laryngeal mask devices. *Anesth Analg.* 2003;97:1189-1191.
18. Twigg SJ, McCormick B, Cook TM. Randomized evaluation of the performance of single-use laryngoscopes in simulated easy and difficult intubation. *Br J Anaesth.* 2003;90:8-13.
19. Annamaneni R, Hodzovic I, Wilkes AR, Latto IP. A comparison of simulated difficult intubation with multiple-use and single-use bougies in a manikin. *Anaesthesia.* 2003;58:45-49.
20. Evans A, Vaughan RS, Hall JE, Mecklenburgh J, Wilkes AR. A comparison of the forces exerted during laryngoscopy using disposable and non-disposable laryngoscope blades. *Anaesthesia.* 2003;58:869-873.
21. Anderson KJ, Bhandal N. The effect of single use laryngoscopy equipment on illumination for tracheal intubation. *Anaesthesia.* 2002;57:773-777.
22. Babb M, Mann S. Disposable laryngoscope blades. *Anaesthesia.* 2002;57:286-288.
23. Jefferson P, Perkins V, Edwards VA, Ball DR. Problems with disposable laryngoscope blades. *Anaesthesia.* 2003;58:385-386, discussion 386.
24. Galinski M, Adnet F, Tran D, Karyo Z, Quintard H, Delettre D. Disposable laryngoscope blades do not interfere with ease of intubation in scheduled general anaesthesia patients. *Eur J Anaesthesiol.* 2003;20:731-735.
25. Cook TM. The classic laryngeal mask airway: a tried and tested airway. What now? *Br J Anaesth.* 2006;96:149-152.

SELF-EVALUATION QUESTIONS

59.1. Which of the following is a known effective method of sterilization in destroying the prion particle?

A. autoclaving (120°C)

B. ultraviolet radiation

C. ionizing radiation

D. sterilization with ethylene oxide

E. none of the above

59.2. All of the following policy issues regarding a difficult airway cart are crucial **EXCEPT**:

A. cart location

B. who is the cart policy manager

C. communications regarding contents

D. maintenance and replacement of contents

E. who is permitted to use the cart

59.3. Since anesthesia practitioners are called to out-of-OR locations to manage airways

A. They are liable for negative outcomes if the equipment they need is not available.

B. They must have input regarding contents of difficult airway carts in locations where they may be called to intervene.

C. They must ensure that policies regarding airway equipment maintenance in out-of-OR locations are in force and followed.

D. Noncompliance in any of the scenarios listed above (including the availability of essential equipment) would be grounds to refuse to participate in airway management in those locations.

E. All of the above.

APPENDIX 59.1

Sample contents of an operating room difficult airway cart

DRAWER #1:Topical anesthesia	ROTIGS Airways (9 cm × 2; 10 cm × 1) Berman Intubating Pharyngeal or Breakaway® Airways (sm, med, lg)—Vital Signs Mucosal Atomization Device (MAD®) (3)—Wolf Tory Medical Mucosal Atomization Device gic (MADgic®) (3)—Wolf Tory Medical Anti-fog (3); Goggles (1); Bite Blocks (2); Med Cups (4) Jackson Crossover Forceps (1) DeVilbiss Atomizer® with O_2 Tubing
	Phenylephrine 0.5% (Neosynephrine®) nasal spray 15 ml (1) 20% Hurricaine gel 6.25 gm (4) Lidocaine 4% aqueous 50 ml bottles (1) Tetracaine 0.45% with epinephrine 1:25,000 (40 $\mu g \cdot ml^{-1}$) (3 × 15 ml bottles) Olympus light source replacement bulb (1) Portex bronchoscope swivel adapter (4) Adult and Pediatric McGill forceps
DRAWER #2:Jet Ventilator	Metered dose inhaler in-line administration adapters (2) Jet ventilator Intravenous needle/catheters for transcricoid insertion (14 and 16 gauge × 2 of each) must be aspiration capable with 3 mL syringe with 7.0-mm ID ETT connector ENK Oxygen Flow Modulator®—Cook 6.0-, 7.0-, and 8.0-mm ID Endotrol® tubes—Mallinckrodt
DRAWER #3: Combitube™ Trachlight™	Small Adult (1) and Regular Adult (1) Combitube™—Sheridan Trachlight™ handles (2) and adult wands (10)
DRAWER #4:LMAs	Fastrach™: #5 × 2; #4 × 1; #3 × 1 LMA Classics™: #1; #1.5; #2; #2.5; #3; #4; #5
DRAWER #5: Surgical airway	Melker Cricothyrotomy Kit®—Cook Retrograde intubation kit
DRAWER #6: Fiberoptics	Bullard laryngoscope Cook Airway Exchange Catheters® (14F × 2; 19F × 2)
Top of cart:	Bronchoscope light source Spare Eschmann Tracheal Tube Introducer
Side cabinet:	3.5 mm pediatric and 5.1 mm bronchoscopes

APPENDIX 59.2

Equipment supplier contact information

The following list of manufacturers of airway equipment is not intended to be exhaustive, nor should be construed to represent any sort of endorsement by the authors.

air-Q® Intubating LMA
Mercury Medical®
11300A-49th Street North
Clearwater, FL 34622-4800
Tel: (800) 237-6418
Fax: (800) 990-6375
http://www.mercurymed.com/

AirTraq (Meditec S.A., Vizcaya, Spain)
Distributor in United States:
Anchor Medical (New York City)
255 West 36th St., Suite 1002
New York, NY 10018
Tel: (212) 643-6208

Distributor in Canada:
Southmedic Inc.
50 Alliance Blvd.,
Barrie, Ontario
Canada L4M 5K3
Tel: (705) 726-9383 × 303
www.southmedic.com

Airway Management Device (AMD™)
Nagor Limited
PO Box 21 Global House
Isle of Man Business Park
Cooil Road Douglas
Isle of Man IM99 1AX
British Isles
Tel: +44 (0) 1624 625556
Fax: +44 (0) 1624 661656

Ambu Laryngeal Mask
Ambu Inc.
6740 Baymeadow Drive
Glen Burnie, Maryland 21060
Tel: (800) 262-8462 or (410) 768-6464
Fax: (800) 262-8673 or (410) 768-3993
www.ambu.com

Angulated Video-Intubation Laryngoscope (AVIL)
Acutronic Medical Systems AG
Fabrik im Schiffli
CH-8816 Hirzel
Schweiz/Switzerland
Tel: ++41 44 729 70 80
Fax: ++41 44 729 70 81

Bivona Tracheostomy Tube
Bivona Medical Technologies Inc.
5700 W 23RD AVE,
Gary, IN 46406-2617
Tel: (219) 989-9150

Beck Airway Airflow Monitor (BAAM)
Alliance Medical
8624 Rte C
PO Box 147
Russelville, MO 65074
Tel: (888) 633-6908
Fax: (800) 425-5633
www.allmed.net

Berman Intubating Pharyngeal Airway (Berman Breakaway Airway)
Vital Signs Inc.
20 Campus Road
Totowa, NJ 07512
Tel: (800) 932-0760
Fax: (973) 790-3307
http://www.vital-signs.com/

Bonfils Retromolar Intubation Fiberscope
Karl Storz Endoscopy-America, Inc.
Attn: Human Resources.
600 Corporate Pointe
Culver City, CA 90230-7600
Fax: (310) 410-5520

Bullard Laryngoscope
Gyrus ACMI Inc.
93 North Pleasant St.
Norwalk, OH 44857
Tel: (508) 804-2600
http://www.acmicorp.com/

C-MAC® Videolaryngoscope
Karl Storz Endoscopy-America, Inc.
Attn: Human Resources.
600 Corporate Pointe
Culver City, CA 90230-7600
Fax: (310) 410-5520

CobraPLA™ (Perilaryngeal Airway™)
Engineered Medical Systems, Inc.
2055 Executive Drive
Indianapolis, IN 46241
Tel: (317) 246-5500
Fax: (317) 246-5501

Combitube™
Tyco Healthcare/Kendall
15 Hampshire St
Mansfield, MA 02048
Tel: (508) 261-8000
Fax: (508) 261-8062

Cook Airway Exchange Catheter
Cook Medical Inc.
PO Box 4195
Bloomington, IN 47402-4195
Tel: (812) 339-2235; (800) 457-4500
Fax: (800) 554-8335
http://www.cookmedical.com/home.do

Cook ILA Intubating LMA
Mercury Medical
11300A-49th Street North
Clearwater, FL 34622-4800
Tel: (800) 237-6418
Fax: (800) 990-6375
http://www.mercurymed.com/

Cricoid Pressure Simulators
Nasco
901 Janesville Avenue
PO Box 901
Fort Atkinson, WI 53538-0901
Tel: (800) 558-9595
Fax: (920) 563-8296
http://www.enasco.com/Static.do?page=contact

Cricothyrotomy (Open) Kits and Needle Cricothyrotomy Devices
Cook Medical Inc.
PO Box 4195
Bloomington, IN 47402-4195
Tel: (812) 339-2235; (800) 457-4500
Fax: (800) 554-8335
http://www.cookmedical.com/home.do

Cricothyrotomy Instruments
Allegiance Healthcare Corp.
V. Meuller division
1435 Lake Cook Road
Deerfield, IL 60015
Tel: (800) 964-5227

DeVilbiss Atomizers
Anthony Products, Inc
7740 Records St
Indianapolis, IN 46226
Tel: (877) 428-1610
Fax: (317) 543-3289
http://www.anthonyproducts.com/contact/contact.htm

Endotracheal Tube Attachment Device (ETAD™)
COS Medical Inc.
3213 Post Woods Drive, Suite B
Atlanta, GA 30339
http://www.continentostomystore.com/

Endotracheal Tube Exchangers (airway exchange catheters)
Cook Medical Inc.
PO Box 4195
Bloomington, IN 47402-4195
Tel: (812) 339-2235; (800) 457-4500
Fax: (800) 554-8335
http://www.cookmedical.com/home.do

Endotrol® Endotracheal Tubes
Mallinckrodt
675 McDonnell Blvd
Hazelwood, MO 63042
Tel: (800) 635-5267
http://www.mallinckrodt.com/contact/contact.html

ENK Oxygen Flow Modulator
Cook Medical Inc.
PO Box 4195
Bloomington, IN 47402-4195
Tel: (812) 339-2235; (800) 457-4500
Fax: (800) 554-8335
http://www.cookmedical.com/home.do

Eschmann Tracheal Tube Introducer (Blue Line® tracheal tube introducer)
SIMS Portex Inc.
10 Bowman Drive
PO Box 0724
Keene, NH 03431
Tel: (800) 258-5361
http://www.portex.com/airway/products/dcategory=General%20Anesthesia

Bronchoscopes and Nasopharyngoscopes
Karl Storz Endoscopy-America, Inc.
Attn: Human Resources.
600 Corporate Pointe
Culver City, CA 90230-7600
Fax: (310) 410-5520

Pentax Precision Instrument Corporation
30 Ramland Road
Orangeburg, NY 10962-2699
Tel: (800) 431-5880
Fax: (845) 365-0822
http://www.pentaxmedical.com/Products/Bronchoscopy.asp

Olympus America Inc.
3500 Corporate Parkway
PO Box 610
Center Valley, PA 18034-0610
Tel: (800) 645-8160
http://www.olympusamerica.com/

Flex-tip (McCoy type) Laryngoscope Blades
Heine USA Ltd.
One Washington Street, Unit 555
Dover, NH 03820
Tel: (800) 367-4872
Fax: (603) 742-7217
http://www.heine.com/

Mercury Medical
11300A-49th Street North
Clearwater, FL 34622-4800
Tel: (800) 237-6418
Fax: (800) 990-6375
http://www.mercurymed.com/

Rusch, Inc.
2450 Meadowbrook Parkway
Duluth, GA 30096
Tel: (800) 553-5214
Fax: (770) 623-1829
http://www.rusch.com/

Flex-Guide Endotracheal Tube Introducer
Green Field Medical Sourcing, Inc.
14141 Highway 290 West Suite 710
Austin, TX 78737
Tel: (512) 894-3002
Fax: (512) 858-1515

Frova Intubating Stylet
Cook Medical Inc.
PO Box 4195
Bloomington, IN 47402-4195
Tel: (812) 339-2235; (800) 457-4500
Fax: (800) 554-8335
http://www.cookmedical.com/home.do

GlideScope® Video Laryngoscope
Verathorn Inc.
20001 North Creek Parkway
Bothell, WA 98011
Tel: (800) 331-2313 (United States & Canada Only);
  (425) 867-1348
Fax: (425) 883-2896

Grandview Laryngoscope Blade
Hartwell Medical
6352 Corte del Abeto, Suite J
Carlsbad, CA 92009-1408
Tel: (800) 633-5900
Fax: (760) 438-2783

Human Patient Simulators (Air Man, Sim Man)
Laerdal Medical Corporation
167 Myers Corners Road, PO Box 1840
Wappingers Falls, NY 12590-8840
Tel: (800) 648-1851
Fax: (800) 227-1143
http://www.laerdal.com/

Jackson Crossover or Jackson Laryngeal Forceps
Surgical Tools
2C Greenmanville Ave
Mystic, CT 06355
Tel: (800) 774-2040
Fax: (860) 536-8532
http://www.surgicaltools.com/

Jet Ventilator
Life-Assist Inc
11277 Sunrise Park
Dr Rancho Cordova, CA 95742
Tel: (800) 824-6016
Fax: (800) 290-9794

King LT™ Airway (Laryngeal Tube Airway)
King Systems Corporation
15011 Herriman Blvd
Noblesville, IN 46060
Tel: (800) 642-5464
http://www.kingsystems.com/Main.htm

Laryngeal Mask Airway, LMA-ProSeal™, LMA-Fastrach™, and LMA-Unique™
LMA North America
9360 Towne Centre Drive, Suite 200
San Diego, CA 92121-3030
Tel: (800) 788-7999
Fax: (858) 622-4130
http://www.lmana.com/prod/components/contact_us.html

LaryVent™
B + P Beatmungs-Produkte GmbH,
Willy-Brandt-Allee 300
Gelsenkirchen, 45891DEU
Tel: +49-209-970770
http://www.masterflex.de

Levitan FPS Scope
Clarus Medical, LLC
1000 Boone Avenue North
Minneapolis, MN 55427
Tel: (763) 525-8403
Fax: (763) 525-8656
http://www.clarus-medical.com/airway-management/airway
  _levitan.htm

MAD® (Mucosal Atomization Device) and MADgic®
Wolf Tory Medical Inc
79 W 4500 South, Suite 16
Salt Lake City, UT 84107
Tel: (888) 380-9808
Fax: (801) 281-0708
www.wolfetory.com

McGrath® Videolaryngoscope
North American Distributor:
LMA North America
9360 Towne Centre Drive, Suite 200
San Diego, CA 92121-3030
Tel: (800) 788-7999
Fax: (858) 622-4130
http://www.lmana.com/prod/components/contact_us.html

Melker Cricothyrotomy Kit
Cook Medical Inc.
PO Box 4195
Bloomington, IN 47402-4195
Tel: (812) 339-2235; (800) 457-4500
Fax: (800) 554-8335
http://www.cookmedical.com/home.do

Metered Dose Inhaler Inline Adapter
DHD Healthcare
1 Madison St Wampsville, NY 13163
Tel: (800) 847-8000
Fax: (315) 363-9462

MLT® Microlaryngeal Tracheal Tube
Mallinckrodt
675 McDonnell Blvd
Hazelwood, MO 63042
Tel: (800) 635-5267
http://www.mallinckrodt.com/contact/contact.html

Pharyngeal Airway Express (PAxpress)
Vital Signs Inc.
20 Campus Road
Totowa, NJ 07512
Tel: (800) 932-0760
Fax: (973) 790-3307
http://www.vital-signs.com/

Pentax AWS Airway Scope
Ambu Inc.
6740 Baymeadow Drive
Glen Burnie, Maryland 21060
Tel: (800) 262-8462 or (410) 768-6464
Fax: (800) 262-8673 or (410) 768-3993
www.ambu.com

Retrograde Intubation Kit
Cook Medical Inc.
PO Box 4195
Bloomington, IN 47402-4195
Tel: (812) 339-2235; (800) 457-4500
Fax: (800) 554-8335
http://www.cookmedical.com/home.do

The Schroeder (Parker Flex-It™ Directional Stylet)
Parker Medical
7275 S. Revere Pkwy, Suite 804
Englewood, CO 80112
Tel: (303) 799-1990
Fax: (303) 799-1996

Sheridan Tube Exchanger
Sheridan Catheter Corp.,
Route 40, Argyle, NY, 12809
Tel: (518) 638-6101
Fax: (518) 638-8493

Shikani Optical Stylet (SOS™)
Clarus Medical, LLC
1000 Boone Avenue North
Minneapolis, MN 55427
Tel: (763) 525-8403
Fax: (763) 525-8656
http://www.clarus-medical.com

Shiley Tracheostomy Tube
Mallinckrodt
675 McDonnell Blvd
Hazelwood, MO 63042
Tel: (800) 635-5267
http://www.mallinckrodt.com/contact/contact.html

Silicone Fluid (Endoscopic Instrument Fluid)
ACMI Corporation
93 North Pleasant St. Norwalk,
OH 44857
Tel: (508) 804-2600
http://www.gyrusacmi.com/user/display.cfm

Streamlined Pharynx Airway Liner (SLIPA™)
ARC Medical Inc.
322 Patterson Ave.,
Scottdale, GA 30079
Tel: (404) 373-8300 ext. 210

StyletScope™
Nihon Kohden America Inc.
90 Icon St.
Foothill Ranch, CA 92610
Tel: (800) 325-0283

Sun Med Intubating Stylet
Mercury Medical
11300A-49th Street North
Clearwater, FL 34622-4800
Tel: (800) 237-6418
Fax: (800) 990-6375
http://www.mercurymed.com/

Trachlight™
Rusch, Inc.
2450 Meadowbrook Parkway
Duluth, GA 30096
Tel: (800) 553-5214
Fax: (770) 623-1829
http://www.rusch.com/

Laerdal Medical Corporation
167 Myers Corners Road, PO Box 1840
Wappingers Falls, NY 12590-8840
Tel: (800) 648-1851
Fax: (800) 227-1143
http://www.laerdal.com/

Trans tracheal Jet Ventilation Sets, Catheters and Equipment
Cook Medical Inc.
PO Box 4195
Bloomington, IN 47402-4195
Tel: (812) 339-2235; (800) 457-4500
Fax: (800) 554-8335
http://www.cookmedical.com/home.do

Truview EVO™ (manufacturer: Truphatek)
North American Distributor:
Teleflex,
Research Triangle Park,
NC 27709
Tel: (866) 246-6990
Fax: (800) 399-1028
www.rusch.com

Universal Cricothyrotomy Kit (both open and Seldinger apparatus)
Cook Medical Inc.
PO Box 4195
Bloomington, IN 47402-4195
Tel: (812) 339-2235; (800) 457-4500
Fax: (800) 554-8335
http://www.cookmedical.com/home.do

UpsherScope™
Mercury Medical
11300A-49th Street North
Clearwater, FL 34622-4800
Tel: (800) 237-6418
Fax: (800) 990-6375
http://www.mercurymed.com/

Video Macintosh (VMAC) Storz (VMS)
Karl Storz Endoscopy-America, Inc.
600 Corporate Pointe
Culver City, CA 90230-7600
Fax: (310) 410-5520

Video-Optical Intubation Stylet (VOIS)
Acutronic Medical Systems AG
Fabrik im Schiffli
CH-8816 Hirzel
Schweiz/Switzerland
Tel: ++41 44 729 70 80
Fax: ++41 44 729 70 81

Viewmax® Laryngoscope Blade
Rusch, Inc.
2450 Meadowbrook Parkway
Duluth, GA 30096
Tel: (800) 553-5214
Fax: (770) 623-1829
http://www.rusch.com/

WuScope System™
Achi Corporation
2168 Ringwood Avenue
San Jose, CA 95131-1720
Tel: (408) 321-9581
Fax: (408) 321-9587
www.achi.com

APPENDIX 59.3

Medication contact supplier information

Tetracaine 1% Aqueous
Abbott Pharmaceuticals
100 Abbott Pk Rd
Abbott Park, IL 60064
Tel: (800) 633-9110
http://www.abbott.com/

Lidocaine 4% Aqueous and Viscous; Lidocaine 5% Ointment
AstraZeneca Pharmaceuticals LP
1800 Concord Pike, PO Box 15437
Wilmington, DE 19850-5437
Tel: (800) 456-3669
http://www.astrazeneca-us.com/products/list.asp

Lidocaine 10% Aerosol Tracheal Spray
Odan Laboratories Ltd
325 Stillview Ave
Point Claire, Quebec
Canada, H9R 2Y6
Tel: (514) 428-1628
Fax: (514) 428-9783
Email: info@odanlab.com
http://www.odanlab.com/

Benzocaine 20% Ointment
Beutlich LP Pharmaceuticals
1541 Shields Dr
Waukegan, IL 60085-8304
Tel: (800) 238-8542
Fax: (847) 473-1122
http://www.beutlich.com/

APPENDIX 59.4

Cart supplier contact information

Armstrong Medical
575 Kinghtsbridge Pkwy
Lincolnshire, IL 60069-0700
Tel: (800) 323-4220
Fax: (847) 913-0138
http://www.armstrongmedical.com/

Blue Bell Bio-Medical
550 Bonneweitz Ave
Van Wert, OH 45891
Tel: (800) 258-3235
Fax: (419) 238-0226
http://www.bluebellcarts.com/

CHAPTER (60)

Documentation of Difficulty and Failure in Airway Management

Lorraine J. Foley, Michael F. Murphy, and Orlando R. Hung

60.1 CASE PRESENTATION

A 39-year-old woman is scheduled for a laparoscopic cholecystectomy under general anesthesia. She is 5 ft 4 in (161 cm), 220 lb (100 kg), with a BMI 38.6 kg·m^{-2}. She denies reflux. On physical examination, she has a Mallampati Class II airway, has 4 cm mouth opening, and a good neck extension. On the 3-3-2 examination she is just less than 3 on mouth, just less than 3 from mandibular to hyoid, and 2 on hyoid to thyroid notch. She has no past surgical history except for a cesarean section under epidural. The patient is placed on standard monitors. Following denitrogenation and induction of anesthesia with 200 mg of propofol, it is determined that she can easily be ventilated by a bag-mask. Rocuronium (40 mg) is administered for muscle relaxation. Direct laryngoscopy is attempted with #3 Macintosh blade. Only a large epiglottis is seen without any change following the application of laryngeal pressure. A #3 Miller blade is then used to lift the epiglottis. But, still no vocal cords are seen. An Eschmann Tracheal Introducer (bougie) is attempted, but passes repeatedly into the esophagus. Bag-mask-ventilation (BMV) remains adequate. Help and the difficult airway cart are summoned. A #3 Intubating Laryngeal Mask Airway (ILMA) is placed, resulting in adequate ventilation. An attempt at blind intubation through the ILMA is unsuccessful. So, a 7.0-mm ID endotracheal tube (ETT) is loaded onto the FAST (Foley fiberoptic airway stylet, Clarus Medical LLC, Minneapolis, MN) and placed through the ILMA. The ILMA is manipulated till vocal cords are visualized and the ETT is placed into trachea without difficulty.

60.2 WHY SHOULD WE DOCUMENT BOTH THE OCCURRENCE AND THE MANAGEMENT OF A DIFFICULT OR FAILED AIRWAY?

As indicated in earlier chapters (most notably Chapter 1), a difficult or failed airway is not the same as a difficult or failed intubation. This distinction is critically important to be able to accurately describe and document an adverse event as important as airway management difficulty and/or failure.

An episode of airway management difficulty and/or failure is an enduring threat to the safety of the patient and a hazard to the airway practitioner (even if only emotionally and medicolegally). From the medicolegal point of view, the medical record is exceedingly important. Thus, it is important that the practitioner documents well.

Although a substantial percentage of difficult airways can be predicted after a routine, yet careful airway examination, unanticipated difficult and failed airways continue to occur. One to three percent of patients undergoing general anesthesia are unanticipated difficult airway/intubations with conventional laryngoscopy.[1,2]

The importance of documentation rests in the prevention of a future disaster. The importance of an accurate verbal, and preferably, a written description of the specific problems encountered is essential so that when these patients return to the health care system, future practitioners do not approach them with trepidation based on vague verbal histories elicited from the patient, nor an inability on the part of the practitioner to access precise documentation of the prior adverse airway event. The written description ought to take two forms: a narrative given to the patient for presentation as needed as well as a well-documented permanent medical record.

The American Society of Anesthesiology Closed Claims Analyses has consistently identified adverse outcomes associated with respiratory events as constituting the single-largest class of injury.[3,4] Of these events in the 1980s, 17% were due to difficult intubation. In an ASA newsletter published in June 1997,[5] Cheney compared the closed claims from the 1970s, 1980s, and 1990s. Again, the three most common respiratory system-related damaging events causing death or brain damage were inadequate ventilation, esophageal intubation, and difficult intubation. A marked reduction among these damaging events was noted over time. Interestingly, while inadequate ventilation fell progressively (22% in 1970s, 15% in 1980s, and only 7% in 1990s) and the incidence of death or brain damage decreased, difficult intubation as a cause of death or brain damage increased from 5% in 1970s to 12% in 1990s. The numbers of claims in 1990s due to difficult intubation were too small to reach statistical significance.

The conclusion is interesting: while the decrease in inadequate ventilation and esophageal intubation may be due to pulse oximetry and end-tidal CO_2 monitoring, difficult intubation is a technical procedure which cannot be prevented by monitoring.

As a result of the Caplan et al analysis of closed claims data from the 1970s and 1980s, the American Society of Anesthesiologists Task Force on the Management of the Difficult Airway published guidelines for management of the difficult airway in 1993, and updated them in 2003.[6,7] The purpose of these guidelines was to reduce the likelihood of adverse outcomes, which include but are not limited to death, brain injury, myocardial injury, and airway trauma.

60.3   HAS THERE EVER BEEN A CONCERTED EFFORT TO ESTABLISH A CENTRAL *DIFFICULT AND FAILED AIRWAY REGISTRY*?

Coincident with the development of these guidelines, an Anesthesia Advisory Council representing anesthesiologists, otolaryngologists, and experts in risk management joined together with the nonprofit Medic Alert Foundation to establish a National Difficult Airway/ Intubation Registry. The major objective of this registry was to develop mechanisms for a uniform documentation and dissemination of critical information related to airway management difficulty and to protect patients. As a result, in 1991, the Anesthesia Advisory Council along with the Medic Alert Foundation established the category "Difficult Airway/Intubation." In 1992, The World Federation of Societies of Anesthesia officially endorsed this initiative and in 1992, the American Academy of Otolaryngology—Head and Neck Surgeons followed suit. Despite these initiatives, the labor intensity of the project for the Medic Alert Foundation led to its demise by the mid 1990s.

60.4   IS THERE ANY EVIDENCE THAT VERBAL ADVICE, MEDICAL RECORD DOCUMENTATION, OR REGISTRIES HAVE ANY EFFECT IN REDUCING THE INCIDENCE OF SUBSEQUENT ADVERSE AIRWAY MANAGEMENT EVENTS?

Two small studies have shown a lower incidence of adverse outcomes associated with a prior knowledge of difficult airway. The first employed The Medic Alert Foundation Registry Database. By February of 1994, a total of 111 patients had been enrolled in the registry from over 30 states within the United States. Preliminary results suggested that knowledge of a prior difficult airway led to the use of fewer airway management techniques, and a lower incidence of adverse outcomes.[8]

In the second study, a computerized In-Hospital Difficult Airway Registry had been developed at the Beth Israel Deaconess Medical Center in Boston, MA.[9] One hundred and twenty nine patients were placed in the registry during the period of April, 1995 and April, 1997. Of these patients, 31 returned at least once to the operating room. Uniform documentation of the prior airway management difficulty was available on the permanent medical record, eliminating the need to rely on the patient's memory. There were no adverse outcomes related to airway management on return to the operating room. Others have also been able to track and warn future anesthesia practitioners by using their Anesthesia Information Management Systems (AIMS).[10,11]

Practice guidelines have been promulgated by anesthesia societies in North America and Europe, recommending communication and documentation of adverse airway management events.[6,7,12,13] In general,[12] broad verbal and written documentation is advisable to prevent future adverse events.

60.5   WHO SHOULD UNDERTAKE THE VERBAL ADVICE AND WRITTEN DOCUMENTATION? WHEN SHOULD THAT OCCUR?

If feasible, patients should be verbally advised in layman's language about the event by the practitioners themselves when the patients are alert and oriented in the post anesthesia care unit, recognizing that this may not always be possible. Importantly, they ought to be quizzed after the explanation to confirm that the gravity of the situation and its details are understood. Because of the residual effects of medications, the complexity of the event and the vagaries of memory, a written narrative must also be given to the patients to take with them so they can show to subsequent practitioners if feasible.

60.6   WHO SHOULD BE ADVISED OF THE EVENT? WHERE SHOULD WE DOCUMENT THE INFORMATION?

Besides the patient, the following should be briefed either verbally or in written form:

- Patient's family members if available.
- Primary care physician should be notified in writing.
- The surgeon should be told at time after the intubation.

A form letter ought to be sent with the patient delineating the precise issues encountered, the methods employed to circumvent the airway difficulties, and advice regarding future management strategies. The practitioner's identifying data and contact information should be included. Similar documentation should be entered in the permanent medical record.

60.7   WHAT SHOULD WE DOCUMENT?

The key elements in documentation are accuracy and consistency of the information recorded. This information is important both for the patient record as well as for future analysis of outcome. A study was conducted by Gallagher et al to identify variation in outcome predictor documentation in out-of-hospital cardiac arrest associated with two different methods of data collection.[14] The investigators showed that differences in methods of collection of cardiac arrest data were associated with a more than twofold variation in the reported incidences of witnessed cardiac arrests. In other words, accuracy and consistency of documentation are critical and they can have a significant impact on the interpretation of patient outcomes.

In documenting an outcome of airway management it is important to report the success and failure of the four basic technical operations (see Chapter 1) if they were employed. For example: Was the BMV difficult? Was the use of the EGD difficult? Was laryngoscopy and intubation difficult? Was laryngoscopy performed with or without laryngeal manipulation? Were other airway adjuncts used? Were other intubation techniques employed? Was cricothyrotomy necessary as a rescue technique? In addition, during laryngoscopy, Laryngeal View Grade Scoring System as proposed by Cormack and Lehane (C/L)[15] or Levitan's Percentage of Glottic Opening (POGO)[16] should also be reported.

While there is no general agreement regarding the information that should be recorded in the patient's chart, the authors believe that the following information ought to be in the note:

Date of operation

Type of operation

Hospital and medical record number

Physical examination that may contribute to the problem: height, weight, Mallampati classification, mouth opening, receding chin, etc.

Medical history that may contribute to the difficult airway: rheumatoid arthritis, diabetes, obesity, obstructive sleep apnea, radiation to the head and neck, etc.

Mask ventilation: easy, difficult, or impossible

Oral or nasal airway size

Type and size of laryngoscope used

Number of attempts at laryngoscopy and intubation, including laryngoscopic view

Alternative airway techniques attempted: if successful or not

Any recommendations

The example for this patient management documentation would be as follows:

Date of Operation: 4/12/05

Type of operation: Laparoscopic cholecystectomy

Winchester Hospital, Winchester MA, Medical Record # 000-00-00

PE: 5 ft 4 in (161 cm), 220 lb (100 kg), with a BMI 38.6 kg·m^{-2}, otherwise healthy normal anatomy

Easy mask ventilation

Attempt 1—Macintosh #3; Grade 3 (C/L) laryngoscopic view, no change with BURP, unsuccessful

Attempt 2—Miller #3; Grade 3 (C/L) laryngoscopic view, Eschmann Tracheal Introducer (bougie) passed, esophageal intubation

Attempt 3—ILMA #3 good ventilation, blind ETT passed, unsuccessful

Attempt 4—ILMA #3, ETT with Foley fiberoptic airway stylet successful

Recommendation for future management: Awake intubation

A suggested sample form letter to be sent with this patient

Dear Sir/Ms,

As we discussed during our postoperative visit, you did very well under anesthesia. However, it was difficult to place the breathing tube into your windpipe. This is known as a difficult intubation. You had also what we call an easy mask ventilation (or not difficult mask ventilation). We wish to emphasize that at no time during this operation was your life at risk.

It will be important for you to inform future practitioners and your primary care physician that we had difficulty placing a breathing tube under anesthesia. You should also inform your relatives of this difficulty in the event that they need to provide this information on your behalf.

Please keep this letter in a safe place for future reference. Registering for the Medic Alert Bracelet would be well advised. Please contact me (phone number) for any further information or questions.

Sincerely,

60.8 SUMMARY

In the event that airway management difficulty or failure of sufficient magnitude as to represent a potential life threat is encountered, the standard of care requires at a minimum that the practitioner advises the patient verbally and in writing, and in the permanent medical record what transpired, the devices and techniques that failed, and succeeded and recommend future airway management strategies.

REFERENCES

1. Rose DK, Cohen MM. The airway: problems and predictions in 18,500 patients. *Can J Anaesth*. 1994;41:372-383.
2. Samsoon GL, Young JR. Difficult tracheal intubation: a retrospective study. *Anaesthesia*. 1987;42:487-490.
3. Caplan RA, Posner KL, Ward RJ, Cheney FW. Adverse respiratory events in anesthesia: a closed claims analysis. *Anesthesiology*. 1990;72:828-833.
4. Peterson GN, Domino KB, Caplan RA, Posner KL, Lee LA, Cheney FW. Management of the difficult airway: a closed claims analysis. *Anesthesiology*. 2005;103:33-39.
5. Cheney FW. Anesthesia patient safety and professional liability continue to improve. *ASA Newslet*. 1997 June;Sect.6.
6. American Society of Anesthesiologists Task Force on Management of the Difficult Airway. Practice guidelines for management of the difficult airway. A report. *Anesthesiology*. 1993;78:597-602.
7. American Society of Anesthesiologists Task Force on Management of the Difficult Airway. Practice guidelines for management of the difficult airway: an updated report. *Anesthesiology*. 2003;98:1269-1277.
8. Mark LJ, Beattie C, Ferrell CL, Trempy G, Dorman T, Schauble JF. The difficult airway: mechanisms for effective dissemination of critical information. *J Clin Anesth*. 1992;4:247-251.
9. Foley L, Sands D, Feinstein D, Park KW. Effect of difficult airway registry on subsequent airway management: experience in the first 2 years of difficult airway registry. *Anesthesiology*. 1998;89:A1220.
10. Atkins RF. Simple method of tracking patients with difficult or failed tracheal intubation. *Anesthesiology*. 1995;83:1373-1374.
11. Pasqual RT, Troianos CA, Phillips CA, 3rd. Difficult airway warning with automated anesthesia recording. *Anesthesiology*. 1996;85:220.
12. Barron FA, Ball DR, Jefferson P, Norrie J. "Airway alerts." How UK anaesthetists organise, document and communicate difficult airway management. *Anaesthesia*. 2003;58:73-77.
13. Crosby ET, Cooper RM, Douglas MJ, et al. The unanticipated difficult airway with recommendations for management. *Can J Anaesth*. 1998;45:757-776.
14. Gallagher EJ, Lombardi G, Gennis P, Treiber M. Methodology-dependent variation in documentation of outcome predictors in out-of-hospital cardiac arrest. *Acad Emerg Med*. 1994;1:423-429.
15. Cormack RS, Lehane J. Difficult tracheal intubation in obstetrics. *Anaesthesia*. 1984;39:1105-1111.
16. Levitan RM, Ochroch EA, Kush S, Shofer FS, Hollander JE. Assessment of airway visualization: validation of the percentage of glottic opening (POGO) scale. *Acad Emerg Med*. 1998;5:919-923.

SELF-EVALUATION QUESTIONS

60.1. Which of the following about the Medic Alert® Bracelet for Difficult Airway is **NOT** true?

A. The World Federation of Societies of Anesthesia and the American Academy of Otolaryngology—Head and Neck Surgery officially endorsed the Medic Alert® Foundation for Difficult Airway.

B. The Medic Alert® Foundation developed a uniform database and specialized patient enrollment form for the Difficult Airway/Intubation category.

C. The major objective of the Medic Alert® Registry was to develop mechanisms for a uniform documentation and dissemination of critical information to maximally protect patients.

D. The Medic Alert® Registry is currently used world wide.

E. The *Difficult Airway/Intubation* has been used as a standardized nomenclature within the Medic Alert® identification since 1992.

60.2. Which of the following information should be documented following the management of an unanticipated difficult or failed airway?

A. date and type of operation

B. anatomic features of the patient on airway examination

C. ability to ventilate using a face mask or an extraglottic device

D. laryngoscopic view and the effectiveness of alternative intubating techniques

E. all of the above

60.3. Following the management of an unanticipated difficult airway, the anesthesia practitioner should inform about the difficult airway to all of the following **EXCEPT**:

A. The patient.

B. The primary care physician.

C. The attending surgeon should be informed immediately following the difficult airway encounter.

D. The Medic Alert® Difficult Airway Registry.

E. A family member who is the caregiver of the patient.

CHAPTER (61)

Teaching and Simulation for Airway Management

Brian K. Ross, Jo Davies, Sara Kim, and Michael F. Murphy

61.1 INTRODUCTION

It is sometimes striking how difficult it is to teach airway management well, and to have the student learn it, even with a comprehensive immersion experience in airway management. This text serves as the syllabus for an airway management education program that places special emphasis on the identification and management of the difficult and failed airway. This program, which has trained over 3000 emergency airway practitioners, has undergone progressive improvement and innovation, and is now called The Difficult Airway Course: Emergency. It is one of a family of educational programs that now includes: The Difficult Airway Course: EMS and The Difficult Airway Course: Anesthesia.

Gas exchange is fundamental to airway management. Thus, an educational program intended to teach airway management must craft educational objectives that support this fundamental goal. These *enabling objectives* are crafted in language typified as: "By the end of this educational program the participant will…" The program of instruction must embrace the knowledge and skills that constitute the standard of care, and, in addition, teach best practices related to the provision of gas exchange for those patients who are unable to do so for themselves.

This chapter serves as a primer for an airway management education program that academic as well as private practice practitioners can apply to their practice to improve both their airway management skills as well as the skills of their health care team. This chapter places special emphasis on the application of simple, easily applied hands-on experiences to improve the identification and management of the difficult and failed airway.

The objectives of a comprehensive airway program should contain five easily identified components. These are:

1. The results of a local needs assessment identifying training issues as well as a focused curriculum.
2. *A cognitive or didactic component*: may be accomplished with either a self-guided reading program or a series of focused lectures.
3. *A skills development component*: a hands-on laboratory that teaches the nuances of the devices identified as the standard of care, and other relevant devices as supported by the local needs assessment, as well as best practice-based evidence or expert consensus.
4. *A practical real-time experience*: an opportunity to put it all together with hands-on cases that simulate a real-life situation.
5. An evaluation process of the program and a self-evaluation process for the participant.

This chapter will focus on providing guidance for the development and execution of an airway management/difficult airway educational program in one's own home institution. The following areas will be discussed:

- The problem.
- The evidence that simulation works, improving patient safety through education, training, and research.
- A serious look at the devices a practitioner might easily use to start a local simulation program.
- A curriculum focused on a needs assessment for your institution and the acquisition of requisite skills.
- A skeleton for a context-sensitive training program—ie, point-of-care or in situ simulation.

61.1.1 What problems are we facing in airway management?

Airway management is the scaffolding upon which the whole practice of anesthesia is built, and is part and parcel of other providers practice, such as emergency physicians, critical care specialists, hospitalists, and prehospital practitioners.[1] Important as excellence in airway management has become, equally critical is the context in which one finds oneself when managing an airway (see Chapter 6). The context is clearly different for each of these provider groups although in practice there is crossover, typically at the scene of an emergency airway. For this reason, airway management training programs for all disciplines must focus on the difficult and failed airway. Physicians, nurses, paramedics, emergency medical technicians (EMTs), and first responders often care for patients who are acutely ill or injured. In these situations, practitioners often find themselves in highly emotionally charged, urgent, high-stakes, high-risk environments.

Despite the multidisciplinary nature of airway management, the ultimate objective in training of all practitioners to be able to effectively manage airways and support gas exchange is the same. The practitioner must know what to do to manage the airway, when to do it, how to do it, when *not* to do certain things and how to get out of trouble when one finds oneself in difficulty. Each of these processes is potentially challenging. Proficient airway management requires one to master a host of anatomical, physiological, pharmacological, and technical aspects. The practitioner must know and understand the normal and pathological anatomy of the airway. These facts must then be integrated into an evaluation process that will lead to the selection of appropriate drugs and devices matching this particular setting. They must then be trained in the use of these drugs and devices. Critical to these decisions is developing the sense as to when might be the best time to intervene and then translate the intervention into real-life situations. A final complication is that frequently things do not go as planned and the practitioner must be able to rescue the situation (and the patient) if the initial plan fails.

Despite the development of new devices, strategies and algorithms to predict, manage, and secure the difficult airway, morbidity and mortality associated with failed gas exchange and airway problems, such as difficult intubation or unrecognized failed intubation remain high. As emphasis has been focused on improving airway management, it has become apparent how difficult it is to teach airway management well, and ensure that the trainee has mastered those skills critical to routine airway instrumentation, as well as those required for difficult and failed airway situations. The problem seems to lay both in the area of adequate skills acquisition as well as in the transfer of these skills and strategies to daily clinical practice. Common methods for airway management training have historically included lecture/cognitive instruction mixed with hands-on sessions with simple intubating mannequins and occasional animal models, or structured curricula in physician training programs.[2] However, since the publication of *To Err is Human*, health care professionals have looked to high reliability industries, such as commercial aviation, for guidance on improving training as well as system safety.[3] One of the most widely adopted aviation-derived approaches is simulation-based skills and team training.

61.2 SIMULATION

61.2.1 Does simulation improve performance?

Medical simulation has become increasingly popular over the last decade as a means for teaching a variety of skills to a broad spectrum of practitioners. However, has it been shown to be effective and does it change practice and improve outcomes? These are difficult measures to quantify given the lack of homogeneity of practitioner's clinical practice.

Do we need evidence that simulation is effective when the reality is that it's becoming less acceptable to perform procedures on patients when the practitioners have had little or no training with the required skills, have not been assessed for proficiency on the skill being employed, and have had no prior experience? The answer is obviously NO. The *see one, do one, teach one* method of training is not appropriate for high-risk but low-frequency events, such as cardiac or respiratory arrest and difficult or failed airway management.

Patients have become increasingly concerned that students, residents, and for that matter, fully trained practitioners, practice on them as they develop the required basic clinical skills or become skilled with new devices as they are introduced. With this change in attitude by patients, clinical medicine has become more focused on patient safety. This has helped to shift the many aspects of clinical skills training from the bedside to arenas where patients are not at risk and the learner is the focus of training. Educators have faced these challenges by restructuring curricula, developing small-group sessions, and increasing self-directed/independent learning opportunities. Nevertheless, a disconnect still exists between the classroom and the clinical environment. Medical simulation has been proposed as a tool to bridge this educational gap. In a meta-analysis recently conducted by Okuda et al, simulation-based training has been demonstrated to lead to improvements in skills.[4] This improved performance was translated into improved medical knowledge, improved performance of basic skills, improved confidence in performance of procedures, improved teamwork and communication performance, improved clinical performance, and improved performance during retesting at a later date. Fewer studies have demonstrated direct improvements in clinical outcomes, but evidence to this effect is slowly accumulating.

Simulation training offers a controlled, safe, and reproducible environment which can be used to train and practice clinical interventions, especially for high-risk and low-frequency events. It has also been shown to be effective in acquiring clinical skills proficiency and improving performance and patient care in real clinical situations.[5] But most importantly, it is through simulation that skills (cognitive as well as psychomotor) acquired in isolation can be translated into life-like clinical settings.

Anecdotally, simulation not only improves performance of skilled tasks but also reduces reaction time in stressful situations with practitioners feeling more confident in their abilities to respond to high-risk but low-frequency events.

Several studies have examined the effectiveness of airway management simulation training. There is a consensus that it improves performance.[5-7] The efficacy appears to last for at least 6 to 8 weeks following initial training but needs to be repeated at intervals of 6 months or less for retention of technical and decision-making skills.[6] Multiple sessions of moderate length, rather than single session of excessive length seem to provide better training experiences and retention of skills. Sessions of 75 to 90 minutes appear optimal.[7]

61.2.2   What are the potential benefits of simulation?

The potential benefits of simulation include:

- No risk to patients.
- Patients with a rare medical condition but *every* trainee needs to see.
- Practice on rare and uncommon but critical events—patients may never see but need to learn to manage.
- Participants can see the outcomes of their decisions and actions.
- Participants can be allowed to make errors—let them walk the plank.
- Identical scenarios can be presented to different clinicians or teams.
- Team training—crew resource management.
- Repetition and feedback to consolidate skills.

Simulation has emerged as a key educational resource in areas where a combination of cognitive and technical factors combines to force the participant to decide the best course of action. The evidence from the literature suggests that simulation enhances performance and that performance enhancement is sustained.[8]

There is also evidence that simulation enhances skills development for airway management skills, reducing the need for actual live patient training.[5,9] This is fortunate in considering the costs of such training, the scarcity of real humans to practice on, and the need to find a surrogate training model, particularly as it is felt that a major cause of high intubation failure rates by airway practitioners is inadequate training and skills maintenance.

Our conclusions support the concept that in-house workshops employing simulation technologies need to be conducted to keep the health care teams that manage airways effective and proficient.

61.2.3   What types of simulation environment are available?

Simulation can be a highly effective approach for the acquisition of knowledge, task and skills proficiency, decision making, and teamwork. It is especially effective in acquiring skills that require eye-hand coordination and ambidextrous maneuvers common to many airway management devices, such as bronchoscopy. This type of training also helps learners prepare to deal with unanticipated rare medical events, develops teamwork and communication skills, increases confidence, and improves performance. Once simulation has produced mastery of fundamental skills, it can expose trainees to difficult situations, abnormalities, and other problems. Advanced simulations can reinforce skills that have been previously learned. Consequently, simulation is not just for new trainees. It can be at least as useful for established practitioners who are constantly challenged to update their skills in response to rapid

changes in clinical practice. Simulation offers the foundation for an interdisciplinary approach to education—equally appropriate for physicians, nurses, emergency medical technicians, therapists, technicians, phlebotomists, and other health professionals.

There are essentially three basic types of simulation environments:

61.2.3.1   Specialized Simulation Center

For those interested in developing their own simulation programs, simulation training can often occur in a specialized simulation center. A simulation center provides a quiet, focused, safe environment where trainees can practice skills, be assessed either individually or as teams, and continue to train until proficiency is attained. However, most practitioners do not have access to such a center.

61.2.3.2   In Situ Simulation Training

In recent years, a new arena for simulation training has emerged; *point-of-care* or what is most recently termed *in situ* training. In situ simulation has evolved as a particular form of simulation, distinct from simulation that is conducted in a simulation center. Patterson et al have published an excellent review on in situ simulation, including the challenges and results.[10]

In situ simulation does not replace simulation conducted in the simulation center. In fact, the objectives of training conducted in a simulation center are likely to be very different from the objectives of in situ simulation. Training based at a simulation center is often related to a curriculum or course and has objectives related to both technical and nontechnical proficiencies (eg, basic suturing skills, central line placement, direct laryngoscopy, endoscopic intubation, communication, and teamwork). On the other hand, in situ simulation allows teams to review and reinforce their skills and to solve problems in the clinical environment.

In situ simulation occurs in the actual clinical environment with participants who are on-duty clinical practitioners during their actual work day. As an educational tool, it promotes experiential learning by training the health care provider in the actual environment in which the practitioner is expected to use these skills. Experiences in simulation labs may accomplish this to some degree, but in situ simulation, by definition, is more closely aligned with the actual work of the health care practitioner and is more likely to achieve success for certain training objectives. It provides a method to improve teamwork, team communication, and safety in high-risk areas. Given that the simulation occurs in the clinical environment, there are opportunities to identify hazards and deficiencies in the clinical systems, the environment, and the practitioner team.

For those institutions that are just beginning to develop simulation programs, in situ simulation offers an opportunity to begin to expose clinical personnel to simulation at considerable cost savings over a *bricks-and-mortar* center.

61.2.3.3   Simulation via Training Programs

Simulation incorporated into specialized airway management training programs is offered in a variety of locations. Examples are those courses offered at national meetings such as the ASA and American College of Emergency Physicians (ACEP); and stand-alone courses such as Street Level Airway Management (SLAM),

Airway Interventions and Management in Emergencies (AIME), and the Difficult Airway Courses (DAC).

61.3 EDUCATIONAL PROGRAM

61.3.1 How do you design an educational program to teach airway management?

It is clear from the educational literature that no single method of education (classroom lecture alone, case studies alone, or skills labs alone) adequately teaches complex cognitive and technical skills, such as airway management. This is consistent with the experience of the authors over decades of education of health care practitioners at all levels. An instructional method that integrates didactic teaching, case studies, and skills development provides the most valuable educational experience. Simulation appears to be an educational technology that might just incorporate all of these methods into one coherent package.

Educational programs to teach airway management would ideally be sensitive to the context in which the practitioner practices, and present cases that they are likely to encounter. Context-sensitive airway management was discussed in Chapter 6. The context also drives the selection of devices and techniques that need to be taught.

The design of the curriculum has to be sensitive to the fact that that airway management in patients if performed badly may have dire consequences. Thus, it is a performance of critical skill. Reason has defined two basic mechanisms whereby practitioners deal with critical incidents[11,12] (see Chapter 2):

1. *A rule-based solution*: In this strategy, on *recognizing the event* for what it is, one identifies and applies a solution that experience has shown will likely be useful in solving the problem. *Recognizing the event* involves a process called "similarity-matching"; based on recognizing that the characteristics of this event is similar to those of past events (ie, pattern recognition). The practitioner then selects the particular solution that is likely to be effective in solving the problem and resolving the threat. This presupposes that the practitioner has had sufficient experience with both the situation and the application of the rule to immediately recognize the problem and to know which rule to apply. This ability constitutes what is called "expertise." Unfortunately, difficult and failed airways are encountered infrequently in practice, and the individual experiences of the vast majority of practitioners are unlikely to have been sufficient to have them considered as experts in managing difficult and failed airways.

2. *A knowledge-based solution*: This is a ground-up, first-principles strategy whereby the practitioner, without substantial past experience with similar situations, attempts to find an appropriate solution. Not surprisingly, such strategies are time consuming, and if forced under pressure of time are more likely to result in failure.

Most airway practitioners, even on a daily basis, do not have sufficient clinical experience with difficult and failed airways to have in their minds a rule-based, organized approach to these airway dilemmas, or the time to build one from first principles (ie, a knowledge-based solution). For this reason a variety of tools such as mnemonics and preformulated airway algorithms have been crafted to aid rapid decision making such that the odds of making correct decisions are enhanced and the risk of making incorrect decisions are minimized (see Chapters 1 and 2). No other environment allows the practice of these tools better than simulation.

It is important, when designing an in-house simulation training experience to follow a formal, albeit simplified, curriculum process. A curriculum expresses in a concrete fashion how the knowledge acquired through the training process will be translated into practice. It also helps identify the actual training needs and gaps in the training process that might exist. Finally, a curriculum forms the instructional content, teaching strategies that one might use to train the selected skill, and helps identify the assessment and evaluation tools and outcome measures.

As one attempts to design an in-house training program for airway management, one must make some decisions:

- Does one need to focus the training on a single skill and a single practitioner (eg, endoscopic intubation)
- Is the focus more on a health care team (eg, difficult airway in a simulation center)
- Or is the focus on the health care team *and* the system in which that team works (eg, an airway rescue device in a specific health care setting—LMA Fastrach in an obstetric suite).

The curriculum development process in each of these scenarios is essentially the same, although the goals and objectives, the actual scenarios, and the assessment metrics may differ.

61.3.2 What are the necessary components in designing a simulation training curriculum for airway management?

A typical, but simplified, training curriculum ought to embrace eight elements:

1. Focused needs assessment
2. Target trainees
3. Prerequisites for training
4. Clear and specific goals and objectives
5. Cognitive component
6. Scenario development—teaching the skill
7. Equipment
8. Outcome assessment

Although this list might look daunting, each element can be satisfied quickly and can result in an effective in-house training experience.

61.3.2.1 Focused Needs Assessment

As one begins to design an in-house airway management training program, it can be stated categorically that the single most critical step in the process is conducting a focused needs assessment. The authors cannot tell you which skills to select for training, but it is logical to select those devices that the practice group has found contextually useful.

Some airway management techniques and devices are so established that they constitute the standard of care and must be taught, such as bag-mask-ventilation (BMV), ventilation using extraglottic devices, laryngoscopy and orotracheal intubation, and cricothyrotomy. That is not to say that they must be taught as first-line interventions, but simply that they must be taught. As one progresses beyond the basic airway interventions, one is struck by the vast array of devices available to the practitioner. The marketplace has been flooded with airway management devices, and novel inventions seem to be introduced almost on a weekly basis. The reason is clear: airway management is difficult and dynamic. The ideal device that is easy to use and guarantees near 100% success has yet to be invented! So, those with expertise in the field must select those devices that are known to deliver an advantage over what currently exists and are supported by scientific evidence when available. Some of the advanced devices and techniques that have found their way into the management of the difficult and failed airway over the past several years include:

- The intubating stylets
- Extraglottic devices
- Rigid and semirigid optical stylets
- Video laryngoscopes
- Flexible endoscopic techniques (eg, bronchoscope)
- Percutaneous and open cricothyrotomy

By scanning this array of devices one begins to appreciate the need for specific training in the use of each. Complicating this task is the fact that at times, a recommended device or technique has particular relevance to a specific practitioner, a particular practice, or a unique practice environment (ie, is context sensitive). The best example is the prehospital environment where sterilization of reuseable devices is not ordinarily possible, rendering an advantage to single use, disposable devices (eg, Glidescope Cobalt® instead of the Glidescope Ranger®; disposable vs reuseable EGDs). Additionally, there are devices that ought not be taught to selected audiences because they may require high frequency of use to maintain competence, are too expensive, or confer little advantage to more simple existing devices or techniques.

61.3.2.2   Target Trainees

It is important to thoughtfully consider the training audience—are they novice or expert physicians, nurse anesthetists, medical/surgical nurses, respiratory therapists, paramedics, etc. This evaluation informs the analysis described in to the following paragraph.

61.3.2.3   Prerequisites for Training

To enable the trainees to focus on the skill central to the training, and to inform the content of the curriculum, it is important that an assessment of individual trainee cognitive knowledge and skill sets be performed prior to the training. This assessment will help target both the cognitive components and the technical components of the actual training session. The goal of the training session is dependent on this analysis to enhance its success.

61.3.2.4   Goals and Objectives

It is important to spend some time on constructing some clear goals and objectives targeted to the knowledge, skills, and attitudes that one wishes the trainee to achieve during the training. Given the unpredictable nature of in situ training, if that is to be incorporated into the session, the curriculum should focus on only one or at most two skill sets (eg, one or two airway rescue devices, one device and team communication, etc). The goals and objectives should be linked to critical action checklists that are sufficiently detailed to ensure the educational/assessment goals are met.

61.3.2.5   Cognitive Component

Nearly every training experience should have embedded within it a cognitive component that ensures the trainees are familiar with and understand such knowledge elements as:

- Required anatomy
- Physiology
- Pharmacology
- Specifics of the device(s)
- Team communication skills (if this is the focus of the training)

These elements can be delivered prior to the training session in lecture-type format, a web-based e-learning module, or in its simplest form a set of assigned readings. However, to be successful, the trainee must have in their possession basic knowledge of the skill/task that they are about to be expected to perform.

61.3.2.6   Scenario Development—Teaching the Skill

As one develops training around a task trainer, there is little need to craft a patient case or a formal training scenario. However, providing context to the trainee as they practice and become proficient with their skills adds to the learning environment. As an example, relating to the trainee instances when one has found the LMA-Fastrach™ beneficial while concomitantly relating the difficulties one found using the device in the clinical setting can add an additional dimension to their understanding of the use of the device.

As one begins to develop an in situ experience, the time spent on scenario development becomes more crucial. The patient history and physical examination, the clinical setting in which the trainee will "find the patient," and the physiological states (ie, vital signs, status of the airway, actions of the other team members) need to be addressed in much more detail. A well-crafted scenario will add realism to the case, elicit emotional responses from the trainee with which they must learn to contend, uncover cognitive decision-making skills or deficits, and finally test the workplace environment in which the trainee practices.

61.3.2.7   Equipment

There is a tendency during simulation experiences to use discarded hospital equipment or equipment that may not be currently employed by the practitioner(s). Training should be conducted using equipment that is in current use. As one moves from task training to in situ training, a detailed equipment list for conducting simulations will need to be generated. Nothing disrupts a simulation session more than not having the usual functional equipment, even the specific types of syringes etc, that the clinicians use. This highlights one of the major advantages of in situ training—the equipment the trainee uses in the simulation is usually the same as that available in day to day practice. Additionally, if an important piece of equipment is missing, the simulation has pointed out a systems error in the actual clinical environment. By correcting this fault, patient care and patient safety will be improved.

61.3.2.8   Outcome Assessment

One should attempt to develop explicit, overt, observable, measurable, and reproducible behaviors the trainee is expected to exhibit by the end of the training. There is a temptation to simply use trainee self-assessment questionnaires, that is, "do you feel you are now more capable of handling an airway emergency?" However, these do not identify the proficiency and skill level of the trainee.

61.3.3   How do you teach fundamental airway skills?

The authors believe that health care practitioners find airway management stressful because some of the fundamental skills that are required in their daily practice are difficult to master and usually poorly taught.

Bag-mask-ventilation (BMV) is one of those skills. It is a skill that is at least as difficult to master as laryngoscopy and intubation. BMV requires a substantial amount of manual dexterity and practice to become proficient, and remain proficient. It remains enigmatic to the authors why BMV has not been relegated to a subsidiary position in basic airway management of the unresponsive patient in favor of easily taught and learned extraglottic devices such as the LMA or King LTS.

Laryngoscopy and orotracheal intubation is renowned as a difficult technique to master. This is backed up by the available literature that identifies roughly 50 orotracheal intubations being necessary to establish competence in the technique, defined as a 90% probability of success.[13] It is a highly nuanced technique that requires detailed step-by-step teaching. The program of instruction must emphasize these nuances (eg, the critical importance of exerting pressure on the hyoepiglottic ligament when performing a curved blade intubation; employing an intubating stylet to facilitate intubation; how BURP is correctly performed; etc). Even the specific manipulations of the endotracheal tube during insertion may be critical to success.

The educational program must identify those details of technique (the tricks) that enhance success (ie, that little maneuver that makes *the last 5%* successful). At the same time, the program of instruction must reinforce true principles of management (eg, leave the dentures in for BMV, but remove them for tracheal intubation) and debunk well-established, but incorrect dogma (eg, smearing KY jelly on a beard makes mask seal during BMV easier).

Virtually all of the devices mentioned in the paragraph 3 of section 61.3.2 require detailed step-by-step instruction with

respect to patient selection, preparation of the device, standard technique, and modifications to the technique in specific situations to achieve success, some more so than others. For example, optical stylets and video laryngoscopes are of limited value in the bloody airway and it is easier to teach and learn how to provide gas exchange to an unresponsive patient with a King LTS than to use BMV. Instruction on BMV is necessarily more intense than Combitube™ insertion because the former is a more difficult technique to master.

61.3.4   What are the advantages and disadvantages in the teaching technologies?

Simulation can take the form of a number of device platforms including screen-based, task-oriented, high-fidelity mannequins, hybrid (to be discussed later), or cadaver/biologic specimen platforms. The location of the simulation may vary from formal bricks and mortar simulation centers to point-of-care or in situ simulation, each of which has its own limitations and benefits:

1. *Screen-based simulators* ordinarily present clinical scenarios designed to teach and reinforce cognitive decision making regarding airway management. However, they are not hands-on, do not teach dexterity or team communication, and so are not optimal for teaching airway *skills*.

2. *Task-oriented simulators* teach skills only. The spectrum ranges from home-made devices (eg, dexterity with a flexible endoscope using an adapted gas can (Figure 61-1.), or more sophisticated

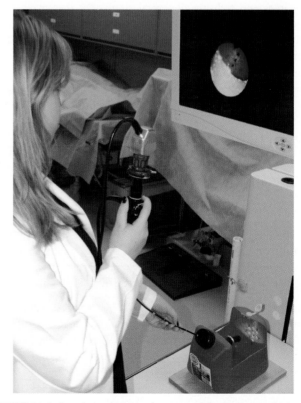

FIGURE 61-1. An adapted gas can being used for fiberoptic dexterity.

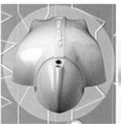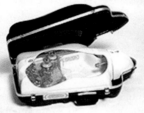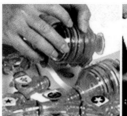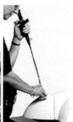

FIGURE 61-2. Dexter Endoscopic Simulator®.

devices such as the Dexter Endoscopic Simulator® (Figure 61-2). However, no team communication or clinical scenarios can be practiced.

3. *High-fidelity simulators* are the computer-controlled, life-sized simulators with adaptable physiology. They are excellent for clinical scenario and team training in a realistic environment such as a virtual OR, but are less useful for individual skills acquisition.

4. *Hybrid simulation* is a combination of high-fidelity simulators with either task-orientated simulators or patient actors.

5. *Cadaver/biologic specimens*: Newly developed techniques of tissue preservation and embalming have enabled the production of cadaver tissues with life-like feel and resilience. These specimens are uniquely suited to airway management training. Biologic tissues can also be employed. Perhaps the best example is the use of pig tracheas to teach surgical airway management, as taught in the Difficult Airway Courses™.

There is a substantial variety of task-orientated and high-fidelity simulators currently in the market. Table 61-1 identifies the names and websites of several companies that make these devices, while Table 61-2 provides more detailed information about a selection of devices, what they can be used for, and an estimate of price. The list is not all inclusive and is devoid of any bias. The authors would recommend that individuals or institutions interested in purchasing any of the simulators contact a company representative to arrange for a demonstration and trial.

However, of all of these technologies, high-fidelity, simulation-based OR team training at the point of care has been identified as a method that best impacts effective teamwork performance in everyday practice.[14]

61.4 SUMMARY

Gas exchange is fundamental to airway management. Educational programs that teach airway management and the use of airway devices must embrace this dictum by designing objectives to achieve this program goal. It is not about the device; it is about how to provide gas exchange to the patient!

Airway management has important and interrelated cognitive and psychomotor skill components. Educational programs that provide an element of didactic teaching, case studies that apply and reinforce the didactic content, skills teaching, and simulation integration in a real-life-simulated environment are best suited to the long-term acquisition of airway management skills.

With this in mind, the authors have attempted to demonstrate the efficacy, value, and relative ease with which airway management training incorporating simulation can be brought into both academic as well as large and small private practices and other training environments. The authors suggest that after identifying training need(s) for their specific practice groups (ie, context-sensitive airway devices), one should then set up a specific training experience using appropriate task trainers to acquire the skills and proficiency level desired. For those who have limited resources, that is, time and money, focused task-oriented skills training sessions employing low-fidelity devices coupled with in situ simulation experiences can add a new dimension to airway management training. Coupling these training platforms enhances the development of proficiency with airway devices and embeds this proficiency in daily clinical practice.

Embracing eight simple curriculum elements permits one to develop a training program that will change and enhance the clinical performance of individuals and teams. Finally, selecting the

TABLE 61-1

Simulator Companies

COMPANY	WEBSITE
Laerdal	http://www.laerdal.com/doc/7423513/Laerdal-Airway-Management.html
Ambu	http://www.ambu.com/COM/All_Products.aspx?ProductID=PROD13907
Simulaids	http://www.simulaids.com/als.htm
VBM-Medical	http://www.vbm-medical.de/cms/101-1-airway-simulators.html
Trucorp	http://www.trucorp.co.uk/sections/default.asp?secid=4&cms=AirSim&cmsid=4&id=4#
METI	http://www.meti.com/products_ps_ecs.htm
Dexter Endoscopy	www.dexterendoscopy.co.nz

TABLE 61-2

Examples of Available Simulation Devices

DEVICE	BAG-MASK-VENTILATION	SUPRAGLOTTIC DEVICES	ENDOTRACHEAL INTUBATION	ENDOSCOPIC INTUBATION (DEXTERITY)	SURGICAL AIRWAY	PRICE
Laerdal						
Laerdal airway management trainer	X	X	X			$$$
Deluxe airway trainer	X	X	X		X	$$$
Cricoids stick simulator					X	$
SimMan	X	X	X	X		$$$$$
Ambu						
Ambu airway management trainer		X	X			$$
Simulaids						
Airway Larry adult airway management trainer	X	X	X			$$
Adult airway management trainer	X	X	X			$$$
VBM-Medical						
Bill	X		X	X	X	$$$
Bill V	X	X	X	X	X	$$$
Frova Crico-Trainer					X	$
Trucorp						
AirSim Standard		X	X		X	$$
AirSim Advanced	X	X	X	X		$$$
AirSim Multi	X		X	X		$$$
METI						
METI ECS	X	X	X	X	X	$$$$$
METI HPS	X	X	X	X	X	$$$$$
Dexter						
Dexter Endoscopy Trainer				X		$$$

$, <$500; $$, $500-$1500; $$$, $1500-$5000; $$$$, $5000-20,000; $$$$$, >$20,000.

most appropriate simulation device(s) has the potential to reduce overall costs and maximize results.

Difficult and failed airway management training demands no less!!

REFERENCES

1. Mason RA. Education and training in airway management. *Br J Anaesth.* 1998;81:305-307.
2. Crosby E, Lane A. Innovations in anesthesia education: the development and implementation of a resident rotation for advanced airway management. *Can J Anaesth.* 2009;56:939-959.
3. Committee on Quality of Health Care in America IoM. *To Err Is Human: Building a Safer Health System.* Washington, DC: National Academy Press; 1999.
4. Okuda Y, Bryson EO, DeMaria S, Jr, et al. The utility of simulation in medical education: what is the evidence? *Mt Sinai J Med.* 2009;76:330-343.
5. Kory PD, Eisen LA, Adachi M, Ribaudo VA, Rosenthal ME, Mayo PH. Initial airway management skills of senior residents: simulation training compared with traditional training. *Chest.* 2007;132:1927-1931.
6. Kuduvalli PM, Jervis A, Tighe SQ, Robin NM. Unanticipated difficult airway management in anaesthetised patients: a prospective study of the effect of mannequin training on management strategies and skill retention. *Anaesthesia.* 2008;63:364-369.
7. Owen H, Plummer JL. Improving learning of a clinical skill: the first year's experience of teaching endotracheal intubation in a clinical simulation facility. *Med Educ.* 2002;36:635-642.
8. Silverman E, Dunkin BJ, Todd SR, et al. Nonsurgical airway management training for surgeons. *J Surg Educ.* 2008;65:101-108.
9. De Lorenzo RA, Abbott CA. Effect of a focused and directed continuing education program on prehospital skill maintenance in key resuscitation areas. *J Emerg Med.* 2007;33:293-297.
10. Patterson M, Blike G, Nadkarni V. In situ simulation: challenges and results. In: Henriksen K, Battles JB, Keyes MA, Grady ML, eds. *Advances in Patient Safety: New Directions and Alternative Approaches.* Vol. 3. *Performance and Tools.* Rockville, MD: Agency for Healthcare Research and Quality; 2008.

11. Murphy MF, Crosby ET. The algorithms. In: Hung OR, Murphy MF, eds. *Difficult and Failed Airway Management*. New York: McGraw Hill; 2008: 15-28.

12. Walls RM. The emergency airway algorithms. In: Walls RM, Murphy MF, eds. *Manual of Emergency Airway Management*. 3rd ed. Philadelphia, PA: Lippincott, Williams and Wilkins; 2008:8-22.

13. Mulcaster JT, Mills J, Hung OR, et al. Laryngoscopic intubation: learning and performance. *Anesthesiology*. 2003;98:23-27.

14. Paige JT, Kozmenko V, Yang T, et al. High-fidelity, simulation-based, interdisciplinary operating room team training at the point of care. *Surgery*. 2009; 145:138-146.

SELF-EVALUATION QUESTIONS

61.1. The objectives of a comprehensive airway management teaching program should contain all of the following components **EXCEPT**:

A. the results of a local needs assessment identifying training issues as well as a focused curriculum

B. a nonexpert instruction model

C. *a cognitive or didactic component*: may be accomplished with either a self-guided reading program or a series of focused lectures

D. *a skills development component*: a *hands-on* lab that teaches the nuances of the devices identified as *the standard of care*, and other relevant devices as supported by the local needs assessment, as well as best practice-based evidence or expert consensus

E. *a practical real-time experience*: an opportunity to *put it all together* with hands-on cases that simulate a real life situation

61.2. The benefits of employing simulation for training airway management include all of the following **EXCEPT**:

A. Simulation poses no risk to patients.

B. It is particularly useful in uncommon but critical events.

C. The available simulators are typically inexpensive and durable.

D. Participants can be allowed to make errors—let them *walk the plank*.

E. Repetition and feedback to consolidate skills are facilitated.

61.3. All of the following concerning the use of simulation to enhance education and training are true **EXCEPT**:

A. Simulation has emerged as a key educational resource in areas where cognitive and technical factors combine to force the participant to judge the best course of action.

B. The evidence from the literature suggests that simulation enhances performance and that performance enhancement is sustained.

C. There is no evidence that simulation enhances skills development for airway management, reducing the need for actual live patient training.

D. Simulation can be a highly effective approach for the acquisition of knowledge, task and skills proficiency, decision making, and teamwork.

E. Simulation training helps learners prepare to deal with unanticipated medical events, develop teamwork and communication skills, increase confidence, and improve performance.

ANSWERS

CHAPTER 1

1.1 (D) While others may play a significant role, the most common factor leading to a failed airway is failure to predict a difficult airway.

1.2 (E) The standard of care is the conduct and skill of an average and prudent practitioner that can be expected by the practitioner's peers and a "reasonable patient," and not the opinions offered by experts.

1.3 (B) The standard of care does not expect the average, reasonable airway practitioner to be an expert and have the expertise in using highly technical airway techniques.

CHAPTER 2

2.1 (A) With the exception of reputable organizations, all are important features of well-designed, clinically useful algorithms.

2.2 (C) The ASA Practice Guidelines are not intended as standards or absolute requirements as the use of practice guidelines cannot guarantee any specific outcome.

2.3 (E) In addition to all the listed weaknesses of the ASA Difficult Airway Algorithm, the algorithm is also unclear that awakening the patient is not always possible.

CHAPTER 3

3.1 (B) The lower border of the quadrangular ligament forms the false vocal cords.

3.2 (C) The maximum effective concentration of topical lidocaine applied to the tongue is 4%.

3.3 (E) Benzocaine is an ester type of local anesthetic which is metabolized to para-aminobenzoic acid. It can also produce methemoglobinemia.

CHAPTER 4

4.1 (C) The ester linkage of remifentanil renders it susceptible to cleavage by nonspecific plasma and tissue esterases.

4.2 (E) In burn victims, extrajunctional receptor sensitization becomes clinically significant at 4 to 5 days postburn. It lasts an indefinite period of time; although the "at risk" period is deemed to have passed at the point healing of the burned area is complete.

4.3 (D) Sugammadex encapsulates and inactivates rocuronium and vecuronium; the resultant complex is excreted in the urine. It does not interact with nicotinic receptors by displacing rocuronium and vecuronium.

CHAPTER 5

5.1 (C) 30 N is more than enough to prevent regurgitation into the pharynx in most patients. Pressures of greater than 30 N (approximately 3 kg, or 7 lb) are unlikely to be necessary. The originally described forces (40 N) would rarely be necessary to prevent gastric regurgitation.

5.2 (D) All of the statements about cricoid pressure and airway techniques are true, including cricoid pressure can also affect ventilation via a face mask.

5.3 (E) All except young children are known factors that increase the risk of aspiration.

CHAPTER 6

6.1 (E) Bag-mask-ventilation, the use of an extraglottic device, tracheal intubation using a Macintosh laryngoscope, and surgical airway are basic techniques in airway management. They all can be used to provide ventilation and oxygenation for this patient.

6.2 (A) In a nonemergency situation, such as in the absence of hypoxemia, a visual technique (direct laryngoscopy) to secure the airway is desirable for this patient as the upper airway anatomy may have been altered. All the other nonvisual or blind techniques should be avoided.

6.3 (E) In an emergency situation, such as in the presence of severe hypoxemia, all airway techniques (both visual and nonvisual or blind techniques) may be considered to rescue the airway while concurrently preparing for a cricothyrotomy.

CHAPTER 7

7.1 (E) All of the above. All of these obstructions may be relieved by a combination of placing an OPA and performing a jaw thrust.

7.2 (D) Performance of a jaw thrust has been shown to be the single most-effective means of relieving a nonpathologic obstruction in the unconscious patient.

7.3 (E) Increasing age is a multifactorial risk factor likely representing a combination of decreased tissue elasticity, neck and jaw mobility, and lack of teeth. Difficult laryngoscopy is an important predictor for DMV.

CHAPTER 8

8.1 (A) To maximize lifting efficacy with minimal muscular effort, it is important to keep the left elbow adducted to your side (roughly the anterior axillary line), not pointing outward. With the elbow in, the handle gripped down low, the forearm is kept straight, and body weight can be used to rock forward slightly so that minimal arm strain occurs.

8.2 (E) All the statements are true with bimanual laryngoscopy.

8.3 (E) All the listed factors are potential causes of mechanical problem while rail-roading an endotracheal tube over a tube introducer into the trachea.

CHAPTER 9

9.1 (E) Laryngospasm, complete airway obstruction, local anesthesia toxicity, laryngeal trauma are potential complications of awake flexible bronchoscopic intubation.

9.2 (E) Presently, there is no reliable method of removing prions from the flexible bronchoscope following its use in a patient with Creutzfeldt-Jakob disease.

9.3 (E) All of the listed steps facilitate advancement of the ensleeved endotracheal tube into the trachea over the flexible bronchoscope.

CHAPTER 10

10.1 (A) While all the other statements are incorrect, the monitor display of the video laryngoscopes does facilitate the recording of the laryngoscopy and intubation.

10.2 (D) While the fiberoptic stylets can be used as stand-alone tools, they are best used as an adjunct to direct laryngoscopy.

10.3 (A) Unlike the flexible bronchoscope which are delicate and are easily damaged, the rigid fiberoptic laryngoscopes are more robust.

CHAPTER 11

11.1 (D) With the exception of blood and secretion, all will affect light-guided intubation using the principle of transillumination.

11.2 (D) The use of a subcricoid puncture, insertion of the guide wire through the "Murphy" eye, passing through the working channel of a flexible bronchoscope, and use of a flexible lightwand have all been shown to improve the success rate of the retrograde intubation.

11.3 (C) While the airway exchange catheter has a hollow lumen with two side ports, the Eschmann Introducer does not.

CHAPTER 12

12.1 (A) The King LT™ is a silicone airway tube which can be used safely in patients with latex allergy.

12.2 (E) It is recommended that the LMA be lubricated with a water-soluble lubricant prior to its use.

12.3 (B) Although the incidence of gastric aspiration associated with the use of LMA is rare, fatal aspiration of gastric content has been reported. Proper assessment for aspiration risk prior to the use of the LMA is imperative. Most airway practitioners would avoid the use of the LMA in patients with a history of hiatal hernia, gastroesophageal reflux, in obstetrical patients, or in patients with a bowel obstruction.

CHAPTER 14

14.1 (D) Rapid-sequence intubation by nonphysician prehospital care providers is supported by the available evidence for critical care prehospital providers.

14.2 (B) All of the statements about "nonparalytic RSI" are correct EXCEPT that "nonparalytic RSI" has not been proven to be safer than "paralytic RSI."

14.3 (C) While the colorimetric end-tidal carbon dioxide determination is effective to confirm tracheal intubation, it is less accurate in identifying correct placement of the ETT in patients with circulatory arrest, with reported false-negative rates as high as 30% to 35%.

CHAPTER 15

15.1 (E) With an appropriate application of MILNS, there is no evidence to suggest that a clinically significant degree of cervical spinal movement is related to tracheal intubation using all the stated airway maneuvers, including the cricoid pressure and external laryngeal manipulation.

15.2 (D) The immediate priority in patient with TBI is oxygenation, due to evidence suggesting that even a single episode of hypoxemia can worsen the prognosis in the patient with TBI.

15.3 (B) Three recent studies suggest that the probability of associated C-spine injury is at least tripled in the head-injured patient with GCS scores of 8 or less.

CHAPTER 16

16.1 (D) Following a motor vehicle crash, scene safety should be ensure before proceeding to manage the airway, breathing, and circulation.

16.2 (E) While EGDs are effective rescue devices for ventilation and oxygenation, not all of them have been well studied in the trauma population.

16.3 (E) The lightwand (Trachlight™) can be used as an airway adjunct on its own or can be combined with other techniques to facilitate tracheal intubation.

CHAPTER 17

17.1 (D) In a patient wearing an open-face helmet, airway management can be performed with the helmet in place and the patient's head can be manually stabilized by an assistant to minimize movement of the head and neck. Direct laryngoscopic intubation under RSI is an acceptable technique to secure the airway.

17.2 (D) In a stable, cooperative patient involved in a high-speed MVC, who is brought to the hospital on a spine board still wearing his full-face style helmet, the most appropriate management is to complete the primary survey assessment, provide oxygen through his helmet if necessary, and complete lateral C-spine x-rays with the helmet in place prior to removing the helmet with the assistance of a skilled colleague.

17.3 (D) In the presence of difficult bag-mask-ventilation (obesity and beard), difficulty in using an EGD (SpO$_2$ on FiO$_2$ 1.00 is 87% with assisted spontaneous ventilation using Combitube™), and repeated failed laryngoscopic intubation, the safest approach is to perform a cricothyrotomy with the Combitube™ in place and the patient breathing spontaneously.

CHAPTER 18

18.1 (C) All the statement about airway management in obese patients are true except that airway obstruction under anesthesia in these obese patients even with the application of a jaw thrust is due to a decrease in the lateral plane and not the anterior-posterior dimension of the velopharynx (nasopharynx).

18.2 (A) All of the listed statement about obstructive sleep apnea (OSA) are true, except that the majority of patients with OSA are not obese.

18.3 (E) All the listed airway techniques are known to be difficult in obese patients with the exception of ventilation using an LMA.

CHAPTER 19

19.1 (C) Bag-mask-ventilation is the ventilation device of choice to attempt to enhance oxygenation in a patient who presents with stridor and oxygen desaturation following a blunt anterior neck trauma. The use of EGDs may be contraindicated in the setting of supraglottic or glottic disruption, or distortion.

19.2 (A) While most practitioners are concerned about a potential cervical spine fracture in patients with a blunt anterior neck trauma, the incidence of a cervical spine injury in this patient population is unclear.

19.3 (E) All of the statements are potential limitations of percutaneous cricothyrotomy in the setting of blunt anterior neck trauma with a concomitant laryngeal fracture.

CHAPTER 20

20.1 (A) An emergency surgical airway, not tracheal intubation, is more appropriate for a patient with an upper airway obstruction.

20.2 (D) Responsibility for ensuring appropriate airway management in the ED should rest primarily with the emergency practitioner of record.

20.3 (E) Delaying airway management at all costs is not an acceptable strategy in managing an unconscious, morbidly obese patient with difficult ventilation and failed laryngoscopic intubation.

CHAPTER 21

21.1 (D) While an increase in mean intrathoracic pressure, tension pneumothorax, hypovolemia, and acute respiratory acidosis may cause hypotension, succinylcholine does not reduce systemic vascular resistance and decrease blood pressure.

21.2 (C) While there is evidence to support the use of magnesium, ketamine, and anticholinergics with respect to the pharmacologic management of asthma in the peri-intubation period, there is no evidence to support the use of lidocaine in acute severe asthma.

21.3 (D) The best way to mechanically ventilate an intubated patient with acute severe asthma is to use small tidal volumes and high peak flow rates.

CHAPTER 22

22.1 (C) Bi-PAP improves ventilation and vital sign more rapidly than CPAP. While all studies show a decrease in intubation rates in those receiving NIVS, no large randomized controls have been done. In addition, meta-analysis of the NIVS shows no significant difference in hospital mortality.

22.2 (E) The underlying disease, respiratory acidosis, positive pressure ventilation, and the use of an induction agent are potential causes of postintubation hypotension in patients with cardiogenic shock.

22.3 (D) Any induction agent, including ketamine and opioids, may result in worsening hypotension, although etomidate has moderate CV stability. But in any patient who is already catecholamine depleted there is still the strong possibility of hypotension. In general, amnesia rather than induction of anesthesia is a better endpoint if one is going to use an induction agent.

CHAPTER 23

23.1 (E) All the statements are correct for a patient with airway burns.

23.2 (C) In the care of a burn patient, as a general rule, it is always better to intubate the trachea early than late as the time course of upper airway swelling leading to total upper airway obstruction is about 12 to 24 hours.

23.3 (E) In patients with burns, the risk of succinylcholine-induced hyperkalemia secondary to extrajunctional receptor sensitization becomes clinically significant at 4 to 5 days postburn. It lasts an indefinite period of time, although the "at risk" period is deemed to have passed at the point healing of the burned area is complete.

CHAPTER 24

24.1 (B) In general, the clinical course of angioedema is unpredictable with respect to the airway.

24.2 (C) Bag-mask-ventilation, the use of extraglottic devices, and tracheal intubation under direct laryngoscopy are likely to be difficult in patients with angioedema. Therefore, tracheal intubation using RSI will be imprudent.

24.3 (A) Fixed laryngeal obstruction with stridor at rest implies a reduction in the caliber of the airway to 4.5 mm or less in diameter.

CHAPTER 25

25.1 (D) In the presence of a decrease in oxygen saturation (high 80%) following a failed RSI attempt, the most appropriate response is to improve attempts at bag-mask-ventilation with improved technique.

25.2 (A) When faced with a "cannot intubate and cannot ventilate" situation (even with the LMA), the most appropriate response is to perform cricothyrotomy.

25.3 (C) The incidence of associated cervical spine fracture with severe blunt facial trauma ranges from 1.0% to 2.6% of patients.

CHAPTER 26

26.1 (C) Ludwig angina is defined as the bilateral cellulitis and edema of the submandibular and sublingual spaces or deep neck infection and edema involving the entire floor of the mouth.

26.2 (E) All the listed airway management strategies may be difficult in patients with Ludwig angina.

26.3 (C) In general, a nonvisual intubating technique, such as intubation using an intubating LMA, should be avoided in managing patients with a Ludwig angina.

CHAPTER 27

27.1 (D) The prolonged use of muscle relaxants in the critically ill patient may contribute to the development of "polyneuropathy of critical illness," a devastating complication with unfavorable patient outcomes.

27.2 (A) Cardiorespiratory depression is a predictable side effect of propofol.

27.3 (C) With the more pliable modern PVC ETTs, more prolonged translaryngeal intubation is well tolerated, and in general, tracheotomy within 14 days of prolonged intubation is desirable.

CHAPTER 28

28.1 (E) Although all of these methods have been used to assess airway edema, none of them has been proven to be a reliable method in assessing airway edema.

28.2 (D) With the exception of muscle relaxation, all of the listed precautions are useful steps to minimize the morbidity associated with jet ventilation through a hollow tube exchanger.

28.3 (E) All of the steps are helpful to reduce airway edema.

CHAPTER 29

29.1 (C) Direct laryngoscopy using a Macintosh laryngoscope is known to be difficult in patients in a halo jacket.

29.2 (E) Likely complications occur during airway exchange are acute airway obstruction and failure to intubate.

29.3 (B) To avoid laryngeal injury, the endotracheal tube should never be advanced over the airway exchange catheter by force.

CHAPTER 30

30.1 (E) All the listed equipment are required to protect the health care providers who are managing a patient with SARS.

30.2 (A) In managing the airway of a patient with SARS, every effort should be made to reduce the risk of aerosolization of SARS droplets (eg, coughing) during the process of intubation. Awake intubation using a flexible bronchoscope should be avoided if at all possible.

30.3 (C) In order to minimize the spread of SARS virus, the patient should be placed in an isolated room, and only those persons required to carry out the intubation should be permitted in the immediate vicinity of the patient. This team may consist of an experienced airway practitioner, respiratory therapist, and an ICU nurse. Additional personnel with airway management expertise who can perform a surgical airway (a surgeon) should stand by outside the room in the event that help is required.

CHAPTER 31

31.1 (D) If ventilation is difficult immediately following the placement of a tracheostomy tube, it is most prudent to remove the tracheostomy tube and advance the indwelling ETT to pass beyond the tracheotomy site (2-4 cm distally) and resume ventilation.

31.2 (D) Tension pneumothorax is one of the known complications of tracheotomy. In the presence of hemodynamic instability, the practitioner should immediately perform a needle decompression in the midclavicular line at the right second intercostal space of the chest.

31.3 (E) Tracheostomy tube change should be done only after the tract is sufficiently mature to minimize the risk of creating a false passage. Following a PDT, the tracheostomy tube change should be done after 7 days as the initial stoma is smaller and only created by a puncture. The practitioner should, therefore, avoid reinserting the tracheostomy tube at bedside 3 days after PDT placement.

CHAPTER 32

32.1 (E) Down syndrome patients are known to have the all these attributes that may lead to failed intubation.

32.2 (D) Even though emergence delirium can occur (incidence varies but may be as high as 10%-30% in adults with a much lower occurrence in children), oral and IM ketamine remains a useful drug in the management of uncooperative patient. Unfortunately, midazolam has not been shown to reduce the incidence of ketamine-induced emergence delirium.

32.3 (A) Ketamine is useful in the management of uncooperative patients, including developmentally delayed individuals and the oral dose is 7.0 mg·kg^{-1}.

CHAPTER 33

33.1 (A) Radiotherapy to the head and neck can produce limited mouth opening, limited cervical spine extension, noncompliant fibrotic soft tissue in the floor of the mouth and pharynx, and alteration of laryngeal anatomy. All airway management techniques, including the surgical airway, can be difficult.

33.2 (E) All techniques to provide oxygenation and ventilation in a patient with a history of radiotherapy to the head and neck can be expected to be challenging.

33.3 (D) In a patient with a history of radiotherapy to the head and neck who presents with evidence of an extremely compromised airway with severe stridor, the most appropriate technique to secure the airway is awake tracheotomy performed under local anesthesia.

CHAPTER 34

34.1 (E) Zone I extends from the level of the clavicles and sternal notch to the cricoid cartilage, Zone II extends from the level of the cricoid cartilage to the angle of the mandible, and Zone III extends from the angle of the mandible to the base of the skull.

34.2 (B) The signs and symptoms of aerodigestive injury include hoarseness or dysphonia, stridor, subcutaneous emphysema or crepitance, dyspnea, dysphagia, hemoptysis, tenderness on palpation of the larynx, and air bubbling from the wound. However, the only hard clinical sign of laryngotracheal injury is air escaping from the neck wound.

34.3 (C) Flexible endoscopy is the investigation of choice for suspected laryngotracheal trauma. Cervical spine and chest x-rays can be done as part of the initial trauma resuscitation. The diagnostic imaging procedure of choice in the evaluation of suspected laryngeal injury is high-resolution CT scanning. However, CT scanning cannot be recommended as a replacement for triple endoscopy in PNI (pharyngolaryngoscopy, esophagoscopy, and bronchoscopy).

CHAPTER 35

35.1 (B) Emergency airway management in a patient lying prone should include BMV, the use of an EGD, the placement of a endotracheal tube, and a surgical airway. But a surgical airway is generally reserved as a last resort.

35.2 (E) All of these techniques are acceptable methods of securing the endotracheal tube (ETT) in a patient with facial hair. However, shaving the beard would require patient's consent.

35.3 (E) While all these methods may provide helpful clues of airway edema, none of them has been proven scientifically to be a reliable method in assessing postoperative airway edema in a patient who has been placed prone for a surgical procedure.

CHAPTER 36

36.1 (C) Both the Univent and double lumen tubes been termed "difficult tubes" because they both have increased rigidity and increased outer diameter, making both difficult to negotiate their way through the glottis.

36.2 (E) All of these can make the change of an SLT for a double lumen tube at the end of the case difficult.

36.3 (C) Ideally, exchange of an SLT for a DLT should be done with an airway exchange catheter and under visual control.

CHAPTER 37

37.1 (A) The literature suggests that the presence of LTH may be associated with obesity, sleep apnea, and previous palatine tonsillectomy.

37.2 (D) LTH is not detectable on routine preoperative physical examination or airway assessment. It is detectable with diagnostic imaging modalities such as plain x-ray, computed tomography, and magnetic resonance imaging as well as with upper airway endoscopy.

37.3 (A) The presence of the LTH at the base of the tongue, and vallecula will prevent proper placement of the laryngoscope blade thus interfering with the basic mechanisms of laryngoscopy.

CHAPTER 38

38.1 (B) The classic clinical signs and symptoms of SVC syndrome are related to upper body venous hypertension. These include facial, neck, and arm swelling, as well as engorgement of the mucous membranes, including those of the upper airway. But, hemoptysis is not a classic clinical sign and symptom of SVC syndrome.

38.2 (E) All the listed airway management strategies may be difficult in patients with a large mediastinal mass and superior vena cava obstruction syndrome.

38.3 (E) Although cardiovascular collapse following induction of GA in adult patients with a mediastinal mass is a rare event, all the listed problems are known complications associated with mediastinal masses and general anesthesia.

CHAPTER 39

39.1 (E) All the statement are true in patients with rheumatoid arthritis.

39.2 (D) If a patient refuses an indicated procedure as part of anesthesia care, every effort should be made to determine that the patient has a reasonable understanding of the issues being discussed and her/his judgment is not based on inaccurate information.

39.3 (B) Impossible BMV has been found to be much less frequent (0.15%), with neck radiation changes as the most significant clinical predictor in addition to male gender, sleep apnea, Mallampati III-IV classification, and presence of a beard.

CHAPTER 40

40.1 (B) The major difference between the ASA Difficult Airway Algorithm and the Failed Airway Algorithm in Chapter 2 of this text is that the ASA algorithm recommends that LMAs and cricothyrotomy be performed sequentially whereas this text recommends that they be performed concurrently. We strongly believe that wasting valuable time attempting a variety of devices or techniques should be avoided at all costs once the failure to maintain oxygenation (CICV) is recognized.

40.2 (D) Although studies have shown that practicing on a mannequin can improve the procedure time and success rate of performing a cricothyrotomy, anesthesia practitioners are generally reluctant to perform cricothyrotomy.

40.3 (A) In general, a difficult mask ventilation can be mitigated by the use of an oral airway and two nasal airways.

CHAPTER 41

41.1 (E) Although several reports recommend caution in the use of succinylcholine in patients with dystrophic epidermolysis bullosa due to concern about a hyperkalemic response, none of the listed medications has been proven to be unsafe to use in these patients.

41.2 (E) Protein deficiency, iron deficiency anemia, and electrolyte disturbances are key features in patients with severe epidermolysis bullosa.

41.3 (B) Patients with DEB have a higher risk of difficult airway. However, successful airway management with the use of BMV, extraglottic devices, and tracheal intubation in patients with DEB have all been reported.

CHAPTER 42

42.1 (D) In 1994, the FDA reversed its earlier relative contraindication to use succinylcholine in children under the age of 16 years decision and downgraded their recommendation to a warning.

42.2 (B) There is no question that damage to the airway can occur with both cuffed and uncuffed tubes. However, there is no evidence today to suggest that cuffed tubes are associated with increased airway injury in children of any age, including less than 2 years of age, compared to uncuffed tubes.

42.3 (D) When emergency intubation is indicated, RSI is the technique of choice in children, as it is in adults. The sequence of events and drug selection for RSI are no different in children than it is in adults. While the effectiveness of cricoid pressure in preventing gastric aspiration remains controversial, cricoid pressure is effective in decreasing gastric insufflation even with ventilation pressures greater than 40 cm H_2O.

CHAPTER 43

43.1 (C) Children with croup tend to be younger, afebrile, and noisy; they have the classic "barking" cough, hoarse stridor, and vocal agitation of the unhappy toddler. Clinical differentiation of croup from supraglottitis is usually based on the slow rate of progression, the absence of respiratory distress, and the clinical or radiological detection of a mass.

43.2 (E) All of the listed management plans are acceptable for a significantly symptomatic pediatric supraglottitis except the surgical airway which is a last resort option.

43.3 (D) All the listed intubation sequences for pediatric supraglottitis are acceptable except the use of extraglottic airway adjuvants, because there is little or no evidence or experience to support their use in the management of supraglottitis.

CHAPTER 44

44.1 (A) Inhalational agents, such as isoflurane, enflurane, and desflurane, are more likely to produce airway irritation on induction and are commonly avoided for the inhalational induction of anesthesia to remove a foreign body from the trachea.

44.2 (B) The use of flexible bronchoscopy (FB) for foreign body removal is not widely practiced. The foreign body cannot be ensheathed within the FB to protect the airway during its removal, potentially increasing the risk of injury to the airway if the object is sharp. It also increases the risk of complete airway obstruction, if the object is dropped as it is retracted proximally.

44.3 (E) Open surgical procedures are seldom required to remove foreign bodies from the airway and a foreign body lodged at the carina should be readily retrieved through a rigid bronchoscope.

CHAPTER 45

45.1 (D) Awake bronchoscopy is not feasible in children.

45.2 (A) Post-tonsillectomy bleeding is an emergency situation that requires urgent fluid resuscitation and operative revision under general anesthesia.

45.3 (E) Ketorolac, ibuprofen, and dexamethasone may increase the risk of bleeding. Morphine may increase the risk of postoperative nausea and vomiting. Hetastarch is used as the initial volume replacement during fluid resuscitation.

CHAPTER 46

46.1 (A) Patients with Robin sequence usually lack a well-developed mentum which makes BMV difficult or impossible. In addition, the presence of glossoptosis and mandibular hypoplasia combine generally make direct laryngoscopy very difficult. However, they generally do not have a small mouth opening and so an appropriately sized oropharyngeal airway, or LMA can often be placed easily to maintain the airway.

46.2 (E) All of the techniques are acceptable airway rescue techniques for the CICV situation in infants less than 1 year of age except the flexible endoscopic intubation which usually takes time to prepare and is not practical in emergency airway management.

46.3 (B) All of the findings are true to indicate increased risk of difficult airway management in a patient with RS except airway obstruction when placed prone. In fact, these patients are usually at their best in the prone position because gravity helps keep the tongue off the roof of the mouth. They may develop varying degrees of obstruction when placed supine.

CHAPTER 47

47.1 (C) All the statements regarding flexible bronchoscopic intubation of the child are true except that general anesthesia and sedation can effectively be achieved via both inhalational and IV routes.

47.2 (C) All the statements regarding the pediatric flexible bronchoscope are true except that the working channel is not very effective for suctioning.

47.3 (E) The major difficulty that one would encounter when using an LMA as a guide to flexible bronchoscopic intubation in a child is the standard ETTs are too short. A long tube, such as the microlaryngeal tube (MLT), is needed for this technique.

CHAPTER 48

48.1 (C) Resuscitation of a child with acute severe head injury begins with airway, breathing, and then circulation.

48.2 (B) All are appropriate for RSI in a 7-year-old with an acute severe head injury except pretreatment with fentanyl which has not been shown to effectively blunt increases in ICP during intubation in children. Furthermore, it should be avoided if hemodynamic instability is suspected.

48.3 (D) In a failed intubation, provided that ventilation is adequate (cannot intubate, can ventilate), an alternative intubating approach is reasonable.

CHAPTER 49

49.1 (A) According to the study reported by Rocke et al, a combination of high Mallampati grade, short neck, protruding maxillary incisors, and receding mandible has been shown to have a high prediction accuracy for a difficult laryngoscopy and intubation in obstetrical population.

49.2 (C) All of the listed gastrointestinal changes associated with pregnancy are true, except that gastric emptying is not delayed during pregnancy.

49.3 (E) Airway edema, swelling, voice change, higher Mallampati grade during labor are known airway changes associated with pregnancy. But these changes do not return to pre-labor state within 12 hours postpartum.

CHAPTER 50

50.1 (D) All of the physiological changes of pregnancy listed are correct except the alveolar-arterial oxygen gradient which is increased in pregnancy. This abnormality can persist in the immediate postpartum period.

50.2 (D) Friable and easily bleeding airway, upper airway edema, pharyngeal narrowing are potential problems of preeclampsia on the parturient airway. Awake intubation using a flexible bronchoscope is an acceptable technique for preeclamptic parturient with an anticipated difficult airway.

50.3 (A) For an obese parturient with severe preeclampsia and a history of difficult laryngoscopic intubation, awake bronchoscopic intubation is the most reasonable technique among these choices.

CHAPTER 51

51.1 (A) While Han et al has shown that the LMA is effective and safe in providing ventilation and oxygenation to healthy, non-obese, fasted parturients for elective cesarean section, it is generally accepted that the LMA should be used only as an emergency rescue device for failed airway management in the parturient undergoing emergency cesarean section.

51.2 (D) It is imprudent to proceed to a third laryngoscopic attempt. BMV should be attempted while maintaining cricoid pressure. If BMV is unsuccessful, even by easing the cricoid pressure, a rescue device, such as an LMA, should be inserted while concurrently prepared for a surgical airway.

51.3 (E) The use of reflux/aspiration prophylaxis together with RSI and cricoid pressure would be the most prudent approach to minimize the risk of regurgitation and aspiration in a healthy parturient undergoing emergency cesarean section.

CHAPTER 52

52.1 (E) According to the US FDA classification for drugs administered to females during pregnancy, most anesthetic and sedating agents fall into the category "C" group, in which risks cannot be ruled out.

52.2 (A) In a "Cannot intubate and cannot ventilate" situation, all of the options are acceptable except to repeat a "failed" technique.

52.3 (E) In a respiratory arrest, the most important management is to restore ventilation and oxygenation immediately.

CHAPTER 53

53.1 (C) Acute appendicitis has significant adverse effects on the maternal and fetal outcome, particularly if peritonitis develops. A delay in diagnosis of appendicitis is likely to increase the risk of morbidity and mortality.

53.2 (B) It has been repeatedly shown that the single most important factor leading to a failed airway is the failure to predict the difficult airway.

53.3 (B) Airway management is context-sensitive. Successful airway management often depends on the interplay between three general categories of modifiers practitioner factors, patient factors; and situational factors. In other words, the degree of mouth opening will determine which device or technique may be useful in securing the airway of this patient.

CHAPTER 54

54.1 (C) According to A Closed Claims Analysis in 2005 by Peterson et al, the majority of claims for difficult airway management (156 out of 179 or 87%) involved perioperative care and 23 claims (13%) involved ectopic locations.

54.2 (C) Although many factors may influence the successful management of the airway in an ectopic location, familiarization of the equipment and the environment beforehand is probably the most important.

54.3 (C) To minimize airway management failure, it is important to establish policies and procedures with respect to the availability of airway management equipment and its maintenance in areas where it is predictable that emergency or urgent airway intervention will occasionally be required.

CHAPTER 55

55.1 (B) Rapid-sequence intubation with induction agent and muscle relaxant in a patient with a neck hematoma is the least safe option. Even with attempted awake intubation or an inhalational induction in the patient with a postsurgical neck hematoma, the risk of complete loss of the airway is always present during the procedure.

55.2 (A) Placing the patient in the sitting or semi-sitting position and administering Heliox may be useful. No benefit has been proven with the use of intravenous steroid or epinephrine aerosols in the setting of a neck hematoma. Administering sedative agents to a patient with obstructing airway pathology may result in complete airway obstruction.

55.3 (C) In the presence of altered or abnormal anatomy (eg, that caused by a neck hematoma), the use of a blind intubation technique (eg, LMA-Fastrach™ intubation) is not recommended.

CHAPTER 56

56.1 (C) Flexible fiberoscopy is not included in WHO guidelines for all levels of facilities, including the district hospitals (level 2 facilities) in all countries.

56.2 (D) There are no international standards in purchasing airway equipment for poorly resourced countries.

56.3 (B) All of the listed methods are common disinfection options in austere environments except ethylene oxide.

CHAPTER 57

57.1 (C) All objects with possible ferromagnetic components should be removed before entering the MRI suite. To avoid burns and fires, electrocardiogram electrodes must be applied at a distance from the imaging area, or should be replaced with special carbon MRI-compatible (not asbestos MRI-compatible) electrodes.

57.2 (A) Apart from small amounts of ferromagnetic materials, such as metallic springs in the cuff inflation valve, the LMA is the only listed airway device that may be used safely in an MRI unit.

57.3 (C) The endotracheal tube is the only listed airway device that is not a known hazard in the MRI suite.

CHAPTER 58

58.1 (B) POPE likely occurs because of an upper airway obstruction (A and D) or laryngospasm (C and E). It is least likely to occur due to difficult laryngoscopic intubation with difficulty with BMV (positive pressure ventilation) between intubation attempts (B).

58.2 (E) Laryngospasm following extubation is best managed by performing an airway-opening maneuver and apply CPAP by mask; if this does not break the laryngospasm within 30 seconds, administer a small dose of IV succinylcholine.

58.3 (B) A retrospective study showed that the majority of POPE cases (63%) occurred following surgery to the aerodigestive tract, suggesting that vigilance be exercised in patients suffering from chronic tonsillar hypertrophy, goiter, and other conditions leading to chronic upper airway obstruction.

CHAPTER 59

59.1 (E) Presently there is no known effective method of sterilization in destroying the prion particle.

59.2 (E) Apart from dictating who can use the airway equipment, all of the points are critical policy issues in designing a difficult airway cart.

59.3 (E) Since anesthesia practitioners are often called to out-of-OR locations to manage the airway, they are liable for negative outcomes if the equipment they need is not available. Therefore, it is critical that they should be involved in the design and maintenance of difficult airway carts. It is the duty of the hospitals and unit management and anesthesia practitioners to understand and embrace this accountability.

CHAPTER 60

60.1 (D) Despite these initiatives, the labor intensity of the project for the Medic Alert Foundation led to its demise by the mid 1990s and so, the Medic Alert Registry is not currently used.

60.2 (E) All the information listed are important following the management of an unanticipated difficult or failed airway.

60.3 (D) All of the listed parties should be notified except the Medic Alert Difficult Airway Registry which does not exist anymore.

CHAPTER 61

61.1 (B) The objectives of a comprehensive airway program should contain five easily identified components (1) local needs assessment; (2) a cognitive or didactic component; (3) a skills development component; (4) a practical real-time experience with hands-on cases that simulate a real life situation; and (5) an evaluation process. But, the use of a nonexpert instruction model is not an objective of an airway program.

61.2 (C) All of them are true benefits of simulation for training airway management, except that simulators are usually quite expensive.

61.3 (C) There is sufficient evidence to suggest that the use of simulation enhances education and training, including skills development for airway management skills, reducing the need for actual live patient training.